Wardlaw's CONTEMPORARY NUTRITION

ELEVENTH EDITION

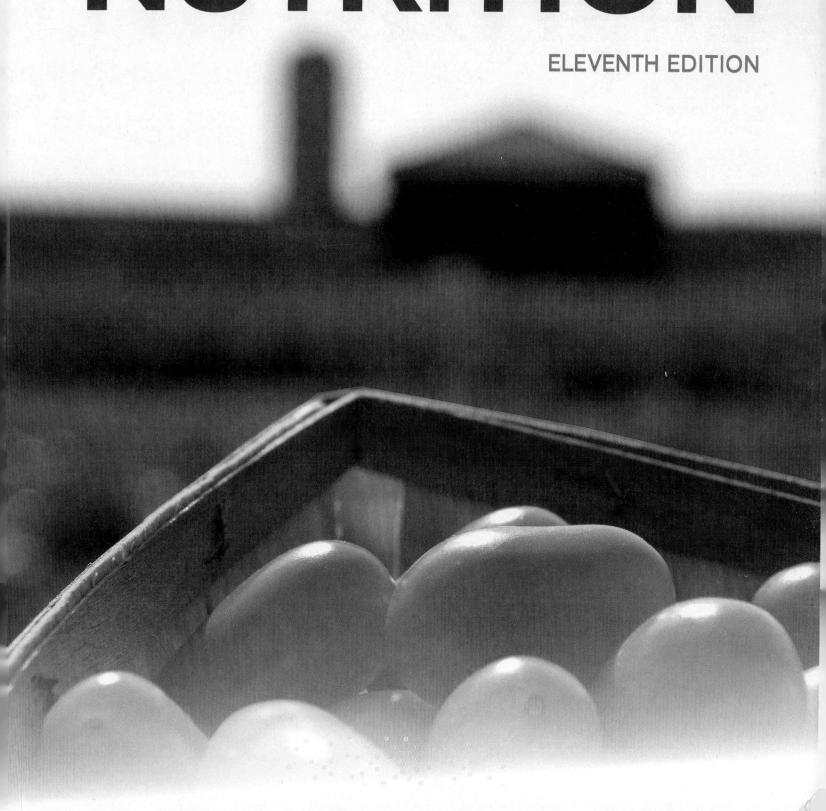

mheducation.com/highered

Brief Contents

About the Cover

The Garden of Hope is a community garden for cancer survivors located at the Waterman Farm at The Ohio State University. Dr. Colleen Spees, co-author of *Wardlaw's Contemporary Nutrition,* leads research efforts at this unique living laboratory that provides cancer survivors and food-insecure families the opportunity to incorporate a Farm-to-Fork approach while harvesting fruits, vegetables, and herbs throughout the growing season.

Tomatoes, like those pictured on the front cover, are considered a "functional food" because they provide health benefits beyond the essential nutrients they contain. Vitamin C and lycopene, a phytochemical in tomatoes, function as powerful antioxidants. Lycopene has also been linked to a reduced risk of stroke, some eye diseases, and certain types of cancer. Tomatoes are also abundant sources of potassium, a mineral often lacking in the American diet. A dietary pattern rich in potassium and low in sodium can lower blood pressure and reduce the risk of heart disease. Nutrients and phytochemicals in tomatoes may also boost the immune system and protect bone health.

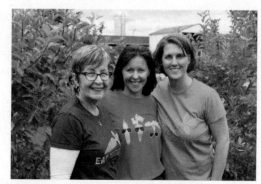

©Briana Zabala

The authors, Anne Smith, Colleen Spees, and Angela Collene at the Garden of Hope.

The eleventh edition of *Wardlaw's Contemporary Nutrition* shows how a primarily plant-based eating pattern—rich in nutrients and phytochemicals—works to support and maintain optimal health throughout life. The new Farm to Fork feature in each chapter outlines the best ways to grow, shop, store, and prepare specific fruits and vegetables to optimize their nutritional value. This comprehensive and evidence-based perspective on nutrition makes learning fun, engaging, and relevant.

Dear Students,

Welcome to the fascinating world of nutrition! Because we all eat several times a day and the choices we make can have a dramatic influence on health, nutrition is our favorite area of science. At the same time, though, the science of nutrition can seem a bit confusing. One reason for all the confusion is that it seems like "good nutrition" is a moving target; different authorities have different ideas of how we should eat, and nutrition recommendations sometimes change! Do carbohydrates cause weight gain? Do I need to limit saturated fat? Should we eat foods that contain gluten? Second, there are so many choices. Did you know that the average supermarket carries about 40,000 food and beverage products? The manufacturers of all those products are vying for your attention, but typically, the most aggressively marketed items are not the healthiest. How can you identify a healthy product? Third, as a nation, we eat many of our meals and snacks away from home. When we eat foods someone else has prepared for us, we surrender control over what is in our food, where the food came from, and how much of it goes on our plates. Undoubtedly, you are interested in what you should be eating and how the food you eat affects you.

__Wardlaw's Contemporary Nutrition__ is designed to accurately convey changing and seemingly conflicting messages to all kinds of students. Our students commonly have misconceptions about nutrition, and many have a limited background in biology or chemistry. We teach complex scientific concepts at a level that will enable you to apply the material to your own life.

This marks the eleventh edition of __Wardlaw's Contemporary Nutrition.__ We are very excited to introduce you to our newest author, Dr. Colleen Spees! Like our other authors, she is a Registered Dietitian Nutritionist, which means she will help you to translate nutrition science into practical advice. At The Ohio State University, Dr. Spees is a valued expert on cancer, nutritional genomics, and food security. We are thrilled to add her unique perspective and contemporary ideas.

As in previous editions, we have written this book to help you make informed choices about the food you eat. We will take you through explanations of the nutrients in food and their relationship to health and make you aware of the multitude of other factors that drive food choices. To guide you, we refer to many reputable research studies, books, policies, and websites throughout the book. With this information at your fingertips, you will be well equipped to make your own informed choices about what and how much to eat. There is much to learn, so let's get started!

Anne Smith
Angela Collene
Colleen Spees

Wardlaw's CONTEMPORARY
NUTRITION

ELEVENTH EDITION

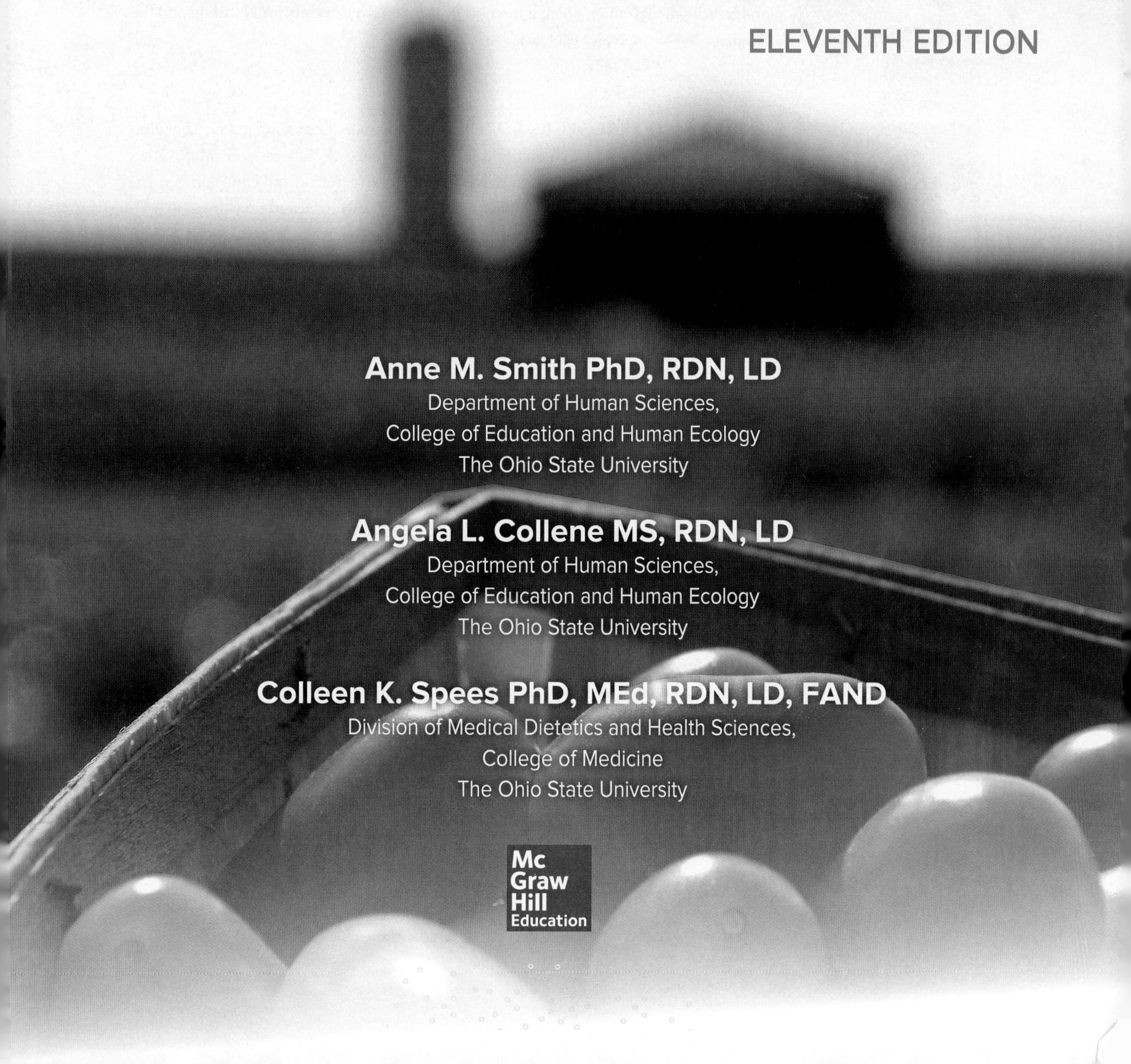

Anne M. Smith PhD, RDN, LD
Department of Human Sciences,
College of Education and Human Ecology
The Ohio State University

Angela L. Collene MS, RDN, LD
Department of Human Sciences,
College of Education and Human Ecology
The Ohio State University

Colleen K. Spees PhD, MEd, RDN, LD, FAND
Division of Medical Dietetics and Health Sciences,
College of Medicine
The Ohio State University

Mc
Graw
Hill
Education

About the Authors

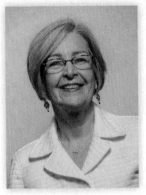

Monty Soungpradith;
©Open Image Studio

ANNE M. SMITH, PhD, RDN, LD, is an associate professor emeritus at The Ohio State University. She was the recipient of the Outstanding Teacher Award from the College of Human Ecology, the Outstanding Dietetic Educator Award from the Ohio Dietetic Association, the Outstanding Faculty Member Award from the Department of Human Nutrition, and the Distinguished Service Award from the College of Education and Human Ecology for her commitment to undergraduate education in nutrition. Dr. Smith's research in the area of vitamin and mineral metabolism has appeared in prominent nutrition journals, and she was awarded the Research Award from the Ohio Agricultural Research and Development Center. She is a member of the American Society for Nutrition and the Academy of Nutrition and Dietetics.

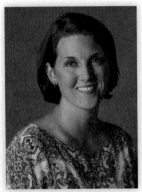

©Tim Klontz, Klontz Photography

ANGELA L. COLLENE, MS, RDN, LD, began her career at her alma mater, The Ohio State University, as a research dietitian for studies related to diabetes and aging. Other professional experiences include community nutrition lecturing and counseling, owner of a personal chef business, and many diverse and rewarding science writing and editing projects. Her interests include novel approaches to glycemic control, weight management, and—quite predictably for the mother of three little girls—maternal and child nutrition. Mrs. Collene currently teaches nutrition at The Ohio State University and Ohio Northern University. She is a member of the Academy of Nutrition and Dietetics.

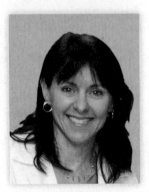

©RALPHOTOSTUDIO

COLLEEN K. SPEES, PhD, MEd, RDN, LD, FAND, is an academic instructor and researcher at The Ohio State University College of Medicine. She earned her Doctorate in Health Sciences at Ohio State with a research focus on Nutritional Genomics and Cancer and her Master's degree in Exercise Science and Health Promotion from Vanderbilt University. Her primary focus of teaching and research involves interventions aimed at providing optimal nutrition for vulnerable populations (http://go.osu.edu/hope). In addition to teaching nutrition at The Ohio State University, Dr. Spees also developed and teaches a graduate level Nutritional Genomics course. She is the recipient of several national awards from the Academy of Nutrition and Dietetics, including the Distinguished Practice Award; Award for Excellence in Oncology Nutrition Research; Outstanding Dietetic Educator Award; Nutrition Informatics Video Challenge Teaching Award; Top Innovator in Education Teaching Award; and has been a Content Expert and Reviewer for the Academy's Nutritional Genomics & Food Security Position Papers. Dr. Spees is also a recognized Fellow of the Academy of Nutrition and Dietetics.

Acknowledgments

It is because of the tireless efforts of a cohesive team of talented professionals that we can bring you the eleventh edition of *Wardlaw's Contemporary Nutrition*. We consider ourselves massively blessed to work with the top-notch staff at McGraw-Hill Education. We are grateful to Marija Magner, Sr. Portfolio Manager, for her strategic leadership and vast knowledge of the higher education market. We thank our award-winning Product Developer, Darlene Schueller, who coordinated the editorial team with her keen eye for detail, strong work ethic, and organizational expertise. We are grateful to our Content Project Manager, Mary Jane Lampe, and her staff for the careful coordination of the numerous production efforts needed to create the very appealing and accurate eleventh edition. We thank Samantha Donisi-Hamm, our Assessment Content Project Manager, for her efforts and assistance. We appreciate the meticulous work of our copyeditor, Marilynn Taylor; proofreaders, Kay J. Brimeyer and Debbie Trilk; and our Content Licensing Specialist, Melissa Homer. We thank our Designer, Tara McDermott, who ensured that every aspect of our work is visually appealing—not just on the printed page but also in a variety of digital formats. Finally, we are indebted to our colleagues, friends, and families for their constant encouragement, honest feedback, and shared passion for the science of nutrition.

Reviewers

In the preparation of each edition, we have been guided by the collective wisdom of reviewers who are excellent teachers. They represent experience in community colleges, liberal arts colleges, institutions, and universities. We have followed their recommendations, while remaining true to our overriding goal of writing a readable, student-centered text.

Roseann Berg
Foothill College

Shawn Bjerke
Minnesota State Community and Technical College

Priscilla Burrow
University of Colorado, Denver

Iveta D. Dinbergs
Middlesex Community College

Virginia B. Gray
California State University Long Beach

Julie Kennel
The Ohio State University

Carol Mack
Erie Community College/North

Sudeep Majumdar
Temple College

Dana Scheunemann
Milwaukee Area Technical College

Shannon Seal
Front Range Community College

James Stevens
Front Range Community College

Dana Wu Wassmer
Cosumnes River College

Student-Informed Reviews

We are very pleased to have been able to incorporate real student data points and input, derived from thousands of our SmartBook® users, to help guide our revision. SmartBook heat maps provided a quick visual snapshot of usage of portions of the text and the relative difficulty students experienced in mastering the content. With these data, we were able to hone not only our text content but also the SmartBook probes.

With the eleventh edition of *Wardlaw's Contemporary Nutrition* we remember its founding author, Gordon M. Wardlaw. Dr. Wardlaw had a passion for the science of nutrition and the research that supports it and demonstrated an exceptional ability to translate scientific principles into practical knowledge. This skill is what made his book truly "contemporary." He was tireless when it came to staying current and relevant to a changing world. It has been a privilege for all of us to join Dr. Wardlaw as coauthors of this textbook. For Anne Smith, he was an extraordinary colleague, mentor, and friend. Angela Collene was blessed to have been one of his graduate students at The Ohio State University, when she first began to assist with revisions to his books. Colleen Spees was a student in Dr. Wardlaw's first nutrition class at The Ohio State University and now holds his previous tenure-track position. Like so many other students, colleagues, and friends, we remember Dr. Wardlaw as a source of vast knowledge, good humor, and inspiration. The best way we know to honor our dear friend and mentor is to carry on his legacy of outstanding textbooks in introductory nutrition. *Wardlaw's Contemporary Nutrition* will continue to evolve and reflect current trends and breakthroughs in nutrition science, but Dr. Wardlaw's fingerprints will remain on every page.

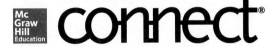 **connect®**

McGraw-Hill Connect® is a highly reliable, easy-to-use homework and learning management solution that utilizes learning science and award-winning adaptive tools to improve student results.

Homework and Adaptive Learning

- Connect's assignments help students contextualize what they've learned through application, so they can better understand the material and think critically.

- Connect will create a personalized study path customized to individual student needs through SmartBook®.

- SmartBook helps students study more efficiently by delivering an interactive reading experience through adaptive highlighting and review.

Connect's Impact on Retention Rates, Pass Rates, and Average Exam Scores

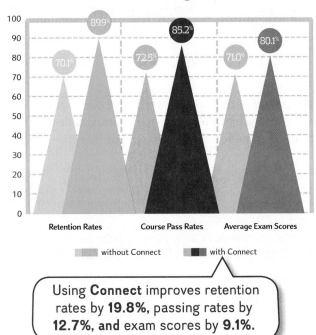

without Connect | with Connect

Using **Connect** improves retention rates by **19.8%**, passing rates by **12.7%, and** exam scores by **9.1%.**

Over **7 billion questions** have been answered, making McGraw-Hill Education products more intelligent, reliable, and precise.

73% of instructors who use **Connect** require it; instructor satisfaction **increases** by 28% when **Connect** is required.

Quality Content and Learning Resources

- Connect content is authored by the world's best subject matter experts, and is available to your class through a simple and intuitive interface.

- The Connect eBook makes it easy for students to access their reading material on smartphones and tablets. They can study on the go and don't need Internet access to use the eBook as a reference, with full functionality.

- Multimedia content such as videos, simulations, and games drive student engagement and critical thinking skills.

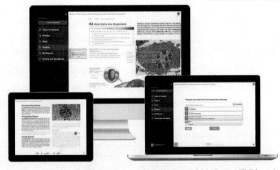

Robust Analytics and Reporting

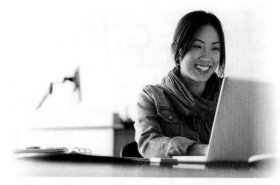

©Hero Images/Getty Images

- Connect Insight® generates easy-to-read reports on individual students, the class as a whole, and on specific assignments.

- The Connect Insight dashboard delivers data on performance, study behavior, and effort. Instructors can quickly identify students who struggle and focus on material that the class has yet to master.

- Connect automatically grades assignments and quizzes, providing easy-to-read reports on individual and class performance.

Impact on Final Course Grade Distribution

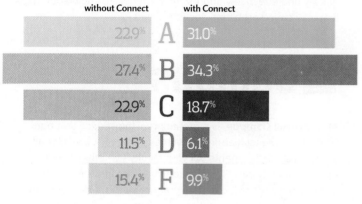

without Connect		with Connect
22.9%	A	31.0%
27.4%	B	34.3%
22.9%	C	18.7%
11.5%	D	6.1%
15.4%	F	9.9%

More students earn **As** and **Bs** when they use **Connect**.

Trusted Service and Support

- Connect integrates with your LMS to provide single sign-on and automatic syncing of grades. Integration with Blackboard®, D2L®, and Canvas also provides automatic syncing of the course calendar and assignment-level linking.

- Connect offers comprehensive service, support, and training throughout every phase of your implementation.

- If you're looking for some guidance on how to use Connect, or want to learn tips and tricks from super users, you can find tutorials as you work. Our Digital Faculty Consultants and Student Ambassadors offer insight into how to achieve the results you want with Connect.

www.mheducation.com/connect

Connecting Teaching and Learning

Dietary Analysis Auto-Graded Assignments Within Connect

One of the challenges many instructors face with teaching nutrition classes is having the time to grade dietary analysis projects. To help overcome that challenge, auto-graded assignments that require students to use NutritionCalc Plus (NCP) and answer questions based on the generated reports have been developed. These assignments were developed and reviewed by faculty who use such assignments in their own teaching. They are designed to be relevant, current, and interesting!

> "The case studies provide a neutral way for my students to explore dietary analysis. My students are engaged by the case study assignments and find them easy to use. The fact that they are auto-graded gives me more time to focus on content development and instruction for my course.
>
> I appreciate how flexible the case study assignments are. I can use the case and the diet plan, and then only assign those questions that best match my learning outcomes. I can also add my own questions to the assignments."
>
> Hannah Thornton, Texas State University

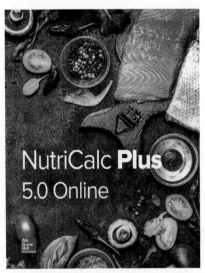

©Victoria Shibut/123RF

NutritionCalc Plus is a powerful dietary analysis tool featuring more than 30,000 foods from the ESHA Research nutrient database, which is comprised of data from the latest USDA Standard Reference database, manufacturer's data, restaurant data, and data from literature sources. NutritionCalc Plus allows users to track food and activities, and then analyze their choices with a robust selection of intuitive reports. The interface was updated to accommodate ADA requirements and modern mobile experience native to today's students.

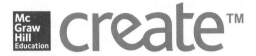

McGraw-Hill Create™ is a self-service website that allows you to create customized course materials using McGraw-Hill Education's comprehensive, cross-disciplinary content and digital products.

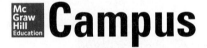

Fueled by LearnSmart—the most widely used and intelligent adaptive learning resource—**LearnSmart® Prep for Nutrition** is designed to get students ready for a forthcoming course by quickly and effectively addressing prerequisite knowledge gaps that may cause problems down the road.

Campus

McGraw-Hill Campus® is a groundbreaking service that puts world-class digital learning resources just a click away for all your faculty and students. All your faculty—whether or not they use a McGraw-Hill Education title—can instantly browse, search, and access the entire library of McGraw-Hill Education instructional resources and services including eBooks, test banks, PowerPoint slides, animations, and learning objects—from any Learning Management System (LMS), at no additional cost to your institution. Users also have single sign-on access to McGraw-Hill Education digital platforms, including Connect, ALEKS®, Create, and Tegrity.

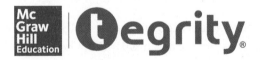

Tegrity® is a fully automated lecture capture solution used in traditional, hybrid, "flipped classes," and online courses to record lessons, lectures, and skills.

Connecting Students to Today's Nutrition

Understanding Our Audience

We have written *Wardlaw's Contemporary Nutrition* assuming that our students have a limited background in college-level biology, chemistry, or physiology. We have been careful to include the essential science foundation needed to adequately comprehend certain topics in nutrition, such as protein synthesis in Chapter 6. The science in this text has been presented in a simple, straightforward manner so that undergraduate students can master the material and apply it to their own lives. The Concept Maps and detailed, annotated figures bring complex topics into view for students from any major.

Featuring the Latest Guidelines and Research

Nutrition is a dynamic field. A vast quantity of research constantly reshapes our knowledge of nutritional science. The eleventh edition has been carefully updated to reflect current scientific understanding, as well as the latest health and nutrition guidelines. For everyday diet planning, students will learn about the *Dietary Guidelines for Americans*, *MyPlate*, and *Healthy People 2020*. In discussions about specific nutrition concerns, the most recent data and recommendations from the Academy of Nutrition and Dietetics, American Heart Association, American Diabetes Association, National Academy of Medicine, and American Psychological Association have been included in this edition.

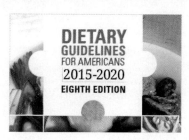

Newsworthy Nutrition, a feature in each chapter, highlights the use of the scientific method in recently published research studies that relate to the chapter topics. In addition, assignable questions in Connect take learning a step further by asking students to read primary literature and apply what they have learned.

Newsworthy Nutrition

Probiotics provide relief from constipation

Up to 25% of adults suffer from functional constipation, a problem characterized by infrequent or difficult bowel movements not due to a physical cause. Typically, functional constipation is treated with medications that can have side effects or lead to dependence. In this study, 40 adults with functional constipation were randomly assigned to receive a daily probiotic supplement containing *Lactobacillus reuteri* or placebo for 4 weeks. By the end of the study period, subjects who received the probiotics reported increased frequency of bowel movements (5.3 per week), compared with subjects who received a placebo (2.7 per week). No adverse effects were reported.

Ask the RDN is a new feature in every chapter that answers questions about topics that may seem to have conflicting viewpoints. This feature will highlight the ability of the RDN to translate the latest scientific findings into easy-to-understand nutrition information.

ASK THE RDN: Who's the Expert?

Dear RDN: *I am interested in making positive changes to my eating pattern to reach a healthy weight and feel better. How can I find a qualified nutrition expert who will give me personalized nutrition advice?*

You have already made a big step toward better nutrition by taking this nutrition course! The information in this textbook is written by authors who are all qualified nutrition experts, namely *registered dietitian nutritionists* (RDN). The textbook and your instructor will provide a solid foundation in nutrition, but be aware that some people call themselves "nutritionists" without qualified training in nutrition. The best approach to finding answers about your personal nutritional state is to consult your primary care provider, **registered dietitian (RD),** or **registered dietitian nutritionist (RDN).** The RD/RDN has been certified by the Commission on Dietetic Registration of the Academy of Nutrition and Dietetics (AND) after completing rigorous classroom and clinical training in nutrition. The RD/RDN must also complete continuing education. The RD credential was recently updated to RDN to better reflect the scope of practice of dietitians. While both titles signify the same credential, we will use RDN when referring to dietitians in this book.

You can begin your search for a local RDN by asking your primary care provider or calling your health insurance company for a referral. You can also find an RDN by using the AND national referral service, called *Find a Registered Dietitian Nutritionist*. This service links consumers with qualified nutrition practitioners who provide reliable, objective nutrition information. Visit the website, www.eatright.org, and click on "Find an Expert." (In Canada, visit the Dietitians of Canada website, www.dietitians.ca, and click on "Find a Dietitian.") Enter your ZIP code or state to display the providers in your area. Select additional specialties that may apply to your specific needs. The website will display a list of providers. A professional with the RD or RDN credential after his or her name is a qualified nutrition expert who is trained to help you separate facts from fads and optimize your health with better food choices. You can trust an RDN to translate the latest scientific findings into easy-to-understand nutrition information.

I hope this answer was helpful. We will use this feature, "Ask the RDN," in every chapter to answer questions about topics that may seem to have conflicting viewpoints.

Your nutrition expert,

Anne M. Smith , PhD, RDN, LD (author)

The *Medicine Cabinet* feature presents information on common medications used to treat diseases that have a nutrition connection. These features highlight the ways medications can affect nutritional status, as well as ways food and nutrients can affect how medications work.

Medicine Cabinet

Some medications may limit vitamin B-12 absorption. Antacids or other medications used to inhibit acid secretions will increase the pH within the stomach, thereby limiting release of B-12 from protein. People who have ulcers or reflux may take these drugs. Metformin, a popular medication for controlling diabetes, may reduce B-12 absorption. With any of these medications, you should check with your primary care provider to see if supplemental B-12 is recommended.

©Peter Dazeley/Photographer's Choice/Getty Images

Connecting with a Personal Focus

Valuing Our Food Supply

In this edition, we introduce a new *Farm to Fork* feature. Each chapter spotlights a food item and traces its path to our plates. Where does it grow? How do you select the most flavorful and nutritious foods? What are the best ways to store and prepare foods to maximize nutritional value?

Applying Nutrition on a Personal Level

Throughout the eleventh edition, we reinforce the fact that each person responds differently to nutrients. To further convey the importance of applying nutrition to their personal lives, we include many examples of people and situations that resonate with college students. We also stress the importance of learning to intelligently sort through the seemingly endless range of nutrition messages to recognize reliable information and to sensibly apply it to their own lives. Our goal is to provide students the tools they need to eat healthfully and make informed nutrition decisions after they complete the class. Many of these features can be assigned and graded through Connect to help students learn and apply the information and engage with the text.

Challenging Students to Think Critically

The pages of *Wardlaw's Contemporary Nutrition* contain numerous opportunities for students to learn more about themselves and their diet and to use their new knowledge of nutrition to improve their health. These pedagogical elements include *Critical Thinking, Ask the RDN, Case Studies, Nutrition and Your Health, What Would You Choose?,* and *Newsworthy Nutrition.* Many of the thought-provoking topics highlighted in these features are expanded upon in the online resources found in Connect.

FARM to FORK **Bananas**

When you enjoy tropical fruits, you are eating globally. The most common tropical fruits are bananas, pineapples, mangos, and papayas—imported from Ecuador, Costa Rica, Mexico, and Hawaii. Bananas are the most consumed fruit in the United States—more than apples and oranges combined!

Grow
- Although bananas grow on "banana palms," bananas do not grow on trees. Banana palms are actually a perennial herb.
- Bananas do not grow from a seed but instead from a bulb or rhizome. After planting a banana palm in a subtropical environment, it can take up to 12 months to literally enjoy the fruits of your labor.
- Because bananas grow in tropical climates, they are not seasonal fruits but rather continue to grow all year long.

Shop
- There are two main categories of bananas. Plantains (or cooking bananas) are starchy, and Cavendish (or dessert bananas) are the sweet, yellow bananas most commonly sold at the supermarket.
- To increase your antioxidant content when eating bananas, look beyond Cavendish bananas. Red bananas and niños, or Lady Fingers, provide greater vitamin C, potassium, calcium, manganese, carotenoids, and zinc than the common Cavendish.

©Corey Hochachka/Design Pics

Store
- Bananas continue to ripen after harvest and are often harvested when immature and green. These bananas will ripen in 5 to 7 days if left at room temperature.
- Store ripe bananas in the refrigerator. Although their skins will turn brown, the flesh will stay fresher for days.

Prep
- Plantains serve as the main carbohydrate source for 20 million individuals globally. Harvested when green, plantains are skinned, then steamed, baked, or fried.
- In the Caribbean, fried plantains are a staple. For a healthier recipe, try baked plantains. Use ripe plantains, spotted with brown or black spots, and slice after peeling. Coat a nonstick baking sheet with cooking spray and lay the plantains in rows. Cook at 450°F for 15 minutes, flipping them frequently.
- Celebrate bananas as the perfect on-the-go snack, lunch box treat, or sliced treat on top of cereal, yogurt, or whole wheat pancakes.

© Shutterstock/Nataliia K

Source: Robinson J. "Tropical Fruits: Make the Most of Eating Globally," in *Eating on the Wild Side.* New York: Little, Brown and Company, 2013.

Rate Your Plate

I. Rate Your Beverage Choices

Water is the key component in the guidelines that have been developed by the Beverage Guidance Panel (Table 9-10). These recommendations give guidance on the health and nutritional benefits as well as the risks of various beverage categories. The basis of the Beverage Guidance System is that fluids should not provide a significant amount of the energy nutrients in a healthy diet. More specifically, the system recommends that beverages provide less than 10% of total calories consumed for a 2200 kcal diet.[24]

TABLE 9-10 ■ The Beverage Guidance System

Level	Category*	Recommended Servings per Day
1	Water	50 fluid ounces (1.7 liters)
2	Tea or coffee, unsweetened	0 to 40 fluid ounces (0 to 1.4 liters)
3	Low-fat and skim milk and soy beverages	0 to 16 fluid ounces (0 to 0.5 liter)
4	Noncalorically sweetened beverages (diet drinks)	0 to 32 fluid ounces (0 to 1 liter)
5	Calorie beverages with some nutrients (100% fruit juices, alcoholic beverages, whole milk, and sports drinks)	0 to 8 fluid ounces 100% fruit juices (0 to 0.25 liter) 0 to 1 alcoholic drink for women 0 to 2 alcoholic drinks for men
6	Calorically sweetened beverages (regular soft drinks)	0 to 8 fluid ounces (0 to 0.25 liter)

*Categories established based on their possible health benefits or risks.
Source: Adapted from Popkin, et al. "A new proposed guidance system for beverage consumption in the United States," *American Journal of Clinical Nutrition* 83:529, 2006

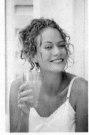
©Hoby Finn/Getty Images

1. Think of all the beverages ... nt to bed. Do your best to recall the types and am...

CASE STUDY **Typical College Student**

Andy is like many other college students. He grew up on a quick bowl of cereal and milk for breakfast and a hamburger, French fries, and cola for lunch, either in the school cafeteria or at a local fast-food restaurant. At dinner, he generally avoided eating any of his salad or vegetables, and by 9:00 P.M. he was deep into bags of chips and cookies. Andy has taken most of these habits to college. He prefers coffee for breakfast and possibly a chocolate bar. Lunch is still mainly a hamburger, French fries, and cola, but pizza and tacos now alternate more frequently than when he was in high school. One thing Andy really likes about the restaurants surrounding campus is that, for a few cents more, he can make his hamburger a double or get extra cheese and pepperoni on his pizza. This helps him stretch his food dollar; searching out large-portion value meals for lunch and dinner has become part of a typical day. Now that he is in college, some of Andy's calories come from alcohol. He will have a beer with dinner a couple nights a week and will binge on a six-pack or more while tailgating before Saturday football games.

Provide Andy some advice about his eating pattern. Start with his positive habits and then provide some constructive criticism, based on what you now know.

Answer the following questions, and as you make suggestions for Andy, think about your favorite food choices, why they are your favorites, and whether these are positive choices.

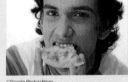
©Dinodia Photos/Almay

What Would You Choose?

You are gearing up to run your first half-marathon in a few weeks. From your long training runs, you know that physical and mental fatigue may set in a few miles before the finish. You've practiced great dietary patterns throughout training but have trouble eating during your runs. You want to try one of those sports nutrition products to help get you through the last few miles. What would you choose to take along during the race to help you make it to the finish line?

a Clif Shot® Turbo energy gel with 100 milligrams caffeine, 22 grams of carbohydrate, and electrolytes

b PowerBar ProteinPlus® energy bar with 23 grams of protein

c Powerade® sports drink with electrolytes, vitamins, and 14 grams of carbohydrate

---

2.8 **Nutrition and Your Health**
Food Labels and Diet Planning

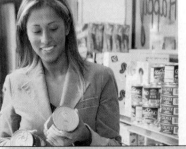

In addition to these required components, manufacturers can choose to list polyunsaturated and monounsaturated fat, potassium, and others. Listing an additional nutrient becomes *required* if the food is fortified with that nutrient or if a claim is made about the health benefits of the specific nutrient.

Remember that the Daily Value is a generic standard used on the food label. The percentage of the Daily Value (% Daily Value or % DV) is usually given for each nutrient per serving. These percentages are based on a 2000-kcal diet and must be adjusted for people who require considerably more or less than 2000 kcal per day with respect to fat and carbohydrate intake. DVs are mostly set at or close to the highest RDA value or related nutrient standard seen in the various age and gender categories for a specific nutrient.

Serving sizes on the Nutrition Facts panel must be consistent among similar foods. This means that all brands of ice cream, for example, must use the same serving size on their label. These serving sizes may differ from those of MyPlate because those on food labels are based on more typical portion sizes. In addition, food claims made on packages must follow legal definitions. A long list of definitions for nutrient claims allowed on food labels is given in Table 2-10. For example, if a product claims to be "low sodium," it must have 140 milligrams of sodium or less per serving.

Connecting to Engaging Visuals

Attractive, Accurate Artwork

Illustrations, photographs, infographics, and tables in the text were created to help students master complex scientific concepts.

- Many illustrations were updated or replaced to inspire student inquiry and comprehension and to promote interest and retention of information. Several were also redesigned to use brighter colors and a more attractive, contemporary style.
- In many figures, color-coding and directional arrows make it easier to follow events and reinforce interrelationships. Process descriptions appear in the body of the figures. This pairing of the action and an explanation walks students step-by-step through the process and increases teaching effectiveness.

The final result is a striking visual program that holds readers' attention and supports the goals of clarity, ease of comprehension, and critical thinking. The attractive layout and design of this edition are clean, bright, and inviting. This creative presentation of the material is geared toward engaging today's visually oriented students.

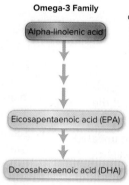

Omega-3 Family

Alpha-linolenic acid

Eicosapentaenoic acid (EPA)

Docosahexaenoic acid (DHA)

Linoleic acid (the essential omega-6 fatty acid) and alpha-linolenic acid (the essential omega-3 fatty acid) must be consumed as part of the diet because the body lacks the enzymes required to make them.

When the essential fatty acids are obtained from the diet, the body can use them to make other, nonessential fatty acids. These eventually give rise to a variety of eicosanoids that regulate body functions.

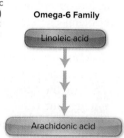

Omega-6 Family

Linoleic acid

Arachidonic acid

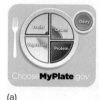

(a)

FIGURE 6-6 ▶ Food sources of protein. (a) The fill of the background color (none, 1/3, 2/3, or completely covered) within each group on MyPlate indicates the average nutrient density for protein in that group. (b) The bar graph shows the protein content of several foods from each food group compared to the RDA for a 70-kilogram male. Overall, the dairy group and the protein group contain many foods that are nutrient-dense sources of protein. The fruits group provides little or no protein (less than 1 gram per serving). Food choices from the vegetables group and grains group provide moderate amounts of protein (2 to 3 grams per serving). The dairy group provides much protein (8 to 10 grams per serving), as does the protein group (7 grams per serving). ©Nutrition data from USDA National Nutrient Database for Standard Reference, Release 26.

(b)

	Food Item and Amount	Protein grams	% RDA for 70 kg Male (56 grams)
Grains	Quinoa, cooked, 1 cup	8.4	15%
	Whole wheat bread, 1 slice	3.5	6%
	White rice, ½ cup	2.1	4%
Vegetables	Edamame, cooked, 1 cup	18.5	33%
	Kidney beans, ½ cup	6.7	12%
	Sweet potato, cooked, medium	2.1	4%
Fruits	Peach, 1 medium	1.4	3%
	Banana, 1 medium	1.3	2%
	Cantaloupe, cubed, 1 cup	1.3	2%
Dairy	Yogurt, Greek, nonfat, 5.3 ounces	13.6	24%
	1% low-fat milk, 1 cup	8.2	15%
	Cheddar cheese, 1 ounce	6.5	12%
Protein	Chicken, breast, roasted, 3 ounces	23.8	43%
	Tuna, canned, 3 ounces	20.1	36%
	Peanuts, 1 ounce	6.9	12%

Connecting with the Latest Updates

Global Changes

- Throughout this new edition we have replaced the term *diet* in most cases with the term *eating pattern* or *dietary pattern*. This reflects the emphasis on "healthy eating patterns" in the *Dietary Guidelines for Americans.* As we discuss healthy eating patterns throughout the text, you will notice more emphasis on the problems of overconsumption of added sugars and less emphasis on problems from the consumption of dietary cholesterol.

- In addition, we have replaced the term *calorie* with *kilocalorie* when referring to specific energy amounts. For example, the Concept Check for Section 1.4 now reads: What are the energy (kilocalorie) values for each of the "energy nutrients?"

- All images of the Nutrition Facts Label have been updated to the new format approved by the U.S. Food and Drug Administration in 2016.

- A new feature, *Ask the RDN (Registered Dietitian Nutritionist)* appears in every chapter and addresses questions we frequently hear students asking about food and nutrition topics covered in the popular media. We use the *Ask the RDN* in Chapter 1 to set the stage, answering the important question "How can I find a qualified nutrition expert who will give me personalized nutrition advice?" Each feature is answered and signed by one of the authors, who are all Registered Dietitian Nutritionists! Along these same lines, we have emphasized RDNs as the nutrition experts throughout the text.

- Another new feature, *Farm to Fork,* appears in every chapter and presents practical information on how to grow, shop for, store, and prepare various fruits and vegetables to obtain and preserve their flavor and nutrients.

- The last section of each chapter, *Nutrition and Your Health,* is now a numbered section (e.g., Section 1.8 in Chapter 1) for easier navigating especially within the digital components of the text.

- The term *physician* or *doctor* has been replaced with *primary care provider,* and references to the Institute of Medicine have been updated to its new name, National Academy of Medicine.

- The Case Study Solutions have been removed from all chapters, so that the *Case Study* can be used as an assignable project. Instructors can time the release of the solutions on Connect.

- *Further Readings* are now superscripted as footnotes in the text.

Chapter-by-Chapter Revisions

Chapter 1: *Nutrition, Food Choices, and Health*

- Figures 1-2 and 1-3 are new and illustrate USDA data from 2014 for vegetable and dairy product consumption, respectively. Figure 1-3 also compares 2014 dairy product consumption with that in 1974.

- Figure 1-4 provides an update on the 10 leading causes of death in the United States in 2014 as reported by the Centers for Disease Control and Prevention in June 2016.

- In Section 1.4 on math concepts, practical examples of metric system conversions have been added. Examples include the conversion of grams of sugar in Greek yogurt to teaspoons and milliliters of water to cups.

- Section 1.6, What Is the Current State of the North American Eating Patterns and Health?, has been updated to reflect recent changes in obesity trends. Figure 1-7 showing the percentage of adults who were obese in 2015 as well as other obesity statistics, has been updated. The most recent report, *F as in Fat: How Obesity Threatens America's Future 2013,* is discussed. The *Newsworthy Nutrition* feature has been updated to "No Decrease in Adult Obesity Rates from 2005 to 2014," summarizing research published in the *Journal of the American Medical Association* in 2016.

- *The Case Study: Typical College Student* has been revised to include alcohol in the dietary pattern.

- The Further Readings have been updated with seven new articles.

Chapter 2: *Designing a Healthy Eating Pattern*

- The *What Would You Choose* feature has been expanded to include snacks as well as beverages and asks which snack combination provides the best amount of calories, nutrients, and energy for an afternoon snack.

- The *Newsworthy Nutrition,* "Effect of healthy eating attitude at the supermarket," is new and is a summary of research published in the *Journal of the Academy of Nutrition and Dietetics* in 2014.

- Significant changes in Chapter 2 revolve around the *Dietary Guidelines for Americans.* In Section 2.2, the entire subsection, Dietary Guidelines—The Basis for Menu Planning, has been revised. To help students understand the political issues surrounding the Guidelines, we have included a discussion of the process used to establish them. Figure 2-1 is adapted from the *Dietary Guidelines* and illustrates typical food choices that can be shifted to more nutrient-dense options. The five foundational guidelines of the *Dietary Guidelines* are outlined and Key Recommendations are illustrated in Figure 2-2.

- The chapter title has changed to *Designing a Healthy Eating Pattern,* and Section 2.2 highlights the Guidelines' new emphasis on "Healthy Eating Patterns" with the following new subsections: Shifting to Healthy Eating Patterns; Importance of Calorie Balance Within Healthy Eating Patterns; Food Components to Include in Your Healthy Eating Pattern; and Food Components to Limit in Your Healthy Eating Pattern. The new Figure 2-3, Comparing current eating patterns in the United States to the *Dietary Guidelines,* is directly from the Guidelines report.

- The *Farm to Fork* feature in Chapter 2 highlights carrots and beets, two colorful vegetables that fit into the Dietary Guideline to eat a variety from all five vegetable subgroups—dark green, red and orange, beans and peas, starchy, and others.

- Several updates have been made to the Section 2.3, MyPlate—A Menu Planning Tool. A new subsection, Build a Healthy Eating Style, includes ideas and tips to help create a healthier eating style. Categories include 1) All Food and Beverage Choices Matter—Focus on Variety, Amount, and Nutrition, 2) Choose an Eating Style Low in Saturated Fat, Sodium, and Added Sugars, 3) Make Small Changes to Create a Healthier Eating Style (introduces the new MyPlate feature, MyWin), and 4) Support Healthy Eating for Everyone.

- Figure 2-6 is an improved illustration of what counts as a serving and the use of standard objects to estimate serving size. Dice have replaced the golf ball as visual cues for items such as butter or peanut butter.

- The focus and caption for Figure 2-7 have been changed to illustrate that all dairy is not the same. This bar graph compares the difference in kilocalories from various types of milks and the added calories from fat and sugar in various milks compared to fat-free milk.

- The *What's Cooking? USDA Mixing Bowl,* an interactive tool for consumers who are ready to make a change and need help with healthy meal planning, cooking, and grocery shopping, has been added to the list of Additional MyPlate Resources.

- Margarine has been deleted and/or replaced with peanut butter in Table 2-7, Putting MyPlate into Practice.

- Section 2.3 includes the new *Ask the RDN* feature, which answers the question of how to follow the Mediterranean Diet eating plan.

- New information on Diet and Nutrition Apps has been added to Section 2.7 and includes a link to the Academy of Nutrition and Dietetics' science-based reviews of the most popular diet and nutrition apps for phones and tablets.

- Section 2.8, Food Labels and Diet Planning, includes a new subsection on Labeling of Food Allergens. Also Figure 2-12 has been updated in accordance with the revised Nutrition Facts Label and includes information about the new line for Added Sugars.

- There are eight new *Further Readings* in Chapter 2.

Chapter 3: *The Human Body: A Nutrition Perspective*

- The new *Farm to Fork* feature describes the benefits of cranberries, which help to prevent infections of the gastrointestinal and urinary tracts.

- Figures 3-8, 3-10, 3-12, 3-14, 3-16, and 3-21 have been updated to an infographic style to more clearly explain key features of the gastrointestinal tract.

- In Section 3.9, the newest taste sensation—oleogustus—is defined, and the *Newsworthy Nutrition* feature has been updated to present recent research on the effects of probiotics on bowel regularity.

- Section 3.11 has been updated with current terminology and the latest statistics on the relationships between nutrition and genetics. Readers will find an expanded and updated collection of web resources for further information on genetics.

- The *Nutrition and Your Health* feature in Section 3.12 includes updated information on treatments for irritable bowel syndrome.

- The new *Ask the RDN* feature explores the question of whether a gluten-free diet is an effective weight-loss method.

- In the *Rate Your Plate* activity, we now provide a link to an interactive tool to generate a medical family tree.

- To provide students with additional resources, Chapter 3 includes 13 new *Further Readings.*

Chapter 4: *Carbohydrates*

- New to Section 4.2, the relationship between gut microbiota and fiber intake are described.

- The new *Farm to Fork* feature focuses on an excellent source of dietary fiber—potatoes!

- In Section 4.3, the idea of consuming fruits and vegetables as juice is discussed as an answer to the *Ask the RDN* question, Is juicing healthier than eating whole fruits or vegetables?

- Also in Section 4.3, energy and sports drinks are added to emphasize these as growing sources of added sugar in the United States.

- Table 4-1 was added to highlight the main differences between whole and refined grains.

- A new table of lactose-containing food sources has been added in Table 4-2.

- *What Are FODMAPs?* is a new information box in Section 4.4 and explains this group of fermentable carbohydrates and lists several websites that provide practical information on foods to avoid and foods to include when restricting FODMAPs.

- The section on glycemic index has been shortened, glycemic load introduced, and an emphasis placed on the role of lifestyle management of glucose control added.

- The "To sugar or not to sugar" content describes the pros and cons of consuming refined sugar and artificial sweeteners.

- Section 4.6 provides a list of the updated *Dietary Guidelines'* recommendations for carbohydrate intake as part of a healthy eating pattern.

- Also featured in Section 4.6 is a new *Newsworthy Nutrition,* "Americans are decreasing consumption of sugar-sweetened beverages," based on research published in 2013.

- The *Nutrition and Your Health* featuring diabetes includes updated information on insulin pumps and highlights the Diabetes Prevention Program.

- The CDC *National Diabetes Statistics Report,* as well as the *Position of the Academy of Nutrition and Dietetics: Health implications of dietary fiber,* have been updated in the *Further Readings* along with eight new articles.

Chapter 5: *Lipids*

- On the whole, Chapter 5 has been reorganized to improve flow of information. Some figures and text *content* have been moved so that all of the information on food sources of lipids appears in Section 5.3 and all of the recommendations for fat intake appear in Section 5.7.

- Throughout the chapter, to reflect updated advice from the *Dietary Guidelines* and the American Heart Association's *Diet and Lifestyle Recommendations,* we emphasize that the quality of fat in the diet is just as important as the total amount of fat in the diet. In addition, we have removed any outdated recommendations about specific limits for dietary cholesterol intake.

- Section 5.1 has been expanded to introduce students to some of the core terminology in the chapter.

- The structures of lipids in Figures 5-1 and 5-4 and the Concept Map are now displayed as ball-and-stick models, which give students a sense of the three-dimensional shape of lipids and how that might affect their functions.

- Figure 5-3 has been revised to more accurately represent the relationships among key omega-3 and omega-6 fatty acids. Likewise, the Lipids Concept Map, now in Section 5.2, has been simplified to show how the various forms of lipids are related to each other.

- In Section 5.3, we point out that partially hydrogenated oils are no longer generally recognized as safe for use in food products.

- Figure 5-5 now combines MyPlate with the bar graph representation of food sources of fat.

- In Section 5.6, we have added a new subsection on the role of lipids in regulating body processes. Information about eicosanoids, which had previously appeared elsewhere in the chapter, is now presented in this section.

- Table 5-5 has been updated with the latest *Diet and Lifestyle Recommendations* from the American Heart Association, which were released in 2013.

- A new Figure 5-17 translates the American Heart Association's *Diet and Lifestyle Recommendations* into practical terms: dinner!

- A new subsection within Section 5.7 summarizes the advice of public health authorities on fish consumption. Also, a new subsection discusses dietary patterns that promote cardiovascular health.

- In Section 5.7, we have included a new *Ask the RDN* feature about the health benefits of coconut oil.

- The content of the *Nutrition and Your Health* section has been simplified to focus less on medical treatments and more on dietary strategies to lower risk for cardiovascular disease.

- Chapter 5 has been updated with 12 new *Further Readings.*

Chapter 6: *Proteins*

- The *What Would You Choose* feature has been updated to focus more on consuming at least 20 to 30 grams of protein at a given meal to optimize muscle protein growth.

- Several updates have been made to Section 6.3, Protein in Foods. Statistics on the consumption of animal products in developing countries have been updated.

- Figure 6-6, Food Sources of Protein, has been reformatted to include information about sources of protein on MyPlate.

- Figure 6-7 is new and illustrates beef, pork, and poultry production in developed and developing countries.

- A new box feature, *Evaluating Protein Quality,* summarizes the new method (Digestible Indispensable Amino Acid Score [DIAAS]) for assessing the quality of dietary proteins that is recommended by the FAO.

- Practical tips on using legumes as a source of protein are listed in the *Farm to Fork* feature.

- Figure 6-10 has been expanded to display eight separate images to represent the eight common food allergens.

- Content on the effects of high protein intakes has been moved to this section.

- The new protein intake recommendations from the *Dietary Guidelines* are outlined in Section 6.6, including the shifts recommended to increase variety in protein food choices and to make more nutrient-dense choices. Section 6.6 also includes a discussion of current research showing that a more equal distribution of protein at each meal is important in maintaining body composition and bone health and in regulating glucose.

- The association between the consumption of high levels of red and processed meat and the increased risk of colorectal cancer, including the findings of the 2015 report of the World Health Organization, is discussed in more detail in Section 6.3.

- New content on meal protein requirements, including discussion of maintaining a more equal distribution of protein at each meal, as well as the increased daily protein intake of > 1.0 g/kg for older adults has been added to Section 6.6, Protein Needs.

- Section 6.6 also includes a discussion of the Paleo Diet™ in the form of an answer to the *Ask the RDN* question: Is the Paleo Diet™ a healthy way to include a good amount of high-quality protein into my eating plan?

- The graphic of "The New American Plate" in Section 6.8 has been replaced with a new photo published by the American Institute for Cancer Research.

- Section 6.8 also includes a new *Newsworthy Nutrition,* "Vegetarian dietary patterns decrease risk of colorectal cancers," based on research published in 2015.

Chapter 7: *Energy Balance and Weight Control*

- The CDC obesity prevalence and trends have been updated throughout to reflect the most current data.

- A new Figure 7-2 includes both youth and adult obesity prevalence.

- The components of a healthy body weight have been revised throughout the chapter to emphasize the importance of dietary patterns and positive lifestyle behaviors in successful weight management and align with the *Dietary Guidelines for Americans.*

- Figure 7-6 highlights the contributions of basal metabolic rate, voluntary activity, and the thermic effect of food to energy output.

- Section 7.3 now includes information about personal body fat scales that include body composition measures that synch with mobile devices for easier tracking.

- Non-HDL cholesterol has been added as a risk factor for nutrition-related chronic disease in Section 7.3.

- Evidence-based updates for Health Problems Associated with Excess Body Fat have been revised in Table 7-2.

- Information on the DEXA-specific software that was developed to assess visceral body fat distribution has now been added in Section 7.3.

- Revisions aligning with the *Dietary Guidelines for Americans* have been made to Table 7-3 to describe factors that encourage excess body fat stores and obesity.

- The weight-loss triad, Figure 7-17, has been updated to emphasize the interrelated components of successful weight-loss.

- Figure 7-18 has been updated to reflect more current characteristics of a sound weight-loss program.

- The Biggest Loser Eating Plan has been added in the new *Ask the RDN* feature in Section 7.5.

- The *Farm to Fork* features amazing stone fruits.

- The *Newsworthy Nutrition* article in Section 7.6 has been updated to document the link between a plant-based dietary pattern and healthy body weight.

- Table 7-5 has been condensed to include most popular physical activities and estimated calorie costs associated with each activity.

- The Section 7.8 title has been altered (Behavioral Strategies for Weight Management) to emphasize the importance of modifiable lifestyle behaviors in successful weight management and control.

- Section 7.8 has also been updated throughout to reflect DGA updates and recommended shifts in dietary patterns to promote a healthy lifestyle. The DGA Strategies for Action with guiding principles and societal efforts help to combat obesity.

- The Blue Zone Power 9 has been added to Section 7.8 to showcase the nine key characteristics of centenarians globally.

- The mindful eating section has been expanded to include the concept of mindless eating—or making the healthier choice the easier choice.

- The title for Table 7-6 has been updated to Behavioral Tactics for Weight Loss.

- Updates to weight-loss medications, recommendations, and contraindications have been made in Section 7.9.

- Information on intermittent fasting has been added to Section 7.9 as a strategy for obesity treatment.

- The AspireAssist weight-loss device has been described in Section 7.9.

- Figure 7-22 has been condensed to reflect details of the most current bariatric procedures in an infographic format.

- Table 7-8 has been created to provide information about the growth of youth bariatrics.

- The *Nutrition and Your Health* section on popular diets has been updated to include the Military Diet, Green Smoothie Cleanse, and a weblink to evidence-based diet plan reviews.

- Table 7-9 now describes the best weight-loss plans of 2016.

- *Further Readings* have been updated with seven new references.

Chapter 8: *Vitamins*

- Vitamin summary tables have been updated to enhance readability and quickly summarize pertinent information on the functions, requirements, food sources, deficiency, and toxicity of the fat and water-soluble vitamins.

- Figure 8-1 has been updated to include vitamins contributing to body defenses and brain health in addition to previous functions.

- An updated section on phytochemicals has been included to reflect current research and updates on these health-promoting plant-based chemicals.
- Carotenoid information has been updated and expanded in Section 8.2.
- Vitamin D and details on doses of sunlight exposure have been added to Section 8.3.
- The new *Ask the RDN* in Section 8.6 features the Raw Food Plant Diet.
- The *What Would You Choose?* feature explores the use of dietary supplements as a source of energy.
- Newly redesigned figures throughout the chapter illustrate food sources of the vitamins with reference to the food groups pictured on MyPlate.
- The discussions of each micronutrient have been reorganized and expanded to touch upon functions, deficiency diseases, food sources, daily requirements, and toxicity in a consistent, easy-to-outline format.
- A new *Newsworthy Nutrition* feature explores the relationship between B vitamins and cognitive function.
- The *Farm to Fork* focuses on crucifers, an excellent source of phytochemicals and vitamins.
- The Top 5 Dietary Supplements has been updated in Section 8.16.
- A new *Newsworthy News* feature has been updated with a study documenting increased emergency department visits for dietary supplement users.
- Websites to evaluate supplement safety have been updated in Section 8.16.
- Figure 8-34 has been updated with the most current data on supplement use.
- The discussion of choline has been revised and expanded to reflect the latest research.
- The new *Nutrition and Your Health* section on nutrition and cancer contains updated statistics and a revised discussion of the progression of cancer. The link between excess body fat and cancer is explored in further detail. In the discussion of cancer prevention, we have emphasized the importance of overall dietary patterns and whole foods rather than individual nutrients.
- The Chapter Summary reflects updates throughout and now includes functional foods. In addition, a new study question on phytochemicals has been added.
- *Further Readings* have been updated to include 10 new articles.

Chapter 9: Water and Minerals

- Section 9.1 has been reorganized with the topic, Electrolytes Regulate Fluid Balance, moved to the end of the section to provide a better transition to the discussion of electrolyte minerals. Figure 9-11 has been enhanced to include the movement of molecules during the change in ion concentrations in the fluid surrounding the cells.

- The discussion of bottled water has been expanded in Section 9.1 with new statistics for the consumption of bottled water in 2014, as well as a link to the Natural Resources Defense Council website where students can read more about bottled water.
- Questions about limiting the amount of salt in the diet are answered in the new *Ask the RDN* feature in Section 9.3, which concludes with a new *Newsworthy Nutrition*, "No Evidence for Extreme Sodium Restrictions for Older Adults," based on research published in 2015.
- Table 9-2, Biological Factors Associated with Bone Status, has been expanded to include estrogen.
- A discussion of the effect of coffee and colas on bone health has been added to Section 9.6 on calcium, in the answer to the *Ask the RDN* question, "Could the caffeine in these drinks be damaging my bones and leading to osteoporosis?"
- Prevalence statistics for 2014 from the National Osteoporosis Foundation have been included, as well as a simplified Figure 9-18 depicting the relationship between peak bone mass and the ultimate risk of developing osteoporosis and related bone fractures.
- You will find more current information on the increasing sales of nondairy milk beverages and the availability of new products such as cashew milk in Section 9.6. Table 9-4 has been expanded with updated values on the nutrient content of nondairy milk beverage.
- The *Further Readings* have been updated with 13 new articles related to water and minerals.
- Table 9-5, Calcium Supplement Comparisons, has been reformatted to better highlight calcium content, forms, cost, and bioavailability and meal timing.
- Garlic and onions, potential sources of selenium, are the focus of this chapter's *Farm to Fork*.
- In Section 9.12, the term *iodine* is now used instead of *iodide* to be consistent with Dietary Reference Intakes. The link between mild iodine deficiency during pregnancy and decreased IQ in offspring is discussed based on recent studies.
- Several updates have been made to Section 9.17 on Minerals and Hypertension. The importance of balancing sodium and potassium to control blood pressure is highlighted in a new *Newsworthy Nutrition*, and medications used to lower blood pressure are now outlined in the *Medicine Cabinet* feature. We recommend the DASH diet and point out that it was named the best overall eating plan for the seventh year in a row on the *U.S. News & World Report's* 2017 Best Diets list.
- *What the Dietitian Chose* includes updates on the class action lawsuits filed by a number of U.S. consumers against the Coca-Cola® Bottling Company for false marketing of its popular vitaminwater® brand.
- There are six new *Further Readings*.

Chapter 10: *Nutrition: Fitness and Sports*

- Sports nutrition advice throughout the chapter has been updated to align with the revised joint position statement on nutrition and athletic performance from the Academy of Nutrition and Dietetics, Dietitians of Canada, and the American College of Sports Medicine, released in 2016.

- Figure 10-1 has been updated to summarize the current mental and physical benefits of physical activity.

- Figures 10-5, 10-7, and 10-8 have been updated to illustrate and simplify the general concepts of energy storage in the chemical bonds of ATP, ATP formation from macronutrients, and the relationship between fuel use and exercise intensity.

- The new *Farm to Fork* features citrus fruits, often consumed by athletes before, during, and after competition.

- The No-Meat Athlete diet is featured in the *Ask the RDN* feature in Section 10.4.

- The role of vitamin D in athletics has been added to Section 10.4.

- The important issue of alcohol and binge drinking related to performance and athletics has been added under the fluid section in 10.4.

- Throughout the chapter, especially in Table 10-4 and Table 10-8, references to sports nutrition products have been updated to reflect the current market.

- In Section 10.4, the discussion of the controversial topic of protein needs of athletes, including the amount and timing of protein intake, has been updated with the latest research.

- The *Newsworthy Nutrition* feature now focuses on research on a link between sports drinks and weight gain among adolescents and young adults.

- Section 10.5 has been updated with the latest statistics and data on commonly used ergogenic aids.

- The *Further Readings* have been updated with 13 new resources on sports nutrition.

Chapter 11: *Eating Disorders*

- In Section 11.2, we have added information about the two subtypes of anorexia nervosa: restricting type and binge eating/purging type. This information reinforces the point that a person with an eating disorder exists on a spectrum of disordered eating behaviors and may migrate from one disorder to another.

- The discussion of physical effects of anorexia nervosa has been updated and expanded.

- In Section 11.3, a new *Newsworthy Nutrition* feature looks at the relationship between bulimia nervosa and binge drinking or substance abuse.

- Section 11.4 has been updated with information on lisdexamfetamine, the first drug to be approved for treatment of binge eating disorder.

- A new *Ask the RDN* feature in Section 11.4 describes the science behind intermittent fasting, but cautions readers that this weight-loss method could be a gateway to disordered eating behavior.

- In Section 11.5, the various types of subthreshold eating disorders are explained in greater detail.

- A new *Farm to Fork* feature shows how an apple a day keeps the doctor away.

- Eighteen new articles have been incorporated into the listing of *Further Readings*.

Chapter 12: *Global Nutrition*

- The chapter title has been changed to *Global Nutrition* to reflect a broader world view of malnutrition and nutrition-related topics.

- Statistics on both domestic and global poverty and hunger from the FAO and U.S. Census Bureau have been updated with the most recent data.

- A new Figure 12-1 highlights the four dimensions of food security, and Figure 12-3 displays the integrated food security phase classifications set by the FAO.

- The prevalences of hunger, nutrient-deficiency diseases, and related health outcomes have been updated to reflect the current literature. The prevalence of regional undernutrition has also been updated in Figure 12-2.

- Updates of the characteristics of users and impact of the federally subsidized nutrition programs, including SNAP, WIC, and Senior Nutrition Services that supply food for people in the United States, has been updated in Section 12.2.

- Section 12.3 now includes expanded information available related to the nutritional impact of war and political unrest in the Middle East and specific to refugees, those internally displaced, or those seeking political or religious asylum.

- Figure 12-6 has been created to highlight the trends in USDA expenditures for food and nutrition assistance.

- An AIDS prevalence figure (12-8) has been added to Section 12.3.

- The *Farm to Fork* feature highlights bananas, often seen as a global staple.

- A section on the Global Hunger Index (GHI), a tool designed to measure and track hunger worldwide, is discussed in Section 12.3. Climate change, the green revolution, and sustainable agriculture and their impact are also expanded in this section.

- The 17 United Nations Sustainable Development Goals, a blueprint for global health, have been updated in the text and Figure 12-9 added.

- Updates of the positive impact of global efforts to combat HIV/AIDS have been added.

- The Non-GMO Project initiative promoting GMO food labeling has been added.

- The *Ask the RDN* features the non-GMO diet.

- A global analysis of GMO crops and pesticide exposure is included in the text and as a *Further Reading*.
- Undernutrition throughout all life stages (pregnancy through older adults) has been updated to reflect current prevalence and associated health outcomes.
- The *Further Readings* include 13 new references.

Chapter 13: *Protecting Our Food Supply*

- Title has been changed to *Protecting Our Food Supply* to better reflect the chapter content, including the safety, security, and sustainability of food.
- Table 13-1, which summarizes the agencies responsible for monitoring the food supply in the United States, has been streamlined to improve readability.
- Information on recent examples of foodborne illness outbreaks has been updated and moved to Tables 13-3 (now alphabetized) and 13-4 on the causes of foodborne illnesses.
- In Section 13.1, bulleted lists are now used to highlight the reasons microorganisms are able to grow rapidly in foods and the consumer and industry trends that are causing an increase in the risk of contracting foodborne illness.
- The discussion of overuse of antibiotics in animal feeds in Section 13.1 has been revised and expanded.
- Figure 13-1, Settings of Norovirus outbreaks from food contamination in the United States in 2009–2012, has been updated.
- In Section 13.3, the subsection on parasites is now titled Protozoan and Helminth Parasites to better reflect the type of parasites discussed.
- Photos have been added to Table 13-6, Types of Food Additives—Sources and Related Health Concerns, to illustrate the types of foods containing specific additives.
- The discussion of the worldwide differences in the approach countries take to the approval of food additives has been expanded in Section 13.4, Food Additives.
- The *Ask the RDN* feature weighs the pros and cons of "clean" eating.
- We have added Table 13-7 to summarize natural substances in foods that can cause foodborne illness and included photos to illustrate foods that may contain these substances.
- Table 13-8 has been revised to include a greater variety of common sources of caffeine.
- Table 13-9 now includes bisphenol A.
- A new margin note in Section 13.6 highlights the ongoing public health crisis that surfaced when high levels of lead were detected in the drinking water in Flint, Michigan.

- Section 13.6, includes updated statistics on the use of pesticides in the United States and information about USDA's Pesticide Data Program.
- Table 13-10 has been updated with the Environmental Working Group's 2016 Dirty Dozen™ and Clean Fifteen.
- Melons are the topic of the *Farm to Fork* feature, including the potential for cantaloupes to harbor bacteria because of their "netted" surface.
- Agroterrorism and food biotechnology are each new topics covered in Section 13.6.
- The topic of sustainability has been greatly expanded, including the potential results of sustainable agriculture, sustainable farming practices, and strategies to reduce your food waste and eat more sustainably.
- The *Newsworthy Nutrition,* "Increase in Foodborne Illnesses Associated with Organic Foods," summarizes new research published in the *Journal of Food Protection* in 2016.
- Statistics on organic food production and farmers markets have been updated in Section 13.7.
- Figure 13-3, Effects of temperature on microbes that cause foodborne illness (Danger Zone), has been moved to Section 13.8, Preventing Foodborne Illness.
- Thirteen new resources have been added to the *Further Readings.*

Chapter 14: *Nutrition During Pregnancy and Breastfeeding*

- The content about nutrition and fertility in Section 14.1 has been organized under the headings, "Hormonal Balance," "Key Nutrients," and "Alcohol."
- *Ask the RDN* reviews *The Fertility Diet.*
- Section 14.3 now includes updated statistics about low birth weight, preterm birth, teenage pregnancy, and prenatal care.
- In several places throughout the chapter, we point out some useful online resources to plan healthy dietary patterns during pregnancy.
- *Farm to Fork* focuses on greens, a good source of folate.
- In Section 14.5, the information about a healthy dietary pattern during pregnancy has been incorporated into a new figure 14-8.
- A new margin note in Section 14.7 summarizes the striking results of a 2016 analysis of the economic benefits of breastfeeding.
- The listing of *Further Readings* now includes 25 updated resources.

Chapter 15: *Nutrition from Infancy Through Adolescence*

- In Table 15-3, the descriptions of infant nutrition products have been updated to reflect the current market.

- In Section 15.2, information about iron supplementation has been updated to reflect the recommendations of the American Academy of Pediatrics.

- Figure 15-2 has been updated to the new food labeling format.

- In Section 15.3, the paragraph on safe preparation and storage of infant formula has been expanded and updated. Information about BPA in baby bottles has been revised.

- A new Table 15-4 presents typical formula intake by infants across a range of ages.

- Updated information from the *Dietary Guidelines for Americans* and American Academy of Pediatrics has been incorporated throughout the recommendations for infant, child, and adolescent dietary planning.

- A new margin note in Section 15.4 highlights current events pertaining to lead contamination of the water supply in Flint, Michigan.

- In Section 15.4, the content on vegetarian diet planning for children has been expanded and revised.

- The new *Farm to Fork* feature is about blueberries, a nutrient-dense snack choice for children.

- A new *Ask the RDN* feature explores the connections between nutrition and autism.

- In Section 15.5, we have included information from the *2016 WHO Report of the Commission on Ending Childhood Obesity.*

- In Section 15.7, information pertaining to food allergies and intolerances has been updated with new statistics and terminology to reflect current medical literature. A new *Newsworthy Nutrition* feature explains the ramifications of the LEAP study for children at risk of peanut allergies.

- Eighteen new resources have been added to the *Further Readings.*

Chapter 16: *Nutrition During Adulthood*

- In Section 16.1, a new *Newsworthy Nutrition* feature highlights research on the relationship between animal protein intake and mortality.

- In Section 16.2, nutrition recommendations for the adult years have been updated to reflect the *Dietary Guidelines for Americans.* In this section, we also present the latest research on protein needs of older adults.

- Figure 16-3 has been updated to match the most recent version of the Nutrition Screening Initiative's Nutrition Checklist for Older Adults, which utilizes the DETERMINE mnemonic.

- Section 16.3 is now called Factors Related to Nutritional Status of Adults and discusses physiological and psychosocial changes that affect nutritional status.

- A margin box introduces the rising popularity of home-delivered meal kits and the most popular services available.

- The *Farm to Fork* feature focuses on grapes, a convenient and widely available fruit.

- Table 16-2 has been revised and expanded to provide more comprehensive array of strategies to cope with the physiological changes of aging.

- In Section 16.3, we have expanded our discussion of nutritional strategies to cope with arthritis. To further expand upon this topic, the new *Ask the RDN* feature reviews the potential benefits of an anti-inflammatory diet.

- Table 16-3 has been updated with the latest research on popular herbal remedies used by American adults. Referrals to some current and relevant online resources pertaining to complementary and alternative medicine are provided.

- A margin box displays the results of a new meta-analysis that found additional benefits of eating 10 a day versus 5 a day for fruits and vegetables.

- In Figure 16-7, we have included the recent MyPlate for Older Adults. Information related to the use of community nutrition services by older Americans has been updated.

- In Section 16.5, we have incorporated new research about alcohol intake and cancer risk. Recommendations regarding alcohol use now reflect the *Dietary Guidelines for Americans.*

- Eighteen recent resources have been added to the *Further Readings.*

Connect Question Banks Updates

- Addition of *Case Studies, Ask the RDN,* and *Farm to Fork* for every chapter as assignable content

- Addition of assignable dietary analysis activities

- NEW assignable content based on *Newsworthy Nutrition* features in the text:

  - Chapter 1: No decrease in adult obesity rates from 2005 to 2014.

  - Chapter 2: Effect of healthy eating attitude at the supermarket.

  - Chapter 3: Probiotics provide relief from constipation.

  - Chapter 4: Americans are decreasing consumption of sugar-sweetened beverages.

  - Chapter 6: Vegetarian dietary patterns decrease risk of colorectal cancers.

- Chapter 7: Plant-based dietary pattern promotes healthy body weight.
- Chapter 8: Increased emergency department visits for dietary supplement users.
- Chapter 9: No evidence for extreme sodium restrictions for older adults & Slash sodium, but step up potassium to control blood pressure.
- Chapter 10: Sports drinks cause weight gain among adolescents and young adults.
- Chapter 11: Substance use among adolescents with eating disorders.
- Chapter 13: Increase in foodborne illnesses associated with organic foods.
- Chapter 15: Early introduction of peanut protein reduces peanut allergy.
- Chapter 16: Low animal protein intake is associated with a major reduction in mortality & Folic acid and vitamin B-12 may prevent cognitive decline.

Instructor Resources Updates

- PowerPoint slides updates to include:
  - *What Would You Choose* from text
  - NEW *Case Studies* from each chapter
  - Accessibility updates
- Updated Teaching Strategies include a variety of classroom discussion topics and activities for student learning. With this edition, we have included many new ideas that make use of digital resources and social media to engage millennial learners. This "buffet" of teaching strategies will provide options that are adaptable for face-to-face, hybrid, or online learning environments.

Contents

Preface iv

Part One: Nutrition: A Key to Health

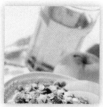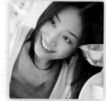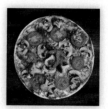

©Corbis/Punchstock   ©BloomImage RF/Getty Images   ©vitals/Shutterstock

Part Two: Energy Nutrients and Energy Balance

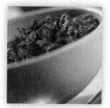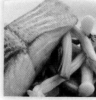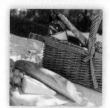

©Medioimages/ Photodisc/Getty Images   ©Ingram Publishing/ SuperStock   ©Pixtal/AGE Fotostock   ©Ingram Publishing

Part Three: Vitamins, Minerals, and Water

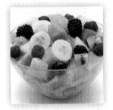 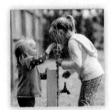

©Nataliia K/Shutterstock   ©Elena Nasledova/Shutterstock

Part Four: Nutrition: Beyond the Nutrients

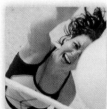
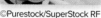
©Purestock/SuperStock RF

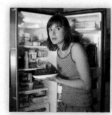
©BananaStock/PunchStock RF

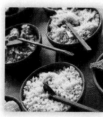
©Nicholas Pitt/Digital
Vision/Getty Images

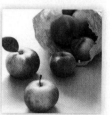
©Lifesize/Getty Images RF

Part Five: Nutrition: A Focus on Life Stages

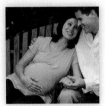
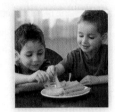
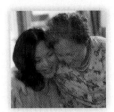

©Getty Images   ©KidStock/BlendImages/GettyImages   ©Digital Vision/PunchStock RF

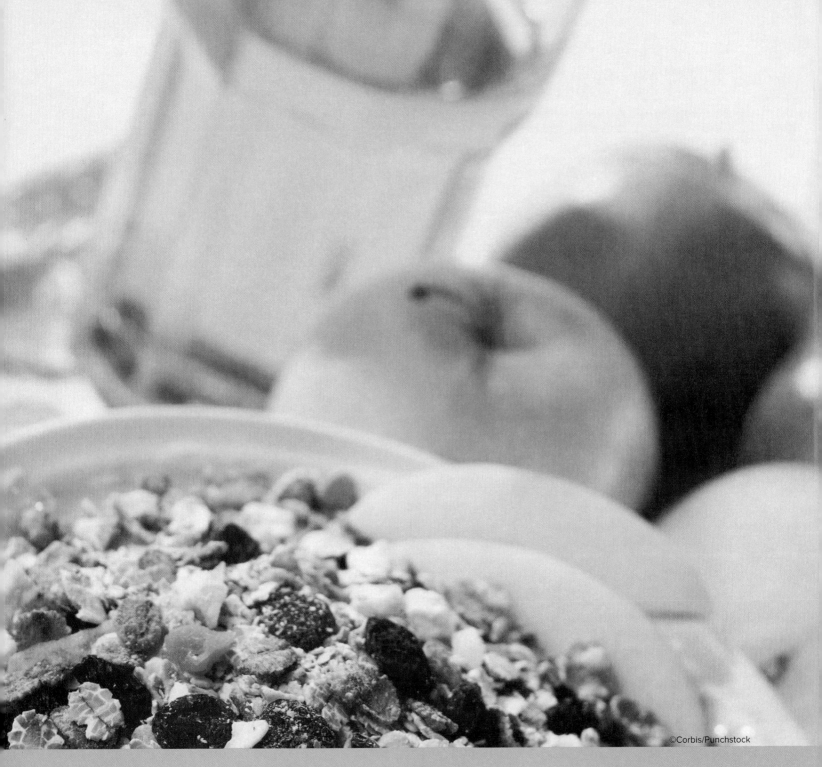

©Corbis/Punchstock

Student Learning Outcomes

Chapter 1 is designed to allow you to:

1.1 Describe how our food choices are affected by the flavor, texture, and appearance of food; routines and habits; early experiences and customs; advertising; nutrition and health concerns; restaurants; social changes; economics; and physiological processes affected by meal size and composition.

1.2 Identify diet and lifestyle factors that contribute to the 15 leading causes of death in North America.

1.3 Define the terms *nutrition, carbohydrate, protein, lipid (fat), alcohol, vitamin, mineral, water, phytochemical, kilocalorie (kcal),* and *fiber.*

1.4 Determine the total calories (kcal) of a food or diet using the weight and calorie content of the energy-yielding nutrients, convert English to metric units, and calculate percentages, such as percent of calories from fat in a diet.

Chapter 1
Nutrition, Food Choices, and Health

What Would You Choose?

We begin each chapter with this activity to get you thinking. We ask you to make a choice that is right for you using the concepts discussed in the chapter. At the end of each chapter, we provide the logic behind what a dietitian would recommend.

You were awake last night until 2:30 A.M. finishing a class project. Unfortunately, your Psychology 101 class meets at 9:00 this morning. When your alarm goes off at 7:30 A.M., you decide to sleep those extra 20 minutes it would take to sit down and enjoy breakfast at the dining hall. What's your best time-saving breakfast option? What factors may hold you back from making the correct choice?

a Skip breakfast but plan to consume a few extra calories at lunch and dinner.

b Eat a low-fat granola bar and iced coffee from the vending machines in your dorm.

c Eat a quick bowl of Wheaties™ with a banana and low-fat milk along with a yogurt, all from your dorm room "pantry."

d Pick up a ham, egg, and cheese bagel to eat during class.

Think about your choice as you read this chapter, then see What the Dietitian Chose at the end of the chapter.

Research has clearly shown that a lifestyle that includes a diet rich in fruits, vegetables, whole grains and lean meat or plant protein, coupled with regular exercise, can enhance our quality of life in the short term and keep us healthy for many years to come. Unfortunately, this healthy lifestyle is not always easy to follow. When it comes to "nutrition," it is clear that some of our diets are out of balance with our metabolism, physiology, and physical activity level.

We begin this chapter with some questions. What influences your daily food choices? How important are factors such as taste, appearance, convenience, or cost? Is nutrition one of the factors you consider? Are your food choices influencing your quality of life and long-term health? By making optimal dietary choices, we can bring the goal of a long, healthy life within reach. This is the primary theme of this chapter and throughout this book.

The ultimate goal of this book is to help you find the best path to good nutrition. The information presented is based on emerging science that is translated into everyday actions that improve health. After completion of your nutrition course, you should understand the knowledge behind the food choices you make and recommend to others. We call this achievement of making food choices that are right for you "nutrition literacy."

1.5 Understand the scientific method as it is used in forming hypotheses and theories in the field of nutrition, including the determination of nutrient needs.

1.6 List the major characteristics of the North American diet, the food habits that often need improvement, and the key "Nutrition and Weight Status" objectives of the *Healthy People 2020* report.

1.7 Describe a basic plan for health promotion and disease prevention and what to expect from good nutrition and a healthy lifestyle.

1.8 Identify food and nutrition issues relevant to college students.

1.1 Why Do You Choose the Food You Eat?

In your lifetime, you will eat about 70,000 meals and 60 tons of food. Many factors—some internal, some external—influence our food choices. This chapter begins with a discussion of these factors and ends with a conversation specifically about eating well as a college student. In between, we examine the powerful effect of eating patterns in determining overall health and take a close look at the general classes of nutrients—as well as the calories—supplied by the food we eat. We also discuss the major characteristics of North American eating patterns, the food habits that often need improvement, and the key "Nutrition and Weight Status" objectives in the *Healthy People 2020* report. A review of the scientific process behind nutrition recommendations is also included, along with an introduction to our "Farm to Fork," "Newsworthy Nutrition," and "Ask the RDN" features that you will see throughout the book.

Understanding what drives us to eat and what affects food choice will help you understand the complexity of factors that influence eating, especially the effects of our routines and food advertising (Fig. 1-1). You can then appreciate why foods may have different meanings to different people and thus why food habits and preferences of others may differ from yours.

WHAT INFLUENCES YOUR FOOD CHOICES?

Food means so much more to us than nourishment—it reflects much of what we think about ourselves. The Bureau of Labor Statistics estimated that in 2015, Americans spent the equivalent of 18 days eating and drinking. If we live to be 80 years old, that will add up to 4 years of eating and drinking. Overall, our daily food choices stem from a complicated mix of biological and social influences (see Fig. 1-1). Let's examine some of the key reasons we choose what we eat.

FIGURE 1-1 ▶ Food choices are affected by many factors. Which have the greatest impact on your food choices?
©Florian Franke/Purestock/Superstock

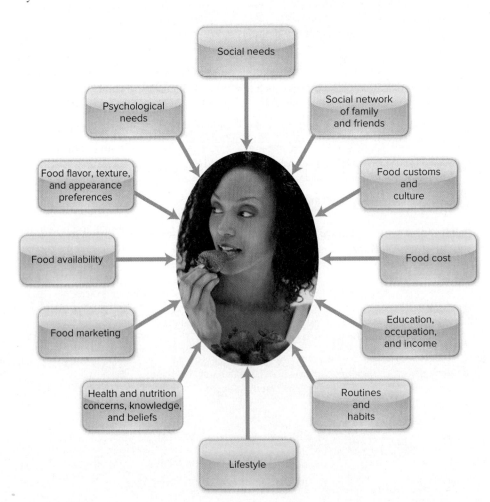

Flavor, texture, and appearance are the most important factors determining our food choices. Creating more flavorful foods that are both healthy and profitable is a major focus of the food industry. The challenge is to combine the "taste" of the foods we prefer with the best nutrition and health characteristics. The good news is that chefs and "food bloggers" are dedicating themselves to creating nutritious food that is also delicious. The results are food that is good for us starting to taste better.

Early influences related to various people, places, and events have a continuing impact on our food choices. Many food customs, including ethnic eating patterns, begin as we are introduced to foods during childhood. Parents can lay a strong foundation knowing that early exposure to food choices during infancy, toddler, and preschool years is important in influencing later health behaviors. Developing healthy patterns during childhood will go a long way to ensure healthy preferences and choices when we are teenagers and adults.

Routines and habits are tied to some food choices. Eating habits, food availability, and convenience strongly influence choices. Most of us eat from a core group of foods with about 100 basic items accounting for 75% of our total food intake. Recent Food Availability and Consumption data from the United States Department of Agriculture (USDA) shows that Americans consume most of their calories from grain products (especially bread, pizza crust, macaroni, and spaghetti) and fats and oils (especially soybean oil). Potatoes and tomatoes are the most commonly consumed vegetables (Fig. 1-2), with French fries and pizza contributing to the high consumption of these two vegetables. The most commonly consumed fruits, oranges and apples, are consumed mostly in juice form. Fluid milk and cheese, especially mozzarella cheese, comprise most of dairy consumption, with fluid milk consumption showing a big decline, while cheese consumption has doubled (Fig. 1-3).

Marketing and advertising are major tools for capturing the food interest of the consumer. Consumers have more food choices than ever and these choices are well advertised in newspapers and magazines, on billboards, radio, and television, and online. The food industry in the United States spends billions on advertising. Some of this advertising is helpful, as it promotes the importance of food components such as calcium and fiber in our diets. However, the food industry also advertises highly sweetened cereals, cookies, snacks, and soft drinks because they bring in the greatest profits. Recent studies indicate that the association between TV advertising of foods and drinks, and childhood obesity is especially prevalent in the United States.[1,2] A recent study, one of the first to show the effect of food advertisements on preschoolers, found that children

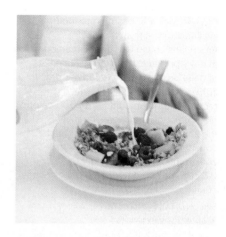

▲ Creating more flavorful foods that are both healthy and profitable is a major focus of the food industry. ©Stockbyte/ PunchStock

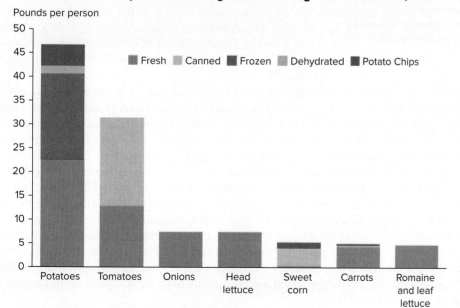

Most commonly consumed vegetables among U.S. consumers, 2014

Pounds per person

Legend: ■ Fresh   ■ Canned   ■ Frozen   ■ Dehydrated   ■ Potato Chips

(Bar chart categories: Potatoes, Tomatoes, Onions, Head lettuce, Sweet corn, Carrots, Romaine and leaf lettuce)

Loss-adjusted food availability data are proxies for consumption.

FIGURE 1-2 ◄ According to food availability data, the favorite vegetables of Americans are potatoes and tomatoes. In 2014, Americans consumed 46.7 pounds per person of potatoes, with half of the consumption as fresh potatoes; 31.4 pounds of tomatoes were consumed in 2014, with 59 percent as canned tomatoes. French fries and pizza contribute to the high consumption of these two vegetables.

Source: USDA, Economic Research Service, Loss-Adjusted Food Availability Data, 2014.

FIGURE 1-3 ▶ According to food availability data from the USDA, Americans consumed a similar amount of dairy products (1.5 cup-equivalents of dairy products per person per day) in 1974 and in 2014. This is half the recommended amount for a 2000-calorie diet. Although the overall quantity is the same, the types of dairy products consumed have changed. Fluid milk consumption deceased from 0.9 to 0.6 cup per person per day, while cheese consumption has doubled.

Source: USDA, Economic Research Service, Loss Adjusted Food Availability Data.

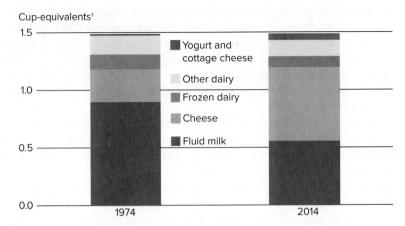

Average U.S. consumption of dairy products, 1974 and 2014

†Based on a 2000-calorie diet. One cup-quivalent for dairy is: 1 cup milk or yogurt; 1½ ounces natural cheese or 2 ounces of processed cheese or ⅓ cup shredded cheese; 1 cup frozen yogurt or 1 ½ cups ice cream; 2 cups cottage cheese. Loss-adjusted food availability data are proxies for consumption. Other dairy includes evaporated milk, condensed milk, dry milk products, half and half, and eggnog.

CRITICAL THINKING

Can healthy choices be legislated? Public health authorities would like to influence health behaviors by banning or taxing unhealthy foods or ingredients; however, industries and many concerned citizens oppose the expanding reach of the government. This struggle gained national attention in the summer of 2014. Mounting evidence for the link between consumption of sugar-sweetened beverages and obesity had prompted the proposal of a ban on the sale of sugary drinks in containers larger than 16 ounces in some establishments. In 2013, the Sugary Drinks Portion Cap Rule, better known as the Soda Ban, was approved by the New York City Board of Health. However, the beverage industry staunchly opposed the ban and the New York Supreme Court invalidated the law. In June 2014, the New York Court of Appeals ruled that this ban overreached the health department's regulatory authority. Whose responsibility is it to determine which foods are good for you?

between the ages of 2 and 5 who watched a show embedded with food advertisements consumed more calories from snacks than those who saw nonfood advertisements. These findings, in children who were eating in the absence of hunger, suggest that exposure to food advertisements may encourage eating behaviors that promote obesity in the very young. Similar findings have been reported previously in older children.[3] Concern for the negative effect of advertising and marketing on the diets and health of children led the Council of Better Business Bureaus to establish the Children's Food and Beverage Advertising Initiative, a self-regulatory program. Participants are 18 of the largest food and beverage companies that represent about 80% of child-directed television food advertising. The Initiative is designed to shift the mix of foods advertised to children to encourage healthier dietary choices and healthy lifestyles.[4] Research also indicates that mass media influences the onset of eating disorders through its depiction of extremely thin models as stereotypes of attractive bodies. Eating disorders will be introduced in Eating Well in College (Section 1.8) and discussed at length in Chapter 11.

Restaurant dining plays a significant role in our food choices. Restaurant food is often calorie dense, in large portions, and of poorer nutritional quality compared to foods made at home. Fast-food and pizza restaurant menus typically emphasize meat, cheese, fried foods, and carbonated beverages. In response to recent consumer demands, restaurants have placed healthier options on their menus, and many are listing nutritional content there, as well. Mandatory posting of the calorie content of restaurant items will go into effect soon as a result of the Affordable Care Act. The law requires chain restaurants with 20 or more locations to post the calorie content of their offerings on menus or menu boards with other nutritional information available upon request. The intent of the law is to provide consumers with clear and consistent nutrition information so that they can make informed and healthful choices. Although many restaurants have already placed calorie information on their menus, the Food and Drug Administration (FDA) extended the date for which establishments must be compliant with the menu labeling rule to May 2018.

Time and convenience have become significant influences affecting food choices. Current lifestyles limit the time available for food preparation.[5] A recent study in Seattle found that individuals who spent the least amount of time cooking were more likely to be working adults who placed a higher priority on convenience than on home-cooked meals. They spent more money eating away from home, especially at fast-food restaurants, suggesting that time is a key ingredient in the development of healthier eating habits.[6] Restaurants and supermarkets have responded to our demanding work schedules and long hours away from home by supplying prepared meals, microwavable entrees, and various quick-prep frozen products.

Cost and economics play a role in our food choices. The 2015 Food and Health Survey indicates that after taste, cost is the number two reason why people choose the food they do. While the average American now spends less on food than in the past, young adults and those with higher incomes spend the most on food. As income increases, so do meals eaten away from home and preferences for foods such as cookies, chocolate, cheese, and meat. Also keep in mind that as calorie intake increases, so does the food bill. Tips for eating well on a college student's budget are discussed in Section 1.8.

Nutrition—or what we think of as "healthy foods"—also directs our food purchases. North Americans who tend to make health-related food choices are often well-educated, middle-class professionals. These same people are generally health oriented, have active lifestyles, and focus on weight control. The recent National Health Interview Survey showed that 74% of women in the study habitually or always read nutrition labels, whereas only 58% of men read labels on food products. Label reading was associated with a lower body mass index (BMI, body weight relative to height), especially in women. Women who read labels had an average body weight 8.6 pounds lower than women who did not read nutrition labels.[7]

WHY ARE YOU SO HUNGRY?

Two drives, **hunger** and **appetite,** influence our desire to eat. These drives differ dramatically. Hunger is primarily our physical, biological drive to eat and is controlled by internal body mechanisms. For example, as foods are digested and absorbed by the stomach and small intestine, these organs send signals to the liver and brain telling us to reduce further food intake.

Appetite, our primarily psychological drive to eat, is affected by many of the external food choice mechanisms we discussed in the last section, such as environmental and psychological factors and social cues and customs (see Fig. 1-1). Appetite can be triggered simply by seeing a tempting dessert or smelling popcorn at the movie theater. Fulfilling either or both drives by eating sufficient food normally brings a state of **satiety,** a feeling of satisfaction that temporarily halts our desire to continue eating.

The *feeding center* and the *satiety center* are in a region of the brain that helps regulate satiety. They work in opposite ways, like a tug-of-war, to promote adequate availability of nutrients at all times. For example, when we haven't eaten for a while, stimulation of the feeding center signals us to eat. As we eat, the nutrient content in the blood rises, and the satiety center is stimulated. This is why we no longer have a strong desire to seek food after a meal. Admittedly, this concept of a tug-of-war between the feeding and satiety centers is an oversimplification of a complex process. The various feeding and satiety messages from body cells to the brain do not single-handedly determine what we eat. We often eat because food comforts us.[8] Almost everyone has encountered a mouthwatering dessert and devoured it, even on a full stomach. It smells, tastes, and looks good. We might eat because it is the right time of day, we are celebrating, or we are seeking emotional comfort to overcome the blues. After a meal, memories of pleasant tastes and feelings reinforce appetite. If stress or depression sends you to the refrigerator, you are mostly seeking comfort, not food calories. Appetite may not be a physical process, but it does influence food intake. We will discuss more about this mechanism, including the effect of meal size and composition on satiety, in Chapter 7 on energy balance and weight control.

hunger The primarily physiological (internal) drive to find and eat food.

appetite The primarily psychological (external) influences that encourage us to find and eat food, often in the absence of obvious hunger.

satiety A state in which there is no longer a desire to eat; a feeling of satisfaction.

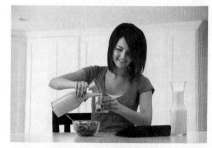

▲ Eating breakfast after sleeping all night is typically a response to hunger signals we are getting from the feeding center in the brain. ©Mike Kemp/Getty Images

PUTTING OUR FOOD CHOICES INTO PERSPECTIVE

The next time you pick up a candy bar or reach for a second helping at a meal, remember the internal and external influences on eating behavior. You should now understand that daily food consumption is a complicated mix of biological and social influences. Body cells, nutrients in the blood, hormones, brain chemicals, and our social and family customs all influence food choices. When food is abundant, appetite—not hunger—more frequently triggers eating. Satiety associated with consuming a meal may reside primarily in our psychological frame of mind. Also, because satiety regulation is not perfect, body weight can fluctuate. We become accustomed to a certain amount of food at a meal. Providing less than that amount leaves us wanting more. One way to use this observation for weight-loss purposes is to train your eye to expect less food by slowly decreasing serving sizes to more appropriate amounts. Your appetite then readjusts as you expect less food. Keep track of what triggers your eating for a few days. Is it primarily hunger or appetite? The Rate Your Plate activity in this chapter also asks you to keep track of what influences your food intake on a daily basis.

✔ CONCEPT CHECK 1.1

1. What are the factors that influence our food choices?
2. How do hunger and appetite differ in the way they influence our desire to eat?
3. What factors influence satiety?

1.2 How Is Nutrition Connected to Good Health?

Fortunately, the foods we eat can support good health in many ways depending on their components. You just learned, however, that lifestyle habits and other factors may have a bigger impact on our food choices than the food components themselves. Unfortunately, many North Americans suffer from diseases that could have been prevented if they had known more about the foods and, more importantly, had applied this knowledge to plan meals and design their eating pattern. We will now look at the effect these choices are having on our health both today and in the future.

WHAT IS NUTRITION?

Nutrition is the science that links foods to health and disease. It includes the processes by which the human organism ingests, digests, absorbs, transports, and excretes food substances.

NUTRIENTS COME FROM FOOD

What is the difference between food and **nutrients?** Food provides the energy (in the form of calories) as well as the materials needed to build and maintain all body cells. Nutrients are the substances obtained from food that are vital for growth and maintenance of a healthy body throughout life. For a substance to be considered an **essential nutrient,** three characteristics are needed:

- First, at least one specific biological function of the nutrient must be identified in the body.
- Second, omission of the nutrient from the diet must lead to a decline in certain biological functions, such as production of blood cells.
- Third, replacing the omitted nutrient in the diet before permanent damage occurs will restore those normal biological functions.

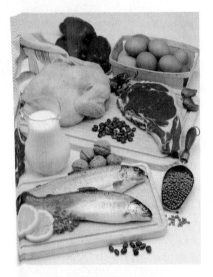

Many foods are rich sources of nutrients. ©Pixtal/AGE Fotostock

nutrients Chemical substances in food that contribute to health, many of which are essential parts of a diet. Nutrients nourish us by providing calories to fulfill energy needs, materials for building body parts, and factors to regulate necessary chemical processes in the body.

essential nutrient In nutritional terms, a substance that, when left out of a diet, leads to signs of poor health. The body either cannot produce this nutrient or cannot produce enough of it to meet its needs. If added back to a diet before permanent damage occurs, the affected aspects of health are restored.

WHY STUDY NUTRITION?

We all may feel like nutrition experts because we all eat several times a day. Nutrition knowledge can be confusing, however, and seem like a moving target. Recommendations may seem to differ depending on their source, and there are so many choices when shopping for food or eating out. We just learned that nutrition is only one of many factors that influence our eating habits. There is a lot to learn, and we know that you are interested in what you should be eating and how the food you eat affects you. Studying nutrition will help you erase any misconceptions you have about food and nutrition and make informed choices about the foods you eat and their relationship to health.

Nutrition is a lifestyle factor that is a key to developing and maintaining an optimal state of health. A poor diet and a sedentary lifestyle are known to be **risk factors** for life-threatening **chronic** diseases such as **cardiovascular (heart) disease, hypertension, diabetes,** and some forms of **cancer.** Together, these and related disorders account for two-thirds of all deaths in North America (Fig. 1-4).[9] Not meeting nutrient needs in younger years makes us more likely to suffer health consequences, such as bone fractures from the disease **osteoporosis,** in later years. At the same time, taking too much of a nutrient—such as a vitamin A supplement—can be harmful. Another dietary problem, drinking too much alcohol, is associated with many health problems.

U.S. government scientists have calculated that a poor diet combined with a lack of sufficient physical activity contributes to hundreds of thousands of fatal cases of cardiovascular disease, cancer, and diabetes each year among adults in the United States. Thus, the combination of poor diet and too little physical activity may be the second leading cause of death in the United States. In addition, **obesity,** which the American Medical Association declared as a disease in 2013, is considered the second leading cause of preventable death in North America (smoking is the first). When they occur together, obesity and smoking cause even more health problems. Obesity and chronic diseases are often preventable. An important key to good health and health care savings is to realize that the cost of prevention, usually when we are children and young adults, is a small fraction of the cost of treating these diseases when we are older.

The good news is that Americans have shown an increased interest in health, fitness, and nutrition that has been associated with long-term decreasing trends for heart disease, cancer, and **stroke** (three of the leading causes of death). Mortality from heart disease, the leading cause of death, has been declining steadily since 1980. As you gain understanding about your nutritional habits and increase your knowledge about optimal nutrition, you will have the opportunity to dramatically reduce your risk for many

risk factors A term used frequently when discussing the factors contributing to the development of a disease. A risk factor is an aspect of our lives, such as heredity, lifestyle choices (e.g., smoking), or nutritional habits.

chronic Long-standing, developing over time. When referring to disease, this term indicates that the disease process, once developed, is slow and lasting. A good example is cardiovascular disease.

cardiovascular disease A general term that refers to any disease of the heart and circulatory system. This disease is generally characterized by the deposition of fatty material in the blood vessels (hardening of the arteries), which in turn can lead to organ damage and death. Also termed coronary heart disease (CHD), as the vessels of the heart are the primary sites of the disease.

hypertension A condition in which blood pressure remains persistently elevated. Obesity, inactivity, alcohol intake, excess salt intake, and genetics may each contribute to the problem.

diabetes A group of diseases characterized by high blood **glucose.** Type 1 diabetes involves insufficient or no release of the hormone insulin by the pancreas and therefore requires daily insulin therapy. Type 2 diabetes results from either insufficient release of insulin or general inability of insulin to act on certain body cells, such as muscle cells. Persons with type 2 diabetes may or may not require insulin therapy.

glucose A six-carbon sugar that exists in a ring form; found as such in blood, and in table sugar bound to fructose; also known as *dextrose,* it is one of the simple sugars.

cancer A condition characterized by uncontrolled growth of abnormal cells.

osteoporosis The presence of a stress-induced fracture or a T-score of −2.5 or lower. The bones are porous and fragile due to low mineral density.

obesity Disorder involving excessive body fat that increases the risk of health problems.

stroke A decrease or loss in blood flow to the brain that results from a blood clot or other change in arteries in the brain. This in turn causes the death of brain tissue. Also called a *cerebrovascular accident.*

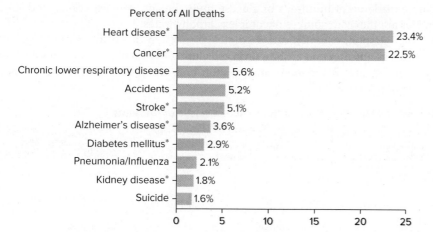

Percent of All Deaths

Cause	Percent
Heart disease*	23.4%
Cancer*	22.5%
Chronic lower respiratory disease	5.6%
Accidents	5.2%
Stroke*	5.1%
Alzheimer's disease*	3.6%
Diabetes mellitus*	2.9%
Pneumonia/Influenza	2.1%
Kidney disease*	1.8%
Suicide	1.6%

FIGURE 1-4 ▲ Ten leading causes of death in the United States.

Source: Centers for Disease Control and Prevention, *National Vital Statistics Report,* Deaths: Leading Causes for 2014, June 30, 2016[9]. Canadian statistics are quite similar.

* Causes of death in which diet plays a part.

carbohydrate A compound containing carbon, hydrogen, and oxygen atoms. Most are known as *sugars, starches,* and *fibers.*

lipid A compound containing much carbon and hydrogen, little oxygen, and sometimes other atoms. Lipids do not dissolve in water and include fats, oils, and cholesterol.

protein Food and body compounds made of more than 100 amino acids; proteins contain carbon, hydrogen, oxygen, nitrogen, and sometimes other atoms in a specific configuration. Proteins contain the form of nitrogen most easily used by the human body.

vitamin An essential organic (carbon-containing) compound needed in small amounts in the diet to help regulate and support chemical reactions and processes in the body.

mineral Element used in the body to promote chemical reactions and to form body structures.

water The universal solvent; chemically, H_2O. The body is composed of about 60% water. Water (fluid) needs are about 9 (women) or 13 (men) cups per day; needs are greater if one exercises heavily.

kilocalorie (kcal) Heat energy needed to raise the temperature of 1000 grams (1 L) of water 1 degree Celsius.

macronutrient A nutrient needed in gram quantities in a diet.

micronutrient A nutrient needed in milligram or microgram quantities in a diet.

simple sugar Monosaccharide or disaccharide in the diet.

complex carbohydrate Carbohydrate composed of many monosaccharide molecules. Examples include glycogen, starch, and fiber.

starch A carbohydrate made of multiple units of glucose attached together in a form the body can digest; also known as *complex carbohydrate.*

cell The structural basis of plant and animal organization. In animals it is bounded by a cell membrane. Cells have the ability to take up compounds from and excrete compounds into their surroundings.

bond A linkage between two atoms formed by the sharing of electrons, or attractions.

common health problems. Recent research has shown that a healthy eating pattern along with other healthy lifestyle factors can protect women from sudden cardiac death. A healthy eating pattern was defined as one with a high proportion of vegetables, fruits, nuts, healthy fats, and fish.[10]

☑ CONCEPT CHECK 1.2

1. How do we define *nutrition?*
2. What are the three leading causes of death in which diet plays a part?

1.3 What Are the Classes and Sources of Nutrients?

To begin the study of nutrition, let's start with an overview of the six classes of nutrients. You are probably already familiar with the terms **carbohydrates, lipids** (fats and oils), **proteins, vitamins,** and **minerals.** These nutrients, plus **water,** make up the six classes of nutrients found in food.

Nutrients can then be assigned to three functional categories: (1) those that primarily provide us with calories to meet energy needs (expressed in **kilocalories [kcal]**); (2) those important for growth, development, and maintenance; and (3) those that act to keep body functions running smoothly. Some function overlap exists among these categories (Table 1-1). The energy-yielding nutrients (carbohydrates, lipids, and protein) along with water are needed in relatively large amounts, so they are called **macronutrients.** Vitamins and minerals are needed in such small amounts in the diet that they are called **micronutrients.**

CARBOHYDRATES

Chemically, carbohydrates can exist in foods as simple sugars and complex carbohydrates. **Simple sugars,** frequently referred to as *sugars,* are relatively small molecules. These sugars are found naturally in fruits, vegetables, and dairy products. Table sugar, known as sucrose, is an example of a simple sugar that is added to many foods we eat. Glucose, also known as blood sugar or dextrose, is an example of a simple sugar in your blood. **Complex carbohydrates** are formed when many simple sugars are joined together. For example, plants store carbohydrates in the form of **starch,** a complex carbohydrate made up of hundreds of glucose units. Breads, cereals, grains, and starchy vegetables are the main sources of complex carbohydrates.

During digestion, complex carbohydrates are broken down into single sugar molecules (such as glucose) and absorbed via **cells** lining the small intestine into the bloodstream (see Chapter 3 for more on digestion and absorption). However, the **bonds**

TABLE 1-1 ■ Major Functions of the Various Classes of Nutrients

Nutrient Classes That Provide Energy	Nutrient Classes That Promote Growth, Development, and Maintenance	Nutrient Classes That Regulate Body Processes
Most carbohydrates	Proteins	Proteins
Proteins	Lipids	Some lipids
Most lipids	Some vitamins	Some vitamins
	Some minerals	Some minerals
	Water	Water

between the sugar molecules in certain complex carbohydrates, called **fiber,** cannot be broken down by human digestive processes. Fiber passes through the small intestine undigested to provide bulk for the stool (feces) formed in the large intestine (colon).

Aside from enjoying their taste, we need sugars and other carbohydrates in our diets primarily to help satisfy the calorie needs of our body cells. Carbohydrates provide a major source of calories for the body, on average 4 kcal per gram. Glucose, a simple sugar that the body can derive from most carbohydrates, is a major source of calories for most cells. When insufficient carbohydrate is consumed, the body is forced to make glucose from proteins—not a healthy alternative. Chapter 4 focuses on carbohydrates.

LIPIDS

Lipids (mostly fats and oils) in the foods we eat also provide energy. Lipids yield more calories per gram than do carbohydrates—on the average, 9 kcal per gram—because of differences in their chemical composition. They are also the main form for energy storage in the body.

Lipids dissolve in certain chemical solvents (e.g., ether and benzene) but not in water. In this book, the more familiar terms *fats* and *oils* will generally be used, rather than *lipids.* Generally, fats are lipids that are solid at room temperature, and oils are lipids that are liquid at room temperature. We obtain fats and oils from animal and plant sources. Animal fats, such as butter or lard, are solid at room temperature. Plant oils, such as corn or olive oil, tend to be liquid at room temperature. To promote heart health, most people would benefit from using more plant oils in place of solid fats (see Chapter 5).

Certain fats are essential nutrients that must come from our diet. These key fats that the body cannot produce, called essential fatty acids, perform several important functions in the body: they help regulate blood pressure and play a role in the synthesis and repair of vital cell parts. However, we need only about 4 tablespoons of a common plant oil (such as olive or soybean oil) each day to supply these essential fatty acids. A serving of fatty fish, such as salmon or tuna, at least twice a week is another healthy source of fats. The unique fatty acids in these fish complement the healthy aspects of common plant oils. This will be explained in greater detail in Chapter 5, which focuses on lipids.

PROTEINS

Proteins are the main structural material in the body. For example, proteins constitute a major part of bone and muscle; they are also important components in blood, body cells, **enzymes,** and immune factors. Proteins can also provide calories for the body—on average, 4 kcal per gram. Typically, however, the body uses little protein for the purpose of meeting daily calorie needs. Proteins are formed when **amino acids** are bonded together. Some of these are essential nutrients.

Protein in our diet comes from animal and plant sources. The animal products meat, poultry, fish, dairy products, and eggs are significant sources of protein in most eating patterns. Beans, grains, and some vegetables are good plant protein sources and are important to include in vegetarian eating patterns.

Most North Americans eat up to two times as much protein as the body needs to maintain health. This amount of extra protein reflects the standard of living and the eating patterns of most North Americans. It is generally not harmful for healthy persons with no evidence of heart or kidney disease, diabetes, or family history of colon cancer or kidney stones. The excess is used for calorie needs and carbohydrate production but ultimately can be converted to and stored as fat. Chapter 6 focuses on proteins.

VITAMINS

The main function of vitamins is to enable many **chemical reactions** to occur in the body. Some of these reactions help release the energy trapped in carbohydrates, lipids, and proteins. Remember, however, that vitamins themselves contain no usable calories for the body.

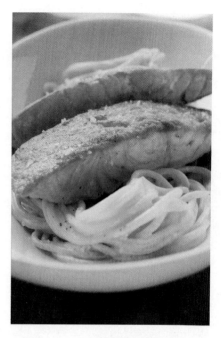

▲ Salmon is a fatty fish that is a healthy source of essential fatty acids.
©FoodCollection

fiber Substances in plant foods not digested in the human stomach or small intestine. These add bulk to feces. Fiber naturally found in foods is also called *dietary fiber.*

enzyme A compound that speeds up the rate of a chemical reaction but is not altered by the reaction. Almost all enzymes are proteins (some are made of genetic material).

amino acid The building block for proteins containing a central carbon atom with nitrogen and other atoms attached.

chemical reaction An interaction between two chemicals that changes both chemicals.

fat-soluble Soluble in fats, oils, or fat solvents.

water-soluble Capable of dissolving in water.

The 13 vitamins are divided into two groups: four are **fat-soluble** because they dissolve in fat (vitamins A, D, E, and K); nine are **water-soluble** because they dissolve in water (the B vitamins and vitamin C). The two groups of vitamins have different sources, functions, and characteristics. Water-soluble vitamins are found mainly in fruits and vegetables, whereas dairy products, nuts, seeds, oils, and breakfast cereals are good sources of fat-soluble vitamins. Cooking destroys water-soluble vitamins much more readily than it does fat-soluble vitamins. Water-soluble vitamins are also excreted from the body much more readily than are fat-soluble vitamins. Thus, the fat-soluble vitamins, especially vitamin A, have the ability to accumulate in excessive amounts in the body, which then can lead to toxicity. Vitamins are discussed in Chapter 8.

MINERALS

inorganic Any substance lacking carbon atoms bonded to hydrogen atoms in the chemical structure.

atom Smallest combining unit of an element, such as iron or calcium. Atoms consist of protons, neutrons, and electrons.

Minerals are structurally simple, **inorganic** substances that do not contain carbon **atoms.** Minerals such as sodium and potassium typically function independently in the body, whereas minerals such as calcium and phosphorus combine to function in tissue, such as bone. Because of their simple structure, minerals are not destroyed during cooking, but they can still be lost if they dissolve in the water used for cooking and that water is then discarded. Minerals are critical players in nervous system functioning, water balance, structural (e.g., skeletal) systems, and many other cellular processes but produce no calories as such for the body.

major mineral Vital to health, a mineral that is required in the diet in amounts greater than 100 milligrams per day.

trace mineral Vital to health, a mineral that is required in the diet in amounts less than 100 milligrams per day.

electrolyte A mineral that separates into positively or negatively charged ions in water. They are able to transmit an electrical current.

The 16 or more essential minerals required in the diet for good health are divided into two groups: **major minerals** and **trace minerals** because dietary needs and concentrations in the body vary enormously. If daily needs are less than 100 milligrams, the mineral is classified as a trace mineral; otherwise, it is a major mineral. Minerals that function based on their electrical charge when dissolved in water are also called **electrolytes;** these include sodium, potassium, and chloride. Many major minerals are found naturally in dairy products and fruits, whereas many trace minerals are found in meats, poultry, fish, and nuts. Minerals are covered in Chapter 9.

WATER

solvent A liquid substance in which other substances dissolve.

Water makes up the sixth class of nutrients. Although sometimes overlooked as a nutrient, water (chemically, H_2O) has numerous vital functions in the body. It acts as a **solvent** and lubricant, as a vehicle for transporting nutrients and waste, and as a medium for temperature regulation and chemical processes. For these reasons, and because the human body is approximately 60% water, the average man should consume about 3 liters—equivalent to 3000 grams or about 13 cups—of water and/or other fluids every day. Women need closer to 2200 grams or about 9 cups per day. Fluid needs vary widely, however, based on differences in body mass and environmental conditions. Because thirst is a late sign of dehydration, urine color can be used as another measure of hydration status. Urine color should be no more yellow than lemonade.

metabolism Chemical processes in the body by which energy is provided in useful forms and vital activities are sustained.

Water is not only available from the obvious sources, but it is also the major component in some foods, such as many fruits and vegetables (e.g., lettuce, grapes, and melons). The body even makes some water as a by-product of **metabolism.** Water is examined in detail in Chapter 9.

OTHER IMPORTANT COMPONENTS IN FOOD

phytochemical A chemical found in plants. Some phytochemicals may contribute to a reduced risk of cancer or cardiovascular disease in people who consume them regularly.

Another group of compounds called **phytochemicals** are found in foods from plant sources, especially within the fruit and vegetable groups. Although these plant components are not considered essential nutrients in the diet, many of these substances provide significant health benefits. Considerable research is focused on various phytochemicals in reducing the risk for certain diseases. For example, evidence from animal and laboratory studies indicates that compounds in blueberries and strawberries prevent the growth of certain cancer cells. Although certain phytochemicals are now available as dietary supplements, research suggests that their health benefits are best obtained through the consumption of whole foods. Foods with high phytochemical content are sometimes called "superfoods" because of the health benefits they are thought to confer. There is no legal definition of the term *superfood,* however, and there is concern that it is being overused in marketing certain foods. Table 1-2 lists some noteworthy phytochemicals with their common food sources. Tomatoes are an important source of phytochemicals and are featured in our new chapter feature, Farm to Fork. Farm to Fork appears in every chapter and presents practical information on how to grow, shop, store, and cook various fruits and vegetables to obtain and preserve their flavor and nutrients. More tips for boosting the phytochemical content of your diet will be discussed in Chapter 2.

Some related compounds under study, such as sphingolipids (meat and dairy products) and conjugated linoleic acid (meat and cheese), are also found in animal products. These are not phytochemicals per se because they are not from plant sources, but they have been shown to have health benefits.

SOURCES OF NUTRIENTS

Now that we know the six classes of nutrients, it is important to understand that the quantities of the various nutrients that people consume in different foods vary widely. On a daily basis, we consume about 500 grams, or about 1 pound, of protein, fat,

TABLE 1-2 ■ **Food Sources of Some Phytochemical Compounds Under Study**

Food Sources	Phytochemical
Garlic, onions, leeks	Allyl sulfides/organosulfurs
Garlic, onions, licorice, legumes	Saponins
Orange, red, and yellow fruits and vegetables (egg yolks are a source as well)	Carotenoids (e.g., lycopene)
Oranges, lemons, grapefruit	Monoterpenes
Chili peppers	Capsaicin
Flaxseed, berries, whole grains	Lignans
Cruciferous vegetables (broccoli, cabbage, kale)	Indoles
Cruciferous vegetables, especially broccoli	Isothiocyanates
Soybeans, other legumes, cucumbers, other fruits and vegetables	Phytosterols
Citrus fruit, onions, apples, grapes, red wine, tea, chocolate, tomatoes	Flavonoids
Soybeans, other legumes	Isoflavones
Tea	Catechins
Blueberries, strawberries, raspberries, grapes, apples, bananas, nuts	Polyphenols
Red, blue, and purple plants (blueberries, eggplant)	Anthocyanosides
Onions, bananas, oranges (small amounts)	Fructooligosaccharides
Grapes, peanuts, red wine	Resveratrol

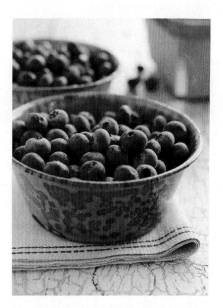

▲ Blueberries are rich in health-promoting phytochemicals. They have been shown to have anticancer effects and therefore could be an important part of dietary cancer prevention strategies. ©Lifesize /Getty Images

FARM to FORK Tomatoes

Grow
- Naturally ripened tomatoes are more nutritious and flavorful than the artificially ripened tomatoes sold in supermarkets. Look for local tomatoes, including heirloom varieties, at nearby farmers' markets.
- Consider growing your own tomatoes, even in containers, to enjoy nutritious varieties harvested at the peak of ripeness.

Shop
- Choose tomatoes with the darkest red color for the most nutrients and highest amount of the phytochemical lycopene.
- Purchase smaller tomatoes for their sweetness and flavor, and the most lycopene and vitamin C per ounce.
- Buy processed tomato products, including canned paste and sauce, for their highly bioavailable lycopene.
- Choose tomato products in glass jars, aseptic-coated paper containers, or BPA-free cans. BPA or bisphenol A, is a synthetic estrogen found in the coatings of some food cans, and has been linked to many health problems.

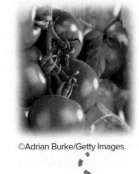
©Adrian Burke/Getty Images

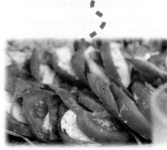
©FoodCollection

Store
- To preserve the flavor of fresh tomatoes, store them stem side up at room temperature. Flavor and aroma quickly decrease when tomatoes are stored in the refrigerator.
- Grape tomatoes should be stored in plastic clamshells to prevent them from drying out.
- Tomatoes are ripe and ready to eat when they are a deep color but still firm. Eat ripe tomatoes within two or three days.

Prep
- Use the whole tomato. The juice contains the flavor enhancer glutamate, and the skin and seeds provide vitamin C and lycopene.
- Snack on nutrition-packed grape tomatoes, and slice or chop them for salads, omelets, sandwiches, or tacos.
- Cooking tomatoes increases the bioavailability of nutrients and phytochemicals.
- Add tomato paste to recipes as a concentrated source of flavor, color, nutrients, and phytochemicals, with no added sugar or salt.

Source: Robinson J: Tomatoes : bringing back their flavor and nutrients. In *Eating on the Wild Side*. New York: Little, Brown and Company, 2013.

and carbohydrate. In contrast, the typical daily mineral intake totals about 20 grams (about 4 teaspoons), and the daily vitamin intake totals less than 300 milligrams (1/15 of a teaspoon). Although we require a gram or so of some minerals, such as calcium and phosphorus, we need only a few milligrams or less of other minerals each day. For example, we need about 10 milligrams of zinc per day, which is just a few specks of the mineral.

The nutrient content of the foods we eat also differs from the nutrient composition of the human body. This is because growth, development, and later maintenance of the human body are directed by the genetic material (DNA) inside body cells. This genetic blueprint determines how each cell uses the essential nutrients to perform body functions. These nutrients can come from a variety of sources. Cells are not concerned about whether available amino acids come from animal or plant sources. The carbohydrate glucose can come from sugars or starches. The food that you eat provides cells with basic materials to function according to the directions supplied by the genetic material **(genes)** housed in body cells. Genetics and nutrition will be discussed in Chapter 3.

gene A specific segment on a chromosome. Genes provide the blueprints for the production of all body proteins.

✓ CONCEPT CHECK 1.3

1. What are the six classes of nutrients?
2. What are the three general functions of nutrients in the body?

1.4 What Math Concepts Will Aid Your Study of Nutrition?

CALORIES

We obtain the energy we need for involuntary body functions and voluntary physical activity from various calorie sources: carbohydrates (4 kcal per gram), fats (9 kcal per gram), and proteins (4 kcal per gram). Foods generally provide more than one calorie source. Plant oils, such as soybean or canola oil, are one exception; these are 100% fat at 9 kcal per gram.

Alcohol is also a potential source of calories, supplying about 7 kcal per gram. It is not considered an essential nutrient, however, because it is not required for human function. Still, alcoholic beverages, such as beer—also rich in carbohydrate—are a contributor of calories to the eating patterns of many adults.

The body releases the energy from the chemical bonds in carbohydrate, protein, and fat (and alcohol) in order to

- build new compounds.
- perform muscular movements.
- promote nerve transmission.
- maintain electrolyte balance within cells.

Chapter 7 describes how that energy is released from the chemical bonds in energy-yielding nutrients and then used by body cells to support the processes just described.

The energy in food is often expressed using the term *calories* on food labels. As defined earlier, a calorie is the amount of heat energy it takes to raise the temperature of 1 gram of water 1 degree Celsius (1°C, centigrade scale). (Chapter 7 has a diagram of the bomb calorimeter that can be used to measure calories in foods.) A calorie is a tiny measure of heat relative to the amount of calories we eat and use. Food energy is more conveniently expressed in terms of the kilocalorie (kcal), which equals 1000 calories. (If the "c" in calories is capitalized, this also signifies kilocalories.) A kilocalorie is the amount of heat energy it takes to raise the temperature of 1000 grams (1 liter) of water 1°C. The abbreviation *kcal* is used throughout this book. On food labels, the word *calorie* (without a capital "C") is also used loosely to mean *kilocalorie.* Any values given on food labels in calories are actually in kilocalories (Fig. 1-5). A suggested intake of 2000 calories per day on a food label is technically 2000 kcal.

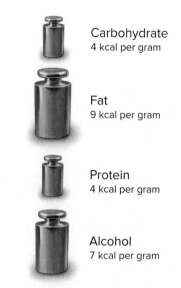

Carbohydrate
4 kcal per gram

Fat
9 kcal per gram

Protein
4 kcal per gram

Alcohol
7 kcal per gram

▲ Calorie content of energy nutrients and alcohol. The weights illustrate their relative energy potential per gram.

alcohol Ethyl alcohol or ethanol (CH_3CH_2OH) is the compound in alcoholic beverages.

WHOLE WHEAT BREAD

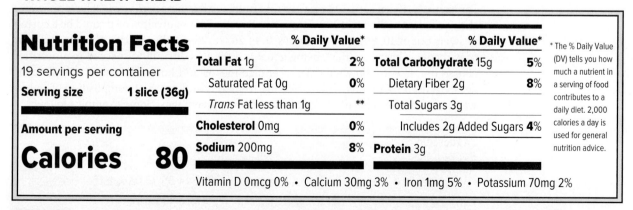

Nutrition Facts

19 servings per container

Serving size   **1 slice (36g)**

Amount per serving

Calories   80

	% Daily Value*
Total Fat 1g	**2%**
Saturated Fat 0g	**0%**
Trans Fat less than 1g	**
Cholesterol 0mg	**0%**
Sodium 200mg	**8%**

	% Daily Value*
Total Carbohydrate 15g	**5%**
Dietary Fiber 2g	**8%**
Total Sugars 3g	
Includes 2g Added Sugars	**4%**
Protein 3g	

* The % Daily Value (DV) tells you how much a nutrient in a serving of food contributes to a daily diet. 2,000 calories a day is used for general nutrition advice.

Vitamin D 0mcg 0% • Calcium 30mg 3% • Iron 1mg 5% • Potassium 70mg 2%

FIGURE 1-5 ▲ Use the nutrient values on the Nutrition Facts panel to calculate calorie content of a food. Based on carbohydrate, fat, and protein content, a serving of this food (whole wheat bread) contains 81 kcal ([15 × 4] + [1 × 9] + [3 × 4] = 81). The label lists 80, suggesting that the calorie value was rounded down.

CALCULATING CALORIES

The calorie estimates for carbohydrate, fat, and protein (4-9-4) can be used to determine calorie content of a food. Consider these foods:

1 Grilled Chicken Sandwich

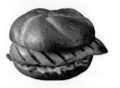

©Burke/Triolo/Brand X Pictures

Carbohydrate	46 grams × 4 = 184 kcal
Fat	14 grams × 9 = 126 kcal
Protein	45 grams × 4 = 180 kcal
Alcohol	0 gram × 7 = 0 kcal
Total	**490 kcal**

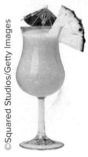

©Squared Studios/Getty Images

8-Ounce Piña Colada

Carbohydrate	57 grams × 4 = 228 kcal
Fat	5 grams × 9 = 45 kcal
Protein	1 gram × 4 = 4 kcal
Alcohol	23 grams × 7 = 161 kcal
Total	**438 kcal**

You can also use the 4-9-4 estimates to determine what portion of total kilocalorie intake is contributed by the various calorie-yielding nutrients. Assume that one day you consume 290 grams of carbohydrates, 60 grams of fat, and 70 grams of protein. This consumption yields a total of 1980 kcal ([290 × 4] + [60 × 9] + [70 × 4] = 1980). The percentage of your total kilocalorie intake derived from each nutrient can then be determined:

$$\% \text{ of kcal as carbohydrate} = (290 \times 4) \div 1980 = 0.59 \,(\times 100 = 59\%)$$
$$\% \text{ of kcal as fat} = (60 \times 9) \div 1980 = 0.27 \,(\times 100 = 27\%)$$
$$\% \text{ of kcal as protein} = (70 \times 4) \div 1980 = 0.14 \,(\times 100 = 14\%)$$

Check your calculations by adding the percentages together. Do they total 100%?

PERCENTAGES

You will use a few mathematical concepts in studying nutrition. Besides performing addition, subtraction, multiplication, and division, you need to know how to calculate percentages and convert English units of measurement to metric units.

The term *percent* (%) refers to a part of the total when the total represents 100 parts. For example, if you earn 80% on your first nutrition examination, you will have answered the equivalent of 80 out of 100 questions correctly. This equivalent also could be 8 correct answers out of 10; 80% also describes 16 of 20 (16/20 = 0.80 or 80%). The decimal form of percents is based on 100% being equal to 1.00. It is difficult to succeed in a nutrition course unless you know what a percentage means and how to calculate one. Percentages are used frequently when referring to menus and nutrient composition. The best way to master this concept is to calculate some percentages. Some examples follow:

Question	Answer
What is 6% of 45?	6% = 0.06, so 0.06 × 45 = 2.7
What percent of 99 is 3?	3/99 = 0.03 or 3% (0.03 × 100)
Joe ate 15% of the adult Recommended Dietary Allowance for iron (RDA = 8 milligrams) at lunch. How many milligrams did he eat?	
	0.15 × 8 milligrams = 1.2 milligrams

THE METRIC SYSTEM

The basic units of the metric system are the meter, which indicates length; the gram, which indicates weight; and the liter, which indicates volume. Appendix F in this textbook lists conversions from the metric system to the English system (pounds, feet, and cups) and vice versa. Here is a brief summary:

A gram (g) is about 1/30 of an ounce (an ounce weighs 28 grams).

5 grams of sugar or salt is about 1 teaspoon.

A pound (lb) weighs 454 grams.

A kilogram (kg) is 1000 grams, equivalent to 2.2 pounds.

To convert weight in pounds to kilograms, divide it by 2.2.

  A 154-pound man weighs 70 kilograms (154/2.2 = 70).

A gram can be divided into 1000 milligrams (mg) or 1,000,000 micrograms (µg or mcg).

  10 milligrams of zinc (approximate adult need) would be a few grains of zinc.

Liters are divided into 1000 units called milliliters (ml); 100 milliliters is a deciliter (dl).

  One teaspoon equals about 5 milliliters (ml), 1 cup is about 240 milliliters, and
  1 quart (4 cups) equals almost 1 liter (L) (0.946 liter to be exact).

A centimeter is 1/100 of a meter; 2.54 centimeters equals 1 inch.

Examples:
You see on the label that a 5.3-ounce (oz) container of Greek yogurt contains
15 grams of sugar. How many teaspoons of sugar does this equal?

Answer: 15 grams ÷ 5 grams/teaspoon = 3 teaspoons of sugar in the 5.3-oz yogurt.

You have heard that you should drink at least 8 cups of water each day. You know
that equals 64 ounces or 2 quarts of water because there are 8 ounces in a cup. The
water bottle you use, however, holds 500 milliliters (ml). How many milliliters or
liters should you drink to equal 64 ounces or 2 quarts?

Answer: 8 cups × 240 ml/cup = 1920 ml = 1.92 liters (almost four 500 ml bottles).

If you plan to work in any scientific field, you will need to learn the metric system. In the field of nutrition, it is important to remember that a kilogram equals 2.2 pounds, an ounce weighs 28 grams, 2.54 centimeters equals 1 inch, and a liter is almost the same as a quart. In addition, know the fractions that the following prefixes represent: micro (1/1,000,000), milli (1/1000), centi (1/100), and kilo (1000).

✓ CONCEPT CHECK 1.4

1. What are the energy (kilocalorie) values for each of the "energy nutrients"?

1.5 How Do We Know What We Know About Nutrition?

The knowledge we have about nutrient needs comes from research. Like other sciences, the research that sets the foundation for nutrition knowledge has developed using the *scientific method,* a testing procedure designed to detect and eliminate error.

THE SCIENTIFIC METHOD

The first step of the scientific method is the observation of a natural phenomenon (Fig. 1-6). Scientists then suggest possible explanations, called **hypotheses,** about its cause. At times, historical events have provided clues to important relationships in nutrition science, such

hypotheses Tentative explanations by a scientist to explain a phenomenon.

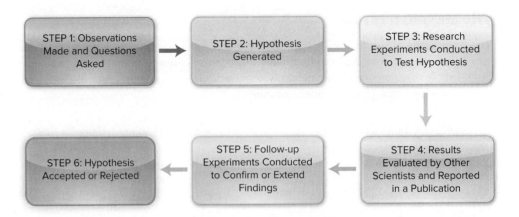

FIGURE 1-6 ▲ The scientific method. Scientists consistently follow these steps when testing all types of hypotheses. Scientists do not accept a nutrition or other scientific hypothesis until it has been thoroughly tested using the scientific method.

scurvy The vitamin C deficiency disease characterized by weakness, fatigue, slow wound healing, bone pain, fractures, sore and bleeding gums, diarrhea, and pinpoint hemorrhages on the skin.

epidemiology The study of how disease rates vary among different population groups.

theory An explanation for a phenomenon that has numerous lines of evidence to support it.

double-blind study An experimental design in which neither the participants nor the researchers are aware of each participant's assignment (test or placebo) or the outcome of the study until it is completed. An independent third party holds the code and the data until the study has been completed.

control group Participants in an experiment who are not given the treatment being tested.

placebo Generally, an inactive medicine or treatment used to disguise the treatments given to the participants in an experiment.

case-control study A study in which individuals who have a disease or condition, such as lung cancer, are compared with individuals who do not have the condition.

peer review Evaluation of work by professionals of similar competence (peers) to the producers of the work to maintain standards of quality and credibility. Scholarly peer review is used to determine if a scientific study is suitable for publication.

as the link between the need for vitamin C and the development of the disease **scurvy** (see Chapter 8). Another approach is for scientists to study diet and disease patterns among various populations, a research method called **epidemiology.**

Thus, hypotheses about the role of diet in various health problems can be suggested by historical and epidemiological findings. *Proving* the role of particular dietary components, however, requires controlled experiments. The data gathered from experiments may either support or refute each hypothesis. If the results of many experiments support a hypothesis, scientists accept the hypothesis as a **theory.** Often, the results from one experiment suggest a new set of questions.

The most rigorous type of controlled experiment follows a study design that is randomized, **double-blind,** and placebo controlled. In this type of study, a group of participants—the experimental group—follows a specific protocol (e.g., consuming a certain food or nutrient), and participants in a corresponding **control group** follow their normal habits or consume a **placebo.** People are randomly assigned to each group. Scientists then observe the experimental group over time to see if there is any effect not found in the control group. A **case-control study** compares individuals who have a disease or condition, such as lung cancer, to individuals who do not have the condition.

TESTING A HYPOTHESIS: CAN A HIGH-FAT DIET CAUSE WEIGHT LOSS?

The following example shows how the scientific method (see Fig. 1-6) was used to test a hypothesis about the effects of low-calorie, high-fat diets on weight loss.

Step 1. Observations Made and Questions Asked. In the mid-1950s, physicians note that in short-term experiments, people eating a low-calorie, high-fat diet lost weight more quickly than people eating a low-calorie, high-carbohydrate diet.

Step 2. Hypothesis Generated. Low-calorie, high-fat diets (e.g., Atkins diet) lead to more weight loss over time than low-calorie, high-carbohydrate diets.

Step 3. Research Experiments Conducted. For 1 year, researchers followed 63 people assigned to either a low-calorie, high-fat diet or a low-calorie, high-carbohydrate diet. At the end of the study, weight loss did not differ significantly between the two groups.

Step 4. Results Evaluated by Other Scientists and Published. A **peer review** indicated that the study was conducted in an unbiased, scientific manner and the results appeared valid. The study was published in *The New England Journal of Medicine* (348:2082, 2003).

Step 5. Follow-up Experiments Conducted to Confirm or Extend the Findings. A study published in 2005 described what happened when 160 people were assigned to a specific diet for a year. One diet was a low-calorie, high-fat diet; the other was a low-calorie, high-carbohydrate diet. Again, at the end of 1 year, weight loss in these two groups did not differ significantly. Peer reviewers indicated that the study was conducted scientifically. It was published in the *Journal of the American Medical Association* (293:43, 2005). A more recent 2-year study compared people who ate one of four reduced-calorie diets that was either low or high in fat, average or high in protein, or low or high in carbohydrates. After 2 years, the amount of weight loss was similar among participants. This study was published in *The New England Journal of Medicine* (360:859, 2009).

Step 6. Accept or Reject Hypothesis? Based on the currently available research studies, the hypothesis is not accepted. Reduced-calorie diets result in weight loss regardless of whether they emphasize fat, protein, or carbohydrate.

TYPES OF EXPERIMENTS

Human experiments provide the most convincing evidence about relationships between nutrients and health, but they are often not practical or ethical to conduct. Thus, much of what we know about human nutritional needs and functions has been gleaned from animal experiments. The use of animal experiments to study the role of nutrition in certain human diseases depends on the availability of an **animal model** in which a disease in laboratory animals closely mimics a particular human disease. Often, if no animal model is available and human experiments are ruled out, scientific knowledge cannot advance beyond what can be learned from epidemiological studies.

Once an experiment is complete, scientists summarize the findings and seek to publish the results in scientific journals. Generally, before articles are published in scientific journals, they are critically peer reviewed by other scientists familiar with the subject, which helps to ensure that only high-quality, objective research findings are published.

Keep in mind that one experiment is never enough to prove a particular hypothesis or provide a basis for nutritional recommendations. Rather, through follow-up studies, the results obtained in one laboratory must be confirmed by similar experiments conducted in other laboratories and, possibly, under varying circumstances. Only then can we really trust and use the results. As shown in Figure 1-7, the more lines of evidence available to support an idea, the more likely it is to be true.

animal model Use of animals to study disease to understand more about human disease.

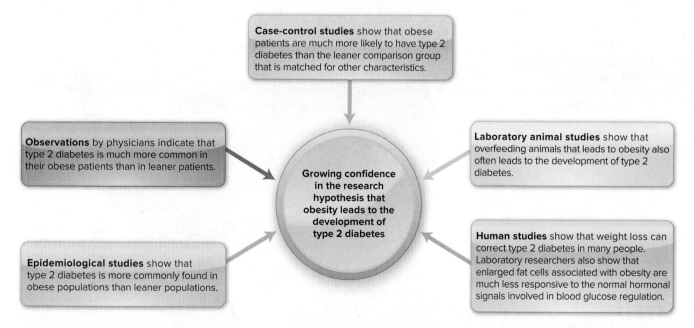

FIGURE 1-7 ▲ Data from a variety of sources can come together to support a research hypothesis. This diagram shows how various types of research data support the hypothesis that obesity leads to the development of type 2 diabetes.

Epidemiological studies may suggest hypotheses, but controlled experiments are needed to rigorously test hypotheses before nutrition recommendations can be made. For example, epidemiologists found that smokers who regularly consumed fruits and vegetables had a lower risk for lung cancer than smokers who ate very few fruits and vegetables. Scientists proposed that beta-carotene, a pigment present in many fruits and vegetables, may be responsible for reducing the damage caused by tobacco smoke in the lungs. However, in double-blind studies of heavy smokers taking beta-carotene in supplements, rather than food, the risk of lung cancer was *higher* for those who took beta-carotene supplements than for those who did not (this is not true for the small amount of beta-carotene found naturally in foods). Soon after these results were reported, two other large studies using beta-carotene supplements were stopped by the federal funding agency on the basis that these supplements are ineffective in preventing both lung cancer and cardiovascular disease.

✓ CONCEPT CHECK 1.5

1. What are the six steps used in the scientific method?

1.6 What Is the Current State of North American Eating Patterns and Health?

DOES OBESITY THREATEN OUR FUTURE?

There is no doubt that the obesity epidemic threatens the future health of Americans. It is estimated that more than 36.5% of adults are currently obese, with *obesity* defined as having an excessive amount of body fat relative to lean tissue. Considered more broadly, two-thirds of adults and one-third of children are overweight or obese. According to the Centers for Disease Control and Prevention (CDC), the average American adult man weighs 195.5 pounds, and the average American adult woman weighs 166.2 pounds. Where you live is also a factor, with obesity rates varying by state. State by state, self-reported obesity data from the CDC (Fig. 1-8) indicates that in 2015, 25 states had an adult obesity rate of 30% or higher and 4 states (Louisiana, Alabama, West Virginia,

FIGURE 1-8 ▶ Percentage of adults who are obese,* by state, 2015.

Source: CDC, Prevalence of Self-Reported Obesity Among U.S. Adults by State and Territory, BRFSS, 2015.

*Body mass index (BMI) > 30, or about 30 pounds overweight for a 5'9" person, based on self-reported weight and height.

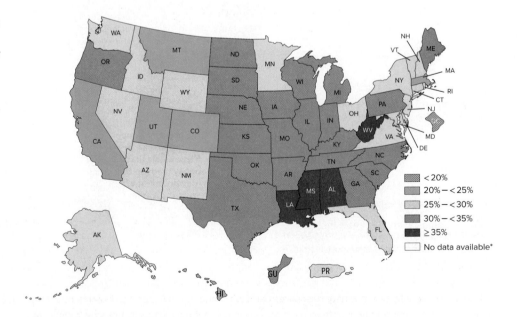

Newsworthy Nutrition

No decrease in adult obesity rates from 2005 to 2014

The prevalence of obesity in the United States is high, with 36.5% of adults estimated to be obese. Despite its high occurrence, an earlier study found that the prevalence of obesity for men and women remained stable between 2003 and 2012. Because of this leveling-off rate, scientists at the National Center for Health Statistics developed a hypothesis that the prevalence of obesity in adults would also have remained stable between 2005 and 2014. The purpose of this study was to analyze trends in adult obesity between 2005 and 2014. The analyses were based on measurements of weight and height in 5455 adults from the 2013–2014 National Health and Nutrition Examination Survey (NHANES) and from 21,013 participants in previous NHANES surveys from 2005 through 2012. For the years 2013–2014, the overall prevalence of obesity was 37.7%; 35.0% of men were obese (BMI ≥ 30) and 5.5% were morbidly obese (BMI ≥ 40); among adult women, 40.4% were obese and 9.9% were morbidly obese. These obesity rates were unchanged over the decade from 2005 through 2014 among men, but there were significant increases among women for overall obesity and for morbid obesity. Based on these results, the authors of this study conclude that other studies are needed to determine the causes of the increases in obesity prevalence.

Source: Flegal KM and others: Trends in Obesity Among Adults in the United States, 2005 to 2014. *Journal of the American Medical Association* 351:2284, 2016.

and Mississippi) have the highest adult obesity rates—over 35%. In 2015, most states with the lowest obesity rates were in the Northeast or the West, and adult obesity rates decreased in four states (Minnesota, Montana, New York, and Ohio). Two states (Kansas and Kentucky) saw increases in obesity rates in 2015, and Louisiana had the highest adult obesity rate at 36.2%.[11] In 2006, only one state was above 30%.

The report *F as in Fat: How Obesity Threatens America's Future 2013*[12] warns that if the incidence of obesity continues to grow at recent rates, the effects on the health and wealth of our nation would be catastrophic by the year 2030. The report calls for a national commitment to the prevention of obesity and outlines a scenario by which a 9% to 14% (depending on the state) reduction of the states' obesity rates by 2030 could greatly decrease obesity-related diseases and health care costs. There is evidence from the National Health and Nutrition Examination Survey (NHANES) conducted over the last decade that the prevalence of obesity has not changed in men but has increased in women. Read more about these results in the Newsworthy Nutrition feature in this section.[13]

It is well documented that this extra weight will continue to have dangerous consequences. In Section 1.2, we pointed out that obesity plays a role in chronic illness, including heart disease, stroke, high blood pressure, high cholesterol, diabetes, arthritis, and certain cancers. It is estimated that obesity kills more than 200,000 Americans a year. Because of its role in so many chronic disorders, obesity is an expensive condition with more than $190 billion spent annually on health care related to obesity. Because of numerous medical conditions, obese individuals are absent from work more often than those of healthy weight. Health economists estimate that obesity-related absenteeism costs employers as much as $6.4 billion a year, whereas loss of on-the-job productivity due to pain, shortness of breath, or other obstacles costs another $30 billion. It has become obvious that the answers to the obesity crisis are not simple. From a nutrition perspective, however, the problem can be clearly stated. Most of us continue to eat too much, especially foods with a high number of calories and a low number of nutrients, and we do not engage in enough physical activity.

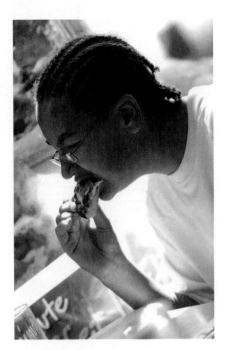

▲ About half the carbohydrate in North American diets comes from simple sugars; the other half comes from starches in foods such as pastas, breads, and potatoes. ©Ingram Publishing

ASSESSING THE CURRENT NORTH AMERICAN EATING PATTERN

With the aim of finding out what North Americans eat, federal agencies conduct surveys to collect data about food and nutrient consumption, as well as connections between diet and health. In the United States, the U.S. Department of Health and Human Services monitors food consumption with the National Health and Nutrition Examination Survey. The NHANES was used in the study highlighted in the Newsworthy Nutrition. In Canada, this information is gathered by Health Canada in conjunction with Agriculture and Agrifood Canada. Survey data from 2009–2012 indicate that North American adults consume about 16% of their calorie intake as proteins, 50% as carbohydrates, and 33% as fats. These percentages, which do not consider alcohol, fall within the ranges recommended by the Food and Nutrition Board (FNB) of the National Academy of Sciences. The FNB advocates that 10% to 35% of calories come from protein, 45% to 65% from carbohydrate, and 20% to 35% from fat. These standards apply to people in both the United States and Canada.

Food-consumption data also indicate that about two-thirds of protein intake is from animal sources for most North Americans, whereas plant sources supply only about one-third. In many other parts of the world, it is just the opposite: plant proteins—from rice, beans, corn, and other grains and vegetables—dominate protein intake. About half the carbohydrate in North American diets comes from simple sugars; the other half comes from starches (such as in pastas, breads, and potatoes). About 60% of dietary fat comes from animal sources and 40% from plant sources.

Evidence of positive changes in dietary habits have begun to appear. Results from the 2011–2012 NHANES show that calories consumed daily by the typical U.S. adult are declining for the first time in over 40 years. One of the most significant declines has been in the amount of sugar-sweetened soda consumed, which has dropped 25% since the late 1990s. Keep in mind that while these changes in calories consumed are a step in the right direction and appear to stem from our growing awareness of the dangers of eating and drinking too much, we often do not choose the foods that will meet all our nutrient needs.

In the next section, we discuss recommendations to consume a variety of nutrient-dense foods within and across the food groups, especially whole grains, fruits, vegetables, low-fat or fat-free milk or milk products, and lean meats and other protein sources. These foods will provide nutrients that are often overlooked, including various B vitamins, vitamin C, vitamin D, vitamin E, calcium, potassium, magnesium, iron, fiber, and many phytochemicals. Daily intake of a balanced multivitamin and mineral supplement is another strategy to help meet nutrient needs but does not make up for a poor eating pattern. Also keep in mind that use of nutrient supplements should be discussed with your health professional to avoid potentially harmful side effects (dietary supplements are discussed in Chapter 8).

Experts also recommend that we pay more attention to balancing calorie intake with needs. An excess intake of calories is usually tied to overindulgence in sugar, fat, and alcoholic beverages. Many North Americans would benefit from a healthier balance of food in their eating patterns. Moderation is the key for some foods that are high in calories from sugar and fat. For other foods, such as fruits and vegetables, increased quantity and variety are warranted. Few adults currently meet the new recommendation to "fill half your plate with fruits and vegetables" promoted in the USDA MyPlate guidelines for total servings of vegetables and fruits.

HEALTH OBJECTIVES FOR THE UNITED STATES FOR THE YEAR 2020

Health promotion and disease prevention have been public health strategies in North America for the past 3 decades. One part of this strategy is *Healthy People 2020,* a report issued in December 2010 by the U.S. Department of Health and Human Services' (DHHS) Public Health Service. Every 10 years, DHHS issues a collection of health objectives for the nation. These objectives are developed by experts in federal agencies and target major public health concerns, setting goals for the coming decade. *Healthy People 2020* sets forth more than 600 health objectives across 42 topic areas and outlines national standards to eliminate health disparities, improve access to health education and quality health care, and strengthen public health services. The vision for 2020 is a society in which all people live long, healthy lives. Important features of *Healthy People 2020* include a focus on creating social and physical environments that promote good health for all and an interactive, personalized website at www.HealthyPeople.gov.

The overarching goals of *Healthy People 2020* are to:

- Attain high-quality, longer lives free of preventable disease, disability, injury, and premature death.
- Achieve health equity, eliminate disparities, and improve health of all groups.
- Create social and physical environments that promote good health for all.
- Promote quality of life, healthy development, and healthy behaviors across all life stages.

Healthy People 2020, like earlier versions, includes nutrition as a specific a topic area. This topic is called Nutrition and Weight Status, and its objectives target individual behaviors, as well as the policies and environments that support these behaviors. Nutrition and weight status are important because a healthful diet helps us reduce our risks for numerous health conditions that burden the public health system, including heart disease, high blood pressure, diabetes, osteoporosis, and some cancers. Good nutrition for children is also emphasized in this report because of its importance for growth and development. The goal of this topic is to promote health and reduce chronic disease risk through the consumption of healthful diets and achievement and maintenance of healthy body weights. This goal also includes increasing household food security and eliminating hunger.

The Nutrition and Weight Status objectives are based on strong science that supports the health benefits of eating a healthful diet and maintaining a healthy body weight. A healthful diet is described as one that includes:

- Consuming a variety of nutrient-dense foods within and across the food groups, especially whole grains, fruits, vegetables, low-fat or fat-free milk or milk products, and lean meats and other protein sources.
- Limiting intake of solid fats, cholesterol, added sugars, sodium (salt), and alcohol.
- Limiting caloric intake to meet caloric needs.

The objectives also emphasize that individual behaviors should be addressed in any efforts to change diet and weight, as well as the policies and environments that support these behaviors in settings such as schools, work sites, health care organizations, and communities.

Table 1-3 lists the six categories of objectives for the Nutrition and Weight Status topic, along with the 22 specific objectives. Table 1-4 provides a more detailed sample of nine specific Nutrition and Weight Status objectives, along with the current status of these objectives and their targets for 2020.

Other new topic areas highlight changes in the health needs of specific segments of the population: early and middle childhood, adolescence, and older adults. Because young people develop habits, including eating and physical activity behaviors, that are likely to persist throughout life, new objectives promote strengthened health education in schools and communities, and fostering an environment in which young people can develop healthy habits. Older adults are the fastest-growing segment of the American population and are at high risk for experiencing the chronic health problems that so severely impact our health care system. The objectives for older adults include improving

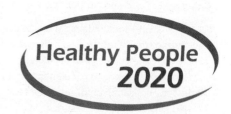

▲ Many nutrition-related objectives are part of the *Healthy People 2020* report. The report outlines health promotion and disease prevention objectives for the United States for the year 2020.

Source: https://www.healthypeople.gov.

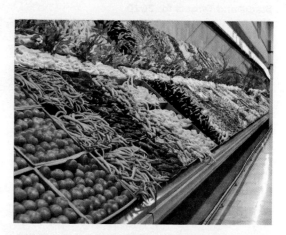

▲ An increase in the consumption of some foods, such as fruits and vegetables, can lead to a healthier balance of food in the North American diet. ©xefstock /Getty Images

TABLE 1-3 ■ *Healthy People 2020:* Nutrition and Weight Status Categories and Objectives

Category 1: Healthier Food Access

1. Increase the number of states with nutrition standards for child care.
2. Increase the proportion of schools that offer nutritious foods and beverages outside of school meals.
3. Increase the number of states that have incentive policies for food retail outlets to provide foods that are encouraged by the Dietary Guidelines for Americans.
4. Increase the proportion of Americans who have retail access to foods recommended by the Dietary Guidelines for Americans.

Category 2: Health Care and Work site Settings

5. Increase the proportion of primary care physicians who measure patients' body mass index (BMI).
6. Increase the proportion of physician office visits that include nutrition or weight counseling or education.
7. Increase the proportion of work sites that offer nutrition and weight-management classes and counseling.

Category 3: Weight Status

8. Increase the proportion of adults who are at a healthy weight.
9. Reduce the proportion of adults who are obese.
10. Reduce the proportion of children and adolescents who are considered obese.
11. Prevent inappropriate weight gain in youth and adults.

Category 4: Food Insecurity

12. Eliminate very low food security among children.
13. Reduce household food insecurity and, in so doing, reduce hunger.

Category 5: Food and Nutrient Consumption

14. Increase the contribution of fruits to the diets of the population ages 2 years and older.
15. Increase the variety and contribution of vegetables to the diets of the population ages 2 years and older.
16. Increase the contribution of whole grains to the diets of the population ages 2 years and older.
17. Reduce consumption of calories from solid fats and added sugars in the population ages 2 years and older.
18. Reduce consumption of saturated fat in the population ages 2 years and older.
19. Reduce consumption of sodium in the population ages 2 years and older.
20. Increase consumption of calcium in the population ages 2 years and older.

Category 6: Iron Deficiency

21. Reduce iron deficiency among young children and females of childbearing age.
22. Reduce iron deficiency among pregnant females.

TABLE 1-4 ■ A Sample of Nutrition and Weight Status Objectives from *Healthy People 2020,* Along with Details About the Current Status and Targets for 2020

	Target	Baseline (2005–08)
Increase the proportion of adults at a healthy weight.	33.9%	30.8%
Reduce the proportion of children and adolescents who are considered obese.	14.6%	16.2%
Increase the contribution of the following to the diets of the population ages 2 years and older (per 1000 calories).		
• Fruits	0.9 cup	0.5 cup
• Total vegetables	1.1 cups	0.8 cup
• Whole grains	0.6 ounce	0.3 ounce
Reduce consumption of calories from solid fats (% total calorie intake).	16.7%	18.9%
Reduce consumption of calories from added sugars (% total calorie intake).	10.8%	15.7%
Increase consumption of calcium in the population ages 2 years and older.	1300 mg	1118 mg
Reduce iron deficiency among females of childbearing age.	9.4%	10.4%

Note: In later chapters, we will explore additional nutrition-related objectives, such as those addressing osteoporosis, various forms of cancer, diabetes prevention and treatment, food allergies, cardiovascular disease, low birth weight, nutrition during pregnancy, breastfeeding, eating disorders, physical activity, and alcohol use.

access to health care, helping older adults to manage their own health conditions, and ensuring proper training and support of professionals and nonprofessionals who care for this population.

A scientifically exciting new topic area in the *Healthy People 2020* report is **genomics.** Nine of the 10 leading causes of death have a strong genetic component. Genetic testing is becoming a valuable tool for improving diagnosis and treatment of chronic diseases, especially for cancers of the breast and colon. In combination with family history, genetic testing can help health care professionals guide patients in treatment options, including lifestyle changes. The relationship between genetics and nutrition will be discussed in Chapter 3.

genomics The study of the function and structure of the complete set of DNA within a single cell of an organism, known as the genome.

✓ CONCEPT CHECK 1.6

1. Surveys indicate that we could improve our diets by focusing on which types of food sources?

2. The consumption of which types of foods should be reduced to attain and maintain good health?

1.7 What Can You Expect from Good Nutrition and a Healthy Lifestyle?

The obesity epidemic and prevalence of chronic diseases in the United States show that something is not right with many of our eating patterns and/or lifestyles. The strong association between obesity and poor health is clear. The reverse is also well documented: when an obese or overweight person loses just 5% to 10% of body weight, that person's risks of many chronic diseases are greatly reduced.

HEALTHY WEIGHT

Because weight gain is one of the greatest lifelong nutrition challenges, we encourage you to seek a lifestyle that will make gaining weight more difficult and maintaining a healthy weight easier. Preventing obesity in the first place is the easiest approach. Unfortunately, many aspects of our society make it hard not to gain weight. The earlier (preferably in childhood) we develop lifestyle habits of good nutrition, regular physical activity, and the avoidance of addictions to salt, fat, sweets, high-calorie foods, and sedentary lifestyles, the better our chances for a long, healthy life. As you enter the workforce, seek out employers who offer wellness programs that encourage weight management and weight loss among their employees. Aim to live in a city or town that has opportunities for physical activity such as bike paths, walking trails, and parks, as well as access to fresh fruits and vegetables through farmers' markets and community gardens. Seek out and join running or walking clubs. Shop at grocery stores that offer a good selection of fruits, vegetables, and other healthy foods. When dining out, choose restaurants that have tasty but healthy options on their menu.

Fortunately, many dietary habits have improved during the past decade. Today, we can choose from a wide variety of food products as a result of continual innovation by food manufacturers. We are eating more breakfast cereals, pizza, pasta entrees, stir-fried meats and vegetables served on rice, salads, tacos, burritos, and fajitas than ever before. Sales of whole milk are down, and sales of fat-free and 1% low-fat milk have increased. Consumption of frozen vegetables rather than canned vegetables is also on the rise. Despite the alarming problem of overweight and obesity, our cultural diversity, varied cuisines, and general lack of nutrient deficiencies should be points of pride for North Americans.

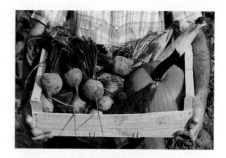

▲ Access to fresh fruits and vegetables through farmers' markets and community gardens is important to a healthy lifestyle. ©Image Source

LONGER, HEALTHIER LIVES

Today, North Americans live longer than ever and enjoy better general health. Deaths from cardiovascular disease, for example, have dropped dramatically since the late 1960s, partly because of better medical care and dietary patterns. Affluence, however, has also led to sedentary lifestyles and high intakes of animal fat, salt, and alcohol. This lifestyle pattern has led to problems such as cardiovascular disease, hypertension, diabetes, and, of course, obesity. Greater efforts are needed by the general public to lower intake of animal fats and to improve variety in our diets, especially from fruits, vegetables, and whole grains. With better technology and greater choices, we can have a much healthier eating pattern today than ever before—if we know what choices to make.

THE TOTAL DIET

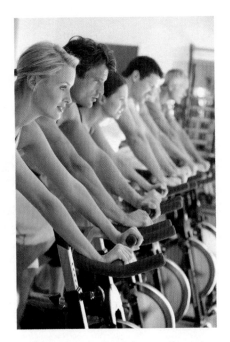

▲ Regular physical activity complements a healthy diet. Whether it is all at once or in segments throughout the day, incorporate 30 to 60 minutes or more of such activity into your daily routine. ©Monkey Business Image/age fotostock

Nutrition experts generally agree that there are no "good" or "bad" foods, but some foods provide relatively few nutrients in comparison to calorie content. In Chapter 2, you will learn that an individual's total diet is the proper focus in a nutritional evaluation. It is the position of the Academy of Nutrition and Dietetics that "the total diet or overall pattern of food eaten is the most important focus of healthy eating."[14] Health experts have prepared many reports and outlined numerous objectives to get us closer to being a "Healthy People" as soon as 2020. In Chapter 2, we will discuss the 'Dietary Guidelines for Americans' that are published every 5 years and the interactive programs available on **ChooseMyPlate.gov.** As you reexamine your nutritional habits, remember your health is largely your responsibility. Your body has a natural ability to heal itself. Offer it what it needs, and it will serve you well. Confusing and conflicting health messages hinder change in our eating patterns.

Prevention of disease is an important investment of one's time, even during the college years. The following recommendations will help promote your health and prevent chronic diseases: (1) consume enough essential nutrients, including fiber, while moderating energy, solid fat, added sugar, and alcohol intake; (2) do adequate, regular physical activity (at least 30 to 60 minutes on most or all days); (3) minimize alcohol intake (no more than two drinks per day for men and one drink for women and all adults age 65 years and older); and (4) do not smoke tobacco cigarettes or cigars. In addition to these recommendations, you can optimize your health by getting adequate sleep (7 to 9 hours per night), consuming sufficient water (9 to 13 cups per day from foods and beverages), reducing stress, using medications prudently, and, of course, abstaining from use of illicit drugs. Having close relationships with others and maintaining a positive outlook on life are also linked to lower risk for disease. Finally, consultation with health care professionals on a regular basis is important. This is because early diagnosis is especially useful for controlling the damaging effects of many diseases. In total, these contribute to maximal health and prevention of the diseases listed. Section 1.8 gives you a "sneak peek" at several nutrition issues relevant to most college students. These issues, including the "freshman 15," vegetarianism, fuel for athletes, eating disorders, and alcohol and binge drinking, also will be covered more fully in later chapters of the book.

☑ CONCEPT CHECK 1.7

1. What are some dietary patterns, physical activities, and lifestyle recommendations for health promotion and disease prevention?

ASK THE RDN: Who's the Expert?

Dear RDN: *I am interested in making positive changes to my eating pattern to reach a healthy weight and feel better. How can I find a qualified nutrition expert who will give me personalized nutrition advice?*

You have already made a big step toward better nutrition by taking this nutrition course! The information in this textbook is written by authors who are all qualified nutrition experts, namely *registered dietitian nutritionists* (RDN). The textbook and your instructor will provide a solid foundation in nutrition, but be aware that some people call themselves "nutritionists" without qualified training in nutrition. The best approach to finding answers about your personal nutritional state is to consult your primary care provider, **registered dietitian (RD),** or **registered dietitian nutritionist (RDN).** The RD/RDN has been certified by the Commission on Dietetic Registration of the Academy of Nutrition and Dietetics (AND) after completing rigorous classroom and clinical training in nutrition. The RD/RDN must also complete continuing education. The RD credential was recently updated to RDN to better reflect the scope of practice of dietitians. While both titles signify the same credential, we will use RDN when referring to dietitians in this book.

You can begin your search for a local RDN by asking your primary care provider or calling your health insurance company for a referral. You can also find an RDN by using the AND national referral service, called *Find a Registered Dietitian Nutritionist.* This service links consumers with qualified nutrition practitioners who provide reliable, objective nutrition information. Visit the website, www.eatright.org, and click on "Find an Expert." (In Canada, visit the Dietitians of Canada website, www.dietitians.ca, and click on "Find a Dietitian.") Enter your ZIP code or state to display the providers in your area. Select additional specialties that may apply to your specific needs. The website will display a list of providers. A professional with the RD or RDN credential after his or her name is a qualified nutrition expert who is trained to help you separate facts from fads and optimize your health with better food choices. You can trust an RDN to translate the latest scientific findings into easy-to-understand nutrition information.

I hope this answer was helpful. We will use this feature, "Ask the RDN," in every chapter to answer questions about topics that may seem to have conflicting viewpoints.

Your nutrition expert,

Anne M. Smith , PhD, RDN, LD (author)

registered dietitian (RD) A person who has completed a baccalaureate degree program approved by the Accreditation Council for Education in Nutrition and Dietetics (ACEND), performed at least 1200 hours of supervised professional practice, passed a registration examination, and complies with continuing education requirements.

registered dietitian nutritionist (RDN) The RDN is the updated credential formerly abbreviated RD. The credential was updated to better reflect the scope of practice of the dietitian and to align with the new name of the professional organization for dietitians, the Academy of Nutrition and Dietetics.

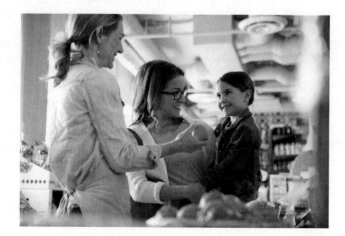

▲ An RD or RDN is a qualified nutrition expert trained to help you separate facts from fads, and optimize your health with better food choices. You can trust an RDN, like this supermarket dietitian, to translate the latest scientific findings into easy-to-understand nutrition information. ©Getty Images

1.8 Nutrition and Your Health

Eating Well in College

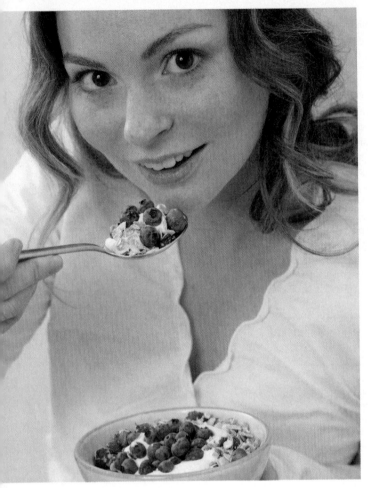

©Food Collection

The college years are a time for freedom and a chance to make personal lifestyle decisions. Studies show that the eating patterns of college students are not optimal. Typically, students fall short of diet recommendations for whole grains, vegetables, fruits, milk, and meat, opting instead to max out on fats, sweets, and alcohol. This information is disturbing because young adulthood is the time when many health behaviors are formed that will persist throughout life.

What is it about the college lifestyle that makes it so difficult to build healthy habits? In this section, we will discuss several topics and provide possible solutions.

Food Choices

College students face changes in academic requirements, interpersonal relationships, and living environments. These stressful situations contribute to poor health behaviors. For example, when you are writing papers and cramming for exams, balanced meals are all too easily replaced by high-fat and high-calorie fast foods, convenience items, and sugary, caffeinated beverages. Physical activity is sacrificed in favor of study time. In a recent study of

college students living on and off campus, two-thirds of the students reported skipping meals, with "no time to prepare" the major reason for this behavior.[15]

Also consider that on campus, you are faced with a wide variety of dining choices. Dining halls, fast-food establishments, bars, and vending machines combine to offer food 24 hours per day. While it is certainly possible to make wise food choices at each of these outlets, the temptations of convenience, taste, and value (i.e., inexpensive, oversized portions) may persuade the college student to select unhealthy options.

Meals and snacks are also times to socialize. You may unintentionally eat a big lunch at noon without regard to hunger if your peers are meeting in the dining hall to catch up. While chatting, it is easy to lose track of portions and to overeat. In addition, food may be a source of familiarity and comfort in a new and stressful place.

Weight Control and the "Freshman 15"

Studies show that most college students gain weight during their first year.[16] The "freshman 15" is a term used to describe the weight gained by students during their first year of college. Although it is becoming evident that most freshmen actually do not gain the 15 pounds, a recent study of over 7000 U.S. college students found that students pack on 2.4 to 3.5 pounds on average during their first year away from home.[17] Very few (just under 10%) of freshmen gained 15 pounds or more, and 25% of freshmen actually lost weight. The research also determined cumulative weight gain over the entire years at college and found that women gained approximately 9 pounds and men, 13 pounds, on average. The two lifestyle factors that made a difference in weight gain among the students were heavy drinking and working during college.

There are several reasons to maintain a healthy weight. Over the long term, risk of chronic diseases goes up as weight increases. In the short term, losing excess weight can improve how you feel and perform. Detecting "flab" around your midsection or feeling that your clothes are getting tighter are two good indicators that you are carrying excess weight. If weight loss is necessary, with some knowledge and perseverance, you can safely lose excess pounds.

Behavioral research clearly demonstrates that setting several small, achievable goals will spur motivation. As you will learn in Chapter 7, body weight is a balancing act between calories in and calories burned. Try keeping track of your calorie consumption for several days and comparing that to your energy needs, based on your age, gender, and activity level. You can use one of the equations presented in Chapter 7, the SuperTracker interactive tools on www.ChooseMyPlate.gov, or the NutritionCalc Plus application in Connect® for this text to estimate your energy needs.

A healthy rate of weight loss is 1 to 2 pounds per week. Greater rates of weight loss will not likely be sustained over time. Remember that the numbers on the scale are not as important as your body composition—the amount of fat in relation to lean mass. In order to lose weight, you must create an energy deficit, either by restricting energy intake below what you need to maintain your current weight or by increasing your physical activity. For an adult with excess weight, an energy deficit of 500 kcal per day will result in weight loss of about 25 pounds over a year's time. As weight is lost, energy needs gradually decrease, such that further deficits will be required to lose additional weight.

CASE STUDY Typical College Student

Andy is like many other college students. He grew up on a quick bowl of cereal and milk for breakfast and a hamburger, French fries, and cola for lunch, either in the school cafeteria or at a local fast-food restaurant. At dinner, he generally avoided eating any of his salad or vegetables, and by 9:00 P.M. he was deep into bags of chips and cookies. Andy has taken most of these habits to college. He prefers coffee for breakfast and possibly a chocolate bar. Lunch is still mainly a hamburger, French fries, and cola, but pizza and tacos now alternate more frequently than when he was in high school. One thing Andy really likes about the restaurants surrounding campus is that, for a few cents more, he can make his hamburger a double or get extra cheese and pepperoni on his pizza. This helps him stretch his food dollar; searching out large-portion value meals for lunch and dinner has become part of a typical day. Now that he is in college, some of Andy's calories come from

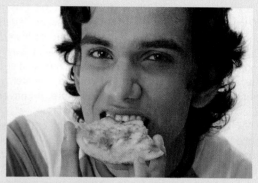

©Dinodia Photos/Almay

alcohol. He will have a beer with dinner a couple nights a week and will binge on a six-pack or more while tailgating before Saturday football games.

Provide Andy some advice about his eating pattern. Start with his positive habits and then provide some constructive criticism, based on what you now know.

Answer the following questions, and as you make suggestions for Andy, think about your favorite food choices, why they are your favorites, and whether these are positive choices.

1. **Start with Andy's positive habits:** What healthy choices are being made when Andy eats at local restaurants?
2. **Now provide some constructive criticism:**
   a. What are some of the negative aspects of items available at fast-food restaurants?
   b. Why is ordering the "value meals" a dangerous habit?
   c. What healthier substitutions could he make at each meal?
   d. List some healthier choices he could make at fast-food restaurants on campus.
   e. What concerns would you share about Andy's weekly alcohol intake?

Complete the Case Study. Responses to these questions can be provided by your instructor.

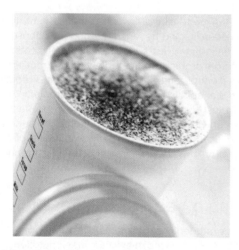

▲ Research has shown that gourmet coffee beverages, such as lattes and cappuccinos, can increase calorie consumption by about 200 kcal per day.[18] ©BananaStock/PunchStock

Although many students skip it, breakfast is the *most* important meal of the day. Starting the day off with a serving of lean protein (e.g., an egg, Canadian bacon, Greek yogurt, or protein shake), a fortified whole grain breakfast cereal, skim milk, and a serving

of fruit puts you on the right path for meeting recommendations for fiber, calcium, and fruit intake. Even though it may seem that coffee gets your brain going in the morning, your brain is fueled best by carbohydrates, not caffeine. Studies also show that eating breakfast prevents overeating later in the day. Read more about the best breakfast choices in the What the Dietitian Chose recommendations at the end of this chapter.

▶ Five Simple Tips to Avert Weight Gain

- **Eat breakfast.** Rev up your metabolism with a protein source such as an egg or Greek yogurt, at least one serving of whole grains such as a breakfast cereal, and a fruit such as a banana.
- **Plan ahead.** Eat a balanced meal or snack every 3 to 4 hours.
- *Limit liquid calories.* Drink water instead of high-calorie soft drinks, fruit juice, alcohol, or coffee; if you drink alcohol, limit it to 1 or 2 drinks per day.
- **Stock the fridge and pantry.** Keep a stash of low-calorie, nutritious snacks such as string cheese, pretzels, light microwave popcorn, and fruit (fresh, canned, or dried).
- **Exercise regularly.** Find a friend to work out with you. Experts recommend 30 minutes of moderate exercise at least 5 days a week.

One of the biggest contributors to weight gain for college students is consuming several hundred calories per day in the form of sugary or alcoholic beverages. One 12-ounce can of regular cola contains about 140 kcal. A 12-ounce can of regular beer has 150 kcal. Consuming gourmet coffee beverages, such as lattes and cappuccinos, can increase average calorie consumption by about 200 kcal per day.[18] Even fruit juices have at least 100 kcal per 8-ounce glass. Furthermore, a 24-ounce mug of a soft drink makes you feel no fuller than an equal volume of water, yet the sugar-sweetened soft drink adds 300 kcal more. A convenient stash of water is the best way to quench your thirst.

Exercise is very important to any weight loss and weight maintenance plan, but sticking with it is hard to do. When you find yourself short on time, exercise is often the first thing that goes. To ensure your success at boosting daily activity, choose activities you enjoy such as working out with friends at the campus recreation center, participating in intramural sports, or taking an activity class such as dancing. Don't forget to include brisk walking to and from classes. For more information on planning an exercise program, see Chapter 10.

Alcohol and Binge Drinking

Excessive alcohol consumption is a big problem on college campuses. Many college students consider drinking alcohol, legally or not, to be a rite of passage into adulthood. On campuses, binge drinking—consuming five or more drinks in a row for men or four drinks or more for women—has become an epidemic. A new level of "extreme drinking" goes far beyond binge drinking. For example, a recent study found that college students consumed an average of 10 drinks during twenty-first birthday celebrations.[19]

The statistics on the impact of binge drinking on college campuses are sobering. In 2013, an estimated 39% of students on college campuses participated in binge drinking. Each year, 1825 college students between the ages of 18 and 24 die from alcohol-related unintentional injuries, including motor vehicle crashes. In addition to deaths and injuries, other problems stemming from binge drinking include unsafe sex and its consequences, long-term health problems, suicides, academic problems, legal troubles, and alcohol abuse or dependence. Twenty percent of college students meet the criteria for alcohol use disorders.

In addition, alcohol consumption definitely contributes to weight gain—by virtue of its own calories and the increased food consumption at events where drinking occurs. If you choose to drink alcohol, do so in moderation—no more than two drinks per day for men and one drink per day for women. Be aware of the warning signs and dangers of alcohol poisoning shown here. Special issues related to alcohol use by adolescents are covered in Chapter 15.

▶ **The warning signs and symptoms of alcohol poisoning:**
- Semiconsciousness or unconsciousness
- Slow respiration of eight or fewer breaths per minute or lapses between breaths of more than 8 seconds
- Cold, clammy, pale, or bluish skin
- Strong odor of alcohol, which usually accompanies these symptoms

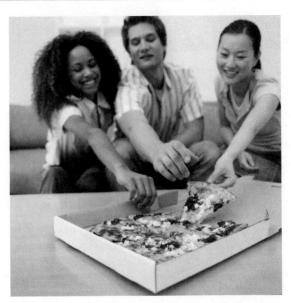
▲ Late-night pizza can add extra calories to the college student's daily intake. ©Stockbyte/PunchStock

Eating Disorders

As many as 30% of college students are at risk of developing an eating disorder. As you will learn in Chapter 11, disordered eating is a mild and short-term change in eating patterns that typically occurs in response to life stress, a desire to change appearance, or a bad habit. Sometimes, disordered eating habits may lead to an eating disorder, such as anorexia nervosa, bulimia nervosa, or binge eating disorder. Chapter 11 includes advice on what to do if you suspect that your roommate or friend is suffering from an eating disorder.

Starving the body also starves the brain, which limits performance in academics and beyond. The negative consequences of disordered eating may last a lifetime. Ultimately, eating disorders do not arise from problems with food but rather from problems with self-esteem, control, and abusive relationships. Frequently, what begins as a diet spirals into a much larger problem. Eating disorders are not just diets gone bad: they require professional intervention. Left unchecked, eating disorders lead to serious adverse effects, such as loss of menstrual periods, thinning of bones, gastrointestinal problems, kidney problems, heart abnormalities, and eventually death.

Choosing a Vegetarian Lifestyle

Many college students experiment with or adopt a vegetarian eating pattern. Plant-based diets can meet nutrition needs and decrease risk of many chronic diseases, but they require appropriate planning at all life stages.

Protein is not typically deficient in vegetarian eating patterns, even with a vegan diet, which contains no animal products. However, vegetarians, and especially vegans, may be at risk for deficiencies of several vitamins and minerals. Consuming a ready-to-eat

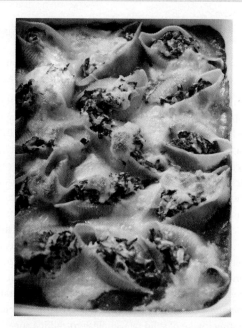

▲ Many students adopt a vegetarian eating pattern during college. Guidelines for planning a nutritious vegetarian eating pattern with items such as this veggie stuffed pasta shells are presented in Chapter 6. ©FoodCollection

breakfast cereal is an easy and inexpensive way to obtain these nutrients. See Chapter 6 for more information on vegetarian food planning.

Restaurants and campus dining services have responded to the growing interest in vegetarian meals by offering a variety of vegetarian options. For optimal health benefits, choose foods that are baked, steamed, or stir-fried rather than deep-fried; select whole grains rather than refined carbohydrates; and consume food fortified with vitamins and minerals. Even if you do not follow a plant-based eating pattern all the time, choosing several plant-based meals each week can help with weight control and boost intake of fiber and beneficial phytochemicals. You will learn in Chapter 2 that the ChooseMyPlate program recommends that the largest portion of your plate be filled with plant foods, including whole grains, fruits, and vegetables.

Fuel for Competition: Student Athletes

Students who compete in sports such as intramural and intercollegiate athletics need to consume more calories and nutrients. Despite an emphasis on a lean physique, athletes at all levels must take care not to severely restrict calories, as this could impact performance and health. Muscles require adequate carbohydrates for fuel, and protein for growth and repair. Fat, as well, is an important source of stored energy for use during exercise. Low energy availability in women may lead to a loss of menstruation (amenorrhea), a condition costly to long-term bone health.

In addition to the calories needed to fuel the body, fluids are essential for health and performance. Water is adequate to replenish losses for events lasting less than 60 minutes; sports drinks are ideal for longer events because they supply carbohydrates to fuel fatigued muscles as well as electrolytes to replenish those lost in perspiration. Intentional fluid losses to "cut weight" for a competition are detrimental to health and performance.

Athletes also should take care not to be wooed by the supplement industry. Simply increasing food intake to meet the energy demands of athletic training should be sufficient to meet most vitamin and mineral needs. As an exception, athletes may be at risk for iron-deficiency anemia. Consuming a balanced multivitamin and mineral supplement is adequate for most people. Individual vitamin, mineral, amino acid, or herbal supplements are not advised, in spite of the hype of supplement makers.

Tips for Eating Well on a College Student's Budget

Because higher education can be hard on the wallet, it is good to know that it is possible to eat well on campus on a budget. If you live on campus, participate in a prepaid campus meal plan. These plans are generally designed to offer great food value with a variety of healthy foods. If you live off campus or have your own kitchen, plan ahead. Packing a lunch from home rather than grabbing lunch on the run will save you money and put you in control of healthy choices. For example, preparing a sandwich at home costs half as much as purchasing one at a fast-food restaurant or deli. (See Table 1-5 for some foods that can be calorie traps.)

Never go grocery shopping on an empty stomach: everything will look good and you'll buy more. Also, go to the store with a list in hand and stick to it, because impulse buys tend to drain your wallet. Buy store-brand rather than name-brand items. Make use of canned and frozen fruits and vegetables; they are just as nutritious as fresh varieties, particularly if you choose low-sodium and low-sugar options. Rather than buying cartons of fruit juice, select cans of fruit juice concentrate and mix with water at home. Likewise, preparing other drinks, such as iced tea, from store-brand powder (look for sugar-free types) will save over gallon jugs or vending machine containers of drinks. Canned (fruits, tuna) and dry (oatmeal) foods can be nutritious and last a long time, so you can avoid throwing out spoiled items. Finally, eggs and peanut butter are inexpensive and simple sources of protein.

TABLE 1-5 ■ Some Calorie Traps for College Students

	Number of Calories
Two handfuls of almonds	500
Two handfuls of granola	330
Personal-size pizza	500 to 600
1 cup of ice cream	300
Two handfuls of frosted cereal	250
Six-pack of regular beer	900

Source: Ann Litt, *The College Student's Guide to Eating Well on Campus,* Revised and Expanded, Tulip Hill Press, Bethesda, MD (2005).

Summary (Numbers refer to numbered sections in the chapter.)

1.1 The flavor, texture, and appearance of foods primarily influence our food choices. Several other factors also help determine food habits and choices: food availability and convenience, early childhood experiences and ethnic customs, nutrition and health concerns, advertising, restaurants, social changes, and economics. A variety of external (appetite-related) forces affect satiety (feeling of satisfaction that halts our desire to continue eating). Hunger cues combine with appetite cues, such as easy availability of food, to promote food intake.

1.2 Nutrition is a lifestyle factor that is a key to developing and maintaining an optimal state of health. A poor eating pattern and a sedentary lifestyle are known to be risk factors for life-threatening chronic diseases such as heart disease, hypertension, diabetes, and cancer. Not meeting nutrient needs in younger years makes us more likely to suffer health consequences in later years. Too much of a nutrient also can be harmful. Drinking too much alcohol is another dietary problem associated with many health problems.

1.3 Nutrition is the study of how the body uses food substances to promote and support growth, maintenance, and reproduction of cells. Nutrients in foods fall into six classes: (1) carbohydrates, (2) lipids (mostly fats and oils), (3) proteins, (4) vitamins, (5) minerals, and (6) water. The first three, along with alcohol, provide calories for the body to use. Phytochemicals are plant chemicals that may contribute to a reduced risk of disease in people who consume them.

1.4 The body transforms the energy contained in carbohydrate, protein, and fat into other forms of energy that in turn allow the body to function. Fat provides, on average, 9 kcal per gram, whereas both protein and carbohydrate provide, on average, 4 kcal per gram. Calculating percentages and converting English units to metric units are important skills needed for the study of nutrition.

1.5 The scientific method is the process for testing the validity of possible explanations of a phenomenon, called hypotheses. Experiments are conducted to either support or refute a specific hypothesis. Once we have enough experimental information to support a specific hypothesis, it then can be called a theory. All of us need to be skeptical of new ideas in the nutrition field, waiting until many lines of experimental evidence support a concept before adopting any suggested dietary practice.

1.6 The obesity problem has worsened, with 36.5% of people in the United States reported to be overweight or obese in 2015. This increase is a result of eating too much, especially foods with a high number of calories and a low number of nutrients, and not engaging in enough physical activity. Results from large nutrition surveys in the United States and Canada suggest that some of us need to concentrate on consuming foods that supply more of certain vitamins, minerals, and fiber. *Healthy People 2020* is a national initiative that includes Nutrition and Weight Status objectives related to eating a healthful diet and maintaining a healthy body weight. A healthful eating pattern includes consuming a variety of nutrient-dense foods within and across the food groups, especially whole grains, fruits, vegetables, low-fat or fat-free milk or milk products, and lean meats and other protein sources; limiting intake of solid fats, cholesterol, added sugars, sodium (salt), and alcohol; and limiting intake of calories to meet energy needs.

1.7 A basic plan for health promotion and disease prevention includes following a varied eating pattern, performing regular physical activity, not smoking, not abusing nutrient supplements (if used), consuming adequate water and other fluids, getting enough sleep, limiting alcohol intake (if consumed), and limiting or appropriately coping with stress. The primary focus of nutrition planning should be on food, not on dietary supplements. The focus on foods to supply nutrient needs avoids the possibility of severe nutrient imbalances.

1.8 Studies show that the eating patterns and other health habits of college students are not optimal. Students fall short of recommendations for servings of grains, vegetables, fruits, milk, and meat, opting instead for fats, sweets, and alcohol. This information is disturbing from a public health standpoint, because young adulthood is the time when many health behaviors are formed and will likely persist throughout life. Issues of particular importance on college campuses are weight control, making healthy meal choices, alcohol and binge drinking, and eating disorders.

Check Your Knowledge (Answers are available at the end of this question set.)

1. Our primary psychological drive to eat that is affected by many external food-choice mechanisms is called
   a. hunger. b. appetite. c. satiety. d. feeding.

2. Energy-yielding nutrients include
   a. vitamins, minerals, and water.
   b. carbohydrates, proteins, and fats.
   c. trace minerals and fat-soluble vitamins.
   d. iron, vitamin C, and potassium.

3. The *essential* nutrients
   a. must be consumed at every meal.
   b. are required for infants but not adults.
   c. can be made in the body when they are needed.
   d. cannot be made by the body and therefore must be consumed to maintain health.

4. Sugars, starches, and dietary fibers are examples of
   a. proteins.   c. carbohydrates.
   b. vitamins.   d. minerals.

5. Which nutrient classes are most important in the regulation of body processes?
   a. Vitamins   c. Minerals
   b. Carbohydrates   d. Both a and c

6. A kcal is a
   a. measure of heat energy.
   b. measure of fat in food.
   c. heating device.
   d. term used to describe the amount of sugar and fat in foods.

7. A food that contains 10 grams of fat would yield _____ kcal.
   a. 40   b. 70   c. 90   d. 120

8. If you consume 300 grams of carbohydrate in a day that you consume 2400 kcal, the carbohydrates will provide _____% of your total energy intake.
   a. 12.5   b. 30   c. 50   d. 60

9. Which of the following is true about North American eating patterns?
   a. Most of our protein comes from plant sources.
   b. About half of the carbohydrates come from simple sugars.
   c. Most of our fats come from plant sources.
   d. Most of our carbohydrates come from starches.

10. A behavior that will decrease the risk of weight gain in college is to
   a. skip breakfast.
   b. drink more liquid calories.
   c. stock your fridge with nutritious snacks.
   d. exercise infrequently.

Study Questions (Numbers refer to Learning Outcomes)

1. Describe the process that controls hunger and satiety in the body. List other factors that influence our food choices. **(LO 1.1)**

2. Describe how your food preferences have been shaped by the following factors:
   a. Exposure to foods at an early age
   b. Advertising (What is the newest food you have tried?)
   c. Eating out
   d. Peer pressure
   e. Economic factors **(LO 1.1)**

3. What products in your supermarket reflect the consumer demand for healthier foods? For convenience? **(LO 1.1)**

4. Name one chronic disease associated with poor nutrition habits. Now list a few corresponding risk factors. **(LO 1.2)**

5. Describe two sources of fat, and explain why the differences are important in terms of overall health. **(LO 1.3)**

6. Identify three ways that water is used in the body. **(LO 1.3)**

7. Explain the concept of calories as it relates to foods. What are the values used to calculate kilocalories from grams of carbohydrate, fat, protein, and alcohol? **(LO 1.4)**

8. A bowl of Panera's broccoli cheddar soup contains 21 grams carbohydrate, 13 grams fat, and 12 grams protein. Calculate the percentage of kilocalories derived from fat. **(LO 1.4)**

9. According to national nutrition surveys, which nutrients tend to be underconsumed by many North Americans? Why do you think this is the case? **(LO 1.6)**

10. List four *Healthy People 2020* objectives for the United States. How would you rate yourself in each area? Why? **(LO 1.6)**

11. List five strategies to avoid weight gain during college. **(LO 1.8)**

What the Dietitian Chose

Even bleary-eyed procrastinators can fuel their bodies for a new day of higher education! *Skipping breakfast is not a smart plan.* After a period of fasting (i.e., overnight), the body and the brain need fuel to operate at peak efficiency. In addition, many research studies demonstrate that eating a sensible breakfast is a good way to control weight. Compared to those who eat breakfast, people who skip breakfast tend to crave higher calorie foods, snack more throughout the day, and eat more at subsequent meals. Consider eating breakfast each day as part of your plan to fend off the "freshman 15."

Grab-and-go food options, such as those available in vending machines or from fast-food establishments, are often high in calories but low in nutrients. For example, a low-fat granola bar has only 100 kcal and 3 grams of fat but offers little else in terms of nutrition. Also, a granola bar is not likely to stave off hunger for very long.

On the other hand, a fast-food breakfast sandwich will probably promote satiety, but its calorie, fat, and sodium contents are too high. This type of sandwich provides 550 kcal, 23 grams of fat (38% of a day's total kilocalories in the sandwich and 35% of the whole day's limit for fat), and 1490 mg sodium (just under the 1500 mg Adequate Intake for this nutrient). A fast-food breakfast sandwich can fit into an otherwise healthy diet on occasion but should not be part of your normal routine. If you stop at the drive-through, choose wisely.

Keeping nutritious but convenient breakfast options accessible is a good strategy for any time-pressed college student. Whole grain,

fortified, ready-to-eat breakfast cereal with fat-free milk is a great choice: it is quick, provides a wide variety of vitamins and minerals, and boosts fiber intake. Adding a source of protein will help to support body processes and maintain fullness for a longer time. Hard-boiled eggs or a handful of dry-roasted nuts provide protein in ready-to-eat form. A cup of low-fat Greek yogurt offers protein with the added benefit of calcium. Fresh and dried fruit are portable and nutritious options for breakfast. Many fruit choices are loaded with potassium and vitamin C, plus they provide fiber. A 1.5-ounce box of raisins, which can be stored for months without a refrigerator, provides about 130 kcal, no fat or cholesterol, very little sodium, 2 grams of fiber, and 320 milligrams of potassium.

So, the bowl of Wheaties with a banana and low-fat milk along with a yogurt, all from your dorm room "pantry," would be the healthiest choice for most.

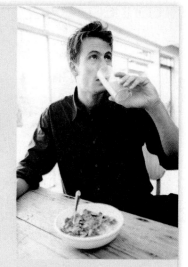

▲ With a little bit of planning, breakfast can be both quick and healthy. ©Stockbyte/Getty Images

Further Readings

1. Andreyeva T and others: Exposure to food advertising on television: Associations with children's fast food and soft drink consumption and obesity. *Economics and Human Biology* 9:221, 2011.

2. Goris JM and others: Television food advertising and the prevalence of childhood overweight and obesity: A multicountry comparison. *Public Health Nutrition* 13:1003, 2010.

3. Emond JA and others: Randomized exposure to food advertisements and eating in the absence of hunger among preschoolers. *Pediatrics* 138: 2361, 2016.

4. Kolish ED and others: *The Children's Food and Beverage Advertising Initiative, A Report on Compliance and Progress During 2014*, Better Business Bureau, December 2015.

5. Blake CE and others: Behavioral contexts, food-choice coping strategies, and dietary quality of a multiethnic sample of employed parents. *Journal of the American Dietetic Association* 111:401, 2011.

6. Monsivais P and others: Time spent on home food preparation and indicators of healthy eating. *American Journal of Preventive Medicine* 47:796, 2014.

7. Loureiro ML and others: The effects of nutritional labels on obesity. *Agricultural Economics* 43:333, 2012.

8. Yanover T and Sacco WP: Eating beyond satiety and body mass index. *Eating Weight Disorders* 3:119, 2008.

9. Kachanek KD and others: Death: Final data for 2014. *National Vital Statistics Reports* 65(4), 2016.

10. Chiuve SE and others: Adherence to a low-risk, healthy lifestyle and risk of sudden cardiac death among women. *Journal of the American Medical Association* 306:6, 2011.

11. Centers for Disease Control and Prevention: *Overweight and obesity 2015.* www.cdc.gov/obesity/data/adult.html. Accessed January 5, 2017.

12. Trust for America's Health: *F as in fat: How obesity threatens America's future, 2013.* Robert Wood Johnson Foundation, August 2013. http:// healthyamericans.org/report/100. Accessed January 6, 2017.

13. Flegal KM and others: Trends in Obesity Among Adults in the United States, 2005 to 2014. *Journal of the American Medical Association* 315:2284, 2016.

14. Academy of Nutrition and Dietetics: Position of the Academy of Nutrition and Dietetics: Total diet approach to healthy eating. *Journal of the Academy of Nutrition and Dietetics* 113:307, 2013.

15. Choi S and Lee Y: Relationship of college students' residence to frequency of meal skipping and snacking pattern. *Journal of the Academy of Nutrition and Dietetics* 112:A24, 2012.

16. Vadeboncoeur C and others: A meta-analysis of weight gain in first year university students: Is freshman 15 a myth? *BioMed Central Obesity* 2:22, 2015.

17. Zagorsky JL and Smith PK: The freshman 15: A critical time for obesity intervention or media myth? *Social Science Quarterly* 92:1389, 2011.

18. Shields DH and others: Gourmet coffee beverage consumption among college women. *Journal of the American Dietetic Association* 104:650, 2004.

19. Brister HA and others: 21st birthday drinking and associated physical consequences and behavioral risks. *Psychology of Addictive Behaviors* 25:573, 2011.

connect To get the most out of your study, visit Connect where you will find NutritionCalc Plus, SmartBook®, and many other dynamic tools.

Rate Your Plate

Source: www.choosemyplate.gov

I. Examine Your Eating Habits More Closely

Choose a day of the week that is typical of your eating pattern. Using the first table found in Appendix C, list all foods and drinks you consumed for 24 hours. In addition, write down the approximate amounts of food you ate in units, such as cups, ounces, teaspoons, and tablespoons. Place the corresponding abbreviation from the list below in the *Reason for Choice* column to indicate why you picked that food or drink. There can be more than one reason for choosing a particular food or drink.

FLVR	Flavor/texture	ADV	Advertisement	PEER	Peers
CONV	Convenience	WTCL	Weight control	NUTR	Nutritive value
EMO	Emotions	HUNG	Hunger	$	Cost
AVA	Availability	FAM	Family/cultural	HLTH	Health

Application

Ask yourself what your most frequent reason is for eating or drinking. To what degree is health or nutritive value a reason for your food choices? Should you make these higher priorities?

II. Observe the Supermarket Explosion

Today's supermarkets carry up to 60,000 items. Think about your last grocery shopping trip and the items you purchased to eat. Following is a list of 20 newer food products added to supermarket shelves. For those items you have tried, use the key from Part I to identify why you chose these products.

_____ Prepackaged salad greens (variety packs other than iceberg lettuce)

_____ Gourmet or sprayable salad oils (e.g., walnut, almond, olive, or sesame oil)

_____ Precooked frozen turkey patties, precooked bacon

_____ Microwavable sandwiches (e.g., Hot Pockets® or frozen sandwiches)

_____ Microwavable meals in a bowl (e.g., mac and cheese or soup)

_____ Refrigerated, precooked pasta (e.g., tortellini or fettucini) and accompanying sauces (e.g., pesto or tomato basil)

_____ Whole grain pasta or rice

_____ Frozen dinners (list your favorite of any of the wide variety)

_____ Bottled waters (flavored or unflavored)

_____ Trendy juices (e.g., draft apple cider, acai, or pomegranate)

_____ Roasted and/or flavored coffees (e.g., beans, ground, instant, or K-Cups)®

_____ Instant hot cereal in a bowl (add water and go!)

_____ "Fast-shake" pancake mix (add water, shake, and ready to cook)

_____ Breakfast bars or cookies (e.g., granola or fruit-flavored bars)

_____ Dried fruit and nut mixes

_____ Meal replacement/fitness products (e.g., "energy" bars, high-protein bars, or sports drinks)

_____ Gluten-free pasta or bread

_____ Low-calorie muffin tops or bagel thins

_____ Packaged yogurt smoothies

_____ Milk substitutes (e.g., rice milk, almond milk, or soy milk)

Finally, identify three new food products not on this list that you have seen in the past year. Discuss the appeal of these products to the North American consumer.

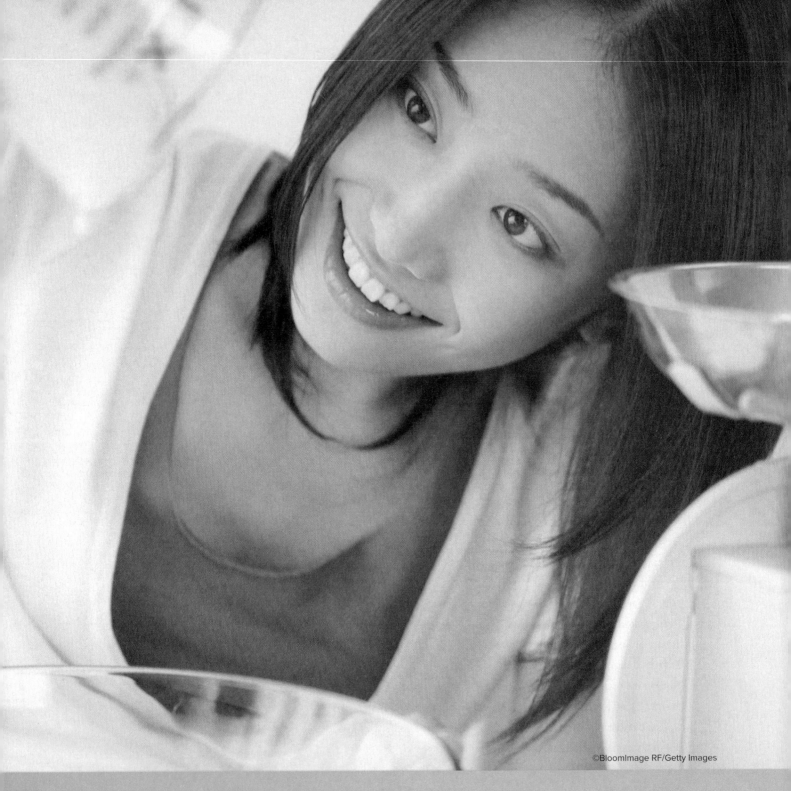

©BloomImage RF/Getty Images

Student Learning Outcomes

Chapter 2 is designed to allow you to:

2.1 Use variety, proportionality, and moderation, as well as nutrient and energy density, to develop a healthy eating pattern.

2.2 List the purpose and key recommendations of the *Dietary Guidelines* and the *Physical Activity Guidelines for Americans*.

2.3 Design a meal that conforms to the MyPlate recommendations as well as to the Mediterranean diet and/or other diet planning guides.

2.4 Describe the three states of nutritional health.

2.5 Outline the measurements used (ABCDEs) in nutritional assessment: **A**nthropometric, **B**iochemical, **C**linical, **D**ietary, and **E**nvironmental status.

Chapter 2
Designing a Healthy Eating Pattern

What Would You Choose?

In between classes, you stop at a nearby convenience store to pick up a cold drink and snack that will quench your thirst and fill your growing stomach. Immediately, you reach for your favorite cola and chips, but the Jones Soda Co.® display with its personalized labels catches your eye. You notice that these sodas are made with pure cane sugar. Is there a nutritional difference between the added sugars in these two types of sodas? Which of the following snack combinations provides the best of calories, nutrients, and energy for an afternoon snack?

a 20-ounce bottle of Coca-Cola® containing high-fructose corn syrup and a 1-ounce bag of potato chips

b 20-ounce bottle of Coke Zero® containing an artificial sweetener and a 1.5-ounce bag of baked potato crisps

c 12-ounce bottle of Jones Soda Co.® Pure Cane Cola Soda and a 1-ounce box of raisins

d ½ pint (8 fluid ounces) of low-fat (1%) chocolate milk and a 1.5-ounce pouch of almonds

e 16-ounce bottle of water and a 3.1-ounce box of M&Ms®

Think about your choice as you read this chapter, then see What the Dietitian Chose at the end of the chapter.

How many times have you heard amazing claims about how healthful certain foods are for you? Many consumers are now focusing more on diet and disease, and food manufacturers are responding with claims that their products have all sorts of health benefits. Hearing claims such as, "Drink pomegranate juice to guard your body against free radicals" makes you think that food manufacturers have all the answers.

Advertising aside, nutrient intakes that are out of balance with our needs—such as excess calories, saturated fat, *trans* fat, salt, alcohol, and sugar intakes—are linked to many leading causes of death in North America, including obesity, hypertension, cardiovascular disease, cancer, liver disease, and type 2 diabetes. Physical inactivity is also too common. In this chapter, you will explore the components of healthy eating and lifestyle patterns—an approach that will minimize your risks of developing nutrition-related diseases. The goal is to provide you with a firm understanding of these concepts before you study the nutrients in detail.

2.6 Describe the specific nutrient recommendation categories within the Dietary Reference Intakes.

2.7 Identify reliable sources of nutrition information.

2.8 Describe the components of the Nutrition Facts panel and the various health claims and label descriptors that are allowed.

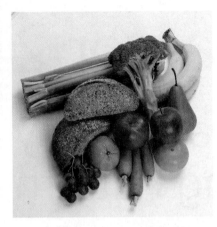

▲ A menu full of fruits, vegetables, and whole grain breads and cereals will help ward off disease and control body weight. ©Ken Karp, photographer/McGraw-Hill Education

phytochemical A chemical found in plants. Some phytochemicals may contribute to a reduced risk of cancer or cardiovascular disease in people who consume them regularly.

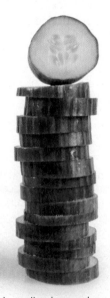

▲ Vegetables such as sliced cucumbers can be added to salads, sandwiches, pizza, tacos, soups, and much more to increase your phytochemical intake. ©Jupiterimages

2.1 A Food Philosophy That Works

You may be surprised that what you should eat to minimize the risk of developing the nutrition-related diseases seen in North America is exactly what you have heard many times before: *Consume a variety of foods balanced by a moderate intake of each food.* Health professionals have recommended the same basic eating and lifestyle pattern for many years:

- Control *how much* you eat.
- Pay attention to *what* you eat: choose more whole grains, fruits, and vegetables.
- Stay physically active.

A healthy eating pattern does not have to mean deprivation and misery; it simply requires some basic nutrition know-how and planning. Actually, eliminating favorite foods typically does not work for "dieters" in the long run. The best plan consists of learning the basics of a healthful eating pattern: variety, moderation, and proportionality. Monitoring total calorie intake is also important for many of us, especially if unwanted weight gain is taking place.

Many nutrition experts agree that there are no exclusively "good" or "bad" foods. Even so, many North Americans have eating patterns that miss the mark when it comes to the foundations of a healthy lifestyle. Eating patterns overloaded with fatty meats, fried foods, sugared soft drinks, and refined starches can result in substantial risk for nutrition-related chronic diseases.

We are more likely to maintain a healthy eating and lifestyle pattern when we emphasize a total diet pattern that is balanced and moderate. Let's now define *variety, moderation,* and *proportionality.* We will also introduce two very important concepts that will help us to make healthy food choices: nutrient density and energy density.

VARIETY MEANS EATING MANY DIFFERENT FOODS

Variety in your dietary pattern means choosing foods from all the food groups and subgroups, rather than eating the "same old thing" day after day. Variety makes meals more interesting and helps ensure that they contain sufficient nutrients. A variety of foods is best because no one food meets all your nutrient needs. For example, meat provides protein and iron but little calcium and no vitamin C. Eggs are a source of protein, but they provide little calcium because the calcium is mostly in the shell. Cow's milk contains calcium but very little iron. None of these foods contains fiber.

One way to balance your eating pattern as you consume a variety of foods is to select foods from each of these five major food groups every day:

- Grains   • Vegetables   • Protein
- Fruits   • Dairy

MyPlate, a food guide plan discussed in Section 2.3, offers a visual reminder and advice to help you make smart choices from each of these food groups. A dinner consisting of a bean burrito, lettuce and tomato salad with oil-and-vinegar dressing, a glass of milk, and an apple covers all groups.

Carrots—a source of fiber and a pigment that forms vitamin A—may be your favorite vegetable. However, if you choose carrots every day as your only vegetable source, you may miss out on other vitamins such as folate. Other vegetables, such as broccoli and asparagus, are rich sources of this nutrient. Hopefully, you're beginning to get a sense of how different foods and food groups vary in the nutrients they contain. For now, just recognize that you need a variety of foods in your eating pattern because the required nutrients are scattered among many foods.

An added bonus of dietary variety, especially within the fruit and vegetable groups, is the inclusion of a rich supply of **phytochemicals.** In Chapter 1 (Table 1-2), we listed many of these substances, which provide significant health benefits (e.g., reducing the risk for cancer). You can't just buy a bottle of phytochemicals: they are generally available only within whole foods. Current multivitamin and mineral supplements contain few or none of these beneficial plant chemicals.

Numerous population studies show reduced cancer risk among people who regularly consume fruits and vegetables.[1] Researchers suspect that some phytochemicals present in fruits and vegetables block the cancer process. Links between cancer and nutrition are described more thoroughly in Chapter 8. Evidence from earlier research studies linked the consumption of fruits and vegetables with a reduced risk of cardiovascular disease. Recent data, however, suggest that it is more important to focus on whole foods and eating patterns rather than individual nutrients or phytochemicals to successfully reduce cardiovascular disease risk.[2]

Foods rich in phytochemicals are now part of a family of foods referred to as **functional foods.** A functional food provides health benefits beyond those supplied by the traditional nutrients it contains. For example, a tomato (highlighted in the Farm to Fork feature in Chapter 1) contains the phytochemical lycopene, so it can be called a functional food.

It will likely take many years for scientists to unravel all of the important effects of the numerous phytochemicals in foods, and it is unlikely that all will ever be available or effective in supplement form. For this reason, leading nutrition and medical experts suggest that an eating pattern rich in fruits, vegetables, and whole grain breads and cereals is the most reliable way to obtain the potential benefits of phytochemicals.

Table 2-1 provides a number of suggestions for including more phytochemicals from fruits, vegetables, and whole grains in your eating pattern, as does the website www.fruitsandveggiesmorematters.org. As you incorporate a wide variety of foods in your eating pattern, be mindful of your total calorie intake.

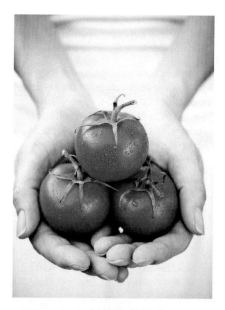

▲ Tomatoes are considered functional foods because they contain phytochemicals such as lycopene that are important for health. ©Sawayasu Tsuji/Getty Images

functional foods Foods that have health benefits beyond basic nutrition.

TABLE 2-1 ■ Tips for Boosting the Phytochemical Content of Your Eating Pattern

- Include vegetables in main and side dishes. Add these to rice, omelets, potato salad, and pastas. Try broccoli or cauliflower florets, mushrooms, peas, carrots, corn, or peppers.

- Look for quick-to-fix whole grain side dishes in the supermarket. Pilafs, couscous, rice mixes, and tabbouleh are just a few that you'll find.

- Choose fruit-filled cookies, such as fig bars, instead of sugar-rich cookies. Use fresh or canned fruit as a topping for pudding, hot or cold cereal, pancakes, and frozen desserts.

- Put raisins, grapes, apple chunks, pineapples, grated carrots, zucchini, or cucumber into coleslaw, chicken salad, or tuna salad.

- Be creative at the salad bar: Add fresh spinach, leaf lettuce, red cabbage, zucchini, yellow squash, cauliflower, peas, mushrooms, or red or yellow peppers to your salad.

- Pack fresh or dried fruit for snacks away from home instead of grabbing a candy bar or going hungry.

- Add slices of cucumber or zucchini, spinach, or carrot slivers to the lettuce and tomato on your sandwiches.

- Each week try one or two vegetarian meals such as beans and rice, vegetable stir-fry, or pasta with tomato sauce.

- If your daily protein intake exceeds the recommended amounts, reduce the meat, fish, or poultry in casseroles, stews, and soups by one-third to one-half and add more vegetables and legumes.

- Choose a snack from a container of fresh vegetables in the refrigerator or from a bowl of fresh fruit.

- Choose fruit or vegetable juices (preferably 100% juice varieties) instead of soft drinks.

- Substitute tea for coffee or soft drinks on a regular basis.

- Switch from crisp head lettuce to looseleaf lettuce, preferably red or dark green.

- Use salsa as a dip for chips in place of creamy dips.

- Choose whole grain breakfast cereals, breads, and crackers.

- In place of salt, add flavor to your plate with onions or herbs such as ginger, rosemary, basil, thyme, garlic, onions, parsley, and chives.

- Incorporate soy products, such as tofu, soy milk, soy protein isolate, and roasted soybeans, into your meals (see Chapter 6).

nutrient density The ratio derived by dividing a food's nutrient content by its calorie content. When the food's contribution to our need for that nutrient exceeds its contribution to our calorie need, the food is considered to have a favorable nutrient density.

PROPORTIONALITY MEANS EATING MORE NUTRIENT-DENSE FOODS

Proportionality, also referred to as balance, is eating more nutrient-dense foods and beverages such as fruits, vegetables, whole grains, and fat-free or low-fat milk products, and fewer foods high in certain types of fat, sugars, cholesterol, and salt, and alcohol. Balance also refers to matching your energy intake (how many total calories you consume) with energy expenditure (calories burned by metabolism and physical activity) over time. A prolonged imbalance between energy intake and energy expenditure leads to fluctuations in body weight.

The **nutrient density** of a food is a characteristic used to determine its nutritional quality. Nutrient density of a food is determined by comparing its protein, vitamin, or mineral content with the amount of calories it provides. A food is deemed nutrient dense if it provides a large amount of a nutrient for a relatively small amount of calories when compared with other food sources. Foods with greater nutrient density are better sources of nutrients. Comparing the nutrient density of different foods is an easy way to estimate their relative nutritional quality.

Generally, nutrient density is determined with respect to individual nutrients. For example, many fruits and vegetables have a high content of vitamin C compared with their modest calorie content; that is, they are nutrient-dense foods for vitamin C. Figure 2-1 shows how typical food choices can be shifted to more nutrient-dense options. The nutrient-dense options are foods that have important nutrients but are not packed with extra calories or sodium.

As noted previously, menu planning should focus on the total dietary pattern, not on the selection of one critical food as the key to an adequate eating pattern.

FIGURE 2-1 ▶ Typical food choices can be shifted to more nutrient-dense options. The nutrient-dense options are foods with important nutrients but that are not packed with extra calories or sodium. Nutrient-dense foods and beverages are naturally lean or low in solid fats and have little or no added solid fats, sugars, refined starches, or sodium.

Source: U.S. Department of Health and Human Services and U.S. Department of Agriculture. *2015–2020 Dietary Guidelines for Americans.* 8th Edition. December 2015. Available at http://health.gov/dietaryguidelines/2015/guidelines/.

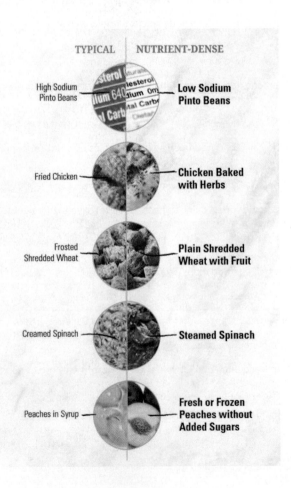

TYPICAL | NUTRIENT-DENSE

High Sodium Pinto Beans — **Low Sodium Pinto Beans**

Fried Chicken — **Chicken Baked with Herbs**

Frosted Shredded Wheat — **Plain Shredded Wheat with Fruit**

Creamed Spinach — **Steamed Spinach**

Peaches in Syrup — **Fresh or Frozen Peaches without Added Sugars**

Many low-cost, nutrient-dense foods—such as fat-free and low-fat milk, lean meats, legumes (beans), oranges, carrots, broccoli, whole wheat bread, and whole grain breakfast cereals—do help balance less nutrient-dense foods such as cookies and potato chips, which many people like to eat. The latter are often called empty-calorie foods because they tend to be high in sugar and/or fat but provide few other nutrients.

Eating nutrient-dense foods is especially important for people who have eating patterns relatively low in calories. This includes some older people and those following weight-loss diets. This is because nutrient needs remain high even though calorie needs may be diminished.

MODERATION REFERS MOSTLY TO PORTION SIZE

Eating in moderation requires paying attention to portion sizes and planning your daily eating pattern so that you do not overconsume any nutrients. It is especially important to choose foods that help you limit intake of animal fat, added sugars, salt, and alcohol. Americans typically consume too much of these food components—and too many calories overall. For example, if you plan to eat a bacon cheeseburger (relatively high in fat, salt, and calories) at lunch, you should eat foods such as fruits and vegetables, including salad greens (less concentrated sources of these nutrients), at other meals that same day. If you prefer whole milk to low-fat or fat-free milk, reduce the fat elsewhere in your meals. Try low-fat salad dressings or use jam rather than butter or margarine on toast. Overall, it is more feasible to consume moderate portions of foods that supply lots of fat, salt, and sugar than to try to eliminate these foods altogether.

Let's be clear that moderation is important for all food components. For example, many North Americans do not consume enough vitamin E, which is found in plant oils, nuts, and some fruits and vegetables. However, taking large doses of vitamin E (e.g., from supplements) can lead to excessive bleeding because of its effects on blood clotting. You *can* get too much of a good thing!

Energy density is a measurement that best describes the calorie content of a food. Energy density of a food is determined by comparing the calorie (kcal) content with the weight of food. A food that is rich in calories but weighs relatively little is considered energy dense. Examples include nuts, cookies, fried foods in general, and even fat-free snacks such as fat-free pretzels. Foods with low energy density include fruits, vegetables, and any food that incorporates lots of water during cooking, such as oatmeal (Table 2-2).

Researchers have shown that eating a meal with many foods of low energy density promotes satiety without contributing many calories.[3,4] This is probably because we typically consume a constant weight of food at a meal rather than a constant number of calories. How this constant weight of food is regulated is not known, but careful laboratory studies show that people consume fewer calories in a meal if most of the food choices are low in energy density, compared with foods high in energy density. An eating pattern low in energy density can aid in losing (or maintaining) weight.

Overall, foods with lots of water and fiber (i.e., low-energy-density foods) contribute few calories even though they help one feel full. Alternatively, foods with high energy density must be eaten in greater amounts to promote fullness. This is one more reason to fill your plate with a variety of fruits, vegetables, and whole grain breads and cereals—a pattern that is typical of many ethnic diets throughout rural areas of the world. Research has shown, however, that consumption of unhealthy diets—in particular, eating fewer fruits and vegetables—is strongly linked to socioeconomic status. Unfortunately, low-energy-density foods, such as fresh fruits and

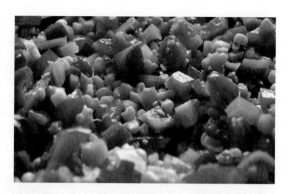

▲ Focus on nutrient-rich foods as you strive to meet your nutrient needs. The more colorful the food on your plate, the greater the content of nutrients and phytochemicals.
©Mary-Jon Ludy, Bowling Green University, Garden of Hope images

energy density A comparison of the calorie (kcal) content of a food with the weight of the food. An energy-dense food is high in calories but weighs very little (e.g., potato chips), whereas a food low in energy density has few calories but weighs a lot (e.g., an orange).

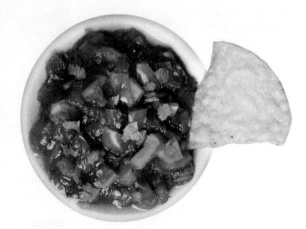

▲ Salsa is full of phytochemicals and a great, very low-energy-density alternative to higher-calorie chip dips. It helps to balance out the high-energy-density tortilla chips. ©D. Hurst/Alamy

TABLE 2-2 ■ **Energy Density of Common Foods (Listed in Relative Order)**

Very Low Energy Density (less than 0.6 kcal per gram)	Low Energy Density (0.6–1.5 kcal per gram)	Medium Energy Density (1.5–4 kcal per gram)	High Energy Density (greater than 4 kcal per gram)
Lettuce	Whole milk	Eggs	Graham crackers
Tomatoes	Oatmeal	Ham	Fat-free sandwich cookies
Strawberries	Cottage cheese	Pumpkin pie	Chocolate
Broccoli	Beans	Whole wheat bread	Chocolate chip cookies
Salsa	Bananas	Bagels	Tortilla chips
Grapefruit	Broiled fish	White bread	Bacon
Fat-free milk	Fat-free yogurt	Raisins	Potato chips
Carrots	Ready-to-eat breakfast cereals with 1% low-fat milk	Cream cheese	Peanuts
Vegetable soup	Plain baked potato	Cake with frosting	Peanut butter
Celery	Cooked rice	Pretzels	Mayonnaise
Cabbage	Spaghetti noodles	Rice cakes	Butter or margarine
Melon			Vegetable oils

Source: Data adapted from Rolls B, *The ultimate volumetrics diet.* New York: HarperCollins, 2012.

Newsworthy Nutrition

Effect of healthy eating attitude at the supermarket

Better access to full-service supermarkets has been associated with healthier eating patterns, including higher consumption of vegetables and fruit. Furthermore, shopping at lower-cost supermarkets has been linked to greater rates of obesity. Improving access to full-service supermarkets, therefore, has become a focus of public health policy. The hypothesis of this study was that shopping at lower-cost supermarkets would be associated with lower diet quality and that this relationship would be explained by socioeconomic status (SES) and attitudes toward healthy foods. The study design was a telephone survey conducted in 2008–2009 and used data from 963 adults in King County, Washington. A food frequency questionnaire was used for dietary intake data, and diet-quality measures were energy density, mean adequacy ratio, and total servings of fruits and vegetables. Data on SES, attitudes toward healthy eating, and supermarket choice (low, medium, or high cost) were also collected. The results found that although shopping at higher-cost supermarkets was associated with higher-quality diets, shoppers with positive attitudes toward healthy eating had equally higher-quality diets, even if they shopped at low-, medium-, or high-cost supermarkets, independent of SES. The authors conclude that shopping at low-cost supermarkets does not prevent consumers from having high-quality diets, as long as they attach importance to good nutrition. To improve diet quality, researchers recommend the promotion of nutrition-education programs for consumers at supermarkets, particularly those catering to low-income groups.

Source: Aggarwal A and others: Positive attitude toward healthy eating predicts higher diet quality at all cost levels of supermarkets. *J Acad Nutr Diet* 2014;114:266.

vegetables, are often more expensive than those that have high energy density. Therefore, the cost of food has been identified as a likely contributor to the socioeconomic patterning in healthy diets.[5] Research into the contribution of food costs to socioeconomic inequalities in diet quality continues. A recent study found that attitudes toward healthy eating are associated with diet quality among shoppers at low-, medium-, and high-cost supermarkets.[6] Read more about this research in the Newsworthy Nutrition feature in this section.

Many foods such as peanut butter are both energy and nutrient dense. Even energy-dense foods can have a place in your dietary pattern, but you will have to plan for them. For example, chocolate is a very energy-dense food, but a small portion at the end of a meal can supply a satisfying finale. In addition, foods with high energy density can help individuals with poor appetites, such as some older people, to maintain or gain weight.

✔ CONCEPT CHECK 2.1

1. What do variety, proportionality, and moderation mean, and how do they work together to result in a healthy eating pattern?
2. How do the concepts of nutrient density and energy density differ?

2.2 Dietary and Physical Activity Guidelines

For well over 100 years, researchers have been translating the science of nutrition into practical dietary advice for people with no special training. Early food guidance systems aimed to reduce risk for nutrient deficiencies, but severe deficiency diseases are no longer common in Western industrialized countries. Marginal deficiencies of calcium, iron, folate and other B vitamins, vitamin C, vitamin D, vitamin E, potassium, magnesium, and fiber are still a problem; but for many North Americans, major health problems stem from overconsumption of one or more of the following: calories, added sugars, saturated fat, *trans* fat, alcohol, and sodium.

The following sections of this chapter describe guidelines and tools for planning healthy lifestyles. You will notice how those core concepts of variety, proportionality, and moderation keep showing up throughout our discussions of the *Dietary Guidelines,* the Physical Activity Guidelines, and MyPlate.

DIETARY GUIDELINES—THE BASIS FOR MENU PLANNING

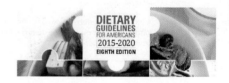

The U.S. Department of Agriculture (USDA) and U.S. Department of Health and Human Services (DHHS) have published *Dietary Guidelines* since 1980.[7] The *Dietary Guidelines* are designed to inform the development of policies and programs for food, nutrition, and health. Although not intended for direct use by the general public, the *Dietary Guidelines* are an important tool for health professionals to use in helping Americans design healthy eating and activity patterns.[8] The federal government uses them to develop nutrition education materials for the public, such as the MyPlate resources.

▲ The latest *Dietary Guidelines* for Americans were published in 2015. U.S. Department of Health and Human Services and U.S. Department of Agriculture. *2015–2020 Dietary Guidelines for Americans.* 8th Edition. December 2015.

The *2015–2020 Dietary Guidelines* were derived from the *Scientific Report of the 2015 Dietary Guidelines Advisory Committee,* written by scientific experts and submitted to the USDA and DHHS in February 2015. The *Scientific Report* was based on the most current evidence from nutrition research. The *Dietary Guidelines* were published in December 2015 after congressional hearings and feedback from federal agencies, industry groups, and the general public. The full *2015–2020 Dietary Guidelines* report contains background on the *Dietary Guidelines,* tables and charts to support the recommendations, and a list of consumer behaviors and key strategies for achieving its recommendations.[9] The aim of the *Dietary Guidelines* is to translate nutrition science into food-based guidelines that will help Americans meet nutrient needs and reduce risk for many chronic diseases. They are not intended for treating disease.

Following are the five foundational guidelines of the *2015–2020 Dietary Guidelines*:

1. **Follow a healthy eating pattern across the lifespan.** All food and beverage choices matter. Choose a healthy eating pattern at an appropriate calorie level to help achieve and maintain a healthy body weight, support nutrient adequacy, and reduce the risk of chronic disease.

2. **Focus on variety, nutrient density, and amount.** To meet nutrient needs within calorie limits, choose a variety of nutrient-dense foods across and within all food groups in recommended amounts.

3. **Limit calories from added sugars and saturated fats and reduce sodium intake.** Consume an eating pattern low in added sugars, saturated fats, and sodium. Cut back on foods and beverages higher in these components to amounts that fit within healthy eating patterns.

4. **Shift to healthier food and beverage choices.** Choose nutrient-dense foods and beverages across and within all food groups in place of less healthy choices. Consider cultural and personal preferences to make these shifts easier to accomplish and maintain.

5. **Support healthy eating patterns for all.** Everyone has a role in helping to create and support healthy eating patterns in multiple settings nationwide, from home to school to work to communities.

The *Dietary Guidelines* are accompanied by Key Recommendations (Fig. 2-2) that provide detail on the elements of healthy eating patterns.

Shifting to Healthy Eating Patterns Healthy eating patterns are the hallmark of the *2015–2020 Dietary Guidelines* and are designed to help people meet the five foundational guidelines and Key Recommendations. The ultimate goal of a healthy eating

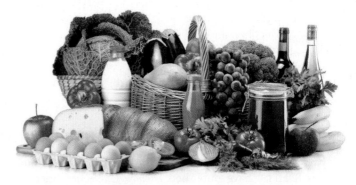

Consume a

healthy eating pattern

*An **eating pattern** represents the totality of all foods and beverages consumed.*

Healthy eating patterns are adaptable to an individual's socio-cultural and personal preferences.

Include . . .

A variety of vegetables from all of the subgroups (dark green, red and orange, beans and peas, starchy, and others)

Fruits, especially whole fruits

Grains, at least half of which are whole grains

Fat-free or low-fat dairy, including milk, yogurt, cheese, and/or fortified soy beverages

A variety of protein foods (seafood, lean meats and poultry, eggs, beans and peas, nuts, seeds, and soy products

Oils

Limit . . .

Added sugars to <10% of daily kcal

Saturated fats to <10% of daily kcal

Sodium to <2,300 milligrams (mg) per day

Alcohol (if consumed at all) to <1 drink per day for women and <2 drinks per day for men

that accounts for all

foods and beverages

*Choose **nutrient-dense** foods.*

Meet your nutritional needs primarily from foods. Fortified foods and dietary supplements may be useful to make up for nutrient shortfalls.

All forms of foods—fresh, canned, dried, and frozen—can be included.

within an

appropriate calorie level

Balance food and beverage intake with physical activity to aid efforts at weight management throughout the lifespan.

FIGURE 2-2 ▲ Key Recommendations from the *2015–2020 Dietary Guidelines for Americans*. ©Getty Images/iStockphoto

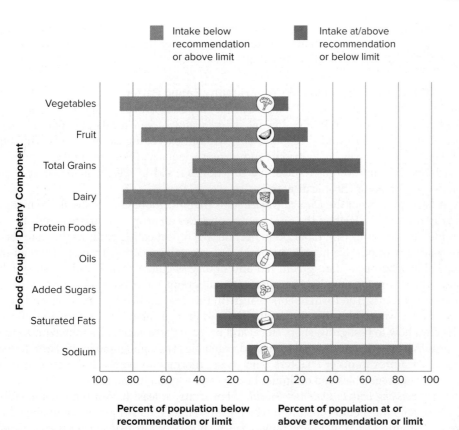

Intake below recommendation or above limit

Intake at/above recommendation or below limit

Percent of population below recommendation or limit

Percent of population at or above recommendation or limit

FIGURE 2-3 ◄ Comparing current eating patterns in the United States to the *Dietary Guidelines.*

Source: *2015–2020 Dietary Guidelines for Americans.* Based on data from U.S. Departmentof Agriculture, Agricultural Research Service and U.S. Department of Health and Human Services, Centers for Disease Control and Prevention. What we eat in America, NHANES 2007–2010 for average intakes by age-sex group. Healthy U.S.-Style Food Patterns, which vary based on age, sex, and activity level, for recommended intakes and limits.

pattern is to support a healthy body weight and help reduce the risk of chronic disease. The *Dietary Guidelines* use the Healthy U.S.-Style Eating Pattern (see Table 2-5 in Section 2.3) to exemplify the specific amounts of food groups and other dietary components that make up healthy eating patterns. It is based on foods Americans typically consume, but in nutrient-dense forms and appropriate amounts. The *Dietary Guidelines* also include the Healthy Mediterranean-Style Eating Pattern and the Healthy Vegetarian Eating Pattern as alternative plans.

Shifts are needed to align current dietary intakes with healthy eating patterns. As seen in Figure 2-3, certain aspects of our eating patterns are close to recommendations, whereas others will require significant improvement. Many Americans have eating patterns that are low in vegetables, fruits, whole grains, dairy, seafood, and oil; and high in refined grains, added sugars, saturated fats, and sodium.

Importance of Calorie Balance Within Healthy Eating Patterns The balance between calories consumed (from foods and beverages) and calories expended (through physical activity and metabolic processes) determines body weight. Consuming too many calories without increasing physical activity will inevitably lead to weight gain, which exacts an enormous toll on individuals and communities. Meeting nutrient needs within calorie limits could alleviate many chronic diseases, especially cardiovascular disease, type 2 diabetes, and osteoporosis. In light of the current epidemic of overweight and obesity, the message of calorie balance within a healthy eating pattern continues to be woven throughout the *Dietary Guidelines,* which encourage all Americans to achieve and maintain a healthy body weight. Knowing how many calories you need each day is a good place to start (Fig. 2-4). Use an online calculator such as Supertracker (www.choosemyplate.gov/tools-supertracker) or NutritionCalc Plus in Connect

	Calorie Range (kcal)		
Children	Sedentary ⟶		Active
2–3 years	1000	⟶	1400
Females			
4–8 years	1200	⟶	1800
9–13	1400	⟶	2200
14–18	1800	⟶	2400
19–30	1800	⟶	2400
31–50	1800	⟶	2200
51+	1600	⟶	2200
Males			
4–8 years	1200	⟶	2000
9–13	1600	⟶	2600
14–18	2000	⟶	3200
19–30	2400	⟶	3000
31–50	2200	⟶	3000
51+	2000	⟶	2800

FIGURE 2-4 ▲ Estimates of calorie (kcal) needs.

Source: *2015–2020 Dietary Guidelines for Americans.*

to calculate your estimated calorie needs. Next, become familiar with the calorie content of foods and beverages. Finally, monitoring weight over time will allow you to see how your food and physical activity choices are balancing out.

Food Components to Include in Your Healthy Eating Pattern To improve nutritional status and overall health, the *Dietary Guidelines* promote the consumption of vegetables, fruits, whole grains, fat-free or low-fat dairy, seafood, lean meats and poultry, eggs, beans and peas, nuts and seeds, and oils, without exceeding calorie needs. This type of dietary pattern will (1) contribute to nutrient adequacy; (2) lower intake of problem nutrients; (3) improve gastrointestinal function; (4) aid in weight management; and (5) decrease risk for chronic diseases.

A basic premise of the *Dietary Guidelines* is that nutritional needs should be met primarily from foods. Each of the food groups provides an array of nutrients, and the recommended amounts (see Table 2-5 in Section 2.3) reflect eating patterns that have been associated with positive health outcomes. For vegetables, eating a variety from all five vegetable subgroups—dark green, red and orange, legumes (beans and peas), starchy, and other—is recommended, because each subgroup contributes different combinations of nutrients. The Farm to Fork feature in this chapter highlights carrots and beets, two colorful vegetables that fit into the red and orange subgroups. Information is provided on how to best grow, shop, store, and prepare these vegetables to maximize their nutritional benefits. Additional fruits and vegetables are highlighted in the Farm to Fork features in other chapters, and more information on the link between fruits and vegetables and optimum health can be found in *Eating on the Wild Side: The Missing Link to Optimum Health.*[10] For fruits, at least half of the recommended amount should come from whole fruits. At least half of grains should be whole grains. Dairy, including milk, yogurt, cheese, or fortified soy beverages, should be fat free or low fat. Protein foods should include several subgroups: seafood, meats, poultry, eggs, nuts, seeds, and soy products, as well as legumes and dairy. Oils are part of healthy eating patterns because they contribute essential fatty acids and vitamin E. In certain cases, fortified foods and dietary supplements may be useful sources of one or more nutrients that otherwise might be consumed in less than recommended amounts.

Food Components to Limit in Your Healthy Eating Pattern Because typical American dietary patterns contain too much added sugars, saturated and *trans* fats, and sodium (see Fig. 2-3), the *Dietary Guidelines* emphasize the need to limit these components. Added sugars and saturated fats are energy dense (high in calories) but provide few essential nutrients. Dietary patterns predominated by these food components especially increase risk for obesity, type 2 diabetes, hypertension, cardiovascular disease, and cancer. Added sugars include sugars and other sweeteners that are added during food processing or cooking. The recommendation is to limit intake of added sugars to less than 10% of total calories per day. Saturated fats are primarily animal fats, such as butter and beef fat. They can be found naturally in foods and are also added during food processing and cooking. Replacing saturated fats with unsaturated fats may reduce risk of cardiovascular disease. Thus, the recommendation is to limit intake of saturated fats to less than 10% of total kilocalories per day. The limit of less than 2300 mg of sodium per day coincides with the Upper Limit for those 14 years and older. Although those who do not drink alcohol should not begin drinking to attain health benefits, moderate alcohol consumption is associated with reduced risk of cardiovascular disease, cognitive decline, and death.

Finally, the *Dietary Guidelines* encourage the use of multiple strategies across all segments of society to promote healthy eating and physical activity behaviors. It is especially important to focus on individuals at the point where they are making food and beverage choices. Table 2-3 provides examples of recommended shifts based on the *Dietary Guidelines*. Diet recommendations for adults have been

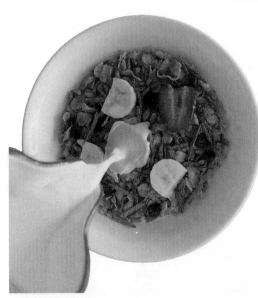

▲ Choose low-sugar, high-fiber cereal with fresh fruit instead of sugary breakfast cereal. Also follow the "Five things to check before you buy breakfast cereal" from NutritionAction.com:[11]

1. Go for whole grains. First two ingredients are whole grain or bran.
2. Check the serving sizes, which range from 30 grams (1 oz) for light cereals to 55 grams (2 oz) for heavy cereals.
3. Choose cereals that do not have more than 1.2 teaspoons (7 grams) of total sugar for light cereals and 2.5 teaspoons (11 grams) for heavy cereals.
4. Get enough unprocessed fiber, such as wheat bran, whole grain wheat, and oats.
5. Look for cereals with less than 2.5 grams of saturated fat.

FARM to FORK Carrots and Beets

Grow
- Carrots and beets are root crops with a wide range of nutrients and flavors.
- The wild ancestor of carrots was purple, but most carrots grown in the United States are orange, a good indicator of the nutrients and other phytochemicals they contain, especially beta-carotene. Farmers are again producing purple carrot varieties, which are sweeter and higher in beta-carotene and the purple pigments, anthocyanins.
- Red beets are high in betalins, phytochemicals that may reduce the risk of cancer and other diseases. Red beet juice has also been shown to better athletic performance.

Shop
- For the freshest and sweetest carrots and beets, buy them with the green tops still attached. They will be at most only a few weeks old. Carrots and beets without tops can be several weeks to months old.
- Refrain from buying baby or frozen carrots. Baby carrots originate from misshapen mature carrots that have been whittled down to a smaller uniform size, and the remaining inner core is not as nutritious as the outer part that is discarded. The peeling, processing, and freeze/thaw cycle of frozen carrots destroys about half of their antioxidant value.
- The processing of beets into canned beets renders them more nutritious with more antioxidant value.

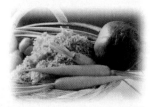

©FoodCollection

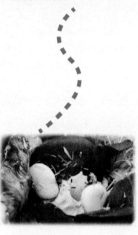

©L. Mouton/PhotoAlto

Store
- Cut the tops off of your fresh carrots so they retain their moisture. To protect carrots from the ethylene gas produced by other fruits and vegetables, store them in a sealed plastic bag in the refrigerator.
- Remove beet greens and store beet roots unwrapped in the crisper drawer of the refrigerator and use them within 2 weeks.

Prep
- Carrots and beets are more nutritious cooked. The heat breaks down cell walls and makes nutrients more bioavailable. Scrub carrots and beets, and cook them whole.

- Carrots can be sautéed or steamed to preserve more nutrients and sweetness. Eat carrots with oil or fat to allow best absorption of the fat-soluble beta-carotene, a precursor of vitamin A.
- Beets can be steamed, microwaved, or roasted. The skin helps retain the water-soluble nutrients while cooking and can be slipped off when cool. Beets will stain hands and surfaces, including wooden cutting boards. Use rubber gloves to avoid beet stains on your hands.
- Eating beets with mustard, horseradish, or vinegar will disguise their earthly flavor.

Source: Robinson J: The Other Root Crops: Carrots, Beets and Sweet Potatoes In *Eating on the Wild Side*. New York: Little, Brown and Company, 2013.

TABLE 2-3 ■ Recommended Eating Pattern Changes Based on the *Dietary Guidelines*

If You Usually Eat This	Try This Instead	Benefits
White bread	Whole wheat bread	• Higher nutrient density, due to less processing • More fiber
Sugary breakfast cereal	Low-sugar, high-fiber cereal with fresh fruit	• Higher nutrient density • More fiber • More phytochemicals
Cheeseburger with French fries	Hamburger and baked beans	• Less saturated fat and *trans* fat • Less cholesterol • More fiber • More phytochemicals
Potato salad	Three-bean salad	• More fiber • More phytochemicals
Doughnut	Bran muffin or bagel with light cream cheese	• More fiber • Less fat
Regular soft drinks	Diet soft drinks	• Fewer calories
Boiled vegetables	Steamed vegetables	• Higher nutrient density, due to reduced loss of water-soluble vitamins
Canned vegetables (typically highly salted)	Fresh or frozen vegetables (add flavor with herbs, spices, or lemon juice)	• Higher nutrient density, due to reduced loss of heat-sensitive vitamins • Lower in sodium

(continued)

TABLE 2-3 ■ (continued)

If You Usually Eat This	Try This Instead	Benefits
Fried meats	Broiled meats	• Less saturated fat
Fatty meats, such as ribs or bacon	Lean meats, such as ground round, chicken, or fish	• Less saturated fat
Whole milk	Low-fat or fat-free milk	• Less saturated fat • Fewer calories • More calcium
Ice cream	Sherbet or frozen yogurt	• Less saturated fat • Fewer calories
Mayonnaise or sour cream salad dressing	Oil-and-vinegar dressings or light creamy dressings	• Less saturated fat • Less cholesterol • Fewer calories
Cookies	Popcorn (air popped with minimal margarine or butter)	• Fewer calories and *trans* fat
Chips	Pretzels	• Less fat

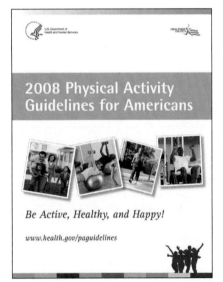

▲ www.health.gov/PAGuidelines/.

issued by other scientific groups such as the American Heart Association, U.S. Surgeon General, National Academy of Sciences, American Cancer Society, Health Canada, and World Health Organization. All are consistent with the spirit of the *Dietary Guidelines.*

PHYSICAL ACTIVITY GUIDELINES FOR AMERICANS

In line with its goal for all Americans to live healthier, more prosperous, and more productive lives, the U.S. Department of Health and Human Services issued its first Physical Activity Guidelines for Americans in 2008 as a complement to the *Dietary Guidelines.*[12] The overarching idea is that regular physical activity—for people of all ages, races, ethnicities, and physical abilities—produces long-term health benefits. The guidelines are truly meant to inform the work of health professionals and policy makers, but consumer materials are available. *Be Active Your Way: A Guide for Adults,* a blog available at www.health.gov, translates the guidelines into consumer-friendly, practical advice.

The key guidelines, listed in Table 2-4, provide measurable physical activity standards for Americans age 6 and older. Specific recommendations (not listed in Table 2-4) also apply to special population groups, including pregnant women, adults with disabilities, and people with chronic medical conditions. For adults, the guidelines emphasize that health benefits occur with at least 150 minutes per week of moderate-intensity physical activity. Adults may accumulate activity throughout the week in a variety of

TABLE 2-4 ■ Selected Recommendations of the *2008 Physical Activity Guidelines for Americans**

Key Guidelines for Children and Adolescents
• Children and adolescents should do 60 minutes or more of physical activity daily.
• Aerobic: Most of the 60 or more minutes a day should be either moderate- or vigorous-intensity aerobic physical activity and should include vigorous-intensity activity at least 3 days a week.
• Muscle strengthening: As part of their 60 or more minutes of daily physical activity, children and adolescents should include muscle-strengthening physical activity on at least 3 days of the week.
• Bone strengthening: As part of their 60 or more minutes of daily physical activity, children and adolescents should include bone-strengthening physical activity on at least 3 days of the week.

- It is important to encourage young people to participate in physical activities that are appropriate for their age, are enjoyable, and offer variety.

Key Guidelines for Adults

- All adults should avoid inactivity. Some physical activity is better than none, and adults who participate in any amount of physical activity gain some health benefits.

- For substantial health benefits, adults should do at least 150 minutes a week of moderate-intensity or 75 minutes a week of vigorous-intensity aerobic physical activity, or an equivalent combination of moderate- and vigorous-intensity aerobic activity. Aerobic activity should be performed in episodes of at least 10 minutes, and preferably, it should be spread throughout the week.

- For additional and more extensive health benefits, adults should increase their aerobic physical activity to 300 minutes a week of moderate-intensity or 150 minutes a week of vigorous-intensity aerobic physical activity, or an equivalent combination of moderate- and vigorous-intensity activity. Additional health benefits are gained by engaging in physical activity beyond this amount.

- Adults should also do muscle-strengthening activities that are moderate or high intensity and involve all major muscle groups on 2 or more days a week, as these activities provide additional health benefits.

Key Guidelines for Safe Physical Activity

To do physical activity safely and reduce the risk of injuries and other adverse events, people should:

- Understand the risks and yet be confident that physical activity is safe for almost everyone.

- Choose to do types of physical activity that are appropriate for their current fitness level and health goals because some activities are safer than others.

- Increase physical activity gradually over time whenever more activity is necessary to meet guidelines or health goals. Inactive people should "start low and go slow" by gradually increasing how often and how long activities are done.

- Protect themselves by using appropriate gear and sports equipment; looking for safe environments; following rules and policies; and making sensible choices about when, where, and how to be active.

- Be followed by a health care provider if they have chronic conditions or symptoms. People with chronic conditions and symptoms should consult their health care provider about the appropriate types and amounts of activity.

*The *2008 Physical Activity Guidelines for Americans* also include recommendations for older adults, pregnant women, adults with disabilities, and people with chronic medical conditions. These are available at www.health.gov.

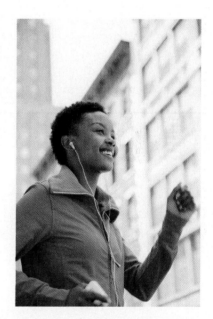

▲ Active means a lifestyle that includes physical activity equivalent to walking more than 3 miles per day at 3 to 4 miles per hour, in addition to the light physical activity associated with typical day-to-day life. ©JGI/Jamie Grill/Blend Images

ways: extended sessions (e.g., 50 minutes on 3 days a week) or in short bursts throughout the week that amount to at least 150 minutes. Children and adolescents should strive to include 60 minutes of physical activity per day. For optimum benefits, include both aerobic and muscle-strengthening activities. Overall, physical activity should be enjoyable and safe for each individual. In 2012, a follow-up report, *Physical Activity Guidelines for Americans Midcourse Report: Strategies to Increase Physical Activity Among Youth,* was published, identifying interventions that can help increase physical activity in youth across a variety of settings. The *Physical Activity Guidelines for Americans, 2nd edition* is expected to be released in late 2018.

✓ CONCEPT CHECK 2.2

1. What are three of the major guidelines of the *2015–2020 Dietary Guidelines for Americans?*

2. How many minutes of moderate-intensity physical activity are advised per week in the *2008 Physical Activity Guidelines for Americans?*

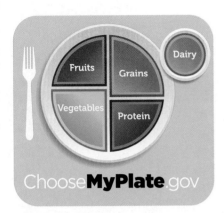

FIGURE 2-5 ▲ MyPlate is a visual representation of the advice contained in the *2015–2020 Dietary Guidelines for Americans.*

Source: ChooseMyPlate.gov

2.3 MyPlate—A Menu-Planning Tool

The titles, food groupings, and shapes of food guides have evolved since the first edition published by the USDA a century ago. The most recent food-guidance systems have provided a means for individualization of dietary advice via online interactive technology available on the Internet.

To keep pace with updated nutrition advice presented by the *Dietary Guidelines for Americans* and *Healthy People 2020* (see Section 1.6), MyPlate was released in 2011 as the leading depiction of healthy eating for Americans (Fig. 2-5). MyPlate, which replaced the familiar MyPyramid, shapes the key recommendations from the *Dietary Guidelines* into an easily recognizable and extremely applicable visual: a place setting.

DISHING UP MyPlate

Although it is not intended to stand alone as a source of dietary advice, MyPlate serves as a reminder of how to build a healthy plate at mealtimes.[13] It emphasizes important areas of the American diet that are in need of improvement. Recall from the discussion of the *Dietary Guidelines* that Americans need to increase the relative proportions of fruits, vegetables, whole grains, and fat-free or low-fat dairy products while simultaneously decreasing consumption of refined grains and high-fat meats.

The MyPlate icon includes five food groups:

- *Fruits* and *vegetables* cover half of the plate. These foods are dense sources of nutrients and health-promoting phytochemicals despite their low calorie contents.
- *Grains* occupy slightly more than one-fourth of the plate. The message to make at least half your grains whole is stressed throughout accompanying consumer-education materials.
- The remaining space on the plate is reserved for sources of **protein.** Specifically, the *2015–2020 Dietary Guidelines* recommend a variety of protein foods, including seafood, lean meats and poultry, eggs, legumes (beans and peas), nuts, seeds, and soy products.
- A cup of *dairy* appears next to the plate. Depending on personalized calorie recommendations, users should have 2 to 3 cups per day of low-fat or fat-free dairy products or other rich sources of calcium.

MyPlate does not display a separate group for fats and oils, as they are mostly incorporated into other foods. MyPlate food guide recommends limiting solid fats and focusing instead on plant oils, which are sources of essential fatty acids and vitamin E.

BUILD A HEALTHY EATING STYLE

MyPlate is designed as a reminder to find your healthy eating style and build it throughout your lifetime. The ChooseMyPlate.gov website provides the following ideas and tips to help you create a healthier eating style that meets your individual needs and improves your health.

All Food and Beverage Choices Matter—Focus on Variety, Amount, and Nutrition

- Focus on making healthy food and beverage choices from all five food groups, including fruits, vegetables, grains, protein foods, and dairy, to get the nutrients you need.
- Eat the right amount of calories for you based on your age, sex, height, weight, and physical activity level.
- Building a healthier eating style can help you avoid overweight and obesity and reduce your risk of diseases such as heart disease, diabetes, and cancer.

Choose an Eating Style Low in Saturated Fat, Sodium, and Added Sugars

- Use Nutrition Facts labels and ingredient lists to find amounts of saturated fat, sodium, and added sugars in the foods and beverages you choose.
- Look for food and drink choices that are lower in saturated fat, sodium, and added sugar.
  - Eating fewer calories from foods high in saturated fat and added sugars can help you manage your calories and prevent overweight and obesity. Most of us eat too many foods that are high in saturated fat and added sugar.
  - Eating foods with less sodium can reduce your risk of high blood pressure.

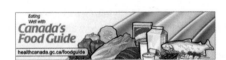

▲ In 1942, Canada released its first set of Official Food Rules. Since then, food guidance has evolved based on nutrition research and the changing needs of the population. Now, Health Canada publishes Canada's Food Guide to Healthy Eating, available at http://www.hc-sc.gc.ca/fn-an/food-guide-aliment/index-eng.php. Source: All rights reserved. Eating Well with Canada's Food Guide. Health Canada, 2011. Reproduced with permission from the Minister of Health, 2014.

Make Small Changes to Create a Healthier Eating Style

*   Think of each change as a personal "win" on your path to living healthier. Each *MyWin* is a change you make to build your healthy eating style. Find little victories that fit into your lifestyle and celebrate them as a *MyWins!*
*   Start with a few of these small changes.
    *   Make half your plate fruits and vegetables.
        *   Focus on whole fruits.
        *   Vary your veggies.
    *   Make half your grains whole grains.
    *   Move to low-fat and fat-free dairy.
    *   Vary your protein routine.
    *   Eat and drink the right amount for you.

Support Healthy Eating for Everyone

*   Create settings where healthy choices are available and affordable to you and others in your community.
*   Professionals, policy makers, partners, industry, families, and individuals can help others in their journey to make healthy eating a part of their lives.

MyPLATE DAILY CHECKLIST

On the ChooseMyPlate.gov website, you will find an interactive tool, *MyPlate Daily Checklist*, that estimates your calorie needs and suggests a food pattern based on your age, gender, height, and weight (Table 2-5). These daily food plans provide useful information for each food group, including recommended daily amounts in common household measures. Modified daily food plans are also available for preschoolers, pregnant or breastfeeding mothers, and those interested in losing weight. Be sure to visit the site to generate your own daily food plan.

The recommended numbers of servings are given in cups for vegetables, fruits, and dairy foods. Grains and protein foods are listed in ounces. How familiar are you with serving-size measurements? Figure 2-6 shows a convenient guide to estimate common serving-size measurements and a description of what counts as a MyPlate serving. Pay close attention to the stated serving size for each choice when following your daily food plan to help control calorie intake.

Common household units are also listed in Appendix F with their metric equivalents. Ounces and fluid ounces differ: ounces are a measure of weight, whereas fluid ounces are a measure of volume.

TABLE 2-5 ■ Healthy U.S.-Style Eating Pattern: Recommended Amounts of Food from Each MyPlate Food Group at 6 Kilocalorie Levels

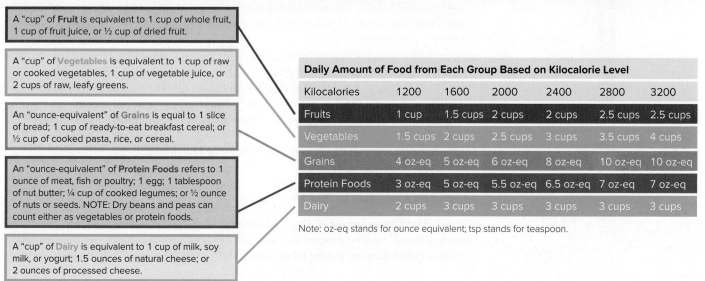

A "cup" of **Fruit** is equivalent to 1 cup of whole fruit, 1 cup of fruit juice, or ½ cup of dried fruit.

A "cup" of **Vegetables** is equivalent to 1 cup of raw or cooked vegetables, 1 cup of vegetable juice, or 2 cups of raw, leafy greens.

An "ounce-equivalent" of **Grains** is equal to 1 slice of bread; 1 cup of ready-to-eat breakfast cereal; or ½ cup of cooked pasta, rice, or cereal.

An "ounce-equivalent" of **Protein Foods** refers to 1 ounce of meat, fish or poultry; 1 egg; 1 tablespoon of nut butter; ¼ cup of cooked legumes; or ½ ounce of nuts or seeds. NOTE: Dry beans and peas can count either as vegetables or protein foods.

A "cup" of **Dairy** is equivalent to 1 cup of milk, soy milk, or yogurt; 1.5 ounces of natural cheese; or 2 ounces of processed cheese.

Daily Amount of Food from Each Group Based on Kilocalorie Level

Kilocalories	1200	1600	2000	2400	2800	3200
Fruits	1 cup	1.5 cups	2 cups	2 cups	2.5 cups	2.5 cups
Vegetables	1.5 cups	2 cups	2.5 cups	3 cups	3.5 cups	4 cups
Grains	4 oz-eq	5 oz-eq	6 oz-eq	8 oz-eq	10 oz-eq	10 oz-eq
Protein Foods	3 oz-eq	5 oz-eq	5.5 oz-eq	6.5 oz-eq	7 oz-eq	7 oz-eq
Dairy	2 cups	3 cups	3 cups	3 cups	3 cups	3 cups

Note: oz-eq stands for ounce equivalent; tsp stands for teaspoon.

Portion sizes

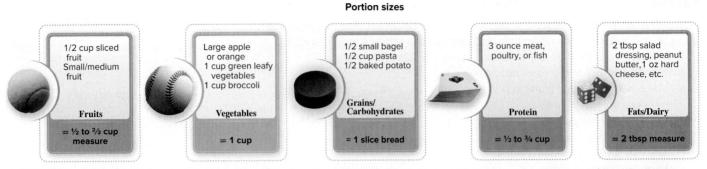

FIGURE 2-6 ▲ A tennis ball, baseball, hockey puck, deck of cards and dice are standard-size objects that make convenient guides for judging serving sizes. ©C Squared Studios/Getty Images (baseball); ©C Squared Studios/Getty Images (tennis ball); ©C Squared Studios/Getty Images (hockey puck); ©Photodisc Collection/Getty Images (deck of cards); ©Ron Chapple Stock/FotoSearch/Glow Images (dice)

MyPlate sets limits for empty calories, which come from saturated fats and/or added sugars. Saturated fats and added sugars add calories to the diet but contribute few nutrients. Saturated fats are solid at room temperature and include butter, beef fat, and shortening. Some saturated fats, such as the marbling in a ribeye steak and the fat in milk (Fig. 2-7), are naturally present in foods. Others, such as the shortening used to make a flaky croissant, are added during food processing or preparation. Added sugars include sugars and syrups that are added to foods during processing or preparation. Examples of foods that are major contributors of empty calories in the American diet are cakes, cookies, pastries, soft drinks, energy drinks, cheese, pizza, ice cream, and processed meats. The MyPlate Daily Checklists available on ChooseMyPlate.gov make some allowance for empty calories throughout the day; depending on total energy needs, allowances range from 120 to 600 kcal per day.

ADDITIONAL MyPLATE RESOURCES

ChooseMyPlate.gov also offers in-depth information regarding the *Dietary Guidelines*, as well as the following additional interactive tools for consumers.

- USDA's 10 Tips Nutrition Education series provides access to one-page printable documents for consumers and health educators. The materials cover over two dozen topics, such as "Kid-friendly veggies and fruits," "Healthy eating for vegetarians," and "Got your dairy today?" The printouts are perfect for posting on a refrigerator, and the suggestions can help you get started toward a healthy dietary pattern.
- The *What's Cooking? USDA Mixing Bowl* is an interactive tool for consumers who are ready to make a change and need help with healthy meal planning, cooking, and grocery shopping. A searchable database includes healthy recipes and options to build a cookbook, print recipe cards, and share recipes via social media.
- Food-A-Pedia allows users to locate calorie and food group information for specific food entries.
- The SuperTracker enables users to self-monitor food and activity.

MENU PLANNING WITH MyPLATE

Overall, MyPlate exemplifies the foundations of a healthy eating pattern you have already learned: variety, proportionality, and moderation. To achieve optimal nutrition, remember the following points when using MyPlate to plan your daily menus:

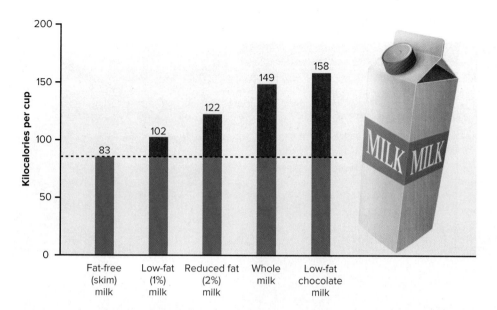

FIGURE 2-7 ◄ Not all dairy is the same. This bar graph compares the difference in kilocalories from various types of milks. The red bars represent the added calories from fat and sugar in various milks compared to fat-free milk.

- The guide does not apply to infants or children under 2 years of age. Daily food plans for children from ages 2 to 8 are based on average height and weight for age and gender.
- Variety is a key to successful implementation of MyPlate. There is no single, perfect food that is absolutely essential to good nutrition. Each food is rich in some nutrients but deficient in at least one essential nutrient. Likewise, no food group is more important than another; each food group makes an important, distinctive contribution to nutritional intake (Table 2-6). Choose foods from each food group and also choose different foods within each food group. For a sample meal plan, see Table 2-7.

Choose Your Foods booklets from the American Diabetes Association offer alternative menu-planning tools. These food lists organize foods based on calorie, protein, carbohydrate, and fat content. The result is a manageable framework for designing diets, especially for treatment of diabetes. For more information on the food lists, see Appendix B.

TABLE 2-6 ■ **Nutrient Contributions of MyPlate Food Groups**

Food Category	Major Nutrient Contributions
Grains	Carbohydrate Vitamins such as thiamin Minerals such as iron Fiber*
Vegetables	Carbohydrate Vitamins such as plant pigments that form vitamin A Minerals such as magnesium Fiber
Fruits	Carbohydrate Vitamins such as folate and vitamin C Minerals such as potassium Fiber
Dairy	Carbohydrate Protein Vitamins such as vitamin D Minerals such as calcium and phosphorus
Protein Foods	Protein Vitamins such as vitamin B-6 Minerals such as iron and zinc

*In whole grain varieties

TABLE 2-7 ■ Putting MyPlate into Practice

Meal	Food Group
Breakfast	
1 small orange	Fruits
¾ cup low-fat granola with ½ cup fat-free milk	Grains / Dairy
½ toasted, small raisin bagel with 2 tsp peanut butter	Grains / Protein
Lunch	
Turkey sandwich	
2 slices whole wheat bread	Grains
2 oz turkey	Protein
2 tsp mustard	
1 small apple	Fruits
2 oatmeal-raisin cookies (small)	Empty calories
3 P.M. Study Break	
6 whole wheat crackers	Grains
1 tbsp peanut butter	Protein
½ cup fat-free milk	Dairy
Dinner	
Tossed salad	
1 cup romaine lettuce	Vegetables
½ cup sliced tomatoes	Vegetables
1½ tbsp Italian dressing	Oils
½ carrot, grated	Vegetables
3 oz broiled salmon	Protein
½ cup rice	Grains
½ cup green beans	Vegetables
Late-Night Snack	
1 cup "light" fruit yogurt	Dairy
Nutrient Breakdown	
1800 kcal	
Carbohydrate	56% of kcal
Protein	18% of kcal
Fat	26% of kcal

This menu meets nutrient needs for all vitamins and minerals for an average adult who needs 1800 kcal. For adolescents, teenagers, and older adults, add one additional serving of milk or other calcium-rich sources.

©Mitch Hrdlicka/Getty Images (top); ©Carolyn Taylor Photography/Getty Images (middle); ©C Squared Studios/Getty Images (bottom)

- The foods within a group may vary widely with respect to nutrients and calories. For example, the calorie content of 3 ounces of baked potato is 98 kcal, whereas that of 3 ounces of potato chips is 470 kcal. With respect to vitamin C, an orange has 70 mg and an apple has 10 mg.
- Choose primarily low-fat and fat-free items from the dairy group. By reducing calorie intake in this way, you can select more items from other food groups. If milk causes intestinal gas and bloating, emphasize yogurt and cheese (see Chapter 4 for details on the problem of lactose intolerance).

- Include plant foods that are good sources of proteins, such as beans and nuts, at least several times a week because many are rich in vitamins (such as vitamin E), minerals (such as magnesium), and fiber.
- For vegetables and fruits, try to include a dark-green or orange vegetable for vitamin A, and a vitamin-C-rich fruit, such as an orange, every day. Do not focus primarily on potatoes (e.g., French fries) for your vegetable choices. Surveys show that fewer than 5% of adults eat a full serving of a dark-green vegetable on any given day. Increased consumption of these foods is important because they contribute vitamins, minerals, fiber, and phytochemicals.
- Choose whole grain varieties of breads, cereals, rice, and pasta because they contribute vitamin E and fiber. A daily serving of a whole grain, ready-to-eat breakfast cereal is an excellent choice because the vitamins (such as vitamin B-6) and minerals (such as zinc) typically added to it, along with fiber, help fill in common nutritional gaps.
- Include some plant oils on a daily basis, such as those in salad dressing, and eat fish at least twice a week. This supplies you with health-promoting essential fatty acids.

LIMITATIONS OF MyPLATE

Although MyPlate will promote important changes in American eating patterns, it has certain limitations. Some critics say that the icon is too simple. For example, it does not immediately provide information about overall calories, serving sizes, or number of servings to choose from each food group. However, many of these details will vary by person. Users will need to access the accompanying materials available on the ChooseMyPlate.gov website to obtain a personally tailored daily food plan.

The MyPlate icon does not address the types of foods to choose within each food group. Making appropriate food choices for weight management and prevention of diet-related chronic diseases requires consumers to have some nutrition knowledge. Fortunately, public health messages and online content related to MyPlate are available to educate Americans.

MyPlate shows how to build a healthy plate at mealtimes, but it does not adequately address the total diet, which in reality includes many snacks between meals. Meal and snack patterns are available in the Daily Checklists for children but not for adults.

As with any public health campaign, it is possible that the people who need it most will overlook the MyPlate message. Educated consumers with access to interactive MyPlate tools likely already comply with many of the *Dietary Guidelines*. Populations with poor diets may be unlikely or unable to access online materials to find their personalized Daily Checklist.

Overall, the MyPlate icon is an attractive and relevant tool that immediately shows us how to build a healthy plate at mealtimes. The strength of MyPlate lies in its simplicity. It conveys the major messages that are needed when shopping, cooking, and eating and can be enhanced with the details provided on the ChooseMyPlate.gov website.

HOW DOES YOUR PLATE RATE?

Regularly comparing your daily food intake with your personalized daily food plan recommendations is a relatively simple way to evaluate the quality of your overall eating pattern. Identify the nutrients that are low in your eating pattern based on the nutrients found in each food group. For example, if you do not consume enough servings from the milk group, your calcium intake is most likely too low. Look for foods that you enjoy that supply calcium, such as calcium-fortified orange juice.

For a more detailed analysis of your current eating pattern, use the SuperTracker tool on ChooseMyPlate.gov or the NutritionCalc Plus function in Connect to compare your food choices to MyPlate. With a detailed dietary analysis, you can compare your intakes of individual nutrients to standards set by the Food and Nutrition Board and clearly see the areas that need improvement. Even small changes to your eating and exercise patterns can have positive results.

Solid fats contribute almost 20% of total calories in the typical American's dietary pattern, but they have little to offer in terms of essential nutrients and dietary fiber. Instead of solid fats, choose foods containing plant oils.

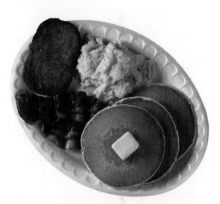

▲ Typical restaurant meals contain oversized portions that do not align with MyPlate. ©Burke/Triolo/Brand X Pictures

Food *quality* is just as important as food *quantity* when it comes to good nutrition. Consider the difference in calorie contents of the following two meals, both of which fit the proportions suggested by MyPlate:

Fried chicken fillet sandwich with mayonnaise on a white sandwich roll, 1 each

French fries, 1 medium order

Apple-filled pastry, 1 each

Whole milk, 1 cup

1293 kcal

Skinless grilled chicken breast, 3 ounces

Brown rice, prepared with olive oil, 1 cup

Steamed green beans, 1 cup

Cubed watermelon, 1 cup

Skim milk, 1 cup

513 kcal

FIGURE 2-8 ▶ The Mediterranean Diet Pyramid is based on dietary patterns from the Mediterranean region, which has low rates of chronic diseases and high life expectancy. Base every meal on fruits, vegetables, whole grains, olive oil, beans, nuts, legumes and seeds; eat fish and seafood at least two times per week; eat poultry and eggs every two days or weekly; eat cheese and yogurt daily to weekly; eat meats and sweets less often; drink water; drink red wine in moderation; be physically active and enjoy meals with others. ©2009 Oldways Preservation & Exchange Trust, *www.oldwayspt.org.* Used by permission

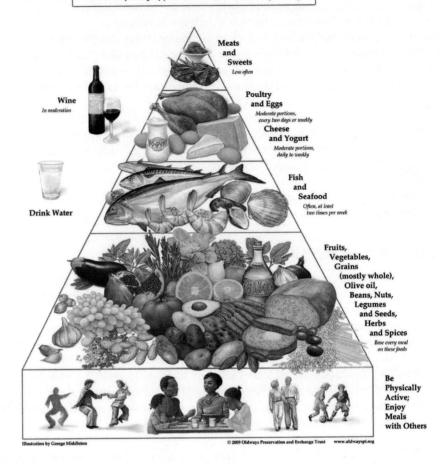

THE MEDITERRANEAN DIET PYRAMID

Updated in 2009, the Mediterranean Diet Pyramid (Fig. 2-8) is a useful alternative to MyPlate. It is based on the dietary patterns of the southern Mediterranean region, which has enjoyed the lowest recorded rates of chronic diseases and the highest adult life expectancy. An abundance of research supports the health benefits of following the Mediterranean Diet.[1,2,14] The *2015–2020 Dietary Guidelines* include the Healthy Mediterranean-Style Eating Pattern, which contains more fruits and seafood and less dairy than the Healthy U.S.-Style Eating Pattern.

Oldways—a respected, international, nonprofit culinary think tank—also publishes the Latin-American Diet Pyramid and was the force behind development of the Whole Grain stamp seen on food packages.

ASK THE RDN   The Mediterranean Diet

Dear RDN: *I know that olives, olive oil, Greek yogurt, and feta cheese are Mediterranean foods, but could you share some more specific tips on how to follow the Mediterranean Diet eating plan?*

The Mediterranean dietary pattern is not limited to Greek and Italian food. As shown on the pyramid in Figure 2-8, foods from plant sources form the foundation of every meal. A variety of fruits and vegetables (other than potatoes) is a big part of this plan. Eat 5 to 10 servings a day, especially of seasonally fresh and locally grown foods. For most produce, each serving is ½ cup cooked or 1 cup raw.

You are right about including olives and olive oil. These and avocados are considered healthy sources of fat, compared to many other plant oils and animal fats. Choose 4 to 6 servings a day—a serving is equal to 1 teaspoon of olive oil, 5 olives, or 1/8 of an avocado. Also include a handful of nuts or seeds daily as good sources of healthy fats, fiber, and protein.

Legumes (beans) are also plant sources of fiber and protein. Eat ½ cup of cooked legumes, including hummus, at least twice a week. You can have bread, but only four small (1-ounce) portions of whole grain bread, pasta, or quinoa each day. A serving of grains is 1 slice of bread or ½ cup of cooked pasta, rice, or cereal. Plenty of herbs and spices, such as basil and oregano, are also used in the Mediterranean eating plan and have antioxidant and anti-inflammatory properties.

As you make your way up the pyramid, eat a 4-ounce serving of fish two to three times a week. Moderate portions (3 to 4 ounces) of lean meat and poultry or 2 eggs are recommended once a week or every few days. Choose low-fat dairy (up to three 1-cup servings a day) from cultured sources such as yogurt or kefir. These are easier to digest and supply beneficial bacteria. Water is the beverage of choice. Moderate drinking of wine (one to two 5-ounce glasses of red wine per day) also has proven health benefits. Finally, remember that regular physical activity that promotes a healthy weight is an important aspect of the Mediterranean lifestyle as well as eating meals with family and friends.

Buon appetito!

Anne M. Smith, PhD, RDN, LD (author)

✔ CONCEPT CHECK 2.3

1. What is the website where you can find all of the tools associated with MyPlate?
2. What are the five major food groups represented on MyPlate?

2.4 States of Nutritional Health

The ultimate intent of the sound nutrition advice found in the *Dietary Guidelines* and the MyPlate food guide is to promote optimal nutritional status for individuals. The amount of each nutrient needed to maintain a state of desirable nutrition is the basis for published dietary intake recommendations. We have already discussed general dietary guidelines and will cover more specific nutrient recommendations in Section 2.6. The body's nutritional health is determined by considering the **nutritional state** of each needed nutrient. Three general categories of nutritional status are recognized: desirable nutrition, undernutrition, and overnutrition. The common term **malnutrition** can refer to either **overnutrition** or **undernutrition.** Neither state is conducive to good health. Furthermore, it is possible to be both overnourished (e.g., consume excess calories) and undernourished (e.g., consume too few essential vitamins and minerals) at the same time.

The amount of each nutrient needed to maintain a state of desirable nutrition is the basis for published dietary intake recommendations.

DESIRABLE NUTRITION

The nutritional state for a particular nutrient is desirable when body tissues have enough of the nutrient to support normal metabolic functions and surplus stores that can be used in times of increased need. A desirable nutritional state can be achieved by obtaining essential nutrients from a variety of foods.

UNDERNUTRITION

Undernutrition occurs when nutrient intake does not meet nutrient needs. At first, any surpluses are put to use; then, as stores are exhausted, health begins to decline. Many nutrients are in high demand due to constant cell loss and regeneration in the body, such

nutritional state The nutritional health of a person as determined by anthropometric measurements (height, weight, circumferences, and so on), biochemical measurements of nutrients or their by-products in blood and urine, a clinical (physical) examination, a dietary analysis, and economic evaluation; also called nutritional status.

malnutrition Failing health that results from longstanding eating practices that do not coincide with nutritional needs.

overnutrition A state in which nutritional intake greatly exceeds the body's needs.

undernutrition Failing health that results from a longstanding dietary intake that is not enough to meet nutritional needs.

FIGURE 2-9 ▶ The general scheme of nutritional status. Green reflects good status, yellow marginal status, and red poor status (undernutrition or overnutrition). This general concept can be applied to all nutrients. Iron was chosen as an example because iron deficiency is the most common nutrient deficiency worldwide.

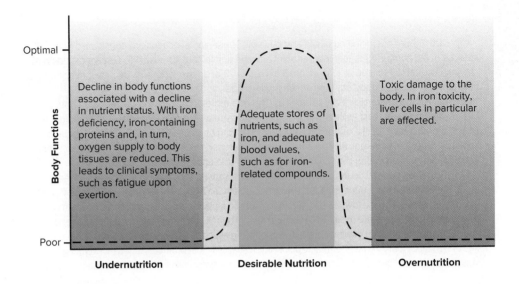

Optimal

Body Functions

Decline in body functions associated with a decline in nutrient status. With iron deficiency, iron-containing proteins and, in turn, oxygen supply to body tissues are reduced. This leads to clinical symptoms, such as fatigue upon exertion.

Adequate stores of nutrients, such as iron, and adequate blood values, such as for iron-related compounds.

Toxic damage to the body. In iron toxicity, liver cells in particular are affected.

Poor

Undernutrition   **Desirable Nutrition**   **Overnutrition**

symptom A change in health status noted by the person with the problem, such as stomach pain.

subclinical Stage of a disease or disorder not severe enough to produce symptoms that can be detected or diagnosed.

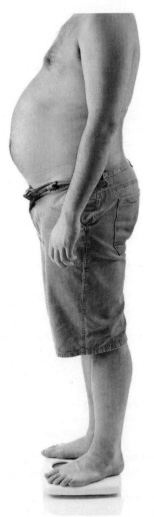

▲ The most common type of overnutrition in North America is the excess intake of calories, which often leads to obesity.
©Ljupco/iStock.com

as in the gastrointestinal tract. For this reason, the stores of certain nutrients, including many of the B vitamins, are exhausted rapidly and therefore require a regular intake. In addition, some women in North America do not consume sufficient iron to compensate for monthly menstrual losses and eventually deplete their iron stores (Fig. 2-9).

Once availability of a nutrient falls sufficiently low, biochemical evidence indicates that the body's metabolic processes have slowed or stopped. At this state of deficiency, there are no outward **symptoms;** thus, it is termed a **subclinical** deficiency. A subclinical deficiency can go on for some time before clinicians are able to detect its effects.

Eventually, clinical symptoms will develop. Clinical evidence of a nutritional deficiency—perhaps in the skin, hair, nails, tongue, or eyes—can occur within months but may take years to develop. Often, clinicians do not detect a problem until a deficiency produces outward symptoms, such as small areas of bruising on the skin from a vitamin C deficiency.

OVERNUTRITION

Prolonged consumption of more nutrients than the body needs can lead to overnutrition. In the short run (e.g., 1 to 2 weeks), overnutrition may cause only a few symptoms, such as stomach distress from excess iron intake. If an excess intake continues, however, some nutrients may accumulate to toxic amounts, which can lead to serious disease. For example, too much vitamin A during pregnancy can cause birth defects.

The most common form of overnutrition in developed nations is an excess intake of calories that leads to obesity. In the long run, outcomes of obesity include other serious diseases, such as type 2 diabetes and certain forms of cancer.

For most vitamins and minerals, the gap between desirable intake and overnutrition is wide. Therefore, even if people take a typical balanced multivitamin and mineral supplement daily, they probably will not receive a harmful dose of any nutrient. The gap between desirable intake and overnutrition is the smallest for vitamin A and the minerals calcium, iron, and copper. Thus, if you take nutrient supplements, keep a close eye on your total vitamin and mineral intake from both food and supplements to avoid toxicity (see Section 8.16 for further advice on use of nutrient supplements).

✔ **CONCEPT CHECK 2.4**

1. What are the main differences between the undernutrition, desirable nutrition, and overnutrition states of nutritional health?

2.5 Measuring Your Nutritional State

To find out how nutritionally fit *you* are, a nutritional assessment—either whole or partial—needs to be performed (Table 2-8). Generally, this is performed by a primary care provider, often with the aid of a registered dietitian nutritionist (RDN).

ANALYZING BACKGROUND FACTORS

Because family health history plays an important role in determining nutritional and health status, it must be carefully recorded and critically analyzed as part of a nutritional assessment. Other related background information includes (1) a medical history, especially for any disease states or treatments that could decrease nutrient absorption or ultimate use; (2) a list of medications taken; (3) a social history (e.g., marital status and living conditions); (4) level of education to determine the degree of complexity that can be used in written materials and oral discussions; and (5) economic status to determine the ability to purchase, transport, and prepare food.

ASSESSING NUTRITIONAL STATUS USING THE ABCDEs

In addition to background factors, four nutritional-assessment categories complete the picture of nutritional status. **Anthropometric assessment** of height, weight (and weight changes), skinfold thicknesses, and body circumferences provides information about the current state of nutrition. Most measures of body composition are easy to obtain and are generally reliable. However, an in-depth examination of nutritional health is impossible without the more expensive process of **biochemical assessment**. This involves the measurement of the concentrations of nutrients and nutrient by-products in the blood, urine, and feces and the activities of specific blood enzymes.

A **clinical assessment** would follow, during which a health professional would search for any physical evidence (e.g., high blood pressure) of diet-related diseases or deficiencies. Then, a close look at the person's eating pattern **(dietary assessment)**, including a record of at least the previous few days' food intake, would help to determine any possible problem areas.

Finally, adding the **environmental assessment** (from the background analysis) provides further details about the living conditions, education level, and ability to purchase and prepare foods needed to maintain health. Now the true nutritional state of a person emerges. Taken together, these five assessments form the ABCDEs of nutritional assessment: anthropometric, biochemical, clinical, dietary, and environmental (Fig. 2-10).

anthropometric assessment Measurement of body weight and the lengths, circumferences, and thicknesses of parts of the body.

biochemical assessment Measurement of biochemical functions (e.g., concentrations of nutrient by-products or enzyme activities in the blood or urine) related to a nutrient's function.

clinical assessment Examination of general appearance of skin, eyes, and tongue; sense of touch; ability to cough and walk; and evidence of rapid hair loss.

dietary assessment Estimation of typical food choices relying mostly on the recounting of one's usual intake or a record of one's previous days' intake.

environmental assessment Includes details about living conditions, education level, and the ability of the person to purchase, transport, and prepare food. The person's weekly budget for food purchases is also a key factor to consider.

TABLE 2-8 ▪ **Conducting an Evaluation of Nutritional Health**

Parameters	Example
Background	Medical history (e.g., current diseases, past surgeries, current weight, weight history, and current medications)
	Social history (e.g., marital status and living conditions)
	Family health history
	Education level
	Economic status
Nutritional	Anthropometric assessment: height, weight, skinfold thickness, arm muscle circumference, and other parameters
	Biochemical (laboratory) assessment of blood and urine: enzyme activities, concentrations of nutrients or their by-products
	Clinical assessment (physical examination): general appearance of skin, eyes, and tongue; sense of touch; ability to walk; and rapid hair loss
	Dietary assessment: usual intake or record of previous days' meals

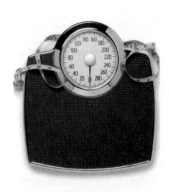

Anthropometric

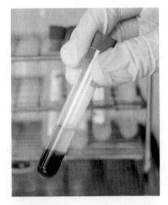

Biochemical

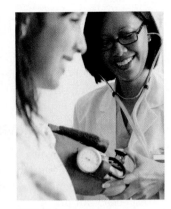

Clinical

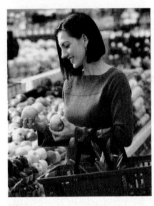

Dietary

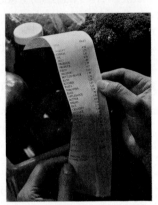

Environmental

A practical example using the ABCDEs for evaluating nutritional status can be illustrated in a person who chronically abuses alcohol. Upon evaluation, the physician notes that this person needs medical attention, including nutrient repletion based on the following nutritional assessment results:

(A) Low weight for height, recent 10-pound weight loss, muscle wasting in the upper body
(B) Low amounts of the vitamins thiamin and folate in the blood
(C) Psychological confusion, facial sores, and uncoordinated movement
(D) Dietary intake of mostly wine and hamburgers for the last week
(E) Currently residing in a homeless shelter; $35 in wallet; unemployed

RECOGNIZING THE LIMITATIONS OF NUTRITIONAL ASSESSMENT

A long time may elapse between the initial development of poor nutritional health and the first clinical evidence of a problem. An eating pattern high in animal and other solid fat often increases blood cholesterol but without producing any clinical evidence for years. However, when the blood vessels become sufficiently blocked by cholesterol and other materials, chest pain during physical activity or a **heart attack** may occur. An active area of nutrition research is the development of better methods for early detection of nutrition-related problems such as heart attack risk.

Another example of a serious health condition with delayed symptoms is low bone density resulting from a calcium deficiency—a particularly relevant issue for adolescent and young adult females. Many young women do not consume the needed amount of calcium but suffer no obvious effects in their younger years; however, the bone structures of these women with low calcium intakes do not reach full potential during the years of growth, making osteoporosis more likely later in life.

heart attack Rapid fall in heart function caused by reduced blood flow through the heart's blood vessels. Often part of the heart dies in the process. Technically called a myocardial infarction.

Furthermore, clinical symptoms of some nutritional deficiencies (e.g., diarrhea, inability to walk normally, and facial sores) are not very specific. These may have causes other than poor nutrition. The long time it takes for symptoms to develop and their potential to be vague often make it difficult to establish a link between an individual's current dietary pattern and nutritional state.

CONCERN ABOUT THE STATE OF YOUR NUTRITIONAL HEALTH IS IMPORTANT

The good news is that people who focus on maintaining nutritional health are apt to enjoy a long, vigorous life. For example, a recent study found that women with a healthy lifestyle had a decreased risk for heart attacks (80% reduction) compared to women without such healthy practices. The healthy habits included:

- Maintained a healthy eating pattern:
  - Varied
  - Included some fish
  - Rich in fiber
  - Low in animal fat and *trans* fat
- Maintained a healthy weight
- Occasionally consumed alcohol in small amounts
- Exercised for at least 30 minutes daily
- Avoided use of tobacco

Should all adults follow this example (with optional use of alcohol)?

> Although nutrition recommendations are often made for the entire healthy population, each of us has individual needs based on our particular health status and genetic background. It would be more appropriate, but also more expensive, if recommendations were made on an individual basis once a person's health status is known.

✓ CONCEPT CHECK 2.5

1. What are the ABCDE steps used in assessing nutritional status?

2.6 Specific Nutrient Standards and Recommendations

The overarching goal of any healthy eating plan is to meet nutrient needs. To begin, we must determine what amount of each essential nutrient is necessary to maintain health. Most of the terms that describe nutrient needs fall under one umbrella term: **Dietary Reference Intakes (DRIs).** The development of DRIs is an ongoing, collaborative effort between the National Academy of Medicine (formerly the Institute of Medicine) in the United States and Health Canada. Included under the DRI umbrella are **Recommended Dietary Allowances (RDAs), Adequate Intakes (AIs), Estimated Energy Requirements (EERs),** and **Tolerable Upper Intake Levels (Upper Levels or ULs).**

As you begin your study of nutrition, all these acronyms can seem like an alphabet soup of abbreviations! To help you understand the meaning of each and the differences among these nutrient standards, some basic knowledge about their use is summarized in Table 2-9.

RECOMMENDED DIETARY ALLOWANCE

A Recommended Dietary Allowance (RDA) is the daily amount of a nutrient that will meet the needs of nearly all individuals (about 97%) in a particular age and gender group. A person can compare his or her daily intake of specific nutrients to the RDA. Although an intake slightly above or below the RDA for a particular nutrient on any given day is no reason for concern, a significant deviation below (about 70%) or above (about three times or more for some nutrients) the RDA for an extended time can eventually result in a deficiency or toxicity of that nutrient, respectively.

Dietary Reference Intakes (DRIs) Term used to encompass nutrient recommendations made by the Food and Nutrition Board of the Institute of Medicine. These include RDAs, AIs, EERs, and ULs.

Recommended Dietary Allowance (RDA) Nutrient intake amount sufficient to meet the needs of 97% to 98% of the individuals in a specific life stage.

Adequate Intake (AI) Nutrient intake amount set for any nutrient for which insufficient research is available to establish an RDA. AIs are based on estimates of intakes that appear to maintain a defined nutritional state in a specific life stage.

Estimated Energy Requirement (EER) Estimate of the energy (kcal) intake needed to match the energy use of an average person in a specific life stage.

Tolerable Upper Intake Level (UL) Maximum chronic daily intake level of a nutrient that is unlikely to cause adverse health effects in almost all people in a specific life stage.

Nutrition Facts

12 servings per container

Serving size	1 donut (about 52g)

Amount per serving

Calories 200

	% Daily Value*
Total Fat 12g	**18%**
Saturated Fat 3g	**15%**
Trans Fat 4g	
Cholesterol 5mg	**1%**
Sodium 95mg	**4%**
Total Carbohydrate 22g	**7%**
Dietary Fiber <1g	**1%**
Total Sugars 12g	
Includes 10g Added Sugars	**20%**
Protein 2g	
Vitamin D 0mcg	0%
Calcium 60mg	6%
Iron 1mg	6%
Potassium 39mg	1%

* The % Daily Value (DV) tells you how much a nutrient in a serving of food contributes to a daily diet. 2,000 calories a day is used for general nutrition advice.

▲ The Daily Value is the nutrient standard used on the Nutrition Facts portion of the food label. The percent Daily Value for each nutrient is based on consuming a 2000-kcal diet. ©David A. Tietz/Editorial Image, LLC

TABLE 2-9 ■ Dietary Reference Intakes and Daily Value

RDA	Recommended Dietary Allowance. Use to evaluate your current intake for a specific nutrient. The further you stray above or below this value, the greater your chances of developing nutritional problems.
AI	Adequate Intake. Use to evaluate your current intake of nutrients but realize that an AI designation implies that further research is required before scientists can establish a more definitive recommendation.
EER	Estimated Energy Requirement. Use to estimate calorie needs of the average person within a specific height, weight, gender, age, and physical activity pattern.
UL	Upper Level. Use to evaluate the highest amount of daily nutrient intake unlikely to cause adverse health effects in the long run in almost all people (97% to 98%) in a population. This number applies to chronic use and is set to protect even very susceptible people in the healthy general population. As intake increases above the Upper Level, the potential for adverse effects generally increases.
DV	Daily Value. Use as a rough guide for comparing the nutrient content of a food to approximate human needs. Typically, the Daily Value used on food labels refers to ages 4 years through adulthood. It is based on a 2000-kcal diet. Some Daily Values also increase slightly with higher calorie intakes (see Fig. 2-12 in Section 2.8 on food labeling).

ADEQUATE INTAKE

An RDA can be set for a nutrient only if there is sufficient information on the human needs for that particular nutrient. Today, there is not enough information on some nutrients, such as chromium, to set such a precise standard as an RDA. For these nutrients, the DRIs include a category called an Adequate Intake (AI). This standard is based on the dietary intakes of people who appear to be maintaining nutritional health. That amount of intake is assumed to be adequate, as no evidence of a nutritional deficiency is apparent.

ESTIMATED ENERGY REQUIREMENT

For calorie needs, we use the Estimated Energy Requirement (EER) instead of an RDA or AI. In contrast to the RDAs, which are set somewhat higher than the average needs for nutrients, the EER is set for the average person. While a slight excess of vitamins and minerals is not harmful, a long-term excess of even a small amount of calories will lead to weight gain. Therefore, the calculation of EER needs to be more specific, taking into account age, gender, height, weight, and physical activity (e.g., sedentary or moderately active). In some cases, the additional calorie needs for growth and lactation are also included (see Chapters 7, 14, and 15 for the specific formulas used). Note that the EER is based on the "average" person. Thus, it can only serve as a starting point for estimating calorie needs.

TOLERABLE UPPER INTAKE LEVEL

A Tolerable Upper Intake Level (Upper Level or UL) has been set for some vitamins and minerals (see Appendix G). The UL is the highest amount of a nutrient unlikely to cause adverse health effects in the long run. As intake exceeds the UL, the risk of ill effects increases. These amounts generally should not be exceeded day after day, as toxicity could develop. For people eating a variety of foods and/or using a balanced multivitamin and mineral supplement, exceeding the UL is unusual. Problems are more likely to arise with eating patterns that promote excessive intakes of a limited variety of foods, with the use of many fortified foods, or with excessive doses of individual vitamins or minerals.

DAILY VALUE

A nutrition standard more relevant to everyday life is the Daily Value (DV). This is a generic standard used on food labels. It is applicable to both genders from 4 years of age through adulthood and is based on consuming a 2000-kcal diet. DVs are mostly set at or close to the highest RDA value or related nutrient standard seen in the various age and gender categories for a specific nutrient and are listed in Appendix A. DVs have been set for vitamins, minerals, protein, and other dietary components. For fat and cholesterol, the DVs represent a maximum level, not a goal one should strive to reach. DVs allow consumers to compare their intake from a specific food to desirable (or maximum) intakes.

HOW SHOULD THESE NUTRIENT STANDARDS BE USED?

As nutrient intake increases, the RDA for the nutrient, if set, is eventually met and a deficient state is no longer present (Fig. 2-11). An individual's needs most likely will be met since RDAs are set high to include almost all people. Related to the RDA concept of meeting an individual's needs are the standards of AI and the EER. These can be used to estimate an individual's needs for some nutrients and calories, respectively. Still, keep in mind that these standards do not share the same degree of accuracy as the RDA. For example, EER may have to be adjusted upward if the individual is very physically active. Finally, as nutrient intake increases above the UL, poor nutritional health is again likely. However, this poor health is due now to the toxic effects of a nutrient, rather than those of a deficiency.

The type of standard set for nutrients depends on the quality of available evidence. A nutrient recommendation backed by lots of experimental research will be expressed as an RDA. For a nutrient that still requires more research, only an AI is presented. We use the EER as a starting point for determining calorie needs. Some nutrients also have a UL if information on toxicity or adverse health effects is available. Periodically, new DRIs become available as expert committees review and interpret the available research.

RDAs and related standards are intended mainly for diet planning. Specifically, an eating pattern should aim to meet the RDA or AI as appropriate and not to exceed the UL over the long term (see Fig. 2-11). Specific RDA, AI, EER, and UL standards are

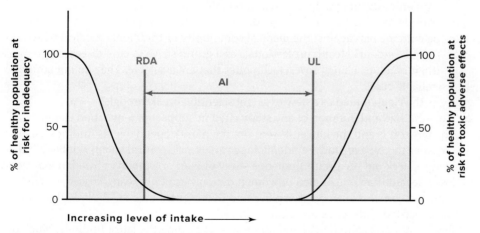

Recommended Dietary Allowance (RDA): The dietary intake level that is sufficient to meet the nutrient requirement of nearly all (97% to 98%) healthy individuals in a particular life stage and gender group. When set for a nutrient, aim for this intake.

Adequate Intake (AI): A recommended intake value based on observed or experimentally determined approximations or estimates of nutrient intake by a group (or groups) of healthy people that is assumed to be adequate; used when an RDA cannot be determined. When set for a nutrient, aim for this intake.

Tolerable Upper Intake Level (Upper Level or UL): The highest level of nutrient intake that is likely to pose no risk of adverse health effects for almost all individuals in the general population. As intake increases above the Upper Level, the risk of adverse effects increases.

FIGURE 2-11 ◄ This figure shows the relationship of the Dietary Reference Intakes (DRIs) to each other and the percentage of the population covered by each. At intakes between the RDA and the UL, the risk of either an inadequate diet or adverse effects from the nutrient in question is close to zero. The UL is then the highest level of nutrient intake likely to pose no risks of adverse health effects to almost all individuals in the general population. At intakes above the UL, the margin of safety to protect against adverse effects is reduced. The AI is set for some nutrients instead of an RDA. There is no established benefit for healthy individuals if they consume nutrient intakes above the RDA or AI.

found in Appendix G. To learn more about these nutrient standards, visit the link for Dietary Guidance at the Food and Nutrition Information Center's website (https://fnic.nal.usda.gov/dietary-guidance/dietary-reference-intakes).

> ☑ **CONCEPT CHECK 2.6**
>
> 1. How do the definitions of RDA and AI differ?
> 2. Which DRI category includes the highest amounts of a nutrient unlikely to cause adverse health effects?

2.7 Evaluating Nutrition Information

The following suggestions should help you make healthful and logical nutrition decisions:

1. Apply the basic principles of nutrition along with the *Dietary Guidelines* for Americans and related resources to any nutrition claim, including those on websites. Do you note any inconsistencies? Do reliable references support the claims? Beware of the following:
   - Testimonials about personal experience
   - Disreputable publication sources
   - Promises of dramatic results (rarely true)
   - Lack of evidence from other scientific studies
2. Examine the background and scientific credentials of the individual, organization, or publication making the nutritional claim. Usually, a reputable author is one whose educational background or present affiliation is with a nationally recognized university or medical center that offers programs or courses in the field of nutrition, medicine, or a closely allied specialty.
3. Be wary if the answer is "Yes" to any of the following questions about a health-related nutrition claim:
   - Are only advantages discussed and possible disadvantages ignored?
   - Are claims made about "curing" disease? Do they sound too good to be true?
   - Is extreme bias against the medical community or traditional medical treatments evident? Health professionals as a group strive to cure diseases in their patients, using proven techniques that are available. They do not ignore reliable cures.
   - Is the claim touted as a new or secret scientific breakthrough?
4. Note the size and duration of any study cited in support of a nutrition claim. The larger it is and the longer it went on, the more dependable its findings. Also consider the type of study: epidemiology versus case-control versus double-blind study. Check out the group studied; a study of men or women in Sweden may be less relevant than one of men or women of Southern European, African, or Hispanic descent, for example. Keep in mind that "contributes to," "is linked to," or "is associated with" does not mean "causes."
5. Beware of news conferences and other hype regarding the latest findings. Much of this will not survive more detailed scientific evaluation.
6. When you meet with a nutrition professional, you should expect that he or she will do the following:
   - Ask questions about your medical history, lifestyle, and current eating habits.
   - Formulate a dietary plan tailored to your needs, as opposed to simply tearing a form from a tablet that could apply to almost anyone.
   - Schedule follow-up visits to track your progress, answer any questions, and help keep you motivated.

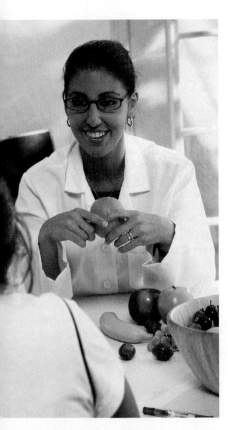

▲ Registered dietitian nutritionists are a reliable source of nutrition advice. ©liquidlibrary/PictureQuest

- Involve family members in the eating plan, when appropriate.
- Consult directly with your primary care provider and readily refer you back to your primary care provider for those health problems a nutrition professional is not trained to treat.

7. Avoid practitioners who prescribe **megadoses** of vitamin and mineral supplements for everyone.
8. Examine product labels carefully. Be skeptical of any promotional information about a product that is not clearly stated on the label. A product is not likely to do something not specifically claimed on its label or package insert (legally part of the label).

Remember from the Ask the RDN in Chapter 1 that the best approach to finding answers about your nutritional state is to consult your primary care provider or registered dietitian nutritionist first.[15] Appendix E also lists many reputable sources of nutrition advice for your use. Overall, nutrition is a rapidly advancing field, and there are always new findings. Finally, the following websites can help you evaluate ongoing nutrition and health claims:

acsh.org
American Council on Science and Health

http://ods.od.nih.gov
National Institutes of Health, Office of Dietary Supplements

www.fda.gov
U.S. Food and Drug Administration

www.ncahf.org
National Council Against Health Fraud

www.quackwatch.org
Quackwatch: Your Guide to Quackery, Health Fraud, and Intelligent Decisions

megadose Large intake of a nutrient well beyond estimates of needs or what would be found in a balanced diet; 2 to 10 times above human needs is typically a starting point.

DIET AND NUTRITION APPS

Science-based reviews of the most popular diet and nutrition apps for phones and tablets are available from the Academy of Nutrition and Dietetics. Food and nutrition experts—registered dietitian nutritionists—have written these reviews of top-rated, free smartphone apps for those looking to lose weight, manage their diabetes, or eat gluten-free foods. Ratings are based on a scale of 1 to 5 stars. The reviews are available at http://www.eatrightpro.org/resources/media/trends-and-reviews/app-reviews.

✓ CONCEPT CHECK 2.7

1. What are some characteristics that suggest that references supporting a nutrition claim are unreliable?
2. What should your expectations be when meeting with a nutrition professional?

2.8 Nutrition and Your Health

Food Labels and Diet Planning

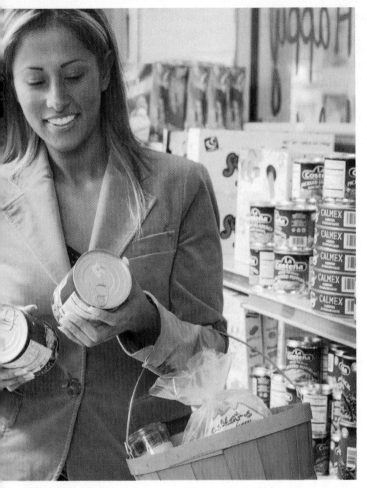

©Photodisc/Getty Images

In addition to these required components, manufacturers can choose to list polyunsaturated and monounsaturated fat, potassium, and others. Listing an additional nutrient becomes *required* if the food is fortified with that nutrient or if a claim is made about the health benefits of the specific nutrient.

Remember that the Daily Value is a generic standard used on the food label. The percentage of the Daily Value (% Daily Value or % DV) is usually given for each nutrient per serving. These percentages are based on a 2000-kcal diet and must be adjusted for people who require considerably more or less than 2000 kcal per day with respect to fat and carbohydrate intake. DVs are mostly set at or close to the highest RDA value or related nutrient standard seen in the various age and gender categories for a specific nutrient.

Serving sizes on the Nutrition Facts panel must be consistent among similar foods. This means that all brands of ice cream, for example, must use the same serving size on their label. These serving sizes may differ from those of MyPlate because those on food labels are based on more typical portion sizes. In addition, food claims made on packages must follow legal definitions. A long list of definitions for nutrient claims allowed on food labels is given in Table 2-10. For example, if a product claims to be "low sodium," it must have 140 milligrams of sodium or less per serving.

Many manufacturers list the Daily Values set for dietary components such as fat, cholesterol, and carbohydrate on the Nutrition Facts panel. This can be useful as a reference point. As noted, they are based on 2000 kcal; if the label is large enough, amounts based on 2500 kcal are listed as well. As mentioned, DVs allow consumers to compare their intake from a specific food to desirable (or maximum) daily intakes.

Changes to Nutrition Labels Approved

For the first time in 20 years, the FDA finalized new rules for the Nutrition Facts panel in May 2016. The changes are designed to promote healthier eating and combat obesity, aiming to help consumers make informed decisions about the foods they eat (Fig. 2-13). Several changes, such as increasing the type size for "Calories," "servings per container," and the "Serving size" declaration, and bolding the number of calories and the "Serving size" declaration, are aimed at making it easier for Americans to know how many calories they are consuming. The Daily Value information for nutrients is being updated and will include the actual amount, in addition to percent Daily Value of vitamin D, calcium, iron and potassium. The Daily Value footnote is changing to better explain the meaning of percent Daily Value. Along with potassium and vitamin D, "Added Sugars" is an addition to the label, whereas calories from fat is being eliminated. These changes to sugar and fat are based on scientific data showing that it is difficult to meet nutrient needs and stay within calorie limits if added sugar is more than 10 percent of total daily calories and that the type of fat is more important than the amount. One of the most significant changes is that serving size information will now more accurately reflect how much is consumed in one sitting. For example, the serving sizes for a soda will go from 8 ounces to 12 ounces, and ice cream will increase from ½ cup to ⅔ cup. To eliminate confusion about the number of servings in a container and calories in

Today, nearly all foods sold in stores must be in a package that has a label containing the following information: the product name, name and address of the manufacturer, amount of product in the package, and ingredients listed in descending order by weight. This food and beverage labeling is monitored in North America by government agencies such as the Food and Drug Administration (FDA) in the United States. The listing of certain food constituents is also required—specifically, on a Nutrition Facts panel (Fig. 2-12). Consumers can use the information in the Nutrition Facts panel to learn more about what they eat. The following components must be listed:

- Total calories (kcal)
- Total fat
- Saturated fat
- *Trans* fat
- Cholesterol
- Sodium
- Total carbohydrate
- Fiber

- Total sugars
- Added sugars
- Protein
- Vitamin A
- Vitamin D
- Calcium
- Iron
- Potassium

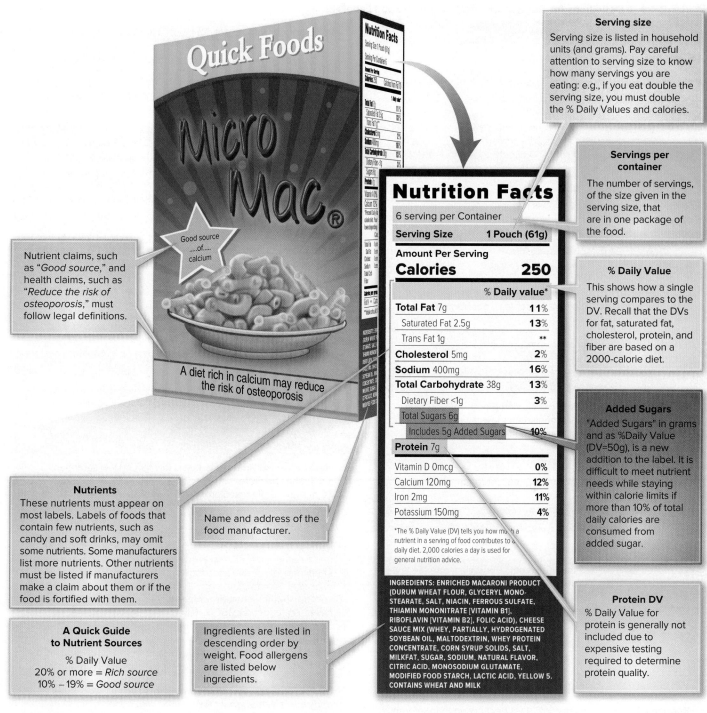

Serving size

Serving size is listed in household units (and grams). Pay careful attention to serving size to know how many servings you are eating: e.g., if you eat double the serving size, you must double the % Daily Values and calories.

Servings per container

The number of servings, of the size given in the serving size, that are in one package of the food.

% Daily Value

This shows how a single serving compares to the DV. Recall that the DVs for fat, saturated fat, cholesterol, protein, and fiber are based on a 2000-calorie diet.

Added Sugars

"Added Sugars" in grams and as %Daily Value (DV=50g), is a new addition to the label. It is difficult to meet nutrient needs while staying within calorie limits if more than 10% of total daily calories are consumed from added sugar.

Protein DV

% Daily Value for protein is generally not included due to expensive testing required to determine protein quality.

Nutrient claims, such as "*Good source*," and health claims, such as "*Reduce the risk of osteoporosis*," must follow legal definitions.

Nutrients

These nutrients must appear on most labels. Labels of foods that contain few nutrients, such as candy and soft drinks, may omit some nutrients. Some manufacturers list more nutrients. Other nutrients must be listed if manufacturers make a claim about them or if the food is fortified with them.

Name and address of the food manufacturer.

A Quick Guide to Nutrient Sources

% Daily Value
20% or more = *Rich source*
10% – 19% = *Good source*

Ingredients are listed in descending order by weight. Food allergens are listed below ingredients.

Nutrition Facts

6 serving per Container

Serving Size	1 Pouch (61g)

Amount Per Serving

Calories	250

% Daily value*

Total Fat 7g	**11**%
Saturated Fat 2.5g	**13**%
Trans Fat 1g	**
Cholesterol 5mg	**2**%
Sodium 400mg	**16**%
Total Carbohydrate 38g	**13**%
Dietary Fiber <1g	**3**%
Total Sugars 6g	
Includes 5g Added Sugars	**10**%
Protein 7g	
Vitamin D 0mcg	0%
Calcium 120mg	12%
Iron 2mg	11%
Potassium 150mg	4%

*The % Daily Value (DV) tells you how much a nutrient in a serving of food contributes to a daily diet. 2,000 calories a day is used for general nutrition advice.

INGREDIENTS: ENRICHED MACARONI PRODUCT (DURUM WHEAT FLOUR, GLYCERYL MONO-STEARATE, SALT, NIACIN, FERROUS SULFATE, THIAMIN MONONITRATE [VITAMIN B1], RIBOFLAVIN [VITAMIN B2], FOLIC ACID), CHEESE SAUCE MIX (WHEY, PARTIALLY, HYDROGENATED SOYBEAN OIL, MALTODEXTRIN, WHEY PROTEIN CONCENTRATE, CORN SYRUP SOLIDS, SALT, MILKFAT, SUGAR, SODIUM, NATURAL FLAVOR, CITRIC ACID, MONOSODIUM GLUTAMATE, MODIFIED FOOD STARCH, LACTIC ACID, YELLOW 5. CONTAINS WHEAT AND MILK

FIGURE 2-12 ▲ Food packages must list product name, name and address of the manufacturer, amount of product in the package, and ingredients. The Nutrition Facts panel is required on virtually all packaged food products. The % Daily Value listed on the label is the percent of the amount of a nutrient needed daily that is provided by a single serving of the product. Canadian food labels use a slightly different group of health claims and label descriptors.

a serving, larger packages, such as a pint of ice cream, will have two columns on the labels, one for "per serving" and one for "per package." Manufacturers with more than $10 million in annual food sales must begin using the new label by July 26, 2018, while others will have an additional year to comply. More information can be found at http://www.fda.gov/Food/-GuidanceRegulation/GuidanceDocumentsRegulatoryInformation/LabelingNutrition/ucm385663.htm.

TABLE 2-10 ■ **Definitions for Nutrient Claims Allowed on Food Labels**

Sugar

- **Sugar free:** less than 0.5 grams (g) per serving.

- **No added sugar; without added sugar:**
- No sugar or sugar-containing ingredient is added during processing.
- If the food doesn't meet the requirements for a low- or reduced-calorie food, the product bears a statement that the food is not low calorie or calorie reduced and directs consumers' attention to the Nutrition Facts panel for further information on sugars and calorie content.

- **Reduced sugar:** at least 25% less sugar per serving than reference food

Calories

- **Calorie free:** fewer than 5 kcal per serving

- **Low calorie:** 40 kcal or less per serving and, if the serving is 30 grams or less or 2 tablespoons or less, per 50 grams of the food

- **Reduced or fewer calories:** at least 25% fewer kcal per serving than reference food

Fiber

- **High fiber:** 5 grams or more per serving (Foods making high-fiber claims must meet the definition for low fat, or the level of total fat must appear next to the high-fiber claim.)

- **Good source of fiber:** 2.5 to 4.9 grams per serving

- **More or added fiber:** at least 2.5 grams more per serving than reference food

Fat

- **Fat free:** less than 0.5 gram of fat per serving

- **Saturated fat free:** less than 0.5 gram per serving, and the level of *trans* fatty acids does not exceed 0.5 gram per serving

- **Low fat:** 3 grams or less per serving and, if the serving is 30 grams or less or 2 tablespoons or less, per 50 grams of the food; 2% milk can no longer be labeled low fat, as it exceeds 3 grams per serving; *reduced fat* will be the term used instead.

- **Low saturated fat:** 1 gram or less per serving and not more than 15% of kcal from saturated fatty acids

- **Reduced or less fat:** at least 25% less per serving than reference food

- **Reduced or less saturated fat:** at least 25% less per serving than reference food

Cholesterol

- **Cholesterol free:** less than 2 milligrams (mg) of cholesterol and 2 grams or less of saturated fat per serving

- **Low cholesterol:** 20 milligrams or less of cholesterol and 2 grams or less of saturated fat per serving or, if the serving is 30 grams or less or 2 tablespoons or less, per 50 grams of the food

- **Reduced or less cholesterol:** at least 25% less cholesterol than reference food and 2 grams or less of saturated fat per serving

Sodium

- **Sodium free:** less than 5 milligrams per serving

- **Very low sodium:** 35 milligrams or less per serving and, if the serving is 30 grams or less or 2 tablespoons or less, per 50 grams of the food

- **Low sodium:** 140 milligrams or less per serving or, if the serving is 30 grams or less or 2 tablespoons or less, per 50 grams of the food

- **Light in sodium:** at least 50% less per serving than reference food

- **Reduced or less sodium:** at least 25% less per serving than reference food

Other Terms

- **Fortified or enriched:** Vitamins and/or minerals have been added to the product in amounts in excess of at least 10% of that normally present in the usual product. *Enriched* generally refers to replacing nutrients lost in processing, whereas *fortified* refers to adding nutrients not originally present in the specific food.

- **Healthy:** An individual food that is low fat and low saturated fat and has no more than 360 to 480 milligrams of sodium or 60 milligrams of cholesterol per serving can be labeled "healthy" if it provides at least 10% of the Daily Value for vitamin A, vitamin C, protein, calcium, iron, or fiber.

- **Light or lite:** The descriptor *light* or *lite* can mean two things: first, that a nutritionally altered product contains one-third fewer kcal or half the fat of reference food (if the food derives 50% or more of its kcal from fat, the reduction must be 50% of the fat) and second, that the sodium content of a low-calorie, low-fat food has been reduced by 50%. In addition, "light in sodium" may be used for foods in which the sodium content has been reduced by at least 50%. The term *light* may still be used to describe such properties as texture and color, as long as the label explains the intent; for example, "light brown sugar" and "light and fluffy."

- **Diet:** A food may be labeled with terms such as *diet, dietetic, artificially sweetened,* or *sweetened with nonnutritive sweetener* only if the claim is not false or misleading. The food can also be labeled *low calorie* or *reduced calorie.*

- **Good source:** *Good source* means that a serving of the food contains 10% to 19% of the Daily Value for a particular nutrient. If 5% or less, it is a *low source.*

- **High:** *High* means that a serving of the food contains 20% or more of the Daily Value for a particular nutrient.

(continued)

TABLE 2-10 ▪ *(continued)*

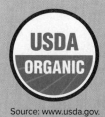

Source: www.usda.gov.

- **Organic:** Federal standards for organic foods allow claims when much of the ingredients do not use chemical fertilizers or pesticides, genetic engineering, sewage sludge, antibiotics, or irradiation in their production. At least 95% of ingredients (by weight) must meet these guidelines to be labeled "organic" on the front of the package. If the front label instead says "made with organic ingredients," only 70% of the ingredients must be organic. For animal products, the animals must graze outdoors, be fed organic feed, and cannot be exposed to large amounts of antibiotics or growth hormones.

- **Natural:** The food must be free of food colors, synthetic flavors, or any other synthetic substance.

The following terms apply only to meat and poultry products regulated by USDA.

- **Extra lean:** less than 5 grams of fat, 2 grams of saturated fat, and 95 milligrams of cholesterol per serving (or 100 grams of an individual food)

- **Lean:** less than 10 grams of fat, 4.5 grams of saturated fat, and 95 milligrams of cholesterol per serving (or 100 grams of an individual food)

Many definitions are from FDA's *Dictionary of Terms,* as established in conjunction with the 1990 Nutrition Labeling and Education Act (NLEA).

USDA Organic seal: Source: https://www.ams.usda.gov/rules-regulations/organic/organic-seal.

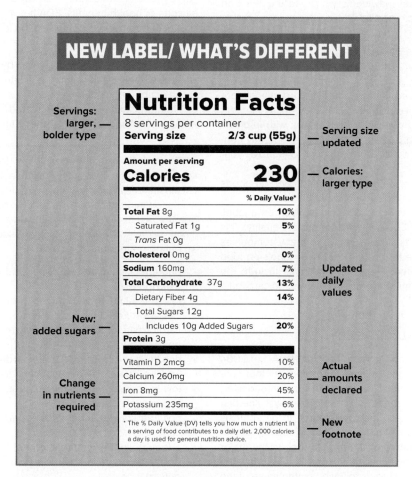

FIGURE 2-13 ▲ New Nutrition Facts label with changes noted.

Source: *FDA: Changes to the Nutrition Facts Label.* http://www.fda.gov/Food/Guidance Regulation/GuidanceDocumentsRegulatoryInformation/LabelingNutrition/ucm385663.htm.

The Nutrition Facts label uses the term *calorie* to express energy content in some cases, but kilocalorie (kcal) values are actually listed.

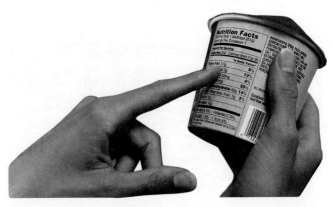

▲ Use the Nutrition Facts label to learn more about the nutrient content of the foods you eat. Nutrient content is expressed as a percent of Daily Value. Canadian food laws and related food labels have a slightly different format. ©Ryan McVay/Getty Images

Menu Planning with Labels

All of the tools discussed in this chapter greatly aid in menu planning. Menu planning can start with MyPlate. The totality of choices made within the groups can then be evaluated using the *Dietary Guidelines*. Individual foods that make up a dietary pattern can be examined more closely using the Daily Values listed on the Nutrition Facts panel of the product. For the most part, these Daily Values are in line with the Recommended Dietary Allowances and related nutrient standards. The Nutrition Facts panel is especially useful in identifying nutrient-dense foods (foods high in a specific nutrient, such as vitamin A but low in the relative amount of calories provided) and the energy-dense foods (foods that fill you up without providing a lot of calories). Generally speaking, the more you learn about and use these tools together, the more they will benefit your diet. Research has shown that individuals who read the Nutrition Facts when shopping for food report healthier nutrient consumption compared to nonusers.[16]

Exceptions to Food Labeling

Foods such as fresh fruits, vegetables, and fish currently are not required to have Nutrition Facts labels. However, many grocers have voluntarily chosen to provide their customers with information about these products on posters or pamphlets that may contain recipes that can assist you in your endeavor to improve your eating pattern.

The % Daily Value for protein is not mandatory on foods because protein deficiency is not a public health concern in the United States. If the % Daily Value for protein is given on a label, FDA requires that the product be analyzed for protein quality. This procedure is expensive and time-consuming, so many companies opt not to list a % Daily Value for protein. However, labels on food for infants and children under 4 years of age must include the % Daily Value for protein, as must the labels on any food carrying a claim about protein content.

LABELING OF FOOD ALLERGENS

The Food Allergen Labeling and Consumer Protection Act of 2004 (FALCPA) requires manufacturers to label food products that contain an ingredient that is or contains protein from a major food allergen. This information can be stated in one of two ways. The first option is to include the name of the food source in parenthesis following the common or usual name of the major food allergen in the list of ingredients if the name of the food source of the major allergen does not appear elsewhere in the ingredient list. The second option is to put the word *Contains* followed by the name of the food source from which the major food allergen is derived immediately after or adjacent to the list of ingredients in type size that is no smaller that the ingredient type size (example: Contains Wheat, Milk, Eggs, and Soy).

Health Claims on Food Labels

As a marketing tool directed toward the health-conscious consumer, food manufacturers like to claim that their products have all sorts of health benefits. FDA has legal oversight over most food products and permits some health claims with certain restrictions. Overall, claims on foods fall into one of four categories:

- Health claims—closely regulated by FDA
- Preliminary health claims—regulated by FDA, but evidence may be scant for the claim
- Nutrient claims—closely regulated by FDA (review Table 2-10)
- Structure/function claims—these are not FDA approved, or necessarily valid

Table 2-10 lists the definitions for nutrient claims on food labels. Currently, FDA limits the use of health messages to specific instances in which there is significant scientific agreement that a relationship exists between a nutrient, food, or food constituent and the disease. The claims allowed at this time may show a link (a "may" or "might" qualifier must be used in the statement) between an eating pattern and the following:

- enough calcium and vitamin D and a reduced risk of osteoporosis.
- low in total fat and a reduced risk of some cancers.
- low in saturated fat and cholesterol and a reduced risk of cardiovascular disease (typically referred to as heart disease on the label).
- rich in fiber—containing grain products, fruits, and vegetables— and a reduced risk of some cancers.
- low in sodium and high in potassium and a reduced risk of hypertension and stroke.
- rich in fruits and vegetables and a reduced risk of some cancers.
- adequate in the synthetic form of the vitamin folate (called folic acid) and a reduced risk of neural tube defects (a type of birth defect).
- sugarless gum and a reduced risk of tooth decay, especially when compared with foods high in sugars and starches.
- rich in fruits, vegetables, and grain products that contain fiber and a reduced risk of cardiovascular disease. Oats (oatmeal,

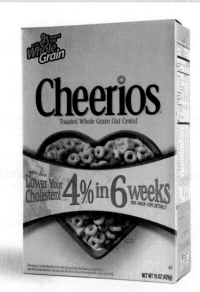

▲ Specific health claims can be made on food labels for whole grain cereals. Cheerios® are made from oats, which can be singled out in reducing the risk of cardiovascular disease as long as the statement also says that the eating pattern should be low in saturated fat and cholesterol. ©Jill Braaten, photographer/McGraw-Hill Education

oat bran, and oat flour) and psyllium are two fiber-rich ingredients that can be singled out in reducing the risk of cardiovascular disease, as long as the statement also says that the diet should be low in saturated fat and cholesterol.

- a diet rich in whole grain foods and other plant foods, as well as low in total fat, saturated fat, and cholesterol, and a reduced risk of cardiovascular disease and certain cancers.
- low in saturated fat and cholesterol that also includes 25 grams of soy protein and a reduced risk of cardiovascular disease. The statement "one serving of the (name of food) provides _____ grams of soy protein" must also appear as part of the health claim.
- fatty acids from oils present in fish and a reduced risk of cardiovascular disease.

- margarines containing plant stanols and sterols and a reduced risk of cardiovascular disease.

In addition, before a health claim can be made for a food product, it must meet two general requirements. First, the food must be a "good source" (before any fortification) of fiber, protein, vitamin A, vitamin C, calcium, or iron. (The legal definition of "good source" appears in Table 2-10.) Second, a single serving of the food product cannot contain more than 13 grams of fat, 4 grams of saturated fat, 60 milligrams of cholesterol, or 480 milligrams of sodium. If a food exceeds any one of these requirements, no health claim can be made for it, despite its other nutritional qualities. For example, even though whole milk is high in calcium, its label can't make the health claim about calcium and osteoporosis because whole milk contains 5 grams of saturated fat per serving. In another example, a health claim regarding fat and cancer can be made only if the product contains 3 grams or less of fat per serving, the standard for low-fat foods.

The FDA's 2003 Consumer Health Information for Better Nutrition Initiative also allows the use of qualified health claims when there is emerging evidence for a relationship between a food, food component, or dietary supplement and reduced risk of a disease or health-related condition. In this case, the evidence is not well enough established to meet the significant scientific agreement standard required for an FDA-authorized health claim. The following are examples of "Qualified Health Claims Subject to Enforcement Discretion." More information can be found at http://www.fda.gov/Food/IngredientsPackagingLabeling/LabelingNutrition/ucm073992.htm.

Qualified claims about cancer risk:
- Tomatoes and/or tomato sauce and prostate, ovarian, gastric, and pancreatic cancers
- Calcium and colon/rectal cancer and calcium and recurrent colon/rectal polyps

Qualified claims about cardiovascular disease risk:
- Nuts and heart disease
- Omega-3 fatty acids and coronary heart disease
- Monounsaturated fatty acids from olive oil and coronary heart disease

CASE STUDY Using the Nutrition Facts Label to Make Food Choices

On her way home from her afternoon nutrition class, Laura stops at the supermarket to pick up a few items she needs for the rest of the week. After picking up bananas, yogurt, bagels, and milk, she heads to the frozen food section to find a quick meal before a busy evening. She is in the mood for pasta and finds two brands of frozen cheese manicotti. Laura remembers to check out the Nutrition Facts panel for the two products to help her choose the healthiest option. Help Laura make the best choice by studying the Nutrition Facts labels for the two brands (Luigi's and Mario's) and answering the following questions.

1. Given that a serving of each product of manicotti weighs the same, which product has the highest energy density?
2. Calculate the calories from fat for each manicotti product. Divide the calories from fat by the total calories for each product. What is the percent calories from fat for Luigi's and Mario's?
3. Calculate the calories from the saturated fat for each manicotti product. For each, what is the percent of the total kilocalories that is saturated fat?
4. Laura sees that the total calories for Mario's manicotti are much lower than the calories for Luigi's. If she ate two packages of Mario's manicotti, how many calories would she consume?
5. How many servings of Luigi's manicotti would Laura need to consume to get 100% of her Daily Value of sodium?
6. The Daily Value for potassium is 4700 milligrams. What is the percent Daily Value for potassium in each manicotti product?
7. Which product has the higher nutrient density for potassium?

Nutrition Facts	
1 servings per container	
Serving size	**1 Package (260g)**
Amount per serving	
Calories	**390**
	% Daily Value*
Total Fat 18g	**27%**
Saturated Fat 9g	**45%**
Trans Fat 2g	
Cholesterol 45mg	**14%**
Sodium 880mg	**36%**
Total Carbohydrate 38g	**14%**
Dietary Fiber	**15%**
Total Sugars 12g	
Includes 10g Added Sugars	**20%**
Protein 17g	
Vitamin D 0mcg	0%
Calcium 400mg	31%
Iron 2mg	11%
Potassium 470mg	10%

* The % Daily Value (DV) tells you how much a nutrient in a serving of food contributes to a daily diet. 2,000 calories a day is used for general nutrition advice.

(a) Luigi's Manicotti

Nutrition Facts	
1 servings per container	
Serving size	**1 Package (260g)**
Amount per serving	
Calories	**230**
	% Daily Value*
Total Fat 4g	**6%**
Saturated Fat 2g	**10%**
Trans Fat 1g	
Cholesterol 15mg	**4%**
Sodium 590mg	**24%**
Total Carbohydrate 28g	**10%**
Dietary Fiber 3g	**12%**
Total Sugars 10g	
Includes 8g Added Sugars	**16%**
Protein 19g	
Vitamin D 0mcg	0%
Calcium 350mg	27%
Iron 1mg	6%
Potassium 280mg	6%

* The % Daily Value (DV) tells you how much a nutrient in a serving of food contributes to a daily diet. 2,000 calories a day is used for general nutrition advice.

(b) Mario's Manicotti

8. The Daily Value for calcium is 1300 milligrams. What is the percent Daily Value in each manicotti product?
9. Which product has the higher nutrient density for calcium?
10. Which of the two brands would you choose? What information on the Nutrition Facts label in the figure contributed to this decision?

Complete the Case Study. Responses to these questions can be provided by your instructor.

Summary (Numbers refer to numbered sections in the chapter.)

2.1 A healthy eating plan is based on consuming a *variety* of foods balanced by a *moderate* intake of each food and will minimize the risk of developing nutrition-related diseases.

Proportionality is eating foods with greater nutrient density and reflects the nutrient content of a food in relation to its calorie content. Nutrient-dense foods are relatively rich in nutrients, in comparison with calorie content.

Energy density of a food is determined by comparing calorie content with the weight of food. A food rich in calories but weighing relatively very little, such as nuts, cookies, fried foods in general, and most snack foods (including fat-free brands), is considered energy dense. Foods with low energy density include fruits, vegetables, and any food that incorporates lots of water during cooking, such as oatmeal.

2.2 *Dietary Guidelines* for Americans have been issued to help improve the health of all Americans ages 2 and older. The guidelines emphasize a healthy eating pattern that includes a variety of vegetables from all of the subgroups, whole fruits, whole grains, fat-free or low-fat dairy, a variety of protein foods, and oils; and limits saturated fats and *trans* fats, added sugars, and sodium.

2.3 MyPlate and accompanying online tools are designed to translate nutrient recommendations into a food plan that exhibits variety, proportionality, and moderation. The best results are obtained by using low-fat or fat-free dairy products, incorporating some vegetable proteins in the dietary pattern in addition to animal-protein foods, including citrus fruits and dark-green vegetables, and emphasizing whole grain breads and cereals.

2.4 A person's nutritional state can be categorized as *desirable nutrition,* in which the body has adequate stores for times of increased needs; *undernutrition,* which may be present with or without clinical symptoms; and *overnutrition,* which can lead to vitamin and mineral toxicities and various chronic diseases.

2.5 Evaluation of nutritional state involves analyzing background factors, as well as anthropometric, biochemical, clinical, dietary, and environmental assessments. It is not always possible to detect nutritional inadequacies via nutritional assessment because symptoms of deficiencies are often nonspecific and may not appear for many years.

2.6 Recommended Dietary Allowances (RDAs) are set for many nutrients. These amounts yield enough of each nutrient to meet the needs of healthy individuals within specific gender and age categories. Adequate Intake (AI) is the standard used when not enough information is available to set a more specific RDA. Estimated Energy Requirements (EERs) set calorie needs for both genders at various ages and physical activity patterns. Tolerable Upper Intake Levels (Upper Levels or ULs) for nutrient intake have been set for some vitamins and minerals. All of these dietary standards fall under the term *Dietary Reference Intakes (DRIs).*

Daily Values are used as a basis for expressing the nutrient content of foods on the Nutrition Facts panel and are based for the most part on the RDAs.

2.7 Apply the basic principles of nutrition to evaluate any nutrition claim. Several indicators of nutrition misinformation include insufficient scientific evidence to support a product claim, lack of credible sources, promises of unbelievable results, or distrust of the medical community. To sort nutrition fact from fiction, seek the advice of a registered dietitian nutritionist.

2.8 Food labels, especially the Nutrition Facts panels, are a useful tool to track your nutrient intake and learn more about the nutritional characteristics of the foods you eat. Changes to the Nutrition Facts panel have been approved recently and include increasing the type size for "Calories," "servings per container," and "Serving size." Any health claims listed must follow FDA-set criteria.

Check Your Knowledge (Answers are available at the end of this question set.)

1. Anthropometric measurements include
   a. height, weight, skinfolds, and body circumferences.
   b. blood concentrations of nutrients.
   c. a diet history of the previous days' intake.
   d. blood levels of enzyme activities.

2. Foods with *high* nutrient density offer the_____nutrients for the_____kilocalories.
   a. least, lowest
   b. least, most
   c. most, lowest
   d. most, most

3. A meal of a bean burrito, cucumber salad, and glass of milk represents foods from all MyPlate food groups except
   a. dairy.
   b. protein.
   c. vegetables.
   d. fruits.

4. The *Dietary Guidelines* for Americans provide advice for Americans
   a. from birth and older.
   b. from age 2 and older.
   c. from age 6 and older.
   d. from age 18 and older.

5. The *2015–2020 Dietary Guidelines* recommend that we increase which of the following foods?
   a. refined grains
   b. whole milk products
   c. seafood
   d. added sugars

6. How many minutes of moderate-intensity physical activity are recommended for adults in the *2008 Physical Activity Guidelines for Americans*?
   a. 150 minutes per week
   b. 60 minutes every day
   c. 50 minutes every day
   d. 30 minutes three days a week

7. The term *Daily Value* is used on
   a. restaurant menus.
   b. food labels.
   c. medical charts.
   d. health claims.

8. The Tolerable Upper Intake Level, or UL, is used to
   a. estimate calorie needs of the average person.
   b. evaluate the highest amount of daily nutrient intake unlikely to cause adverse health effects.
   c. evaluate your current intake for a specific nutrient.
   d. compare the nutrient content of a food to approximate human needs.

9. The current food label must list
   a. a picture of the product.
   b. a uniform and realistic serving size.
   c. the RDA for each age group.
   d. ingredients alphabetically.

10. The most common type of undernutrition in industrialized nations, such as the United States, is
    a. anorexia.
    b. protein deficiency.
    c. obesity.
    d. iron deficiency.

Answer Key: 1. a (LO 2.5), 2. c (LO 2.1), 3. d (LO 2.3),
4. b (LO 2.2), 5. c (LO 2.2), 6. a (LO 2.2),
7. b (LO 2.8), 8. b (LO 2.6), 9. b (LO 2.8), 10. d (LO 2.4)

Study Questions (Numbers refer to Learning Outcomes)

1. How would you explain the concepts of nutrient density and energy density to a fourth-grade class? (**LO 2.1**)

2. Describe the intent of the *Dietary Guidelines* for Americans. Based on the discussion of the *Dietary Guidelines* for Americans, suggest two key dietary changes the typical North American adult should consider making. (**LO 2.2**)

3. What changes to your eating pattern would you need to make to comply with the healthy eating guidelines exemplified by MyPlate on a regular basis? (**LO 2.3**)

4. Describe what would happen to the status of a nutrient in the body for a person who transitions from an overnourished to an undernourished state. (**LO 2.4**)

5. What steps would you follow to evaluate the nutritional state of an undernourished person? (**LO 2.5**)

6. How do RDAs and AIs differ from Daily Values in intention and application? (**LO 2.6**)

7. What would you list as the top five sources of reliable nutrition information? What makes these sources reliable? (**LO 2.7**)

8. Dietitians encourage all people to read labels on food packages to learn more about what they eat. What four nutrients could easily be tracked in your diet if you read the Nutrition Facts panels regularly on food products? (**LO 2.8**)

9. Define the USDA definition for the term *organic*. (**LO 2.8**)

10. List some specific health claims that can be made on food labels. (**LO 2.8**)

What the Dietitian Chose

It is smart to reach for a carbohydrate-containing beverage and snack when you need quick energy. Some of us also rely on caffeine in drinks to give us a boost. Many beverages on the market contain high concentrations of carbohydrate as "added sugar." Excessive sugar intake has been linked to several adverse health conditions. The major sources of added sugars are sodas, energy drinks, and sports drinks.

The main issue here is the abundance of empty calories supplied by soft drinks. Studies show that liquid calories do not promote satiety in the same way as food calories do. Excess calories from any source will lead to weight gain over time.

For these empty calories, portion size is a concern. A 20-ounce bottle of regular cola contains about 68 grams (about 15 teaspoons) of sweeteners. Both types of soft drink provide about 250 kcal. In terms of a soft drink, a 12-ounce soda, such as the Jones Root Beer Soda,® will have proportionally less sugar (48 grams) due to its smaller volume. If you consume one soft drink per day or less, the type of sweetener is not likely to make a big difference. If you consume several soft drinks per day, you would be better off choosing a beverage that does not contain calories, such as diet cola or water. Beverages with artificial sweeteners, such as Coke Zero,® typically are calorie free and therefore provide you with no energy when you need a boost. You may feel a temporary lift from the caffeine in some of these products. Water is the perfect drink to restore fluid losses and prevent dehydration, but it contains no calories for energy.

Your best choice when needing a quick energy boost in this case is low-fat chocolate milk. The nutrient-dense chocolate milk not only provides less sugar than the sodas on our list, but it is also the best source of total nutrition. Most convenience stores sell chocolate milk in pint bottles or half-pint (8-ounce) cartons (similar to those served in school cafeterias). The 8-ounce carton of chocolate milk provides a good amount of kilocalories (150 kcal) as well as 8 grams of protein, 2.5 grams of fat, and 25 grams of sugar. It also provides calcium (290 milligrams), vitamin A (490 IU), and vitamin D (2.8 micrograms), as well as other vitamins and minerals. A pint bottle (16 ounces) would provide twice the amount of kilocalories and other nutrients. In addition, the chocolate provides a source of caffeine that you may be looking for.

The same criteria of nutrient density should be used when choosing a snack. While all of the snack choices provide an appropriate amount of calories, they differ significantly in their saturated fat, sugar, and sodium contents. The potato chips (160 kcal) contain unnecessary saturated fat (1.5 grams) and sodium (170 milligrams), and provide only 2 grams of protein, as do the potato crisps (120 kcal, 135 milligrams sodium). The raisins (90 kcal) are high in sugar (20 grams) and lowest in protein

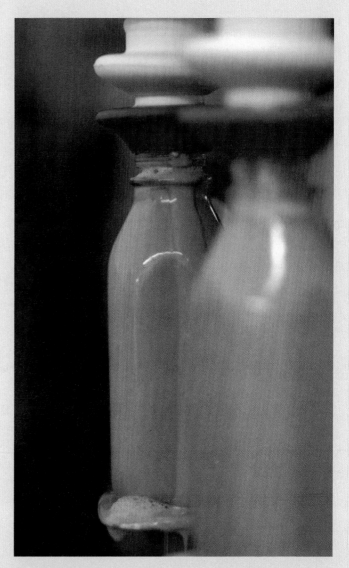

▲ Chocolate milk is a very nutritious beverage that provides protein, vitamins, and minerals, along with calories. ©Real Food by Warren Diggles/Alamy

(1 gram). Although the M&Ms® provide the most calories (240 kcal) and are paired with the no-calorie water, they also provide the most saturated fat (6 g) and sugar (30 g) and only 2 grams of protein. The pouch of almonds scores the highest in nutrient density, providing 100 kcal, 4 grams of protein, 2 grams of fiber, and no sodium, and is a perfect complement to the chocolate milk.

Further Readings

1. Schwingshackl L and Hoffmann G: Does a Mediterranean-type diet reduce cancer risk? *Curr Nutr Rep* 2016;5:9.

2. Alissa EM and Ferns GA. Dietary fruits and vegetables and cardiovascular diseases risk. *Crit Rev Food Sci Nutr* 2017;57:1950.

3. Perez-Escamilla R and others: Dietary energy density and body weight in adults and children: A systematic review. *J Acad Nutr Diet* 2012;112:671.

4. Rolls B, Hermann M: *The Ultimate Volumetrics Diet: Smart, Simple, Science-Based Strategies for Losing Weight and Keeping It Off.* New York: HarperCollins, 2012.

5. Pechey R and Monsivais P: Socioeconomic inequalities in the healthiness of food choices: Exploring the contributions of food expenditures. *Prev Med* 2016;88:203.

6. Aggarwal A and others: Positive attitude toward healthy eating predicts higher diet quality at all cost levels of supermarkets. *J Acad Nutr Diet* 2014;114:266.

7. Watts ML and others: The art of translating nutritional science into dietary guidance: History and evolution of the *Dietary Guidelines* for Americans. *Nutr Rev* 2011;69:404.

8. Ivens BJ and others: Translating the *Dietary Guidelines* to promote behavior change: Perspectives from the Food and Nutrition Science Solutions Joint Task Force. *J Acad Nutr Diet* 2016;116:1697.

9. U.S. Department of Health and Human Services and U.S. Department of Agriculture: *2015–2020 Dietary Guidelines for Americans. 8th Edition.* December 2015. Available at http://health.gov/dietaryguidelines/2015/guidelines/ (Accessed January 15, 2017).

10. Robinson J: *Eating on the Wild Side: The Missing Link to Optimum Health.* New York: Little, Brown and Company, 2013.

11. Moyer L: Five things to check before you buy breakfast cereal. Our tips for finding the healthiest cereal. Nutrition Action.com http://www.nutritionaction.com/daily/what-to-eat/five-things-to-check-before-you-buy-breakfast-cereal/ Posted December 5, 2016.

12. U.S. Department of Health and Human Services: *2008 Physical Activity Guidelines for Americans.* 2008. www.health.gov/PAGuidelines/. (Updated/accessed January 18, 2017).

13. U.S. Department of Agriculture: USDA's MyPlate. July 2015. www.choosemyplate.gov. (Accessed January 15, 2017).

14. Chiuve SE and others: Adherence to a low risk, healthy lifestyle and risk of sudden cardiac death among women. *J Amer Med Asso* 2011;306:62.

15. Academy of Nutrition and Dietetics: Practice Paper of the Academy of Nutrition and Dietetics: Communicating accurate food and nutrition information. *J Acad Nutr Diet* 2012;112:759.

16. Ollberding NJ and others: Food label use and its relation to dietary intake among U.S. adults. *J Amer Diet Asso* 2010;110:1233.

connect To get the most out of your study, visit Connect where you will find NutritionCalc Plus, SmartBook®, and many other dynamic tools.

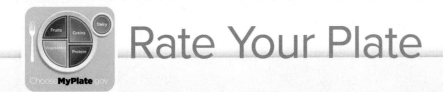

Rate Your Plate

Does Your Diet Compare to MyPlate?

Using your food-intake record from Chapter 1, place each food item in the appropriate group of the accompanying MyPlate chart. That is, for each food item, indicate how many servings it contributes to each group based on the amount you ate. Many of your food choices may contribute to more than one group. For example, spaghetti with meat sauce contributes to three categories: grains, vegetables, and proteins. After entering all the values, add the number of servings consumed in each group. Finally, compare your total in each food group with the recommended number of servings shown in Table 2-5 or obtained from the ChooseMyPlate.gov website. Enter a minus sign (–) if your total falls below the recommendation or a plus sign (+) if it equals or exceeds the recommendation.

Indicate the number of servings from MyPlate that each food yields:

Food or Beverage	Amount Eaten	Grains	Vegetables	Fruits	Dairy	Protein
Group totals						
Recommended servings						
Shortages/overages in numbers of servings						

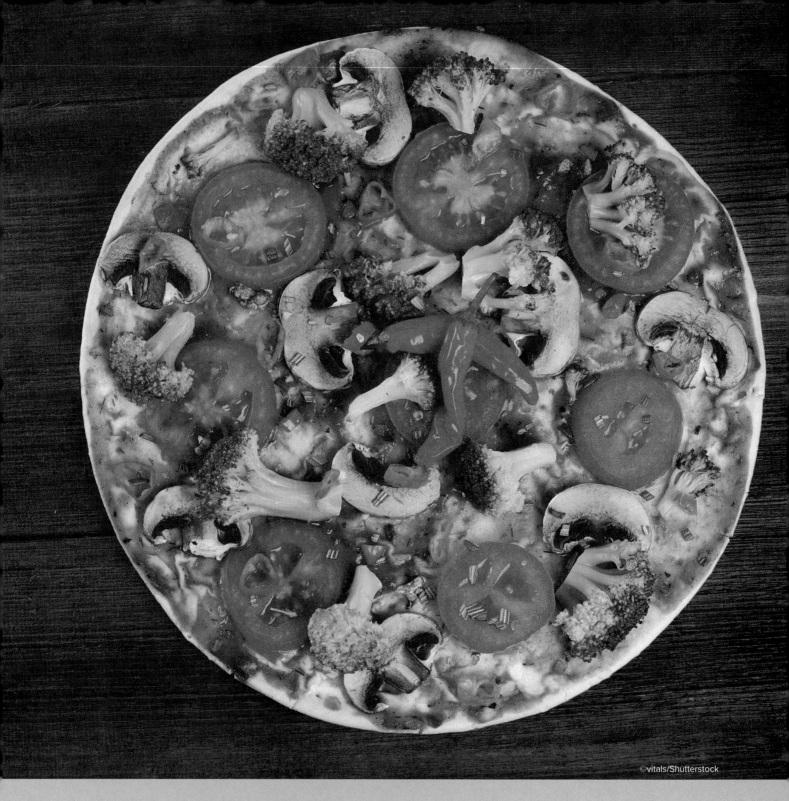

Student Learning Outcomes

Chapter 3 is designed to allow you to:

3.1 Understand some basic roles of nutrients in human physiology.

3.2 Identify the functions of the common cellular components.

3.3 Define *tissue*, *organ*, and *organ system*.

3.4 Identify the role of the cardiovascular and lymphatic systems in nutrition.

3.5 List basic characteristics of the nervous system and its role in nutrition.

3.6 List basic characteristics of the endocrine system, especially the pancreas, and its role in nutrition.

3.7 List basic characteristics of the immune system and its role in nutrition.

Chapter 3

The Human Body: A Nutrition Perspective

What Would You Choose?

For spring break, you are volunteering to help build a house with Habitat for Humanity. You are carpooling with some friends and staying in a retreat house. Unfortunately, the travel, budget, living accommodations, and your building schedule won't allow for home-cooked meals this week. Being out of your normal routine and relying on fast-food sandwiches and pizza have left you feeling constipated. This reminds you that you will need to make smarter choices at fast-food establishments. To decrease your constipation, which menu combination would you choose from a pizza buffet?

a 2 slices of pepperoni pizza and 2 cups of tossed salad

b 2 slices of veggie pizza and 1 cup of bean and pasta soup

c 2 slices of ham and pineapple pizza and 1 cup of pasta with Alfredo sauce

d 2 slices of cheese pizza and 1 garlic breadstick with marinara sauce

Think about your choices as you read this chapter, then see What the Dietitian Chose at the end of the chapter.

Merely eating food won't nourish you. You must first digest the food by breaking it down into usable forms of the essential nutrients that can be absorbed into the bloodstream. Once nutrients are taken up by the bloodstream, they can be distributed to and used by body cells.

We rarely think about digesting and absorbing foods. Except for a few voluntary responses—such as deciding what and when to eat, how well to chew food, and when to eliminate the remains—most digestion and absorption processes control themselves. We don't consciously decide when the pancreas will secrete digestive substances into the small intestine or how quickly foodstuffs will be propelled down the intestinal tract. Hormones and nerve impulses control these functions. Your only awareness of these involuntary responses may be a hunger pang right before lunch or a "full" feeling after eating that last slice of pizza.

You've learned about cells, tissues, and organs before, but now let's look at the human body from a nutrition perspective. Refresh your memory of the basic anatomy (structure) and physiology (function) of the circulatory system, nervous system, endocrine system, immune system, and urinary system. In particular, as you focus on the digestive system, you will gain an in-depth understanding of how the food you eat nourishes your body.

3.8 Outline the overall processes of digestion and absorption in the mouth, stomach, small intestine, and large intestine, as well as the roles played by the liver, gallbladder, and pancreas.

3.9 List basic characteristics of the urinary system and its role in nutrition.

3.10 Understand the importance of the body storage areas for nutrients.

3.11 Understand the emerging field of nutritional genomics.

3.12 Identify the major nutrition-related gastrointestinal health problems and approaches to treatment.

3.1 Nutrition's Role in Human Physiology

The everyday function of the human body relies on the coordination of many complex organ systems. Together, these systems are composed of trillions of cells. Each cell is a self-contained, living entity. Cells of the same type normally join together to form **tissues,** such as muscle tissue. One, two, or more tissues then combine in a particular way to form more complex structures called **organs.** All organs contribute to nutritional health, and a person's overall nutritional state determines how well each organ functions. At a still higher level of coordination, several organs that work together form an **organ system,** such as the digestive system.

Chemical processes (reactions) occur constantly in every living cell; the production of new substances is balanced by the breakdown of older ones. An example is the constant formation and degradation of bone. For this turnover of substances to occur, cells require a continuous supply of energy derived from dietary carbohydrate, protein, and/or fat. Cells also need water; building supplies, especially protein and minerals; and chemical regulators, such as the vitamins. Almost all cells also need a steady supply of oxygen. These substances enable the tissues, made of individual cells, to function properly.

Getting an adequate supply of all nutrients to the body's cells begins with a healthy diet. To ensure optimal use of nutrients, the body's cells, tissues, organs, and organ systems also must work efficiently.

This chapter covers the anatomy and physiology of the cell and major organ systems, especially as they relate to human nutrition. In later chapters, you will examine the intricacies of each of the essential nutrients, but let us start out by admiring the "big picture" of the human body.

tissues Collections of cells adapted to perform a specific function.

organ A group of tissues designed to perform a specific function; for example, the heart, which contains muscle tissue, nerve tissue, and so on.

organ system A collection of organs that work together to perform an overall function.

> ✓ **CONCEPT CHECK 3.1**
>
> 1. Discuss the levels of organization of the human body.
> 2. Describe three ways essential nutrients support cell functions.

3.2 The Cell: Structure, Function, and Metabolism

The cell is the basic structural and functional component of life. Living organisms are made of many different kinds of cells specialized to perform particular functions, and all cells are derived from preexisting cells. In the human body, all cells have certain common features. These cells have membranes and **organelles** that perform specialized functions (Fig. 3-1). There are at least 15 different organelles, but the nutritional relevance of just six of the organelles will be examined here. Metabolism, the chemical processes that take place in body cells, is also discussed.

organelles Compartments, particles, or filaments that perform specialized functions within a cell.

CELL (PLASMA) MEMBRANE

There is an outside and inside to every cell, separated by the cell (plasma) membrane. (Please note that animal cells do not have cell walls.) The cell membrane itself is not an organelle, but it holds the cellular contents (cytoplasm and organelles) together and regulates the flow of substances into and out of the cell. Cell-to-cell communication also occurs by way of this membrane.

The cell membrane, illustrated in Figure 3-1(b), is a lipid bilayer (or double membrane) of **phospholipids** with their water-soluble heads facing both the interior and the exterior of the cell. Their water-insoluble tails are tucked into the interior of the cell membrane.

phospholipid Any of a class of fat-related substances that contain phosphorus, fatty acids, and a nitrogen-containing component. Phospholipids are an essential part of every cell.

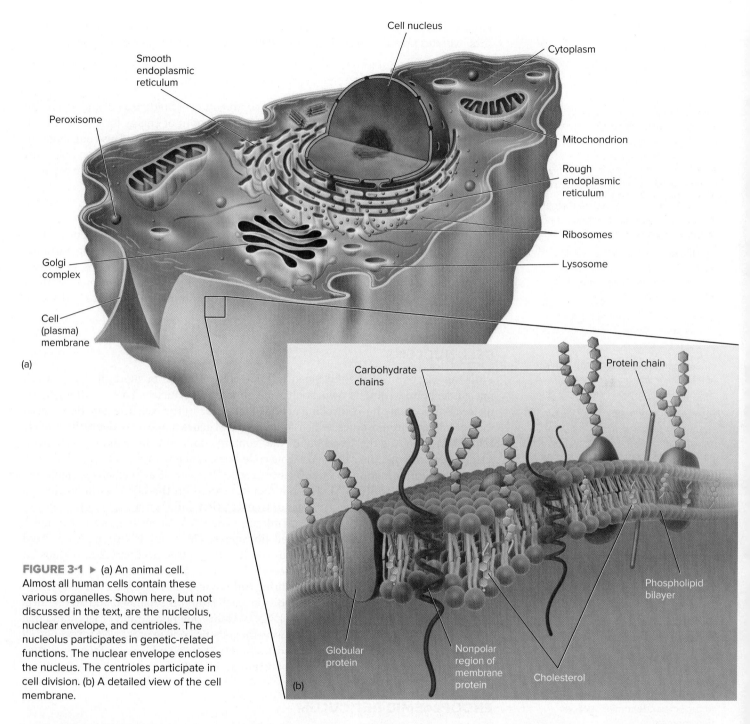

FIGURE 3-1 ▶ (a) An animal cell. Almost all human cells contain these various organelles. Shown here, but not discussed in the text, are the nucleolus, nuclear envelope, and centrioles. The nucleolus participates in genetic-related functions. The nuclear envelope encloses the nucleus. The centrioles participate in cell division. (b) A detailed view of the cell membrane.

Cholesterol is another component of the cell membrane. It is fat soluble, so it is embedded within the bilayer. This cholesterol provides rigidity and thus stability to the membrane.

Some of these proteins provide structural support, while others function as **enzymes** to regulate chemical reactions (see Section 3.9 for more about enzymes). Other proteins serve as transport vehicles. They may shuttle substances across the membrane or act as gates that open and close to control the flow of various particles into and out of the cell. Still other proteins on the outside surface of the membrane act as receptors, snagging essential substances that the cell needs and drawing them into the cell.

In addition to lipids and proteins, the membrane also contains carbohydrates that mark the exterior of the cell. These carbohydrates are combined with either protein or fat, and they help send messages to the cell's organelles and act as identification markers

cholesterol A waxy lipid found in all body cells. It has a structure containing multiple chemical rings that is found only in foods that contain animal products.

enzyme A compound that speeds the rate of a chemical reaction but is not altered by the reaction. Almost all enzymes are proteins.

for the cell. In addition, they detect invaders and initiate defensive actions. In sum, these carbohydrates provide tags that are important to cellular identity and interaction.

CYTOPLASM

The **cytoplasm** (also known as cytosol) is the combination of fluid material and organelles within the cell, not including the nucleus. A small amount of energy for use by the cell can be produced by chemical processes that occur in the cytoplasm. This contributes to the survival of all cells and is the sole source of energy production in red blood cells. This energy production is called **anaerobic** metabolism because it does not require oxygen.

MITOCHONDRIA

Mitochondria are sometimes called the "power plants" or the "powerhouse" of the cell. These organelles are capable of converting the food energy in energy-yielding nutrients (carbohydrate, protein, and fat) to a form of energy that cells can use. This is an **aerobic** process that uses the oxygen we inhale, along with water, enzymes, and some vitamins and minerals. Except for red blood cells, all cells contain mitochondria; only the size, shape, and quantity vary.

CELL NUCLEUS

With the exception of the red blood cell, all cells have one or more nuclei. The **cell nucleus** is bounded by its own double membrane. The nucleus contains the genetic material responsible for controlling actions that occur in the cell. The genetic material includes many **chromosomes,** which contain several **genes** made up of **deoxyribonucleic acid (DNA).** DNA is the "code book" that contains directions for making substances, specifically proteins, the cell needs. This code book remains in the nucleus of the cell but sends its information to other cell organelles by way of a "messenger" molecule called **ribonucleic acid (RNA).** The information stored on the DNA in the nucleus is copied onto RNA through the process of **transcription** and then moves out to the cytoplasm through pores in the nuclear membrane. The RNA carries the transcribed DNA code to protein-synthesizing sites called **ribosomes.** There, the RNA template is used in the process of **translation** to make a specific protein (see Section 6.2 for details on protein synthesis). Altogether, this process is known as **gene expression.**

All of the DNA in a cell is copied during cell replication. DNA is a double-stranded molecule, and when the cell begins to divide, each strand is separated and an identical copy of each is made. Thus, each new DNA contains one new strand of DNA and one strand from the original DNA. In this way, the genetic code is preserved from one cell generation to the next. (The mitochondria contain their own DNA, so they reproduce themselves within a cell independent of action in the cell's nucleus.)

ENDOPLASMIC RETICULUM

The outer membrane of the cell nucleus is continuous with a network of tubes called the **endoplasmic reticulum (ER).** Part of the endoplasmic reticulum (termed the rough [as opposed to smooth] ER) contains the ribosomes, where the RNA code is translated into proteins during protein synthesis. Many of these proteins play a central role in human nutrition. Parts of the endoplasmic reticulum are also involved in lipid synthesis, detoxification of toxic substances, and calcium storage and release in the cell.

GOLGI COMPLEX

The **Golgi complex** is a packaging site for proteins used in the cytoplasm or exported from the cell. It consists of sacs within the cytoplasm in which proteins are "packaged" as **secretory vesicles** for secretion by the cell.

cytoplasm The fluid and organelles (except the nucleus) in a cell; also called cytosol.

mitochondria Organelles that are the main sites of energy production in a cell. They contain the pathway for oxidizing fat for fuel, among other metabolic pathways.

cell nucleus Membrane-bound organelle that contains the genetic information (DNA) for protein synthesis and cell replication.

chromosome A single, large DNA molecule and its associated proteins; contains many genes to store and transmit genetic information.

gene A specific segment on a chromosome. Genes provide the blueprint for the production of cell proteins.

deoxyribonucleic acid (DNA) The site of hereditary information in cells; DNA directs the synthesis of cell proteins.

ribonucleic acid (RNA) The single-stranded nucleic acid involved in the transcription of genetic information and translation of that information into protein structure.

transcription Process by which genetic information stored as DNA within the nucleus is copied to RNA during protein synthesis.

ribosomes Cytoplasmic particles that mediate the linking together of amino acids to form proteins; may exist freely in the cytoplasm or attached to endoplasmic reticulum.

translation Process by which genetic information copied into RNA dictates the amino acid sequence to form a protein.

gene expression Use of DNA information on a gene to produce a protein. Thought to be a major determinant of cell development.

endoplasmic reticulum (ER) An organelle composed of a network of canals running through the cytoplasm. Part of the endoplasmic reticulum contains ribosomes.

Golgi complex The cell organelle near the nucleus that processes newly synthesized protein for secretion or distribution to other organelles.

secretory vesicles Membrane-bound vesicles produced by the Golgi complex; contain protein and other compounds to be secreted by the cell.

LYSOSOMES

Lysosomes are the cell's digestive system. They are sacs that contain enzymes for the digestion of foreign material. Sometimes known as "suicide bags," they are responsible for digesting worn-out or damaged cell components. Certain cells associated with immune functions contain many lysosomes.

PEROXISOMES

Peroxisomes contain enzymes that detoxify harmful chemicals. Peroxisomes get their name from the fact that hydrogen peroxide (H_2O_2) is formed as a result of such enzyme action. Peroxisomes also contain a protective enzyme called **catalase,** which prevents excessive accumulation of hydrogen peroxide in the cell, which would be very damaging. Peroxisomes also play a minor role in metabolizing one possible source of energy for cells—alcohol.

CELL METABOLISM

Metabolism refers to the entire collection of chemical processes involved in maintaining life. It encompasses all the sequences of chemical reactions that occur in the body's cells. These biochemical reactions take place in the cell cytoplasm and organelles that we have just discussed. They enable us to release and use energy from foods, synthesize one substance from another, and prepare waste products for excretion.

The reactions of metabolism that take place within your body can be categorized into one of two types. One type of reaction, *anabolic,* puts different molecules together and, therefore, requires energy. The other type of reaction, *catabolic,* takes molecules apart and, therefore, releases energy. The metabolism of carbohydrates, proteins, and fats yields energy. Vitamins and minerals contribute to the enzyme activity that supports metabolic reactions in the cell.

The metabolism of energy production begins in the cytoplasm with the initial anaerobic breakdown of glucose. The remaining aerobic steps of energy production take place in the mitochondria. Ultimately, the cells of the body use these interconnected processes to convert the energy found in food to energy stored in the high-energy compound **adenosine triphosphate (ATP).** You will learn more about energy metabolism in Chapter 10.

lysosome A cellular organelle that contains digestive enzymes for use inside the cell for turnover of cell parts.

peroxisome A cell organelle that destroys toxic products within the cell.

catalase Enzyme that catalyzes the decomposition of hydrogen peroxide into water and oxygen.

adenosine triphosphate (ATP) The main energy currency for cells. ATP energy is used to promote ion pumping, enzyme activity, and muscular contraction.

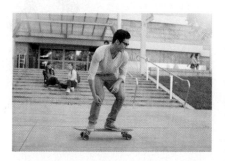

▲ Where do you get the energy to work and play? Your cells use the energy stored in the chemical bonds of carbohydrates, fats, and proteins to generate ATP. ©Sam Edwards/Getty Images

✓ CONCEPT CHECK 3.2

1. What is an organelle?
2. Choose three organelles and explain their relevance to human nutrition.
3. What is the difference between anabolic and catabolic reactions?
4. What is ATP?

3.3 Body Systems

As noted earlier, when groups of similar cells work together to accomplish a specialized task, the arrangement is referred to as a tissue. Humans are composed of four primary types of tissue: **epithelial, connective, muscle,** and **nervous** tissue. Epithelial tissue is composed of cells that cover surfaces both inside and outside the body. For example, the lining of the respiratory tract is made up of epithelial cells. Epithelial cells secrete important substances, absorb nutrients, and excrete waste. Connective tissue supports and protects the body, stores fat, and produces blood cells. Muscle tissue is designed for movement. Nervous tissue found in the brain and spinal cord is designed for communication. These four types of tissues then go on to form various organs and, ultimately, organ systems (Fig. 3-2).

epithelial tissue The surface cells that line the outside of the body and all external passages within it.

connective tissue Protein tissue that holds different structures in the body together. Some body structures are made up of connective tissue—notably, tendons and cartilage. Connective tissue also forms part of bone and the nonmuscular structures of arteries and veins.

muscle tissue A type of tissue adapted to contract to cause movement.

nervous tissue Tissue composed of highly branched, elongated cells that transport nerve impulses from one part of the body to another.

Cardiovascular System

Major components
heart, blood vessels, and blood

Functions
• Carries blood and regulates blood supply

• Transports nutrients, waste products, hormones, and gases (oxygen and carbon dioxide) throughout the body

• Regulates blood pressure

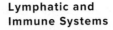

Lymphatic and Immune Systems

Major lymphatic components
lymph, lymphocytes, lymphatic vessels, and lymph nodes

Major immune components
white blood cells, lymph vessels and nodes, spleen, thymus gland, and other lymph tissues

Lymphatic functions
• Removes foreign substances from blood and lymph

• Maintains tissue fluid balance

• Aids fat absorption

Immune functions
• Provides defense against pathogens

• Formation of white blood cells

Urinary System

Major components
kidneys, urinary bladder, and the ducts that carry urine

Functions
• Removes waste products from the blood and forms urine

• Regulates blood acid–base (pH) balance, overall chemical balance, and water balance

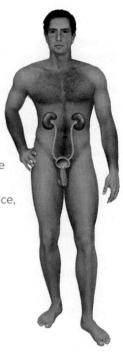

Nervous System

Major components
brain, spinal cord, nerves, and sensory receptors

Functions
• Detects and interprets sensation

• Controls movements, physiological, and intellectual functions

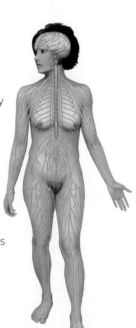

Endocrine System

Major components
endocrine glands, such as the pituitary, thyroid, and adrenal glands; hypothalamus; and pancreas

Functions
• Regulates metabolism, growth, reproduction, and many other functions by producing and releasing hormones

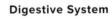

Digestive System

Major components
mouth, esophagus, stomach, intestines, and accessory organs (liver, gallbladder, and pancreas)

Functions
• Performs the mechanical and chemical processes of digestion of food, absorption of nutrients, and elimination of wastes

• Assists the immune system by destroying some pathogens and forming a barrier against foreign materials

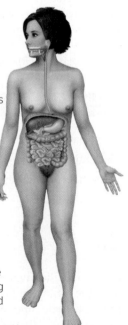

FIGURE 3-2 ▲ Organ systems of the body. ©McGraw-Hill Education

Integumentary System

Major components
skin, hair, nails, and sweat glands

Functions
- Protects the body
- Regulates body temperature
- Prevents water loss
- Produces vitamin D

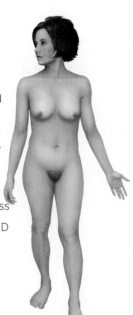

Skeletal System

Major components
bones, cartilage, ligaments, and joints

Functions
- Protects organs
- Supports body weight
- Allows body movement
- Produces blood cells
- Stores minerals

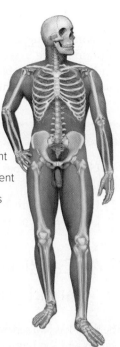

Muscular System

Major components
smooth, cardiac, and skeletal muscle

Functions
- Produces body movement, heartbeat, and body heat
- Propels food in the digestive tract
- Maintains posture

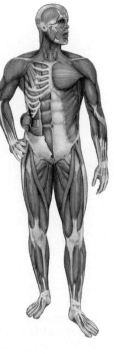

Respiratory System

Major components
lungs and respiratory passages

Functions
- Exchanges gases (oxygen and carbon dioxide) between the blood and the air
- Regulates blood acid–base (pH) balance

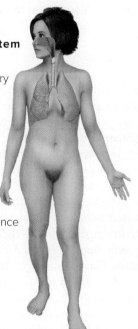

Reproductive System

Major components
gonads (ovaries and testes), genitals, and breasts

Functions
- Performs the processes of sexual maturation and reproduction
- Influences sexual functions and behaviors
- Produces human milk to nourish an infant

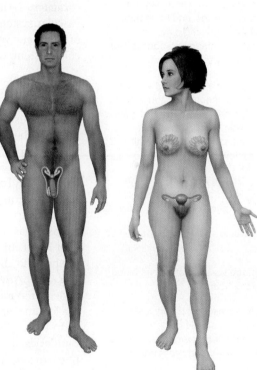

FIGURE 3-2 ▲ *(Continued)*

Sometimes organs within a system can serve another system. For example, the basic function of the digestive system is to convert the food we eat into absorbable nutrients. At the same time, the digestive system serves the immune system by preventing dangerous pathogens from invading and causing illness in the body. As you study nutrition, you will note the multiple roles played by many organs (see Fig. 3-2).

The main objective of this chapter is to understand the actions of nutrients as they affect different cells, tissues, organs, and organ systems. As we explore several key organ systems—cardiovascular, lymphatic, urinary, nervous, endocrine, immune, and digestive systems—look for the ways each system both *affects* and *is affected by* nutrition.

Also in this chapter, we introduce the study of interactions between genetics and nutrition. Throughout this book, discussions will point out how you can personalize nutrition advice based on your genetic background. In this way, you can identify and avoid some controllable risk factors that would contribute to development of genetically linked diseases present in your family.

✔ CONCEPT CHECK 3.3

1. List the four types of tissues, and give an example of where you could find each in the body.
2. Examine Figure 3-2. Provide three examples of ways the organs of one system support the functions of another system.

3.4 Cardiovascular System and Lymphatic System

cardiovascular system The body system consisting of the heart, blood vessels, and blood. This system transports nutrients, waste products, gases, and hormones throughout the body and plays an important role in immune responses and regulation of body temperature.

lymphatic system A system of vessels and lymph that accepts fluid surrounding cells and large particles, such as products of fat absorption. Lymph eventually passes into the bloodstream from the lymphatic system.

lymph A clear fluid that flows through lymph vessels; carries most forms of fat after their absorption by the small intestine.

plasma The fluid, extracellular portion of blood.

artery A blood vessel that carries blood away from the heart.

capillary A microscopic blood vessel that connects the smallest arteries and veins; site of nutrient, oxygen, and waste exchange between body cells and the blood.

vein A blood vessel that carries blood to the heart.

The body has two separate organ systems that circulate fluids in the body: the **cardiovascular system** and the **lymphatic system.** Some texts group these two systems together as the *circulatory system,* but each system has distinct components and functions. The cardiovascular system consists of the heart and blood vessels. The lymphatic system consists of lymphatic vessels and a number of lymph tissues. Blood flows through the cardiovascular system, while **lymph** flows through the lymphatic system.

CARDIOVASCULAR SYSTEM

The heart is a muscular pump that normally contracts and relaxes 50 to 90 times per minute when the body is at rest. This continual pumping, measured by taking your pulse, keeps blood moving through the blood vessels. The blood that flows through the cardiovascular system is composed of **plasma,** red blood cells, white blood cells, platelets, and many other substances. It travels two basic routes. In the first route, blood circulates from the right side of the heart, through the lungs, and then back to the heart. In the lungs, blood picks up oxygen and releases carbon dioxide. After this exchange of gases has taken place, blood is said to be *oxygenated* and returns to the left side of your heart. In the second route, the oxygenated blood circulates from the left side of the heart to all other body cells, eventually returning back to the right side of the heart (Fig. 3-3). After blood has circulated throughout the body, it is *deoxygenated.* (As you review anatomy diagrams in this book, recognize that *left* and *right* designations refer to the left and right sides of your body, not of the diagram in front of you.)

In the cardiovascular system, blood leaves the heart via **arteries,** which branch into **capillaries,** a network of tiny blood vessels that are just one cell layer thick. Exchange of nutrients, oxygen, and waste products between the blood and cells occurs through the tiny, weblike pores of the capillaries (Fig. 3-4). The blood then returns to the heart via the **veins.**

The cardiovascular system facilitates the exchange of oxygen, nutrients, and wastes between the body's internal and external environments. Other functions include delivery of hormones to their target cells, maintenance of a constant body temperature, and distribution of white blood cells throughout the body to protect against pathogens as part of the immune system (see Section 3.8).

Portal Circulation in the Gastrointestinal Tract Once absorbed through the stomach or intestinal wall, nutrients reach one of two destinations. Some nutrients are taken up by cells in the intestines and portions of the stomach to nourish those organs. Most of these water-soluble nutrients from recently eaten foods, however, are transferred into

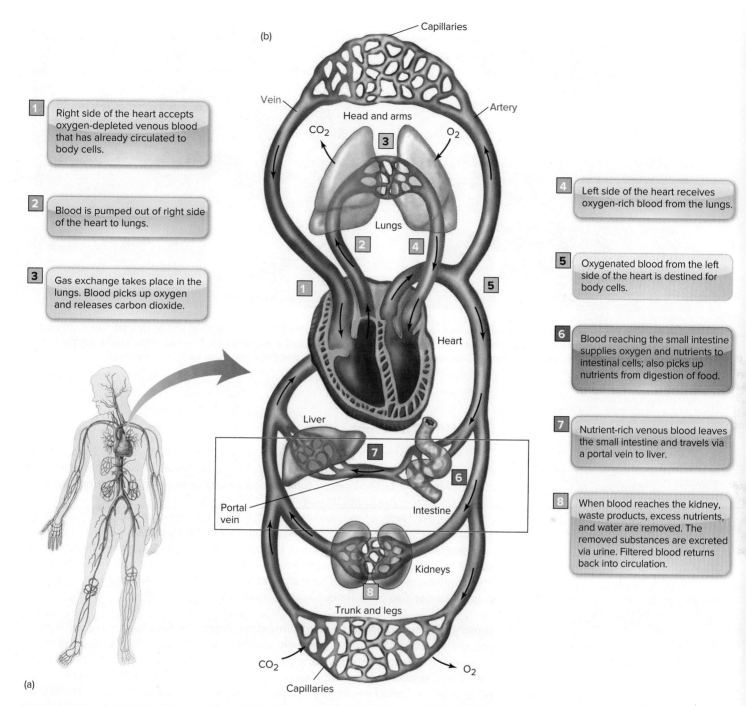

1 Right side of the heart accepts oxygen-depleted venous blood that has already circulated to body cells.

2 Blood is pumped out of right side of the heart to lungs.

3 Gas exchange takes place in the lungs. Blood picks up oxygen and releases carbon dioxide.

4 Left side of the heart receives oxygen-rich blood from the lungs.

5 Oxygenated blood from the left side of the heart is destined for body cells.

6 Blood reaching the small intestine supplies oxygen and nutrients to intestinal cells; also picks up nutrients from digestion of food.

7 Nutrient-rich venous blood leaves the small intestine and travels via a portal vein to liver.

8 When blood reaches the kidney, waste products, excess nutrients, and water are removed. The removed substances are excreted via urine. Filtered blood returns back into circulation.

FIGURE 3-3 ▲ Blood circulation through the body. (a) The heart and some examples of the major arteries and veins of the cardiovascular system. (b) The paths that blood takes from the heart to the lungs (1–3), back to the heart (4), and through the rest of the body (5–8). The red color indicates blood richer in oxygen; blue is for blood carrying more carbon dioxide. Keep in mind that arteries and veins go to all parts of the body.

the **hepatic portal circulation.** (The term *hepatic* refers to the liver. There are other portal systems in physiology, but the simpler terms *portal circulation* or *portal vein* usually refer to hepatic portal circulation.) To enter portal circulation, the nutrients pass from the intestinal capillaries into veins that eventually merge into a very large vein called the **hepatic portal vein.** Unlike most veins in the body—which carry blood back to the heart—this portal vein leads directly to the liver. This enables the liver to process absorbed nutrients before they enter the general circulation of the bloodstream. Overall, hepatic portal circulation represents a special form of circulation in the cardiovascular system.

hepatic portal circulation The portion of the circulatory system that uses a large vein (portal vein) to carry nutrient-rich blood from capillaries in the intestines and portions of the stomach to the liver.

hepatic portal vein Large vein that carries absorbed nutrients from the gastrointestinal tract to the liver.

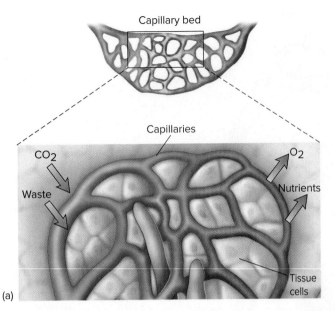
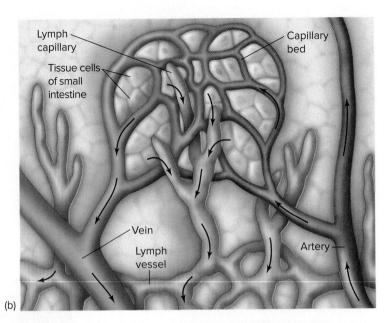

FIGURE 3-4 ▲ Capillary and lymph vessels. (a) Exchange of oxygen (O_2) and nutrients for carbon dioxide (CO_2) and other waste products occurs between the capillaries and the surrounding tissue cells. (b) Lymph vessels are also present in capillary beds, such as in the small intestine. Lymph vessels in the small intestine are also called *lacteals.* The lymph vessels have closed ends and are important for fat absorption.

LYMPHATIC SYSTEM

The lymphatic system consists of a network of lymphatic vessels and the fluid (lymph) that moves through them. The lymph vessels take up excess fluid that collects between cells and return it to the bloodstream. Lymph is similar to blood, consisting largely of blood plasma that has found its way out of capillaries and into the spaces between cells. It contains a full array of the various white blood cells that play an important role in the immune system. However, neither red blood cells nor platelets are present. Lymph is collected in tiny lymph vessels all over the body and moves through even larger vessels until it eventually enters the cardiovascular system through major veins near the heart. The lymphatic system does not have a pump (like the heart); its flow is driven by muscle contractions arising from normal body movements.

lacteal Lymphatic vessel that absorbs fats from the small intestine.

Lymphatic Circulation in the Gastrointestinal Tract The lymphatic vessels that serve the gastrointestinal tract are specifically known as **lacteals.** Besides contributing to the defense of the body against invading pathogens, lacteals play an important role in nutrition. These vessels pick up and transport the majority of products of fat digestion and fat absorption. These fat-related products are too large to enter the bloodstream directly and therefore are generally emptied into the bloodstream only after passing through the lymphatic system.

✓ CONCEPT CHECK 3.4

1. Describe how nutrients, oxygen, and wastes are exchanged between the body's internal and external environments.
2. What is hepatic portal circulation?
3. Which nutrients are absorbed into the lymph? Why?

FARM to FORK   Cranberries

Grow
- Cranberries grow in bogs. Growers sometimes flood the bogs to harvest cranberries, knocking them off their vines with special farm equipment, then quickly collecting the berries when they float to the surface.
- Cold temperatures actually increase the sugar content of the berries, making them less tart.
- Fresh cranberries are widely available during the winter months, but the frozen or dried varieties are quite nutritious and can be enjoyed throughout the year.

Shop
- Look for firm berries with the deepest red color. The red pigments (anthocyanins) are powerful cancer-fighting phytochemicals!
- Food manufacturers add sugars to dried cranberries. Choose varieties that are made with less sugar.
- Although it doesn't pack quite the same disease-fighting punch as fresh cranberries, cranberry juice may be beneficial for preventing or reducing infections in the GI and urinary tracts. Phytochemicals in cranberries may impede the ability of some bacteria to adhere to epithelial tissue and grow. Choose 100% cranberry juice rather than cocktails or juice blends and look for brands with less added sugar.

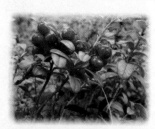

©F1 ONLINE/SuperStock

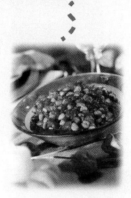

©Pixtal/AGE Fotostock

Store
- Fresh cranberries can be stored in the refrigerator for 1 week. They should be kept in the crisper drawer in a perforated bag (i.e., the original packaging) to maintain optimal water content and exposure to air.
- If you don't plan to eat fresh cranberries within 1 week of purchase, freezing the berries is the best option to preserve nutrients.

Cook
- Add dried cranberries to salads or trail mix to add a dose of antioxidants as well as flavor. In recipes, pairing cranberries with sweeter fruits, such as apples and pears, can strike a nice balance between sweet and tart.
- Fresh, frozen, or dried cranberries make a colorful addition to baked goods, but for maximum health benefits, enjoy cranberries raw. Cooking the berries greatly reduces their antioxidant content.

Source: Robinson J: Strawberries, cranberries, and raspberries: Three of our most nutritious fruits. In *Eating on the Wild Side*. New York: Little, Brown and Company, 2013.

3.5 Urinary System

The **urinary system** is composed of two kidneys, one on each side of the spinal column. Each kidney is connected to the bladder by a **ureter**. The bladder is emptied by way of the **urethra** (Fig. 3-5). The main function of the kidneys is to remove waste from the body. The kidneys are constantly filtering blood to control its composition. This results in the formation of urine, which is composed of water, dissolved waste products of metabolism such as **urea**, and excess or unneeded water-soluble vitamins and various minerals.

Together with the lungs, the kidneys also maintain the acid–base balance (**pH**) of the blood. The kidneys contribute to bone health because they convert a form of vitamin D into its active hormone form. The kidneys also produce a hormone that stimulates red blood cell synthesis (**erythropoietin;** see Section 10.6 for information on misuse of this hormone by some athletes). During times of fasting, the kidneys even produce glucose from certain amino acids. Thus, the kidneys perform many important functions related to nutrition.

The proper function of the kidneys is closely tied to the strength of the cardiovascular system, particularly its ability to maintain adequate blood pressure, and the consumption of sufficient fluid. Uncontrolled diabetes, hypertension, and drug abuse are harmful to the kidneys. See Farm to Fork in this section to learn how some phytochemicals in cranberries may protect the health of the urinary system.

urinary system The body system consisting of the kidneys, urinary bladder, and the ducts that carry urine. This system removes waste products from the circulatory system and regulates blood acid–base balance, overall chemical balance, and water balance in the body.

ureter Tube that transports urine from the kidney to the urinary bladder.

urethra Tube that transports urine from the urinary bladder to the outside of the body.

urea Nitrogenous waste product of protein metabolism; major source of nitrogen in the urine.

pH A measure of relative acidity or alkalinity of a solution. The pH scale is 0 to 14. A pH of 7 is neutral; a pH below 7 is acidic; a pH above 7 is alkaline.

erythropoietin A hormone secreted mostly by the kidneys that enhances red blood cell synthesis and stimulates red blood cell release from bone marrow.

FIGURE 3-5 ▶ Organs of the urinary system. The kidneys (1), bean-shaped organs located on either side of the spinal column, filter waste from the blood and form urine, which is transported to the bladder by the ureters (2) and stored in the bladder (3) as urine. The urethra (4) transports the urine to outside the body. The urinary system of the female is shown. The male's urinary system is the same, except that the urethra extends through the penis.

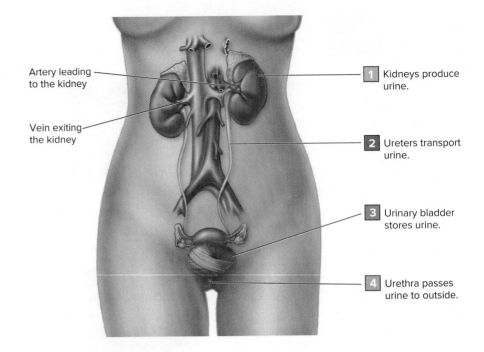

Artery leading to the kidney

Vein exiting the kidney

1 Kidneys produce urine.

2 Ureters transport urine.

3 Urinary bladder stores urine.

4 Urethra passes urine to outside.

☑ **CONCEPT CHECK 3.5**

1. List three functions of the kidneys.
2. Trace the path of waste products out of the body.

3.6 Nervous System

nervous system The body system consisting of the brain, spinal cord, nerves, and sensory receptors. This system detects sensations, directs movements, and controls physiological and intellectual functions.

The **nervous system** is a regulatory system that centrally controls most body functions. The nervous system can detect changes occurring in various organs and the external environment and initiate corrective action when needed to maintain a constant internal body environment. The nervous system also regulates activities that change almost instantly, such as voluntary muscle contractions and the body's response to stress or danger. The body has many receptors that receive information about what is happening within the body and in the outside environment. For the most part, these receptors are found in our eyes, ears, skin, nose, and stomach. We act on information from these receptors via the nervous system.

neuron The structural and functional unit of the nervous system. Consists of a cell body, dendrites, and an axon.

The basic structural and functional unit of the nervous system is the **neuron.** Neurons are elongated, highly branched cells. The body contains about 100 billion neurons. Neurons respond to electrical and chemical signals, conduct electrical impulses, and release chemical regulators. Overall, neurons allow us to perceive what is occurring in our environment, engage in learning, store vital information in memory, and control the body's voluntary (and involuntary) actions.

The brain stores information, reacts to incoming information, solves problems, and generates thoughts. In addition, the brain plans a course of action based on the other sensory inputs. Responses to the stimuli are carried out mostly through the rest of the nervous system. Nutrition and brain health will be discussed in Section 16.3.

Simply put, the nervous system receives information through stimulation of various receptors, processes this information, and sends out signals through its various branches for an action that needs to be taken. Actual transmission of the signal occurs through a change in the concentration of two nutrients, sodium and potassium, in the neuron. There is an influx of sodium into the neuron and a loss of potassium as the message is sent. Concentrations of these minerals are then restored to normal amounts in the neuron after the signal passes, making it ready to conduct another message. You will learn more about the functions of these electrolyte minerals in Chapter 9.

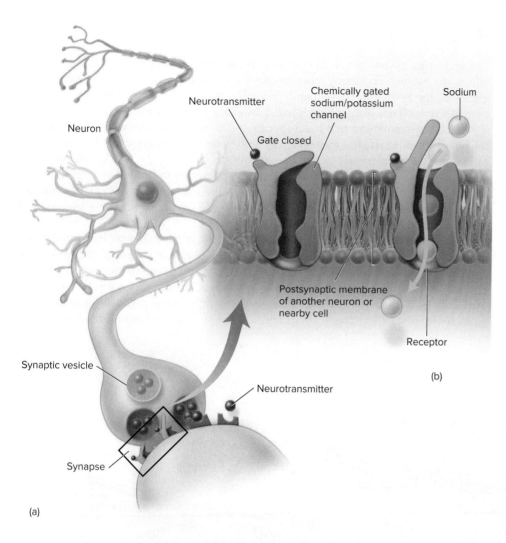

FIGURE 3-6 ◀ Transmission of a message from one neuron to another neuron or to another type of cell relies on neurotransmitters. Figure (a) shows how vesicles containing neurotransmitters, formed within the neuron, fuse with the membrane of the neuron and the neurotransmitter is released into the synapse. Enlarged in (b), the neurotransmitter then binds to the receptors on the nearby neuron (or cell). In this way, the message is transmitted from one neuron to another or to the cell that ultimately performs the action directed by the message.

When the signal must bridge a gap **(synapse)** between the branches of different neurons, the message is generally converted into a chemical signal called a **neurotransmitter.** The neurotransmitter is then released into the gap, and its target may be another neuron or another type of cell, such as a muscle cell (Fig. 3-6). If the signal is sent to another neuron, this allows it to continue on to its final destination. The neurotransmitters used in this process are often made from common nutrients found in foods such as amino acids. The amino acid tryptophan is converted to the neurotransmitter serotonin, and the amino acid tyrosine is converted to the neurotransmitters **norepinephrine** and **epinephrine** (also called *adrenaline*).

Other nutrients also play a role in the nervous system. Calcium is needed for the release of neurotransmitters from neurons. Vitamin B-12 plays a role in the formation of the **myelin** sheath, which provides insulation around specific parts of most neurons. Finally, a regular supply of carbohydrate in the form of glucose is important for supplying fuel for the brain. The brain can use other energy sources but generally relies on glucose.

synapse The space between one neuron and another neuron (or cell).

neurotransmitter A compound made by a nerve cell that allows for communication between it and other cells.

norepinephrine A neurotransmitter from nerve endings and a hormone from the adrenal gland. It is released in times of stress and is involved in hunger regulation, blood glucose regulation, and other body processes.

epinephrine A hormone also known as *adrenaline;* it is released by the adrenal glands at times of stress. It acts to increase glycogen breakdown in the liver, among other functions.

myelin A combination of lipids and proteins that covers nerve fibers.

✓ CONCEPT CHECK 3.6

1. Why are sodium and potassium important for the work of the nervous system?
2. How are signals transmitted between one neuron and the next? Why are amino acids important in this process?
3. Which nutrient is the brain's preferred source of energy?

3.7 Endocrine System

endocrine system The body system consisting of the various glands and the hormones these glands secrete. This system has major regulatory functions in the body, such as reproduction and cell metabolism.

endocrine gland A hormone-producing gland.

insulin A hormone produced by the pancreas. Insulin allows for the movement of glucose from the blood into body cells and signals the synthesis of glycogen.

The **endocrine system** plays a major role in the regulation of metabolism, reproduction, water balance, and many other functions by producing hormones in the **endocrine glands** of the body and subsequently releasing them into the blood (Table 3-1). The term *hormone* comes from a Greek word, meaning "to stir or excite." A true hormone is a regulatory compound that has a specific site of synthesis from which it then enters the bloodstream to reach target cells. Hormones are the messengers of the body. They can be *permissive* (turn on), *antagonistic* (turn off), or *synergistic* (work in cooperation with another hormone) in performing a task. Some compounds must undergo chemical changes before they can function as hormones. For example, vitamin D, synthesized in the skin or obtained from food, is converted into an active hormone by chemical changes made in the liver and kidneys.

The hormone **insulin,** synthesized in and released from the pancreas, helps control the amount of glucose in the blood (Fig. 3-7). When the amount of glucose in the blood rises above normal (usually after a meal), insulin is released and travels to the muscle, adipose, and liver cells of the body. Among its many functions, insulin allows for the movement of glucose from the blood into muscle and adipose cells. In the liver cells, insulin causes an increase in stored glycogen by stimulating the synthesis of glycogen from glucose.

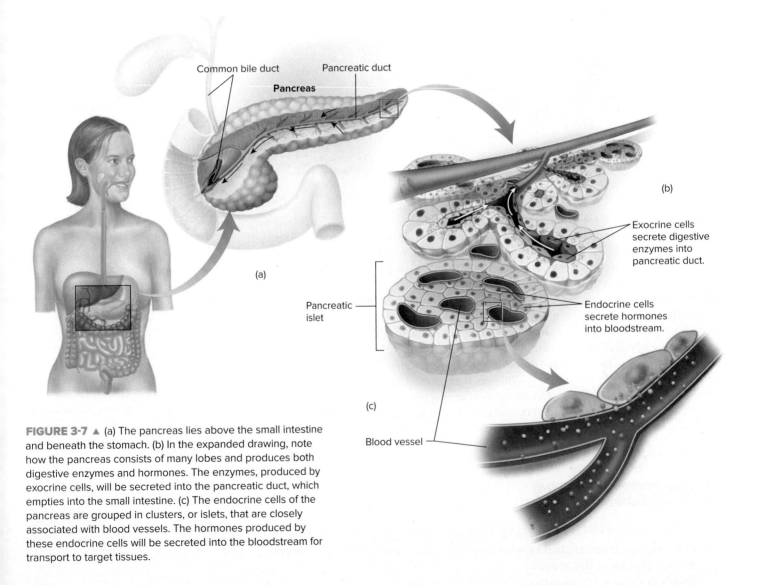

FIGURE 3-7 ▲ (a) The pancreas lies above the small intestine and beneath the stomach. (b) In the expanded drawing, note how the pancreas consists of many lobes and produces both digestive enzymes and hormones. The enzymes, produced by exocrine cells, will be secreted into the pancreatic duct, which empties into the small intestine. (c) The endocrine cells of the pancreas are grouped in clusters, or islets, that are closely associated with blood vessels. The hormones produced by these endocrine cells will be secreted into the bloodstream for transport to target tissues.

TABLE 3-1 ■ Some Hormones of the Endocrine System with Nutritional Significance

Hormone	Gland/Organ	Target	Effect	Role in Nutrition
Insulin	Pancreas	Adipose, muscle, and liver cells	Decreased blood glucose	Uptake and storage of glucose, fat, and amino acids by cells
Glucagon	Pancreas	Liver	Increased blood glucose	Release of glucose from liver stores, synthesis of glucose from amino acids, release of fat from adipose tissue
Epinephrine, Norepinephrine	Adrenal glands	Heart, blood vessels, brain, lungs	Increased body metabolism and blood glucose	Release of glucose and fat into the blood
Growth hormone	Pituitary gland	Most cells	Promotion of amino acid uptake by cells, increased blood glucose	Promotion of protein synthesis and growth, increased fat use for energy
Thyroid hormones	Thyroid gland	Most organs	Increased oxygen consumption, overall growth, development of the nervous system	Protein synthesis, increased body metabolism

Once a sufficient amount of glucose has been cleared from the blood, the production of insulin lessens. The hormones epinephrine, norepinephrine, glucagon, and growth hormone have just the opposite effect on blood glucose. They all cause an increase in blood glucose through a variety of actions (see Table 3-1). **Thyroid hormones,** synthesized in and released from the thyroid gland, help to control the body's rate of metabolism. Other hormones are especially important in regulating digestive processes (see Section 3.9).

Hormones are not taken up by all cells in the body but only by those with the correct **receptor** protein. These binding sites, which generally are found on the cell membrane, are highly specific for a certain hormone. The hormone attaches to its receptor on the cell membrane. This binding activates additional compounds called second messengers within the cell to carry out the assigned task. This is true of insulin. A few hormones can penetrate the cell membrane and eventually bind to receptors on the DNA in the nucleus (e.g., thyroid hormone and estrogen).

thyroid hormones Hormones produced by the thyroid gland that regulate growth and metabolic rate.

receptor A site in a cell at which compounds (such as hormones) bind. Cells that contain receptors for a specific compound are partially controlled by that compound.

✓ CONCEPT CHECK 3.7

1. Examine Figure 3-7. What are the endocrine roles of the pancreas? What are the exocrine roles of the pancreas?
2. What effect does insulin have on the storage of nutrients?
3. List at least three hormones that tend to increase blood sugar.
4. If a person has hypothyroidism, the thyroid gland produces low levels of thyroid hormone. Will a person with hypothyroidism tend to lose weight or gain weight? Explain your answer.

3.8 Immune System

The immune system provides a very clear example of the interrelationship between nutrition status and organ system function. In developing nations, where food shortages are common, malnutrition increases susceptibility to infectious diseases, such as diarrheal disease. Cells throughout the body—skin and intestinal cells—work in concert with the cells and tissues of the immune system to defend the body against infection.

We are born with some aspects of immune function, such as physical and chemical barriers against infection, the inflammatory response, and the ability of some **white blood cells** to engulf microorganisms by **phagocytosis.** These are termed **nonspecific (innate) immunity** because they protect the body against invasion by any microorganism.

white blood cells One of the formed elements of the circulating blood system; also called *leukocytes*. White blood cells are able to squeeze through intracellular spaces and migrate. They phagocytize bacteria, fungi, and viruses, as well as detoxify proteins that may result from allergic reactions, cellular injury, and other immune system cells.

phagocytosis A process in which a cell forms an indentation, and solid particles enter the indentation and are engulfed by the cell.

nonspecific immunity Defenses that stop the invasion of pathogens; requires no previous encounter with a pathogen; also called *innate immunity*.

The skin and the intestinal cells support the immune system by forming an important barrier against invading microorganisms. If the integrity of either one of these barriers is compromised, microorganisms can invade the body and cause illness. Substances secreted by the skin and intestinal cells can also destroy pathogens.

If the body's nonspecific immune defenses are unable to block a microorganism's entry into the bloodstream, cells and chemicals involved in **specific (adaptive) immunity** will identify and destroy the invading pathogen. Specific immunity involves the process by which certain white blood cells produce **antibodies** (also called **immunoglobulins**) that target specific microorganisms or foreign proteins (known as **antigens**). After initial exposure to an antigen, a "memory" is created such that a second exposure to the substance will produce a more vigorous and rapid attack.

The turnover of many cells of the immune system is quite rapid—only a few hours or days. The constant resynthesis of cells requires steady nutrient intake. Nutrients that are important for the health of the immune system include essential fatty acids (Chapter 5), protein (Chapter 6), vitamins A, C, D, and some B vitamins (Chapter 8), and iron, copper, and zinc (Chapter 9).

specific immunity Function of white blood cells directed at specific antigens; also called *adaptive immunity.*

antibody Blood protein that binds foreign proteins found in the body.

antigen Any substance that induces a state of sensitivity and/or resistance to microorganisms or toxic substances after a lag period; a foreign substance that stimulates a specific aspect of the immune system.

digestive system System consisting of the gastrointestinal tract and accessory structures (liver, gallbladder, and pancreas). This system performs the mechanical and chemical processes of digestion, absorption of nutrients, and elimination of wastes.

digestion Process by which large ingested molecules are mechanically and chemically broken down to produce basic nutrients that can be absorbed across the wall of the GI tract.

absorption The process by which substances are taken up from the GI tract and enter the bloodstream or the lymph.

gastrointestinal (GI) tract The main sites in the body used for digestion and absorption of nutrients. It consists of the mouth, esophagus, stomach, small intestine, large intestine, rectum, and anus. Also called the *digestive tract.*

lumen The hollow opening inside a tube, such as the GI tract.

✔ CONCEPT CHECK 3.8

1. Contrast nonspecific (innate) and specific (adaptive) immunity.
2. What are the roles of antigens and antibodies in the immune response?
3. List three nutrients that support the immune system.

3.9 Digestive System

The foods and beverages we consume, for the most part, must undergo extensive alteration by the **digestive system** to provide us with usable nutrients. The processes of **digestion** and **absorption** take place in a long tube that is open at both ends and extends from the mouth to the anus. This tube is called the **gastrointestinal (GI) tract** (Fig. 3-8). The open space inside the GI tract is called the **lumen.** Nutrients from the food we eat must pass through the walls of the GI tract—from the lumen through the cells lining the GI tract—to be absorbed into the bloodstream. The organs that make up the GI tract, as well as some additional accessory organs located nearby, are collectively known as the digestive system.

In the digestive system, food is broken down mechanically and chemically. Mechanical digestion takes place as soon as you begin chewing your food and continues as muscular contractions simultaneously mix and move food through the length of the GI tract.

Chemical digestion refers to the chemical breakdown of foods by acid and enzymes secreted into the GI tract. Enzymes are a key part of digestion. Each enzyme is specific to one type of chemical process. For example, the enzyme that recognizes and digests table sugar (sucrose) ignores milk sugar (lactose). Besides working on only specific types of chemicals, enzymes are sensitive to acidic and alkaline conditions, temperature, and the types of vitamins and minerals they require to function. Digestive enzymes that work in the acidic environment of the stomach do not work well in the alkaline environment of the small intestine. The pancreas and small intestine produce most of the digestive enzymes; however, the mouth and the stomach also contribute their own enzymes to the process of digestion. The organs of the digestive system are able to fine-tune the production of each type of digestive enzyme in response to the nutritional makeup and amount of food consumed. Overall, the enzymes of the digestive system work together to hasten the breakdown of ingested food into absorbable nutrients (Fig. 3-9).

As food moves along the GI tract, nutrients are absorbed. In addition to nutrients from the food we eat, the bacteria that live in the large intestine produce some vitamins (vitamin K and biotin) that can be absorbed. By the time the meal contents reach

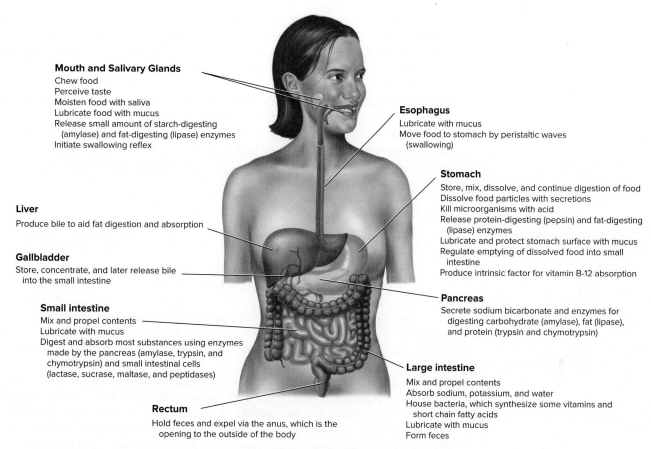

Mouth and Salivary Glands
Chew food
Perceive taste
Moisten food with saliva
Lubricate food with mucus
Release small amount of starch-digesting
    (amylase) and fat-digesting (lipase) enzymes
Initiate swallowing reflex

Esophagus
Lubricate with mucus
Move food to stomach by peristaltic waves
    (swallowing)

Stomach
Store, mix, dissolve, and continue digestion of food
Dissolve food particles with secretions
Kill microorganisms with acid
Release protein-digesting (pepsin) and fat-digesting
    (lipase) enzymes
Lubricate and protect stomach surface with mucus
Regulate emptying of dissolved food into small
    intestine
Produce intrinsic factor for vitamin B-12 absorption

Liver
Produce bile to aid fat digestion and absorption

Gallbladder
Store, concentrate, and later release bile
    into the small intestine

Pancreas
Secrete sodium bicarbonate and enzymes for
    digesting carbohydrate (amylase), fat (lipase),
    and protein (trypsin and chymotrypsin)

Small intestine
Mix and propel contents
Lubricate with mucus
Digest and absorb most substances using enzymes
    made by the pancreas (amylase, trypsin, and
    chymotrypsin) and small intestinal cells
    (lactase, sucrase, maltase, and peptidases)

Large intestine
Mix and propel contents
Absorb sodium, potassium, and water
House bacteria, which synthesize some vitamins and
    short chain fatty acids
Lubricate with mucus
Form feces

Rectum
Hold feces and expel via the anus, which is the
    opening to the outside of the body

FIGURE 3-8 ▲ Physiology of the GI tract. Many organs cooperate in a regulated fashion to allow the digestion and absorption of nutrients in foods. Partially digested food spends about 2 to 3 hours in the stomach (longer for large meals). Passage through the small intestine takes 3 to 10 hours, followed by up to 72 hours in the large intestine. On average, digestion and absorption of a meal takes about 2 days. Food matter tends to pass more quickly through the GI tract of men than women.

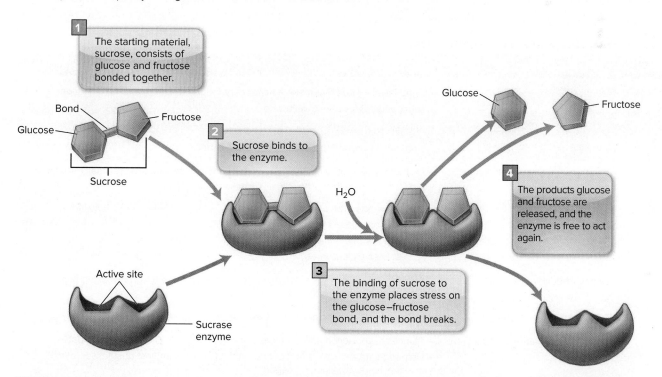

FIGURE 3-9 ▲ A model of enzyme action. The enzyme sucrase splits the sugar sucrose into two simpler sugars, glucose and fructose. (Note that sometimes energy input is needed to make reactions occur.)

the large intestine, most of the usable nutrients have been absorbed. What remains is waste. The final role of the digestive system is elimination of wastes.

Most of the processes of digestion and absorption are under autonomic control; that is, they are involuntary. Almost all of the functions involved in digestion and absorption are controlled by signals from the nervous system, hormones from the endocrine system, and hormone-like compounds. Many common ailments arise from problems with the digestive system. Several of these digestive problems are discussed in Section 3.12.

The digestive system is composed of six separate organs; each organ performs one (or more) specific job(s). Let's look briefly at the role of each organ. These organs are shown in Figure 3-8. More detailed descriptions of digestive processes will be provided in later chapters as each nutrient is introduced.

MOUTH

The mouth performs many functions in the digestion of food. Besides chewing food to reduce it to smaller particles, the mouth also senses the taste of the foods we consume. The tongue, through the use of its taste buds, identifies foods on the basis of their specific flavor(s). Sweet, sour, salty, bitter, **umami,** and **oleogustus** comprise the primary taste sensations we experience. Surprisingly, the nose and our sense of smell greatly contribute to our ability to sense the taste of food. When we chew a food, chemicals are released that stimulate the nasal passages. Thus, it makes perfect sense that when we have a cold and our nose is stuffed up and congested, even our favorite foods will not taste as good as they normally do.

The taste of food, or the anticipation of it, signals the rest of the GI tract to prepare for the digestion of food. Once in the mouth, mechanical and chemical digestion begins. Salivary glands produce **saliva,** which functions as a solvent so that food particles can be further separated and tasted. In addition, saliva contains a starch-digesting enzyme, salivary **amylase** (see Section 4.4 for more on starch-digesting enzymes) and a fat-digesting enzyme, **lipase** (see Section 5.4). **Mucus,** another component of saliva, makes it easy to swallow a mouthful of food. The food then travels to the esophagus. The important secretions and products of digestion are listed in Table 3-2.

umami A brothy, meaty, savory flavor in some foods. Monosodium glutamate enhances this flavor when added to foods.

oleogustus A taste for fat. The presence of fatty acids in foods stimulates taste receptors in the mouth; this sensation is unpleasant.

amylase Starch-digesting enzyme produced by the salivary glands and the pancreas.

lipase Fat-digesting enzyme produced by the salivary glands, stomach, and pancreas.

bile acid A compound produced by the liver. Bile acids are the main component of bile, which aids in emulsification of fat during digestion in the small intestine.

TABLE 3-2 ■ Important Secretions of the Digestive Tract

Secretion	Site of Production	Purpose
Saliva	Mouth	• Contains enzymes that make a minor contribution to starch and fat digestion • Lubrication of food for swallowing
Mucus	Mouth, esophagus, stomach, small intestine, large intestine	• Protects GI tract cells • Lubricates food as it travels through the GI tract
Enzymes	Mouth, stomach, small intestine, pancreas	• Promote digestion of carbohydrates, fats, and proteins into forms small enough for absorption (examples: amylases, lipases, proteases)
Acid	Stomach	• Promotes digestion of protein • Destroys pathogens • Solubilizes some minerals • Activates some enzymes
Bile	Liver (stored in gallbladder)	• Aids fat digestion in the small intestine by suspending fat in water using **bile acids,** cholesterol, and phospholipids
Bicarbonate	Pancreas, small intestine	• Neutralizes stomach acid when it reaches the small intestine
Hormones	Stomach, small intestine, pancreas	• Stimulate production and/or release of acid, enzymes, bile, and bicarbonate • Help regulate peristalsis and overall GI tract flow (examples: gastrin, secretin, insulin, cholecystokinin, glucagon)
Intrinsic factor	Stomach	• Facilitates absorption of vitamin B-12 in the small intestine

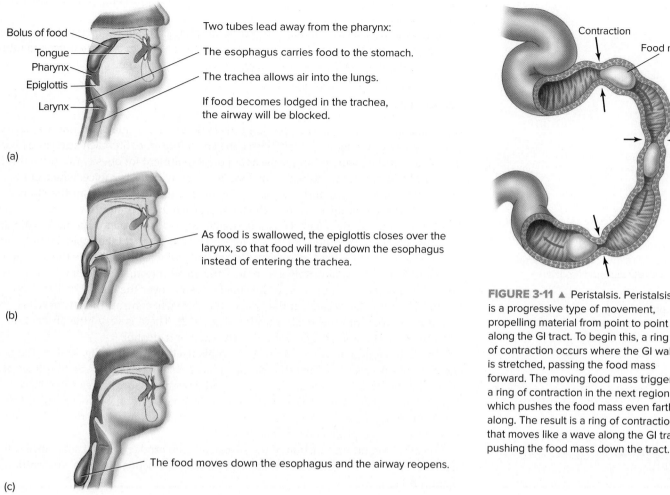

Bolus of food
Tongue
Pharynx
Epiglottis
Larynx

Two tubes lead away from the pharynx:

The esophagus carries food to the stomach.

The trachea allows air into the lungs.

If food becomes lodged in the trachea, the airway will be blocked.

(a)

As food is swallowed, the epiglottis closes over the larynx, so that food will travel down the esophagus instead of entering the trachea.

(b)

The food moves down the esophagus and the airway reopens.

(c)

FIGURE 3-10 ▲ The process of swallowing.

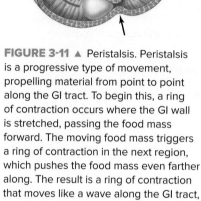

Contraction

Food mass

FIGURE 3-11 ▲ Peristalsis. Peristalsis is a progressive type of movement, propelling material from point to point along the GI tract. To begin this, a ring of contraction occurs where the GI wall is stretched, passing the food mass forward. The moving food mass triggers a ring of contraction in the next region, which pushes the food mass even farther along. The result is a ring of contraction that moves like a wave along the GI tract, pushing the food mass down the tract.

ESOPHAGUS

The **esophagus** is a long tube that connects the **pharynx** with the stomach. Near the pharynx is a flap of tissue (called the **epiglottis**) that prevents the **bolus** of swallowed food from entering the **trachea** (windpipe) (Fig. 3-10). During swallowing, food lands on the epiglottis, folding it down to cover the opening of the trachea. Breathing also stops automatically. These responses ensure that swallowed food will only travel down the esophagus. If food instead travels down the trachea, choking may occur (the victim will not be able to speak, cough, or breathe). A group of techniques to treat a choking person is called the Heimlich maneuver (see www.heimlichinstitute .org for details).

At the top of the esophagus, nerve fibers release signals to tell the GI tract that food has been consumed. This results in an increase in GI muscle action, called **peristalsis.** These continual waves of muscle contractions, followed by muscle relaxation, force the food along the digestive tract from the esophagus onward (Fig. 3-11).

At the end of the esophagus is the **lower esophageal sphincter,** a muscle that constricts (closes) after food enters the stomach. The main function of sphincters is to prevent the backflow of GI tract contents. Sphincters respond to various stimuli, such as signals from the nervous system, hormones, acidic conditions, and pressure that builds up around the sphincter. The primary function of the lower esophageal sphincter is to prevent the acidic contents of the stomach from flowing back up into the esophagus.

esophagus A tube in the GI tract that connects the pharynx with the stomach.

pharynx The organ of the digestive tract and respiratory tract located at the back of the oral and nasal cavities, commonly known as the throat.

epiglottis The flap that folds down over the trachea during swallowing.

bolus A moistened mass of food swallowed from the oral cavity into the pharynx.

trachea The airway that extends from the throat, down the neck, to the lungs. Also called the *windpipe*.

peristalsis A coordinated muscular contraction used to propel food down the gastrointestinal tract.

lower esophageal sphincter A circular muscle that constricts the opening of the esophagus to the stomach. Also called the *gastroesophageal sphincter* or the *cardiac sphincter.*

Dysfunction of this sphincter can cause some of the health problems we will discuss in Section 3.12.

No digestion or absorption occurs in the esophagus; it serves merely to transport food from the mouth to the stomach. The cells of the esophagus secrete mucus to lubricate the passage of food, but no digestive enzymes are produced.

STOMACH

The stomach is a large sac that can hold up to 4 cups (or 1 quart) of food for several hours until all of the food is able to enter the small intestine. Stomach size varies individually and can be reduced surgically as a radical treatment for obesity (more on this in Section 7.9). While in the stomach, the food is mixed with gastric juice, which contains water, hydrochloric acid, and enzymes. (*Gastric* is a term pertaining to the stomach.) The acid in the gastric juice destroys the biological activity of proteins, converts inactive digestive enzymes to their active form, partially digests food protein, and makes dietary minerals soluble so that they can be absorbed. The mixing that takes place in the stomach produces a watery food mixture, called **chyme,** which slowly leaves the stomach a teaspoon (5 milliliters) at a time and enters the small intestine. Following a meal, the stomach contents are emptied into the small intestine over the course of 1 to 4 hours. The **pyloric sphincter,** located at the base of the stomach, controls the rate at which the chyme is released into the small intestine (Fig. 3-12). There is very little absorption of nutrients from the stomach, except for some water and alcohol.

You might wonder how the stomach prevents itself from being digested by the acid and enzymes it produces. First, the stomach has a thick layer of mucus that lines and protects it. Second, the production of acid and enzymes also requires the release of a specific hormone (gastrin). This release happens primarily when we are eating or thinking about eating. Last, as the concentration of acid in the stomach increases, hormonal control causes acid production to taper off.

One other important function of the stomach is the production of a substance called **intrinsic factor.** This vital proteinlike compound is essential for the absorption of vitamin B-12.

SMALL INTESTINE

The small intestine is considered "small" because its diameter is only 1 inch (2.5 centimeters). It is actually quite long—about 10 feet (3 meters), beginning at the stomach and extending to the large intestine (Fig. 3-13). The three parts of the small intestine are the **duodenum** (first 10 inches), the **jejunum** (second 4 feet), and the **ileum** (last 5 feet). Most of the digestion and absorption of food occurs in the small intestine. As chyme moves from the stomach into the first part of the small intestine, it is still very acidic. You just learned that the stomach secretes a thick layer of mucus to protect itself from the strong acid. However, if the small intestine were coated with mucus, digestion and absorption would be very limited. Therefore, the pancreas and intestinal cells secrete bicarbonate to neutralize the acid. The neutral pH also optimizes the activity of the digestive enzymes that work in the small intestine. Muscular contractions move the chyme through the small intestine and thoroughly mix food particles with digestive juices (review Fig. 3-11). These juices contain many enzymes that break down carbohydrates, protein, fat, and some vitamins into absorbable units.

The physical structure of the small intestine is very important to the body's ability to digest and absorb the nutrients it needs. The lining of the small intestine is called the mucosa and is folded many times; within these folds are fingerlike projections called **villi.** These "fingers" are constantly moving, which helps them trap food to enhance absorption. Each individual villus (singular) is made up of many **absorptive cells** (also called enterocytes), and the mucosal surface of each of these cells is folded even further into **microvilli.** The combined folds, villi, and microvilli in the small intestine increase its surface area 600 times beyond that of a simple tube (see Fig. 3-13).

chyme A mixture of stomach secretions and partially digested food.

pyloric sphincter Ring of smooth muscle between the stomach and the small intestine.

intrinsic factor A proteinlike compound produced by the stomach that enhances vitamin B-12 absorption in the ileum.

duodenum First segment of the small intestine that receives chyme from the stomach and digestive juices from the pancreas and gallbladder. This is the site of most chemical digestion of nutrients; approximately 10 inches in length.

jejunum Middle segment of the small intestine; approximately 4 feet in length.

ileum Last segment of the small intestine; approximately 5 feet in length.

villi (singular, villus) The fingerlike protrusions into the small intestine that participate in digestion and absorption of food.

absorptive cells Also known as *enterocytes;* the intestinal cells that line the villi and participate in nutrient absorption.

microvilli Extensive folds on the muscosal surface of the absorptive cells.

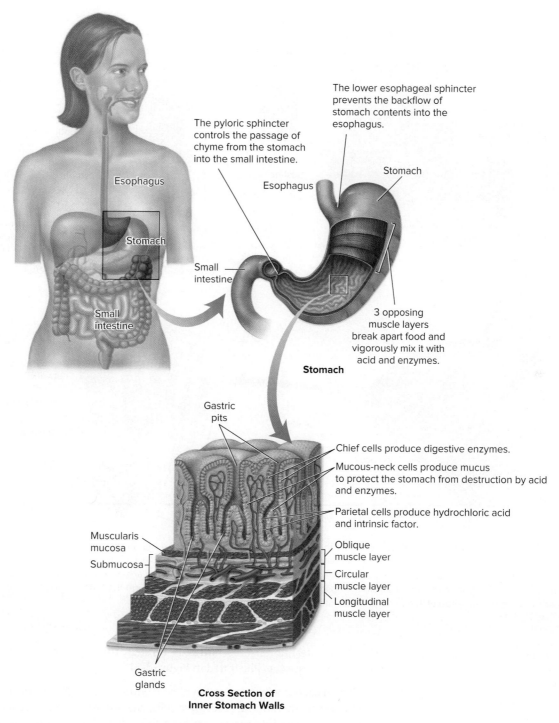

The lower esophageal sphincter prevents the backflow of stomach contents into the esophagus.

The pyloric sphincter controls the passage of chyme from the stomach into the small intestine.

Esophagus

Esophagus

Stomach

Small intestine

Small intestine

3 opposing muscle layers break apart food and vigorously mix it with acid and enzymes.

Stomach

Gastric pits

Chief cells produce digestive enzymes.

Mucous-neck cells produce mucus to protect the stomach from destruction by acid and enzymes.

Parietal cells produce hydrochloric acid and intrinsic factor.

Muscularis mucosa

Submucosa

Oblique muscle layer

Circular muscle layer

Longitudinal muscle layer

Gastric glands

Cross Section of Inner Stomach Walls

FIGURE 3-12 ▲ Physiology of the stomach.

The absorptive cells have a short life. New intestinal absorptive cells are constantly produced in the crypts of the small intestinal lining (see Fig. 3-13) and appear daily along the surface of each villus. This is probably because absorptive cells are subjected to a harsh environment, so renewal of the intestinal cell lining is necessary. This rapid cell turnover leads to high nutrient needs for the small intestine. Fortunately, many of the old cells can be broken down and have their parts reused. The health of the cells is further enhanced by various hormones and other substances that participate in or are produced as part of the digestive process.

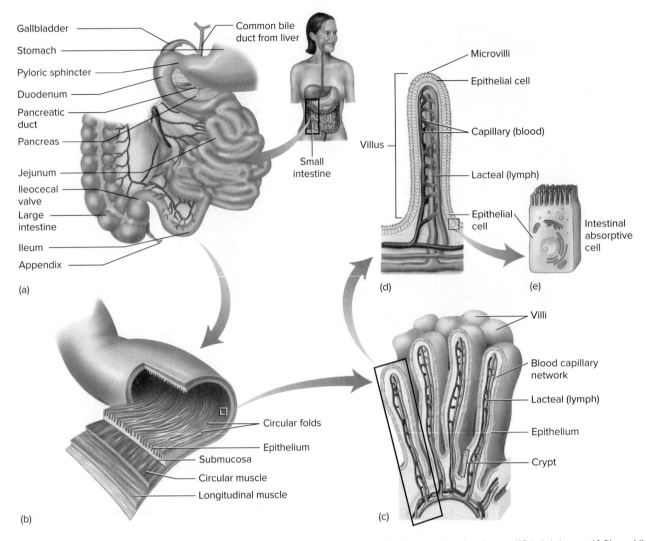

FIGURE 3-13 ▲ Organization of the small intestine. (a) The three parts of the small intestine are the duodenum (10 in.), jejunum (4 ft), and ileum (5 ft). (b) Several layers of muscle work together to mix and propel chyme through the small intestine. (c) The highly folded lining of the small intestine increases the surface area for absorption up to 600 times that of a simple tube. (d) The villi are covered with absorptive cells. Capillaries and lacteals inside each villus transport nutrients from the absorptive cells of the small intestine through the blood and lymph. (e) The mucosal side of the absorptive cells is covered with microvilli, which maximize nutrient absorption.

passive diffusion Movement of a substance across a semipermeable membrane from an area of higher solute concentration to an area of lower solute concentration. This type of transport does not require a carrier and does not require energy.

facilitated diffusion Movement of a substance across a semipermeable membrane from an area of higher solute concentration to an area of lower solute concentration. This type of transport does not require energy, but it does require a carrier.

active absorption Movement of a substance across a semipermeable membrane from an area of lower solute concentration to an area of higher solute concentration. This type of transport requires energy and a carrier.

The small intestine absorbs nutrients through the intestinal wall through various means and processes, as illustrated in Figure 3-14.

- **Passive diffusion:** When the nutrient concentration is higher in the lumen of the small intestine than in the absorptive cells, the difference in nutrient concentration drives the nutrient into the absorptive cells by diffusion. Fats, water, and some minerals are examples of nutrients that move down a concentration gradient to be absorbed by passive diffusion.
- **Facilitated diffusion:** Some compounds require a carrier protein to follow a concentration gradient into absorptive cells. This type of absorption is called facilitated diffusion. Fructose is one example of a compound that makes use of such a carrier to allow for facilitated diffusion.
- **Active absorption:** In addition to the need for a carrier protein, some nutrients also require energy input to move from the lumen of the small intestine into the absorptive cells. This mechanism makes it possible for cells to take up nutrients even when they are consumed in low concentrations (i.e., against a concentration gradient). Some sugars, such as glucose, are actively absorbed, as are amino acids.

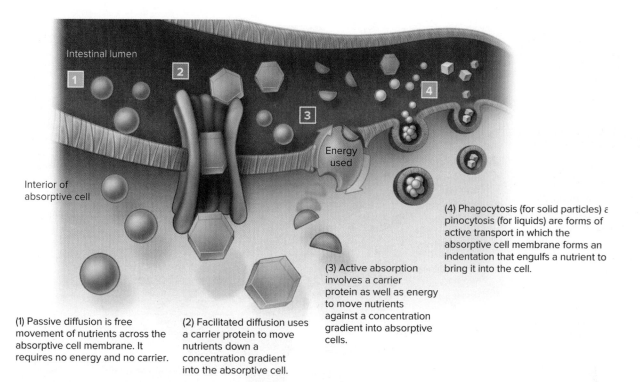

Intestinal lumen

Interior of
absorptive cell

Energy
used

(4) Phagocytosis (for solid particles) and
pinocytosis (for liquids) are forms of
active transport in which the
absorptive cell membrane forms an
indentation that engulfs a nutrient to
bring it into the cell.

(3) Active absorption
involves a carrier
protein as well as energy
to move nutrients
against a concentration
gradient into absorptive
cells.

(1) Passive diffusion is free
movement of nutrients across the
absorptive cell membrane. It
requires no energy and no carrier.

(2) Facilitated diffusion uses
a carrier protein to move
nutrients down a
concentration gradient
into the absorptive cell.

FIGURE 3-14 ▲ Nutrient absorption relies on four major absorptive processes.

- **Phagocytosis** and **pinocytosis:** In a further means of active absorption, absorptive cells literally engulf compounds (phagocytosis) or liquids (pinocytosis). A cell membrane can form an indentation of itself so that when particles or fluids move into the indentation, the cell membrane surrounds and engulfs them. This process is used when an infant absorbs immune substances from human milk (see Section 14.7).

Once absorbed, water-soluble compounds such as glucose and amino acids are transported by the capillaries to the hepatic portal vein, which leads directly to the liver. Most fats are absorbed into the lymph vessels, which eventually empty into the bloodstream (review Figs. 3-3 and 3-4).

Undigested food cannot be absorbed into cells of the small intestine. Any undigested food that reaches the end of the small intestine must pass through the **ileocecal sphincter** on the way to the large intestine (Fig. 3-15). This sphincter prevents the contents of the large intestine from reentering the small intestine.

LARGE INTESTINE

When the contents of the small intestine enter the large intestine, the material that is left bears little resemblance to the food that was originally eaten. Under normal circumstances, only a minor amount (5%) of carbohydrate, protein, and fat escapes absorption to reach the large intestine (Table 3-3).

The large intestine (sometimes called the *colon*) can be subdivided into five main segments: the **cecum, ascending colon, transverse colon, descending colon,** and **sigmoid colon** (see Fig. 3-15). Physiologically, the large intestine differs from the small intestine in that there are no villi or digestive enzymes. The absence of villi means that little absorption takes place in the large intestine in comparison to the small intestine. Nutrients absorbed from the large intestine include water, some vitamins, some fatty acids, and the minerals sodium and potassium. Unlike the small intestine, the large intestine has a number of mucus-producing cells. The mucus secreted by these cells functions to hold the feces together and protect the large intestine from the bacterial activity within it.

phagocytosis A process in which a cell forms an indentation, and solid particles enter the indentation and are engulfed by the cell.

pinocytosis A process in which a cell forms an indentation, and fluid enters the indentation and is engulfed by the cell.

ileocecal sphincter The ring of smooth muscle between the end of the small intestine and the beginning of the large intestine.

cecum A pouch at the first part of the large intestine that houses many bacteria.

ascending colon Segment of the large intestine that carries feces from the cecum, up the right side of the abdomen, to the transverse colon.

transverse colon Segment of the large intestine that carries feces from the ascending colon, from right to left across the top of the abdomen, to the descending colon.

descending colon Segment of the large intestine that carries feces from the transverse colon, down the left side of the abdomen, to the sigmoid colon.

sigmoid colon Last segment of the large intestine that carries feces from the descending colon to the rectum.

FIGURE 3-15 ► The parts of the large intestine include the cecum, ascending colon, transverse colon, descending colon, and sigmoid colon. Overall, the large intestine is about 3 ½ feet (1.1 meters) long.

CRITICAL THINKING

The authors of some popular (fad) diet books contend that eating certain combinations of foods, such as meats and fruits together, hinders the digestive processes. Based on what you have learned so far about the enzymes and digestion, does this sound accurate?

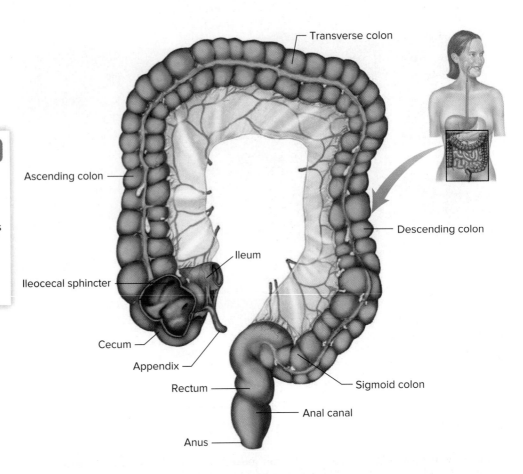

TABLE 3-3 ■ **Major Sites of Absorption Along the GI Tract**

Organ	Primary Nutrients Absorbed
Stomach	Alcohol (20% of total)
	Water (minor amount)
Small intestine	Calcium, magnesium, iron, and other minerals
	Glucose
	Amino acids
	Fats
	Vitamins
	Water (70% to 90% of total)
	Alcohol (80% of total)
	Bile acids
Large intestine	Sodium
	Potassium
	Some fatty acids
	Gases
	Water (10% to 30% of total)

Newsworthy Nutrition

Probiotics provide relief from constipation

Up to 25% of adults suffer from functional constipation, a problem characterized by infrequent or difficult bowel movements not due to a physical cause. Typically, functional constipation is treated with medications that can have side effects or lead to dependence. In this study, 40 adults with functional constipation were randomly assigned to receive a daily probiotic supplement containing *Lactobacillus reuteri* or placebo for 4 weeks. By the end of the study period, subjects who received the probiotics reported increased frequency of bowel movements (5.3 per week), compared with subjects who received a placebo (2.7 per week). No adverse effects were reported. This study demonstrated that taking a probiotic supplement can significantly increase the frequency of bowel movements among adults with functional constipation.

Source: Ojetti V and others: The effect of *Lactobacillus reuteri* supplementation in adults with chronic functional constipation: A randomized, double-blind, placebo-controlled trial. *Journal of Gastrointestinal and Liver Diseases* 23(4):387, 2014.

The large intestine is home to a large population of bacteria (over 500 different species). While the stomach and small intestine have some bacterial activity, the large intestine is the organ most heavily colonized with bacteria. Starting at infancy, the diet influences the type of bacteria in our digestive tracts. The number and type of bacteria in the human colon recently has become of great interest. Research has shown that intestinal bacteria play a significant role in the maintenance of health, especially health of the colon. It is speculated that higher levels of beneficial organisms can reduce the activity of disease-causing bacteria. This is another illustration of the GI tract working as an important immune organ. The strains *bifidobacteria* and *lactobacilli* are typically associated with health, whereas *clostridia* are considered problematic. Bacteria in the large intestine are able to break down some of the remaining food products that enter the large intestine, such as the milk sugar lactose (in lactose-intolerant people), and some components of fiber. Some of the products of bacterial metabolism in the large intestine, which include various fatty acids and gases, can be absorbed.

Foods containing certain live microorganisms such as *lactobacilli* have been linked to some health benefits, such as improving intestinal tract health. These microorganisms are called **probiotics** because once consumed, they take up residence in the large intestine and confer health benefits. You can find these probiotic microorganisms in certain forms of fluid milk, fermented milk, and yogurt, and in pill form.[1, 2] A related term is **prebiotic**. Prebiotics are substances that increase growth of probiotic microorganisms. One example is fructooligosaccharides (see Table 1-3 in Chapter 1 for dietary sources). The beneficial organisms of the large intestine and their use as probiotics are highlighted in Newsworthy Nutrition in this section.

Some water remains in the material that enters the large intestine because the small intestine absorbs only 70% to 90% of the fluid it receives, which includes large amounts of GI-tract secretions produced during digestion. The remnants of a meal also contain some minerals and some fiber. Because water is removed from the large intestine, its contents become semisolid by the time they have passed through the first two-thirds of it. What remains in the **feces,** besides water and undigested fiber, is tough connective tissues (from animal foods); bacteria from the large intestine; and some body wastes, such as parts of dead intestinal cells.

RECTUM

The feces or *stool* remains in the last portion of the large intestine, the **rectum,** until muscular movements push it into the **anus** to be eliminated. The presence of feces in the rectum stimulates elimination. The anus contains two **anal sphincters** (internal and

probiotic Live microorganisms that, when administered in adequate amounts, confer health benefits on the host.

prebiotic Selectively fermented ingredient that results in specific changes in the composition and/or activity of the gastrointestinal microbiota, thus conferring benefits upon the host.

feces Mass of water, fiber, tough connective tissues, bacterial cells, and sloughed intestinal cells that passes through the large intestine and is excreted through the anus; also called *stool*.

rectum Terminal portion of the large intestine.

anus Last portion of the GI tract; serves as an outlet for the digestive system.

anal sphincters A group of two sphincters (inner and outer) that help control expulsion of feces from the body.

external), one of which is under voluntary control (external sphincter). Relaxation of this sphincter allows for elimination.

ACCESSORY ORGANS

gallbladder An organ attached to the underside of the liver; site of bile storage, concentration, and eventual secretion.

The liver, **gallbladder,** and pancreas work with the GI tract and are considered accessory organs to the process of digestion (review Fig. 3-8). These accessory organs are not part of the GI tract through which food passes, but they play necessary roles in the process of digestion. These organs secrete digestive fluids into the GI tract and enable the process of breaking food down into absorbable nutrients.

bile A liver secretion stored in the gallbladder and released through the common bile duct into the first segment of the small intestine. It is essential for the digestion and absorption of fat.

Liver and Gallbladder The liver produces a substance called **bile.** The bile is stored and concentrated in the gallbladder until the gallbladder receives a hormonal signal to release the bile. This signal is induced by the presence of fat in the small intestine. Bile is released and delivered to the duodenum via a tube called the bile duct (Fig. 3-16).

In action, bile is like soap. Components of the bile enable large portions of fat to break into smaller bits so that they can be suspended in water (Chapter 5 will cover this process in detail). Interestingly, some of the bile constituents can be "recycled" in a process known as **enterohepatic circulation.** These components of bile are reabsorbed from the small intestine, returned to the liver via the portal vein, and reused.

enterohepatic circulation A continual recycling of compounds such as bile acids between the small intestine and the liver.

In addition to bile, the liver releases a number of other substances that travel with the bile to the gallbladder and end up in the small intestine and eventually in the large intestine for excretion. The liver functions in this manner to remove unwanted substances from the blood. (Other by-products are excreted via the urine; see Section 3.5.)

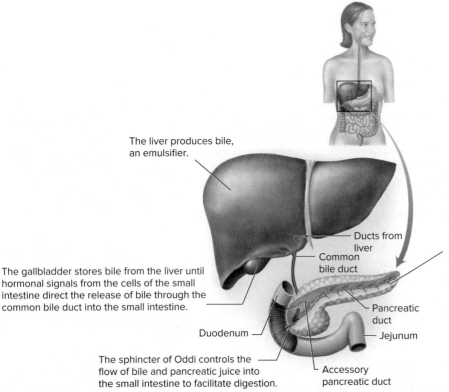

The liver produces bile, an emulsifier.

The gallbladder stores bile from the liver until hormonal signals from the cells of the small intestine direct the release of bile through the common bile duct into the small intestine.

The sphincter of Oddi controls the flow of bile and pancreatic juice into the small intestine to facilitate digestion.

Ducts from liver

Common bile duct

Duodenum

Accessory pancreatic duct

Pancreatic duct

Jejunum

The pancreas produces pancreatic juice, which contains water, bicarbonate, and digestive enzymes. Pancreatic juice is released through the pancreatic duct, which joins with the common bile duct, to flow into the small intestine in response to hormonal signals from the cells of the small intestine.

FIGURE 3-16 ▲ Although food does not come into contact with these accessory organs, the liver, gallbladder, and pancreas are important for digestion.

Pancreas The pancreas has both endocrine and digestive functions. As a gland of the endocrine system, the pancreas manufactures hormones—insulin and glucagon—that are secreted into the blood to regulate blood glucose levels (review Fig. 3-7). As an organ of the digestive system, it produces "pancreatic juice," a mixture of water, bicarbonate, and a variety of digestive enzymes capable of breaking apart carbohydrates, proteins, and fats into small fragments. Bicarbonate is a base that neutralizes the acidic chyme as it moves from the stomach into the duodenum. As noted earlier, the small intestine does not have a protective layer of mucus because mucus would impede nutrient absorption. Instead, the neutralizing capacity of bicarbonate from the pancreas protects the walls of the small intestine from erosion by acid, which would otherwise lead to the formation of an ulcer (see Section 3.12).

✓ CONCEPT CHECK 3.9

1. Choose three secretions of the digestive system. Where is each secreted? What is the role of each in the process of digestion?
2. What are enzymes? Is bile an enzyme?
3. How do mucus and surface area affect absorption?
4. Which absorptive processes use energy? How does *concentration gradient* factor into this?
5. What did you have for lunch today? Trace the path of your meal through the digestive system. Where is each nutrient broken down as it passes through the GI tract? Where is each absorbed?

3.10 Nutrient Storage Capabilities

The human body must maintain reserves of nutrients; otherwise, we would need to eat continuously. Storage capacity varies for each different nutrient. Most fat is stored in **adipose tissue.** Short-term storage of carbohydrate occurs in muscle and liver in the form of glycogen. The blood maintains a small reserve of glucose and amino acids. Many vitamins and minerals are stored in the liver, whereas other nutrient stores are found in other sites in the body.

When people do not meet their needs for certain nutrients, blood levels of these nutrients can be maintained by breaking down body tissues. For example, calcium is taken from bone and protein is taken from muscle. In cases of long-term deficiency, these nutrient losses weaken and harm these tissues.

Many people believe that if too much of a nutrient is obtained—for example, from a vitamin or mineral supplement—only what is needed is stored and the rest is excreted by the body. Though true for some nutrients, such as vitamin C, the large dosages of other nutrients frequently found in supplements, such as vitamin A and iron, can cause harmful side effects because they are not readily excreted. This is one reason why obtaining your nutrients primarily (or exclusively) from a balanced diet is the safest means to acquire the building blocks you need to maintain the good health of all organ systems.

adipose tissue Connective tissue made up of cells that store fat and also cushions and insulates the body.

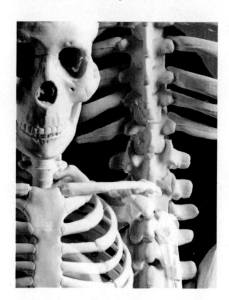

▲ The skeletal system provides a reserve of calcium for day-to-day needs when dietary intake is inadequate. Long-term use of this reserve, however, reduces bone strength. ©Jason Reed/Ryan McVay/Getty Images

✓ CONCEPT CHECK 3.10

1. What is the body's most efficient form of energy storage?
2. Why is it important to consume nutrients daily?
3. When it comes to vitamins and minerals, is consuming more than the RDA or AI a good way to ensure optimal nutrition status? Why or why not?

3.11 Nutrition and Genetics

Once nutrients and other dietary components are taken up by cells, they may interact with our genes and affect gene expression. The growth, development, and maintenance of cells, and ultimately of the entire organism, are directed by genetic mechanisms present in the cells. Each gene essentially represents instructions for a recipe, noting the ingredients (nucleic acids forming amino acids) and how these ingredients are arranged (to create proteins). The products (proteins) of all the recipes in the cookbook (the human genome) make up the human organism. The genome and the **epigenome** control the expression of genes and determine individual traits such as eye color and susceptibility to many diseases. **Epigenetics** refers to changes in gene expression caused by mechanisms other than changes in the underlying DNA sequence. While our genome contains the code for the proteins that can be made by our bodies, our epigenome is an extra layer of instructions that influences gene activity. In many cases, environmental and dietary factors can alter the epigenome.

The causes of chronic diseases are complex and include both genetic and environmental components. Through research, our understanding of the links between nutrition and genetics is becoming clearer. Genetic discoveries are leading to new drugs that target disease processes at the molecular level as well as affordable genetic tests that predict our risk for disease.

THE EMERGING FIELD OF NUTRITIONAL GENOMICS

In the near future, the accessibility of genetic information will enhance the ability of health professionals to personalize nutrition recommendations that can optimize nutritional status and improve the outcomes of nutrition-related diseases. Collectively, the interactions between genetics and nutrition are known as **nutritional genomics.** It is evident that nutritional status can both *affect* and *be affected by* an individual's genetic makeup. **Nutrigenetics** is the branch of nutritional genomics that examines how variations in genes can affect nutritional health. For example, the efficiency of absorption, metabolism, and excretion of a particular nutrient is controlled by genes. On the other hand, **nutrigenomics** refers to the many ways dietary components affect gene expression—particularly as it relates to development and treatment of nutrition-related diseases, such as cardiovascular disease. Let us examine each of these branches of nutritional genomics more closely.

In Section 2.6, you learned how Dietary Reference Intakes are set. Recall that nutrient recommendations, such as RDAs, are not absolute but are actually estimates of a level of intake that is likely to meet the needs of most (97% to 98%) of the population. For example, the RDA for folic acid (a B vitamin) is 400 micrograms per day. For most of the population, consuming 400 micrograms per day of folic acid from foods or supplemental sources will supply enough of the vitamin to optimize its function in body processes, such as the formation of red blood cells and metabolism of amino acids. There are certain subgroups of the population, however, for whom 400 micrograms of folic acid is not sufficient. These people have a genetic variation that alters the production of an enzyme necessary for amino acid metabolism, so their dietary requirements for folic acid may be as much as 10 times higher than the RDA. Nutrigenetics researchers are actively examining how genetic variations like this can affect individual nutrient requirements, how we can identify these people, and how we can personalize nutrition advice based on this knowledge.[3]

With nutrigenomics, researchers are interested in finding out how nutrients or other dietary components can influence gene expression, particularly as it relates to development of chronic diseases. Traditionally, nutrition and lifestyle recommendations have been based on the results of observational or experimental research that links diet to disease within the population as a whole. Nutrigenomics research now highlights the fallacy of a "one-size-fits-all" approach to nutrition interventions for disease prevention

---

epigenome A network of chemical compounds surrounding DNA that modify the genome without altering the DNA sequences and have a role in determining which genes are active (expressed) or inactive (silenced) in a particular cell.

epigenetics Heritable changes in gene function that are independent of DNA sequence. For example, malnutrition during pregnancy may modify gene expression in the fetus and affect long-term body weight regulation in the offspring.

Nutrition and genetics interact in various ways:

- Genes dictate much of our individual nutrient requirements.
- Genes may make us more susceptible or resistant to certain nutrition-related diseases.
- Nutrients and other dietary components can affect gene expression.

nutritional genomics Study of interactions between nutrition and genetics; includes nutrigenetics and nutrigenomics.

nutrigenetics Study of the effects of genes on nutritional health, such as variations in nutrient requirements and responsiveness to dietary modifications.

nutrigenomics Study of how food impacts health through its interaction with our genes and its subsequent effect on gene expression.

and management. It is becoming clear that generalized nutrition recommendations may not apply to all individuals within a population group. Nutrients or other compounds in the diet can turn certain genes on or off (like a light switch), thus manipulating the production of proteins that can affect—positively or negatively—the development or progression of diseases. Current areas of research include obesity, diabetes, cardiovascular disease, celiac disease, cancer, osteoporosis, and Alzheimer's disease. With a better understanding of the interactions between genes and our diet, it will not be long before dietary recommendations can be tailored to help those with genetically linked diseases.

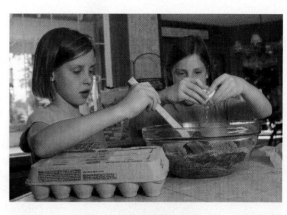

▲ Studies of twins have provided strong evidence for the interaction between genes and diet and their combined effects on disease risk. ©mylife photos/Alamy

NUTRITIONAL DISEASES WITH A GENETIC LINK

Studies of families, including those with identical twins and adopted children, provide strong support for the effects of genetics in various disorders. In fact, family history is considered to be an important risk factor in the development of many nutrition-related diseases.

Cardiovascular Disease There is strong evidence that cardiovascular disease is the result of gene–environment interactions. About one of every 500 people in North America has a defective gene that greatly delays cholesterol removal from the bloodstream. Another genetic variation can lead to elevated blood levels of an amino acid, called homocysteine, which increases cardiovascular disease risk. As discussed in Section 1.2, elevated blood cholesterol is one of the risk factors for development of cardiovascular disease. Discoveries of gene–diet interactions related to management of blood lipids will allow for personalized treatment plans for medications and nutrition therapy to reduce disease risk and improve health outcomes. Although dietary modifications are important and can make a difference, medications and even surgery are often needed to fully address these problems.

Obesity Most obese North Americans have at least one obese parent. This strongly suggests a genetic link. Findings from many human studies suggest that a variety of genes (likely 60 or more) are involved in the regulation of body weight. For example, specific gene variations have been linked to the propensity to overeat and alterations in metabolism.

   Still, although some individuals may be genetically predisposed to store body fat, whether they do so depends on how many calories they consume relative to their needs. A common concept in nutrition is that *nurture*—how people live and the environmental factors that influence them—allows *nature*—each person's genetic potential—to be expressed. Although not every person with a genetic tendency toward obesity becomes obese, those genetically predisposed to weight gain have a higher lifetime risk than individuals without a genetic predisposition to obesity.

Diabetes Both of the two common types of diabetes—type 1 and type 2—are influenced by genetics. Evidence for these genetic links comes from studies of families, including twins, and from the high incidence of diabetes among certain population groups (e.g., South Asians or Pima Indians). Diabetes, in fact, is a complex disease with more than 200 genes identified as possible causes. Only sensitive and expensive testing can identify who is at greatest risk. Type 2 diabetes is the most common form of diabetes (90% of all cases) and is linked to obesity. Typically, type 2 diabetes is diagnosed after a person becomes obese, not before. In this case, nurture affects nature.

Cancer Approximately 10% of cancers have a genetic link. Approximately 90% of cancers are related to environmental and lifestyle factors. Body weight and dietary patterns have been estimated to account for approximately 60% of all cancers. Other environmental influences on cancer risk include tobacco, sedentary lifestyles, family history, viruses, radiation, and toxic exposures.

CRITICAL THINKING

Wesley notices that at family gatherings, his parents, uncles, aunts, and older siblings typically drink excessive amounts of alcohol. His father has been arrested for driving while intoxicated, as has one of his aunts. Two of his uncles died before the age of 60 from alcohol use disorders. As Wesley approaches the age of legal drinking, he wonders if he is destined to fall into the pattern of heavy drinking. What advice would you give to Wesley concerning his future use of alcohol?

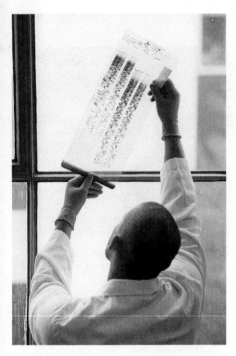

▲ Genetic testing for disease susceptibility will be more common in the future as the genes that increase the risk of developing various diseases are isolated and decoded. ©Rob Meinychuk/Getty Images

YOUR GENETIC PROFILE

From this discussion, you can see that your genes can greatly influence your risk of developing certain diseases. By recognizing your potential for developing a particular disease, you can avoid behaviors and exposures that further raise your risk. How can you figure out your genetic profile? Genetic testing can be valuable if it confirms that you carry a genetic mutation associated with a disease and might alter the course of treatment. Testing is also of interest when you do not know your family medical history or there are gaps in your family tree. Depending on the gene of interest, it typically costs under $1000 to have your DNA sequenced to reveal potential susceptibility for diseases or disorders. Many genetic tests are now covered by health insurance plans. The Genetic Information Nondiscrimination Act, which became a law in May 2008, prohibits health insurers from raising premiums or denying coverage based on genetic information. DNA testing includes providing a DNA sample (blood, saliva, hair). Areas of interest in the genome are sequenced and read in a process known as genotyping. If you are considering genetic testing, it is best to consult a Certified Genetic Counselor. You can find one at nsgc.org.

Many of the genes involved in common diseases, such as diabetes, are still unknown. Although there are genetic tests available for some diseases, your family history of certain diseases is still a much better indicator of your genetic profile and risk of disease. Put together a family tree of illnesses and deaths by compiling a few key facts on your primary relatives: siblings, parents, aunts and uncles, and grandparents, as suggested in the Rate Your Plate section. In general, the greater number of your relatives who had a genetically transmitted disease and the closer they are related to you, the greater your risk. If there is a significant family history of a certain disease, lifestyle changes may be appropriate. For example, women with a family history of breast cancer should avoid becoming overweight or obese, minimize alcohol use, and continue regular checkups.

Figure 3-17 shows an example of a medical family tree (also called a *genogram*). Risk is high when two or more first-degree relatives in a family have a specific disease (first-degree relatives include one's biological parents, siblings, and offspring) or when a first-degree relative develops a disease before the age of 50 to 60 years. In the family depicted in Figure 3-17, prostate cancer killed the man's father. Knowing this, the man should be tested regularly for prostate cancer. His sisters should have frequent mammograms and breast exams because their mother died of breast cancer. Because heart attack and stroke are also common in the family, all the children should adopt a lifestyle that minimizes the risk of developing these conditions, such as avoiding excessive animal fat and salt intake. Colon cancer is also evident, so careful screening throughout life is important.

Information about our genetic makeup should increasingly influence our dietary and lifestyle choices. Throughout this text, we will discuss "controllable" risk factors that could contribute to development of genetically linked diseases present in your family. This information will help you personalize nutrition advice based on your genetic background and identify and avoid the risk factors that could lead to the diseases present in your family.

PERSONALIZING NUTRITION ADVICE

Nutrition professionals already recognize that dietary advice must be tailored to personal and cultural preferences. Research is now paving the way for even more personalized nutrition that incorporates the results of genetic testing to determine which eating pattern will work most effectively for each person. There are genetic tests available for at least 1500 diseases and conditions. Many companies—most of them online—are already offering dietary advice and supplements based on direct-to-consumer genetic tests.

As we discussed in Section 2.7 caution is always needed when evaluating nutrition information and claims. Some DNA-testing companies are responsible organizations, but many are not. Marketing schemes may belittle the science of genetics to consumers. Even though there have been some great advancements in nutritional genomics in

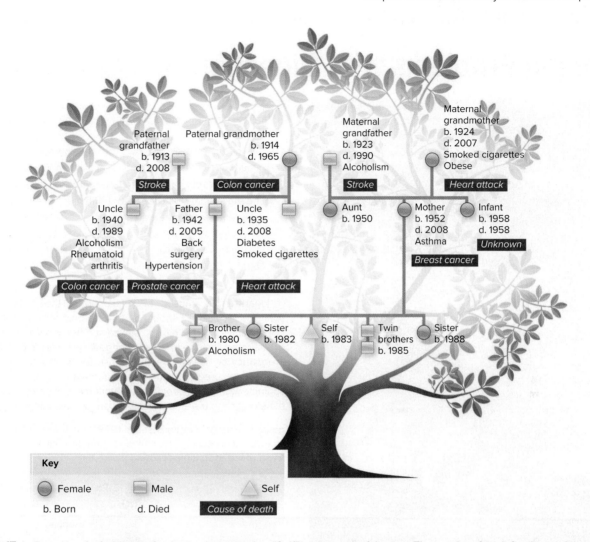

FIGURE 3-17 ▲ Example of a family tree for Justin, designated as "Self" at the trunk of the tree. The gender of each family member is identified by color (blue squares for males and orange circles for females). Dates of birth (b) and death (d) are listed below each family member. If deceased, the cause of death is highlighted using white text against a red background. Other medical conditions the family members experienced are noted beneath each name. Create your own family tree of frequent diseases using the diagram in Rate Your Plate or the interactive tool available at https://familyhistory.hhs.gov/FHH/html/index.html. Then show your family tree to your health care provider to get a more complete picture of what the information means for your health.

recent years, there is still much to learn. Not only is the science of nutritional genomics in its infancy, but application of this technology will require advanced training for health practitioners. Most health professionals agree that genetic testing complements carefully planned nutrient recommendations and dietary guidelines, but on its own, it is not quite ready for "prime time."

This chapter's review of human anatomy, physiology, and genetics from a nutrition perspective sets the stage for a more in-depth look at the nutrients in Chapters 4 through 9. As you learn about recommendations for specific nutrients or prevention of diseases, keep in mind that individual variations in genetic profiles will prove to be important considerations when tailoring nutrition advice.

✓ CONCEPT CHECK 3.11

1. What is the difference between nutrigenetics and nutrigenomics?
2. List two nutrition-related diseases that are strongly affected by genetics.
3. Predict how nutritional genomics will affect nutrition recommendations in the future.

3.12 Nutrition and Your Health

Common Problems with Digestion

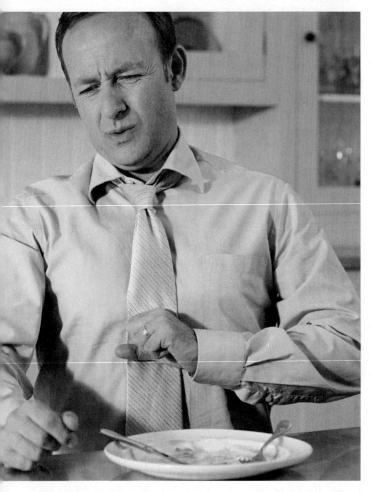

©Image Source

When suffering from persistent heartburn or GERD, see a doctor if you have

- difficulty swallowing or pain when swallowing.
- heartburn that has persisted for more than 10 years.
- initial onset of heartburn after age 50.
- heartburn that resists treatment with medications.
- sudden, unexplained weight loss.
- chest pain.
- blood loss or anemia.
- blood in stool or vomit.

Heartburn is caused by relaxation of the gastroesophageal sphincter. Typically, it should be relaxed only during swallowing, but in individuals with GERD, it is relaxed at other times as well. Increased pressure against the lower esophageal sphincter (e.g., as a result of pregnancy or obesity) heightens risk for heartburn. The hormonal changes of pregnancy also tend to relax the lower esophageal sphincter. For some people, slow movement of gastric contents from the stomach to the small intestine complicates the problem.

gastroesophageal reflux disease (GERD) Disease that results from stomach acid backing up into the esophagus. The acid irritates the lining of the esophagus, causing pain.

Without fanfare, the digestive system does the important work of extracting nutrients from the food you eat to supply the needs of your body's trillions of cells. It is not until something goes awry that you notice digestion at all. In this section, you learn about nutritional strategies to cope with heartburn, ulcers, constipation, hemorrhoids, irritable bowel syndrome (IBS), diarrhea, gallstones, and celiac disease. Three other digestive disorders—lactose maldigestion, diverticulosis, and cystic fibrosis—will be discussed in Section 4.4 and Section 5.6.

Heartburn

About half of North American adults experience occasional heartburn, also known as acid reflux (Fig. 3-18). This gnawing pain in the upper chest is caused by the movement of acid from the stomach into the esophagus. Unlike the stomach, the esophagus has very little mucus to protect it, so acid quickly erodes the lining of this organ. Acid reflux symptoms may include pain, nausea, gagging, cough, or hoarseness. The recurrent and therefore more serious form of the problem is called **gastroesophageal reflux disease (GERD).** GERD is diagnosed when symptoms occur two or more times per week.

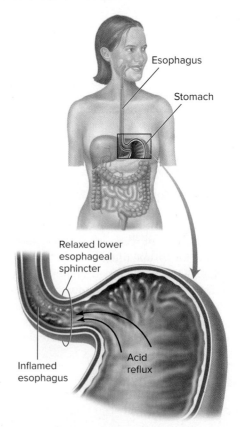

FIGURE 3-18 ▲ Heartburn is a sign of reflux of stomach acid into the esophagus.

If left untreated, heartburn can damage the lining of the esophagus, leading to chronic esophageal inflammation and an increased risk of esophageal cancer. Heartburn sufferers should follow the general recommendations given in Table 3-4. For occasional heartburn, quick relief can be found with over-the-counter (OTC) antacids. Taking antacids will reduce the acid in the stomach but will not stop the acid reflux. For more persistent (few days a week or everyday) heartburn or GERD, H$_2$ blockers or **proton pump inhibitors (PPIs)** may be needed (see the Medicine Cabinet feature in this section). PPIs provide long-lasting relief by reducing stomach acid production and should be taken before the first meal of the day because they take longer to work. Medications that improve GI **motility** may also be useful. If the proper medications are not effective at controlling GERD, surgery may be needed to strengthen the weakened esophageal sphincter.[4]

Ulcers

A peptic **ulcer** occurs when the lining of the esophagus, stomach, or small intestine is eroded by the acid secreted by stomach cells (Fig. 3-19). A disruption of the layer of mucus that usually protects the stomach allows acid and protein-digesting enzymes to damage the stomach lining. Acid can also erode the lining of the esophagus and the first part of the small intestine, the duodenum. This can cause pain, blood loss, and even **perforation.** At any given time, about 4.5 million people in the United States are affected by peptic ulcers. In young people, most ulcers occur in the small intestine, whereas in older people, they occur primarily in the stomach.

proton pump inhibitor A medication that inhibits the ability of gastric cells to secrete hydrogen ions.

motility Generally, the ability to move spontaneously. It also refers to movement of food through the GI tract.

ulcer Erosion of the tissue lining, usually in the stomach or the upper small intestine. As a group, these are generally referred to as peptic ulcers.

perforation A hole made by boring or piercing. With reference to the gastrointestinal tract, the hole is in the wall of the esophagus, stomach, intestine, rectum, or gallbladder. Complications include bleeding and infection.

TABLE 3-4 ■ Nutrition and Lifestyle Recommendations for Care of Heartburn and Peptic Ulcers

	Heartburn	Peptic Ulcers
Avoid smoking.	√	√
Avoid large doses of aspirin, ibuprofen, and other NSAID compounds unless a physician advises otherwise.[a]	√	√
Achieve or maintain a healthy body weight.	√	√
Eat small, low-fat meals.	√	√
Limit alcohol consumption.	√	√
Limit consumption of caffeine (e.g., coffee, some soft drinks).	√	√
Consume a nutritionally complete diet with adequate fiber (see Section 4.3 for sources of fiber).	√	√
Avoid foods that worsen symptoms.[b]		
• Acidic foods (e.g., orange juice, tomato products)	√	√
• Highly spiced foods (e.g., chili, cayenne, and black pepper)	√	√
• Foods that relax the lower esophageal sphincter (e.g., peppermint, spearmint, chocolate)	√	
• Carbonated beverages	√	√
• Onions and garlic	√	
Avoid tight-fitting clothing.	√	
Elevate the head of the bed 6 to 8 inches.	√	
Avoid eating at least 3 to 4 hours before lying down.	√	
Wash hands often and follow food safety guidelines (see Section 13.8).		√

[a] For people who must use these medications, FDA has approved an NSAID combined with a medication to reduce gastric damage. The medication reduces gastric acid production and enhances mucus secretion.

[b] These foods do not *cause* heartburn or ulcers, but they may irritate sites of existing damage in the esophagus or stomach.

CASE STUDY Gastroesophageal Reflux Disease

Caitlin is a 20-year-old college sophomore. Over the last few months, she has been experiencing regular bouts of heartburn. This usually happens after a large lunch or dinner. Occasionally, she has even bent down after dinner to pick up something and had some stomach contents travel back up her esophagus and into her mouth. This especially frightened Caitlin, so she visited the University Health Center.

The nurse practitioner at the center told Caitlin it was good that she came in for a checkup because she suspects Caitlin has a disease called gastroesophageal reflux disease. She tells Caitlin that this can lead to serious problems, such as a rare form of cancer, if not controlled. She provides Caitlin with a pamphlet describing GERD and schedules an appointment with a physician for further evaluation.

1. What dietary and lifestyle habits may have contributed to Caitlin's symptoms of GERD?
2. What is the dietary and lifestyle management advice that will help Caitlin cope with this health problem?
3. What types of medications have been especially useful for treating this problem?
4. Overall, how will Caitlin cope with this health problem, and will it ever go away?
5. Why is management of GERD so important?

Complete the Case Study. Responses to these questions can be provided by your instructor.

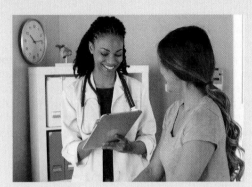

▲ Caitlin was wise to see a health professional about her persistent heartburn. ©Shutterstock/ Rocketclips, Inc.

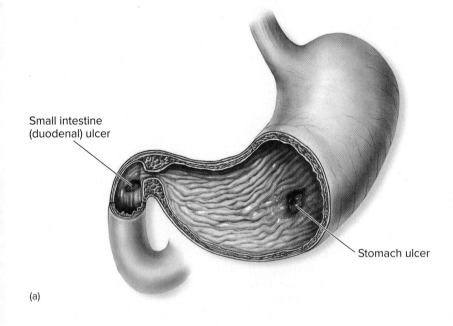

(a)

Small intestine (duodenal) ulcer

Stomach ulcer

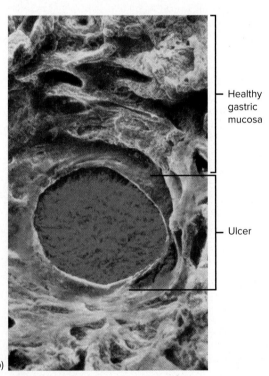

Healthy gastric mucosa

Ulcer

(b)

FIGURE 3-19 ▲ (a) A peptic ulcer in the stomach or small intestine. *H. pylori* bacteria and NSAIDs (e.g., aspirin) cause ulcers by impairing mucosal defense, especially in the stomach. Smoking, genetics, and stress also can impair mucosal defense or cause an increase in the release of pepsin and stomach acid. (b) Close-up of a stomach ulcer. This needs to be treated or eventual perforation of the stomach is possible.
©J. James/Science Source

How do you know if you have a peptic ulcer? Some people experience no symptoms at all, but most notice stomach pain about 2 hours after eating. Stomach acid acting on a meal irritates the ulcer after most of the meal has moved from the site of the ulcer. Other symptoms may include weight loss, lack of appetite, nausea and vomiting, or bloating. Vomiting blood or what looks like coffee grounds and the appearance of black, tarry stools are signs of bleeding in the GI tract. Any evidence of GI bleeding warrants immediate medical attention.

The two chief culprits of peptic ulcer disease are infection of the stomach by the acid-resistant bacteria, *Helicobacter pylori* (*H. pylori*), and heavy use of medications that impair mucus production by the stomach. Conditions that cause excessive stomach acid production also play a role. In addition, cigarette smoking is known to cause ulcers, increase ulcer complications such as bleeding, and lead to ulcer treatment failure.

H. pylori bacteria is found in more than 80% of patients with stomach and duodenal ulcers.[5] The bacteria is common but results in ulcer disease in only 10% to 15% of those infected. Although the mechanism by which *H. pylori* causes ulcers is not well understood, treatment of the infection with antibiotics heals the ulcers and prevents their recurrence. Two Australian physicians were awarded the Nobel Prize in 2005 "for their discovery of the bacterium *H. pylori* and its role in gastritis and peptic ulcer disease."

Nonsteroidal anti-inflammatory drugs (NSAIDs) are medications for painful inflammatory conditions such as arthritis. Aspirin, ibuprofen, and naproxen are the most commonly used types. NSAIDs reduce the mucus secreted by the stomach. Newer medications, called "COX-2 inhibitors" (e.g., celecoxib [Celebrex]),® have been used as a replacement for NSAIDs because they are less likely to cause stomach ulcers. They do offer some advantages over NSAIDs, but they may not be totally safe for some people, especially those with a history of cardiovascular disease or strokes.

The primary risk associated with an ulcer is the possibility that it will erode entirely through the stomach or intestinal wall. The GI contents could then spill into the body cavities, causing a massive infection. In addition, an ulcer may damage a blood vessel, leading to substantial blood loss. For these reasons, it is important to never ignore the early warning signs of ulcer development, which include a persistent gnawing or burning near the stomach that may occur immediately following a meal or awaken you at night.

Today, a combination approach is used for ulcer therapy.[6] People infected with *H. pylori* are given antibiotics and stomach acid-blocking medications (see the Medicine Cabinet feature in this section). There is a 90% cure rate for *H. pylori* infections in the first week of this treatment. Recurrence is unlikely if the infection is cured, but an incomplete cure almost certainly leads to repeated ulcer formation.

Are dietary changes effective for prevention or treatment of peptic ulcers? Many people think that eating spicy or acidic foods can cause ulcers. Contrary to popular belief, these foods do not cause ulcers. However, once an ulcer has developed, these foods may irritate damaged tissues. Thus, for some people, avoidance of spicy or acidic foods may help to relieve symptoms.

In the past, milk and cream were thought to help cure ulcers. Clinicians now know that milk and cream are two of the worst foods for a person with ulcers because the calcium in these foods stimulates acid secretion and actually inhibits ulcer healing.

Medicine Cabinet

Proton pump inhibitors (PPIs) are medications that inhibit the ability of gastric cells to secrete hydrogen ions and thus reduce acid production. Low doses of this class of medications may be available without a prescription. Because stomach acid is important for the absorption of vitamin B-12, prolonged use of PPIs could impair vitamin B-12 status.

Examples:

- Omeprazole (Prilosec OTC)®
- Lansoprazole (Prevacid)®
- Rabeprazole (Aciphex)®
- Esomeprazole (Nexium)®

H₂ blockers impede the stimulating effect of histamine on acid-producing cells in the stomach.

Examples:

- Cimetidine (Tagamet)®
- Ranitidine (Zantac)®
- Nizatidine (Axid)®
- Famotidine (Pepcid)®

©Peter Dazeley/Photographer's Choice/Getty Images

Overall, medical treatment of *H. pylori* infection has so revolutionized ulcer therapy that dietary changes are of minor importance. People with ulcers should refrain from smoking and minimize the use of NSAIDs. Current dietary therapy approaches simply recommend avoidance of foods that tend to worsen ulcer symptoms (see Table 3-4).

Constipation

Constipation, difficult or infrequent evacuation of the bowels, is commonly reported by adults. Slow movement of fecal material through the large intestine causes constipation. More fluid is absorbed during the extended time the feces stay in the large intestine, so the feces become dry and hard.

Constipation can result when people regularly ignore their normal bowel reflexes for long periods. People may ignore normal urges when it is inconvenient to interrupt occupational or social activities. Muscle spasms of an irritated large intestine can also slow the movement of feces and contribute to constipation. Calcium or iron supplements and medications such as antacids can also cause constipation.

NSAIDs Nonsteroidal anti-inflammatory drugs; include aspirin, ibuprofen (Advil),® and naproxen (Aleve).®

constipation A condition characterized by infrequent bowel movements (i.e., fewer than three bowel movements per week).

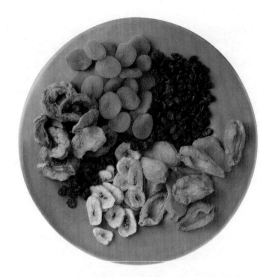

▲ Dried fruits are a natural source of fiber and can help prevent constipation when consumed with an adequate amount of fluid.
©C Squared Studios/Getty Images

Fiber and fluid are the best strategies for treating mild cases of constipation.[7] Whole grain breads and cereals, beans, and dried fruits are excellent sources of fiber. Fiber stimulates peristalsis by drawing water into the large intestine and helping to form a bulky, soft fecal output. Additional fluid should be consumed to facilitate fiber's action in the large intestine. Also, people with constipation may need to develop more regular bowel habits; allowing the same time each day for a bowel movement can help to train the large intestine to respond routinely. Finally, relaxation facilitates regular bowel movements, as does regular physical activity.

Laxatives can lessen constipation. Some laxatives work by irritating the intestinal nerve junctions to stimulate peristalsis, while others that contain fiber draw water into the intestine to enlarge fecal output. The larger output stretches the peristaltic muscles, making them rebound and then constrict. Regular use of laxatives, however, should be supervised by a physician. Overall, the bulk-forming fiber laxatives are the safest to use.

CRITICAL THINKING

Amelia has heard that taking laxatives after overeating prevents deposition of body fat from excess calorie intake. Laxatives hasten emptying of the large intestine and increase fluid losses. Based on what you have learned about digestion and absorption of nutrients, do you think Amelia can count on laxatives to prevent fat gain from excess calorie intake?

---

laxative A medication or other substance that stimulates evacuation of the intestinal tract.

hemorrhoid A pronounced swelling of a large vein, particularly veins found in the anal region.

FODMAPs **F**ermentable **o**ligosacchardes, **d**isaccharides, **m**onosaccharides, **a**nd **p**olyols. These carbohydrates may be poorly digested and lead to GI symptoms such as bloating, gas, and diarrhea in some people.

Hemorrhoids

Hemorrhoids, also called *piles,* are swollen veins of the rectum and anus. The blood vessels in this area are subject to intense pressure, especially during bowel movements. Added stress to the vessels from pregnancy, obesity, prolonged sitting, violent coughing or sneezing, or straining during bowel movements (particularly with constipation) can lead to a hemorrhoid.

Hemorrhoids can develop unnoticed until a strained bowel movement precipitates symptoms. Itching (caused by moisture in the anal canal), swelling, and irritation are the most common symptoms. Pain, if present, is usually aching and steady. Bleeding may result from a hemorrhoid and appear in the toilet as a bright red streak in the feces. The sensation of a mass in the anal canal after a bowel movement is a symptom of an internal hemorrhoid that protrudes through the anus.

Anyone can develop a hemorrhoid, and about half of adults over age 50 do. Diet, lifestyle, and heredity may contribute to the problem. For example, a low-fiber diet can lead to hemorrhoids as a result of straining during bowel movements. If you think you have a hemorrhoid, you should consult your physician. Rectal bleeding, although usually caused by hemorrhoids, may also indicate other problems, such as cancer.

A physician may suggest a variety of self-care measures for hemorrhoids. Pain can be lessened by applying warm, soft compresses or sitting in a tub of warm water for 15 to 20 minutes. Dietary recommendations are the same as those for treating constipation, emphasizing the need to consume adequate fiber and fluid. OTC remedies, such as Preparation H,® can also offer relief from symptoms.

Irritable Bowel Syndrome

An estimated 10% to 15% of adults have irritable bowel syndrome (IBS), characterized by a combination of cramps, gassiness, bloating, and irregular bowel function (diarrhea, constipation, or alternating episodes of both). It is about twice as common in women as it is in men. The disease leads to about 3.5 million visits to physicians in the United States each year.

Symptoms associated with IBS include visible abdominal distention, pain relief after a bowel movement, increased stool frequency, loose stools with pain onset, mucus in stool, and a feeling of incomplete elimination after a bowel movement. Although IBS can be uncomfortable and upsetting, it is harmless as it carries no risk for cancer or other serious digestive problems.

It is difficult to pinpoint an exact cause for IBS. Recent studies indicate that alterations in some of the hormones that regulate the movement of food matter through the GI tract may be to blame. Also, inflammatory responses in the GI tract could be involved for some people with IBS. The majority of people who suffer from IBS perceive that their symptoms are food related, but there is little evidence of actual food allergies or intolerances. When it comes to specific foods, poorly digested carbohydrates are a prime suspect (see the discussion of **FODMAPs** in Chapter 4).[8] Fructose, sugar alcohols, and other carbohydrates may lead to diarrhea or excessive gas if they reach the large intestine undigested. Depression and stress are also associated with IBS; up to 50% of sufferers report a history of verbal or sexual abuse.

Given the diversity of symptoms and possible causes, therapy must be individualized. Medications that target nerves or alter the bacterial population in the GI tract may help people who suffer from frequent diarrhea. For IBS patients whose primary complaint is constipation, medications are available to stimulate peristalsis or block abdominal pain.

Medications may be expensive and some have side effects. Therefore, dietary strategies to cope with IBS are of great interest. Increasing **soluble fiber** (e.g., oats, apples, legumes) may be helpful for some people with IBS, but **insoluble fiber** (e.g., whole grains, vegetables) seems to worsen symptoms (see Section 4.2). Elimination diets that focus on avoiding dairy products and gas-forming foods, such as legumes, certain vegetables (cabbage, beans, and broccoli), and some fruits (grapes, raisins, cherries, and cantaloupe), can alleviate symptoms. Probiotics and peppermint oil have been shown to decrease symptoms of IBS and improve overall quality of life.[9, 10] The patient should limit or eliminate caffeine-containing foods and beverages. Low-fat and more frequent, small meals may help because large meals can trigger contractions of the large intestine. Other strategies include a reduction in stress, psychological counseling, and antidepressant medications. Hypnosis has been shown to relieve symptoms in severe cases.

Following a diet that eliminates certain foods or entire food groups can limit nutritional adequacy. Indeed, research indicates that intakes of some nutrients, including calcium and vitamin A, are inadequate among people with IBS. For help with dietary monitoring, identifying problem foods, and planning a nutritionally adequate diet, a registered dietitian nutritionist can be a valuable resource for a person with IBS.

Diarrhea

Diarrhea is defined as increased fluidity, frequency, or amount of bowel movements compared to a person's usual pattern. Most cases of diarrhea are of short duration and result from viral or bacterial infections. These microorganisms produce substances that cause the intestinal cells to secrete fluid rather than absorb fluid. Another form of diarrhea can be caused by consumption of substances that are not readily absorbed, such as sorbitol, a sugar alcohol found in sugarless gum (see Section 4.3) or large amounts of a high-fiber source such as bran. When consumed in large amounts, the unabsorbed substance draws water into the intestines, leading to diarrhea.

The goal of diet therapy for any form of diarrhea is to prevent dehydration. Increasing intake of water and **electrolytes** is the first line of defense against dehydration. Prompt treatment of dehydration—within 24 to 48 hours—is critical, especially for infants and older adults (see Section 15.2 and Section 16.2). Diarrhea that lasts more than 7 days in adults should be investigated by a physician as it can be a sign of a more serious intestinal disease, especially if there is also blood in the stool.

For diarrhea caused by infection, dietary changes (besides increased fluid intake) are usually not necessary. Some sources recommend temporarily decreasing intake of caffeine, fat, fiber, and poorly absorbed carbohydrates, but other sources show that maintaining a regular diet speeds recovery. Foods containing probiotics may assist recovery. For diarrhea caused by a poorly absorbed substance, such as excess sugar alcohols or lactose, avoidance of the offending substance is the key to relief.[11]

Gallstones

Gallstones are a major cause of illness and surgery, affecting 10% to 20% of U.S. adults. Gallstones are pieces of solid material that develop in the gallbladder when substances in the

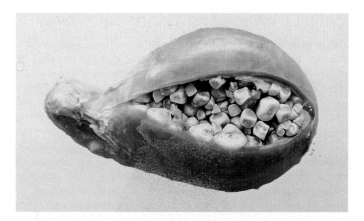

FIGURE 3-20 ▲ Gallbladder and gallstones seen after surgical removal from the body. Size and composition of the stones vary from one case to another. ©The Sydney Morning Herald/Getty Images

bile—primarily cholesterol (80% of gallstones)—form crystal-like particles. They may be as small as a grain of sand or as large as a golf ball (Fig. 3-20). These stones are caused by a combination of factors, with excess weight being the primary modifiable factor, especially among women. Other factors include genetic background (e.g., Native Americans), advanced age (>60 years), pregnancy, reduced activity of the gallbladder (contracts less than normal), altered bile composition (e.g., too much cholesterol or not enough bile salts), diabetes, and diet (e.g., low-fiber diets). In addition, gallstones may develop during rapid weight loss or prolonged fasting (as the liver metabolizes more fat, it secretes more cholesterol into the bile).

Attacks due to gallstones are characterized by intermittent pain in the upper right abdomen, gas and bloating, nausea or vomiting, or other health problems. Medications are available to dissolve gallstones, but these take a long time to work, and the recurrence of gallstones after therapy is common. Therefore, surgical removal of the gallbladder is the most common method for treating gallstones (500,000 surgeries per year in the United States).

The best prevention strategy is to avoid becoming overweight, especially for women. Avoiding rapid weight loss (>3 pounds per week), limiting animal protein and focusing more on plant protein intake (especially nuts), and following a high-fiber diet can help as well. Regular physical activity is also recommended, as is moderate to no caffeine and alcohol intake.[12]

soluble fiber A fiber that is readily fermented by bacteria in the large intestine; also called *viscous fiber*.

insoluble fiber A fiber that is not easily metabolized by intestinal bacteria; also called *nonfermentable fiber*.

diarrhea Increased fluidity, frequency, or amount of bowel movements (i.e., three or more loose stools per day).

electrolyte A mineral that separates into positively or negatively charged ions in water. They are able to transmit an electrical current.

Celiac Disease and Gluten Sensitivity

Celiac disease (sometimes called *celiac sprue*) affects about 1% of the U.S. population. Development of celiac disease depends on two factors: a genetic predisposition and dietary exposure to a protein called **gluten.** Gluten is a type of protein found in certain grains: wheat, rye, and barley. Protein-digesting enzymes in the GI tract break down some of the bonds in gluten, but digestion is incomplete. These partially digested proteins can be absorbed into the cells lining the small intestine. When people with a genetic predisposition for celiac disease are exposed to these small proteins from gluten, they experience an inflammatory reaction. Although many people think celiac disease is a food allergy, it is actually an *autoimmune* response: the immune system attacks and destroys its own cells. (You will learn more about food allergies in Section 6.3 and Section 15.7.)

The immune response that occurs after exposure to gluten targets the cells of the small intestine, causing a flattening of the villi, which thereby reduces the absorptive surface (Fig. 3-21). The production of some digestive enzymes is decreased, and the ability of the small intestine to absorb nutrients is impaired. Malabsorption leads to a variety of GI complaints: diarrhea, bloating, cramps, and flatulence. In fact, it is common for celiac disease to be misdiagnosed as IBS. However, the pathology underlying celiac disease has far worse consequences than IBS. Over time, malabsorption of nutrients can lead to fatigue, weight loss (or poor growth in children), anemia, infertility, and even bone loss.[13]

If celiac disease is suspected, the first step in making a formal diagnosis is a blood test for the presence of antibodies to gluten. This may be followed by one or more biopsies of the small intestine to confirm the pathological defects. There is also a genetic test for celiac disease, but having the gene does not always predict development of the disease.

Strict dietary avoidance of food products containing wheat, rye, and barley is the only proven way to manage the disease.[14] On food labels, food manufacturers must identify the presence of wheat (one of eight major food allergens). However, rye and barley are not as easy to spot. Therefore, people following a gluten-free diet must learn to carefully interpret the list of ingredients to identify sources of gluten. Within the grains group, rice, potato flour, cornmeal, buckwheat, arrowroot, and soy are gluten free, but ingredients such as wheat, rye, barley, bran, graham flour, semolina, spelt, and malt are sources of gluten and must be avoided. Oats do not traditionally contain gluten, but contamination in the field or during food processing could introduce gluten into this grain as well.

People with celiac disease quickly learn that wheat, barley, and rye can be hidden ingredients in any food group. Wheat and its derivatives are used to thicken sauces and condiments, as flavoring agents in dairy products and many other processed foods, and in breading for deep-fried vegetables and meats. It is helpful that many food manufacturers now voluntarily disclose the presence or absence of gluten in their products. However, not all products clearly identify gluten. Dining out is yet another challenge: even a dusting of wheat flour can have adverse effects for a person with celiac disease.

After several weeks on a gluten-free diet, the small intestinal lining regenerates, GI symptoms subside, and nutrient absorption improves. So far, the gluten-free diet is the only proven way to manage celiac disease, but research on other treatments is underway. Food scientists are working toward developing strains of wheat, barley, and rye that do not contain gluten. From a gastroenterological perspective, other approaches are to supply digestive enzymes that will break down the gluten proteins before they stimulate an autoimmune response and to use polymers that will bind to gluten in the GI tract and prevent it from being absorbed. From an immunological perspective, researchers are looking at medications that could block immune responses that damage the small intestine.

A related issue is **nonceliac gluten sensitivity (NCGS),** sometimes called *gluten intolerance.* Some people experience symptoms of celiac disease after ingestion of gluten, but they do not have the small intestinal pathology of celiac disease, nor do they express the antibodies typical of celiac disease. Some reports indicate that for each person who is diagnosed with celiac disease, as many as six others have NCGS. Aside from GI symptoms, patients with NCGS may also report fatigue, headache, muscle and joint pain, and/or sleep disorders. Symptoms subside with a gluten-free diet but reappear when gluten is reintroduced. The medical community recognizes NCGS as a verifiable condition, but the immunological mechanism that causes it is not well understood. There is no diagnostic test for the condition—only the effectiveness of the

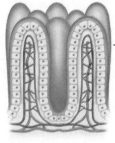

← Normal small intestinal cells. Note the intact villi, which increase the surface area of the small intestine to maximize nutrient absorption.

(a)

Damaged small intestinal → cells of a person with untreated celiac disease. See how the villi appear flattened. The damaged cells cannot absorb nutrients efficiently.

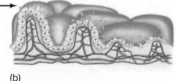

(b)

FIGURE 3-21 ▲ Biopsy findings in patients with and without celiac disease. (a) Normal small intestinal cells. Note the intact villi, which increase the surface area of the small intestine to maximize nutrient absorption. (b) The small intestinal cells of a person with celiac disease. The villi appear flattened. (a, b): ©guniita/123RF

celiac disease Chronic, immune-mediated disease precipitated by exposure to dietary gluten in genetically predisposed people.

gluten Poorly digested protein found in wheat, barley, and rye.

nonceliac gluten sensitivity (NCGS) One or more of a variety of immune-related conditions with symptoms similar to celiac disease that are precipitated by the ingestion of gluten in people who do not have celiac disease.

gluten-free diet in alleviating symptoms. Many questions remain: Is NCGS a permanent condition? Is there a level of gluten intake that would not trigger symptoms? It seems that there are multiple immunological reactions to gluten that are predicted by different genetic traits.[15]

Overall, the prevalence and awareness of celiac disease and NCGS seem to be on the rise. A cause for the increased prevalence has not been pinpointed, but some scientists speculate that changes in wheat production or widespread use of wheat in the food supply may be to blame. Others suspect that an infection or exposure to some environmental toxin could lead to gluten sensitization.

Summary

The conditions discussed here can be very serious, possibly leading to malnutrition, internal bleeding, and life-threatening infections. It is important to seek competent medical advice if you or someone you know suspects a GI disorder. However, you should feel empowered to know that you can control some risks and complement medical treatment with nutrition and other lifestyle changes. Overall, keeping body weight within a healthy range, meeting recommendations for fiber and fluid intake, and avoiding tobacco and overuse of NSAID medications are useful strategies that can help you cope with several common disorders of the GI tract.

ASK THE RDN   Gluten-Free Diet

Dear RDN: *I have heard that a gluten-free diet is a healthier choice. Will a gluten-free diet help me lose weight?*

The media is brimming with popular advice to eliminate wheat and other grains from the diet, promising everything from a clear mind to a trim waistline. For individuals with celiac disease and nonceliac gluten sensitivity, avoiding gluten is a health priority. It will likely correct gastrointestinal complications and a range of other symptoms such as fatigue and body pain. Weight loss, however, is not one of the benefits of a gluten-free diet.

The only reason a gluten-free diet might induce weight loss is because it can be restrictive. For the person who regularly overconsumes bread, pasta, pizza, and baked goods, eliminating all sources of gluten could limit these food choices, thus leading to weight loss. Important point: Weight loss is the result of a calorie deficit, not the lack of gluten. Now, with the increased availability of gluten-free options in grocery stores and restaurants, you will soon realize that a gluten-free diet may not be that restrictive after all.

In fact, you may actually *gain* weight on a gluten-free diet. For a person with celiac disease, as the small intestine heals, nutrient absorption will increase and appetite will likely improve. In addition, many gluten-free products contain more calories than their wheat-based counterparts. To compensate for losses of taste and texture, some gluten-free products incorporate extra fat or sugar. For example, a typical slice of whole-grain wheat bread is about 80 kcal; some brands of gluten-free bread provide as many as 140 kcal per slice. Keep in mind that the "Gluten-Free" claim does not make a food healthy!

Lastly, grains are an important part of a balanced diet. They provide calories, of course, but they also supply dietary fiber and essential vitamins and minerals. Wheat flour is fortified with thiamin, niacin, riboflavin, folic acid, and iron. So, if you are planning to try a gluten-free diet, work with a registered dietitian nutritionist to ensure that your diet meets your nutrient needs. Choose whole gluten-free grains and unprocessed fruits and vegetables to replace wheat and balance calories to avoid weight gain.

With a grain of truth,

Angela Collene, MS, RDN, LD (author)

Summary (Numbers refer to numbered sections in the chapter.)

3.1 Cells join together to make up tissues, tissues unite to form organs, and organs work together as an organ system.

3.2 The basic structural unit of the human body is the cell. Almost all cells contain the same organelles, but cell structure varies according to the type of job cells must perform.

3.3 Epithelial, connective, muscle, and nervous tissues are the four primary types of tissues in the human body. Each type of organ system is affected by nutrient intake.

3.4 From the cells of the GI tract, water-soluble nutrients are absorbed into capillaries and fat-soluble nutrients are absorbed into lymph vessels, which eventually connect to the bloodstream. Blood delivers nutrients and oxygen to cells and picks up waste as it circulates around the body.

3.5 The urinary system, including the kidneys, is responsible for filtering the blood, removing body waste, and maintaining the chemical composition of the blood.

3.6 The nervous system allows for communication and regulation. Vitamin B-12 is part of the insulation that surrounds neurons. Transmission of nerve impulses relies on sodium and potassium. Neurotransmitters are made from amino acids.

3.7 The endocrine system produces hormones—protein-based chemical messengers—to regulate metabolic reactions and the levels of nutrients in the blood.

3.8 With assistance from the skin and the gastrointestinal tract, the immune system protects the body from pathogens. Optimal immune system function relies on protein; essential fatty acids; vitamins A, C, and D; some B vitamins; and the minerals iron, zinc, and copper.

3.9 The GI tract consists of the mouth, esophagus, stomach, small intestine, large intestine (colon), rectum, and anus.

Spaced along the GI tract are sphincters that regulate the flow of food matter. Peristalsis is the movement of food matter along the GI tract. Nerves, hormones, and other substances control the activity of sphincters and peristaltic muscles.

Digestive enzymes are secreted by the mouth, stomach, small intestine, and pancreas. Little digestion and absorption occur in the stomach or large intestine, but some protein is digested in the stomach.

Most absorption occurs through the cells of the villi, which line the small intestine. Absorptive processes include passive diffusion, facilitated diffusion, active transport, phagocytosis, and pinocytosis.

Some water and mineral absorption takes place in the large intestine. Some constituents of undigested carbohydrates are broken down by bacteria in the large intestine. Some of these products are absorbed; remaining undigested materials are eliminated in the feces.

The liver, gallbladder, and pancreas participate in digestion and absorption. Products from these organs, such as enzymes and bile, enter the small intestine and help in digesting protein, fat, and carbohydrate.

3.10 Limited stores of nutrients are present in the blood for immediate use. Some nutrients, such as minerals and fat-soluble vitamins, can be stored extensively in bone, adipose, and liver tissues. Excessive storage of nutrients can be toxic. Conversely, breakdown of vital tissues can supply nutrients in times of need, but continued breakdown eventually leads to ill health.

3.11 Nutritional genomics includes the study of how genes influence nutritional status (nutrigenetics) and how nutrients and other dietary components influence gene expression (nutrigenomics). Genograms and gene testing can be useful tools for identifying prevalence for disease. Personalized nutritional prescriptions can then be applied to promote optimal health.

3.12 Common GI tract diseases, such as heartburn, constipation, and irritable bowel syndrome, can be treated with a combination of diet changes and medications.

Check Your Knowledge (Answers are available at the end of this question set.)

1. The stomach is protected from digesting itself by producing
   a. bicarbonate.
   b. a thick layer of mucus.
   c. hydroxyl ions to neutralize acid.
   d. antipepsin that destroys enzymes.

2. The lower esophageal sphincter is located between the
   a. stomach and esophagus.
   b. stomach and duodenum.
   c. ileum and the cecum.
   d. colon and the anus.

3. A muscular contraction that propels food down the GI tract is called
   a. a sphincter.
   b. enterohepatic circulation.
   c. gravitational pull.
   d. peristalsis.

4. Bicarbonate ions (HCO_3^-) from the pancreas
   a. neutralize acid in the stomach.
   b. are synthesized in the pyloric sphincter.
   c. neutralize bile in the duodenum.
   d. neutralize acid in the duodenum.

5. Most digestive processes occur in the
   a. mouth.
   b. stomach.
   c. small intestine.
   d. large intestine.
   e. liver.

6. Bile is formed in the _____ and stored in the _____.
   a. stomach, pancreas
   b. duodenum, kidney
   c. liver, gallbladder
   d. gallbladder, liver

7. Much of the digestion that occurs in the large intestine is caused by
   a. lipase.
   b. pepsin.
   c. saliva.
   d. bacteria.

8. Treatment of ulcers may include
   a. H₂ blockers.
   b. proton pump inhibitors.
   c. antibiotics.
   d. all of these.

9. The study of how food impacts health through interaction with genes is
   a. nutrigenomics.
   b. epidemiology.
   c. immunology.
   d. nutrigenetics.

10. Energy production that takes place in the cytoplasm is anaerobic metabolism because it does not require
    a. water.
    b. oxygen.
    c. anabolic steroids.
    d. aerobic bacteria.

Answer Key: 1. b (LO 3.8), 2. a (LO 3.8), 3. d (LO 3.8) 4. d (LO 3.8), 5. c (LO 3.8), 6. c (LO 3.8), 7. d (LO 3.8), 8. d (LO 3.12), 9. a (LO 3.11), 10. b (LO 3.2)

Study Questions (Numbers refer to Learning Outcomes)

1. Identify at least one function of the 12 organ systems related to nutrition. **(LO 3.3)**

2. Draw and label parts of the cell, and explain the function of each organelle as it relates to human nutrition. **(LO 3.2)**

3. Trace the flow of blood from the right side of the heart and back to the same site. How is blood routed through the small intestine? Which class of nutrients enters the body via the blood? Via the lymph? **(LO 3.4)**

4. Explain why the small intestine is better suited than the other GI tract organs to carry out the absorptive process. **(LO 3.8)**

5. Identify the six basic tastes. Give an example of one food that exemplifies each of these basic taste sensations. **(LO 3.8)**

6. What is one role of acid in the process of digestion? Where is it secreted? **(LO 3.8)**

7. Contrast the processes of active absorption and passive diffusion of nutrients. **(LO 3.8)**

8. Identify two accessory organs that empty their contents into the small intestine. How do the digestive substances secreted by these organs contribute to the digestion of food? **(LO 3.8)**

9. In which organ systems would the following substances be found? chyme **(LO 3.8)**, plasma **(LO 3.4)**, lymph **(LO 3.4)**, urine **(LO 3.9)**

10. Describe the nutrition-related diseases for which genetics or family history is considered to be an important risk factor. **(LO 3.11)**

What the Dietitian Chose

Constipation results from slow movement of fecal material through the large intestine. Increasing fiber and water in your diet can often relieve constipation without the aid of an over-the-counter laxative. To boost your fiber intake, choose whole grains, fruits, vegetables, and legumes (beans). This can be a tough task when most of the menu options you will find in fast-food restaurants and convenience stores are low in fiber.

As you select your pizza, look for slices with extra vegetables or fruit. This will increase the fiber content by about 1 gram per slice. Pizza with whole grain crust would add another 1 gram of fiber per slice. These are small improvements, so you will probably still need to look for additional fiber sources.

What about your side dish? Unless they are made with whole grains, the pasta and breadsticks will not add much fiber to your meal. A breadstick and a cup of pasta with Alfredo sauce provide about 1 and 2 grams of fiber, respectively. These carbohydrate-rich add-ons are supplying extra calories and would be better off skipped. The salad provides about 1 to 3 grams of fiber, depending on its size and ingredients. The core ingredients of tossed salad—lettuce, cucumbers, tomato—are mostly water and not particularly high in fiber. Toppings such as cheese, egg, or diced meat will not help relieve constipation. Instead, dried fruit (e.g., dried cranberries or raisins) and nuts supply some additional fiber.

An even better choice, however, is the soup! A cup of bean and pasta soup is just what the doctor ordered to help relieve constipation. It provides about 6 grams of fiber and some extra water, as well.

Lastly, be sure to drink plenty of water. Dehydration is an often overlooked cause of constipation. Water helps lubricate the digestive tract and adds bulk to the feces when absorbed by fiber in the large intestine.

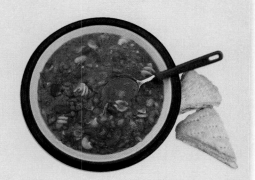

▲ Whole grain pasta and beans used in salads and soups are good sources of fiber that can prevent intestinal issues such as constipation. ©Ingram Publishing/Alamy

Further Readings

1. Bull MJ and Plummer NT: Part 1: The human gut microbiome in health and disease. *Integrative Medicine* 13:17, 2014.

2. Bull MJ and Plummer NT: Part 2: Treatments for chronic gastrointestinal disease and gut dysbiosis. *Integrative Medicine* 14:25, 2015.

3. Kamp, KM and others: Position of the Academy of Nutrition and Dietetics: Nutritional genomics. *Journal of the Academy of Nutrition and Dietetics* 114:299, 2014.

4. National Digestive Diseases Information Clearinghouse: Acid reflux (GER and GERD) in adults. 2014. Available at https://www.niddk.nih .gov/health-information/digestive-diseases/acid-reflux-ger-gerd-adults. (Accessed January 12, 2017).

5. Hunt RH and others: The stomach in health and disease. *Gut* 64:1650, 2015.

6. National Digestive Diseases Information Clearinghouse: Peptic ulcers (stomach ulcers). 2014. Available at https://www.niddk.nih.gov/health-information/digestive-diseases/peptic-ulcers-stomach-ulcers. (Accessed January 12, 2017).

7. National Digestive Diseases Information Clearinghouse: Constipation. 2014. Available at https://www.niddk.nih.gov/health-information/ digestive-diseases/constipation. (Accessed January 12, 2017).

8. Dugum M, Barco K, and Garg S. Managing irritable bowel syndrome: The low-FODMAP diet. *Cleveland Clinic Journal of Medicine* 83:655, 2016.

9. Schoenfeld PS: Advances in IBS 2016: A review of current and emerging data. *Gastroenterology and Hepatology* 12:3, 2016.

10. National Digestive Diseases Information Clearinghouse: Irritable bowel syndrome. 2015. Available at https://www.niddk.nih.gov/health-information/digestive-diseases/irritable-bowel-syndrome. (Accessed January 12, 2017).

11. National Digestive Diseases Information Clearinghouse: Diarrhea. 2016. Available at https://www.niddk.nih.gov/health-information/digestive-diseases/diarrhea. (Accessed January 12, 2017).

12. National Digestive Diseases Information Clearinghouse: Gallstones. 2013. Available at https://www.niddk.nih.gov/health-information/digestive-diseases/gallstones. (Accessed January 12, 2017).

13. Lebwohl B and others: Celiac disease and non-celiac gluten sensitivity. *BMJ* 351:h4347, 2015.

14. Keller M: The gluten-free journey. *Today's Dietitian* 15:24, 2013.

15. Zelman K: Is gluten sensitivity real? New research causes new thinking. *Food and Nutrition Magazine* Sept/Oct 2015:16, 2015.

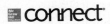 **To get the most out of your study, visit Connect where you will find NutritionCalc Plus, SmartBook®, and many other dynamic tools.**

Rate Your Plate

Source: www.choosemyplate.gov

I. Are You Taking Care of Your Digestive Tract?

People need to think about the health of their own digestive tract. There are symptoms we need to notice, as well as habits we need to practice to protect it. The following assessment is designed to help you examine your habits and symptoms associated with the health of your digestive tract. Put a *Y* in the blank to the left of the question to indicate yes and an *N* to indicate no.

_____ 1. Are you currently experiencing greater than normal stress and tension?

_____ 2. Do you have a family history of digestive tract problems (e.g., ulcers, hemorrhoids, recurrent heartburn, and constipation)?

_____ 3. Do you experience pain in your stomach region about 2 hours after you eat?

_____ 4. Do you smoke cigarettes?

_____ 5. Do you take aspirin frequently?

_____ 6. Do you have heartburn at least once per week?

_____ 7. Do you commonly lie down after eating a large meal?

_____ 8. Do you drink alcoholic beverages more than 2 or 3 times per day?

_____ 9. Do you experience abdominal pain, bloating, or gas 1 ½ to 2 hours after consuming milk products?

_____ 10. Do you often have to strain while having a bowel movement?

_____ 11. Do you consume less than 9 (women) or 13 (men) cups of a combination of water and other fluids per day?

_____ 12. Do you perform physical activity for less than 60 minutes on most or all days of the week (e.g., jog, swim, walk briskly, row, and stair climb)?

_____ 13. Do you eat a diet relatively low in fiber? (Recall that significant fiber is found in whole fruits, vegetables, legumes, nuts and seeds, whole grain breads, and whole grain cereals.)

_____ 14. Do you frequently have diarrhea?

_____ 15. Do you frequently use laxatives or antacids?

Add up the number of yes answers and record the total. If your score is from 8 to 15, your habits and symptoms put you at risk for experiencing future digestive tract problems. Take particular note of the habits to which you answered yes. Consider trying to cooperate more with your digestive tract.

II. Create Your Family Tree for Health-Related Concerns

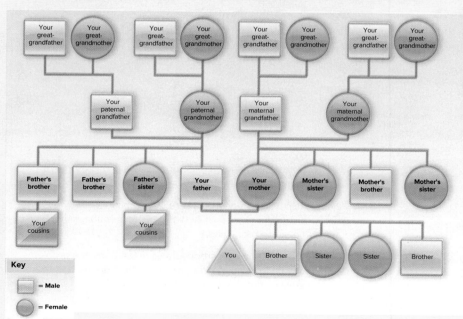

Adapt this diagram to your family tree. Under each heading, list year born, year died (if applicable), major diseases that developed during the person's lifetime, and cause of death (if applicable). Figure 3-17 shows one such example. You may also use the interactive tool available at https://familyhistory.hhs.gov/FHH/html/index.html to generate a medical family tree.

You are likely to be at risk for any diseases listed. Creating a plan for preventing such diseases when possible, especially those that developed in your family members before age 50 to 60 years, is advised. Speak with your physician about any concerns arising from this exercise.

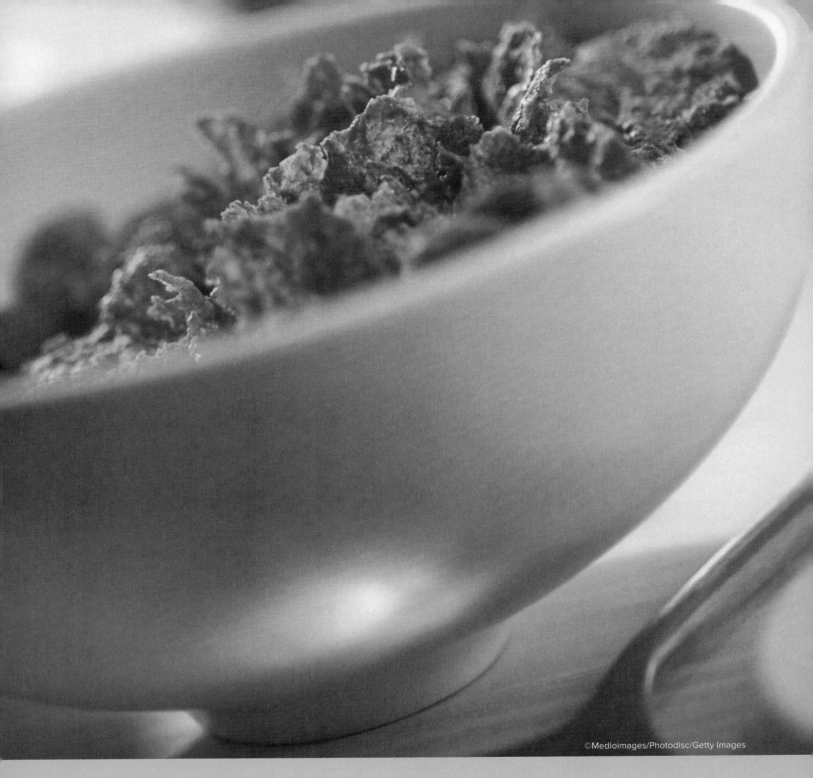

Student Learning Outcomes

Chapter 4 is designed to allow you to:

4.1 Explain the most important nutritional role of carbohydrates and how they are created.

4.2 Identify the basic structures of the major carbohydrates: monosaccharides, disaccharides, polysaccharides (e.g., starches), and fiber.

4.3 Describe food sources of carbohydrates and list some alternative sweeteners.

4.4 Explain how carbohydrates are taken in and used by the body, including the processes of digestion, absorption, metabolism, and glucose regulation.

4.5 List the functions of carbohydrates in the body, the problems that result from not eating enough carbohydrates, and the beneficial effects of fiber on the body.

Chapter 4
Carbohydrates

Think about your choice as you read this chapter, then see What the Dietitian Chose at the end of the chapter.

What Would You Choose?

It is lunchtime and you have a 30-minute break between classes. You stop at Doug's Deli for a quick sandwich. In making a sandwich choice, you remember the importance of the MyPlate food pattern and that several of the food groups provide sources of carbohydrates. All of the sandwiches provide about 350 kcal. The fiber content ranges from about 1 gram to about 7.5 grams. Which sandwich would you choose to maximize the number of servings from a variety of healthy carbohydrate sources?

a Turkey and Swiss on rye with tomato slices, sliced cucumbers, romaine lettuce, and mustard

b Ham and Swiss on sourdough made with extra-lean ham and mayonnaise

c Tuna salad on whole wheat made with tuna, grated carrots, onions, and mayonnaise and served with romaine lettuce, and cucumber slices

d Hotdog on a white bun with relish, mustard, and ketchup

e Soy burger on whole wheat English muffin with tomato, pickle slices, romaine lettuce, and mayonnaise

f Peanut butter and jelly on soft white bread made with strawberry jelly and smooth peanut butter

Think about your choice as you read this chapter, then see What the Dietitian Chose at the end of the chapter.

What did you eat to obtain the energy you are using right now? Chapters 4 through 6 will examine this question by focusing on the main nutrients the human body uses for fuel. These nutrients are carbohydrates (4 kcal per gram) and fats and oils (9 kcal per gram). Although protein (4 kcal per gram) *can* be used for energy needs, the body typically reserves this nutrient for other key processes.

It is likely that you have recently consumed fruits, vegetables, dairy, cereal, breads, and pasta. These foods all supply carbohydrates. Although some carbohydrate sources are more beneficial than others, carbohydrates should contribute to a significant portion of our dietary patterns. Many people think carbohydrate-rich foods cause weight gain, but pound for pound, carbohydrates supply less calories than fats and oils. Furthermore, high-carbohydrate foods, especially fiber-rich foods such as fruits, vegetables, whole grains and legumes, provide many important health benefits in addition to the calories they contain. Almost all carbohydrate-rich foods, except pure sugars, provide essential nutrients and should generally constitute 45% to 65% of our daily calorie intake. Now, let's take a closer look at carbohydrates.

4.6 State the RDA for carbohydrate and various guidelines for carbohydrate intake.

4.7 Identify the consequences of diabetes, and explain appropriate dietary measures that will reduce the adverse effects of this chronic disease.

4.1 Carbohydrates—Our Most Important Energy Source

glycogen A carbohydrate made of multiple units of glucose with a highly branched structure. It is the storage form of glucose in humans and is synthesized (and stored) in the liver and muscles.

photosynthesis Process by which plants use energy from the sun to synthesize energy-yielding compounds, such as glucose.

glucose A six-carbon sugar that exists in a ring form; found in blood and in table sugar bound to fructose; also known as *dextrose*, it is one of the simple sugars.

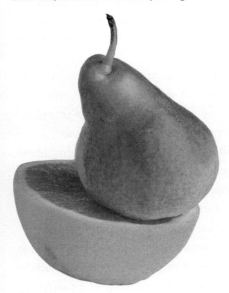

▲ Whole fruits, such as oranges and pears, are excellent sources of carbohydrates, especially dietary fiber.
©John Foxx/Imagestate

Carbohydrates are a main fuel source for some cells, especially those in the brain, nervous system, and red blood cells. Muscles also rely on a dependable supply of carbohydrates to fuel intense physical activity. Carbohydrates provide approximately 4 kcal per gram and are a readily available fuel for all cells, in the form of both blood glucose and **glycogen** stored in the liver and muscles. The glycogen stored in the liver can be used to maintain blood glucose concentrations in times when you have not eaten for several hours or the food you eat does not supply enough carbohydrates. Regular intake of carbohydrates is important because liver glycogen stores are depleted in about 18 hours if no carbohydrates are consumed. After that point, the body is forced to produce carbohydrates, either from the breakdown of protein or fat stores, depending on dietary patterns. This can lead to health problems, including the loss of muscle tissue. To obtain adequate energy, the Food and Nutrition Board of the National Academy of Medicine recommends that 45% to 65% of the calories we consume each day come from carbohydrates (see the Acceptable Macronutrient Distribution Range table in the DRI charts in Appendix G).

Despite their important role as a calorie source, some forms of carbohydrate promote health more than others. As you will see in this chapter, whole grain products have greater health benefits than refined and highly processed forms of carbohydrate. Choosing whole grain carbohydrate sources and limiting the intake of refined carbohydrate sources, contributes to a healthier dietary pattern. Although it is difficult to eat so little carbohydrate that body fuel needs are not met, it is easy to overconsume the simple carbohydrates, namely sugars, that contribute to health risks. Let's explore this concept further as we learn about carbohydrates in detail.

Green plants synthesize most of the carbohydrates in our foods. Leaves capture the sun's solar energy in their cells and transform it into chemical energy. This energy is then stored in the chemical bonds of the carbohydrate glucose as it is produced from carbon dioxide in the air and water in the soil. This complex process is called **photosynthesis** (Fig. 4-1).

$$6 \text{ carbon dioxide} + 6 \text{ water} + \text{solar energy} \rightarrow \text{glucose} + 6 \text{ oxygen}$$
$$(CO_2) \qquad\qquad (H_2O) \qquad\qquad\qquad (C_6H_{12}O_6) \qquad (O_2)$$

Translated into English, this reads: 6 molecules of carbon dioxide combine with 6 molecules of water combined with the sun's energy form 1 molecule of **glucose** and release 6 molecules of oxygen into the air. Converting solar energy into chemical bonds in the sugar is a key part of the process.

FIGURE 4-1 ▶ A summary of photosynthesis. Plants use carbon dioxide, water, and the sun's energy to produce glucose (sugar). Glucose is then stored in the plant and can undergo further metabolism to form starch and fiber in the plant. With the addition of nitrogen from soil or air, glucose can also be transformed into protein.

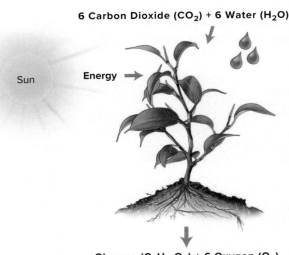

6 Carbon Dioxide (CO_2) + 6 Water (H_2O)

Sun

Energy →

Glucose ($C_6H_{12}O_6$) + 6 Oxygen (O_2)

1. Why are carbohydrates considered our most valuable energy source?

4.2 Forms of Carbohydrates

As the name suggests, most carbohydrate molecules are composed of carbon, hydrogen, and oxygen atoms. Simple forms of carbohydrates are called **sugars.** Larger, more complex forms are primarily called either **starches** or **fibers,** depending on their digestibility. Starches are digestible, whereas fibers are not. The *Carbohydrate Concept Map* at the end of this section summarizes the forms and characteristics of carbohydrates.

Simple carbohydrates contain only one or two sugar units and are called monosaccharides and disaccharides, respectively. On the new food label, sugars are labeled as *Total Sugars* with *Added Sugars* listed as a subcategory below it.

MONOSACCHARIDES—GLUCOSE, FRUCTOSE, AND GALACTOSE

Monosaccharides are the **simple sugar** units (*mono* means "one") that serve as the basic unit of all carbohydrate structures. The most common monosaccharides in foods are glucose, fructose, and galactose (Fig. 4-2).

Glucose is the major monosaccharide found in the body. Glucose is also known as *dextrose,* and glucose in the bloodstream may be called *blood sugar.* Glucose is an important source of energy for human cells, although few foods contain glucose as their primary carbohydrate source. Most glucose comes from the digestion of starches and **sucrose** (common table sugar) from our food. Sucrose is made up of the monosaccharides glucose and fructose. For the most part, sugars and other carbohydrates in foods are eventually converted into glucose in the liver. This glucose then becomes available to serve as a source of fuel for cells.

Fructose, also called *fruit sugar,* is another monosaccharide. Fructose is found naturally in fruits and forms half of each sucrose molecule. After it is consumed, fructose is absorbed by the small intestine and then transported to the liver, where it is quickly metabolized. Much is converted to glucose, but the remaining goes on to form other compounds, such as fat, if fructose is consumed in excessive amounts. Most of the free fructose in the food we eat comes from the use of **high-fructose corn syrup (HFCS)** in soft drinks, candies, jams, jellies, and many other fruit products and desserts (see discussion on nutritive sweeteners in Section 4.3).

The sugar **galactose** has nearly the same structure as glucose. Large quantities of pure galactose do not exist in nature. Instead, galactose is usually found bonded to glucose in **lactose,** a sugar found in milk and other milk products. During digestion, lactose is broken down to galactose and glucose and then absorbed. When galactose arrives at the liver, it is either transformed into glucose or further metabolized into glycogen, depending on the body's energy needs at the time. This is a good example of the body transforming nutrients to be used by the body in other forms as needed. Much of the galactose in the diet is metabolized to glucose. When required for milk production in the mammary gland of a lactating woman, galactose is resynthesized from glucose to help

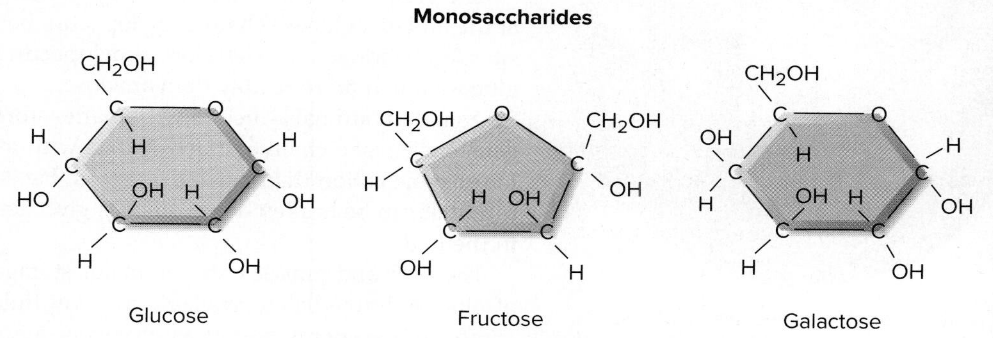

sugar A simple carbohydrate with the chemical composition $(CH_2O)\,n$. The basic unit of all sugars is *glucose*.

starch A carbohydrate made of multiple units of glucose attached together in a form the body can digest; also known as *complex carbohydrate*.

fiber Indigestible substances in plant foods that add bulk to feces. Fiber naturally found in foods is also called *dietary fiber.*

monosaccharide Simple sugar, such as glucose, that is not broken down further during digestion.

simple sugar Monosaccharide or disaccharide in the diet. These simple carbohydrates are broken down and digested very quickly. Most contain refined sugars and very few essential vitamins and minerals.

sucrose Disaccharide composed of fructose bonded to glucose; also known as *table sugar.*

fructose A six-carbon monosaccharide that usually exists in a ring form; found in fruits and honey; also known as *fruit sugar.*

high-fructose corn syrup (HFCS) Corn syrup that has been manufactured to contain between 42% and 90% fructose.

galactose A six-carbon monosaccharide that usually exists in a ring form; closely related to glucose.

lactose Glucose bonded to galactose; also known as *milk sugar.*

Monosaccharides

FIGURE 4-2 ▲ Chemical forms of the important monosaccharides.

Disaccharides

Sucrose: glucose + fructose
Lactose: glucose + galactose
Maltose: glucose + glucose

FIGURE 4-3 ▲ Chemical form of the disaccharide sucrose.

disaccharide Class of sugars formed by the chemical bonding of two monosaccharides.

maltose A disaccharide consisting of glucose bonded to glucose.

fermentation The conversion of carbohydrates to alcohols, acids, and carbon dioxide without the use of oxygen.

polysaccharides Carbohydrates containing many glucose units, from 10 to 1000 or more.

amylose A digestible straight-chain type of starch composed of glucose units.

amylopectin A digestible branched-chain type of starch composed of glucose units.

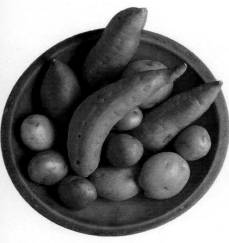

▲ Root vegetables such as potatoes, yams, and tapioca are high in amylopectin starch. ©C Squared Studios/Getty Images

form the milk sugar lactose. Although milk consumption is recommended for lactating mothers, this amazing process produces milk for the baby even if mom doesn't consume milk!

DISACCHARIDES: SUCROSE, LACTOSE, AND MALTOSE

Disaccharides are formed when two monosaccharides combine (*di* means "two"). The disaccharides in food are sucrose, lactose, and **maltose.** All contain glucose.

Sucrose forms when the two sugars, glucose and fructose, bond together (Fig. 4-3). Sucrose is found naturally in sugarcane, sugar beets, honey, and maple sugar. These products are processed to varying degrees to make brown, white, and powdered sugars.

Lactose forms when glucose bonds with galactose during the synthesis of milk. Therefore, our major food source for lactose is milk products. Section 4.4 on lactose maldigestion and lactose intolerance discusses the problems that result when a person can't readily digest lactose.

Maltose results when starch is broken down to just two glucose molecules bonded together. Maltose plays an important role in the beer and liquor industry. In the production of these alcoholic beverages, starches are converted to simpler carbohydrates by enzymes present in the grains. The products of this are then mixed with yeast cells in the absence of oxygen. The yeast cells convert most of the sugars to alcohol (ethanol) and carbon dioxide through a process called **fermentation.** Very little maltose remains in the final product. Small amounts of maltose can be found in some foods, including fruits, vegetables, and breads. Most maltose that we digest (in the small intestine) is produced during our own digestion of starch.

COMPLEX CARBOHYDRATES

In many foods, numerous single-sugar units are bonded together to form a chain known as a polysaccharide (*poly* means "many"). **Polysaccharides,** also called *complex carbohydrates* or *starch,* may contain 1000 or more glucose units and are found chiefly in grains, vegetables, and fruits. When the Nutrition Facts panel on food labels lists *Total Carbohydrates,* this primarily refers to starch content.

Plants store carbohydrates in two forms of starch digestible by humans: **amylose** and **amylopectin.** Amylose, a long, straight chain of glucose units, comprises about 20% of the digestible starch found in vegetables, beans, breads, pasta, and rice. Amylopectin has a highly branched-chain structure and makes up the remaining 80% of digestible starches in the diet (Fig. 4-4). Cellulose (a fiber) is another complex carbohydrate in plants. Although similar to amylose, it cannot be digested by humans, as discussed in Section 4.3.

The enzymes that break down starches to glucose and other related sugars act only at the end of a glucose chain. Amylopectin, because it is branched, provides many more sites (ends) for action. Therefore, amylopectin is digested more rapidly and raises blood glucose much more readily than amylose.

As noted, animals—including humans—store glucose in the form of glycogen. Glycogen consists of a chain of glucose units with many branches, providing even more sites for enzyme action than amylopectin (see Fig. 4-4). Because of its highly branched structure that can be broken down quickly, glycogen is an ideal storage form of carbohydrate in the body.

The liver and muscles are the major storage sites for glycogen. Because the amount of glucose immediately available in body fluids can provide only about 120 kcal, the carbohydrate energy stored as glycogen—amounting to about 1800 kcal—is extremely important. Of this 1800 kcal, liver glycogen (about 400 kcal) can readily contribute to

FIGURE 4-4 ▼ Some common starches, amylose and amylopectin, and glycogen. We consume essentially no glycogen. All glycogen found in the body is produced by our cells, primarily in the liver and muscles.

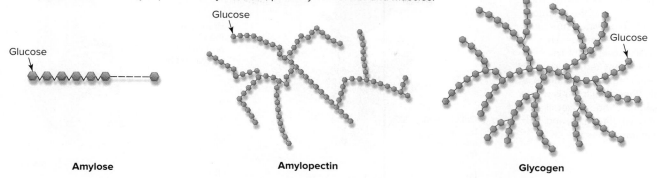

blood glucose. Muscle glycogen stores (about 1400 kcal) cannot raise blood glucose but instead supply glucose for muscle use, especially during high-intensity and endurance exercise. Although animals store glycogen in their muscles, animal products such as meats, fish, and poultry are not good sources of carbohydrates because glycogen stores quickly degrade after the animal dies.

FIBER

Fiber is mainly made up of polysaccharides, but fibers differ from starches insofar as the chemical bonds that join the individual sugar units cannot be digested by human enzymes in the gastrointestinal (GI) tract. This prevents the small intestine from absorbing the sugars because they cannot be released from the various fibers. Fiber is not a single substance but a group of substances with similar characteristics. The group is composed of the carbohydrates **cellulose, hemicelluloses, pectins, gums,** and **mucilages,** as well as the noncarbohydrate **lignin.** In total, these constitute all the non-starch polysaccharides in foods. Nutrition Facts labels combine the individual forms of fiber together under the term **dietary fiber.**

Cellulose, hemicelluloses, and lignin form the structural parts of plants. Bran layers form the outer covering of all grains and are rich in hemicelluloses and lignin. (The woody fibers in broccoli are partly lignin.) **Whole grains** (i.e., unrefined) are good sources of bran fiber (Fig. 4-5). Because the majority of these fibers neither readily dissolve in water nor are easily metabolized by intestinal bacteria, they are called **insoluble** or *nonfermentable fibers.* Insoluble fiber is found in wheat bran, nuts, fruit skins, and some vegetables. Insoluble fiber acts as a natural laxative because it speeds up the transit time of food through the GI tract.

Pectins, gums, and mucilages are contained around and inside plant cells. These fibers either dissolve or absorb water and are therefore called **soluble** or *viscous fibers.* They also are readily fermented by bacteria in the large intestine. These fibers are primarily found in beans, oats, oat bran, and some fruits and vegetables. Soluble fiber slows the rate of absorption by attracting water into the GI tract, reduces blood cholesterol, and controls blood glucose.

Most foods contain mixtures of soluble and insoluble fibers. Food labels do not generally distinguish between the two types, but manufacturers have the option to do so. The definition of fiber has recently been expanded to include: (1) *dietary fiber,* which describes the nondigestible carbohydrates and lignin that are naturally occurring and intact in plants; and (2) **functional fiber,** which consists of the isolated nondigestible carbohydrates that are added to food because they have beneficial physiological effects in human beings. The commercially produced functional or isolated fibers include resistant starch, polydextrose, indigestible dextrins, and inulin, which is one of the most popular varieties currently added to products. The health benefits of many of these fibers are still unclear and are therefore a hot discussion topic.[1,2]

The role of the gut microbiota in human health is a growing area of research. Dietary fiber is an important substrate for the gut microbiota, so dietary fiber alterations have an

cellulose An undigestible, nonfermentable, straight-chain polysaccharide made of glucose molecules.

hemicellulose A nonfermentable fiber containing xylose, galactose, glucose, and other monosaccharides bonded together.

pectin A soluble fiber containing chains of galacturonic acid and other monosaccharides; characteristically found between plant cell walls.

gums Polysaccharides occurring naturally that cause an increase in solubility; used as thickeners, gels, emulsifiers, and stabilizers.

mucilage A soluble fiber consisting of chains of galactose, mannose, and other monosaccharides; characteristically found in seaweed.

lignin A nonfermentable fiber made up of a multi-ringed alcohol (noncarbohydrate) structure.

dietary fiber Fiber found in food.

whole grains Grains containing the entire seed of the plant, including the bran, germ, and endosperm (starchy interior). Examples are whole wheat bread and brown rice.

insoluble fiber A fiber that is not easily metabolized by intestinal bacteria; also called *nonfermentable fiber.*

soluble fiber A fiber that is readily fermented by bacteria in the large intestine; also called *viscous fiber.*

functional fiber Fiber added to foods that has been shown to provide health benefits.

FIGURE 4-5 ▶ Soluble (viscous) and insoluble (nonfermentable) fiber. (a) The skin of an apple consists of the insoluble fiber cellulose, which provides structure for the fruit. The soluble fiber pectin *glues* the fruit cells together. (b) The outside layer of a wheat kernel is made of layers of bran—primarily hemicellulose, a nonfermentable fiber—making this whole grain a good source of fiber. Overall, fruits, vegetables, whole grains, and beans are rich in fiber.

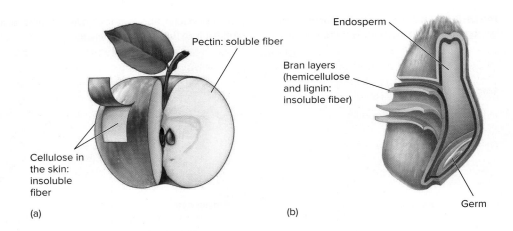

▶ This Carbohydrate Concept Map summarizes the various forms and characteristics of the simple and complex carbohydrates.

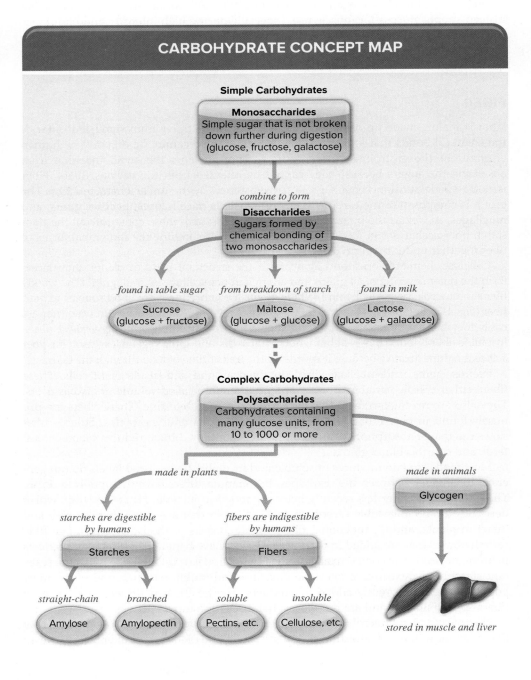

immediate and direct impact on gut microbes. In addition, other compounds in foods containing fiber, such as *flavonoids*, may also modulate the gut microbiota. Gut microbiota is intimately linked to immune function. Therefore, dietary fiber may also impact immune function by way of the gut microbiota. Additional research on dietary fiber and gut microbiota is needed to better understand this link and the potential impact on health outcomes. Many of these fibers fall into a category of functional fiber called the **prebiotics.** Prebiotics include a group of short-chain carbohydrates or oligosaccharides, resistant to digestion but fermented by bacteria in the colon. *Probiotics* promote the growth of helpful bacteria in the gut that improves the host's health.

prebiotic Selectively fermented ingredient that results in specific changes in the composition and/or activity of the gastrointestinal microbiota, thus conferring benefits upon the host.

✅ CONCEPT CHECK 4.2

1. What are the specific names and definitions of the monosaccharides and disaccharides, and what happens to them when they are digested and absorbed?
2. What is a polysaccharide and what are the differences between the plant polysaccharides?
3. What is the name of the storage form of glucose and its locations in the body?
4. What makes fiber a very different kind of carbohydrate, and what is the difference between soluble, insoluble, and functional fiber?

4.3 Carbohydrates in Foods

Four of the groups on MyPlate—grains, vegetables, fruits, and dairy—contain the most nutrient-dense sources of carbohydrates (Fig. 4-6). A healthy, carbohydrate-rich dietary pattern emphasizes a variety of foods from these groups. Most dietary carbohydrate comes from starches. Because plants store glucose in the form of starches, plant-based foods (beans, potatoes, and the grains used to make breads, cereals, and pasta) are the best sources of starch. A dietary pattern rich in these starches also provides many micronutrients, phytochemicals, and fiber along with the carbohydrates. Soluble fibers (pectin, gums, and mucilages) are found in the skins and flesh of many fruits and berries; as thickeners and stabilizers in jams, yogurts, sauces, and fillings; and in products that contain psyllium and seaweed. Fiber is also available as a supplement or as an additive to certain foods (functional fiber) such that individuals with relatively low intakes of natural dietary fiber can still obtain the health benefits of fiber.

Unfortunately, the top carbohydrate sources for U.S. adults in recent years include sugar-sweetened beverages (including energy and sports drinks), followed by yeast breads and rolls, and pastries (cakes, cookies, quick bread, pie). Remember that these foods are on the *Dietary Guidelines* list of foods and food components to reduce. Many North Americans are starting to take a closer look at their carbohydrate sources and improve them from a nutritional standpoint by including more whole grain versions of breads, pasta, rice, and cereals, as well as fruits and vegetables. The decline in soft drink consumption in the United States over the past 11 years is particularly encouraging with shoppers turning to water, energy drinks, and coffee instead. The annual per capita consumption of soft drinks in the United States continues to drop from its highest level in 1985 (currently, it is 43.8 gallons of soft drinks consumed per person per year in 2014). This drop in soda consumption is responsible for a reduction of 79 kcal per day for the average American child.

It is important to understand the percentage of calories from carbohydrates when planning a healthy dietary pattern. The food sources that yield the highest percentage of calories from carbohydrates are table sugar, honey, jam, jelly, fruit, and plain baked potatoes (Fig. 4-6). Cornflakes, rice, bread, and noodles are next, all containing at least 75% of calories as carbohydrates. Foods with moderate amounts of carbohydrate calories are peas, broccoli, oatmeal, dry beans and other legumes, cream pies, French fries, and fat-free milk. In these foods, the carbohydrate content is diluted either by protein, as in

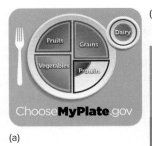

Food Item and Amount	Carbohydrates (grams)	% RDA for Adult Males and Females (130 grams)
Grains		
Cooked rice, ½ cup	22	17%
Spaghetti noodles, ½ cup	19	15%
Seven-grain bread, 1 slice	12	9%
Vegetables		
Baked potato, 1 each	51	39%
Cooked corn, ½ cup	21	16%
Cooked carrots, ½ cup	8	6%
Fruits		
Banana, 1 each	28	22%
Orange, 1 medium	16	12%
Pineapple chunks, ½ cup	10	8%
Dairy		
Light yogurt, 1 cup	19	15%
2% millk, 1 cup	14	11%
Fat-free millk, 1 cup	12	9%
Protein		
Kidney beans, ½ cup	19	15%
Chickpeas, ¼ cup	9	7%
Peanuts, 1 oz	6	5%
Empty calories		
Soda pop, 12 fluid oz	51	39%
Plain M&Ms, ½ oz	30	23%
Energy drink, 8 fluid oz	30	23%

FIGURE 4-6 ▲ Food sources of carbohydrates. (a) The fill of the background color (none, 1/3, 2/3, or completely covered) within each group on MyPlate indicates the average nutrient density for carbohydrate in that group. (b) The bar graph shows the carbohydrate content of several foods in each group compared to the RDA for adult males and females. Overall, the richest sources of carbohydrates are empty calories (sugar-sweetened beverages), starchy vegetables (potatoes), and fruit.

Sources: *Nutrition data from USDA National Database for Standard Reference, Release 26;* www.choosemyplate.gov

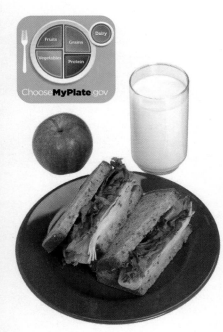

▲ How does this lunch of a turkey, cheese, lettuce, and tomato sandwich on whole grain bread with an apple and a glass of low-fat milk compare to MyPlate? ©McGraw-Hill Education/Ken Karp, photographer

the case of fat-free milk, or by fat, as in the case of cream pies. Foods with essentially no carbohydrates include beef, eggs, chicken, fish, vegetable oils, butter, and margarine.

WHOLE GRAINS

The *Dietary Guidelines* recommend that we consume at least half of all grains as whole grains; increase whole grain intake by replacing refined grains with whole grains; and limit the consumption of foods that contain refined grains, especially refined grain foods that contain solid fats, added sugars, and sodium. The *Dietary Guidelines* define whole grain as the entire grain seed or kernel made of three components: bran, germ, and endosperm. When the term *whole grain* is used on a food package, it also means that the product contains a minimum of 51% whole grain ingredients by weight per serving. Examples of whole grains include whole wheat flour, bulgur (cracked wheat), oatmeal, whole cornmeal, and brown rice. Although most Americans consume enough grains, very few are whole grains. *At least half* of all the grains eaten should be whole grains. In contrast, refined grains have been milled, a process that removes the bran and germ. This process gives grains a finer texture and improves their shelf life, but it also removes dietary fiber, iron, and many B vitamins (Table 4-1). Some examples of refined grain products are white flour, de-germed cornmeal, white bread, and white rice.

TABLE 4-1 ■ Characteristics of Refined and Whole Grains

Refined Grains	Whole Grains
Contains endosperm only	Contains all components of grain (bran, germ, and endosperm)
Increased blood glucose response	Complex carbohydrate with slower glucose response
Lower in fiber	Higher in fiber
Lighter texture	Denser texture
Typically less expensive	Typically more expensive
Lower in nutrient density but enriched	Higher in vitamins, minerals, and antioxidants

Is White Whole Wheat Really Whole Grain?

White whole wheat is a whole grain. It has the nutritional benefits of whole wheat but a milder taste, softer texture, and the lighter color of white bread. Traditional whole wheat is made from red wheat, which has a darker color and strongly flavored phenolic compounds. Switching to white whole wheat may be an acceptable option for those who prefer the taste and texture of white bread.

Although more fiber is one of the primary advantages of whole grains, many benefits of whole grains are thought to be due to the combined effects of several compounds. These compounds include fiber, minerals, trace minerals, vitamins, carotenoids, and other phytochemicals. These are mainly contained in the bran and germ parts of the grains. The *Dietary Guidelines* recommend consuming two to three servings of whole grains per day. Several studies have shown that this is enough to impart numerous health benefits, including reducing risks of cardiovascular disease, diabetes, metabolic syndrome, some cancers, and obesity.

It is estimated that 95% of people don't meet the whole grain recommendation that at least half of all grains consumed be whole grains. Although Americans like grains and consume almost 7 ounces daily, less than 1 ounce is typically whole grain. The reasons Americans are reluctant to consume whole grains include preferences in the taste, texture, cost, and availability of whole grains, compared to products made with refined flour.

In addition to our preference for refined grains, many consumers who are trying to choose a whole grain product are very confused by the deceptive marketing messages on the labels of grain products. For example, a label that says a cereal is *made with whole grains* does not guarantee that the cereal contains 100% whole grain. Terms such as *cracked wheat bread, stoneground wheat, enriched wheat flour, 12-grain bread,* and *multigrain* are confusing because these products may contain little to no whole grain. Multigrain cereals may contain multiple grains, but many of them may be refined with just a small amount of whole grains added to a substantial amount of refined grains. Some *whole grain breads* are white bread in disguise because brown coloring is added to enriched white flour.[3]

With all of the confusing buzzwords, it is crucial to look beyond the front-of-the-package marketing claims and examine the list of ingredients. To confirm that products contain 100% whole grain, look for *whole* as the first word on the ingredient list. Sugary breakfast cereals that claim to be whole grain may list the first ingredient as a whole grain such as corn, rice, oat, or wheat, but then the next several ingredients may be various forms of sugar that together weigh more than the whole grain.[4,5]

Although whole grains make up only about 10% to 15% of grains on the grocery shelves, it is getting easier to find whole wheat products and other whole grain pastas. See Table 4-2 for information on several whole grains that are available, including their potential health benefits. To help simplify the process of finding whole grain foods, the Whole Grains Council developed the Whole Grain stamp for food manufacturers to use on grain products (image to right). The Whole Grain stamp is on over 10,500 different products and in over 44 countries. Choosing products with the 100% whole grain stamp will help us reach the minimum goal of getting 3 ounce equivalents of whole grains per day.[3] Schools are doing their part to increase whole grain consumption by children by meeting requirements of the USDA's Healthy, Hunger-Free Kids Act. Foods must contain at least 50% whole grains to meet the whole grain–rich criteria for the federal school breakfast and lunch programs.

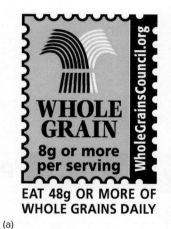

(a)

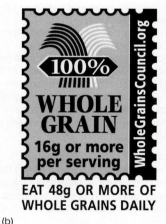

(b)

▲ The Whole Grains Council developed the Whole Grain stamp for use on grain products to identify whole grain foods. There are two versions of the stamp. (a) The basic stamp is used if a product contains at least 8 grams (a half serving) of whole grain, but it may also contain some refined grain. (b) The 100% stamp is used if all grain ingredients are whole grains and there is a minimum of 16 grams (a full serving) of whole grain per serving.

Source: WholeGrainCouncil.org.

VEGETABLES

Vegetables are a valuable source of carbohydrates in the form of starch and fiber. They are naturally low in fat and calories and come packed with many other nutrients vital for health, including potassium, folate, vitamin A, and vitamin C. Potatoes, as featured in this chapter's *Farm to Fork*, contain many nutrients as well as a healthy dose of fiber. Eating the recommended amount of vegetables has been shown to reduce the risk of several chronic diseases. As we discussed with whole grains, the fiber in vegetables may reduce the risk of heart disease, obesity, cancer, and type 2 diabetes. Within the MyPlate guidelines, any vegetable or 100% vegetable juice counts as a member of the vegetables group. Vegetables are organized into five subgroups (dark-green vegetables, starchy vegetables, red and orange vegetables, beans and peas, and other vegetables) based on their nutrient content. Vegetable choices should be selected from among the vegetable subgroups but may be raw or cooked; fresh, frozen, canned, or dried/dehydrated; and whole, cut up, or mashed. Although it is not necessary to eat vegetables from each subgroup daily, the amounts listed from each subgroup should be eaten over a week as a way to add variety, improve intake of key nutrients, and reach your daily intake recommendation.

The amount of vegetables you need depends on your age, sex, and level of physical activity. For example, recommended total daily amounts for women age 19 to 50 years of age are 2 ½ cups. In general, 1 cup of raw or cooked vegetables or vegetable juice or 2 cups of raw leafy greens can be considered as "1 cup equivalent" from the vegetables group. Recommended weekly amounts from each vegetable subgroup are given as amounts to eat weekly. For example, the recommendations for women age 19 to 50 years

FARM to FORK   Potatoes

Grow

- Potatoes are one of the most productive crops around the world. This is good news because the average American eats more than 130 pounds of potatoes each year!
- Thankfully, potatoes can be easily grown in most climates with little maintenance.
- For the best results, plant one seed potato in the bottom third of a gallon container. As the plant grows, mound more soil/compost mix around stem until you reach the top of the vessel. Stop watering for 2 weeks after the foliage dies.
- Harvest by hand, allow to dry for one day, then brush off soil, wash, and enjoy!

Shop

- "New" potatoes (harvested early in the season) have thin skins and a waxy flesh. They cause a slower rise in blood glucose than "old" potatoes (harvested late in the season), which have thick skins and are typically used for baking.
- Of the most common varieties, Russett potatoes have the most phytochemicals. They are good sources of potassium, vitamin C, and several B vitamins.
- Try colorful novelty potatoes (red, blue, and black-skinned) with deep-colored flesh to get a more varied boost of phytochemicals.
- Consider buying organic potatoes to reduce pesticide residues.

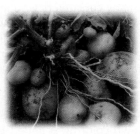

©D Leonis/Getty Images

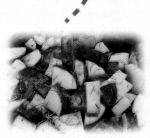

©Peter Madril

Store

- Store "new" potatoes in the refrigerator and eat within 1 week of purchase.
- "Old" potatoes can be stored for months in a cool, dark, well-ventilated location.

Prep

- Scrub potatoes before cooking, and eat with the skins to increase nutrient consumption by up to 50%.
- Most varieties of potatoes contain rapidly digested starch, which causes a sharp rise in blood glucose.
- For those concerned with blood glucose control, leftovers are better! Cook potatoes, refrigerate overnight, then reheat and eat them the next day. The cooler temperatures, postcooking, change the structure of the starch, which will delay a sharp rise in blood glucose.
- To add flavor and nutrients, opt for toppings such as yogurt, vegetarian chili, salsa, herbs, and spices.
- Sadly, much of the U.S. potato consumption is in the form of French fries and potato chips. Try to limit consumption of these potato products and aim for less highly processed potatoes.

Source: Robinson J: Potatoes: From wild to fries. In *Eating on the Wild Side*. New York: Little, Brown and Company, 2013.

TABLE 4-2 ■ **Know Your Whole Grains**

Grain	Characteristics	How to Spot Whole Grain	Health Benefits
Barley	Highest in fiber with a tough hull which is difficult to remove without losing some of the bran; very slow cooking	Look for whole barley, hulled barley, or hull-less barley. Pearled barley is not technically a whole grain.	Barley fiber may lower cholesterol even more effectively than oat fiber.
Buckwheat	High levels of the antioxidant rutin and a high level of protein	If buckwheat is on ingredient list, it is almost always whole buckwheat.	Rutin improves circulation and prevents LDL cholesterol from blocking blood vessels.
Corn	Known for its sweet flavor	Avoid labels that say *degerminated* and look for the words *whole corn.*	Corn has highest level of antioxidants of any grain or vegetable.
Oats	High in protein, often popular for breakfast	*Oats, oatmeal,* or *oat groats* on an ingredient list are almost always whole oats. Steel-cut oats contain the entire oat kernel. In the U.S., most oats are steamed and flattened to produce *old-fashioned* or regular oats, quick oats, and instant oats.	Oat fiber is especially effective in lowering cholesterol.
Quinoa	Rich in high-quality protein, this is a small, light-colored round grain.	*Quinoa* on ingredient list almost always means whole quinoa.	Quinoa is a protein that contains all the essential amino acids.
Rice	Many whole grain varieties, including brown, black, purple, or red. Brown rice is lower in fiber than most other whole grains but rich in many nutrients. White rice is refined.	Brown rice is always whole grain, as are most other colored rices, such as black rice or red rice.	One of the most easily digested grains; rice is ideal for those on a restricted diet or who are gluten intolerant.
Rye	Unusual among grains for the high level of fiber in its endosperm—not just in its bran	Look for whole rye or rye berries in the ingredient list.	Rye fiber promotes a rapid feeling of fullness. Rye products generally have a lower glycemic index than products made from most other grains, making them a good choice for diabetics.
Wheat	Dominates the grains we eat because it contains large amounts of gluten, a stretchy protein that enables bakers to create risen breads	Look for the term *whole wheat* (in Canada, for the term *whole grain whole wheat*).	Studies of *whole grains* attest to the benefits of whole wheat, including reduced risk of stroke, type 2 diabetes, heart disease, inflammatory disease, asthma, better weight maintenance and healthier blood pressure.

Source: Adapted from the Whole Grains Council, Whole grains A to Z, at http://wholegrainscouncil.org/whole-grains-101/whole-grains-a-to-z.

are 1 ½ cups of dark-green vegetables, 5 ½ cups of red and orange vegetables, 1 ½ cups of beans and peas, 5 cups of starchy vegetables, and 4 cups of other vegetables such as cauliflower or mushrooms.

FRUITS

Fruits provide carbohydrates primarily in the form of natural sugar and fiber. Eating fruits provides health benefits similar to those discussed for vegetables; people who eat more fruits as part of an overall healthy dietary pattern are more likely to have a reduced risk of several chronic diseases. Dietary fiber from fruits helps reduce blood cholesterol levels, may lower risk of heart disease, and is important for proper bowel function. The fiber in fruits helps with weight maintenance by providing a feeling of fullness with fewer calories. Remember that whole or cut-up fruits are a great source of dietary fiber, compared to fruit juices that contain little or no fiber.

ASK THE RDN | Juicing

Dear RDN: *Is juicing healthier than eating whole fruits or vegetables?*

Juicing has become a popular way to consume fruits and vegetables and can be a fun way to drink the fruits and vegetables you do not enjoy eating. It is also a smart way to get your vitamins and minerals if you have gas or cramping when you eat fiber-rich produce. The good news is that most of the vitamins, minerals, and phytochemicals remain in the juice that is extracted from the fruits and vegetables during the juicing process. Also, you control the amount of added sugars and preservatives in the end product. The downside of the juicing process is that the natural fiber found in whole fruits and vegetables is typically lost. Thus, the juice is not healthier than whole fruit. In fact, there is no scientific evidence to support claims that juice extracts provide any health benefits or that nutrients are better absorbed from juice. Remember that juices from both fruits and vegetables contain a significant amount of natural sugar and juicing concentrates the sugar and calories. If consumed in excess, those calories can quickly add up! For example, juicing three apples will result in 40 grams of sugar and 200 calories. To make your juice healthier, add some of the pulp back to obtain valuable fiber that can help you feel full. Even better, instead of a juicer, you can use an extractor (e.g., NutriBullet®), which pulverizes fruits, vegetables, and nuts into the consistency of juice. Finally, keep sugar, calories, and fiber content in mind when buying ready-made juices at trendy juice bars.

To your health,

Anne M. Smith, PhD, RDN, LD (author)

DAIRY

Foods in the dairy group provide carbohydrates in the form of lactose. Dairy products also provide other key nutrients, including calcium, potassium, vitamin D, and protein, which are responsible for many health benefits, especially improved bone health. While calcium-fortified soy milk (soy beverage) is part of the dairy group, foods made from milk that are primarily fat, such as cream cheese, cream, and butter, are not part of this group. The lactose content of dairy products varies somewhat (Table 4-3). Some individuals experience the condition of lactose intolerance and maldigestion when they consume high-lactose foods (further discussed in Section 4.4). The amount of food you need to eat from the dairy group depends on your age, with the recommended daily amounts being 3 cups for all males and females 9 years and older. Typically, 1 cup of milk, yogurt, or soy milk (soy beverage), 1 ½ ounces of natural cheese, or 2 ounces of processed cheese is considered as "1 cup equivalent" from the dairy group.

TABLE 4-3 ▪ **Lactose in Common Dairy Foods**

Food Product	Lactose (grams)
Cheese (1 oz, American, Swiss)	1
Cheese (1 oz, cheddar, brie)	0
Cottage cheese (1/2 cup)	3
Ice cream (1/2 cup)	6
Lactaid® milk (1 cup)	0
Milk (1 cup, skim/2%/whole)	12
Sour cream (1/2 cup)	4
Yogurt (8 oz, Greek)	5
Yogurt (8 oz container, 12 g protein)	15

Source: USDA, ARS National Agriculture Library: Nutrient Data Laboratory. Lactose may vary by brand. Read labels carefully.

NUTRITIVE SWEETENERS

The various substances that impart sweetness to foods fall into two broad classes: nutritive sweeteners, which can provide calories for the body, and alternative sweeteners, which, for the most part, provide no calories.[7] Alternative sweeteners are much sweeter on a per-gram basis than the nutritive sweeteners. The taste and sweetness of sucrose make it the benchmark against which all other sweeteners are measured. Sucrose is obtained from sugarcane and sugar beet plants. Both sugars and sugar alcohols provide calories along with sweetness. Sugars are found in many different food products, whereas sugar alcohols have rather limited uses.

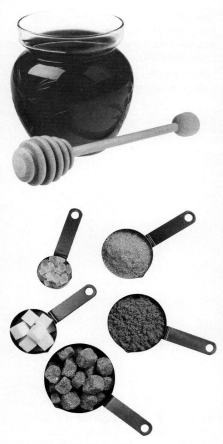

Sugars. All of the monosaccharides (glucose, fructose, and galactose) and disaccharides (sucrose, lactose, and maltose) discussed earlier are designated *nutritive sweeteners* because they provide calories. Many forms of sugar, including those naturally present in food and those added during processing or preparation, add up to an average intake of about 28 teaspoons of total sugar per day. The *Dietary Guidelines* recommend that we reduce the intake of calories from added sugars. Added sugars are defined as caloric sweeteners added to foods during processing or preparation or before consumption. It is estimated that Americans consume an average of 20 teaspoons of added sugar per day, far exceeding the recommendation of no more than 6 to 9 teaspoons daily for adults. Data from a recent National Health and Nutrition Examination Survey (NHANES) indicate that 14.6% of our total energy intake is from added sugar and that 60% of it comes from sugar-sweetened beverages, grain-based desserts, and fruit drinks. Keep in mind the *Dietary Guidelines* recommend a dietary pattern that has less than 10% of calories from added sugar.

High-fructose corn syrup (HFCS) is a sweetener used in a wide variety of foods, from soft drinks to barbecue sauce. It is called *high-fructose* corn syrup because it contains 55% fructose, compared to sucrose, which contains only 50% fructose. HFCS is made by an enzymatic process that converts some of the glucose in cornstarch into fructose, which tastes sweeter than glucose. In the United States, corn is abundant and inexpensive compared to sugarcane or sugar beets, much of which is imported. Food manufacturers prefer HFCS because of its low cost and broad range of food-processing applications, and because it is easy to transport, has better shelf stability, and improves food properties. An average American consumes about 25 pounds of HFCS each year. There has been much confusion and controversy surrounding the use and possible health effects of HFCS. After extensive review, the scientific community has concluded that there are no metabolic or endocrine response differences between HFCS and sucrose related to obesity or any other adverse health outcome.[7]

▲ There are many forms of sugar on the market. Together they contribute to our daily intake of approximately 100 grams (20 teaspoons) of sugar in our diets. ©Burke/Triolo Productions/Getty Images (honey jar); ©C Squared Studios/Getty Images (measuring spoons)

In addition to sucrose and HFCS, brown sugar, turbinado sugar, honey, maple syrup, agave nectar, and other sugars are also added to foods. Brown sugar is essentially sucrose containing some molasses that is not completely removed from the sucrose during processing or is added to the sucrose crystals. Turbinado sugar is a partially refined version of raw sucrose that is often marketed as *raw sugar*. Maple syrup is made by boiling down and concentrating the sap from sugar maple trees. Because pure maple syrup is expensive, most pancake syrup is primarily corn syrup and HFCS with maple flavor added.

Honey is a product of plant nectar that has been altered by bee enzymes. The enzymes break down much of the nectar's sucrose into fructose and glucose. Honey offers essentially the same nutritional value as other simple sugars—a source of energy and little else. However, honey is not safe for infants because it can contain spores of the bacterium *Clostridium botulinum* that causes fatal foodborne illness. Unlike the acidic environment of an adult's stomach, which inhibits the growth of the bacteria, an infant's stomach does not produce much acid, making infants more susceptible to the threat that this bacterium poses.

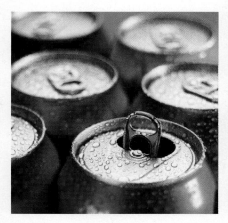

▲ Soft drinks are typical sources of either sugars or alternative sweeteners, depending on the type of soft drink chosen. ©BananaStock/PunchStock

Sugar Alcohols. Food manufacturers and consumers have numerous options for obtaining sweetness while using less sugar and calories. Sugar alcohols are carbohydrates with a chemical structure that partially resembles both sugar and alcohol, but they don't contain ethanol. They are incompletely absorbed and metabolized by the body, and

sorbitol Alcohol derivative of glucose that yields about 3 kcal/g but is slowly absorbed from the small intestine; used in some sugarless gums and dietetic foods.

xylitol Alcohol derivative of the five-carbon monosaccharide xylose.

consequently contribute fewer calories than most sugars. This allows people with diabetes to enjoy the flavor of sweetness while controlling sugars; they also provide noncaloric or very-low-calorie sugar substitutes for persons trying to lose (or control) body weight.

Sugar alcohols, or polyols, such as **sorbitol** and **xylitol,** are used as nutritive sweeteners but contribute fewer calories (about 2.6 kcal per gram) than sugars. They are also absorbed and metabolized to glucose more slowly than are simple sugars. Because of this, they remain in the intestinal tract for a longer time and in large quantities, can cause diarrhea. In fact, any product that may be consumed in amounts that result in a daily ingestion of 50 grams or more of sugar alcohols must bear the statement, *Excess consumption may have a laxative effect* on the label.

Sugar alcohols must be listed on labels. If only one sugar alcohol is used in a product, its name must be listed; however, if two or more are used in one product, they are grouped together under the heading *sugar alcohols.* The caloric value of each sugar alcohol used in a food product is calculated so that when one reads the total amount of calories a product provides, it includes the sugar alcohols in the overall amount.

Sugar alcohols are used in sugarless gum, breath mints, and candy. Unlike sucrose, sugar alcohols are not readily metabolized by bacteria to acids in the mouth and thus do not promote tooth decay.

ALTERNATIVE SWEETENERS

Alternative, or artificial, *nonnutritive* sweeteners yield little or no calories when consumed in amounts typically used in food products. They also are not metabolized by bacteria in the mouth, so they do not promote dental caries. A growing number of alternative sweeteners are currently available in the United States, resulting in a $1.2 billion industry.[6]

Acceptable Daily Intake (ADI) Estimate of the amount of a sweetener that an individual can safely consume daily over a lifetime. ADIs are given as milligrams per kilogram of body weight per day.

For each sweetener, the FDA determines an **Acceptable Daily Intake (ADI)** guideline. ADIs are set at a level 100 times less than the level at which no harmful effects were noted in animal studies. Current evidence suggests that alternative sweeteners can be used safely by adults and children, and are considered safe during pregnancy. Note that large, long-term studies have yet to be conducted in humans.

saccharin Alternative sweetener that yields no energy to the body; 200 to 700 times sweeter than sucrose.

Saccharin The oldest alternative sweetener, **saccharin** represents about half of the alternative sweetener market in North America (typically packaged in pink packets, including Sweet 'N Low).® The FDA lists the ADI for saccharin at 5 milligrams per kilogram, or the equivalent of 9 to 12 packets of the sweetener.

aspartame Alternative sweetener made of two amino acids and methanol; about 200 times sweeter than sucrose.

Aspartame. Aspartame is in widespread use throughout the world (typically packaged in blue packets, including Equal).® It has been approved for use in more than 90 countries, and its use has been endorsed by the World Health Organization, the American Medical Association, the American Diabetes Association, among other reputable scientific groups.

The components of aspartame are the amino acids phenylalanine and aspartic acid, along with methanol. Recall that amino acids are the building blocks of proteins, so aspartame is more like a protein than a carbohydrate. Like protein, aspartame yields about 4 kcal per gram, but because it is about 200 times sweeter than sucrose, only a small amount is needed to obtain the desired sweetness. Like other proteins, however, aspartame is not heat-stable and would lose its sweetness if exposed to excessive heat. Aspartame is used in beverages, gelatin desserts, chewing gum, and toppings.

The ADI of aspartame is 50 milligrams per kilogram of body weight. This is equivalent to about 18 cans of aspartame-containing diet soft drinks or 8 packets of Equal. Aspartame appears to be safe for pregnant women and children, but some scientists suggest cautious use by these groups, especially young children, who need ample calories to grow.

phenylketonuria (PKU) Disease caused by a genetic defect in the liver's ability to metabolize the amino acid phenylalanine into the amino acid tyrosine; untreated, toxic by-products of phenylalanine build up in the body and lead to brain damage and severe health issues.

sucralose Alternative sweetener that has chlorines in place of 3 hydroxyl (—OH) groups on sucrose; 600 times sweeter than sucrose.

Persons with an uncommon disease called **phenylketonuria (PKU),** which interferes with the metabolism of phenylalanine, should avoid aspartame because of its high phenylalanine content. People with PKU will find a mandatory warning label on products containing aspartame (see label for sugarless gum).

Sucralose. Sucralose (Splenda)® is made by adding three chlorine molecules to sucrose. It cannot be broken down or absorbed, so it yields no calories, and it is about 600 times sweeter than table sugar. It can be used in cooking and baking because it does not break down under high heat conditions. Sucralose is approved as an additive to foods such as soft drinks, gum, baked goods, syrups, gelatins, frozen dairy desserts such as ice cream, jams, processed fruits, and fruit juices, and for tabletop use. The ADI for sucralose is 5 milligrams per kilogram (about 30 packets of Splenda or 6 cans of diet soda for an adult).

Neotame. Neotame was approved by the FDA for use as a general-purpose sweetener but is used in few foods. Depending on its food application, Neotame is approximately 7000 to 13,000 times sweeter than table sugar. Neotame is heat-stable and can be used as a tabletop sweetener as well as in cooking. Neotame is safe for use by the general population, including children, pregnant and lactating women, and people with diabetes. Although similar to aspartame, neotame does not require labeling for people with PKU because it is not broken down in the body to individual amino acid components.

Acesulfame-K. Acesulfame-K is an organic acid linked to potassium (K) and is 200 times sweeter than sucrose. It is sold as Sunette® and can be used in baking. In the United States, it is currently approved for use as a general-purpose sweetener. The ADI for acesulfame-K is 15 milligrams per kilogram, or the equivalent of 6 cans of diet soda.

Stevia. Stevia, sold as Truvia® and Sweet Leaf,® is an alternative sweetener derived from a South American plant. Stevia extracts are 200 to 400 times sweeter than sucrose but provide no energy. It has been used in teas and as a sweetener in Japan since the 1970s, and stevia is considered generally recognized as safe (GRAS) for use in foods.

Luo Han Guo. Luo han guo is an extract of the monk fruit. It was approved by the FDA and is sold as the sweeteners Nectresse™ and Monk Fruit in the Raw.™ Luo han guo is between 100 to 250 times sweeter than sucrose.

Advantame. In May 2014, the FDA announced that a new food additive, advantame, is safe for use as a general-purpose sweetener and flavor enhancer in food. Advantame is stable at higher temperatures and can be used as a tabletop sweetener as well as in cooking. Chemically, advantame is similar to aspartame but is much sweeter. Because only a small amount is needed to achieve the same level of sweetness (it is 20,000 times sweeter than sucrose), foods that contain advantame do not need to include alerts for people with PKU.

To Sugar or Not to Sugar . . . That Is the Question! There is much controversy surrounding which is a healthier option—consuming diet soft drinks or *natural* sugar-sweetened beverages. Like most of the field of nutrition, the answer is: There is NO simple answer! In several recent studies, high consumption of artificial sweeteners has been linked with appetite alterations, obesity promotion, and even changes in gut microbes. On the other hand, we have definitive scientific evidence that large quantities of refined sugars (such as those found in soda, and sports and energy drinks), is related to dental caries, obesity-related chronic disease, and even alterations in brain function. Until we know more, RDNs recommend consuming any beverages, other than WATER, in moderation.[6]

✓ CONCEPT CHECK 4.3

1. Which food groups are the primary sources of carbohydrate in our diets?
2. What specific foods contain the highest percentage of calories from carbohydrates?
3. What are the common nutritive sweeteners?
4. Which alternative sweeteners are approved for use in food?

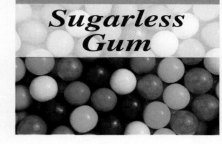

INGREDIENTS: SORBITOL, GUM BASE, MANNITOL, GLYCEROL, HYDROGENATED GLUCOSE SYRUP, XYLITOL, ARTIFICIAL AND NATURAL FLAVORS, ASPARTAME, RED 40, YELLOW 6 AND BHT (TO MAINTAIN FRESHNESS). PHENYLKETONURICS: CONTAINS PHENYLALANINE.

Sugarless Gum

▲ Sugar alcohols and the alternative sweetener aspartame are used to sweeten this product. Note the warning for people with phenylketonuria (PKU) that this product is made with aspartame and, thus, contains phenylalanine. ©Nancy R. Cohen/Getty Images

neotame General-purpose, nonnutritive sweetener that is approximately 7000 to 13,000 times sweeter than table sugar. It has a chemical structure similar to aspartame.

acesulfame-K Alternative sweetener that yields no energy to the body; 200 times sweeter than sucrose.

stevia Alternative sweetener derived from South American shrub; 200 to 400 times sweeter than sucrose.

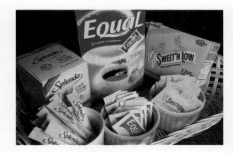

▲ A variety of alternative sweeteners are available. ©McGraw-Hill Education/Jill Braaten, photographer

4.4 Making Carbohydrates Available for Body Use

As discussed in Chapter 3, simply eating a food does not supply nutrients to body cells. Digestion and absorption must occur first.

STARCH AND SUGAR DIGESTION

Food preparation can be viewed as the start of carbohydrate digestion because cooking softens tough connective structures in the fibrous parts of plants, such as broccoli stalks. When starches are heated, the starch granules swell as they soak up water, making them much easier to digest. All of these effects of cooking generally make carbohydrate-containing foods easier to chew, swallow, and break down during digestion.

The enzymatic digestion of starch begins in the mouth, when the saliva, which contains an enzyme called salivary **amylase,** mixes with carbohydrate-containing food products during the chewing of food. This amylase immediately breaks down starch into many smaller units, primarily disaccharides, such as maltose (Fig. 4-7). You can taste this conversion while chewing a saltine cracker. Prolonged chewing of the cracker causes it to taste sweeter as some starch breaks down into the sweeter disaccharides, such as maltose. Usually, food is in the mouth for such a short amount of time that this phase of digestion is negligible. In addition, once the food moves down the esophagus and reaches the stomach, the acidic environment inactivates salivary amylase.

When the carbohydrates reach the small intestine, the more alkaline environment of the intestine is better suited for further carbohydrate digestion. The pancreas releases enzymes, such as pancreatic amylase, to aid the last stage of starch digestion. After amylase action, the original carbohydrates in a food are now present in the small intestine as the monosaccharides glucose and fructose, originally present as such in food, and disaccharides (maltose from starch breakdown, lactose mainly from dairy products, and sucrose from food and added at the table).

The disaccharides are digested to their single monosaccharide units once they reach the wall of the small intestine, where the specialized enzymes on the absorptive cells digest each disaccharide into monosaccharides. The enzyme **maltase** acts on maltose to produce two glucose molecules. **Sucrase** acts on sucrose to produce glucose and fructose. **Lactase** acts on lactose to produce glucose and galactose.

LACTOSE MALDIGESTION AND LACTOSE INTOLERANCE

Deficient production of the enzyme lactase will impair the digestion of lactose. The most common form of this condition is **primary lactose maldigestion,** a normal pattern of physiology that often begins to develop around ages 3 to 5 years. This primary form of lactose maldigestion is estimated to be present in about 75% of the world's population, although not all of these individuals experience symptoms. **Secondary lactose maldigestion** is a temporary condition in which lactase production is decreased in response to another condition, such as intestinal diarrhea. Rarely, lactase production is absent from birth, a condition known as **congenital lactase deficiency.** Any of these types of lactose maldigestion can lead to symptoms of gas, abdominal bloating, cramps, and diarrhea when lactose is consumed. The bloating and gas are caused by bacterial fermentation of lactose in the large intestine. The diarrhea is caused by undigested lactose in the large intestine as it draws water from the circulatory system into the large intestine. When significant symptoms develop after lactose intake, it is then called **lactose intolerance.** It is important to note that lactose maldigestion and resultant lactose intolerance are not equivalent to a milk allergy.

In North America, only about 25% of adults show signs of decreased lactose digestion in the small intestine. Asian Americans, African-Americans, and Latino/Hispanic

amylase Starch-digesting enzyme produced by the salivary glands and the pancreas.

maltase An enzyme made by absorptive cells of the small intestine; this enzyme digests maltose to two glucoses.

sucrase An enzyme made by absorptive cells of the small intestine; this enzyme digests sucrose to glucose and fructose.

lactase An enzyme made by absorptive cells of the small intestine; this enzyme digests lactose to glucose and galactose.

primary lactose maldigestion Develops at about age 3 to 5 years when the production of the enzyme lactase decreases.

secondary lactose maldigestion Occurs when production of the enzyme lactase declines for unknown reasons. When significant symptoms develop after lactose intake, it is then called *lactose intolerance.*

congenital lactase deficiency Birth defect resulting in the inability to produce lactase, such that a lactose-free diet is required from birth.

lactose intolerance A condition in which symptoms such as abdominal gas and bloating appear as a result of severe lactose maldigestion.

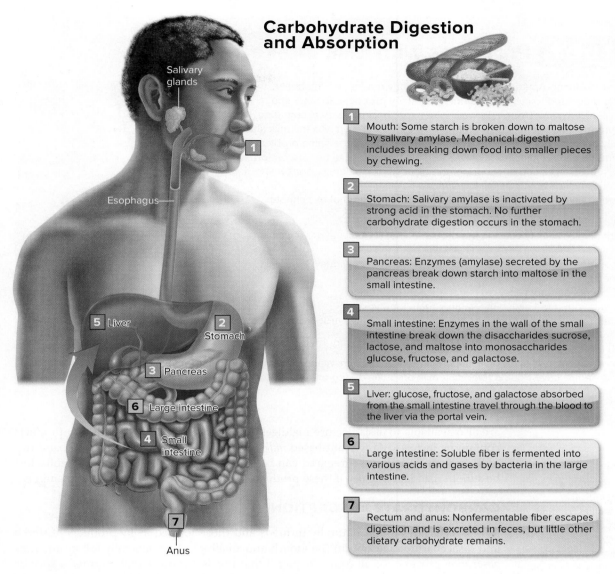

Carbohydrate Digestion and Absorption

Salivary glands

Esophagus

5 Liver

2 Stomach

3 Pancreas

6 Large intestine

4 Small intestine

7

Anus

1 Mouth: Some starch is broken down to maltose by salivary amylase. Mechanical digestion includes breaking down food into smaller pieces by chewing.

2 Stomach: Salivary amylase is inactivated by strong acid in the stomach. No further carbohydrate digestion occurs in the stomach.

3 Pancreas: Enzymes (amylase) secreted by the pancreas break down starch into maltose in the small intestine.

4 Small intestine: Enzymes in the wall of the small intestine break down the disaccharides sucrose, lactose, and maltose into monosaccharides glucose, fructose, and galactose.

5 Liver: glucose, fructose, and galactose absorbed from the small intestine travel through the blood to the liver via the portal vein.

6 Large intestine: Soluble fiber is fermented into various acids and gases by bacteria in the large intestine.

7 Rectum and anus: Nonfermentable fiber escapes digestion and is excreted in feces, but little other dietary carbohydrate remains.

FIGURE 4-7 ◄ Carbohydrate digestion and absorption. Enzymes made by the mouth, pancreas, and small intestine participate in the process of digestion. Most carbohydrate digestion and absorption take place in the small intestine. Chapter 3 covered the physiology of digestion and absorption in detail.

Americans are the population groups most likely to suffer lactose maldigestion, and the occurrence increases as people age. Many of these individuals can still consume moderate amounts of lactose with minimal or no gastrointestinal discomfort because of eventual lactose breakdown by bacteria in the large intestine. Studies have shown that nearly all individuals with decreased lactase production can tolerate ½ to 1 cup of milk with meals and that most individuals adapt to intestinal gas production resulting from the fermentation of lactose by bacteria in the large intestine. Thus, it is unnecessary for these people to totally restrict or avoid their intake of lactose-containing foods, such as milk and milk products, which are important for maintaining bone health. Obtaining enough calcium and vitamin D from the diet is much easier if milk and milk products are included in a diet.

Combining lactose-containing foods with other foods also helps because certain properties of foods can have positive effects on rates of digestion. For example, fat in a meal slows digestion, leaving more time for lactase action. Hard cheese and yogurt are also more easily tolerated than milk. Much of the lactose is lost during the production of cheese, and the active bacteria cultures in yogurt digest the lactose with their lactase. In addition, products such as lactose-free or lactose-reduced milk (Lactaid® and Dairy Ease)® are made by treating regular milk with the lactase enzyme. Lactase supplements

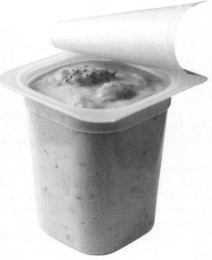

▲ Use of yogurt helps lactose maldigesters meet calcium needs.
©Ingram Publishing/SuperStock

CASE STUDY Problems with Milk Intake

Myeshia is a 19-year-old African-American female who recently read about the health benefits of calcium and decided to increase her intake of dairy products. To start, she drank a cup of 1% milk at lunch. Not long afterward, she experienced bloating, cramping, and increased gas production. She suspected that the culprit of this pain was the milk she consumed, especially because her parents and her sister complain of the same problem. She wanted to determine if other milk products were, in fact, the cause of her discomfort, so the next day she substituted a cup of yogurt for the glass of milk at lunch. Consuming the yogurt did not cause any pain.

Answer the following questions and check your response at the end of this chapter.

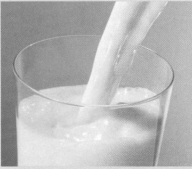

©NOBUHIRO ASADA/Shutterstock

1. Why did Myeshia believe that she was sensitive to milk?
2. What component of milk is likely causing the problems that Myeshia experiences after drinking milk?
3. Why does this component cause intestinal discomfort in some individuals?
4. What is the name of this condition?
5. What groups of people are most likely to experience this condition?
6. Why did consuming yogurt not cause the same effects for Myeshia?
7. Are there any other products on the market that can replace regular milk or otherwise alleviate symptoms for individuals with this problem?
8. Can people with this condition ever drink regular milk?
9. What other foods should Myeshia include to supply calcium, potassium, vitamin A, and vitamin D that are typically found in cow's milk?
10. Why do some individuals have trouble tolerating milk products during or immediately after an intestinal viral infection?

What Are FODMAPs?

You learned in Section 3.12, that a group of carbohydrates known as FODMAPs (fermentable oligo-, di-, and monosaccharides and polyols) may cause gastrointestinal symptoms such as gas, bloating, and diarrhea in some people. The FODMAPs include fructose, lactose, fructans (in wheat, onions, and garlic), galactans (in legumes), and polyols (sugar alcohols, see Section 4.3). Some individuals are poor digesters of FODMAPs. These carbohydrates reach the large intestine without being digested. They draw water into the digestive tract and undergo fermentation by the bacteria that reside in the large intestine, leading to bloating and gas. Following a low-FODMAP dietary pattern may be the key to relief for many people with irritable bowel syndrome. It is important to work with a gastroenterologist and RDN when limiting FODMAPs. Ideally, you should eliminate only those foods that trigger digestive problems; overly restrictive dietary patterns can lead to nutrient inadequacies. The following website provides practical information on foods to avoid and foods to include when restricting FODMAPs: https://patienteducation.osumc.edu/documents/lowfodmapdiet.pdf.

are also available to assist lactose maldigesters when they decide to consume products containing lactose. Many plant-based *milks*, including soy milk, almond milk, and rice milk, are naturally lactose-free and can be used as an alternative to regular milk. Just be sure to read labels to see if these products are fortified with calcium and vitamin D.

CARBOHYDRATE ABSORPTION

Monosaccharides found naturally in foods and those formed as by-products of starch and disaccharide digestion in the mouth and small intestine generally follow an *active absorption* process. Recall from Chapter 3 that this is a process that requires a specific carrier and energy input for the substance to be taken up by the absorptive cells in the small intestine. Glucose and its close relative, galactose, undergo active absorption. They are pumped into the absorptive cells along with sodium.

Fructose is taken up by the absorptive cells via *facilitated diffusion*. In this case, a carrier is used, but no energy input is needed. This absorptive process is thus slower than that seen with glucose or galactose. So, large doses of fructose are not readily absorbed and can contribute to diarrhea as the monosaccharide remains in the small intestine and attracts water.

Once glucose, galactose, and fructose enter the absorptive cells, some fructose is metabolized into glucose. The single sugars in the absorptive cells are then transferred to the portal vein that goes directly to the liver. The liver then metabolizes those sugars by transforming the monosaccharides galactose and fructose into glucose and:

- releases it directly into the bloodstream for transport to organs such as the brain, muscles, kidneys, and adipose tissues;
- produces glycogen for storage of carbohydrate; and,
- produces fat when carbohydrates are consumed in high amounts and overall calorie needs are exceeded.

Unless an individual has a disease that causes malabsorption or an intolerance to a carbohydrate such as lactose (or fructose), only a minor amount of some sugars (about 10%) escapes digestion. Any undigested carbohydrate travels to the large intestine and is fermented there by bacteria. The acids and gases produced by bacterial metabolism of the undigested carbohydrate are absorbed into the bloodstream. Scientists suspect that some of these products of bacterial metabolism promote the health of the large intestine by providing it with a source of calories.

FIBER AND INTESTINAL HEALTH

Bacteria in the large intestine ferment soluble fibers into such products as acids and gases. The acids, once absorbed, also provide calories for the body. In this way, soluble fibers provide about 1.5 kcal per gram. Although the intestinal gas (flatulence) produced by this bacterial fermentation is not harmful, it can be painful and sometimes embarrassing. Over time, however, the body tends to adapt to a high-fiber dietary pattern, eventually producing less gas. Many gas-forming foods are good sources of soluble fiber.

Because insoluble fiber is an indigestible carbohydrate, it remains in the intestinal tract and supplies bulk to the feces, making elimination much easier. When enough fiber is consumed, the stool is large and soft because many types of plant fibers attract water. The larger size stimulates the intestinal muscles to contract, which aids elimination. Consequently, less pressure is necessary to expel the stool. When too little fiber is eaten, the opposite can occur: very little water is present in the feces, making it small and hard. Constipation may result, which forces one to exert excessive pressure in the large intestine during defecation. This high pressure can force parts of the large intestine (colon) wall out from between the surrounding bands of muscle, forming many small pouches called **diverticula** (Fig. 4-8). **Hemorrhoids** (discussed in Section 3.12) may also result from excessive straining during defecation. In about 80% of people affected with diverticula, no symptoms are present. The asymptomatic form of this disease is called **diverticulosis.** If feces (and bacteria) become trapped within diverticuli, they may become inflamed or infected, a painful condition known as **diverticulitis.** In the short term, intake of fiber then should be reduced to limit further bacterial activity. Once the inflammation subsides, a high-fiber diet is recommended to ease stool elimination and reduce the risk of a future attack.

Very high intakes of fiber—for example, 60 grams per day—can also pose some health risks and therefore should be followed only under the guidance of a primary care provider. Increased fluid intake is extremely important with a high-fiber diet. Inadequate fluid intake can leave the stool very hard and painful to eliminate. In more severe cases, the combination of excess fiber and insufficient fluid may contribute to blockages in the intestine, which may require surgery. Aside from problems with the passage of materials through the gastrointestinal tract, a high-fiber diet may also decrease the availability of nutrients. Certain components of fiber may bind to essential minerals, blocking them from being absorbed. For example, when fiber is consumed in large amounts, zinc and iron absorption may be hindered.

Many population studies have shown a link between increased fiber intake and a decrease in colon cancer development. Most research on diet and colon cancer focuses on the potential preventive effects of fruits, vegetables, whole grain breads and cereals, and beans. It is more advisable to increase fiber intake by using fiber-rich foods than by relying on fiber supplements. Overall, the health benefits to the colon that stem from a high-fiber dietary pattern are partially due to the nutrients that are commonly present in most high-fiber foods, such as vitamins, minerals, phytochemicals, and, in some cases, essential fatty acids.

diverticula Pouches that protrude through the exterior wall of the large intestine.

hemorrhoid A pronounced swelling of a large vein, particularly veins found in the anal region.

diverticulosis The condition of having many diverticula in the large intestine.

diverticulitis Inflammation of the diverticula caused by acids produced by bacterial metabolism inside the diverticula.

✓ CONCEPT CHECK 4.4

1. In what form are carbohydrates absorbed, and what happens to these compounds after absorption?

2. What are the names and locations of the enzymes that digest carbohydrates?

3. Why do some individuals feel discomfort after they consume large amounts of lactose? How can they avoid these symptoms?

4. What are the beneficial effects of fiber in the intestinal tract?

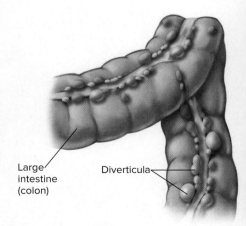

Large intestine (colon) — Diverticula

FIGURE 4-8 ▲ Diverticula in the large intestine. A low-fiber dietary pattern increases the risk of developing diverticula. About one-third of people over age 45 and two-thirds over age 85 have diverticulosis.

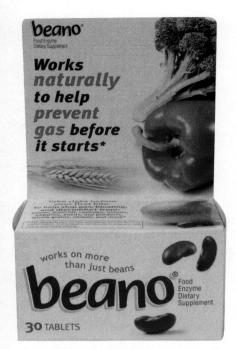

▲ Beano® is a dietary supplement that contains natural digestive enzymes. Such products can be used to reduce intestinal gas produced by bacterial metabolism of undigested carbohydrates in beans and some vegetables in the large intestine. ©McGraw-Hill Education/Mark Dierker, photographer

ketone bodies Partial breakdown products of fat that contain three or four carbons.

ketosis The condition of having a high concentration of ketone bodies and related breakdown products in the bloodstream and tissues.

4.5 Putting Carbohydrates to Work in the Body

As discussed, all of the digestible carbohydrate that we eat is eventually converted into glucose. Glucose then goes on to function in body metabolism. The other sugars can generally be converted into glucose, and the starches are broken down to yield glucose, so the functions described here apply to most carbohydrates. The functions of glucose in the body start with supplying calories to fuel the body.

PROVIDING ENERGY

The main function of glucose is to supply calories for use by the body. Certain tissues in the body, such as red blood cells, can use only glucose and other simple carbohydrate forms for fuel. Most parts of the brain and central nervous system also derive energy only from glucose, unless the diet contains almost no available glucose. In that case, the brain can use partial breakdown products of fat—called **ketone bodies**—for energy needs. Other body cells, including muscle cells, can use simple carbohydrates as fuel, but many of these cells can also use fat or protein for energy needs.

A dietary pattern that supplies enough digestible carbohydrates to prevent breakdown of proteins for energy needs is considered *protein sparing.* Under normal circumstances, digestible carbohydrates in the diet end up as blood glucose, and protein is reserved for functions such as building and maintaining muscles and vital organs. However, if you don't eat enough carbohydrates, your body is forced to make glucose from body proteins, draining the pool of amino acids available in cells for other critical functions. During long-term starvation, the continuous withdrawal of proteins from the muscles, heart, liver, kidneys, and other vital organs can result in weakness, poor function, and even failure of body systems.

The wasting of protein that occurs during long-term fasting can be life threatening. This has prompted companies that make formulas for rapid weight loss to include sufficient carbohydrates in the products to decrease protein breakdown and thereby protect vital tissues and organs, including the heart. Most of these very-low-calorie products are powders that can be mixed with different types of fluids and are consumed five or six times per day. When considering any weight-loss products, be sure that your total diet provides at least the RDA for carbohydrate.

In addition to the loss of protein, when you don't eat enough carbohydrates, the metabolism of fats is inefficient. In the absence of adequate carbohydrates, fats are not broken down completely in metabolism and instead form ketone bodies. This condition, known as **ketosis,** should be avoided because it disturbs the body's normal acid–base balance and leads to other health problems. This is a good reason to question the long-term safety of the low-carbohydrate diets that have been popular.

REGULATING BLOOD GLUCOSE

Under normal circumstances, a person's blood glucose concentration is regulated within a narrow range. When carbohydrates are digested and taken up by the absorptive cells of the small intestine, the resulting monosaccharides are transported directly to the liver. One of the liver's roles, then, is to guard against excess glucose entering the bloodstream after a meal. The liver works together with the pancreas to regulate blood glucose.

When the concentration of glucose in the blood is high, such as during and immediately after a meal, the pancreas releases the hormone insulin into the bloodstream. Insulin delivers two different messages to various body cells to cause the level of glucose in the blood to fall. First, insulin directs the liver to store glucose as glycogen. Second, insulin directs muscle, adipose, and other cells to remove glucose from the bloodstream by taking it into those cells. By triggering both glycogen synthesis in the liver and glucose movement out of the bloodstream into certain cells, insulin keeps the concentration of glucose from rising too high in the blood (Fig. 4-9).

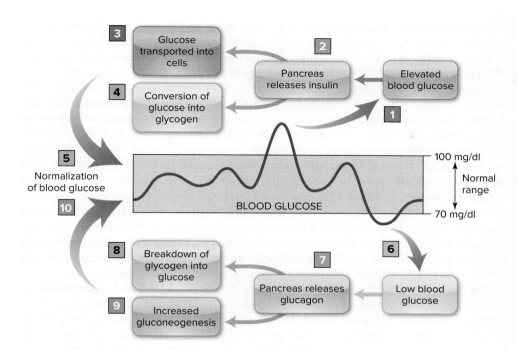

FIGURE 4-9 ◄ Regulation of blood glucose. Insulin and glucagon are key factors in controlling blood glucose. When blood glucose rises above the normal range of 70 to 100 milligrams per deciliter (mg/dl) and blood glucose becomes elevated (1), insulin is released from the pancreas (2) to lower it (3) and (4) blood glucose then falls back into the normal range (5). Inversely, when blood glucose falls below the normal range (6), glucagon is released (7), which has the opposite effect of insulin (8) and (9) this then restores blood glucose to the normal range (10). Other hormones, such as epinephrine, norepinephrine, cortisol, and growth hormone, also contribute to blood glucose regulation.

On the other hand, when a person has not eaten for a few hours and blood glucose begins to fall, the pancreas releases the hormone **glucagon.** This hormone has the opposite effect of insulin. It prompts the breakdown of liver glycogen into glucose and the generation of glucose from noncarbohydrate substances, which is then released into the bloodstream to keep blood glucose from falling too low.

A different mechanism increases blood glucose during times of stress. Epinephrine (adrenaline) is the hormone responsible for the *flight or fight* response. Epinephrine is released in large amounts from the adrenal glands (located on top of each kidney) in response to a perceived threat, such as a car approaching head-on. These hormones cause glycogen in the liver to be quickly broken down into glucose. The resulting rapid flood of glucose from the liver into the bloodstream helps fuel quick mental and physical reactions.

This complex regulatory system is responsible for maintaining blood glucose within an acceptable range. It provides a safeguard against extremely high blood glucose **(hyperglycemia)** or low blood glucose **(hypoglycemia).** In essence, the actions of insulin on blood glucose are balanced by the actions of glucagon, epinephrine, and other hormones. If hormonal balance is not maintained, major changes in blood glucose concentrations occur. The disease type 1 diabetes is an example of the underproduction of insulin. The failure of blood glucose regulation will be discussed in Section 4.7.

Lifestyle Management and Blood Glucose Control. Continued evidence supports lifestyle management techniques to improve blood glucose control. Directly aligning with the *Dietary Guidelines*, individuals are encouraged to consume a primarily plant-based dietary pattern rich in carbohydrates from vegetables, whole grains, fruits, legumes, and dairy products. Fat quality (selecting monounsaturated and polyunsaturated fats over *trans* fats and saturated fats) has been found to be more important than fat quantity. Recommendations also encourage limiting or avoiding intakes of sugar-sweetened beverages, reducing sodium to less than 2300 mg per day, and eating fatty fish at least two times (2 servings) per week. Note that dietary patterns that align to the majority of these guidelines include the Mediterranean, vegan, vegetarian, low-fat, low-carb, and DASH diets. To be safe, individuals with inadequate blood glucose control or diagnosed with prediabetes or diabetes should work closely with a RDN and endocrinologist to obtain individualized lifestyle recommendations. If insulin is prescribed, it may be necessary to count carbohydrates, protein, and fat until insulin dosing and blood glucose levels are controlled (see Section 4.7).

glucagon A hormone made by the pancreas that stimulates the breakdown of glycogen in the liver into glucose; this ends up increasing blood glucose. Glucagon also increases the generation of glucose from noncarbohydrate substances.

hyperglycemia High blood glucose, above 125 milligrams per 100 milliliters of blood.

hypoglycemia Low blood glucose, below 40 to 50 milligrams per 100 milliliters of blood for nondiabetics.

glycemic index (GI) The blood glucose response of a given food, compared to a standard (typically, glucose or white bread). Glycemic index is influenced by starch structure, fiber content, food processing, physical structure, and macronutrients in the meal such as fat.

glycemic load (GL) A measure of both the quality (GI value) and quantity (grams per serving) of a carbohydrate in a meal.

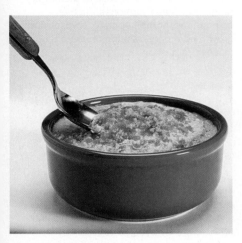

▲ Oatmeal is a rich source of soluble fiber. The FDA allows a health claim for the benefits of oatmeal to lower blood cholesterol because of the effects of this soluble fiber. ©John A. Rizzo/Getty Images

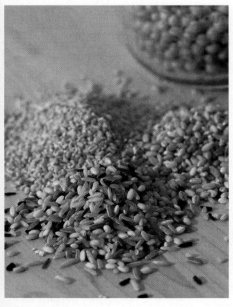

▲ Whole grains contain all three parts of the kernel: bran, germ, and endosperm. ©Nancy R. Cohen/Getty Images

The Glycemic Index and Blood Glucose. Our bodies react uniquely to different sources of carbohydrates. For example, a serving of a high-fiber food, such as black beans, results in lower blood glucose levels compared to the same size serving of mashed potatoes. The effects of various foods on blood glucose are important to know because foods that result in a high blood glucose cause a large release of insulin from the pancreas. When this type of high insulin output occurs frequently, it leads to many deleterious effects on the body. Some of these undesirable effects are high blood triglycerides, increased fat deposition in the adipose tissue, increased tendency for blood to clot, increased fat synthesis in the liver, and a more rapid return of hunger after a meal (insulin rapidly lowers the macronutrients in the blood as it stimulates their storage, signaling hunger). Over time, this increase in insulin output may also cause the muscles to become resistant to the action of insulin and eventually lead to type 2 diabetes in some people.

The **glycemic index (GI)** is a measurement of how the carbohydrate in a food raises blood glucose and has been used as a measure for planning diets for diabetics. Glycemic index is a ratio of the blood glucose response to a given food compared to the response to a reference such as glucose or white bread. Foods are ranked based on this comparison with a high GI food raising blood glucose more than a medium or low GI food.

The GI of a food is influenced by starch structure, fiber content, and food processing. Keep in mind that the GI value only describes the type, not the amount, of carbohydrate in a food. The **glycemic load (GL)** measures both the quality and quantity of carbohydrates in meals. This measure has also been used in meal planning. Portion sizes are important to manage, to control blood glucose and maintain weight. Maintaining a healthy body weight and performing regular physical activity further reduces the effects of a high GI dietary pattern.

FIBER: REDUCING CHOLESTEROL ABSORPTION AND OBESITY RISK

Aside from its role in maintaining bowel regularity, the consumption of fiber has many additional health benefits. A high intake of soluble fiber also inhibits absorption of cholesterol and cholesterol-rich bile acids from the small intestine, thereby reducing blood cholesterol and possibly reducing the risk of cardiovascular disease and gallstones. Recall that good sources of soluble fiber are apples, bananas, oranges, carrots, barley, oats, and kidney beans. The beneficial bacteria in the large intestine degrade soluble fiber and produce certain fatty acids that probably also reduce cholesterol synthesis in the liver. In addition, the slower glucose absorption that occurs with diets high in soluble fiber is linked to a decrease in insulin release. One of the effects of insulin is to stimulate cholesterol synthesis in the liver, so this reduction in insulin may contribute to the ability of soluble fiber to lower blood cholesterol. Overall, a fiber-rich diet containing fruits, vegetables, beans, and whole grains is advocated as part of a strategy to reduce risk of cardiovascular disease (i.e., coronary heart disease and stroke). Again, this is something that a low-carbohydrate dietary pattern cannot promise.

A diet high in fiber helps control weight and reduces the risk of developing obesity.[8] Due to their bulky nature, high-fiber foods require more time to chew and thus fill us up without yielding many calories. Increasing intake of foods rich in fiber is one strategy for feeling satisfied or full after a meal (review the discussion of energy density in Section 2.1).

✓ CONCEPT CHECK 4.5

1. What is the primary role of carbohydrates in the body?
2. How does the body respond when too little carbohydrate is consumed?
3. What are the mechanisms by which blood glucose levels are maintained within a narrow range?
4. What are some of the important functions of fiber?

4.6 Carbohydrate Needs

The RDA for carbohydrates is 130 grams per day for adults. This is based on the amount needed to supply adequate glucose for the brain and nervous system, without having to rely on ketone bodies from incomplete fat breakdown as a calorie source. Somewhat exceeding this amount is fine; the Food and Nutrition Board recommends that carbohydrate intake should range from 45% to 65% of total calorie intake. The Nutrition Facts panel on food labels uses 60% of calorie intake as the standard for recommended carbohydrate intake. This would be 300 grams of carbohydrate when consuming a 2000-calorie diet.

Survey data from the USDA indicate that carbohydrates are available for the average American in greater amounts (256 grams per day) than any other component in the food system. Recommendations for carbohydrate consumption, however, emphasize the type of carbohydrates we should consume rather than just the total amount. Experts agree that one's carbohydrate intake should be based primarily on fruits, vegetables, whole grain breads and cereals, and beans, rather than on refined grains, potatoes, and sugars.

The *Dietary Guidelines* for Americans recommend that we choose fiber-rich fruits, vegetables, and whole grains often. More specifically, 3 or more ounce equivalents of grains—roughly one-half of one's grains—should be whole. Whole grain is defined as the entire grain seed or kernel made of three components: the bran, germ, and endosperm, which must be in nearly the same relative proportions as the original grain if cracked, crushed, or flaked.[4,5]

HOW MUCH FIBER DO WE NEED?

An Adequate Intake for fiber has been set based on the ability of fiber to reduce risk of disease. The Adequate Intake for fiber for adults is 25 grams per day for women and 38 grams per day for men. The goal is to provide at least 14 grams per 1000 kcal in a diet. After age 50, the Adequate Intake falls to 21 grams per day and 30 grams per day, respectively. The Daily Value used for fiber on food and supplement labels is 25 grams for a 2000-kcal diet. In North America, fiber intake remains well below the recommended values (approximately 17 grams per day and less than one serving per day for whole grains). This low intake is attributed to the lack of knowledge on the benefits of whole grains and the inability to recognize whole grain products at the time of purchase. Thus, most of us could benefit from increasing our fiber intake. At least three ounce equivalents of whole grains per day are recommended. Eating a high-fiber cereal (at least 3 grams of fiber per serving) for breakfast is one easy way to increase fiber intake (Fig. 4-10).[1,2]

The Rate Your Plate exercise shows a diet containing 25 or 38 grams of fiber within moderate calorie intakes. Diets to meet the fiber recommendations are possible and enjoyable if you incorporate plenty of whole wheat bread, fruits, vegetables, and beans. Use the Rate Your Plate exercise to estimate the fiber content of your diet and determine *your* fiber score.

Remember that excessively high intakes of fiber can be unhealthy and that fluid intake must be increased with a high-fiber diet. A high-fiber diet may also decrease the absorption of essential minerals, especially zinc and iron.

In the final analysis, keep in mind that any nutrient can lead to health problems when consumed in excess. High carbohydrate, high fiber, and low fat do not mean zero calories. Carbohydrates help moderate calorie intake in comparison with fats, but high-carbohydrate foods also contribute to total calorie intake.

HOW MUCH SUGAR IS TOO MUCH?

The main problems with consuming an excess amount of sugar are that it provides empty calories and increases the risk for dental decay, weight gain, and other health issues.

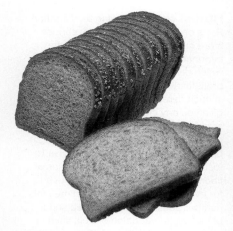

▲ When buying a bread labeled as *wheat bread*, most people think they are buying a whole wheat product. Because the flour is from the wheat plant, manufacturers can correctly list enriched white (refined) flour as wheat flour on food labels; however, if *whole wheat flour* is not listed first on the ingredient list, then the product is not primarily a whole wheat bread and thus does not contain as much fiber as it could. Careful reading of labels is important in the search for more fiber. Look for *100% whole grain* or *whole wheat* flour on the label for breads that are an excellent source of fiber. ©Getty Images

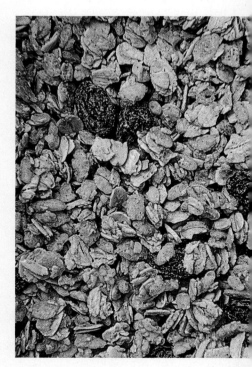

▲ Whole grain foods, such as granola, are excellent sources of fiber but often contain saturated fat and a concentrated source of calories. Reading labels is key! ©Brand X Pictures/PunchStock

FIGURE 4-10 ▶ Reading the Nutrition Facts on food labels helps us choose more nutritious foods. Based on the information from these nutrition labels, which cereal is the better choice for breakfast? Consider the amount of fiber in each cereal. Did the ingredients lists give you any clues? (Note: Ingredients are always listed in descending order by weight on a label.) When choosing a breakfast cereal, it is generally wise to focus on those that are rich sources of fiber. Sugar content can also be used for evaluation; however, sometimes this number does not reflect added sugar but simply the addition of fruit, such as raisins, thus complicating the evaluation.

Nutrition Facts

10 servings per container

Serving size: 1 cup (55g/2.0 oz.)

Amount per serving	Cereal	Cereal with ½ Cup Vitamins A & D Skim Milk
Calories	**170**	**210**

	% Daily Value**	
Total Fat 1.0g*	2%	2%
Sat. Fat 0g	0%	0%
Trans Fat 0g		*
Cholesterol 0mg	0%	0%
Sodium 300mg	13%	15%
Potassium 340mg	10%	16%
Total Carbohydrate 43g	14%	16%
Dietary Fiber 7g	28%	28%
Total Sugars 16g		
Includes 10g Added Sugars	20%	20%
Protein 4g		
Vitamin D 1mcg, 2.5mcg	10%	25%
Calcium 20mg, 120mg	2%	12%
Iron 12mg, 12mg	65%	65%
Potassium 225mg, 402 mg	6%	11%
Vitamin A 225mcg, 300mcg	15%	20%
Vitamin C 12mg, 13mg	20%	22%
Thiamin 0.3mg, 0,5mg	25%	30%
Riboflavin 0.4mg, 0.6mg	25%	35%
Niacin 5mg, 5mg	25%	25%
Vitamin B$_6$ 0.5mg, 0.5mg	25%	25%
Folic acid 120mcg, 120mcg	30%	30%
Vitamin B$_{12}$ 1.5mcg, 2.1mcg	25%	35%
Phosphorus 200mg, 300mg	20%	30%
Magnesium 80mg, 100mg	20%	25%
Zinc 3.7mg, 3,7mg	25%	25%
Copper 0.2mg, 0.2mg	10%	10%

* Amount in cereal. One half cup skim milk contributes an additional 40 calories, 65mg sodium, 6g total carbohydrate (6g sugars), and 4g protein.

** The % Daily Value (DV) tells you how much a nutrient in a serving of food contributes to a daily diet. 2,000 calories a day is used for general nutrition advice.

Nutrition Facts

17 servings per container

Serving size: ¾ cup (30g)

Amount per serving	Cereal	Cereal with ½ Cup Skim Milk
Calories	**170**	**210**

	% Daily Value**	
Total Fat 0g*	0%	1%
Saturated Fat 0g	0%	1%
Trans Fat 0g		*
Cholesterol 0mg	0%	1%
Sodium 60mg	2%	4%
Potassium 80mg	2%	8%
Total Carbohydrate 35g	9%	11%
Dietary Fiber 1g	4%	4%
Total Sugars 20g		
Includes 15g Added Sugars	30%	30%
Protein 3g		
Vitamin D 1mcg, 2mcg	10%	20%
Calcium 0mg, 150mg	0%	15%
Iron 1.8mg, 1.8mg	10%	10%
Potassium 95mg, 272 mg	3%	8%
Vitamin A 375mcg, 450mcg	25%	30%
Vitamin C 0mg,1.2mg	0%	2%
Thiamin 0.3mg, 0.3mg	25%	25%
Riboflavin 0.4mg, 0.6mg	25%	35%
Niacin 5mg, 5mg	25%	25%
Vitamin B$_6$ 0.5mg, 0.5mg	25%	25%
Folic acid 100mcg, 100mcg	25%	25%
Vitamin B$_{12}$ 1.5mcg, 1.8mcg	25%	30%
Phosphorus 40mg, 150mg	4%	15%
Magnesium 16mg, 32mg	4%	8%
Zinc 1.5mg, 1.5mg	10%	10%
Copper 0.04mg, 0.04mg	2%	2%

* Amount in Cereal. One-half cup skim milk contributes an additional 65mg sodium, 6g total carbohydrate (6g sugars), and 4g protein.

** The % Daily Value (DV) tells you how much a nutrient in a serving of food contributes to a daily diet. 2,000 calories a day is used for general nutrition advice.

Diet Quality Declines When Sugar Intake Is Excessive. Overcrowding the diet with sweet treats can leave little room for important, nutrient-dense foods, such as fruits and vegetables. Children and teenagers are at the highest risk for consuming too many empty calories in place of nutrients essential for growth. Many children and teenagers are drinking an excess of sugar-sweetened soft drinks and other sugar-containing beverages, including energy and sports drinks, and much less milk than ever before.

Replacing sugar-laden drinks for milk can compromise bone health because milk contains calcium and vitamin D, which are both essential for bone health.

With regard to sugar intake, an upper limit of 25% of total calorie intake from *added sugars* has been set by the Food and Nutrition Board. Remember that *added sugars* are sugars added to foods during processing and preparation. Dietary patterns that go beyond this upper limit are likely to be deficient in vitamins and minerals. The World Health Organization (WHO) continues to reiterate a *strong recommendation* that added sugars provide no more than 10% of total daily calorie intake. A moderate intake of about 10% of calorie intake corresponds to a maximum of approximately 50 grams (or 12 teaspoons) of sugars per day, based on a 2000 kcal diet. Because of the association between excessive consumption of sugars and several metabolic abnormalities and adverse health conditions, the American Heart Association recommends reductions in the intake of added sugars such that the upper limit of intake for most American women is no more than 100 kcal (25 grams) per day from added sugars and no more than 150 kcal (37.5 grams) per day for most American men.[9] In 2014, the WHO proposed a similar *conditional recommendation* that a sugar intake of less than 5% of daily calories (25 grams for an adult of normal BMI) should be the target in order to avoid health risks such as weight gain and tooth decay.

Most of the sugars we eat come from foods and beverages to which sugar has been added during processing and/or manufacturing. The Food Consumption Survey data indicates that the average daily intake of added sugars for American adults was 84 grams and for children was 77 grams, amounting to about 15% of calorie intake. Major sources of added sugars include soft drinks, cakes, cookies, fruit drinks, and dairy desserts such as ice cream (Fig. 4-11). Table 4-4 lists suggestions to limit sources of added sugars, including sweet desserts such as cakes, cookies, and ice cream (full and reduced fat). Also limit low-fat and fat-free snack products, which typically contain lots of added sugar to produce an acceptable taste but resulting in a high-calorie food with as many or more calories than the high-fat food product it was designed to replace.

> The *Dietary Guidelines* for Americans provide the following recommendations regarding carbohydrate intake as part of a healthy eating pattern while staying within calorie needs:
>
> - Include a variety of vegetables from all of the subgroups—dark green, red and orange, legumes (beans and peas), starchy, and other.
> - Include fruits, especially whole fruits.
> - Include grains, at least half of which are whole grains.
> - Limit intake of calories from added sugars to less than 10% per day.

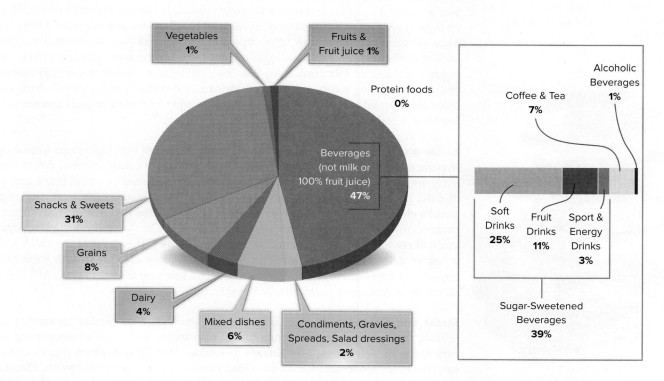

FIGURE 4-11 ▲ Sources of added sugars in the diets of the U.S. population age 2 years and older. Source: What We Eat in America (WWEIA) Food Category Analyses for the 2015 Dietary Guidelines Advisory Committee. Estimates based on day 1 dietary recalls from *WWEIA, NHANES 2009–2010*.

TABLE 4-4 ■ Suggestions for Reducing Added Sugar Intake

At the Grocery Store

- Read the ingredients list on food labels. Look for all forms of added sugars. Added sugars are often hidden in tomato sauce, crackers, condiments, and salad dressings. Sugar also hides under names like high fructose corn syrup, invert sugar, sucrose, dried cane syrup, brown rice syrup, honey, molasses, and maple syrup. These can be listed separately on ingredients lists and add up!
- Buy unsweetened versions of foods typically high in sugar such as cereals, applesauce, yogurt, and canned fruit (in heavy syrup). Look for foods labeled no added *sugar* or *unsweetened*.
- Buy nuts and unsweetened dried fruits to replace candy for snacks.

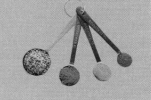

In the Kitchen

- Reduce the sugar in foods prepared at home. Try low-sugar recipes or adjust the sugar on your own. The amount of sugar can be decreased in recipes for foods such as pancakes, waffles, cookies, and cakes that will still taste great. Start by reducing the sugar gradually until you've decreased it by one-third or more.
- Add sweetness to foods with flavors and spices such as vanilla, citrus zest, cinnamon, cardamom, coriander, nutmeg, ginger, and mace.

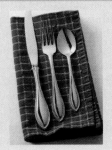

At the Table

- Choose fewer foods high in sugar, such as prepared baked goods and sweet desserts. Reach for fresh fruit instead of cookies or candy for dessert and between-meal snacks.
- Include more protein such as eggs and turkey, and healthy fats such as nuts, seeds, and olive oil to decrease the desire for sugar.
- Add less sugar to foods such as coffee, tea, cereal, and fruit. Reduce the use of white and brown sugars, honey, molasses, syrups, jams, and jellies. Cut back gradually to a quarter or half the amount. Resist using sugar alternatives, which can confuse the body's taste for sweets.
- Substitute water for sugared soft drinks, sweet tea, coffee drinks, energy drinks, punches, and fruit juices.

©Stockbyte/Getty Images (top); ©Stockbrokerextra Images/Photolibrary (middle); ©McGraw-Hill Education/Jack Holtel, photographer (bottom)

An excess intake of sugar-sweetened beverages has recently been linked to a risk for both weight gain and type 2 diabetes in adults.

Supersizing sugar-rich beverages has also become common and has led to more sugar consumption; for example, in the 1950s, a typical serving size of a soft drink was a 6.5-ounce bottle, and now a 20-ounce plastic bottle is a typical serving. This one change in serving size contributes an extra 162 kcal to the diet—all from added sugars. Most convenience stores now offer cups that will hold 64 ounces of soft drink. Health messages about the sugary beverages appear to be having some positive effects, resulting in a decrease in soft drink sales over the past decade. Market research indicates that youth are choosing more water, energy drinks, and coffee in place of soft drinks. Read more about trends in added sugar consumption and the decline in soda consumption in the Newsworthy Nutrition in this section.[10]

Sugar and Hyperactivity. There is a widespread notion that high sugar intake causes hyperactivity in children, typically part of the syndrome called *attention deficit hyperactivity disorder (ADHD)*. However, several well-controlled studies found that sugar in the diet did not affect children's behavior. Some researchers suggest that expecting sugar to affect a child can influence parents' interpretation of what they see. A study of parents' perceptions showed that parents who believe a child's behavior is affected by sugar are more likely to perceive their child as hyperactive when they believe the child just had a sugary drink. Experts recommend that other factors associated with hyperactivity, including temperament, emotional disturbances, learning disorders (e.g., ADHD), overstimulation, and sleep problems, be considered.

Sugar and Oral Health. Sugars in the diet (and starches readily fermented in the mouth, such as crackers and white bread) also increase the risk of developing **dental caries.** Recall that caries, also known as cavities, are formed when sugars and other carbohydrates are metabolized into acids by bacteria that live in the mouth. These acids dissolve the tooth enamel and underlying structure. Bacteria also use the sugars to make plaque, a sticky substance that both adheres acid-producing bacteria to teeth and diminishes the acid-neutralizing effect of saliva.

▲ Cookies and cakes are top contributors of simple carbohydrate sources for U.S. adults. ©Brand X Pictures/PunchStock

Newsworthy Nutrition

Americans Are Decreasing Consumption of Sugar-Sweetened Beverages

Sugar-sweetened beverages (SSBs) are high in added sugars and calories, and have few, if any, nutrients. Consumption of SSBs has been associated with dental caries and risk factors of cardiovascular disease and obesity. Reducing SSB consumption, therefore, has been recommended to promote optimal health. The objective of this study was to examine trends in SSB consumption among youth and adults in the United States. This design was a large cross-sectional study of the energy intake from SSBs of 22,367 youth aged 2 to 19 years and 29,133 adults aged 20 years of older using dietary data from NHANES between 1999 and 2010. SSBs included soda, fruit drinks, sports and energy drinks, sweetened coffee and tea, and other sweetened beverages. The location and meal occasion of SSB consumption was also examined. The results of this study indicate that between 1999–2000 and 2009–2010, the intake of calories from SSBs decreased from 223 to 155 kcal per day for youth and from 196 to 151 kcal per day for adults. During the 12-year study, SSB consumption decreased both in the home and away from home and with both meals and snacks. The percentage of total energy from SSBs also decreased to 8% among youth and 7% among adults in 2009–2010. The authors conclude from their analysis that there is a declining trend in SSB consumption among youth and adults in the United States.

Source: Kit BK and others: Trends in sugar-sweetened beverage consumption among youth and adults in the United States: 1999–2010. *American Journal of Clinical Nutrition* 98:180, 2013.

The worst offenders in terms of promoting dental caries are sticky and gummy foods high in sugars, such as caramel and gummies, because they stick to the teeth and supply the bacteria with a long-lived carbohydrate source. For this reason, snacking regularly on sugary foods is likely to cause caries because it gives the bacteria on the teeth a steady source of carbohydrates from which to continually make acid. Frequent consumption of liquid sugar sources (e.g., fruit juices, soda, sports beverages, energy drinks, and even many smoothies) can also cause dental caries. Chewing sugar-laden gum between meals is a prime example of a poor dental habit. Still, sugar-containing foods are not the only foods that promote acid production by bacteria in the mouth. As mentioned, if starch-containing foods (e.g., crackers and bread) are held in the mouth for a long time, the starch will be broken down to sugars by enzymes in the mouth; bacteria can then produce acid from these sugars. Overall, the sugar and starch contents of a food and its ability to remain in the mouth largely determine its potential to cause caries.

Fluoridated water and toothpaste are major factors in the prevention of dental caries in North American children due to fluoride's tooth-strengthening effect (see Chapter 9). Research has also indicated that certain foods—such as cheese, peanuts, and sugar-free chewing gum—can help reduce the amount of acid on teeth. In addition, rinsing the mouth after meals, drinking plenty of water, and eating healthy snacks reduces the acidity in the mouth. Certainly, good nutrition, habits that do not present an overwhelming challenge to oral health (e.g., chewing sugar-free gum), and routine visits to the dentist all contribute to improved dental health.

dental caries Erosions in the surface of a tooth caused by acids made by bacteria as they metabolize sugars.

CRITICAL THINKING

John and Mike are identical twins who like the same games, sports, and foods. However, John likes to chew sugar-free gum and Mike doesn't. At their last dental visit, John had no cavities but Mike had two. Mike wants to know why John, who chews sugar-free gum after eating, doesn't have cavities and he does. How would you explain this to him?

✓ CONCEPT CHECK 4.6

1. What is the recommended intake of total carbohydrate per day, and how do typical dietary intakes compare?

2. How much fiber is recommended each day?

3. How can we reduce our consumption of added sugars?

4. What is the link between sugar and oral health?

Diabetes—When Blood Glucose Regulation Fails

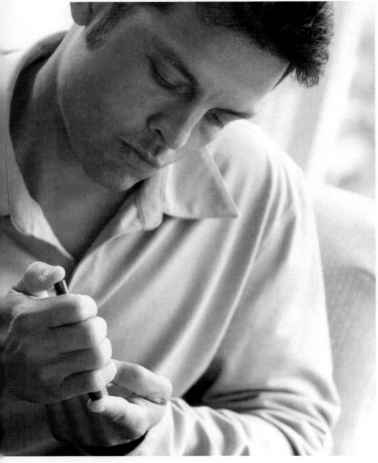

©BananaStock/Photolibrary

Improper regulation of blood glucose results in either *hypergly-cemia* (high blood glucose) or *hypoglycemia* (low blood glucose). High blood glucose is most commonly associated with diabetes (technically, *diabetes mellitus*), a disease that affects 29 million adults, or 9% of the North American population 20 years or older.[12] It is estimated that over 28%, or 8 million of these people do not know that they have the disease. Diabetes remains the seventh leading cause of death in the United States. Diabetes is currently increasing in epidemic proportions in the United States, with 1.4 million new cases diagnosed in people 18 years or older in 2012. The American Diabetes Association (ADA) recommends test-ing fasting blood glucose in adults over age 45 every 3 years to screen for diabetes. Diabetes was diagnosed for decades using a fasting blood glucose of 126 milligrams per 100 milliliters of blood or greater. In 2010, the ADA began using hemoglobin A1c (HbA1c) test to diagnose diabetes with a threshold of greater than 6.5%. The HbA1c is a more sensitive, long-term indicator of poor blood glucose control than the fasting blood glucose level. When blood glucose is too high, the glucose builds up in the blood and com-bines with hemoglobin (protein in red blood cells), making it gly-cated. The amount of glycated hemoglobin, or HbA1c, reflects the last several weeks or months of blood glucose levels.[11]

Diabetes

There are two major forms of diabetes: **type 1** (formerly called insulin-dependent or juvenile-onset diabetes) and **type 2 diabetes** (formerly called noninsulin-dependent or adult-onset diabetes) (Table 4-5). The change in names to type 1 and type 2 diabetes stems from the fact that many type 2 diabetics eventually must also rely on insulin injections as a part of their treatment. In addition, many children today have type 2 diabetes. A third form, called ges-tational diabetes, occurs in some pregnant women (see Chapter 18). It is usually treated with an insulin regimen and diet, and resolves after delivery of the baby. However, women who have gestational diabetes during pregnancy are at high risk for developing type 2 diabetes later in life.

Traditional symptoms of diabetes are excessive urination, exces-sive thirst, and excessive hunger. No one symptom is diagnostic of diabetes, and other symptoms—such as unexplained weight loss, exhaustion, blurred vision, tingling in hands and feet, frequent infections, poor wound healing, and impotence—often accompany traditional symptoms.

Type 1 Diabetes

Type 1 diabetes often begins in late childhood, around age 10 to 14 years, but can occur at any age. Approximately 1.3 million Ameri-cans have type 1 diabetes, and an estimated 40,000 people will be diagnosed with the disease each year in the United States. Children usually are admitted to the hospital with abnormally high blood glucose after eating, as well as evidence of ketosis.

The onset of type 1 diabetes is generally associated with decreased release of insulin from the pancreas. As insulin in the blood declines, blood glucose increases, especially after eating. Figure 4-12 shows a typical glucose response observed in a patient with this form of diabetes after consuming about 75 grams of glu-cose. When blood glucose levels are high, the kidneys let excess glucose spill into the urine, resulting in frequent urination that is high in sugar.

Most cases of type 1 diabetes begin with an immune system disorder, which causes destruction of the insulin-producing cells in the pancreas. The disease may stem from genetic, autoimmune, or environmental factors. Most likely, a virus or protein foreign to the body sets off the destruction. In response to their damage, the affected pancreatic cells release other proteins, which stimulate a more aggressive attack. Eventually, the pancreas loses its ability to synthesize insulin, and the clinical stage of the disease begins. Hyperglycemia and other symptoms develop slowly and only after 90% or more of the insulin-secreting cells have been destroyed. HbA1c, fasting blood glucose, or an oral glucose tolerance test can be used to diagnose diabetes. Remember that HbA1c is

type 1 diabetes A form of diabetes characterized by total insulin deficiency due to destruction of insulin-producing cells of the pancreas. Insulin therapy is required.

type 2 diabetes A form of diabetes characterized by insulin resistance and often associated with obesity. Insulin therapy can be used but is often not required.

TABLE 4-5 ■ **Comparison of Type 1 and Type 2 Diabetes**

	Type 1 Diabetes	Type 2 Diabetes
Occurrence	5% to 10% of cases of diabetes	90% to 95% of cases of diabetes
Cause	Autoimmune destruction of the pancreas	Insulin resistance
Risk factors	Moderate genetic predisposition	Strong genetic predisposition Obesity and physical inactivity Ethnicity Metabolic syndrome Prediabetes
Characteristics	Distinct symptoms (frequent thirst, hunger, and urination) Ketosis Weight loss	Mild symptoms, especially in early phases of the disease (fatigue and nighttime urination) No ketosis generally
Treatment	Insulin Diet Exercise	Diet Exercise Oral medications to lower blood glucose Insulin (in advanced cases)
Complications	Cardiovascular disease Kidney disease Nerve disease Blindness Infections	Cardiovascular disease Kidney disease Nerve damage Blindness Infections
Monitoring	Blood glucose Urine ketones HbA1c*	Blood glucose HbA1c

*Hemoglobin A1c.

the recommended measure because over time, blood glucose attaches to hemoglobin in red blood cells, especially when blood glucose remains elevated. A HbA1c value of over 7% indicates poor blood glucose control.

Type 1 diabetes is treated primarily by insulin therapy, either with injections or with an *insulin infusion pump*. The pump dispenses insulin at a steady rate into the body, with greater amounts delivered after each meal. Advantages of using an insulin pump include eliminating individual insulin injections; delivering insulin more accurately than injections; improved stabilization of blood glucose levels; enabling more dietary and physical activity flexibility; reducing severe low blood glucose episodes; and eliminating unpredictable effects of intermediate- or long-acting insulin. Now, an amazing innovation is showing great promise for management of type 1 diabetes. The *bionic pancreas* is a novel device that would fully automate blood glucose tracking and adjust the hormonal response accordingly. Several biotech companies are testing models.[12]

Dietary therapy includes balancing carbohydrate intake with the insulin regimen and physical activity schedule to manage blood glucose levels. The amount and timing of carbohydrates eaten should be consistent from day to day to maintain blood glucose control. Insulin should be adjusted to match carbohydrate intake in

Symptoms of Diabetes

The symptoms of diabetes may occur suddenly and include one or more of the following:

- Extreme thirst
- Frequent urination
- Drowsiness, lethargy
- Sudden vision changes
- Increased appetite
- Sudden weight loss
- Sugar in urine
- Fruity, sweet odor on breath
- Heavy, labored breathing
- Stupor, unconsciousness

persons who adjust their mealtime insulin doses or who are using an insulin pump. There are several methods available to estimate carbohydrate content of foods, including carbohydrate counting, exchange lists, and the glycemic index and glycemic load of foods.[13,14] If one does not eat often enough, the injected insulin can

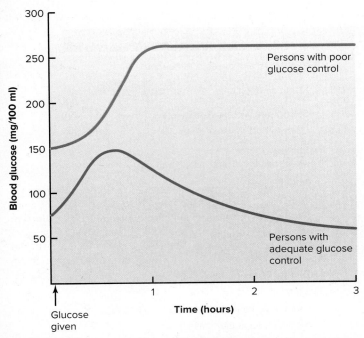

FIGURE 4-12 ▲ Glucose tolerance test. A comparison of blood glucose concentrations after a 75-gram glucose load displaying a healthy blood glucose response (in blue) and a dysfunctional response (in red).

cause a severe drop in blood glucose or hypoglycemia because it acts on whatever glucose is available. The diet should be moderate in simple carbohydrates, include ample fiber and unsaturated fat but be low in both animal and *trans* fats, and supply an amount of calories in balance with needs. Providing adequate calories and nutrients to promote growth and development in children is crucial for young diabetics.[11,14,15]

The hormone imbalances that occur in people with untreated type 1 diabetes—primarily, not enough insulin—lead to mobilization of body fat, taken up by liver cells. Ketosis is the result because the fat is partially broken down to ketone bodies. Ketone bodies can rise excessively in the blood and eventually spill into the urine. These pull sodium and potassium ions as well as water into the urine. This series of events also causes frequent urination and can contribute to a chain reaction that eventually leads to dehydration, ion imbalance, coma, and even death, especially in patients with poorly controlled type 1 diabetes. Treatment includes provision of insulin, fluids, and minerals such as sodium and potassium.

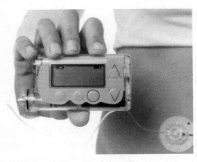

▲ Insulin pumps alleviate the discomfort of injecting insulin under the skin multiple times per day. ©Oscar Gimeno Baldo/Alamy

Several degenerative complications, including cardiovascular disease, blindness, kidney disease, and nerve damage, result from poor blood glucose regulation, specifically long-term hyperglycemia. The high blood sugar concentration physically deteriorates small blood vessels (capillaries) and nerves. When improper nerve stimulation occurs in the intestinal tract, intermittent diarrhea and constipation result. Because of nerve deterioration in the extremities, many people with diabetes lose the sensation of pain associated with injuries or infections. They do not have as much pain, so they often delay treatment of hand or foot problems. This delay, combined with a rich environment for bacterial growth (bacteria thrive on glucose), sets the stage for damage and death of tissues in the extremities, sometimes leading to the need for amputation of feet and legs. Elevated blood glucose also leads to glucose binding (known as glycation) to proteins and fats in the body, forming what are called *advanced glycation endproducts (AGEs)*. These have been shown to be toxic to cells, especially those of the immune system and kidneys.

Current research has shown that aggressive treatment directed at keeping blood glucose within the normal range can slow the development of blood vessel and nerve complications of diabetes. Maintaining near-normal HbA1c (6% or less) greatly reduces the risk of death and developing other diseases in people with diabetes. A person with diabetes must work closely with a primary care provider and registered dietitian nutritionist to make the correct alterations in diet and medications and to perform physical activity safely. Physical activity enhances glucose uptake by muscles independent of insulin action, which in turn can lower blood glucose. This outcome is beneficial, but people with type 1 diabetes need to be aware of their blood glucose response to physical activity and compensate appropriately to avoid hypoglycemia.

Type 2 Diabetes

Type 2 diabetes usually begins after age 30. This is the most common type of diabetes, accounting for about 90% to 95% of the cases diagnosed in North America. The disease is progressive and is present, in many cases, long before it is diagnosed. Hyperglycemia develops slowly such that the classic symptoms are not noticed in the early stages of the disease, even though the risk for complications is rising. Risk factors for type 2 diabetes are both genetic and environmental and include a family history of diabetes; older age; obesity, especially intra-abdominal obesity; physical inactivity; prior history of gestational diabetes; prediabetes; and race or ethnicity. Latino/Hispanic Americans, African-Americans, Asian Americans, Native Americans, and Pacific Islanders are at particular risk. The overall number of people affected is also on the rise, primarily because of widespread inactivity and obesity in our population. There has been a substantial increase in type 2 diabetes in children, due mostly to an increase in body fatness in this population (coupled with limited physical activity).

Type 2 diabetes arises when the insulin receptors on the cell surfaces of certain body tissues, especially muscle and fat tissue, become *insulin resistant*. During the onset of the disease, there is an abundance of insulin, but it is not used properly and blood glucose is not readily transferred into cells. The person develops high blood glucose as a result of the glucose remaining in the bloodstream. As the pancreas attempts to increase insulin output to compensate, the beta cells in the pancreas lose the ability to produce sufficient quantities of the hormone. As the disease

Often people with type 2 diabetes did not develop the disease suddenly. It may develop for years before symptoms are noticed. Prediabetes is a condition in which the concentration of blood glucose drifts up higher than normal. By the time symptoms are noticeable, organs and tissues may already be damaged. Simple tests of your fasting blood glucose level or HbA1c can determine if you are prediabetic. Early detection of diabetes risk can help prevent diabetes if you make lifestyle changes. If you have a family history of diabetes or if your habits (being physically inactive and overweight, and having a poor dietary pattern) put you at risk, it is important to discover if your blood glucose is still in the prediabetic stage. Prediabetes, also called *impaired fasting glucose,* is diagnosed if the fasting blood glucose is 100 to 125 milligrams per deciliter or the HbA1c is 5.7% to 6.4%.

The Diabetes Prevention Plan (DPP) was a large, multisite study designed to improve glucose control and prevent the onset of diabetes. The DPP found that participants who lost even a modest amount of weight via dietary and physical activity changes sharply reduced their chances of developing diabetes. More impressive is that the DPP lifestyle intervention had health outcomes that were better than those in the medication-treated cohort.[16]

develops, pancreatic function can fail, leading to reduced insulin output. Because of the genetic link for type 2 diabetes, those who have a family history should schedule regular diabetes screening and be careful to avoid risk factors such as obesity and inactivity.

Many cases of type 2 diabetes (about 90%) are associated with overweight and obesity (especially with fat located in the abdominal region), but high blood glucose is not directly caused by the obesity. In fact, some lean people also develop this type of diabetes. Obesity associated with oversized adipose cells increases the risk for insulin resistance by the body as more fat is added to these cells during weight gain.

Because type 2 diabetes is linked to obesity, achieving a healthy weight should be a primary goal of treatment, with even limited weight loss leading to better blood glucose regulation. Although many cases of type 2 diabetes can be relieved by reducing excess adipose tissue stores, many people struggle to lose weight. They remain affected with diabetes and may experience the degenerative complications seen in the type 1 form of the disease. Ketosis, however, is not usually seen in type 2 diabetes. Glucose-lowering medications and insulin are used as needed in patients with type 2 diabetes. New classes of drugs that mimic gut hormones are helping diabetic patients overcome the chronic problems that conventional treatments alone have been unable to control.

Regular patterns of meals and physical activity are important elements of therapy for type 2 diabetes. Physical activity helps the muscles take up more glucose. Medical nutrition therapy should emphasize overall calorie control, increased intakes of fiber-rich foods and fish, and reduced intakes of added sugars and solid fats. Distributing carbohydrates throughout the day helps minimize the high and low swings in blood glucose concentrations. As in type 1 diabetes, it is critical that discussions include a RDN and primary care provider to create a tailored lifestyle management plan to meet the needs of each individual.[17] It is also important to consume the recommended 25 to 38 grams of fiber, with emphasis on soluble fiber sources, which will help regulate glucose.

Although sugar does not have to be completely eliminated, persons with diabetes will benefit from adhering to the recommendation to reduce consumption of added sugars. If sugar is included in the meal plan, it should be substituted for other carbohydrate sources. Because persons with diabetes are at increased risk of cardiovascular disease, heart-healthy choices should also be included in the diabetic meal plan.

Hypoglycemia

People with diabetes who are taking insulin sometimes have hypoglycemia if they do not eat frequently enough. The first signs of diabetic hypoglycemia include shakiness, sweating, palpitations, anxiety, and hunger. Later symptoms are the result of insufficient glucose reaching the brain and include mental confusion, extreme fatigue, seizures, and unconsciousness. Symptoms should be treated immediately with consumption of glucose or food containing carbohydrate.

Metabolic Syndrome

Metabolic syndrome is characterized by the presence of several risk factors for diabetes and cardiovascular disease. A person with metabolic syndrome must have at least three of the following metabolic risk factors (or be on medication to treat these risk factors) to be diagnosed with metabolic syndrome: a large waistline from abdominal obesity (accumulation of fat around and within the midsection), high blood triglycerides, low HDL or *good* cholesterol,

For more information on diabetes, consult the following websites: www.diabetes.org and www.ndep.nih.gov.

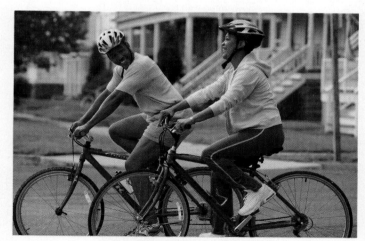

▲ Regular exercise is a key part of a plan to prevent (and control) type 2 diabetes.[15] ©Ariel Skelley/Blend Images LLC

metabolic syndrome A condition in which a person has poor blood glucose regulation, hypertension, increased blood triglycerides, and other health problems. This condition is usually accompanied by obesity, lack of physical activity, and a diet high in refined carbohydrates. Also called *Syndrome X.*

hypertension, and high fasting blood glucose (Fig. 4-13). Each aspect of metabolic syndrome is a unique health problem with its own treatment. In metabolic syndrome, however, these risk factors are clustered together, making a person twice as likely to develop cardiovascular disease and five times more likely to develop diabetes.

It is generally accepted that one key element unifies all the aspects of metabolic syndrome: *insulin resistance.* As you learned, insulin is a hormone that directs tissues to pull glucose out of the blood and into cells for storage or fuel. With insulin resistance, the pancreas produces plenty of insulin, but the cells of the body do not respond to it effectively. Instead, excess glucose stays in the bloodstream. For a while, the pancreas may be able to compensate for the resistance of cells to insulin by overproducing insulin. Over time, however, the pancreas is unable to keep up the accelerated insulin production, and blood glucose levels remain elevated. With metabolic syndrome, blood glucose is not high enough to be classified as diabetes (≥ 126 mg/dl), but without intervention, it is likely to get worse and eventually lead to diabetes.

Genetics and aging contribute to the development of insulin resistance and the other elements of metabolic syndrome, but

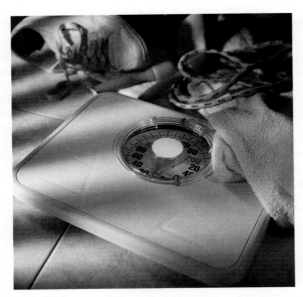

▲ Decreasing body weight and increasing physical activity are interventions to help prevent metabolic syndrome. ©Dynamic Graphics/ JupiterImages

environmental factors such as diet and activity play an important role. Obesity, particularly abdominal obesity, is highly related to insulin resistance. More than half of adults in the United States are overweight, 30% are obese, and these numbers continue to climb year after year. Increases in body weight among children and adolescents are of great concern because childhood obesity places them at high risk for these health problems. This increase in body weight has precipitated a dramatic surge in cardiovascular disease and diabetes risk: an estimated 50 million Americans now have metabolic syndrome.

The insulin resistance that precedes and contributes to type 2 diabetes also leads to several other components of the metabolic syndrome. The chief culprits contributing to the high blood triglycerides of metabolic syndrome are large meals rich in simple sugars and refined starches and low in fiber, coupled with little to no physical activity. Nutrition and lifestyle changes are key strategies in addressing all of the unhealthy conditions of metabolic syndrome as a whole. Suggested interventions include:

- Decrease body weight. Even small improvements (e.g., 3% to 5% weight loss) for overweight and obese individuals can lessen disease risk. The most successful weight-loss and weight-maintenance programs include moderate dietary restriction combined with physical activity.
- Increase physical activity. To alleviate risks for chronic diseases, the *Dietary Guidelines* recommend at least 150 minutes of moderate-intensity physical activity each week.
- Limit solid fat consumption, especially animal and *trans* fat sources. We will explore the different types and sources of fats and their effects in Chapter 5.

**Metabolic Syndrome
Risk Indicators**

For a patient to be diagnosed with metabolic syndrome, he or she must have **three** of the five risk factors listed below.

- *High blood pressure*
  130/85 mmHg or higher

- *Low HDL cholesterol*
  - Men with HDL level less than 40 mg/dl

  - Women with HDL level less than 50 mg/dl

- *Elevated glucose*
  Fasting level of 100 mg/dl or higher

- *Elevated triglycerides (blood fat)*
  150 mg/dl or higher

- *Abdominal obesity*
  - Men with waist circumference greater than 40 inches

  - Women with waist circumference greater than 35 inches

FIGURE 4-13 ▲ Metabolic syndrome is characterized by the presence of several risk factors for diabetes and cardiovascular disease.

Summary (Numbers refer to numbered sections in the chapter.)

4.1 Carbohydrates are created in plants through photosynthesis. They are our main fuel source for body cells. Refined and highly processed products lack many of the health benefits provided by the carbohydrates found in whole grains, beans, fruits, and vegetables.

4.2 The common monosaccharides in food are glucose, fructose, and galactose. Once these are absorbed from the small intestine and delivered to the liver, much of the fructose and galactose is converted into glucose.

The major disaccharides are sucrose (glucose + fructose), maltose (glucose + glucose), and lactose (glucose + galactose). When digested, these yield their component monosaccharides.

One major group of polysaccharides consists of storage forms of glucose: starches in plants and glycogen in humans. These can be broken down by human digestive enzymes, releasing the glucose units. The main plant starches—straight-chain amylose and branched-chain amylopectin—are digested by enzymes in the mouth and small intestine. In humans, glycogen is synthesized in the liver and muscle tissue from glucose. Under the influence of hormones, liver glycogen is readily broken down to glucose, which can enter the bloodstream to fuel necessary cells.

Fiber is composed primarily of the polysaccharides cellulose, hemicellulose, pectin, gum, and mucilage, as well as the noncarbohydrate lignins. These substances are not broken down by human digestive enzymes. Soluble (also called viscous) fiber, however, is fermented by bacteria in the large intestine.

4.3 Table sugar, honey, jelly, fruit, and plain baked potatoes are some of the most concentrated sources of carbohydrates. Other high-carbohydrate foods, such as pie and fat-free milk, are diluted by either fat or protein. Nutritive sweeteners in food include sucrose, high-fructose corn syrup, brown sugar, and maple syrup. Several alternative sweeteners approved for use by the FDA include saccharin, aspartame, sucralose, neotame, and acesulfame-K.

4.4 Some starch digestion occurs in the mouth with assistance from the enzyme amylase. Carbohydrate digestion is completed in the small intestine. Some plant fibers are digested by the bacteria present in the large intestine; undigested plant fibers become part of the feces. Monosaccharides in the intestinal contents mostly follow an active absorption process. They are then transported via the portal vein that leads directly to the liver.

The ability to digest lactose often diminishes with age. Lactose maldigestion also can develop early in childhood and is most common among people of African, Asian, or Hispanic descent. Undigested lactose travels to the large intestine, resulting in such symptoms as abdominal gas, pain, and diarrhea. The occurrence of severe symptoms after consuming lactose is called lactose intolerance. Most people with lactose maldigestion can tolerate cheese, yogurt, and moderate amounts of milk.

4.5 Carbohydrates provide calories (4 kcal per gram), protect against wasteful use of food and body protein for energy, and prevent ketosis. The RDA for carbohydrate is 130 grams per day. If carbohydrate intake is inadequate for the body's needs, protein is metabolized to provide glucose for energy needs. However, the price is loss of body protein, ketosis, and eventually a general body weakening. For this reason, low-carbohydrate diets are not recommended for extended periods.

Blood glucose concentration is regulated within a narrow range of 70 to 99 milligrams per deciliter. Insulin and glucagon are hormones that control blood glucose concentration. When we eat a meal, insulin promotes glucose uptake by cells. When fasting, glucagon promotes glucose release from glycogen stores in the liver.

Insoluble (also called nonfermentable) fiber provides mass to the feces, thus easing elimination. In high doses, soluble fiber can help control blood glucose in individuals with diabetes and lower blood cholesterol.

4.6 A goal of about half of calories as complex carbohydrates is a good one, with about 45% to 65% of total calories coming from carbohydrates in general. Foods to consume align with the *Dietary Guidelines*, which encourage fiber-rich fruits, vegetables, and whole grains. Specifically, 3 or more ounce equivalents of grains, roughly one-half of one's grains, should be whole.

Moderating sugar intake, especially between meals, reduces the risk of dental caries. Alternative sweeteners, such as aspartame, aid in reducing intake of sugars.

4.7 Diabetes is characterized by a persistent high blood glucose concentration. Regular physical activity and a balanced meal plan that emphasizes fiber and limits added sugars and solid fats are helpful in treating both type 1 and type 2 diabetes. Insulin is the main medication employed: it is required in type 1 diabetes and may be used in type 2 diabetes.

Check Your Knowledge (Answers are available at the end of this question set.)

1. Dietary fiber
   a. raises blood cholesterol levels.
   b. speeds up transit time for food through the digestive tract.
   c. causes diverticulosis.
   d. causes constipation.

2. When the pancreas detects excess glucose, it releases the
   a. enzyme amylase.
   b. monosaccharide glucose.
   c. hormone insulin.
   d. hormone glucagon.

3. Cellulose is a(n)
   a. indigestible fiber.
   b. simple carbohydrate.
   c. energy-yielding nutrient.
   d. animal polysaccharide.

4. Digested white sugar is broken into _____ and _____.
   a. glucose, lactose
   b. glucose, fructose
   c. sucrose, maltose
   d. fructose, sucrose

5. Starch is a
   a. complex carbohydrate.
   b. fiber.
   c. simple carbohydrate.
   d. gluten.

6. Fiber content of the diet can be increased by adding
   a. fresh fruits.
   b. fish and poultry.
   c. eggs.
   d. whole grains and cereals.
   e. both a and d.

7. Which form of diabetes is most common?
   a. type 1
   b. type 2
   c. type 3
   d. gestational

8. The recommended daily intake for fiber is approximately _____ grams.
   a. 5 to 10
   b. 25 to 38
   c. 75 to 100
   d. 200 to 400

9. Lactose intolerance is the result of
   a. drinking high-fat milk.
   b. eating a large amount of yogurt.
   c. low lactase activity.
   d. a high-fiber diet.

10. One of the components of metabolic syndrome is
    a. high HDL.
    b. high waist circumference.
    c. low blood sugar.
    d. low blood pressure.

Answer Key: 1. b (LO 4.5), 2. c (LO 4.5), 3. a (LO 4.2), 4. b (LO 4.2), 5. a (LO 4.2), 6. e (LO 4.3), 7. b (LO 4.7), 8. b (LO 4.6), 9. c (LO 4.4), 10. b (LO 4.7)

Study Questions (Numbers refer to Learning Outcomes)

1. Why do we need carbohydrates in the diet? **(LO 4.3)**

2. What are the three major monosaccharides and the three major disaccharides? Describe how each plays a part in the human diet. **(LO 4.2)**

3. Why are some foods that are high in carbohydrates, such as cookies and fat-free milk, not considered to be concentrated sources of carbohydrates? **(LO 4.3)**

4. Describe the digestion of the various types of carbohydrates in the body. **(LO 4.4)**

5. Describe the reason why some people are unable to tolerate high intakes of milk. **(LO 4.4)**

6. List three alternatives to simple sugars for adding sweetness to the diet without adding calories. **(LO 4.3)**

7. Outline the basic steps in blood glucose regulation, including the roles of insulin and glucagon. **(LO 4.5)**

8. What are the important roles that fiber plays in the diet? **(LO 4.5)**

9. Summarize current carbohydrate intake recommendations. **(LO 4.6)**

10. What, if any, are the proven ill effects of excessive sugar in the diet? **(LO 4.6)**

What the Dietitian Chose

Sandwiches can be a great option for a quick lunch that includes several, if not all, of the food groups on MyPlate. The challenge arises in incorporating vegetables and fruits, often missing from quick lunches, into this meal. All of the sandwiches on this menu provide 1 ½ to 2 ½ ounces of protein. The hot dog and the peanut butter sandwich are the lowest, at 1 ½ ounces, and the soy burger is the highest with 2 ½ ounces of protein.

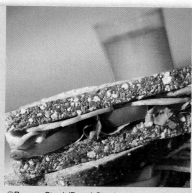
©BananaStock/PunchStock

Additionally, we want to consider the nutritional quality of the grains, protein, and dairy items. All of the sandwiches on this menu provide 1 ½ to 2 ½ ounces of protein with the hot dog having the lowest and soy have the highest protein content. If we evaluate the sandwiches based on their carbohydrate sources, we see that only three of the sandwiches offer servings of vegetables. The addition of two tomato slices, four slices of cucumber or pickles, and two lettuce leaves to the turkey sandwich and the soy burger provides ¾ cup of vegetables to each. The tuna salad sandwich provides the most vegetables, 1 ¼ cups from the carrots and onions in the tuna salad and the two leaves of lettuce, and four cucumber slices added to the sandwich.

Although we see strawberry jelly on the peanut butter sandwich, jelly does not count as a fruit serving and instead provides 32 kcal (~ 10% of total calories in the sandwich) from added sugars.

As we move to the grains aspect of MyPlate, we note the tuna salad on whole wheat and the soy burger on a whole wheat English muffin both offer 2 ounces of whole grain for this quick lunch. The combination of vegetables and whole grain provides a significant amount of dietary fiber. The tuna salad sandwich has 7 grams and the soy burger has 7.5 grams of dietary fiber, which is close to 30% of the daily recommendation of 25 to 38 grams per day. The soy burger on whole wheat also has the benefit of having both soluble fiber from the soybean and insoluble fiber from the whole wheat. The peanut butter sandwich also provides 3 grams of primarily soluble fiber from the peanut butter.

The turkey and Swiss is also a good choice with 4 grams of fiber, and it provides a ¾-cup serving of dairy. Unfortunately, the rye is not necessarily a whole grain bread. The ham and Swiss provides 2 ounces of lean protein and ¾ cup of dairy but provides only 1.5 grams of fiber because it is on sourdough bread made from refined white flour. It is also low on the list of choices because of its high sodium content (about 1100 milligrams).

Although it is sometimes described as America's favorite, the hot dog on a white bun has the least to offer nutritionally. It provides the lowest amount of grain at 1 ½ ounces, and the grain is refined. It also has the lowest protein content at 1 ½ ounces and offers only 1 gram of fiber. It is high in sodium at over 700 milligrams and contains 6 grams of animal fat.

In summary, the dietitian would choose either the meatless soy burger or the tuna salad sandwich to maximize the number of servings from a variety of healthy carbohydrate sources including vegetables and whole grains.

Further Readings

1. Hall M: Fiber facts about cereal. *Today's Dietitian* 2012; 14(12):30.

2. Position of the Academy of Nutrition and Dietetics: Health implications of dietary fiber. *J Acad Nutr Diet* 115:1861, 2015.

3. Getz L: Deciphering whole grain food labels: Separating fact from fiction. *Today's Dietitian* 2012; 14(6):44.

4. Schaeffer J: Boosting whole grain consumption. *Today's Dietitian* 2013; 15(2):33.

5. Webb D: Whole grain goodness. *Today's Dietitian* 2012; 14(9):56.

6. Position of the Academy of Nutrition and Dietetics: Use of nutritive and nonnutritive sweeteners. *J Acad Nutr Diet* 2012; 112:739.

7. Rippe JM, Angelopoulos TJ: Sucrose, high-fructose corn syrup, and fructose, their metabolism and potential health effects: What do we really know? *Advances in Nutrition* 2013; 4:236.

8. Cho SS and others: Consumption of cereal fiber, mixtures of whole grains and bran, and whole grains and risk reduction in type 2 diabetes, obesity, and cardiovascular disease. *Am J Clin Nutr* 2013; ajcn-067629.

9. Johnson RK and others: Dietary sugars intake and cardiovascular health: A scientific statement from the American Heart Association. *Circulation* 2009; 120(11):1011.

10. Malik VS and others: Sugar-sweetened beverages and weight gain in children and adults: A systematic review and meta-analysis. *Am J Clin Nutr* 2013; 98.4: 1084–1102.

11. Standards of medical care in diabetes 2017: Summary of revisions. *Diabetes Care* 2017;40(Suppl. 1):S4–S5 (DOI: 10.2337/dc17-S003).

12. Russell SJ and others: Outpatient glycemic control with a bionic pancreas in type 1 diabetes. *New Engl J Med* 2014; 371.4: 313–325.

13. Centers for Disease Control and Prevention: *National Diabetes Statistics Report, 2016.* Atlanta, GA: U.S. Department of Health and Human Services, Centers for Disease Control and Prevention, 2014.

14. Young-Hyman D and others: Psychosocial care for people with diabetes: A position statement of the American Diabetes Association. *Diabetes Care* 2016; 39.12: 2126–2140.

15. American Diabetes Association. Standards of medical care for patients with diabetes mellitus. *P R Health Sci J* 2013; 20.2.

16. Ma J and others: Translating the Diabetes Prevention Program lifestyle intervention for weight loss into primary care: A randomized trial. *JAMA Intern Med* 2013; 173.2: 113–121.

17. Evert AB and others: Nutrition therapy recommendations for the management of adults with diabetes. *Diabetes Care* 2014; Suppl 1:S120–S143.

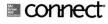

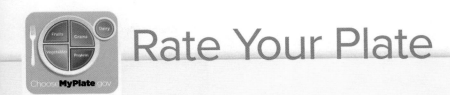

Rate Your Plate

Estimate Your Fiber Intake

Review the sample menus shown in Table 4-6. The first menu contains 1600 kcal and 25 grams of fiber (AI for women); the second menu contains 2100 kcal and 38 grams of fiber (AI for men).

TABLE 4-6 ■ **Sample Menus Containing 1600 kcal with 25 Grams of Fiber and 2000 kcal with 38 Grams of Fiber***

Menu	25 Grams of Fiber			38 Grams of Fiber		
	Serving Size	Carbohydrate Content (g)	Fiber Content (g)	Serving Size	Carbohydrate Content (g)	Fiber Content (g)
Breakfast						
Muesli cereal	1 cup	60	6	1 cup	60	6
Raspberries	½ cup	11	2	½ cup	11	2
Whole wheat toast	1 slice	13	2	2 slices	26	4
Margarine	1 tsp	0	0	1 tsp	0	0
Orange juice	1 cup	28	0	1 cup	28	0
1% milk	1 cup	24	0	1 cup	24	0
Coffee	1 cup	0	0	1 cup	0	0
Lunch						
Bean and vegetable burrito	2 small	50	4.5	3 small	75	7
Guacamole	¼ cup	5	4	¼ cup	5	4
Monterey Jack cheese	1 oz	0	0	1 oz	0	0
Pear (with skin)	1	25	4	1	25	4
Carrot sticks	—	—	—	¾ cup	6	3
Sparkling water	2 cups	0	0	2 cups	0	0
Dinner						
Grilled chicken (no skin)	3 oz	0	0	3 oz	0	0
Salad		7	3	½ cup	19	6
Red cabbage	½ cup					
Romaine	½ cup			½ cup		
Peach slices	¼ cup			1 cup		
Toasted almonds	—	—	—	½ oz	3	2
Fat-free salad dressing	2 tbsp	0	0	2 tbsp	0	0
1% milk	1 cup	24	0	1 cup	24	0
Total		247	25		306	38

diet is based on MyPlate breakdown of approximate energy content: carbohydrate, 58%; protein, 12%; and fat, 30%.

ce/Corbis (breakfast); ©BananaStock/PunchStock (lunch); ©Ingram Publishing/Superstock (dinner)

To roughly estimate your daily fiber consumption, determine the number of servings that you ate yesterday from each food category listed here. If you are not meeting your fiber needs, how could you do so? Multiply the serving amount by the value listed and then add up the total amount of fiber.

Food	Servings	Grams
Vegetables		
(serving size: 1 cup raw leafy greens or 1/2 cup other vegetables)	_____ × 2	_____
Fruits		
(serving size: 1 whole fruit, 1/2 grapefruit, 1/2 cup berries or cubed fruit, and 1/4 cup dried fruit)	_____ × 2.5	_____
Beans, lentils, split peas		
(serving size: 1/2 cup cooked)	_____ × 7	_____
Nuts, seeds		
(serving size: 1/4 cup; 2 tbsp peanut butter)	_____ × 2.5	_____
Whole grains		
(serving size: 1 slice whole wheat bread; 1/2 cup whole wheat pasta, brown rice, or other whole grain; and 1/2 each bran or whole grain muffin)	_____ × 2.5	_____
Refined grains		
(serving size: 1 slice bread, 1/2 cup pasta, rice, or other processed grains; and 1/2 each refined bagels or muffins)	_____ × 1	_____
Breakfast cereals		
(serving size: check package for serving size and amount of fiber per serving)	_____ × grams of fiber per serving	_____
Total Grams of Fiber =		_____

Source: Adapted from Fiber: Strands of protection. *Consumer Reports on Health,* p. 1, August 1999.

How does your total fiber intake for yesterday compare with the general recommendation of 25 to 38 grams of fiber per day for women and men, respectively?

If you are not meeting your needs, how could you improve your fiber intake?

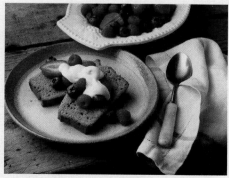

▲ This dessert is an excellent source of fiber from 2 slices of whole wheat banana bread (7 grams) with ½ cup of berries (1.8 grams) and 2 ounces of yogurt for a total of 8.8 grams of fiber. ©Kevin Sanchez/Cole Group/Getty Images

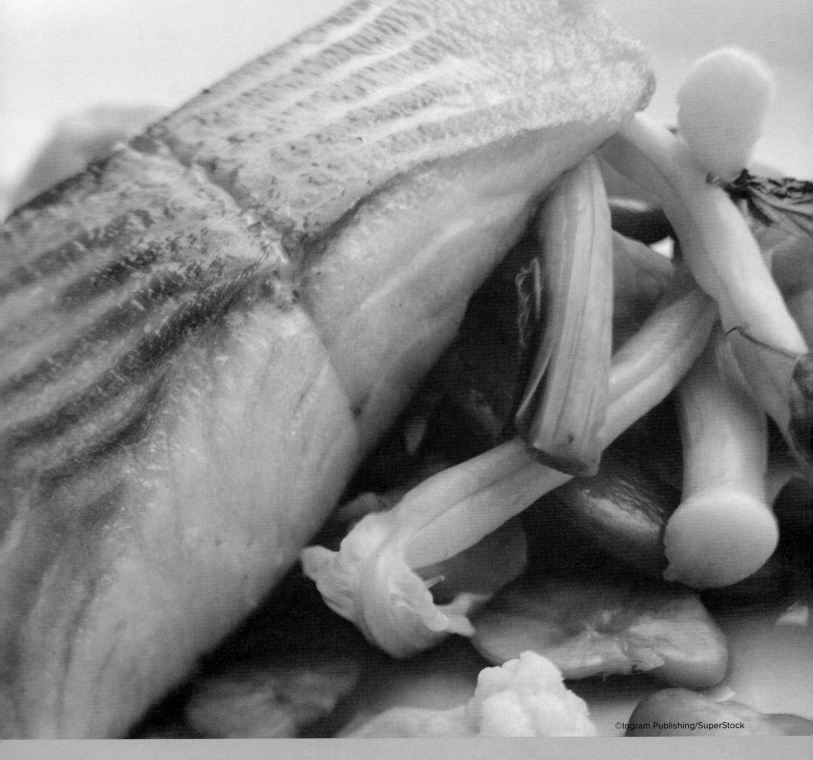

Student Learning Outcomes

Chapter 5 is designed to allow you to:

5.1 Understand the common properties of lipids.

5.2 Describe the structures of the three forms of lipids: fatty acids, phospholipids, and sterols.

5.3 Discuss the importance of the essential fatty acids.

5.4 Identify food sources of saturated, monounsaturated, polyunsaturated and *trans* fatty acids; phospholipids; and cholesterol.

5.5 Explain how lipids are digested and absorbed.

5.6 Name the lipoproteins and classify them according to their functions.

5.7 Describe the functions of the various forms of lipids in the body.

Chapter 5
Lipids

What Would You Choose?

Several of your friends are getting together for a cookout, and you have volunteered to be the grill master. Hamburgers will be the main "protein" portion of your meal. (Remember the size of that group on MyPlate?) You have heard that eating red meat is bad for your heart. Is all red meat bad for your heart? In the meat section of the grocery store, you see several varieties of ground beef. Which of the following types of ground beef would you choose for heart health?

a Ground round

b Ground chuck

c Ground sirloin

d Ground beef

Think about your choice as you read this chapter, then see What the Dietitian Chose at the end of the chapter.

Lipids are energy dense! Per gram, fats yield more than twice as much energy as carbohydrates or protein. Consumption of certain types of fats also contributes to the risk of cardiovascular disease. For these reasons, some concern about fat intake is warranted. Lipids do play vital roles, however, both in the body and in foods. Their presence in the diet is essential to good health. In fact, lipids found in seafood, such as the salmon pictured here, have been linked to *lower* risk for several chronic diseases. In general, lipids should comprise 20% to 35% of an adult's total calorie intake.

Humans can survive with very little fat in their diet. In fact, the body's need for the essential fatty acids can be met by daily consumption of only about 2 to 4 tablespoons of plant oil and two servings of fatty fish such as salmon or tuna per week. However, humans can thrive with a much more liberal fat intake. The Food and Nutrition Board suggests that fat intake can be as high as 35% of calories consumed for an adult. Some experts suggest that an intake as high as 40% of calories is appropriate as long as the predominant type of fat is a healthy one, such as olive oil. After learning more about lipids—fats, oils, and related compounds—in this chapter, you can decide for yourself how much fat you want to consume.

Let us look at lipids in detail—their forms, functions, and food sources. In this chapter, you will see how lipids are digested and absorbed and how specific types of lipids can influence the risk for certain diseases.

5.8 Explain current recommendations for fat intake.

5.9 Characterize the relationship between lipids and cardiovascular disease.

triglyceride The major form of lipid in the body and in food. It is composed of three fatty acids bonded to glycerol.

phospholipid Any of a class of fat-related substances that contain phosphorus, fatty acids, and a nitrogen-containing component. Phospholipids are an essential part of every cell.

sterol A compound containing a multi-ring (steroid) structure and a hydroxyl group (—OH). Cholesterol is a typical example.

glycerol A three-carbon alcohol used to form triglycerides.

cholesterol A waxy lipid found in all body cells. It has a structure containing multiple chemical rings that is found only in foods of animal origin.

acid group In chemistry, a functional group that consists of a carbon atom that shares bonds with two oxygen atoms. This is the site where fatty acids are linked to glycerol to form triglycerides.

methyl group In chemistry, a carbon atom that shares bonds with three hydrogen atoms. The methyl group is the omega end of a fatty acid.

saturated fatty acid A fatty acid containing no carbon-carbon double bonds.

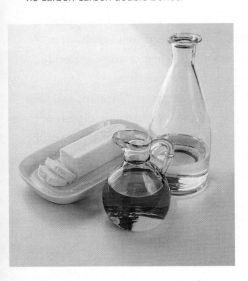

▲ Foods that are rich in saturated fatty acids, such as butter, are solid at room temperature, whereas foods that are rich in unsaturated fatty acids such as olive and corn oil, are liquid at room temperature. ©Tetra Images/Getty Images

5.1 Lipids: Common Properties

Lipids are composed primarily of the elements carbon and hydrogen; they contain fewer oxygen atoms than do carbohydrates. Chemical energy can be derived from breakdown of all those carbon-hydrogen bonds, so lipids yield more than twice as much energy (9 kcal per gram) as carbohydrates or proteins (4 kcal per gram).

Lipid is a generic term that includes **triglycerides, phospholipids,** and **sterols.** Food experts, such as chefs, refer to lipids that are solid at room temperature as *fats,* while lipids that are liquid at room temperature are called *oils.* Most people use the word *fat* to refer to all lipids because they do not realize that there is a difference. To simplify our discussion, this chapter primarily uses the term *fat.* When necessary for clarity, the name of a specific lipid, such as cholesterol, will be used. This word use is consistent with the way many people use these terms.

As a class of nutrients, lipids share one main characteristic: they do not readily dissolve in water. Think of an oil-and-vinegar salad dressing. The oil is not soluble in the water-based vinegar; on standing, the two separate into distinct layers, with oil on the top and vinegar on the bottom.

As you will learn in Section 5.2, the chemical structures of lipids are diverse. Triglycerides are the most common type of lipid found in the body and in foods. Each triglyceride molecule consists of three fatty acids bonded to **glycerol.** Phospholipids and sterols (including **cholesterol**) are also classified as lipids, although their structures can be quite different from the structure of triglycerides. All of these lipid compounds are described in this chapter.

✓ CONCEPT CHECK 5.1

1. What is the common property that all lipid compounds share?

5.2 Lipids: Triglycerides, Phospholipids, and Sterols

FATTY ACIDS AND TRIGLYCERIDES

Fatty Acids: The Simplest Form of Lipids Triglycerides are the primary form of lipids in the body and in foods. Fatty acids are found in triglycerides. A fatty acid is basically a long chain of carbons bonded together and flanked by hydrogens. At one end of the molecule (the alpha end) is an **acid group.** At the other end (the omega end) is a **methyl group** (Fig. 5-1).

Fats in foods are not composed of a single type of fatty acid. Rather, each dietary fat, or triglyceride, is a complex mixture of many different fatty acids, the combination of which provides each food its unique taste and smell.

Fatty acids can be saturated or unsaturated with hydrogen. Chemically speaking, a carbon atom can form four bonds. Within the carbon chain of a fatty acid, each carbon bonds to two other carbons and to hydrogens. The carbons that make up the chain of a **saturated fatty acid** are all connected to each other by single bonds. This allows the maximum number of hydrogens to be bound. Just as a sponge can be saturated (full) with water, a saturated fatty acid, such as stearic acid, is saturated with hydrogen [see Fig. 5-1(a)]. The saturated fatty acids are very straight and linear and therefore can pack very close together. This close packing or stacking of saturated fat molecules makes them solidify at room temperature.

Animal fats are high in saturated fatty acids and remain solid at room temperature. A good example is the solid fat surrounding a piece of uncooked steak. Chicken fat, semi-solid at room temperature, contains less saturated fat than beef fat. However, in some

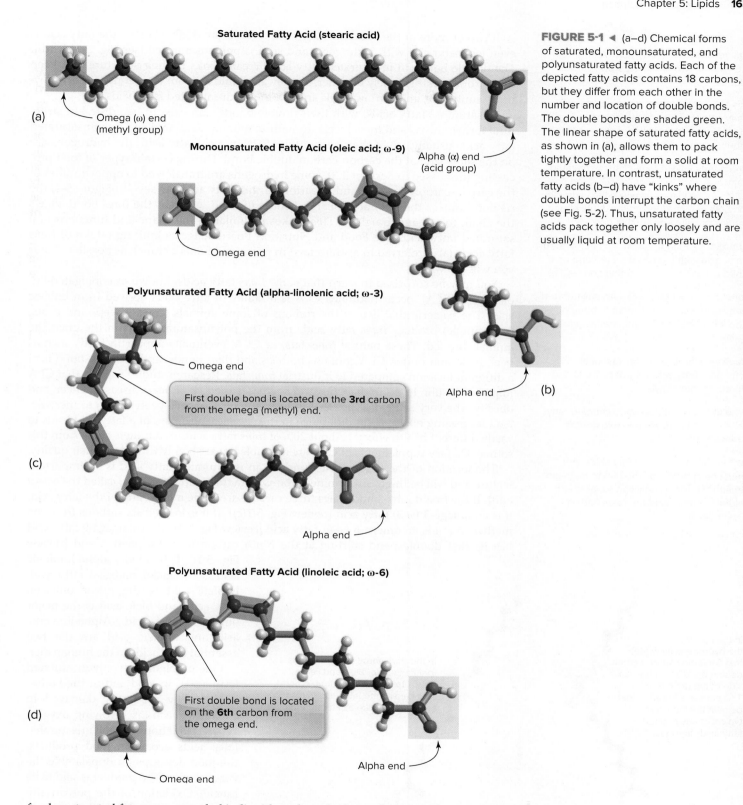

Saturated Fatty Acid (stearic acid)

(a)

Omega (ω) end
(methyl group)

Alpha (α) end
(acid group)

Monounsaturated Fatty Acid (oleic acid; ω-9)

Omega end

Alpha end

(b)

Polyunsaturated Fatty Acid (alpha-linolenic acid; ω-3)

Omega end

First double bond is located on the **3rd** carbon from the omega (methyl) end.

(c)

Alpha end

Polyunsaturated Fatty Acid (linoleic acid; ω-6)

First double bond is located on the **6th** carbon from the omega end.

(d)

Alpha end

Omega end

FIGURE 5-1 ◄ (a–d) Chemical forms of saturated, monounsaturated, and polyunsaturated fatty acids. Each of the depicted fatty acids contains 18 carbons, but they differ from each other in the number and location of double bonds. The double bonds are shaded green. The linear shape of saturated fatty acids, as shown in (a), allows them to pack tightly together and form a solid at room temperature. In contrast, unsaturated fatty acids (b–d) have "kinks" where double bonds interrupt the carbon chain (see Fig. 5-2). Thus, unsaturated fatty acids pack together only loosely and are usually liquid at room temperature.

foods, saturated fats are suspended in liquid, such as the butterfat in whole milk, so the solid nature of these fats at room temperature is less apparent.

If the carbon chain of a fatty acid contains a double bond, those carbons in the chain have fewer bonds to share with hydrogen, and the chain is said to be *unsaturated*. A fatty acid with only one double bond is **monounsaturated** [see Fig. 5-1(b)]. Canola oil, olive oil, and avocados contain a high percentage of monounsaturated fatty acids (see Farm to Fork).

monounsaturated fatty acid A fatty acid containing one carbon-carbon double bond.

polyunsaturated fatty acid A fatty acid containing two or more carbon-carbon double bonds.

cis fatty acid A form of an unsaturated fatty acid that has the hydrogens lying on the same side of the carbon-carbon double bond.

trans fatty acid A form of an unsaturated fatty acid, usually a monounsaturated one when found in food, in which the hydrogens on both carbons forming the double bond lie on opposite sides of that bond.

omega-3 (ω-3) fatty acid An unsaturated fatty acid with the first double bond on the third carbon from the methyl end ($-CH_3$).

omega-6 (ω-6) fatty acid An unsaturated fatty acid with the first double bond on the sixth carbon from the methyl end ($-CH_3$).

alpha-linolenic acid An essential omega-3 fatty acid with 18 carbons and three double bonds.

linoleic acid An essential omega-6 fatty acid with 18 carbons and two double bonds.

essential fatty acids Fatty acids that must be supplied by the diet to maintain health. Currently, only linoleic acid and alpha-linolenic acid are classified as essential.

If two or more of the bonds between the carbons are double bonds, the fatty acid is even less saturated with hydrogens, and so it is **polyunsaturated** [see Fig. 5-1(c), (d)]. The double bonds in unsaturated fatty acids create kinks in their structure that keep them from packing closely together, so they are liquid at room temperature. Corn, soybean, sunflower, and safflower oils are rich in polyunsaturated fatty acids.

Unsaturated fatty acids, with their double bonds, can exist in two different structural forms: the *cis* and *trans* forms. In nature, monounsaturated and polyunsaturated fatty acids usually are in the *cis* form (Fig. 5-2). In a **cis fatty acid,** the hydrogens are on the same side of the carbon-carbon double bond. During certain types of food processing (discussed in Section 5.3), some hydrogens are transferred to opposite sides of the carbon-carbon double bond, creating a **trans fatty acid.** As seen in Figure 5-2, the *cis* bond causes the fatty acid's carbon chain to bend, whereas the *trans* bond allows the chain to remain straighter. This makes it similar to the shape and functions of a saturated fatty acid. The Food and Nutrition Board suggests limiting intake of *trans* fatty acids (also referred to as *trans* fats) in processed foods as much as possible. Later you will see why.

You may be surprised to learn that some *trans* fatty acids, known as conjugated linoleic acid (CLA), occur naturally. CLA is a family of fatty acids derived from linoleic acid. The bacteria that live in the rumens of some animals (cows, sheep, and goats, for example) produce *trans* fatty acids from the polyunsaturated fats in the grass the animals are fed. These natural *trans* fats, or CLA, eventually appear in foods such as beef, milk, and butter. CLA contains both *cis* and *trans* bonds, and the *trans* bond is in a different location compared to industrial *trans* fats. Research studies suggest that CLA improves insulin levels in diabetics and decreases the risk of heart disease, cancer, and obesity—the very same diseases that industrial *trans* fats have been shown to increase. Isn't it amazing how a slight difference in the chemical structure of a fatty acid leads to vastly different health effects? About 20% of *trans* fatty acids in our diets come from this source. Dietary supplements of CLA are available but are highly variable in their quality.

The location of the first double bond on an unsaturated fatty acid is an important feature and will be three, six, or nine carbons from the methyl end (also called the *omega* end). If the first double bond starts three carbons from the methyl end of the fatty acid, it is an **omega-3 (ω-3) fatty acid** [review Fig. 5-1(c)]. If it is located six carbons from the methyl end, it is an **omega-6 (ω-6) fatty acid** [review Fig. 5-1(d)]. An omega-9 fatty acid has its first double bond starting at the ninth carbon from the methyl end [review Fig. 5-1(b)]. In foods, **alpha-linolenic acid** is the major omega-3 fatty acid, **linoleic acid** is the major omega-6 fatty acid, and **oleic acid** is the major omega-9 fatty acid. Alpha-linolenic acid and linoleic acid are the two **essential fatty acids** in the human diet.

One problem with polyunsaturated fatty acids—in food and in the body—is that they are easily damaged in chemical reactions involving oxygen. When oxidation of polyunsaturated fatty acids occurs in food products, the food develops an unpalatable flavor and odor. The product is said to be **rancid.** Oxidation of the polyunsaturated fatty acids in the body can cause inflammation and tissue damage. This process is thought to contribute to aging, atherosclerosis, and cancer. Fortunately, antioxidants such as

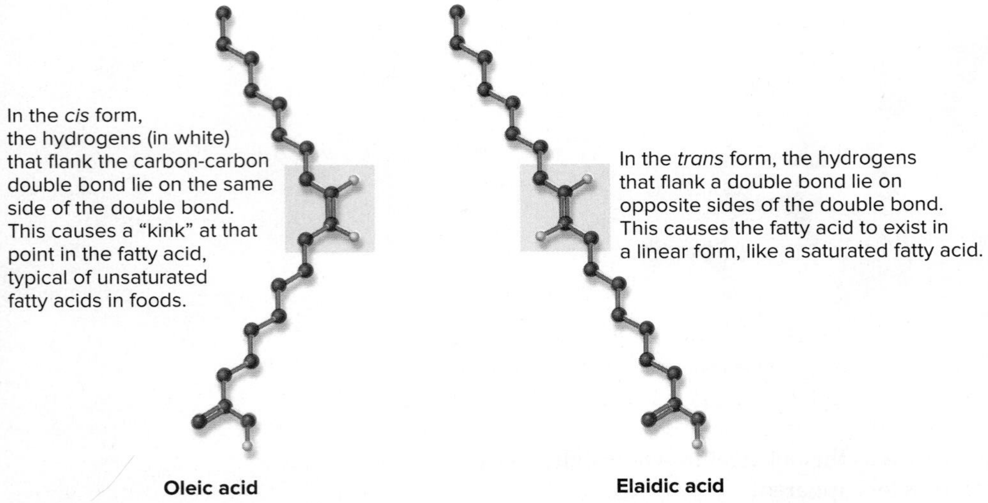

In the *cis* form, the hydrogens (in white) that flank the carbon-carbon double bond lie on the same side of the double bond. This causes a "kink" at that point in the fatty acid, typical of unsaturated fatty acids in foods.

In the *trans* form, the hydrogens that flank a double bond lie on opposite sides of the double bond. This causes the fatty acid to exist in a linear form, like a saturated fatty acid.

Oleic acid

Elaidic acid

FIGURE 5-2 ▲ *Cis* and *trans* fatty acids. *Cis* fatty acids are much more common in foods than *trans* fatty acids. The latter are primarily found in foods containing partially hydrogenated fats, notably stick margarine, shortening, and deep-fat fried foods.

vitamin E halt the process of oxidation. Many of the dietary recommendations for fat intake aim to decrease the likelihood of these harmful oxidation reactions.

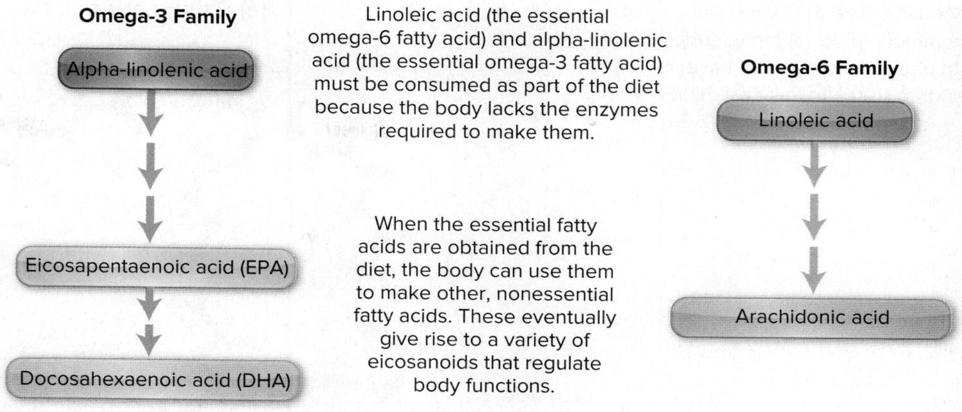

Essential Fatty Acids The various classes of lipids have diverse functions in the body and are necessary for health. Of all the types of lipids found in foods, however, only two polyunsaturated fatty acids are essential in the human diet. Linoleic acid (an omega-6 fatty acid) and alpha-linolenic acid (an omega-3 fatty acid) are called *essential* fatty acids because

Omega-3 Family

Alpha-linolenic acid

↓

Eicosapentaenoic acid (EPA)

↓

Docosahexaenoic acid (DHA)

Linoleic acid (the essential omega-6 fatty acid) and alpha-linolenic acid (the essential omega-3 fatty acid) must be consumed as part of the diet because the body lacks the enzymes required to make them.

When the essential fatty acids are obtained from the diet, the body can use them to make other, nonessential fatty acids. These eventually give rise to a variety of eicosanoids that regulate body functions.

Omega-6 Family

Linoleic acid

↓

Arachidonic acid

FIGURE 5-3 ▲ The essential fatty acid (EFA) family.

we must obtain them from foods to maintain health. The essential fatty acids form parts of vital body structures, perform important roles in immune system function and vision, help form cell membranes, and produce **eicosanoids,** which are involved in practically all important functions in the body.

Many fatty acids that serve important functions in the body are derived from the essential fatty acids (Fig. 5-3). Human enzymes convert the two essential fatty acids to other long-chain polyunsaturated fatty acids, such as **eicosapentaenoic acid (EPA)** and **docosahexaenoic acid (DHA),** which are particularly important for proper function of the brain and nervous system. EPA is needed for concentration and vision and is converted into a powerful anti-inflammatory agent. Because of its role in brain structure, DHA is especially important during pregnancy for fetal brain and nervous system development.

If humans fail to consume enough essential fatty acids, their skin becomes flaky and itchy, and diarrhea and other symptoms such as infections often are seen. Growth and wound healing may be restricted.

Triglycerides The lipids in foods and in body structures are mostly in the form of triglycerides. Although some fatty acids are transported in the bloodstream attached to proteins, most fatty acids in the body are part of triglycerides.

Triglycerides contain a simple three-carbon alcohol, called glycerol, which serves as a backbone for the three attached fatty acids [Fig. 5-4(a)]. Removing one fatty acid from a triglyceride forms a **diglyceride.** Removing two fatty acids from a triglyceride forms a **monoglyceride.** Later you will see that before most dietary fats are absorbed, the two outer fatty acids are typically removed from the triglyceride during digestion in the small intestine. This produces a mixture of fatty acids and monoglycerides that can be absorbed into the intestinal cells. After absorption, the fatty acids and monoglycerides are mostly reformed into triglycerides inside body cells.

PHOSPHOLIPIDS

Phospholipids are another class of lipids. Like triglycerides, they are built on a backbone of glycerol. However, at least one fatty acid is replaced with a compound containing phosphorus (and often other elements, such as nitrogen) [see Fig. 5-4(b)]. Many types of phospholipids exist in the body, especially in the brain. They are an important part of cell membranes. **Lecithin** is a common example of a phospholipid. Various forms of phospholipids are found in body cells, and they participate in fat digestion, absorption, and transport. The body is able to produce all the phospholipids it needs. Even though lecithin is sold as a dietary supplement and is used as an additive in many foods, phospholipids are not essential components of the diet.

eicosanoids A class of hormone compounds, including the prostaglandins, derived from the essential polyunsaturated fatty acids. These signaling compounds are involved in cellular activity that affects practically all important functions in the body.

eicosapentaenoic acid (EPA) An omega-3 fatty acid with 20 carbons and five carbon-carbon double bonds. It is present in large amounts in fatty fish and is slowly synthesized in the body from alpha-linolenic acid.

docosahexaenoic acid (DHA) An omega-3 fatty acid with 22 carbons and six carbon-carbon double bonds. It is present in large amounts in fatty fish and is slowly synthesized in the body from alpha-linolenic acid. DHA is especially present in the retina and brain.

diglyceride A breakdown product of a triglyceride consisting of two fatty acids bonded to a glycerol backbone.

monoglyceride A breakdown product of a triglyceride consisting of one fatty acid attached to a glycerol backbone.

lecithin A group of phospholipid compounds that are major components of cell membranes.

FIGURE 5-4 ▶ Chemical forms of common lipids: (a) triglyceride, (b) phospholipid (in this case, lecithin), and (c) sterol (in this case, cholesterol).

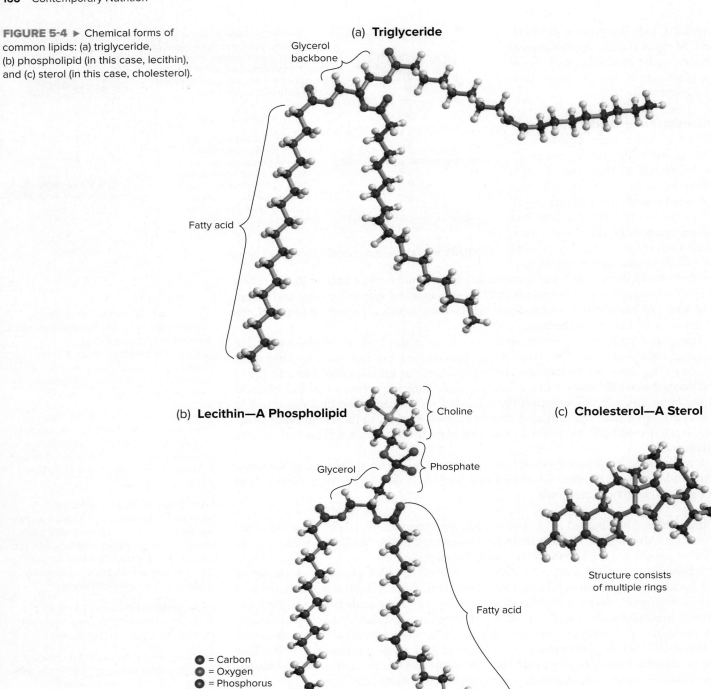

(a) **Triglyceride**

Glycerol backbone

Fatty acid

(b) **Lecithin—A Phospholipid**

Choline

Glycerol

Phosphate

Fatty acid

= Carbon
= Oxygen
= Phosphorus
= Nitrogen

(c) **Cholesterol—A Sterol**

Structure consists of multiple rings

STEROLS

Sterols are a class of lipids characterized by a multi-ringed structure that makes them structurally and functionally different from the other lipids already discussed [see Fig. 5-4(c)]. The most common example of a sterol is cholesterol. This waxy substance does not look like the other lipids discussed so far, but it is classified as a lipid because it does not readily

LIPIDS CONCEPT MAP

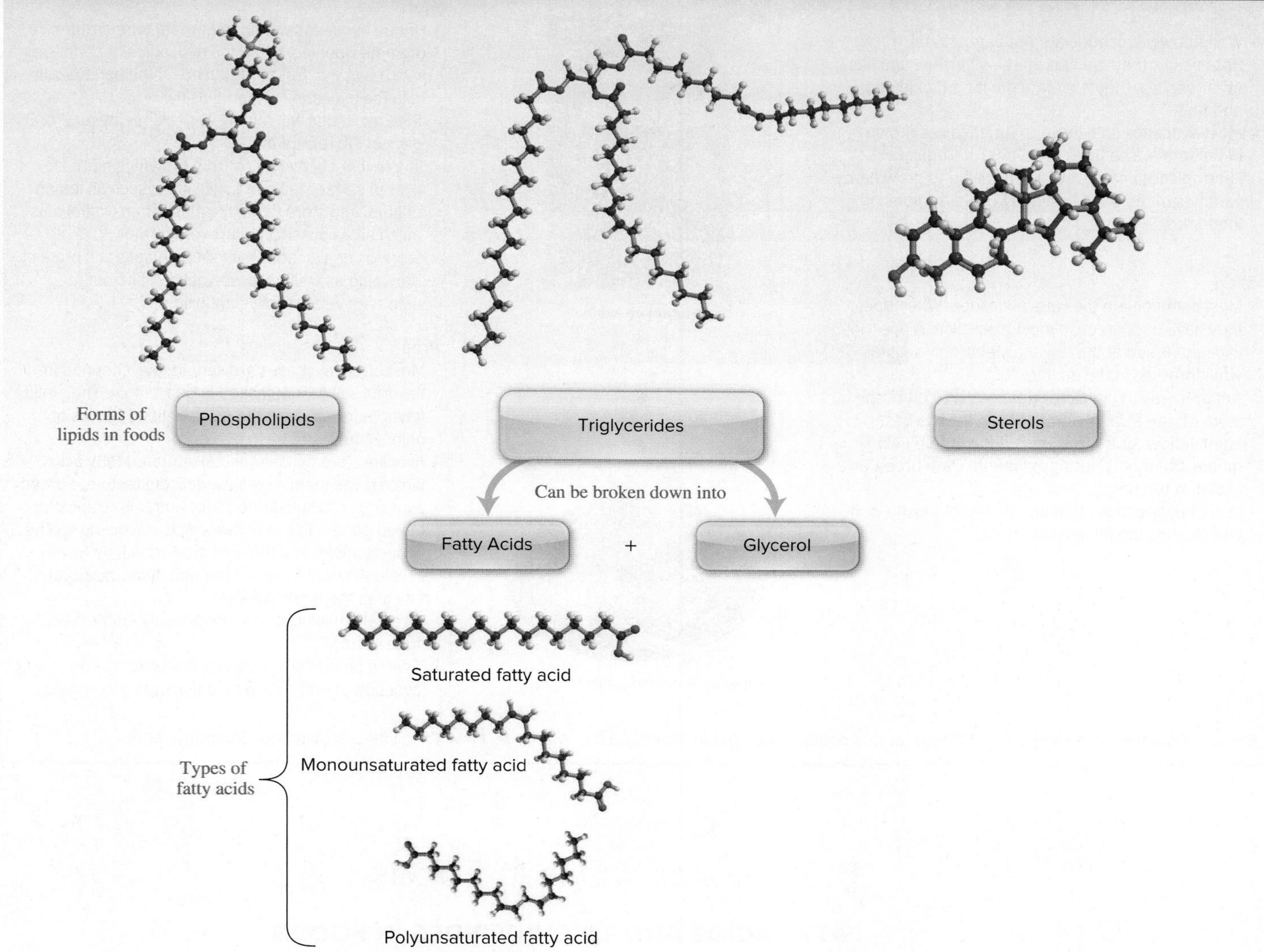

Forms of lipids in foods

Phospholipids

Triglycerides

Sterols

Can be broken down into

Fatty Acids + Glycerol

Saturated fatty acid

Monounsaturated fatty acid

Types of fatty acids

Polyunsaturated fatty acid

dissolve in water. Among other functions, cholesterol is used to form certain hormones and bile acids, and is incorporated into cell structures. The body can make all the cholesterol it needs, so sterols are not essential components of the diet.

The Lipids Concept Map above summarizes the various forms of lipids.

✓ CONCEPT CHECK 5.2

1. Name three structural forms of lipids.
2. What is the structural difference between saturated and unsaturated fatty acids?
3. What is the structural difference between omega-3 and omega-6 fatty acids?
4. Which two fatty acids are essential?
5. How do triglycerides differ from phospholipids?
6. What are the main functions of cholesterol in the body?

FARM to FORK   Avocados

Grow

- Who knew? Avocados are not vegetables! Botanically, they are classified as berries, and like other berries, they are loaded with antioxidants and fiber.
- Most avocados sold in North America are grown in California. The trees grow best in tropical or subtropical climates, but it is possible to grow hardy varieties of the plant in slightly cooler regions or indoors.

Shop

- Most common are the Hass avocados. When ripe, they have dark green, almost black skin. A ripe avocado is soft at the top and yields only slightly when pressed in the middle.
- Another way to check for ripeness is to pluck the stem off the fruit. A vibrant green flesh is best. Light yellow (or if the stem is difficult to pluck) means the fruit is not ripe enough. Dark green or brown is too ripe.
- Don't buy avocados that are dented or mushy, or if you can feel the pit moving inside.

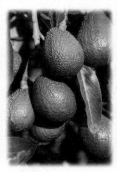

©imagebroker/Alamy

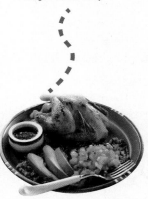

©Ingram Publishing/Alamy

Store

- Unripe avocados will ripen at room temperature. To promote ripening, place the avocado in a paper bag with a banana. Gases produced by the banana will help the avocado to ripen quickly.
- Ripe avocados will remain at peak quality for 2 or 3 days in the refrigerator.
- To prevent cut avocados from browning, sprinkle the cut surface with an acidic juice, such as lemon or lime, and store them in a plastic bag (remove as much air as possible) in the refrigerator.
- Storing cut avocados with sliced onions will prevent browning as well because volatile oils from the onion are very effective antioxidants.

Prep

- Most often, avocados are served raw, chopped in flavorful salsas, or mashed in guacamole. Their mild flavor pairs well with the more defined flavors of onion, citrus, and fresh herbs.
- Avocados are rich in monounsaturated fatty acids, which gives them a creamy, delicate texture. Pureed avocados can substitute 1:1 for butter in recipes for baked goods. The mild flavor of the avocado will be imperceptible, and the final product will be lower in calories but higher in fiber and monounsaturated fats than the original recipe.
- Use half an avocado as a deliciously edible bowl for tuna salad.
- Search online for trendy ways to bake an egg in an avocado or grill it up with lean meats and veggies.

Source: Robinson J: Artichoke, asparagus, and avocados: indulge! In *Eating on the Wild Side.* New York: Little, Brown and Company, 2013.

5.3 Fats and Oils in Foods

FATTY ACIDS AND TRIGLYCERIDES IN FOODS

Lipids (in the form of triglycerides) are abundant in the North American diet. The foods highest in fat (and therefore energy density) include salad oils and spreads such as butter, margarine, and mayonnaise. All of these foods contain close to 100% of calories as fat.

Other high-fat foods include nuts, bologna, avocados, and bacon, which have about 80% of calories as fat (Fig. 5-5). Next, peanut butter and cheddar cheese have about 75% of calories from fat. Marbled steak and hamburgers (ground chuck) have about 60% of calories from fat, and chocolate bars, ice cream, doughnuts, and whole milk have about 50% of calories as fat. Eggs, pumpkin pie, and cupcakes have 35%, as do lean cuts of meat such as top round, ground round, and sirloin. Bread contains about 15% of calories as fat. Foods such as cornflakes, sugar, and fat-free milk have essentially no fat. Figure 5-5 shows examples of food sources of fat.

While you certainly should monitor the *total amount* of fat, the *type* of fat in foods is another important consideration when it comes to selecting a dietary pattern that promotes optimal health. Remember that triglycerides are composed of a mixture of fatty acids of various lengths and degrees of saturation. Overall, a fat or an oil is classified as saturated, monounsaturated, or polyunsaturated based on the type of fatty acids present in the greatest concentration (Fig. 5-6). Fats in foods that contain primarily saturated fatty acids are solid at room temperature, especially if the fatty acids have long

▲ Dairy products are a primary contributor of saturated fat to our diets. ©D. Hurst/Alamy

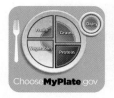

FIGURE 5-5 ◄ Sources of fats from MyPlate. The fill of the background color (none, 1/3, 2/3, or completely covered) within each group in the plate indicates the average nutrient density for fat in that group. The fruit group and vegetable group are generally low in fat. In the other groups, both high-fat and low-fat choices are available. Careful reading of food labels can help you choose lower fat versions of some foods. In general, any type of frying adds significant amounts of fat to a product, as with French fries and fried chicken.

Source: www.choosemyplate.gov

(a)

(b)

Food Item and Amount	Fat (grams)	% AHA Recommendation (65 grams)
Croissant, 1 medium	12	18%
Snack crackers, 1 ounce	7	11%
Whole wheat bread, 1 slice	1	2%
French fries, 1 small serving	16	25%
Spinach, cooked, 1 cup	0.5	< 1%
Acorn squash, baked, 1 cup	0.3	< 1%
Avocado, ½ cup	11	17%
Blueberries 1 cup	0.5	< 1%
Orange juice, 1 cup	0.3	< 1%
Cheddar cheese, 1 ounce	10	15%
Whole milk, 1 cup	8	12%
Whole-milk yogurt, 8 ounces	7	11%
Mixed nuts, 1 ounce	16	25%
Hamburger with bun, 1 each	12	18%
Chicken breast with skin, 2 ounces	7	11%
Canola oil, 1 teaspoon	4.5	7%
Margarine, 1 teaspoon	4	6%
Butter, 1 teaspoon	4	6%

carbon chains (i.e., a **long-chain fatty acid**), as opposed to shorter versions. In contrast, fats containing primarily polyunsaturated or monounsaturated fatty acids (regardless of the length of the carbon chain) are usually liquid at room temperature. Almost all fatty acids in the body and in foods are long-chain fatty acids.

Animal fats are the chief contributors of saturated fatty acids to the North American diet. About 40% to 60% of total fat in dairy and meat products is in the form of saturated fatty acids. Palm oil and coconut oil are two plant oils that are rich sources of saturated fatty acids.

Aside from palm oil and coconut oil, most plant oils are rich in unsaturated fatty acids, ranging from 73% to 94% of total fat. The major sources of monounsaturated fatty acids in the diet are canola oil, olive oil, and peanut oil. Corn, cottonseed, sunflower, soybean, and safflower oils contain mostly polyunsaturated fatty acids (54% to 77%).

Food Sources of Essential Fatty Acids Rich food sources of linoleic acid—the essential omega-6 fatty acid—include safflower, sunflower, corn, and cottonseed oils, as well as nuts and seeds. In the North American diet, chicken is the leading source of linoleic acid, simply because it is so frequently consumed.

long-chain fatty acid A fatty acid that contains 12 or more carbons.

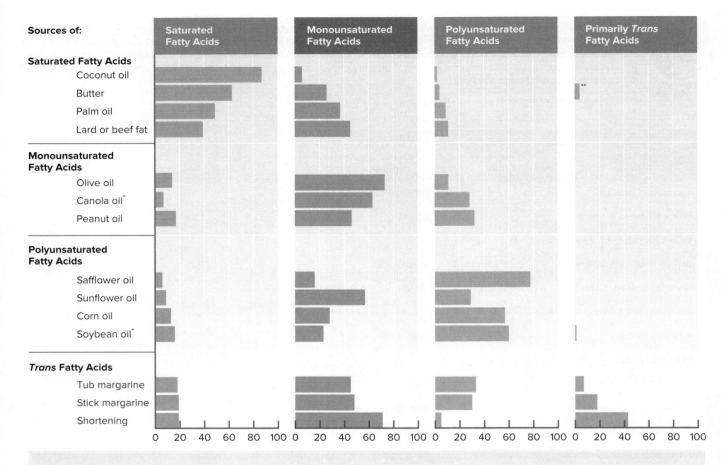

Sources of:	Saturated Fatty Acids	Monounsaturated Fatty Acids	Polyunsaturated Fatty Acids	Primarily *Trans* Fatty Acids

Saturated Fatty Acids
- Coconut oil
- Butter
- Palm oil
- Lard or beef fat

Monounsaturated Fatty Acids
- Olive oil
- Canola oil*
- Peanut oil

Polyunsaturated Fatty Acids
- Safflower oil
- Sunflower oil
- Corn oil
- Soybean oil*

***Trans* Fatty Acids**
- Tub margarine
- Stick margarine
- Shortening

0 20 40 60 80 100   0 20 40 60 80 100   0 20 40 60 80 100   0 20 40 60 80 100

*Rich source of the omega-3 fatty acid alpha-linolenic acid (7% and 12% of total fatty acid content for soybean oil and canola oil, respectively).

**The natural *trans* fatty acids in butter are not harmful and may even have health-promoting properties, such as preventing certain forms of cancer.

FIGURE 5-6 ▲ Saturated, monounsaturated, polyunsaturated, and *trans* fatty acid composition of common fats and oils (expressed as percent of all fatty acids in the product).

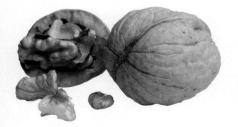

▲ Walnuts are one of the richest plant sources of the omega-3 fatty acid, alpha-linolenic acid, and are a good source of plant sterols. ©lynx/iconotec.com/Glow Images

Two nutrient-dense food sources of alpha-linolenic acid (the essential omega-3 fatty acid) are flax seeds and walnuts.[1] Flax seeds can be purchased in many natural food stores rather inexpensively. These need to be chewed thoroughly, or they will pass through the GI tract undigested. Many people find it easier to grind them in a coffee grinder before eating them. Flax seed oil is also available, but it turns rancid very quickly, especially if not refrigerated. Compared to other nuts and seeds, walnuts are one of the richest sources of alpha-linolenic acid (2.6 grams per 1-ounce serving or 14 walnut halves). In addition, walnuts are a rich source of plant sterols known to inhibit intestinal absorption of cholesterol. Other rich food sources of alpha-linolenic acid include oils from perilla seeds, chia seeds, canola, and soybeans.

Omega-3 Fatty Acids in Fish Looking at Figure 5-3, you can see that eicosapentaenoic acid (EPA) and docosahexaenoic acid (DHA) can be made in the body, so they are not essential fatty acids. However, by consuming food sources of EPA and DHA, you effectively skip a few rather slow and inefficient steps in the conversion of alpha-linolenic acid to EPA and DHA. These two omega-3 fatty acids are naturally found in fatty fish such as salmon, tuna, sardines, anchovies, striped bass, catfish, herring, mackerel, trout, and halibut. The *Dietary Guidelines for Americans* and recommendations from the American Heart Association encourage us to consume two servings of fatty fish per week for optimal cardiovascular health (see Section 5.7). An EPA/DHA supplement is useful for people who do not regularly consume fatty fish.

A word of caution: some types of fish can be a source of mercury, which is toxic in high amounts, especially during gestation, infancy, and early childhood (see Section 13.6). Fish species that are highest in mercury include shark, swordfish, king mackerel, tilefish, marlin, orange roughy, and bigeye, or ahi, tuna. Salmon, sardines, herring, and albacore or yellowfin tuna are better choices because they are lower in mercury, yet still provide heart-healthy omega-3 fatty acids. To limit exposure to mercury, vary your choices rather than always eating the same species of fish and limit overall intake to 12 ounces per week (two to three meals of fish or shellfish per week). Overall, research indicates that the benefits of fish intake, especially in reducing the risk of cardiovascular disease, outweigh the possible risks of mercury contamination.

FOOD SOURCES OF PHOSPHOLIPIDS

Wheat germ, peanuts, egg yolks, soybeans, and organ meats are rich sources of phospholipids. Phospholipids such as lecithin, a component of egg yolks, are often added to salad dressing. Lecithin is used as an **emulsifier** in these and other products because of its ability to keep mixtures of lipids and water from separating (Fig. 5-7). Emulsifiers are added to salad dressings to keep the vegetable oil suspended in water. Eggs added to cake batters likewise emulsify the fat with the milk.

FOOD SOURCES OF STEROLS

Cholesterol is found only in animal foods (Table 5-1). One large egg yolk contains about 185 milligrams of cholesterol. Eggs, meats, and whole milk are our main dietary sources of cholesterol. Foods of plant origin are naturally cholesterol free, but they may contain plant sterols. Some plant sterols have blood cholesterol-lowering properties (refer to the discussion in Section 5.8 on medical interventions to lower blood lipids).

Omega-3 Fatty Acids in Fish (grams per 3-ounce serving):	
Atlantic salmon	1.8
Anchovy	1.7
Sardines	1.4
Rainbow trout	1.0
Coho salmon	0.9
Bluefish	0.8
Striped bass	0.8
Tuna, white, canned	0.7
Halibut	0.4
Catfish, channel	0.2

Recommended omega-3 fatty acid (alpha-linolenic acid) intake per day:	
Men	1.6 grams
Women	1.1 grams

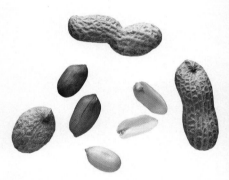

▲ Peanuts are a source of lecithins, as are wheat germ and egg yolks. ©C Squared Studios/Getty Images

emulsifier A compound that can suspend fat in water by isolating individual fat droplets, using a shell of water molecules or other substances to prevent the fat from coalescing.

Emulsifiers and Agitation in Salad Dressing

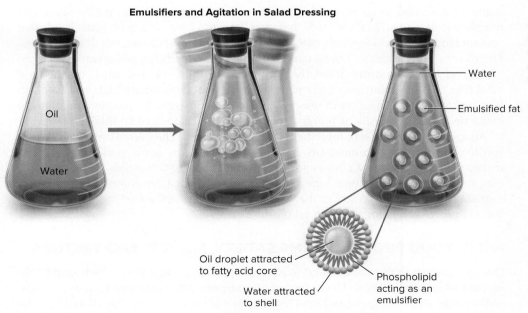

Oil

Water

Water

Emulsified fat

Oil droplet attracted to fatty acid core

Water attracted to shell

Phospholipid acting as an emulsifier

FIGURE 5-7 ▲ Emulsifiers in action. Emulsifiers prevent many brands of salad dressings and other condiments from separating into layers of water and fat. Emulsifiers attract fatty acids inside and have a water-attracting group on the outside. Add them to salad dressing, shake well, and they hold the oil in the dressing away from the water. Emulsification is important in both food production and fat digestion/absorption.

TABLE 5-1 ■ Cholesterol Content of Foods

3 oz beef brains	2635 mg
3 oz beef liver	337 mg
1 large egg yolk*	185 mg
3 oz shrimp	166 mg
3 oz beef*	75 mg
3 oz pork loin, roasted	75 mg
3 oz chicken or turkey (white meat)*	75 mg
1 cup ice cream	63 mg
3 oz trout	60 mg
3 oz tuna	45 mg
3 oz hot dog	38 mg
1 oz cheddar cheese*	30 mg
1 cup whole milk*	24 mg
1 cup 1% milk	12 mg
1 cup fat-free milk	5 mg
1 large egg white	0 mg

*Leading dietary sources of cholesterol in American diets.

USING FOOD LABELS TO IDENTIFY FAT

Some fat discussed so far is obvious: butter on bread, mayonnaise in potato salad, and marbling in raw meat. In some foods, however, fat is not immediately obvious. Foods that contain hidden fat include whole milk, pastries, cookies, cake, cheese, hot dogs, crackers, French fries, and ice cream. The fat (and calories) in these foods can add up rather quickly!

A good way to find out about the fat content of the foods you eat is on the food label (Fig. 5-8). The Nutrition Facts panel displays total fat, saturated fat, and *trans* fat. You can use that information to select foods that comply with the recommendations of major health authorities, which urge Americans to limit saturated fat intake.

Also, check out the list of ingredients on the food label. The ingredients list can alert you to the presence of animal fats (e.g., bacon, beef, ham, lamb, pork, chicken, and turkey fats), dairy fats (e.g., butter and cream), egg and egg-yolk solids, nuts, vegetable oils, and partially hydrogenated shortening or vegetable oil. Conveniently, the label lists ingredients by order of weight in the product. If fat is one of the first ingredients listed, you are probably looking at a high-fat product.

FAT IN FOOD PROVIDES SOME SATIETY, FLAVOR, AND TEXTURE

Does fat promote satiety? Fats tend to slow the process of digestion, which could help you to feel full after a meal. However, fats also improve the flavor and texture of foods, so they may stimulate increased food intake. Fat's effect on satiety may depend on the size and saturation of the fatty acids in foods. What everyone knows for sure is that fats contain more than twice the calories of carbohydrates and proteins. Therefore, a high-fat meal is likely to be a high-calorie meal.

Fat provides texture in foods. If you have ever taken a bite of high-quality milk chocolate, you probably agree that the feel of fat melting on the tongue is good. The fat in

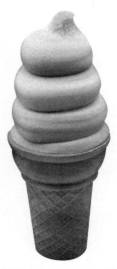

▲ Fat replacements such as gum fiber are typically seen in soft serve ice cream.
©Ingram Publishing/Alamy

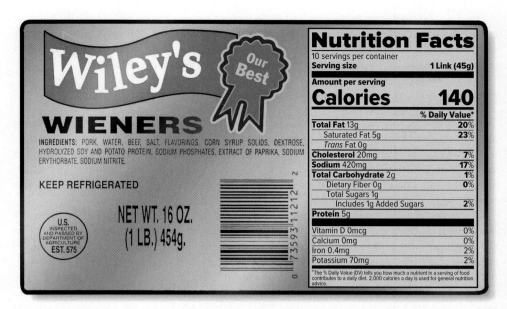

Definitions for Nutrient Claims About Fat and Cholesterol on Food Labels

Fat

- **Fat free:** less than 0.5 gram of fat per serving
- **Saturated fat free:** less than 0.5 gram per serving, and the level of *trans* fatty acids does not exceed 0.5 gram per serving
- **Low fat:** 3 grams or less per serving and, if the serving is 30 grams or less or 2 tablespoons or less, per 50 grams of the food; 2% milk cannot be labeled low fat, as it exceeds 3 grams per serving. *Reduced fat* is used instead.
- **Low saturated fat:** 1 gram or less per serving and not more than 15% of calories from saturated fatty acids
- **Reduced or less fat:** at least 25% less per serving than reference food
- **Reduced or less saturated fat:** at least 25% less per serving than reference food

Cholesterol

- **Cholesterol free:** less than 2 milligrams of cholesterol and 2 grams or less of saturated fat per serving
- **Low cholesterol:** 20 milligrams or less of cholesterol and 2 grams or less of saturated fat per serving and, if the serving is 30 grams or less or 2 tablespoons or less, per 50 grams of the food
- **Reduced or less cholesterol:** at least 25% less cholesterol and 2 grams or less of saturated fat per serving than reference food

FIGURE 5-8 ▲ Reading labels helps locate hidden fat. Who would think that wieners (hot dogs) can contain about 85% of food calories as fat? Looking at the hot dog does not suggest that almost all of its food calories come from fat, but the label shows otherwise. Let us do the math: 13 grams total fat × 9 kcal per gram of fat = 120 kcal from fat; 120 kcal/140 kcal per link = 0.86 or 86% kcal from fat.

milk also provides a richness that fat-free milk lacks. The most tender cuts of meat are high in fat, visible as the marbling of meat. In addition, fat carries flavors in foods. Heating spices in oil intensifies the flavors of an Indian curry or a Mexican dish. You can see why reduced-fat foods seem less appealing than their full-fat counterparts!

FAT-REPLACEMENT STRATEGIES FOR REDUCED-FAT FOODS

Manufacturers have introduced reduced-fat versions of numerous food products. The fat content of these alternatives ranges from 0% in fat-free Fig Newtons to about 75% of the original fat content in other products. However, the total calorie content of most fat-reduced products is not substantially lower than that of the regular products. Generally, when fat is removed from a product, something must be added—commonly, sugars—in its place. It is difficult to reduce both the fat and sugar contents of a product at the same time and maintain flavor and texture. For this reason, many reduced-fat products (e.g., cakes and cookies) are still energy dense. Use the Nutrition Facts panel on the food label to choose the portion size that fits into your daily calorie needs.

To lower the fat in foods, manufacturers may replace some of the fat with water, protein (Simplesse,® Dairy-Lo),® or forms of carbohydrates such as starch derivatives (Z-trim),® fiber (Maltrin,® Stellar,™ Oatrim), and gums. In reduced-fat margarines, water replaces some of the fat. While regular margarines are 80% fat by weight (11 grams per tablespoon), some reduced-fat margarines are as low as 30% fat by weight (4 grams per tablespoon). When used in recipes, the extra water added to these margarines can cause texture and volume changes in the finished product. Cookbooks can suggest alterations in recipes to compensate for the increased water content of these products.

Manufacturers also may use engineered fats, such as olestra (Olean)® and salatrim (Benefat),® that are made with fat and sucrose (table sugar) but that provide few or no calories because they cannot be digested and/or absorbed well. The main problem with the fat replacer olestra is that it can bind the fat-soluble vitamins and reduce their absorption.

Canada has not approved the use of olestra in food products; the United States is the sole country that permits the use of this fat substitute in foods.

To date, fat replacements have had little impact on our diets. This is partly because currently approved fat replacements lack versatility and are not used extensively by manufacturers. In addition, fat replacements are not practical for use in the foods that provide the most fat in our diets: beef, cheese, whole milk, and pastries.

RANCIDITY LIMITS SHELF LIFE OF FOODS

Decomposing oils emit a disagreeable odor and taste sour and stale. Stale potato chips are a good example. The double bonds in unsaturated fatty acids break down, producing rancid by-products. Ultraviolet light, oxygen, and heat (as in deep-fat frying) can break double bonds and, in turn, destroy the structure of polyunsaturated fatty acids. Saturated fats and *trans* fats can more readily resist these effects because they contain fewer carbon-carbon double bonds.

Rancidity is not a major problem for consumers because the odor and taste generally discourage us from eating enough to become sick. However, rancidity is a problem for the food industry and restaurant business because it reduces a product's shelf life. To increase shelf life, manufacturers often add partially hydrogenated plant oils to products. Foods most likely to become rancid are deep-fried foods and those with a large amount of exposed surface. Polyunsaturated oils are a good choice for products such as salad dressings, whereas more saturated fats are best for high-heat cooking. The fat in fish is also susceptible to rancidity because it is highly polyunsaturated.

Antioxidants such as vitamin E help protect foods against rancidity by guarding against fat breakdown. The vitamin E naturally occurring in plant oils reduces the breakdown of double bonds in fatty acids. When food manufacturers want to prevent rancidity in polyunsaturated fats, they often add the synthetic antioxidants **BHA** and **BHT** or vitamin C to products that contain fat, such as salad dressings and cake mixes. Manufacturers also tightly seal products and use other methods to reduce oxygen levels inside packages.

BHA, BHT Butylated hydroxyanisole and butylated hydroxytoluene: two common synthetic antioxidants added to foods.

hydrogenation The addition of hydrogen to a carbon-carbon double bond, producing a single carbon-carbon bond with two hydrogens attached to each carbon.

HYDROGENATION OF FATTY ACIDS IN FOOD PRODUCTION INCREASES *TRANS* FATTY ACID CONTENT

As mentioned previously, most foods that are rich in long-chain saturated fatty acids are solid at room temperature, and those that are rich in unsaturated fatty acids are liquid at room temperature. In the production of some foods, solid fats work better than liquid oils. In pie crust, for example, solid fats yield a flaky product, whereas crusts made with liquid oils tend to be greasy and more crumbly. If oils with unsaturated fatty acids are used to replace solid fats, they often must be made more saturated (with hydrogen), as this solidifies the vegetable oils into shortenings and margarines. Hydrogen is added by bubbling hydrogen gas under pressure into liquid vegetable oils in a process called **hydrogenation** (Fig. 5-9). The fatty acids are not fully hydrogenated to the saturated fatty acid form, as this would make the product too hard and brittle. Partial hydrogenation—leaving some monounsaturated fatty acids—creates a semisolid product.

The process of hydrogenation produces *trans* fatty acids, which were described in Section 5.2. Most natural monounsaturated and polyunsaturated fatty acids exist in the *cis* form, causing a bend in the carbon chain, whereas the straighter carbon forms of *trans* fat more closely resemble saturated fatty acids. This may be the mechanism whereby *trans* fat increases the risk for heart disease. Studies also indicate that *trans* fats increase overall inflammation in the body, which is not healthful. Thus, the *Dietary Guidelines for Americans,* the American Heart Association, and the Food and Nutrition Board each recommend minimal *trans* fat intake.

Partially hydrogenated soybean oil—rich in *trans* fat—became the major fat in food processing when manufacturers eliminated the tropical oils

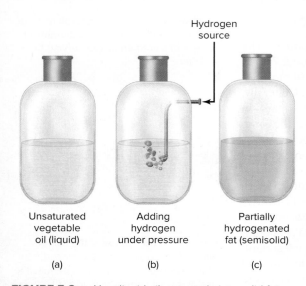

Hydrogen source

Unsaturated vegetable oil (liquid)	Adding hydrogen under pressure	Partially hydrogenated fat (semisolid)
(a)	(b)	(c)

FIGURE 5-9 ▲ How liquid oils are made into solid fats. (a) Unsaturated fatty acids are present in liquid form in large metal tanks. (b) Hydrogens are added (hydrogenation), changing some carbon-carbon double bonds to single bonds and producing some *trans* fatty acids. (c) The partially hydrogenated product is likely to be used in margarine, shortening, or for deep-fat frying.

TABLE 5-2 ■ Main Sources of Fatty Acids and Their State at Room Temperature

Type and Health Effects	Main Sources	State at Room Temperature
Saturated Fatty Acids Tend to increase blood levels of cholesterol		
Long-chain	Lard; fat in beef, pork, and lamb	Solid
Medium-and short-chain	Milk fat (butter), coconut oil, palm oil, palm kernel oil	Soft or liquid
Monounsaturated Fatty Acids Tend to decrease blood levels of cholesterol	Olive oil, canola oil, peanut oil	Liquid
Polyunsaturated Fatty Acids Tend to decrease blood levels of cholesterol	Sunflower oil, corn oil, safflower oil, fish oil	Liquid
Essential Fatty Acids Omega-3: alpha-linolenic acid Reduces inflammation responses, blood clotting, and plasma triglycerides	Cold-water fish (salmon, tuna, sardines, mackerel), walnuts, flaxseed, hemp oil, canola oil, soybean oil, chia seeds, and perilla oil	Liquid
Omega-6: linoleic acid Regulates blood pressure and increases blood clotting	Beef, poultry, safflower oil, sunflower oil, corn oil	Solid to liquid
Trans **Fatty Acids** Increase blood cholesterol more than saturated fat	Margarine (squeeze, tub, stick), shortening	Soft to very solid

rich in saturated fat (palm, palm olein, and coconut). While foods made with partially hydrogenated oil were becoming popular, there was very little known about the *trans* fats they contained and their harmful effects. It was not until the 1990s that scientists began identifying the adverse health effects of *trans* fats. Currently, *trans* fat intake in North America amounts to 3 to 4 grams per day. Table 5-2 includes typical sources of *trans* fat.

The American Heart Association strongly advises that we avoid food sources of *trans* fats, such as foods prepared with partially hydrogenated oils. The FDA has taken action to make consumers more aware of the amounts of *trans* fat in foods. Since 2006, federal regulations have required the disclosure of *trans* fat content on food packages (review Fig. 5-8). Food labels in Canada also must list *trans* fat content. In 2015, the FDA determined that partially hydrogenated oils—the main sources of *trans* fats in the diet—are no longer "generally recognized as safe" for use in human food products.[2] North American companies have already been responding to consumer demands by creating products that are free of *trans* fat. For example, Promise,® Smart Balance,® and Fleischmann's® margarines are free of *trans* fat (less than 0.5 gram per serving) compared to typical margarines. By 2018, most *trans* fats will be eliminated from food products.

To minimize *trans* fat intake, a general guideline is to limit consumption of fried (especially deep-fat fried) food items, any pastries or flaky bread products (such as pie crusts, crackers, croissants, and biscuits), and cookies. Most importantly, use little or no stick margarine or shortening. Instead, substitute vegetable oils and softer tub margarines (whose labels

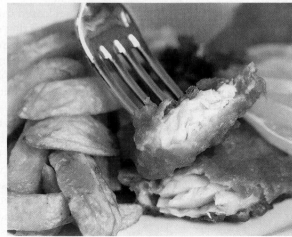

▲ Fried foods can be a rich source of *trans* fats. Reducing the intake of these foods can help lower blood lipid levels. ©Getty Images/Digital Vision

Nut Butters: Are They "Good" Fat?

Nut butters are plant products, so they are naturally cholesterol free and provide 2 or 3 grams of fiber, which can lower blood cholesterol. Nuts are also a good source of unsaturated fats. Two tablespoons of peanut butter provide about 12 grams of unsaturated fats and only 3 grams of saturated fat. As you've learned, monounsaturated and polyunsaturated fats tend to lower blood cholesterol levels. To steer clear of *trans* fats, be on the lookout for partially hydrogenated oils in the list of ingredients. These have been used in some products to increase shelf life, although food manufacturers are gradually phasing them out. Lastly, check the sugar content. Nut butters naturally contain 1 or 2 grams of sugar, but processed varieties (e.g., cinnamon swirl) may contain up to 9 grams of sugar. Reap the most heart-health benefits by choosing natural nut butters and controlling the size of your portion.

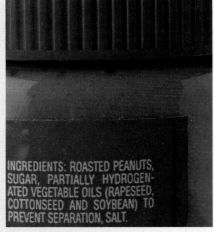

INGREDIENTS: ROASTED PEANUTS, SUGAR, PARTIALLY HYDROGEN-ATED VEGETABLE OILS (RAPESEED, COTTONSEED AND SOYBEAN) TO PREVENT SEPARATION, SALT.

©Elite Images/McGraw-Hill Education

lipase Fat-digesting enzyme produced by the salivary glands, stomach, and pancreas.

list vegetable oil or water as the first ingredient). Avoid deep-fat frying any food in shortening. Substitute baking, panfrying, broiling, steaming, grilling, or deep-fat frying in unhydrogenated oils with high "smoke points," meaning they do not break down at deep-frying temperatures. Peanut, safflower, sunflower, and canola oils are good choices. Replace nondairy creamers with reduced-fat or fat-free milk, as most nondairy creamers are rich in partially hydrogenated vegetable oils. Finally, read the ingredients on food labels, using the previous tips to estimate *trans* fat content. If partially hydrogenated vegetable oil is one of the first three ingredients on the label, you can assume that there is a significant amount of *trans* fat in the product.

✔ CONCEPT CHECK 5.3

1. Which foods are the most fat dense (> 60% total calories as fat)?
2. Where is cholesterol found in the food supply?
3. Which types of fat are used as emulsifiers, and what is their function in food?
4. What are some strategies used to produce reduced-fat foods?
5. How do fats become rancid, and how can this be prevented?
6. What happens to unsaturated fats during the process of hydrogenation?
7. What regulations are in place to educate and protect the public from *trans* fats in foods?

5.4 Making Lipids Available for Body Use

It is no secret that fats and oils make foods more appealing. Their presence in foods adds flavor, moistness, and texture. What happens to lipids once they are eaten? Let us take a closer look at the digestion, absorption, and uses of lipids in the body.

DIGESTION

In the first phase of fat digestion, the stomach (and salivary glands to some extent) secretes the enzyme **lipase.** Salivary lipase and gastric lipase act primarily on triglycerides that have fatty acids with short chain lengths, such as those found in butterfat. The action of these lipase enzymes, however, is dwarfed by that of the lipase enzyme that is released from the pancreas to digest fats in the small intestine. Most of the triglycerides in the diet contain fatty acids with longer chain lengths and are generally not digested until they reach the small intestine (Fig. 5-10).

In the small intestine, triglycerides are broken down by lipase into smaller products, namely monoglycerides (glycerol backbones with a single fatty acid attached) and fatty acids. Under the right circumstances, digestion is rapid and thorough. The "right" circumstances depend on the presence of bile from the gallbladder. Bile acids (components of bile) act to emulsify fats in the watery digestive juices. Emulsification improves digestion and absorption because it separates large fat globules into smaller ones, thereby increasing the total surface area for lipase action (Fig. 5-11). What happens to the bile acids after their work in fat digestion is complete? They get recycled! After participating in fat digestion, most bile acids are absorbed in the last segment of the small intestine and transported back to the liver. Through this process, approximately 98% of bile acids are recycled. Only 1% to 2% of bile acids end up in the large intestine to be eliminated in the feces.

Phospholipid digestion is similar to triglyceride digestion. Enzymes from the pancreas and cells in the wall of the small intestine digest phospholipids. The eventual products are glycerol, fatty acids, and the remaining phosphorus-containing parts.

Fat Digestion and Absorption

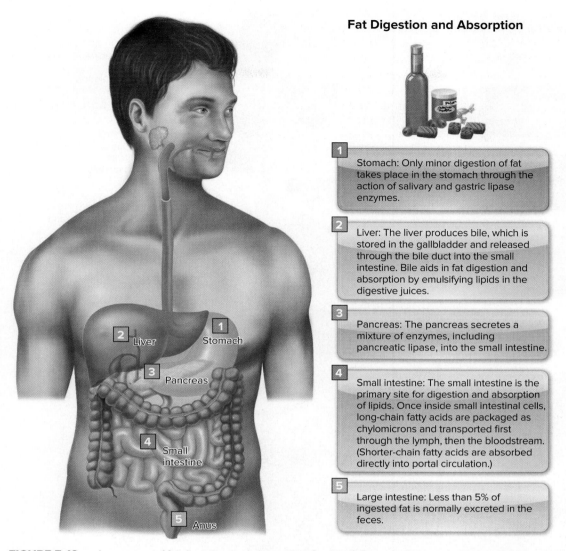

1 Stomach: Only minor digestion of fat takes place in the stomach through the action of salivary and gastric lipase enzymes.

2 Liver: The liver produces bile, which is stored in the gallbladder and released through the bile duct into the small intestine. Bile aids in fat digestion and absorption by emulsifying lipids in the digestive juices.

3 Pancreas: The pancreas secretes a mixture of enzymes, including pancreatic lipase, into the small intestine.

4 Small intestine: The small intestine is the primary site for digestion and absorption of lipids. Once inside small intestinal cells, long-chain fatty acids are packaged as chylomicrons and transported first through the lymph, then the bloodstream. (Shorter-chain fatty acids are absorbed directly into portal circulation.)

5 Large intestine: Less than 5% of ingested fat is normally excreted in the feces.

FIGURE 5-10 ▲ A summary of fat digestion and absorption. Section 3.9 covered general aspects of this process.

With regard to cholesterol digestion, any cholesterol with a fatty acid attached is broken down to free cholesterol and fatty acids by enzymes released from the pancreas. Any fatty acids that are part of these structures could be broken down to yield energy, but contribution to overall calorie intake is miniscule compared to the energy stored in triglycerides.

ABSORPTION

The products of fat digestion in the small intestine are fatty acids and monoglycerides. These products diffuse into the absorptive cells of the small intestine. About 95% of dietary fat is absorbed in this way. The chain length of fatty acids dictates how they will be distributed to the rest of the body. If the chain length of a fatty acid is less than 12 carbon atoms, it is relatively soluble in water and small enough to be absorbed into the capillaries and transported via the portal vein directly to the liver. Longer chain fatty acids are too large to be absorbed directly into portal circulation. These larger products of fat digestion are reformed into triglycerides within the absorptive cells of the small intestine and eventually enter circulation via the lymphatic system.

If the gallbladder is surgically removed (e.g., in cases of gallstone formation), bile will enter the small intestine directly from the liver. Moderate amounts of fat can still be digested adequately, but some people experience loose stools after eating high-fat meals because some fat reaches the large intestine unabsorbed.

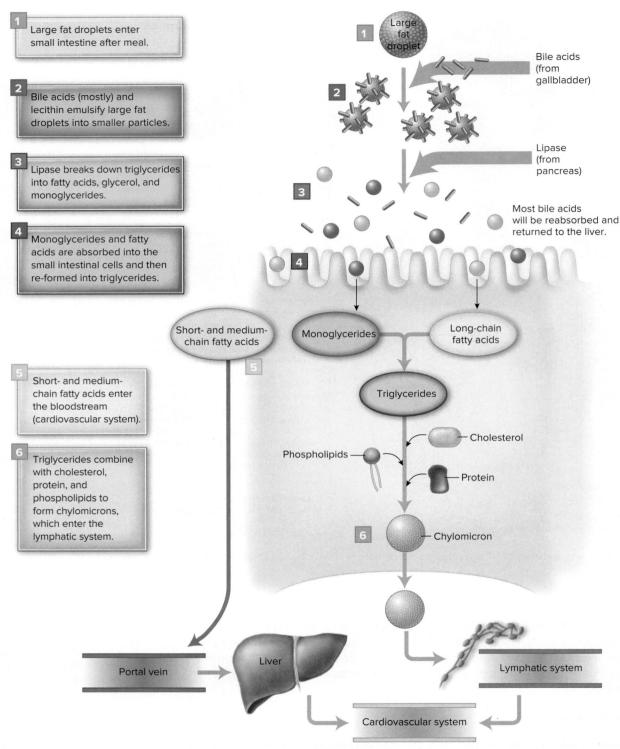

1. Large fat droplets enter small intestine after meal.

2. Bile acids (mostly) and lecithin emulsify large fat droplets into smaller particles.

3. Lipase breaks down triglycerides into fatty acids, glycerol, and monoglycerides.

4. Monoglycerides and fatty acids are absorbed into the small intestinal cells and then re-formed into triglycerides.

5. Short- and medium-chain fatty acids enter the bloodstream (cardiovascular system).

6. Triglycerides combine with cholesterol, protein, and phospholipids to form chylomicrons, which enter the lymphatic system.

Large fat droplet

Bile acids (from gallbladder)

Lipase (from pancreas)

Most bile acids will be reabsorbed and returned to the liver.

Short- and medium-chain fatty acids

Monoglycerides

Long-chain fatty acids

Triglycerides

Cholesterol

Phospholipids

Protein

Chylomicron

Portal vein

Liver

Lymphatic system

Cardiovascular system

FIGURE 5-11 ▲ Bile acids facilitate the digestion of triglycerides by emulsifying fat droplets in the chyme in the small intestine. This allows for efficient action of pancreatic lipase and subsequent absorption of monoglycerides and fatty acids into the mucosal cells of the small intestine.

✓ CONCEPT CHECK 5.4

1. What enzymes are responsible for digestion of triglycerides?
2. What are the end products of fat digestion?
3. What are the differences between the absorption of long- versus short-chain fatty acids?

5.5 Carrying Lipids in the Bloodstream

As noted earlier, fat and water do not mix easily. This incompatibility presents a challenge for the transport of fats through the blood and lymph, which are mostly water. **Lipoproteins** serve as vehicles for transport of lipids from the small intestine and liver to the body tissues (Table 5-3). They are found in the bloodstream and contain a core of lipids with a shell composed of protein, phospholipids, and cholesterol (Fig. 5-12).

Lipoproteins are classified into four groups—chylomicrons, VLDL, LDL, and HDL—based on their densities. Lipids are less dense than proteins. Therefore, lipoproteins that contain a large percentage of lipids in comparison to protein are less dense than those depleted of lipids (Fig. 5-13).

CHYLOMICRONS TRANSPORT DIETARY FATS

As you learned in Section 5.4, digestion of dietary fats results in a mixture of glycerol, monoglycerides, and fatty acids. Once these products are absorbed by the cells of the small intestine, they are reassembled into triglycerides. Then, the intestinal cells package the triglycerides into **chylomicrons,** which enter the lymphatic system and eventually the bloodstream. Chylomicrons are the largest of the lipoproteins; they are loaded with dietary fat and originate only from the intestinal cells. Like the other lipoproteins, chylomicrons are composed of large droplets of lipid surrounded by a thin, water-soluble shell of phospholipids, cholesterol, and protein (see Fig. 5-13). The water-soluble shell around a chylomicron allows the lipid to float freely in the lymph and blood, which are both water based. Some of the proteins in the shell may also help other cells identify the lipoprotein as a chylomicron.

Once a chylomicron enters the bloodstream, the triglycerides in its core are broken down into fatty acids and glycerol by yet another lipase enzyme. This one is called **lipoprotein lipase,** and it is attached to the inside walls of the blood vessels. As soon as the fatty acids are released to the bloodstream, they are absorbed by nearby cells. The remaining glycerol backbone circulates back to the liver. Muscle cells can immediately use the absorbed fatty acids for fuel. Adipose cells, on the other hand, tend to reassemble the fatty acids into triglycerides for storage.

What happens to the rest of the chylomicron after triglycerides have been removed? The leftover materials are called **chylomicron remnants.** Chylomicron remnants are removed from circulation by the liver, and their components are recycled to make other lipoproteins and bile acids.

VLDLs and LDLs TRANSPORT LIPIDS FROM THE LIVER TO THE BODY CELLS

The liver takes up various lipids from the blood. The liver also is the manufacturing site for lipids and cholesterol. The raw materials for lipid and cholesterol synthesis include free fatty acids taken up from the bloodstream, as well as carbon and hydrogen derived

lipoprotein A compound found in the bloodstream containing a core of lipids with a shell composed of protein, phospholipids, and cholesterol.

chylomicron Lipoprotein made of dietary fats surrounded by a shell of cholesterol, phospholipids, and protein. Chylomicrons are formed in the absorptive cells of the small intestine after fat absorption and travel through the lymphatic system to the bloodstream.

lipoprotein lipase An enzyme attached to the cells that form the inner lining of blood vessels; it breaks down triglycerides into free fatty acids and glycerol.

chylomicron remnant Lipoprotein that remains after triglycerides have been removed from a chylomicron; composed of protein, phospholipids, and cholesterol.

TABLE 5-3 ■ Composition and Roles of the Major Lipoproteins in the Blood

Lipoprotein	Primary Component	Key Role
Chylomicron	Triglyceride	Carries dietary fat from the small intestine to cells
VLDL	Triglyceride	Carries lipids made and taken up by the liver to cells
LDL	Cholesterol	Carries cholesterol made by the liver and from other sources to cells
HDL	Protein	Contributes to cholesterol removal from cells and, in turn, excretion of it from the body

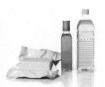
©Torbjorn Lagerwall/Alamy

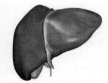
©MedicalRF.com

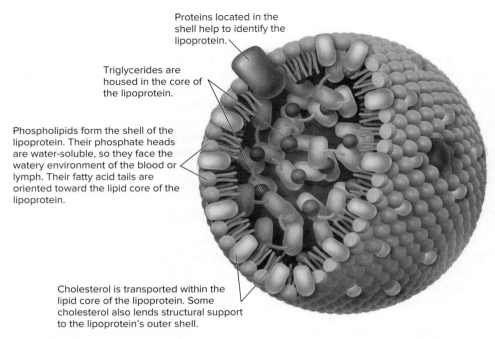

Proteins located in the shell help to identify the lipoprotein.

Triglycerides are housed in the core of the lipoprotein.

Phospholipids form the shell of the lipoprotein. Their phosphate heads are water-soluble, so they face the watery environment of the blood or lymph. Their fatty acid tails are oriented toward the lipid core of the lipoprotein.

Cholesterol is transported within the lipid core of the lipoprotein. Some cholesterol also lends structural support to the lipoprotein's outer shell.

FIGURE 5-12 ▲ The structure of a lipoprotein (specifically, LDL). This structure allows fats to circulate in the water-based bloodstream. Various lipoproteins are found in the bloodstream.

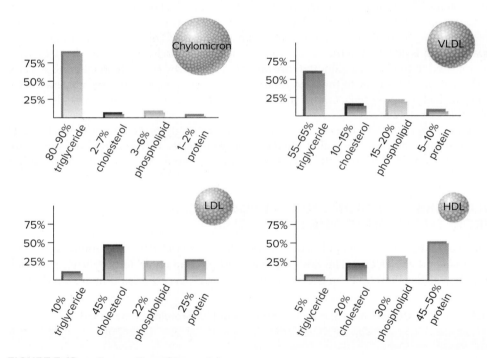

FIGURE 5-13 ▲ Composition of lipoproteins.

from carbohydrates, protein, and alcohol. The liver then must package the lipids it makes into lipoproteins for transport in the blood to body tissues.

First in our discussion of lipoproteins made by the liver are **very-low-density lipoproteins (VLDL).** These particles are composed of cholesterol and triglycerides surrounded by a water-soluble shell of phospholipids and protein. VLDLs are rich in triglycerides and thus are very low in density (Fig. 5-13). Once in the bloodstream,

very-low-density lipoprotein (VLDL) The lipoprotein created in the liver that carries cholesterol and lipids that have been taken up or newly synthesized by the liver.

lipoprotein lipase on the inner surface of the blood vessels breaks down the triglycerides into fatty acids and glycerol. Fatty acids and glycerol are released from the VLDL into the bloodstream and are taken up by the body cells.

As its triglycerides are released, the VLDL becomes proportionately more dense. Much of what eventually remains of the VLDL particle is then called **low-density lipoprotein (LDL).** Primarily composed of cholesterol, the role of LDL is to transport cholesterol to tissues. LDL particles are taken up from the bloodstream by specific receptors on cells, especially liver cells, and are then broken down. The cholesterol and protein components of LDL provide some of the building blocks necessary for cell growth and development, such as synthesis of cell membranes and hormones.

low-density lipoprotein (LDL) The lipoprotein in the blood containing primarily cholesterol; elevated LDL is strongly linked to cardiovascular disease risk.

HDLS REMOVE CHOLESTEROL FROM THE BLOOD

The final group of lipoproteins, **high-density lipoproteins (HDL),** is a critical and beneficial participant in this process of lipid transport. Its high proportion of protein makes it the densest lipoprotein. The liver and intestine produce most of the HDL in the blood. It roams the bloodstream, picking up cholesterol from dying cells and other sources. HDL donates the cholesterol primarily to other lipoproteins for transport back to the liver to be excreted. Some HDL travels directly back to the liver.

high-density lipoprotein (HDL) The lipoprotein in the blood that picks up cholesterol from dying cells and other sources and transfers it to the other lipoproteins in the bloodstream, as well as directly to the liver; low HDL increases the risk for cardiovascular disease.

"GOOD" AND "BAD" CHOLESTEROL IN THE BLOODSTREAM

HDL and LDL are often described as "good" and "bad" cholesterol, respectively. Many studies demonstrate that the amount of HDL in the bloodstream can closely predict the risk for cardiovascular disease. Risk increases with low HDL because little cholesterol is transported back to the liver and excreted. Women tend to have high amounts of HDL, especially before **menopause,** compared to men. High amounts of HDL slow the development of cardiovascular disease, so any cholesterol carried by HDL can be considered "good" cholesterol.

menopause The cessation of the menstrual cycle in women, usually beginning at about 50 years of age.

On the other hand, LDL is sometimes considered "bad" cholesterol. In our discussion of LDL, you learned that it is taken up by receptors on various cells. If LDL is not readily cleared from the bloodstream, **scavenger cells** in the arteries take up the lipoprotein, leading to a buildup of cholesterol in the blood vessels. This buildup, known as **atherosclerosis,** greatly increases the risk for cardiovascular disease. Low amounts of LDL are needed as part of routine body functions, but a high level of LDL cholesterol is a risk factor for cardiovascular disease. Read more about the link between LDL and cardiovascular disease in Section 5.8.

scavenger cells Specific form of white blood cells that can bury themselves in the artery wall and accumulate LDL. As these cells take up LDL, they contribute to the development of atherosclerosis.

atherosclerosis A buildup of fatty material (plaque) in the arteries, including those surrounding the heart.

Here is an important point: the cholesterol in foods is not designated as "good" or "bad." It is only after cholesterol has been made or processed by the liver that it shows up in the bloodstream as part of LDL or HDL. Dietary patterns can certainly affect the lipoproteins in your blood. The cholesterol in your diet does not have a very big impact on the levels of LDL and HDL in the blood. However, dietary patterns that are low in saturated and *trans* fats tend to lower total cholesterol, particularly LDL.

CONCEPT CHECK 5.5

1. Describe how the structure of lipoproteins allows fats to be transported through the watery environment of the lymph and blood.
2. How are dietary fats packaged in the small intestine and transported?
3. Where are VLDLs made and what do they contain?
4. Where do LDLs originate and what is their destination?
5. Why are HDLs considered "good" cholesterol?

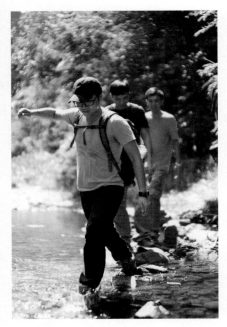

▲ When at rest or during light activity, the muscles use mostly fatty acids for fuel. ©Flickr RF/@mr.jerry/Getty Images

5.6 Roles of Lipids in the Body

Many key functions of fat in the body require the use of fatty acids in the form of triglycerides. Triglycerides are used for energy storage, insulation, and transportation of fat-soluble vitamins.

PROVIDING ENERGY

Triglycerides contained in the diet and stored in adipose tissue provide the fatty acids that are the main fuel for muscles while at rest and during light activity. Muscles use a mixture of fat and carbohydrates for fuel. (Protein is a minor fuel source.) During low-intensity exercise, more fatty acids are used; as exercise intensity increases, more carbohydrates are used. Other body tissues also use fatty acids for energy needs. Overall, about half of the energy used by the entire body at rest and during light activity comes from fatty acids. When considering the whole body, the use of fatty acids by skeletal and heart muscle is balanced by the use of glucose by the nervous system and red blood cells. Recall from Section 4.5 that cells need a supply of carbohydrate to efficiently process fatty acids for fuel. The details about how we burn fat as a fuel will be discussed in Section 10.3.

STORING ENERGY FOR LATER USE

We store energy mainly in the form of triglycerides. The body's ability to store fat is essentially limitless. Its fat storage sites, adipose cells (Fig. 5-14), can increase about 50 times in weight. If the amount of fat to be stored exceeds the ability of the existing cells to expand, the body can form new adipose cells.

An important advantage of using triglycerides to store energy in the body is that they are energy dense. Recall that these yield, on average, 9 kcal per gram, whereas proteins and carbohydrates yield only about 4 kcal per gram. In addition, triglycerides are chemically stable, so they are not likely to react with other cell constituents, making them a safe form for storing energy. Finally, when it comes to storage, triglycerides are space savers. Adipose cells contain about 80% lipid and only 20% water and protein. When we store triglycerides in adipose cells, we store little else. In contrast, muscle tissue is about 73% water. What if we had to store energy as muscle tissue? Body weight linked to energy storage would increase dramatically. The same would be true if we stored energy primarily as glycogen, as about 3 grams of water are stored for every gram of glycogen.

INSULATING AND PROTECTING THE BODY

The insulating layer of fat just beneath the skin is made mostly of triglycerides. Fat tissue also surrounds and protects some organs (e.g., kidneys) from injury. We usually do not notice the important insulating function of fat tissue because we wear clothes and add more as needed. A layer of insulating fat is important in animals living in cold climates. Polar bears, walruses, and whales all build a thick layer of fat tissue around themselves to insulate against cold-weather environments. The extra fat also provides energy storage for times when food is scarce.

TRANSPORTING FAT-SOLUBLE VITAMINS

Triglycerides and other fats in food carry fat-soluble vitamins to the small intestine and aid their absorption. People who absorb fat poorly, such as those with the disease cystic fibrosis, are at risk for deficiencies of fat-soluble vitamins, especially vitamin K. A similar risk comes from taking mineral oil as a laxative at mealtimes. The body cannot digest or absorb mineral oil, so the undigested oil carries the fat-soluble vitamins from the meal into the feces, where they are eliminated. Recall that the main problem with the fat replacer olestra is that it can bind the fat-soluble vitamins and reduce their absorption. Unabsorbed fatty acids can bind minerals, such as calcium and magnesium, and draw them into the stool for elimination. In this way, fat malabsorption can harm mineral status as well.

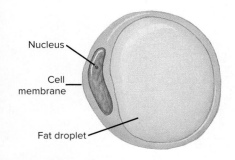

Nucleus

Cell membrane

Fat droplet

FIGURE 5-14 ▲ An adipose cell.

REGULATING BODY PROCESSES

The lipids are potent regulators of chemical processes within the body. Sterols are important in the synthesis of hormones, including estrogen, testosterone, and the active form of vitamin D. Individual fatty acids also orchestrate many aspects of human metabolism. As you learned in Section 5.2, the essential omega-3 and omega-6 fatty acids can be converted in the body into other fatty acids, which give rise to eicosanoids. Eicosanoids act as chemical messengers that direct growth and development, immune function, and the work of the central nervous system. The essential omega-3 fatty acid, alpha-linolenic acid, can be converted into EPA and DHA in the body. Eicosanoids made from these omega-3 fatty acids tend to decrease blood clotting and inflammatory processes in the body. This is in contrast to the pro-inflammatory effects of omega-6 fatty acids. The omega-6 parent fat, linoleic acid, is converted by the body into **arachidonic acid (AA).** Arachidonic acid has some important functions in the body, but when omega-6 fatty acids are consumed in excess, arachidonic acid can contribute to inflammatory conditions such as arthritis, blood clotting, and other cardiovascular problems.

arachidonic acid (AA) An omega-6 fatty acid made from linoleic acid with 20 carbon atoms and four carbon-carbon double bonds.

Some studies show that people who eat fish at least twice a week (total weekly intake of 8 ounces) run lower risks for heart attack than do people who rarely eat fish. In these cases, the omega-3 fatty acids in fish oil are probably acting to reduce blood clotting. As will be covered in detail in Section 5.8, blood clots are part of the heart attack process. In addition, omega-3 fatty acids have a favorable effect on heart rhythm. Consequently, the risk of heart attack decreases with the consumption of omega-3 fatty acids from fish, especially for people already at high risk.

Recognize that excessive intakes of omega-3 fatty acids can be unhealthy, too! Certain groups of people, such as the Greenlandic Inuit, eat so much seafood that their normal blood-clotting ability can be impaired. This increases the risk for uncontrolled bleeding and may cause **hemorrhagic stroke.** An excessive intake of long-chain fatty acids in seafood can also depress immune function, resulting in more infections.

hemorrhagic stroke Damage to part of the brain resulting from rupture of a blood vessel and subsequent bleeding within or over the internal surface of the brain.

PHOSPHOLIPIDS IN THE BODY

The structure of phospholipids—with their water-soluble phosphate heads and their fat-soluble fatty acid tails—gives them the unique ability to be simultaneously soluble in water and fat. In cell membranes, this property allows phospholipids to form a bilayer. A cell membrane looks much like a sea of phospholipids with protein "islands" (Fig. 5-15). The phosphate heads face the watery environment inside (cytosol) or outside the cell, while the fatty acid tails form the interior of the cell membrane. The proteins form receptors for hormones, function as enzymes, and act as transporters for nutrients. Some cholesterol is also present in the membrane.

Phospholipids also participate in fat digestion. They work as emulsifiers, which enable a fat to be suspended in water. Think of phospholipids as bridges between the oil and water. Along with bile acids, phospholipids help to break apart large droplets of fat into tiny oil droplets so that digestive enzymes can perform the work of breaking down the fats in a meal.

Last but not least, phospholipids are very important to proper function of the nervous system. Sphingomyelin is a phospholipid that surrounds and protects nerve cells. It participates in cell-to-cell communication within the nervous system.

CHOLESTEROL IN THE BODY

Cholesterol plays many vital roles in the body. It is used to make some important hormones, such as estrogen, testosterone, and the vitamin D hormone. Cholesterol is an essential structural component of cells and the outer layer of the lipoprotein particles that transport lipids in the blood. The cholesterol content of the heart, liver, kidney, and brain is high, reflecting its critical role in these organs. Cholesterol is also the building block of bile acids, which are needed for fat digestion.

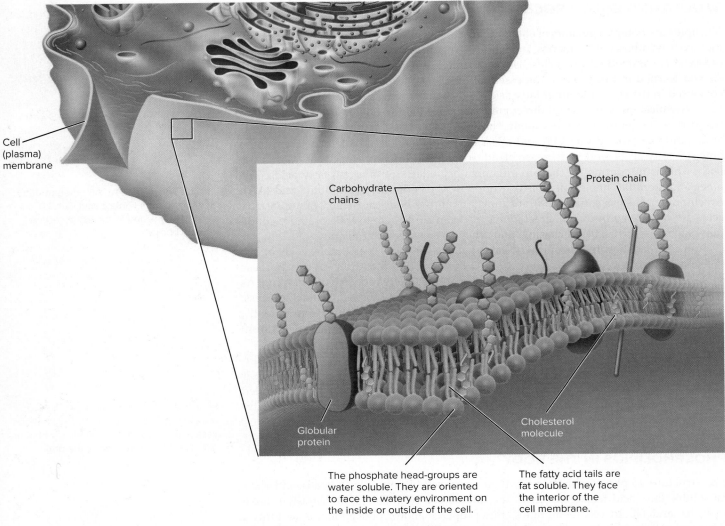

Cell (plasma) membrane

Carbohydrate chains

Protein chain

Globular protein

Cholesterol molecule

The phosphate head-groups are water soluble. They are oriented to face the watery environment on the inside or outside of the cell.

The fatty acid tails are fat soluble. They face the interior of the cell membrane.

FIGURE 5-15 ▶ The phospholipid bilayer. Phospholipids are the main components of cell membranes, forming a double layer (bilayer) of lipid.

About two-thirds of the cholesterol circulating through your body is made by body cells; the remaining one-third comes from the diet. Most of the time, cholesterol synthesis by the body is well regulated: if you eat more dietary cholesterol, the liver synthesizes less cholesterol. Each day, your body's cells produce approximately 875 milligrams of cholesterol. Of this amount, about 400 milligrams are used to make new bile acids to replenish those lost in the feces, and about 50 milligrams are used to make hormones. In addition to all the cholesterol cells make, we consume about 180 to 325 milligrams of cholesterol per day from animal-derived food products, with men consuming the higher amount compared to women. Absorption of cholesterol from food ranges from about 40% to 65%. The relationship between dietary cholesterol and cardiovascular disease risk will be discussed in Section 5.8.

✔ CONCEPT CHECK 5.6

1. What are the functions of triglycerides in the body?
2. Where are phospholipids found in the body?
3. What are some compounds that are made from cholesterol in the body?

5.7 Recommendations for Fat Intake

There is no RDA for total fat intake for adults, although there is an Adequate Intake set for total fat for infants (see Section 15.2). The *Dietary Guidelines for Americans* and the Food and Nutrition Board recommend that total fat intake should be 20% to 35% of total calories, which equates to 44 to 78 grams per day for a person who consumes 2000 kcal daily.

Regarding essential fatty acids, the Food and Nutrition Board has issued recommendations for linoleic acid and alpha-linolenic acid. Table 5-4 lists the AIs for adults. To meet our dietary requirements for essential fatty acids, we only need to consume 2 to 4 tablespoons of plant oil each day, which equates to roughly 5% of our total calories. We can easily get that much from cooking oils, salad dressings, nuts and seeds, vegetables, and whole grain breads. Even a low-fat diet will provide enough essential fatty acids if it follows a balanced plan such as MyPlate.

EATING FOR HEART HEALTH

The most specific recommendations for fat intake come from the American Heart Association (AHA).[3] Many North Americans are at risk for developing cardiovascular disease, so AHA promotes dietary and lifestyle goals aimed at reducing this risk. The AHA diet and lifestyle goals for cardiovascular disease risk reduction for the general public include aiming for an overall healthy eating pattern; appropriate body weight; and a desirable blood cholesterol profile, blood pressure, and blood glucose level. In Table 5-5, a more detailed list of recommendations is provided for those who currently are at high risk or have cardiovascular disease.

TABLE 5-4 ■ Food and Nutrition Board Recommendations for Essential Fatty Acids

	Men (g/d)	Women (g/d)
Linoleic acid (omega-6)	17 (3.6 tsp)	12 (2.6 tsp)
Alpha-linolenic acid (omega-3)	1.6 (0.35 tsp)	1.1 (0.24 tsp)

The advice to consume 20% to 35% of calories as fat does not apply to infants and toddlers below the age of 2 years. These youngsters are forming new tissue that requires fat, especially in the brain, so their intake of fat and cholesterol should not be greatly restricted.

TABLE 5-5 ■ American Heart Association's *Diet and Lifestyle Recommendations*

Use up at least as many calories as you take in.

Eat a variety of nutritious foods from all the food groups, including:
- A variety of fruits and vegetables
- Whole grains
- Low-fat dairy products
- Skinless poultry and fish
- Nuts and legumes
- Nontropical vegetable oils

Eat less of the nutrient-poor foods:
- Limit foods and beverages that are high in calories but low in nutrients.
- Limit the amount of saturated fat, *trans* fat, and sodium you eat.

As you make daily food choices, base your eating pattern on these recommendations:
- Eat a variety of fresh, frozen, and canned fruits and vegetables without high-calorie sauces or added salt and sugars.
- Choose fiber-rich whole grains for most grain servings.
- Choose poultry and fish without the skin and prepare them in healthy ways.
- Eat a variety of fish (especially those rich in omega-3 fatty acids) at least twice a week.
- Select fat-free and low-fat dairy products.
- Avoid foods containing partially hydrogenated vegetable oils to reduce *trans* fat in your diet.
- Limit saturated fat and *trans* fat and replace them with monounsaturated and polyunsaturated fats. If you need to lower blood cholesterol, reduce saturated fats to no more than 5% to 6% of total calories.
- Cut back on beverages and foods with added sugars.
- Choose foods with less sodium and prepare foods with little or no salt.
- If you drink alcohol, drink in moderation (no more than 1 drink per day for women and no more than 2 drinks per day for men).
- Follow the AHA recommendations when you eat out and keep an eye on portion sizes.

Source: Eckel RH, et al.: 2013 AHA/ACC guideline on lifestyle management to reduce cardiovascular risk: A report of the American College of Cardiology/American Heart Association Task Force on Practice Guidelines. *Circulation* 129:S76, 2013.

To reduce risk for cardiovascular disease, the AHA recommends reducing *trans* fat and limiting saturated fat to no more than 5% to 6% of total calories. These are the primary fatty acids that raise LDL. Table 5-6 is an example of a diet that adheres to 20% or 30% of calories as fat. Compare these recommendations to the actual dietary intake patterns of these fats by North Americans: 33% of calories from total fat, with about 13% of calories from saturated fat each day.

Please note that the latest guidelines set no specific limits on dietary cholesterol. This is because dietary cholesterol intake has little impact on blood cholesterol levels. Instead, evidence shows that saturated fat and *trans* fat have the greatest impact on blood lipids. That doesn't mean you should eat limitless quantities of cholesterol-rich foods! As it turns out, rich food sources of cholesterol are usually sources of saturated fat, as well. Thus, as you reduce the saturated fat in your diet, you will likely reduce your cholesterol intake, too.

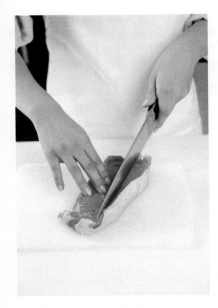

▲ Trimming the visible fat from meats can help reduce saturated fat intake, but you cannot remove the marbling (streaks of fat running through the meat). Limit portion size to 3 ounces and choose leaner cuts of meat to help keep your blood cholesterol levels in check.
©Chris Stein/Getty Images RF

TABLE 5-6 ■ Daily Menu Examples Containing 2000 kcal and 30% or 20% of Calories as Fat

30% of Calories as Fat		20% of Calories as Fat	
Food	Fat (grams)	Food	Fat (grams)
Breakfast			
Orange juice, 1 cup	0.5	Same	0.5
Shredded wheat, ¾ cup	0.5	Shredded wheat, 1 cup	0.7
Toasted whole grain bagel	1.1	Same	1.1
Peanut butter, 3 teaspoons	8.0	Same	8.0
1% low-fat milk, 1 cup	2.5	Fat-free milk, 1 cup	0.6
Lunch			
Whole wheat bread, 2 slices	2.4	Same	2.4
Roast beef, 2 ounces	4.9	Light turkey roll, 2 ounces	0.9
Mustard, 3 teaspoons	0.6	Same	0.6
Swiss cheese, 2 slices	15.6	Swiss cheese, 1 slice	7.8
Lettuce	—	Same	—
Tomato	—	Same	—
Oatmeal cookie, 1	3.3	Oatmeal cookie, 2	6.6
Snack			
Apple	—	Same	—
Dinner			
Chicken tenders frozen meal	18.0	Fat-free chicken tenders	—
Carrots, ½ cup	—	Same	—
Dinner roll, 1	2.0	Same	2.0
Olive oil, 1.5 teaspoons	6.8	Same	6.8
Banana	0.6	Same	0.6
1% low-fat milk, 1 cup	2.5	Fat-free milk, 1 cup	0.6
Snack			
Raisins, 2 teaspoons	—	Raisins, ½ cup	—
Air-popped popcorn, 3 cups	1.0	Air-popped popcorn, 6 cups	2.0
Parmesan cheese, 2 tablespoons	2.8	Same	2.8
Totals	**73.1**		**44.0**

Newsworthy Nutrition

Mediterranean diet decreases risk of cardiovascular disease

Based on earlier observations of an inverse relationship between adherence to the Mediterranean diet and risk of cardiovascular disease, the effect of the Mediterranean diet pattern on the primary prevention of cardiovascular disease events was studied in Spain, using a randomized multicenter trial design. Participants (7447 persons, 55 to 80 years, 57% women) were at high cardiovascular risk but had no cardiovascular disease at the beginning of the study and were randomly assigned to either a Mediterranean diet supplemented with extra-virgin olive oil; a Mediterranean diet supplemented with mixed nuts; or a control diet with advice to reduce dietary fat. Participants were followed for a median of 4.8 years and assessed for the occurrence of the following major cardiovascular events: myocardial infarction, stroke, or death from cardiovascular causes. There was good adherence to the interventions for the two Mediterranean-diet groups. At least one major cardiovascular event occurred in 288 participants. This included 96 events for the group assigned to a Mediterranean diet with extra-virgin olive oil and 83 events for the group assigned to a Mediterranean diet with nuts versus 109 events for the control group. The authors concluded that a Mediterranean diet, unrestricted in calories but supplemented with extra-virgin olive oil or nuts, resulted in a substantial reduction in the incidence of major cardiovascular events among persons at high cardiovascular risk. These results, therefore, support the benefits of the Mediterranean diet for the prevention of cardiovascular disease.

Source: Estruch R, et al. "Primary prevention of cardiovascular disease with a Mediterranean diet," *N Engl J Med* 368:1279–1290, 2013.

RECOMMENDATIONS FOR FISH CONSUMPTION

The *Dietary Guidelines* and the American Heart Association's *Diet and Lifestyle Recommendations* encourage Americans to eat 2 or more servings of fatty fish each week. Fish is not only a rich source of omega-3 fatty acids but also a valuable source of protein and trace elements that may provide protective effects for the cardiovascular system. Broiled or baked fish is recommended rather than fried fish because frying may increase the ratio of omega-6 to omega-3 fatty acids and may produce *trans* fatty acids and oxidized lipid products that may increase cardiovascular disease risk.

Although consuming fish is thought to have greater benefits, fish oil capsules can be safely substituted for fish if a person does not like fish. Generally, about 1 gram of omega-3 fatty acids (about three capsules) from fish oil per day is recommended, especially for people with evidence of cardiovascular disease. The American Heart Association also recently suggested that fish oil supplements (providing 2 to 4 grams of omega-3 fatty acids per day) could be employed to treat elevated blood triglycerides. However, fish oil capsules should be limited for individuals who have bleeding disorders, take anticoagulant medications, or anticipate surgery because they may increase risk of uncontrollable bleeding and hemorrhagic stroke. Thus, for fish oil capsules, as well as other dietary supplements, it is important to follow a physician's recommendations. Remember that fish oil supplements are not regulated by the FDA; the quality of these supplements is not standardized, and contaminants naturally present in the fish oil may not have been removed.

DIETARY PATTERNS THAT PROMOTE CARDIOVASCULAR HEALTH

In recent years, the Mediterranean diet (see the Newsworthy Nutrition in the section) has attracted a lot of attention because of the lower rates of chronic diseases seen among people following such a diet plan.[5,6] Reduction of cardiovascular disease has been one

Do fish oil capsules leave a nasty taste in your mouth? Freezing fish oil capsules before consumption, using enteric-coated capsules, and using capsules with vitamin E will reduce the fishy aftertaste.

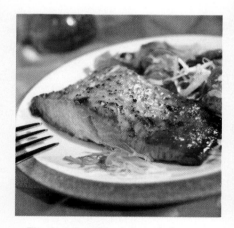

▲ The American Heart Association recommends eating fatty fish such as salmon at least twice a week. As a source of omega-3 fatty acids, fish is a heart-healthy alternative to other animal sources of protein, which can be high in saturated fat and cholesterol. ©Purestock/SuperStock

of the most consistent results of the Mediterranean diet. The major sources of fat in the Mediterranean diet include liberal amounts of olive oil compared to a small amount of animal fat (from animal flesh, eggs, and dairy products). In contrast, major sources of fat in the typical North American diet include animal flesh, whole milk, pastries, cheese, margarine, and mayonnaise. While dietary fat sources definitely play a role in prevention of chronic disease, it is important to remember that other aspects of one's lifestyle also contribute to disease risk. People who follow a Mediterranean diet also tend to consume moderate alcohol (usually in the form of red wine, which contains many antioxidants), eat plenty of whole grains and few refined carbohydrates, and are also more physically active than typical North Americans.[7]

An alternative plan for reduction of cardiovascular disease is Dr. Dean Ornish's purely vegetarian **(vegan)** diet plan.[8] This diet is very low in fat, including only a scant quantity of vegetable oil used in cooking and the small amount of oils present in plant foods. Individuals restricting fat intake to 20% of calories should be monitored by a physician, as the resulting increase in carbohydrate intake can increase blood triglycerides in some people, which is not a healthful change. Over time, however, the initial problem of high blood triglycerides on a low-fat diet may self-correct. Among people following

vegan A person who eats only plant foods.

ASK THE RDN   Coconut Oil

Dear RDN: My friend at the health food store said I should start using coconut oil in my cooking because it has all kinds of health benefits. Is coconut oil a good choice?

Recently, coconut oil has been promoted for weight loss, heart health, cancer protection, and brain health. Indeed, there is some interesting research on the health effects of the particular fatty acids in coconut oil. At this point, however, there is little evidence to back up the claims that coconut oil is a miracle cure for anything.

Coconut oil is highly saturated. In fact, nearly 90% of the fatty acids in coconut oil are saturated, which is even more than butter or beef fat. This makes for a desirable product: it has that "melt in your mouth" quality and it is very shelf stable, which is attractive for food manufacturers and consumers alike. How do saturated fats impact your health? In this chapter, you have seen the recommendations from all the major health authorities urging Americans to limit their intakes of saturated fat. This is because saturated fatty acids have been shown to increase blood levels of LDL cholesterol, which are linked to atherosclerosis. Proponents of coconut oil point to research showing that the fatty acids in coconut oil, while they do raise LDL, also raise HDL levels. Recently, the American Heart Association advised against the use of coconut oil (and other sources of saturated fatty acids) because of these effects on LDL levels.[4]

When it comes to weight loss, the producers of coconut oil focus on the size of the fatty acids in their product. Most dietary fats are long-chain fatty acids. About 60% of the fatty acids in coconut oil, however, are medium-chain fatty acids, which are more likely to be burned as fuel and less likely to be stored in adipose tissue. Does coconut oil help you lose weight? There are two small human studies that show a decrease in waist circumference with coconut oil, but there is not yet enough evidence to promote coconut oil as a weight-loss aid.

If you like coconut oil, *use it in moderation.* Like any dietary fat, coconut oil is a dense source of calories. Simply adding coconut oil to your dietary pattern is not a wise choice because those extra fat calories can quickly add up. Extra calories from any source inevitably lead to weight gain. Use it instead of butter or margarine, aiming to keep your total intake of saturated fat less than 10% of total calories. Most of the time, though, choose unsaturated plant oils, which have proven benefits for heart health. Coconut oil is not a cure-all, but it can be included as part of an overall healthy dietary pattern that meets your calorie needs.

Yours in health,

Angela Collene, MS, RDN, LD (author)

the Ornish plan, blood triglycerides initially increased but within a year fell to normal values as long as the individuals emphasized high-fiber carbohydrate sources, controlled (or improved) body weight, and followed a regular exercise program.

FAT *QUALITY* VERSUS FAT *QUANTITY*

Weight control is a vitally important way to minimize risk for a variety of chronic diseases. Because it is a dense source of calories, many people seek to limit fat intake as a way to manage body weight. However, it is important to recognize that excess calories from any source—fat, carbohydrates, or protein—contribute to weight gain. If weight loss is needed, understand that your overall calorie intake is more important than the specific ratio of carbohydrates, fats, and protein in your diet.

As you have learned, the general consensus among nutrition experts is that fat should comprise 20% to 35% of total calories. When it comes to improving your dietary pattern, it is usually not necessary to drastically lower the *quantity* of fat in your diet. However, we should aim to choose more foods that provide omega-3 fatty acids, while choosing fewer sources of saturated and *trans* fats.[9] In short, most Americans need to improve their fat *quality*.

Simply selecting the reduced-fat versions of pastries, cookies, and cakes will not improve the quality of your diet. Often, extra sugar or salt has been added to these foods to compensate for losses of taste and texture. Instead, focus your efforts on choosing plant sources of fat more often than animal sources (Table 5-7). Fruits, vegetables, and whole grains are usually low in total fat and saturated fat; the (mostly unsaturated) fats they do provide are accompanied by vitamin E, vitamin K, and a variety of health-promoting phytochemicals.[4]

TABLE 5-7 ■ **Tips for Cutting Back on Saturated Fats and *Trans* Fats**

	Eat Less of These Foods	Eat More of These Foods
Grains	• Pasta dishes with cheese or cream sauces • Croissants • Pastries • Doughnuts • Pie crust	• Whole grain breads • Whole grain pasta • Brown rice • Air-popped popcorn
Vegetables	• French fries • Potato chips • Vegetables cooked in butter, cheese, or cream sauces	• Fresh, frozen, baked, or steamed vegetables
Fruit	• Fruit pies	• Fresh, frozen, or canned fruits
Dairy	• Whole milk • Ice cream • High-fat cheese • Cheesecake	• Fat-free and reduced-fat milk • Low-fat frozen desserts (e.g., yogurt, sherbet, and ice milk) • Reduced-fat/part-skim cheese
Protein	• Bacon • Sausage • Organ meats (e.g., liver) • Egg yolks	• Fish • Skinless poultry • Lean cuts of meat (with fat trimmed away) • Soy products • Egg whites/egg substitutes
Fat and Oils	• Butter • Lard • Stick margarine	• Plant oils • Tub margarine (with no *trans* fat)

CASE STUDY Planning a Heart-Healthy Diet

Jackie is a 21-year-old, health-conscious individual majoring in business. She recently learned that a diet high in saturated fat can contribute to high blood cholesterol and that exercise is beneficial for the heart. Jackie now takes a brisk 30-minute walk each morning before going to class, and she has started to cut as much fat out of her diet as she can, replacing it mostly with carbohydrates. A typical day for Jackie now begins with a 2-cup bowl of Fruity Pebbles™ with 1 cup of skim milk and ½ cup of apple juice. For lunch, she might pack a turkey sandwich on white bread with lettuce, tomato, and mustard; a 1-ounce package of fat-free pretzels; and five reduced-fat vanilla wafers. Dinner could be a 2-cup portion of pasta with some olive oil and garlic mixed in, and a small iceberg lettuce salad with lemon juice squeezed over it. Her snacks are usually baked chips, low-fat cookies, fat-free frozen yogurt, or fat-free pretzels. She drinks five diet soft drinks throughout the day as her main beverage.

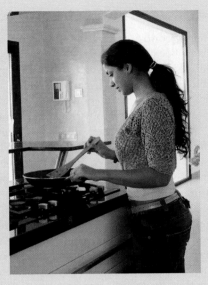

▲ Are there important food groups missing from Jackie's new diet plan?
©Stuart Pearce/Pixtal/AGE Fotostock

1. Is there much fat left in Jackie's new diet plan? Is it necessary for her to drastically lower her fat intake?
2. What types of fat should Jackie try to consume? Why are these types of fat the most desirable?
3. What types of foods has Jackie used to replace the fat in her diet?
4. What food groups are missing from her new diet plan? How many servings should she be including from these food groups?
5. Is Jackie's new exercise routine appropriate?

Complete the Case Study. Responses to these questions can be provided by your instructor.

✓ CONCEPT CHECK 5.7

1. How does the percent of calories as fat in the North American diet compare to recommendations?
2. Describe the current recommendations for saturated fat and *trans* fat intake.
3. What are the key features of the Mediterranean diet?

5.8 Nutrition and Your Health

Lipids and Cardiovascular Disease

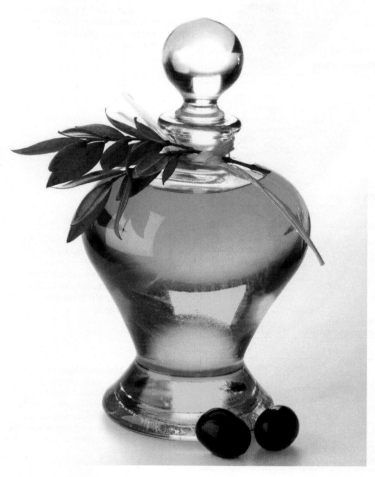

©Foodcollection

The typical forms of cardiovascular disease—coronary heart disease and strokes—are associated with inadequate blood circulation in the heart and brain related to buildup of this plaque. Blood supplies the heart muscle, brain, and other body organs with oxygen and nutrients. When blood flow via the coronary arteries surrounding the heart is interrupted, the heart muscle can be damaged. A heart attack, or **myocardial infarction,** may result (review Fig. 5-16). This may cause the heart to beat irregularly or to stop. About 25% of people do not survive their first heart attack. Similarly, if blood flow to parts of the brain is interrupted long enough, part of the brain dies, causing a **cerebrovascular accident,** or stroke.

Sometimes, a heart attack can strike with the sudden force of a sledgehammer, with pain radiating up the neck or down the arm. Other times, it can sneak up at night, masquerading as indigestion, with slight pain or pressure in the chest. Crushing chest pain is a more common symptom in men.[11] Many times, the symptoms are so subtle in women that death occurs before she or the health professional realizes that a heart attack is taking place. If there is any suspicion that a heart attack is taking place, the person should first call 911 and then chew an aspirin (325 milligrams) thoroughly. Aspirin helps to reduce the blood clotting that leads to a heart attack.

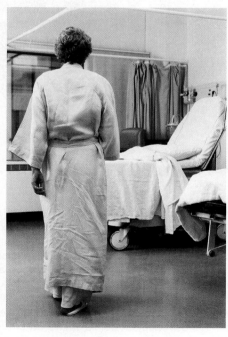

▲ Cardiovascular disease kills more women than any other disease.
©image100/PunchStock

Cardiovascular disease is the major killer of North Americans. It typically involves the coronary arteries and, thus, frequently the term *coronary heart disease (CHD)* or *coronary artery disease (CAD)* is used. Each year, about 610,000 people die of coronary heart disease in the United States. About 735,000 people in the United States have a heart attack each year. Women generally lag about 10 years behind men in developing the disease. Still, it eventually kills more women than any other disease. The cost of coronary heart disease alone is $108.9 billion each year, which includes the costs of health care services, medications, and lost productivity.[10]

Development of Cardiovascular Disease

The symptoms of cardiovascular disease develop over many years and often do not become obvious until old age. Nonetheless, autopsies of young adults under 20 years of age have shown that many of them had atherosclerotic **plaque** in their arteries (Fig. 5-16). This finding indicates that plaque buildup can begin in childhood and continue throughout life, although it usually goes undetected for some time.[11]

plaque A cholesterol-rich substance deposited in the blood vessels; it contains various white blood cells, smooth muscle cells, various proteins, cholesterol and other lipids, and eventually calcium.

myocardial infarction Death of part of the heart muscle. Also termed a *heart attack.*

cerebrovascular accident (CVA) Death of part of the brain tissue due typically to a blood clot. Also termed a *stroke.*

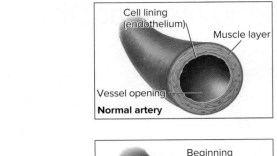

A healthy blood vessel is smooth and flexible. Blood can easily move through the vessel and it is able to stretch to accommodate changes in blood pressure throughout the course of a day.

Normal artery — Cell lining (endothelium), Muscle layer, Vessel opening

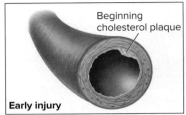

Injury to an artery wall begins the process of plaque formation. Possible causes for injury include smoking, diabetes, high blood pressure, high blood cholesterol, or infection.

Early injury — Beginning cholesterol plaque

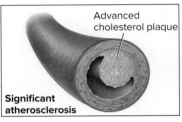

The initial injury is followed by a progressive buildup of plaque in the artery walls. The plaque consists of fatty materials (e.g., oxidized LDL), platelets, and minerals. Over time, the blood vessel narrows.

Significant atherosclerosis — Advanced cholesterol plaque

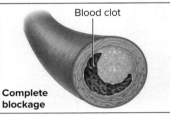

A blood clot becomes lodged in the narrow blood vessel, blocking or greatly restricting blood flow to tissues. Nutrients and oxygen cannot reach the tissue, so it is damaged and may die. A heart attack results when this occurs in a blood vessel that supplies the heart muscle.

Complete blockage — Blood clot

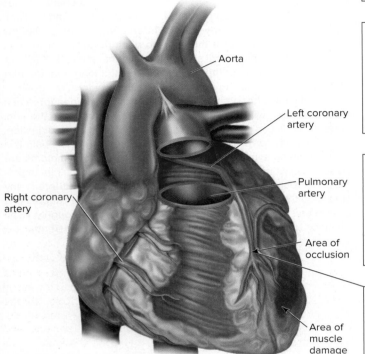

Aorta, Left coronary artery, Pulmonary artery, Right coronary artery, Area of occlusion, Area of muscle damage

FIGURE 5-16 ▲ How atherosclerosis leads to heart attack.

Atherosclerosis probably first develops to repair damage in a vessel lining. A healthy blood vessel is smooth and flexible so that blood can easily move through it. What happens to cause damage to a blood vessel? Likely culprits include smoking, diabetes, high blood pressure, high blood cholesterol, infection—basically any process that causes inflammation in the body. (A laboratory test for C-reactive protein in the blood is used to detect inflammation.) Atherosclerosis can be seen in arteries throughout the body. The damage develops especially at points where an artery branches into two smaller vessels. A great deal of stress is placed on the vessel walls at these points due to changes in blood flow.

Once blood vessel damage has occurred, plaque continues to build up at the site of initial damage. The rate of plaque buildup is directly related to the amount of LDL in the blood. Specifically, oxidized LDL appears to be responsible for plaque formation. Oxidized LDL has undergone changes that make it more likely to be taken up by scavenger cells in the arterial wall. The body also sends white blood cells called macrophages to the location of the cholesterol accumulation on the blood vessel wall. In an attempt to destroy it, the macrophage surrounds the fatty deposit and

produces lipid-loaded **foam cells.** Over years, the blood vessels stiffen, so they cannot dilate or constrict to accommodate normal changes in blood pressure throughout the day. In addition, the buildup of plaque can restrict or block blood flow. Some plaques can become unstable and tear away from the artery. If they rupture, a blood clot will form inside the artery, and within minutes, blood flow is cut off, resulting in a heart attack or stroke.

Blood clotting is a normal and necessary process that prevents blood loss in case of injury. Some people, however, develop disorders in which their blood forms clots too frequently. In areas of the blood vessels that are already partially blocked by plaque, a blood clot can cut off blood flow, leading to tissue damage or death. More than 95% of heart attacks are caused by total blockage of the coronary arteries due to a blood clot forming in an area of the artery already partially blocked by plaque.

foam cells Lipid-loaded white blood cells that have surrounded large amounts of a fatty substance, usually cholesterol, on the blood vessel walls.

Typical warning signs of a heart attack:

- Intense, prolonged chest pain or pressure, sometimes radiating to other parts of the upper body (men and women)
- Shortness of breath (men and women)
- Sweating (men and women)
- Nausea and vomiting (especially women)
- Dizziness (especially women)
- Weakness (men and women)
- Jaw, neck, and shoulder pain (especially women)
- Irregular heartbeat (men and women)

Factors that typically bring on a heart attack in a person already at risk include dehydration; acute emotional stress (such as firing an employee); strenuous physical activity when not otherwise physically fit (shoveling snow, for example); waking during the night or getting up in the morning (linked to an abrupt increase in stress); and consuming large, high-fat meals (increases blood clotting).

Risk Factors for Cardiovascular Disease

For a person at low risk of cardiovascular disease, the advice of health experts is to consume a balanced diet, perform regular physical activity, have a complete fasting lipoprotein analysis performed at age 20 or beyond, and reevaluate risk factors every 5 years.

How do you know if you are at risk? Risk factors include:

- ***Total blood cholesterol over 200 milligrams per 1 deciliter of blood*** (200 mg/dl; 1 deciliter equals 100 milliliters). Risk is especially high when total cholesterol is at or over 240 mg/dl and LDL-cholesterol readings are over 130 to 160 mg/dl. (The terms *LDL cholesterol* and *HDL cholesterol* are used when expressing the blood concentration because it is the cholesterol content of these lipoproteins that is measured.)
- ***Smoking.*** Smoking is the main cause of about 20% of cardiovascular disease deaths. Smoking greatly increases the expression of a person's genetically linked risk for cardiovascular disease, even if one's blood lipids are low. Smoking also makes blood more likely to clot. Even secondhand smoke has been implicated as a risk factor. Among women, the combination of smoking and oral contraceptive use particularly increases risk.
- ***Hypertension.*** **Systolic blood pressure** over 139 (millimeters of mercury) and **diastolic blood pressure** over 89 indicate hypertension. Healthy blood pressure values are less than 120 and 80, respectively. (Treatment of hypertension is reviewed in Section 9.9.)
- ***Diabetes.*** Diabetes virtually guarantees development of cardiovascular disease. Insulin increases cholesterol synthesis in the liver, in turn increasing LDL in the bloodstream. This disease negates any female advantage.[12]
- ***HDL cholesterol*** under 40 mg/dl, especially when the ratio of total cholesterol to HDL cholesterol is greater than 4:1 (3.5:1 or less is optimal). A value of 60 mg/dl or more is especially protective. Before menopause, women often have high HDL, which affords them some protection against cardiovascular disease. However, smoking and diabetes negate any protective effect, and after menopause, their risk for cardiovascular disease is similar to that for men.

Healthy People 2020 has set a goal of reducing death from coronary heart disease by 20%, compared with today's incidence.

- ***Age.*** Men over 45 years and women over 55 years are at heightened risk.
- ***Family history*** of cardiovascular disease, especially before age 50 increases risk. Some cases of cardiovascular disease are due to genetic defects that are unrelated to lifestyle.
- ***Blood triglycerides*** 200 mg/dl or greater in the fasting state increase risk. Triglyceride levels less than 100 mg/dl are optimal.
- ***Obesity*** (especially fat accumulation in the waist) increases risk in a variety of ways. Typical weight gain seen in adults is a chief contributor to the increase in LDL seen with aging. Obesity is related to insulin resistance, creating a diabetes-like state and ultimately the disease itself. It also increases overall inflammation throughout the body.
- ***Inactivity.*** Exercise conditions the arteries to adapt to physical stress. Regular exercise also improves insulin action in the body. The corresponding reduction in insulin output leads to a reduction in lipoprotein synthesis in the liver.

The term *risk factor* is not equivalent to "cause of disease"; nevertheless, the more of these risk factors one has, the greater the chances of ultimately developing cardiovascular disease. A good example is the **metabolic syndrome,** discussed in Section 4.7. A person with the metabolic syndrome would have abdominal obesity, high blood triglycerides, low HDL cholesterol, hypertension, poor blood glucose regulation (i.e., high fasting blood glucose), and increased blood clotting. This profile raises the risk for cardiovascular disease considerably. On a positive note, cardiovascular disease is rare in populations that have low LDL cholesterol, normal blood pressure, and do not smoke or have diabetes. By minimizing these risk factors, as well as following the dietary recommendations of the American Heart Association in Section 5.7 and staying physically active, one will most likely reduce many of the other controllable risk factors listed. In other words, develop and follow a total lifestyle plan. Medications may also be added to lower blood lipids, as discussed later in this section.

Lifestyle Modifications to Prevent Cardiovascular Disease

In Section 5.7, you read about recommendations to modify fat intake to promote heart health. For the general population, the *Dietary Guidelines* and the American Heart Association recommend limiting saturated fat intake to 10% of total kilocalories and avoiding *trans* fats. For people at risk of cardiovascular disease, the American Heart Association recommends restricting saturated

systolic blood pressure The pressure in the arterial blood vessels associated with the pumping of blood from the heart.

diastolic blood pressure The pressure in the arterial blood vessels when the heart is between beats.

metabolic syndrome A condition in which a person has poor blood glucose regulation, hypertension, increased blood triglycerides, and other health problems. This condition is usually accompanied by obesity, lack of physical activity, and a diet high in refined carbohydrates. Also called Syndrome X.

fat intake even further to 5% to 6% of total kilocalories. These recommendations are based on scientific evidence that links saturated and *trans* fat intake to higher levels of LDL, which promote plaque formation in blood vessels.[13]

Even while cutting back on saturated and *trans* fat, overall fat intake should generally fall within the range of 20% to 35% of total kilocalories. This means you shouldn't simply cut fat out of your diet. Rather, you should choose unsaturated sources of fat, such as fatty fish, plant oils, nuts, and seeds, instead of foods rich in saturated fats. The omega-3 fatty acids in fish are particularly helpful for promoting heart health.

Remember that eating for heart health involves more than just fat! Over the past few decades, evidence has accumulated that excessive intakes of added sugars have contributed to the high rate of cardiovascular disease. This is why it's important to replace saturated fat with unsaturated fat, rather than with simple carbohydrates. Excessive intakes of refined carbohydrates and added sugars promote high levels of insulin, inflammation, and increased blood cholesterol. As you just read, uncontrolled blood sugar among people with diabetes is a significant risk factor for cardiovascular disease. Review recommendations for healthy carbohydrate choices in Section 4.3.

You also read about the dangers of **oxidized** LDL—the form of LDL that contributes to plaque formation. Nutrients and phytochemicals that have **antioxidant** properties may reduce LDL oxidation. Fruits and vegetables are particularly rich in these compounds. Eating fruits and vegetables regularly is one positive step

we can make to reduce plaque buildup and slow the progression of cardiovascular disease. Some fruits and vegetables particularly helpful in this regard include legumes (beans), nuts, dried plums (prunes), raisins, berries, plums, apples, cherries, oranges, grapes, spinach, broccoli, red bell peppers, and onions. Tea, coffee, and dark chocolate are also sources of antioxidants. Please note that *foods* are the best choices for antioxidants. The American Heart Association does not support use of antioxidant supplements (such as vitamin E) to reduce cardiovascular disease risk. This is because large-scale studies have shown no decrease in cardiovascular disease risk with use of antioxidant supplements.

Some plants contain natural cholesterol-lowering compounds called plant stanols or plant sterols. Some rich food sources of plant sterols include wheat germ, sesame seeds, pistachios, and sunflower seeds. These compounds have been clinically shown to reduce LDL (bad) cholesterol, and products that contain these natural cholesterol reducers are backed by the following FDA-approved health claim: *Foods containing at least 0.4 gram per serving of plant sterols, eaten twice a day with meals for a daily*

oxidize In the most basic sense, the loss of an electron or gain of an oxygen by a chemical substance. This change typically alters the shape and/or function of the substance.

antioxidant A substance that has the ability to prevent or repair the damage caused by oxidation.

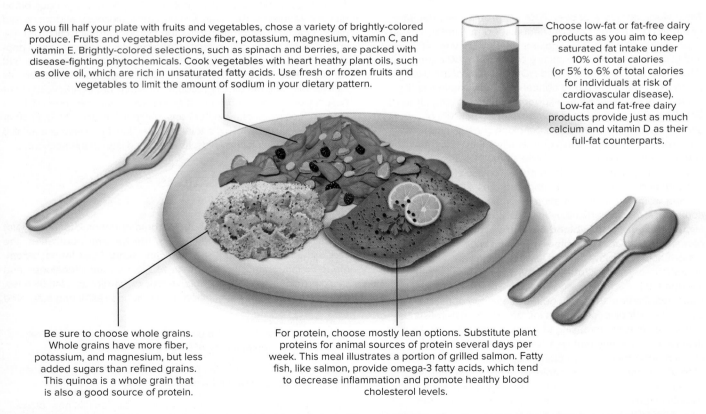

As you fill half your plate with fruits and vegetables, chose a variety of brightly-colored produce. Fruits and vegetables provide fiber, potassium, magnesium, vitamin C, and vitamin E. Brightly-colored selections, such as spinach and berries, are packed with disease-fighting phytochemicals. Cook vegetables with heart heathy plant oils, such as olive oil, which are rich in unsaturated fatty acids. Use fresh or frozen fruits and vegetables to limit the amount of sodium in your dietary pattern.

Choose low-fat or fat-free dairy products as you aim to keep saturated fat intake under 10% of total calories (or 5% to 6% of total calories for individuals at risk of cardiovascular disease). Low-fat and fat-free dairy products provide just as much calcium and vitamin D as their full-fat counterparts.

Be sure to choose whole grains. Whole grains have more fiber, potassium, and magnesium, but less added sugars than refined grains. This quinoa is a whole grain that is also a good source of protein.

For protein, choose mostly lean options. Substitute plant proteins for animal sources of protein several days per week. This meal illustrates a portion of grilled salmon. Fatty fish, like salmon, provide omega-3 fatty acids, which tend to decrease inflammation and promote healthy blood cholesterol levels.

FIGURE 5-17 ▲ Use MyPlate with the American Heart Association's *Diet and Lifestyle Recommendations* to build a heart healthy meal. Complement your plan for heart-healthy eating with an active lifestyle.

total intake of at least 0.8 gram, as part of a diet low in saturated fat and cholesterol, may reduce the risk of heart disease. Coro-Wise® is a leading brand of plant sterols. Products such as Smart Balance® margarines and Minute Maid Heart Wise® orange juice contain these plant sterols. The plant sterols work by reducing cholesterol absorption in the small intestine and lowering its return to the liver. The liver responds by taking up more cholesterol from the blood so it can continue to make bile acids. Studies show that 2 to 5 grams of plant sterols per day can reduce total blood cholesterol by 8% to 10% and LDL cholesterol by 9% to 14% (similar to what is seen with some cholesterol-lowering drugs).[14]

Besides dietary changes, exercise is an important way to modify risk for cardiovascular disease. Exercising for at least 45 minutes four times a week can increase HDL by about 5 mg/dl. Both regular aerobic exercise and resistance exercise are recommended. A person with existing cardiovascular disease should seek physician approval before starting such a program, as should older adults.[15] The diet and lifestyle recommendations described above are summarized in Figure 5-17.

> Two approaches have been shown to cause reversal of atherosclerosis in the body. One employs a vegan diet and other lifestyle changes that are part of the Dr. Dean Ornish program. The other employs aggressive LDL-lowering with medications.

Medications to Lower Blood Lipids

For some people, diet and lifestyle changes are simply not enough to lower blood cholesterol. Fortunately, medications offer a more aggressive approach to treating high cholesterol.

> *Healthy People 2020* has set a goal of reducing total blood cholesterol among adults from the average of 198 mg/dl to 178 mg/dl, as well as reducing the percentage of adults with high blood cholesterol from 15% to 13.5%.

Cholesterol-lowering medications may be appropriate for individuals who are at heightened risk for cardiovascular disease. Some factors to take into consideration include clinical evidence of atherosclerosis (see Fig. 5-16), very high LDL levels, or pre-existing diabetes or hypertension.

Medications work to lower blood cholesterol in several ways. Examples are listed in the Medicine Cabinet feature in this section. Keep in mind that medications may lead to adverse effects, especially on liver function, so physician monitoring is required. In addition, the cost of treatment with one of these drugs can vary widely, from as little as $12 per month to more than $500.[14]

Surgical Treatment for Cardiovascular Disease

The two most common surgical treatments for coronary artery blockage are percutaneous transluminal coronary angioplasty

Medicine Cabinet

Aspirin. Most common medication recommended to prevent heart attacks in people with coronary artery disease by helping to maintain blood flow to the heart

Statins. Most frequently prescribed cholesterol-lowering drugs that block a liver enzyme involved in cholesterol synthesis and thus reduce the amount of cholesterol in the blood. Examples: simvastatin (Zocor),® atorvastatin (Lipitor),® androsuvastatin (Crestor)®

Selective Cholesterol Absorption Inhibitors. Just as the name would suggest, these drugs keep cholesterol from being absorbed from the small intestine. Cholesterol will still be produced by the liver, but the contribution from dietary cholesterol is minimized. Example: ezetimibe (Zetia)®

Resins. These medications bind to bile acids in the intestine and are excreted in the feces, reducing their supply. This stimulates the liver to produce more bile acids, which uses more cholesterol and causes a decrease in blood cholesterol levels. Examples: cholestyramine (Questran)® and colesevelam (Welchol)®

Fibrates. These drugs lower blood triglycerides by decreasing the production of triglycerides by the liver. Example: gemfibrozil (Lopid)®

Niacin. A megadose of nicotinic acid, a form of the B-vitamin niacin, can help to increase HDL and lower triglyceride levels. Example: Niaspan®

Combination Drugs. Some pharmaceutical companies combine medications with different mechanisms of action. A statin drug (simvastatin) has been combined with another drug (ezetimibe) and is marketed as Vytorin.® While the statin reduces the cholesterol made by the liver, the ezetimibe helps to block the absorption of cholesterol from food.[15]

©Peter Dazeley/Photographer's Choice/Getty Images

(PTCA) and coronary artery bypass graft (CABG). PTCA involves the insertion of a balloon catheter into an artery. Once it is advanced to the area of the blockage, the balloon is expanded to crush the buildup of plaque. Afterward, the blood vessel may be held open with metal mesh, called a stent. CABG involves the relocation of a large vein—from the leg, for example—to bypass the blocked blood vessel.

> For more information on cardiovascular disease, see the website of the American Heart Association at www.heart.org or the heart disease section of Healthfinder at healthfinder.gov. This is a site created by the U.S. government for consumers. In addition, visit the website www.nhlbi.nih.gov.

Summary (Numbers refer to numbered sections in the chapter.)

5.1 Lipids are a group of compounds that do not dissolve in water. Fatty acids are the simplest form of lipids. There are three fatty acids on every triglyceride, the most common type of lipid found in the body and foods. Phospholipids and sterols are two other classes of lipids in food and our bodies.

5.2 Saturated fatty acids contain no carbon-carbon double bonds, monounsaturated fatty acids contain one carbon-carbon double bond, and polyunsaturated fatty acids contain two or more carbon-carbon double bonds in the carbon chain. In omega-3 polyunsaturated fatty acids, the first of the carbon-carbon double bonds is located three carbons from the methyl end of the carbon chain. In omega-6 polyunsaturated fatty acids, the first carbon-carbon double bond counting from the methyl end occurs at the sixth carbon. The essential fatty acids are linoleic acid (an omega-6 fatty acid) and alpha-linolenic acid (an omega-3 fatty acid). These must be included in the diet to maintain health. The hormonelike compounds produced from omega-3 fatty acids tend to reduce blood clotting, blood pressure, and inflammatory responses in the body. Those produced from omega-6 fatty acids tend to increase blood clotting.

Triglycerides are formed from a glycerol backbone with three fatty acids. Triglycerides rich in long-chain saturated fatty acids tend to be solid at room temperature, whereas those rich in monounsaturated and polyunsaturated fatty acids are liquid at room temperature. Triglycerides are the major form of fat in both food and the body. They allow for efficient energy storage, protect certain organs, transport fat-soluble vitamins, and help insulate the body.

5.3 Foods rich in fat include salad oils, butter, margarine, and mayonnaise. Nuts, bologna, avocados, and bacon are also high in fat, as are peanut butter and cheddar cheese. Steak and hamburger are moderate in fat content, as is whole milk. Many grain products and fruits and vegetables in general are low in fat.

Fats and oils have several functions as components of foods. Fats add flavor and texture to foods and provide some satiety after meals. Some phospholipids are used in foods as emulsifiers, which suspend fat in water.

When fatty acids break down, food becomes rancid, resulting in a foul odor and unpleasant flavor. Hydrogenation is the process of converting carbon-carbon double bonds into single bonds by adding hydrogen at the point of unsaturation. The partial hydrogenation of fatty acids in vegetable oils changes the oils to semisolid fats and helps in food formulation and reduces rancidity. Hydrogenation also increases *trans* fatty acid content. High amounts of *trans* fat in the diet are discouraged, as these increase LDL and reduce HDL.

5.4 Fat digestion takes place primarily in the small intestine. Lipase enzyme released from the pancreas digests long-chain triglycerides into monoglycerides (glycerol backbones with single fatty acids attached) and fatty acids. The breakdown products are then taken up by the absorptive cells of the small intestine. These products are mostly remade into triglycerides inside intestinal cells and eventually enter the lymphatic system before they pass into the bloodstream.

5.5 Lipids are carried in the bloodstream by various lipoproteins, which consist of a lipid core encased in a shell of protein, cholesterol, and phospholipids. Chylomicrons are released from intestinal cells and carry lipids arising from dietary intake. Very-low-density lipoprotein (VLDL) and low-density lipoprotein (LDL) carry lipids both taken up by and synthesized in the liver. High-density lipoprotein (HDL) picks up cholesterol from cells and facilitates its transport back to the liver.

5.6 Triglycerides are used for energy storage, insulation, and transportation of fat-soluble vitamins. Phospholipids are derivatives of triglycerides in which one or two of the fatty acids are replaced by phosphorus-containing compounds. Phospholipids are important parts of cell membranes, and some act as emulsifiers.

Cholesterol forms vital biological compounds, such as hormones, cell membranes, and bile acids. Cells in the body make cholesterol whether we eat it or not. It is not a necessary part of an adult's diet.

5.7 There is currently no RDA for fat for adults. Plant oils should contribute at least 5% of total calories to achieve the Adequate Intakes proposed for essential fatty acids (linoleic acid and alpha-linolenic acid). Fatty fish are a rich source of omega-3 fatty acids and should be consumed at least twice per week.

Many health agencies and scientific groups suggest a fat intake of no more than 30% to 35% of total calories. Some health experts advocate an even further reduction to 20% of calorie intake for some people to maintain a normal LDL value, but such a diet requires professional guidance. If fat intake exceeds 30% of total calories, the diet should emphasize monounsaturated fat. The typical North American diet contains about 33% of total calories as fat.

5.8 In the blood, elevated amounts of LDL and low amounts of HDL are strong predictors of risk for cardiovascular disease. Additional risk factors for the disease are smoking, hypertension, diabetes, obesity, and inactivity. Lifestyle modifications to improve heart health include limiting saturated fat; choosing fish and plant oils instead of food sources of saturated fats; limiting added sugar intake; consuming plenty of fruits, vegetables and whole grains to obtain antioxidants; incorporating plant sterols; and exercising regularly.

Check Your Knowledge (Answers are available at the end of this question set.)

1. Margarine usually is made by a process called _____, in which hydrogen atoms are added to carbon-carbon double bonds in the polyunsaturated fatty acids found in vegetable oils.
   a. saturation
   b. esterification
   c. isomerization
   d. hydrogenation

2. Fatty acids that cause a decrease in blood clotting are
   a. omega-3 fatty acids.
   b. omega-6 fatty acids.
   c. omega-9 fatty acids.
   d. prostacyclins.

3. Cholesterol is
   a. an essential nutrient.
   b. found in foods of plant origin.
   c. an important part of human cell membranes.
   d. all of the above.

4. Which of the following groups of foods are rich sources of saturated fatty acids?
   a. Olive oil, peanut oil, canola oil
   b. Palm oil, palm kernel oil, coconut oil
   c. Safflower oil, corn oil, soybean oil
   d. All of the above

5. Lipoproteins are important for
   a. transport of fats in the blood and lymphatic system.
   b. synthesis of triglycerides.
   c. synthesis of adipose tissue.
   d. enzyme production.

6. Which of the following foods is the best source of omega-3 fatty acids?
   a. Fatty fish
   b. Peanut butter
   c. Lard and shortenings
   d. Beef and other red meats

7. Immediately after a meal, newly digested and absorbed dietary fats appear in the lymph and then the blood as part of which of the following?
   a. LDL
   b. HDL
   c. Chylomicrons
   d. Cholesterol

8. High blood concentrations of _____ decrease the risk for cardiovascular disease.
   a. low-density lipoproteins
   b. chylomicrons
   c. high-density lipoproteins
   d. cholesterol

9. Phospholipids such as lecithin are used extensively in food preparation because they
   a. provide the agreeable feel of fat melting on the tongue.
   b. are excellent emulsifiers.
   c. carry fat-soluble vitamins.
   d. impart delicate flavors.

10. The main form of lipid found in the food we eat is
    a. cholesterol.
    b. phospholipids.
    c. triglycerides.
    d. plant sterols.

Answer Key: 1. d (LO 5.4), 2. a (LO 5.3), 3. c (LO 5.7), 4. b (LO 5.4), 5. a (LO 5.6), 6. a (LO 5.4), 7. c (LO 5.6), 8. c (LO 5.6), 9. b (LO 5.7), 10. c (LO 5.2)

What the Dietitian Chose

With heart health in mind, you will want to choose the ground meat with the lowest fat, saturated fat, and cholesterol. Check the Nutrition Facts panel, if available, to compare the lipid content of various products. Look for cuts of meat with "round " or "loin" in the name for lowest fat content.

USDA allows up to 30% fat (by weight) in raw ground beef, so the cut of beef makes a difference. Regular ground beef typically contains the most fat (about 20% to 30% fat). Next comes ground chuck (about 15% fat), followed by ground round (about 10% fat), and ground sirloin (about 3% fat). Table 5-8 shows a further breakdown of the fat content of varieties of ground beef. Based on this information, you can see that the ground sirloin will give you the leanest burgers.

The ground sirloin, however, will also be the most expensive variety of ground beef. You may, therefore, want to take

TABLE 5-8 ■ Calorie, Fat, and Cholesterol Content of Types of Ground Beef

	Energy (kcal)	Total Fat (g)	Saturated Fat (g)	Cholesterol (mg)
Regular ground beef, 3.5 ounces cooked	273	18	7	82
Ground chuck, 3.5 ounces cooked	232	14	5	86
Ground round, 3.5 ounces cooked	204	11	4	82
Ground sirloin, 3.5 ounces cooked	164	6	3	76

(continued)

advantage of the fact that ground beef loses a lot of fat during cooking—as much as 50% for the highest fat products. Typically, regular ground beef is the least expensive product. As the percent lean increases, so does price.

For foods in which the ground beef will be shaped, then cooked (e.g., hamburger patties, meatballs, or meatloaf), bake, grill, or broil the ground meat on a rack so that fat will drain from the product as it cooks, then let the cooked product rest on paper towels for 1 minute after cooking. For recipes that incorporate browned ground beef into a mixed dish (e.g., casseroles or spaghetti sauce), brown ground beef, crumbling as you cook, then blot with paper towels or rinse under warm water to achieve a final cooked product with nearly the same fat content as the ground round. Using the rinsing method, 100 grams (about 3.5 ounces) of ground beef yields a final product with just 4 grams of fat. Because a greater percentage of the starting product is lost during cooking, you will end up with less meat in the final product. However, this is not such a big deal because most Americans consume two to three times as much protein as they need. To further enhance the heart healthiness of mixed dishes,

replace some of that lost product with beans. Chili or tacos would be excellent recipes to try with this method.

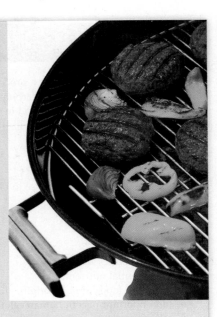

▶ Whereas the more expensive ground round and ground sirloin will give you lowest-fat burgers to start, the less expensive regular ground beef or ground chuck burgers will lose fat while cooking. You will therefore want to consider both fat content and cost when making your choice. ©Comstock/PunchStock

Study Questions (Numbers refer to Learning Outcomes)

1. Name a common property of all lipids. **(LO 5.1)**

2. Describe the chemical structures of saturated and polyunsaturated fatty acids and their different effects in both food and the human body. **(LO 5.2)**

3. Relate the need for omega-3 fatty acids in the diet to the recommendation to consume fatty fish at least twice a week. **(LO 5.8)**

4. Describe the structures, origins, and roles of the four major blood lipoproteins. **(LO 5.6)**

5. What are the recommendations from various health care organizations regarding fat intake? What does this mean in terms of food choices? **(LO 5.8)**

6. What are two important attributes of fat in food? How are these different from the general functions of lipids in the human body? **(LO 5.7)**

7. Describe the significance of and possible uses for reduced-fat foods. **(LO 5.4)**

8. Does the total cholesterol concentration in the bloodstream tell the whole story with respect to cardiovascular disease risk? **(LO 5.9)**

9. List the main risk factors for the development of cardiovascular disease. **(LO 5.9)**

10. Describe three lifestyle changes to decrease the risk of cardiovascular disease development. **(LO 5.9)**

Further Readings

1. Kris-Etherton PM and Fleming JA: Emerging nutrition science on fatty acids and cardiovascular disease: Nutritionists' perspectives. *Adv Nutr* 2015; 6:326S.

2. Food and Drug Administration: Talking about *trans* fat: What you need to know. *Food Facts.* June 2015. http://www.fda.gov/downloads/Food/IngredientsPackagingLabeling/UCM239579.pdf. (Accessed February 7, 2017).

3. Eckel RH and others: 2013 AHA/ACC guideline on lifestyle management to reduce cardiovascular risk: A report of the American College of Cardiology/American Heart Association Task Force on Practice Guidelines. *Circulation* 2013; 129:S76.

4. Sacks FM and others: Dietary fats and cardiovascular disease: A presidential advisory from the American Heart Association. *Circulation* 2017; 135, e1.

5. Estruch R and others: Primary prevention of cardiovascular disease with a Mediterranean diet. *N Engl J Med* 2013; 368:1279–1290.

6. Shen J and others: Mediterranean dietary patterns and cardiovascular health. *Annu Rev Nutr* 2015; 35:425.

7. Dennett C: Key ingredients of the Mediterranean Diet—the nutritious sum of delicious parts. *Today's Dietitian* 2016; 18(5):28.

8. Palmer S: Low-fat vegan diets. *Today's Dietitian* 2016; 18(10):20.

9. Vannice G and others: Position of the Academy of Nutrition and Dietetics: Dietary fatty acids for healthy adults. *J Acad Nutr Diet* 2014; 114:136.

10. Centers for Disease Control and Prevention: Heart disease fact sheet. 2015. https://www.cdc.gov/dhdsp/data_statistics/fact_sheets/docs/fs_heart_disease.pdf. (Accessed February 7, 2017).

11. Schaeffer J: Prevent heart disease: How to dispel the five common heart-health myths with clients and set the record straight. *Today's Dietitian* 2013; 15(2):20.

12. Fox CS and others: Update on prevention of cardiovascular disease in adults with type 2 diabetes mellitus in light of recent evidence: A scientific statement from the American Heart Association and the American Diabetes Association. *Diabetes Care* 2015; 38:1777.

13. McCulloch M: Saturated fat: Not so bad or just bad science? *Today's Dietitian* 2014; 16(11):32.

14. National Center for Health Research: *A guide to cholesterol medication.* 2016. http://center4research.org/medical-care-for-adults/your-medicine-cabinet/a-guide-to-cholesterol-medication/. (Accessed February 7, 2017).

15. Riccardi G and others: How well can we control dyslipidemias through lifestyle modifications? *Curr Cardiol Rep* 2016; 18:66.

connect To get the most out of your study, visit Connect where you will find NutritionCalc Plus, SmartBook®, and many other dynamic tools.

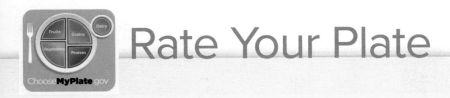

Rate Your Plate

I. Choosing Foods for Heart Health

Instructions: The foods listed in column A tend to be high in saturated fat, *trans* fatty acids, cholesterol, and total fat. Fill in column B with alternative foods that are generally low in these dietary components. After filling in your ideas, see our suggestions for column B for foods that will reduce your risk of cardiovascular disease.

Column A		Column B
Bacon and eggs	or	
Doughnut or sweet roll	or	
Breakfast sausage	or	
Whole milk	or	
Cheeseburger	or	
French fries	or	
Ground chuck	or	
Soup with cream base	or	
Macaroni and cheese	or	
Cream/fruit pie	or	
Cream-filled cookies	or	
Ice cream	or	
Butter or stick margarine	or	

Ready-to-eat whole grain breakfast cereal
Whole wheat roll, bagel, or bread
Fruit
Reduced-fat, low-fat, or fat-free milk
Turkey sandwich, no cheese
Plain baked potato with salsa
Ground round
Soup with broth base
Macaroni with marinara sauce
Graham crackers
Granola bar
Frozen yogurt, sherbet, or reduced-fat ice cream
Vegetable oils or soft margarine in a tub

II. Applying the Nutrition Facts Label to Your Daily Food Choices

Imagine that you are at the supermarket looking for a quick snack to help you keep your energy up during afternoons. In the snack section, you settle on two choices [see labels (a) and (b)]. Evaluate the products using the accompanying table.

Compare the nutrients in each product by completing this list. For each serving, which product is lower in each of the following?

Calories	(a)	(b)	no difference
Calories from Fat	(a)	(b)	no difference
Total Fat	(a)	(b)	no difference
Saturated Fat	(a)	(b)	no difference
Trans Fat	(a)	(b)	no difference
Cholesterol	(a)	(b)	no difference
Sodium	(a)	(b)	no difference
Total Carbohydrates	(a)	(b)	no difference
Dietary Fiber	(a)	(b)	no difference
Sugars	(a)	(b)	no difference
Protein	(a)	(b)	no difference
Iron	(a)	(b)	no difference

Which package has more servings per container?

	(a)	(b)	no difference

(a)

Nutrition Facts

6 servings per container

Serving size   **2 bars (42g)**

Amount per serving

Calories   180

% Daily Value*

Total Fat 6g	**9%**
Saturated Fat 0.5g	**3%**
Trans Fat 0g	
Cholesterol 0mg	**0%**
Sodium 160mg	**7%**
Total Carbohydrate 29g	**10%**
Dietary Fiber 2g	**8%**
Total Sugars 11g	
Includes 8g Added Sugars	**16%**
Protein 4g	
Iron 1mg	6%
Potassium 100mg	3%

Not a significant source of vitamin D and calcium.

*The % Daily Value (DV) tells you how much a nutrient in a serving of food contributes to a daily diet. 2,000 calories a day is used for general nutrition advice.

INGREDIENTS: WHOLE GRAIN ROLLED OATS, SUGAR, CANOLA OIL, CRISP RICE WITH SOY PROTEIN (RICE FLOUR, SOY PROTEIN CONCENTRATE, SUGAR, MALT, SALT), HONEY, BROWN SUGAR SYRUP, HIGH FRUCTOSE CORN SYRUP, SALT, SOY LECITHIN, BAKING SODA, NATURAL FLAVOR, PEANUT FLOUR, ALMOND FLOUR, HAZELNUT FLOUR, WALNUT FLOUR, PECAN FLOUR.

(b)

Nutrition Facts

12 servings per container

Serving size   **2 cookies (38g)**

Amount per serving

Calories   180

% Daily Value*

Total Fat 7g	**11%**
Saturated Fat 2g	**10%**
Trans Fat 2g	
Cholesterol 0mg	**0%**
Sodium 100mg	**4%**
Total Carbohydrate 26g	**9%**
Dietary Fiber 1g	**4%**
Total Sugars 12g	**4%**
Includes 10g Added Sugars	**20%**
Protein 2g	
Iron 0.4mg	2%
Potassium 75mg	2%

Not a significant source of vitamin D and calcium.

*The % Daily Value (DV) tells you how much a nutrient in a serving of food contributes to a daily diet. 2,000 calories a day is used for general nutrition advice.

INGREDIENTS: ENRICHED FLOUR (WHEAT FLOUR, NIACIN, REDUCED IRON, THIAMINE MONONITRATE, RIBOFLAVIN, FOLIC ACID), SUGAR, VEGETABLE OIL SHORTENING (PARTIALLY HYDROGENATED SOYBEAN, COCONUT, COTTONSEED, CORN AND/OR SAFFLOWER AND/OR CANOLA OIL), CORN SYRUP, HIGH FRUCTOSE CORN SYRUP, WHEY (A MILK INGREDIENT), CORN STARCH, SALT, SKIM MILK, LEAVENING (BAKING SODA, AMMONIUM BICARBONATE), ARTIFICIAL FLAVOR, SOYBEAN LECITHIN, COLOR (CONTAINING FD&C YELLOW #5 LAKE).

1. Which of the two brands would you choose?

    _____

    _____

2. What information on the Nutrition Facts labels contributed to your decision?

    _____

    _____

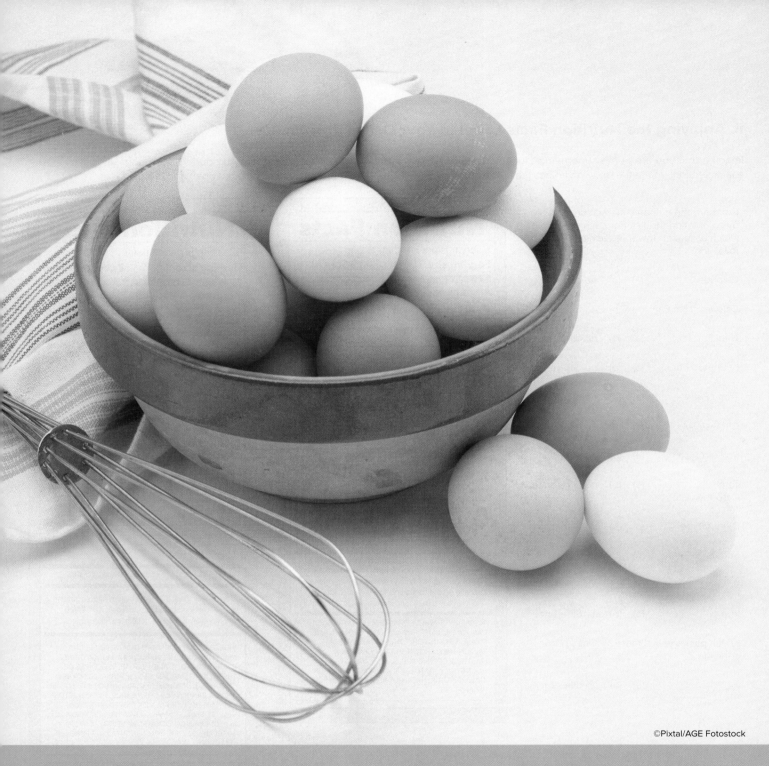

©Pixtal/AGE Fotostock

Student Learning Outcomes

Chapter 6 is designed to allow you to:

6.1 Distinguish between essential and nonessential amino acids, and explain why adequate amounts of each of the essential amino acids are required for protein synthesis.

6.2 Describe how amino acids form proteins.

6.3 Identify food sources of protein, distinguish between high-quality and low-quality proteins, and describe the concept of complementary proteins.

6.4 Describe how protein is digested, absorbed, and metabolized in the body.

6.5 List the primary functions of protein in the body.

Chapter 6
Proteins

What Would You Choose?

About 6 weeks ago at the start of the semester, you began a workout program including lifting weights at the student recreation center. You are disappointed that you have not seen the results you were anticipating. You can lift more now than you could when you started, but you were hoping to firm and define the muscles in your arms, back, and abs. You are wondering if you need more protein. You have seen numerous advertisements for protein and amino acid supplements, but they are expensive. What would you choose as the optimal dietary protein pattern to support your weight-training regimen?

- **a** Take individual amino acid supplements.

- **b** Consume protein in small meals, including taking whey protein supplements throughout the day.

- **c** Eat most of your protein (about 60%) as animal protein during your evening meal.

- **d** Consume a diet that provides 35% of calories as protein distributed at three meals with at least 30 grams of protein from a variety of sources at each meal.

Think about your choice as you read this chapter, then see What the Dietitian Chose at the end of the chapter.

Consuming enough protein is vital for maintaining health. Proteins form important structures in the body, make up a key part of the blood, help regulate many body functions, and can fuel body cells.

Although North Americans generally eat more protein than is needed to maintain health the timing of our protein consumption during the day may not be optimal for health. Our daily protein intake comes primarily at the evening meal and mostly from animal sources, such as meat, poultry, fish, eggs, milk, and cheese. In contrast, in the developing world, eating patterns can be deficient in protein.

Eating patterns that are mostly vegetarian still predominate in much of Asia and areas of Africa, and many North Americans practice some form of vegetarianism. In fact, North Americans are encouraged to consume a greater portion of their food, including protein, from plant sources. Over the years, plant sources of protein such as nuts, seeds, and legumes have been sidelined by meats. Sources of plant proteins, however, offer a wealth of nutritional benefits—from lowering blood cholesterol to preventing certain forms of cancer.

We can benefit from eating more plant sources of proteins, but it takes some knowledge to get the right quantity and quality of protein at each meal to meet protein needs. This chapter takes a close look at protein, including the distribution of our protein intake throughout the day and the benefits of plant proteins in our eating patterns. It will also examine the benefits and potential risks of vegetarian eating patterns. Let's see why a detailed study of protein is worth your attention.

6.6 Apply current recommendations for protein intake to determine protein needs for healthy adults, and describe what is meant by positive protein balance, negative protein balance, and protein equilibrium.

6.7 Describe how protein-calorie malnutrition eventually can lead to disease in the body.

6.8 Develop healthy plant-based eating patterns that meet the body's nutritional needs.

6.1 Amino Acids—Building Blocks of Proteins

protein Food and body compounds made of more than 100 amino acids; proteins contain carbon, hydrogen, oxygen, nitrogen, and sometimes other atoms in a specific configuration. Proteins contain the form of nitrogen most easily used by the human body.

amino acid The building block for proteins containing a central carbon atom with nitrogen and other atoms attached.

Thousands of substances in the body are made of **protein.** Aside from water, proteins form the major part of lean body tissue, totaling about 17% of body weight. **Amino acids** are compounds that serve as the building blocks for proteins. They are chemically unique in that they contain nitrogen along with carbon, oxygen, and hydrogen. Plants combine nitrogen from the soil with carbon and other elements to form amino acids. They then link these amino acids together to make proteins. Proteins are thus an essential part of a healthy eating pattern because they supply nitrogen in a form we can readily use, namely, amino acids. Using simpler forms of nitrogen is, for the most part, impossible for humans.

Proteins are crucial to the *regulation* and *maintenance* of the body. Body functions such as blood clotting, fluid balance, hormone and enzyme production, visual processes, transport of many substances in the bloodstream, and cell repair require specific proteins. The body makes proteins in many configurations and sizes so that they can serve these greatly varied functions. Formation of these body proteins begins with amino acids from both the protein-containing foods we eat and those synthesized from other compounds within the body. Proteins can also be broken down to *supply energy* for the body—on average, 4 kcal per gram.

Your body uses 20 different amino acids to function (Table 6-1). Although all of these commonly found amino acids are important, 11 (alanine, arginine, asparagine, aspartic acid, cysteine, glutamic acid, glutamine, glycine, proline, serine, and tyrosine) are considered **nonessential** with respect to our eating patterns. All tissues have some ability to make the nonessential amino acids as long as the right ingredients are present—the key factor being nitrogen that is already part of another amino acid. Therefore, it is not essential that these amino acids be consumed.

Amino acids are formed mostly of carbon, hydrogen, oxygen, and nitrogen. Figure 6-1 shows the structure of a generic amino acid and two examples of specific amino acids. The various amino acids used to make proteins are slight variations of generic amino acid with different chemical makeups (see Appendix D). Each amino acid has an "acid" group, an "amino" group, and a "side" or R group specific to the amino acid.

The R group on some amino acids has a branched shape, like a tree. These so-called **branched-chain amino acids** are leucine, isoleucine, and valine. The branched-chain amino acids are the primary amino acids that promote and signal protein synthesis and turnover in muscles. Whey protein (from milk) is popular among strength-training athletes because it is particularly rich in branched-chain amino acids (see Section 14.4).

TABLE 6-1 ■ **Classification of Amino Acids**

Essential Amino Acids	Nonessential Amino Acids
Histidine	Alanine
Isoleucine*	Arginine
Leucine*	Asparagine
Lysine	Aspartic acid
Methionine	Cysteine
Phenylalanine	Glutamic acid
Threonine	Glutamine
Tryptophan	Glycine
Valine*	Proline
	Serine
	Tyrosine

*A branched-chain amino acid.

nonessential amino acids Amino acids that can be synthesized by a healthy body in sufficient amounts; there are 11 nonessential amino acids. These are also called *dispensable amino acids*.

branched-chain amino acids Amino acids with a branching carbon backbone; these are leucine, isoleucine, and valine. All are essential amino acids.

ESSENTIAL AMINO ACIDS

The nine amino acids (histidine, isoleucine, leucine, lysine, methionine, phenylalanine, threonine, tryptophan, and valine) the body cannot make in sufficient amounts or at

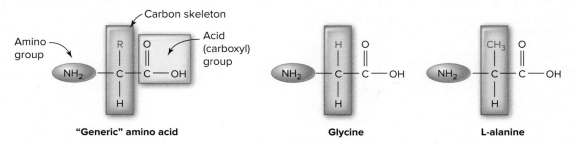

FIGURE 6-1 ▲ Amino acid structure. The side chain (R) differentiates glycine (H) and alanine (CH$_3$).

all are known as **essential.** The essential amino acids must be obtained from foods because body cells cannot make the needed carbon-based foundation of the amino acid, cannot put a nitrogen group on the needed carbon-based foundation, or just cannot do the whole process fast enough to meet body needs. If you do not eat enough essential amino acids, your body first struggles to conserve what essential amino acids it can. However, eventually your body slows production of new proteins until at some point, you will break protein down faster than you can make it. When that happens, health deteriorates.

Animal sources of protein, such as meat and dairy products, and plant sources of protein, such as beans, nuts, and seeds, can supply us with an adequate amount of both the essential and nonessential amino acid building blocks needed to maintain good health. Both nonessential and essential amino acids are present in foods that contain protein.

The essential amino acid in smallest supply in a food or meal in relation to body needs becomes the limiting factor or **limiting amino acid** because it limits the amount of protein the body can synthesize. Typically, 50% of the amino acids in dietary proteins are essential. Fortunately, adults need only about 11% of their total protein requirement to be supplied by them.

The estimated requirements for essential amino acids for infants and preschool children are greater (40% of total protein intake) because of the needs of rapid growth and development; however, in later childhood, the need drops to 20%. Dietary plans designed for infants and young children need to take this into account to make sure enough high-quality proteins are present. Providing animal sources of protein, such as human milk or cow's milk-based formula for infants, or cow's milk for children, helps ensure this. A major health risk for infants and children occurs in famine situations in which only one type of cereal grain, such as rice, is available, increasing the probability that one or more of the nine essential amino acids are lacking in the total diet. This is discussed further in Section 6.7 on protein-calorie malnutrition (PCM).

Conditionally Essential Amino Acids Some of the nonessential amino acids, which are usually synthesized in the body, can become essential during times of rapid growth, disease, or metabolic stress. For example, the need for amino acids to promote healing during recovery from surgery or burns is so high that the activity of enzymes that synthesize nonessential amino acids cannot keep up with demands. Arginine and glutamine are two examples of **conditionally essential amino acids.**

The disease phenylketonuria (PKU) is an example of a genetic disorder in which a nonessential amino acid becomes conditionally essential. A person with PKU has a limited ability to metabolize the essential amino acid phenylalanine. Normally, the body uses an enzyme to convert much of our dietary phenylalanine intake into tyrosine. In PKU-diagnosed persons, the activity of the enzyme used in processing phenylalanine to tyrosine is insufficient. The results are that (1) tyrosine becomes essential (it must be obtained from the diet); whereas (2) phenylalanine from the diet builds up to toxic levels in the blood. Elevated phenylalanine disrupts brain function, leading to mental retardation. PKU is treated with a special diet that limits phenylalanine.

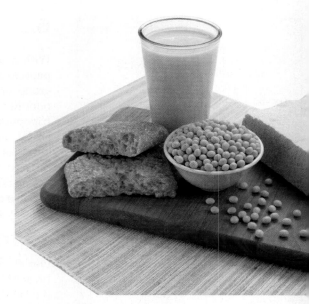

▲ Soy products such as soy milk, tofu, soy bread, and soybeans themselves provide a plant source of all the essential amino acids. ©Mitch Hrdlicka/Getty Images

essential amino acids The amino acids that cannot be synthesized by humans in sufficient amounts or at all and therefore must be included in the diet; there are nine essential amino acids. These are also called *indispensable amino acids.*

limiting amino acid The essential amino acid in lowest concentration in a food or diet relative to body needs.

conditionally essential amino acids Amino acids that must be made from essential amino acids if insufficient amounts are eaten.

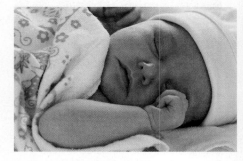

▲ All newborns are tested for phenylketonuria within the first few days of life using blood collected by a heel prick during the routine newborn screening. If PKU is diagnosed, the special diet should begin as soon as possible after birth to ensure normal brain development. ©Corbis/PictureQuest

✔ **CONCEPT CHECK 6.1**

1. What is the basic structure of an amino acid?

2. What is the difference between the essential and nonessestial amino acids?

3. What are some examples of conditions in which a nonessential amino acid becomes essential?

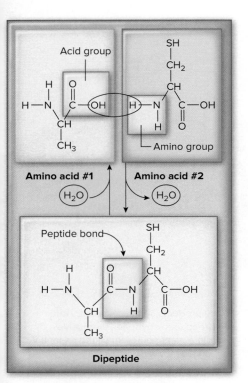

FIGURE 6-2 ▲ Peptide bonds link amino acids. The synthesis of a peptide bond is a dehydration reaction in which a molecule of water is removed. When peptide bonds are broken (as in digestion), a molecule of water is added (hydrolysis).

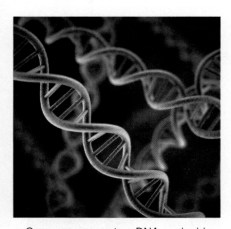

▲ Genes are present on DNA—a double-stranded helix. The cell nucleus contains most of the DNA in the body. DNA can be compared to a "cookbook" that contains the "recipes" (genes) for the synthesis of all proteins that cells need to make. Because the cookbook cannot leave the nucleus to get to the "cooks" (the ribosomes), the recipes for proteins must be transcribed into a form (mRNA) that can leave the nucleus. The amino acids that form a protein can be equated to the "ingredients" required for the recipe.
©Andrey Prokhorov/Getty Images

6.2 Protein Synthesis and Organization

Within body cells, amino acids are linked together by chemical bonds—technically called **peptide bonds**—to form proteins (Fig. 6-2). Peptide bonds form between the amino group of one amino acid and the acid (carboxyl) group of another. Through peptide bonding of amino acids, cells can synthesize dipeptides (joining of two amino acids), tripeptides (joining of three amino acids), oligopeptides (joining of four to nine amino acids), and **polypeptides** (joining of 10 or more amino acids). Most proteins are polypeptides ranging from about 50 to 2000 amino acids. The body can synthesize many different proteins by linking together the 20 common types of amino acids with peptide bonds. These bonds are difficult to break, but heat, acids, enzymes, and other agents are able to do so during cooking and chemical digestion.

PROTEIN SYNTHESIS

Our discussion of protein synthesis begins with deoxyribonucleic acid (DNA). DNA is present in the nucleus of the cell and contains coded instructions for protein synthesis (i.e., which specific amino acids are to be placed in a protein and in which order). Recall from Chapter 3 that DNA is a double-stranded molecule.

Protein synthesis, however, takes place in the cytoplasm of the cell, not in the nucleus (Fig. 6-3). Thus, the DNA code used for synthesis of a specific protein must be transferred from the nucleus to the cytoplasm to allow for protein synthesis. This transfer is the job of messenger RNA (mRNA). During transcription, enzymes in the nucleus first read the code (a gene) on a DNA base sequence that encodes one or more proteins and then *transcribe* that information into a single-stranded mRNA molecule (Fig. 6-3) that is ready to leave the nucleus.

Once in the cytoplasm, mRNA travels to the ribosomes. The ribosomes read the mRNA code and *translate* those instructions to produce a specific protein. During translation, amino acids are added one at a time to the growing polypeptide chain, according to the instructions on the mRNA. Another key participant in protein synthesis, transfer RNA (tRNA), is responsible for bringing the specific amino acids to the ribosomes as needed during protein synthesis (review Fig. 6-3). Energy input is required to add each amino acid to the chain, making protein synthesis "costly" in terms of calorie use.

Once synthesis of a polypeptide is complete, it twists and folds into the appropriate three-dimensional shape of the intended protein. These structural changes occur based on specific interactions among the amino acids on the polypeptide chain. Some polypeptides, such as the hormone insulin, also undergo further changes in the cell before they are functional.

PROTEIN ORGANIZATION

Through the bonding together of the 20 common types of amino acids into various combinations, the body synthesizes thousands of different proteins. The sequential order of the amino acids then ultimately determines the protein's shape. An important point is that only correctly positioned amino acids can interact and fold properly to form the intended shape for the protein. The resulting unique, three-dimensional form, such as that shown for the protein hemoglobin in Figure 6-4, goes on to dictate the function of each particular protein. If it lacks the proper structure, a protein cannot function.

The relationship between DNA and the proteins eventually produced by a cell is very important. If the DNA code contains errors, this is a genetic defect and an incorrect mRNA will be produced. The ribosomes will then read this incorrect message, and an incorrect amino acid will be added, resulting in an incorrect polypeptide chain being produced. Genetic engineering has begun to be used to correct gene defects in humans by placing the correct DNA code in the nucleus so that the correct protein can be made by the ribosomes.

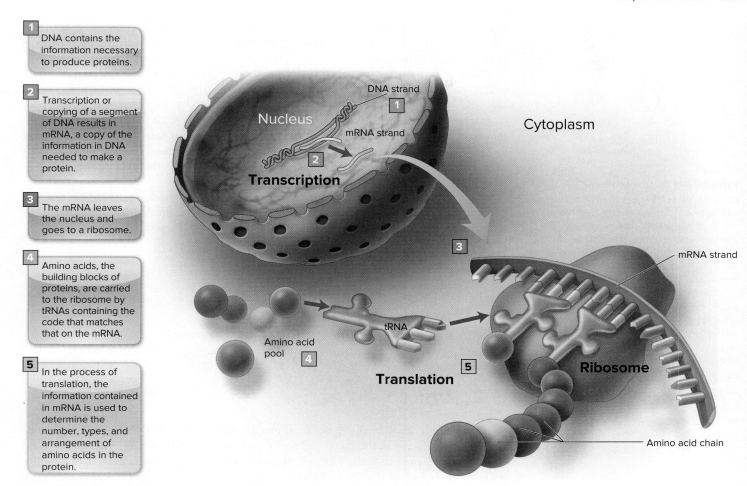

1. DNA contains the information necessary to produce proteins.

2. Transcription or copying of a segment of DNA results in mRNA, a copy of the information in DNA needed to make a protein.

3. The mRNA leaves the nucleus and goes to a ribosome.

4. Amino acids, the building blocks of proteins, are carried to the ribosome by tRNAs containing the code that matches that on the mRNA.

5. In the process of translation, the information contained in mRNA is used to determine the number, types, and arrangement of amino acids in the protein.

Nucleus — DNA strand — mRNA strand — **Transcription** — Cytoplasm — mRNA strand — Amino acid pool — tRNA — **Translation** — **Ribosome** — Amino acid chain

FIGURE 6-3 ▲ Protein synthesis (simplified). Once the mRNA is fully read, the amino acids have been connected into the polypeptide, which is released into the cytoplasm. It generally is then processed further to become a functioning cell protein.

peptide bond A chemical bond formed between amino acids in a protein.

polypeptide A group of 10 to 2000 or more amino acids bonded together to form proteins.

Sickle cell disease (also called **sickle cell anemia**) is one example of a genetic disease in which amino acids are out of order on a protein. In North America, people of African descent are especially prone to this genetic disease. Sickle cell anemia is not a nutritional disease but is caused by a mutation in the genetic code for hemoglobin, the protein depicted in Figure 6-4 that carries oxygen in red blood cells. The mutation causes the amino acid glutamic acid to be replaced with the amino acid valine. This error produces a profound change in hemoglobin structure. It can no longer form the shape needed to carry oxygen efficiently inside the red blood cell. Instead of forming normal circular disks, the red blood cells collapse into crescent (or sickle) shapes (see Fig. 6-5). Sickle red blood cells become hard and sticky, which causes them to clog blood flow and break apart. This can cause severe bone and joint pain, abdominal pain, headache, convulsions, paralysis, and even death due to the lack of oxygen.

These life-threatening symptoms are caused by a minute, but critical, error in amino acid order. It results from a defect in a person's genetic blueprint, DNA, inherited from one's parents. A defect in the DNA can dictate that a wrong amino acid will be built into the sequence of the body proteins. Many other diseases, including cancer, also stem from errors in the DNA code.

DENATURATION OF PROTEINS

Changing the shape of a protein often destroys its ability to function normally such that it loses its biological activity. Exposure to acid or alkaline substances, heat, or agitation

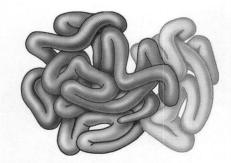

FIGURE 6-4 ▲ Protein organization. Proteins often form a coiled shape, as shown by this drawing of the blood protein hemoglobin. This shape is dictated by the order of the amino acids in the protein chain. To get an idea of its size, consider that each teaspoon (5 milliliters) of blood contains about 10^{18} hemoglobin molecules. (One billion is 10^9.)

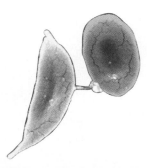

FIGURE 6-5 ▲ An example of the consequences of errors in DNA coding of proteins. A normal circular red blood cell is shown on the right along with an abnormal sickle-shaped red blood cell on the left. ©CDC/Sickle Cell Foundation of Georgia: Jackie George, Beverly Sinclair/photo by Janice Haney Carr

sickle cell disease (sickle cell anemia) An illness that results from a malformation of the red blood cell because of an incorrect structure in part of its hemoglobin protein chains.

denaturation Alteration of a protein's three-dimensional structure, usually because of treatment by heat, enzymes, acid or alkaline solutions, or agitation.

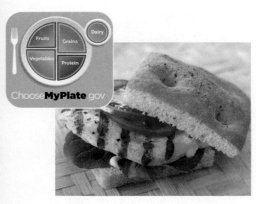

▲ This grilled chicken (protein) sandwich with lettuce and tomato (vegetables) on foccacia bread (grains) completes three section of MyPlate. Which sections are missing? ©Ingram Publishing/SuperStock; https// www.choosemyplate.gov

(e.g., whipping egg whites) can alter a protein's structure, leaving it uncoiled or otherwise deformed. This process of altering the three-dimensional structure of a protein is called **denaturation** (see Fig. 6-11).

Denaturation of dietary proteins does not alter their nutritional value and is a necessary part of digestion and other body processes. The heat produced during cooking starts the denaturation of some proteins. After food is ingested, the secretion of stomach acid denatures many forms of proteins in foods such as some bacterial proteins, plant hormones, and many active enzymes, making it safer to eat. Denaturation enhances digestion because the unraveling increases exposure of the polypeptide chain to digestive enzymes. Denaturing proteins in some foods can also reduce their tendencies to cause allergic reactions.

Recognize that we need the amino acids, especially essential ones, supplied by proteins in the diet—not the intact proteins themselves. We dismantle ingested dietary proteins and use the amino acid building blocks to assemble the proteins we need.

✓ CONCEPT CHECK 6.2

1. What is the role of DNA in protein synthesis?
2. What are the steps of protein synthesis?
3. Why is the amino acid order within a protein important?
4. What are some of the ways a protein can become denatured?

6.3 Protein in Foods

Protein is found in all of the major food groups, but much of the protein we eat comes from animal sources in the dairy and protein sections of MyPlate (Fig. 6-6). The top five contributors of protein to the North American diet have traditionally been beef, poultry, milk, white bread, and cheese. Food consumption surveys have revealed, however, a steady drop in U.S. meat and poultry consumption. According to the USDA, the average American consumed 202 pounds of red meat and poultry in 2014, 8% less than in 2004. This decrease was primarily related to a sharp drop in beef consumption. In 2014, the U.S. beef consumption per person of 54.2 pounds, was down 18% from 10 years ago and down about 30% from 1980. The downward trend seems to be a result of the rising cost of beef as well as conscious decisions to eat less red meat for health, environmental, and social reasons.

While the consumption of animal products has declined in the United States, world meat and dairy consumption has increased greatly.[1] World meat consumption increased from 11 kg per person in 2005 to 13.5 kg per person in 2015. It is particularly interesting that the demand for meat, eggs, and dairy products has increased in developing nations at a dramatic rate (Fig. 6.7). The greatest increases in consumption are occurring in East and Southeast Asia. In 2013, Asia produced 131.5 million tons of meat, accounting for close to 43% of world output of 308.5 million tons.[1] Dairy production and consumption have also soared in China and India over the past few decades. Overall, these increases in demand and consumption have had a substantial impact on agriculture because of the significant increase in the farm animal population over the past three decades. The "factory farms" that have developed have a significant environmental impact because of the large amount of land and water used, and the high level of waste produced.[2] These negative effects are in addition to the adverse health implications of consuming a diet high in animal products. It is predicted that the increasing intake of meat and dairy will have profound impacts on our agricultural and ecological resources, and our ability to provide food in the future. Because the Mediterranean diet is recognized as being low in meat, rich in fresh fruit and vegetables, and low in added sugar and saturated fatty acids, it is recommended as a sustainable alternative dietary pattern.[3] It has been advocated by the United Nations Food and Agricultural Organization (FAO) and could be a starting point for discussing the creation of policies to support sustainable food production.

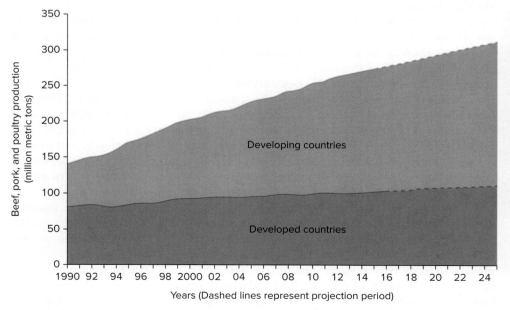

	Food Item and Amount	Protein grams	% RDA for 70-kg Male (56 grams)
Grains	Quinoa, cooked, 1 cup	8.4	15%
	Whole wheat bread, 1 slice	3.5	6%
	White rice, ½ cup	2.1	4%
Vegetables	Edamame, cooked, 1 cup	18.5	33%
	Kidney beans, ½ cup	6.7	12%
	Sweet potato, cooked, medium	2.1	4%
Fruits	Peach, 1 medium	1.4	3%
	Banana, 1 medium	1.3	2%
	Cantaloupe, cubed, 1 cup	1.3	2%
Dairy	Yogurt, Greek, nonfat, 5.3 ounces	13.6	24%
	1% low-fat milk, 1 cup	8.2	15%
	Cheddar cheese, 1 ounce	6.5	12%
Protein	Chicken breast, roasted 3 ounces	23.8	43%
	Tuna, canned, 3 ounces	20.1	36%
	Peanuts, 1 ounce	6.9	12%

FIGURE 6-6 ▲ Food sources of protein. (a) The fill of the background color (none, 1/3, 2/3, or completely covered) within each group on MyPlate indicates the average nutrient density for protein in that group. (b) The bar graph shows the protein content of several foods from each food group compared to the RDA for a 70-kilogram male. Overall, the dairy group and the protein group contain many foods that are nutrient-dense sources of protein. The fruits group provides little or no protein (less than 1 gram per serving). Food choices from the vegetables group and grains group provide moderate amounts of protein (2 to 3 grams per serving). The dairy group provides much protein (8 to 10 grams per serving), as does the protein group (7 grams per serving). ©Nutrition data from USDA National Nutrient Database for Standard Reference, Release 26.

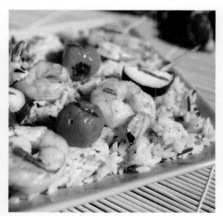

▲ Small amounts of animal protein in a meal easily add up to meet daily protein needs when mixed with grains and vegetables. ©Purestock/SuperStock

FIGURE 6-7 ▲ Beef, pork, and poultry production in developed and developing countries from 1990 to 2016 and projected through 2024. Meat production has been rapidly expanding in developing countries.

Evaluating Protein Quality

Having accurate information to evaluate a food's ability to deliver nutrition is essential to creating a sustainable diet to meet the needs of the growing global population. An important part of this information is an accurate measure of the amounts of amino acids absorbed by the body and the contribution of an individual protein source to human amino acid and nitrogen requirements.

In 2013, the FAO recommended a new, advanced method [the Digestible Indispensable Amino Acid Score (DIAAS)] for assessing the quality of dietary proteins.[4] DIAAS determines amino acid digestibility at the end of the small intestine, which more accurately measures the amounts of amino acids absorbed by the body and the protein's contribution to human amino acid and nitrogen requirements.

The DIAAS method allows researchers to differentiate protein sources by their ability to supply amino acids for use by the body. For example, the DIAAS method has demonstrated the higher bioavailability of dairy proteins when compared to plant-based protein sources, with whole milk powder having a DIAAS score of 1.22, compared to scores of 0.64 for peas and 0.40 for wheat.[4]

PROTEIN QUALITY OF FOODS

The quality of proteins can differ greatly according to their origin (animal or plant), their individual amino acid composition, and their level of amino acid bioactivity. With the rapid increase in the world population happening simultaneously with a decline in agricultural resources such as land and water, it is more important than ever to understand the true quality of our protein foods. Scientists have been working on more accurate techniques to assess protein quality of foods, and a description of the state of the methodology is summarized in the box "Evaluating Protein Quality."

Animal proteins contain ample amounts of all nine essential amino acids. Gelatin—made from the animal protein collagen—is an exception because it is low in essential amino acids. With a few exceptions such as soy protein and quinoa seed, plant proteins do not match our need for essential amino acids as precisely as animal proteins. Many plant proteins, especially those found in grains, are low in one or more of the nine essential amino acids.

"High-quality proteins" are those that are readily digestible and contain the essential amino acids in quantities that human require. As you might expect, humans are able to use proteins from any single animal source more efficiently to support growth and maintenance than from any single plant source. For this reason, animal proteins (except gelatin) are considered **high-quality** (also called **complete**) **proteins,** which contain sufficient amounts of the nine essential amino acids. The majority of individual plant sources of proteins are considered **lower-quality** (also called **incomplete**) **proteins** because their amino acid patterns can be quite different from ours. Thus, a single plant protein source, such as corn alone, cannot easily support human growth and maintenance. To obtain a sufficient amount of essential amino acids, a variety of plant proteins needs to be consumed because each plant protein lacks adequate amounts of one or more essential amino acids.

When only lower-quality protein foods are consumed, the amount of the essential amino acids needed for protein synthesis may not be obtained. Therefore, a greater amount of lower-quality protein is needed to meet the demands of protein synthesis, compared to high-quality proteins. Once any of the nine essential amino acids in the plant protein we have eaten is used up, further protein synthesis becomes impossible. Because the depletion of just one of the essential amino acids prevents protein synthesis, the process illustrates the *all-or-none principle:* either all essential amino acids are available, or none can be used. The remaining amino acids would then be used for energy needs or converted into carbohydrate or fat.

high-quality (complete) proteins Dietary proteins that contain ample amounts of all nine essential amino acids.

lower-quality (incomplete) proteins Dietary proteins that are low in or lack one or more essential amino acids.

CRITICAL THINKING

Evan, a vegetarian, has heard of the "all-or-none principle" of protein synthesis but does not understand how this principle applies to protein synthesis in the body. He asks you, "How important is this nutritional concept for meal planning?" How would you answer his question?

When two or more protein sources are combined in a meal or snack to compensate for deficiencies in their essential amino acid contents, the proteins are called **complementary proteins.** Meals with a variety of protein sources generally result in a complementary protein pattern. Many legumes, for example, are deficient in the essential amino acid methionine, whereas grains are limited in lysine. Eating a combination of legumes and grains, such as beans and rice, will supply the body with adequate amounts of all essential amino acids (Fig. 6-8). Likewise vegetables, which are limited in methionine, can be combined with nuts, which are limited in lysine. With these combinations, healthy adults should have little concern about obtaining enough of all nine essential amino acids. Even when following a plant-based dietary pattern, complementary proteins need not be consumed at the same meal. Meeting amino acid needs over the course of a day is a reasonable goal because there is a ready supply of amino acids present in body cells and in the blood (see Fig. 6-14).

In general, many North Americans should consume a higher proportion of plant sources of protein than they currently do. Plant foods contribute fewer calories than most animal products, but supply an ample amount of protein (Fig. 6-9). Plant sources of proteins, especially legumes and nuts, are a heart-healthy alternative to animal proteins because they contain very little saturated fat, aside from that added during processing or cooking.

A CLOSER LOOK AT SOURCES OF PROTEINS

Plant Proteins Per gram of protein, plant foods provide more magnesium, fiber, folate, vitamin E, iron (absorption is increased by the vitamin C also present), and zinc than animal sources of protein, and some calcium. Also, phytochemicals from these foods are implicated in prevention of a wide variety of chronic diseases.

Legumes are a plant family with pods that contain a single row of seeds. Examples include garden and black-eyed peas, kidney beans, great northern beans, lentils, soybeans, and peanuts. Dried varieties of the mature legume seeds—what we know as beans—also make an impressive contribution to the protein, vitamin, mineral, and fiber content of a meal.[5] A ½-cup serving of legumes provides 100 to 150 kcal, 5 to 10 grams of protein, less than 1 gram of fat, and about 5 grams of fiber. Recall from Chapter 4 that consumption of beans can lead to intestinal gas because our bodies lack the enzymes to break down certain carbohydrates in beans. Gas production can be decreased by soaking dry beans in water to leach the indigestible carbohydrates into the water, which then can be disposed. Read more about legumes in the Farm to Fork feature in this chapter.

Nuts and seeds are also excellent sources of plant protein. Commonly consumed nuts include almonds, pistachios, walnuts, and pecans. The defining characteristic of a nut is that it grows on a tree. Remember that peanuts, because they grow underground, are legumes. Seeds, including pumpkin, sesame, and sunflower seeds, are similar to nuts in nutrient composition. A 1-ounce serving of nuts or seeds generally supplies 160 to 190 kcal, 6 to 10 grams of protein, and 14 to 19 grams of fat. Although they are a dense source of calories, nuts and seeds make a powerful contribution to health when consumed in moderation.

In summary, plant proteins are a nutritious alternative to animal proteins. They are inexpensive, versatile, tasty, a colorful addition to your plate, and beneficial to health beyond their contribution of protein to the diet. Learning to substitute plant proteins in

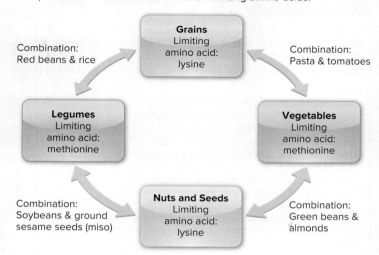

FIGURE 6-8 ▼ Plant group combinations in which the proteins complement each other based on their limiting amino acids.

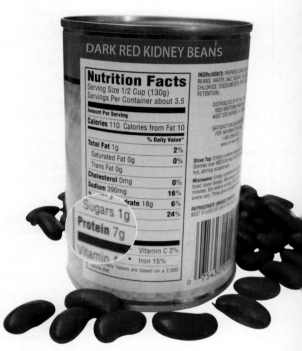

FIGURE 6-9 ▲ Legumes are rich sources of protein. These kidney beans provide a significant amount of protein per serving: 7 grams per 1/2 cup. ©Mark Dierker, photographer/McGraw-Hill Education

complementary proteins Two food protein sources that make up for each other's inadequate supply of specific essential amino acids; together, they yield a sufficient amount of all nine and so provide high-quality (complete) protein for the diet.

FARM to FORK Legumes

Legumes are seeds that grow in pods and include beans, peas, and lentils. Beans have an oval or kidney shape, while peas are round, and lentils are flat disks. Legumes are typically "shelled" before eating.

Grow
- Legumes have a mutually beneficial relationship with bacteria in the soil. The bacteria take gaseous nitrogen from the air in the soil and feed this nitrogen to the legumes. Legumes are environmentally friendly, providing carbohydrates to the bacteria and nitrogen to support plants growing nearby.
- Pole beans can grow tall on trellises, making the most of limited garden spaces, and you can even grow them in containers.
- If you stagger the planting of beans, you can enjoy usable amounts of beans throughout the growing season.

Shop
- Look for multicolored legumes—kidney beans, black beans, yellow peas, black-eyed peas, and lentils—to obtain abundant and varied phytochemicals. If you're having a hard time finding colorful varieties, look in the ethnic foods section of your local grocery store.
- Buy canned beans. The heat during the canning process increases their nutritional value.
- Choose fresh or frozen pod peas to get the most fiber and antioxidants. Canned peas have lost up to 50% of their antioxidant content.
- To prevent dried beans from drying out further, keep them in a food-safe storage container with a tight sealing lid. Remove any broken beans or rocks and place the container in a cool, dry place away from sunlight.

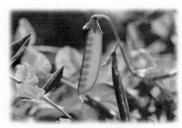

©ASO FUJITA/age fotostock

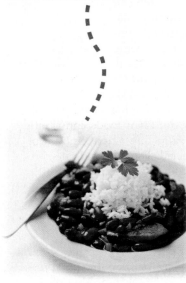

©Digital Vision/age fotostock

Store
- Store fresh beans in a moisture-proof, airtight container for several days to maintain freshness. Beans tend to get tough quickly after harvest.
- Canned beans remain highly nutritious over a long shelf life.

Prep
- Soak dry beans in water overnight prior to cooking. Discarding the water will help to reduce the flatulence that often occurs after eating legumes.
- During cooking, more than half of the antioxidants in dried beans will be leached into cooking water. Consuming this water or allowing the cooked beans to soak for 1 hour after cooking will help retain much of the nutrient content.
- Cooking beans in a pressure cooker saves time, produces a tender product, and retains the most nutrients of any cooking method.
- For the greatest convenience, use canned beans in cooking because they are higher in antioxidant content than fresh beans. Canned beans, however, are typically high in sodium, so drain and rinse them under cold water to remove nearly half of the sodium.
- Legumes are low in the essential amino acid methionine. To plan a diet that provides all of the essential amino acids, combine legumes with whole grains, which are a good source of methionine.

Source: Robinson J: Legumes: Beans, Peas and Lentils. In *Eating on the Wild Side: The Missing Link to Optimum Health.* Little, Brown and Company, NY, 2013.

place of less healthy foods is one way to reduce your risk for many diseases. The impact of plant proteins on health will be discussed in Section 6.9.

Animal Proteins Dietary patterns that include high protein intakes are typically of concern only when these intakes rely heavily on animal sources of protein. A high animal-protein diet is not recommended by the Dietary Guidelines for Americans or the American Heart Association because of their potential to increase the risk for cardiovascular and other diseases. Eating patterns rich in animal products are most likely low in beneficial substances found in plant sources, including fiber, some vitamins (e.g., folate), some minerals (e.g., magnesium), and phytochemicals, and are high in substances such as saturated fat.

Although meat is one of the richest sources of protein, excessive intake of red meat, especially processed forms, has been linked to colon cancer. A 2015 report of the World Health Organization confirmed that consumption of high levels of red and processed meat is associated with an increased risk of colorectal cancer.[6] The report, based on the review of more than 800 studies, indicated that reducing consumption of processed meats can reduce the risk of colorectal cancer. Experts concluded that each 50-gram portion of processed meat eaten daily increases the risk of colorectal cancer by 18%.

An association also has been found between red meat consumption and deaths caused by cardiovascular disease and cancer.[7,8] This connection could be caused by the curing agents used to process meats such as ham and salami, as well as substances that

Newsworthy Nutrition

Red meat consumption linked to deaths

Red meat, a major source of protein and fat in most diets, has been associated with an increased risk of several chronic diseases, leading researchers to hypothesize that red meat consumption is associated with an increase in early deaths. This study assessed meat consumption and causes of death from two prospective studies that included 37,698 men from the Health Professionals Follow-up Study (1986–2008) and 83,644 women from the Nurses' Health Study (1980–2008) who were free of cardiovascular disease (CVD) and cancer when the study began. During the study, there were 23,926 deaths, including 5910 caused by CVD and 9464 caused by cancer. Consumption of both unprocessed and processed red meat was associated with an increased risk of total, CVD, and cancer deaths in men and women. Substituting one serving per day of other healthy protein sources (including fish, poultry, nuts, legumes, low-fat dairy, and whole grains) for one serving per day of red meat was associated with a 7% to 19% lower mortality risk. They also estimated that 9.3% of deaths in men and 7.6% in women could be prevented at the end of the study if all the individuals consumed less than one-half serving per day (approximately 42 grams per day) of red meat. These results support the hypothesis that red meat consumption is associated with an increased risk of total and early deaths from CVD and cancer.

Source: Pan, A., et al. "Red meat consumption and mortality: Results from two prospective cohort studies," *Archives of Internal Medicine* 172:555, 2012.

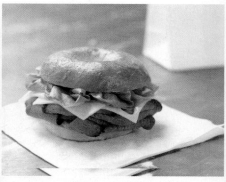

▲ Animal-protein foods, such as roast beef (2 ounces) and Swiss cheese (1 ounce) on a bagel (3.5 inches), are typically our main sources of protein in the North American diet. This sandwich provides 332 kcal and 31 grams of protein.
©Ingram Publishing/SuperStock

form during cooking of meats at high temperatures (see the Newsworthy Nutrition in this section). Any type of meat should be trimmed of all visible fat before cooking, especially grilling. The excessive fat or low-fiber contents of diets high in red meat may also be a contributing factor. Because of these concerns, some nutrition experts suggest we focus more on poultry, fish, nuts, legumes, and seeds to meet protein needs.

Red and processed meat has also been shown to be associated with increased risk of kidney disease.[9] Some researchers have expressed concern that a high-protein intake in general may overburden the kidneys by forcing them to excrete the extra nitrogen as urea. Also, animal proteins may contribute to kidney stone formation in certain individuals. A high-protein diet is not recommended for persons preserving kidney function such as those who have diabetes, early signs of kidney disease, or only one functioning kidney. There is some evidence that low-protein diets are helpful in slowing the decline in kidney function somewhat. High-protein diets increase urine output, which can lead to dehydration, especially in athletes.

FOOD PROTEIN ALLERGIES

Allergies occur when the immune system reacts to what it thinks is a foreign protein. In the case of food allergies, the immune system mistakes a food protein for a harmful invader. Overall, food allergies occur in up to 8% of children 4 years of age or younger and in up to 2% of adults. Eight foods account for 90% of food-related allergies (soy, peanuts, tree nuts, wheat, milk, eggs, fish, and shellfish; Fig. 6-10). The allergic reactions can range from a mild intolerance to fatal allergic reactions. Introducing allergenic foods such as peanut butter and eggs to infants as young as 4 to 6 months old is a new approach to combating food allergies that will be discussed further in Section 15.7.

☑ CONCEPT CHECK 6.3

1. What types of foods contain high-quality proteins?
2. Why are complementary proteins important when pairing plant food sources?
3. What are the eight foods responsible for most food allergies?

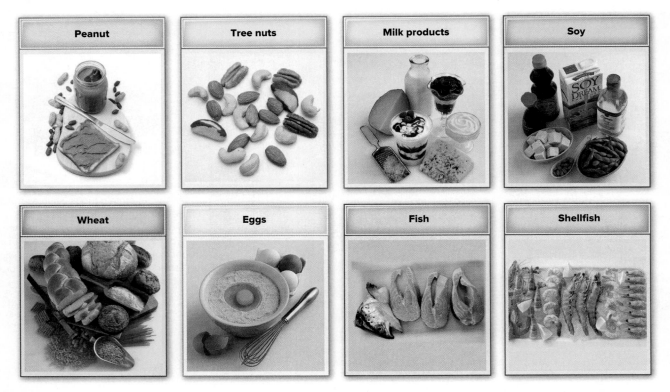

FIGURE 6-10 ▲ Most common food allergens. ©Igor Dutina/iStockphoto/Getty Images (peanut); ©Image Source/Glow Images (tree nuts); Photos courtesy of Dennis Gottlieb (milk products); Photos courtesy of Dennis Gottlieb (soy); Photos courtesy of Dennis Gottlieb (wheat); Photos courtesy of Dennis Gottlieb (eggs); ©Pixtal/AGE Fotostock (fish); ©FoodCollection (shellfish)

6.4 Protein Digestion and Absorption

As with carbohydrate digestion, protein digestion begins with the cooking of food. Cooking unfolds (denatures) proteins (Fig. 6-11) and softens tough connective tissue in meat. Cooking also makes many protein-rich foods easier to chew and swallow, and facilitates their breakdown during later digestion and absorption. Cooking also makes many protein-rich foods, such as meats, eggs, fish, and poultry, much safer to eat.

DIGESTION

The enzymatic digestion of protein begins in the stomach (Fig. 6-12). Proteins are first denatured by stomach acid. **Pepsin,** a major stomach enzyme for digesting proteins, then goes to work on the unraveled polypeptide chains. Pepsin breaks the polypeptide into shorter chains of amino acids because it can break only a few of the many peptide bonds found in these large molecules. The release of pepsin is controlled by the hormone gastrin. Thinking about food or chewing food stimulates gastrin release in the stomach. Gastrin then stimulates the stomach to produce acid and release pepsin.

The partially digested proteins move from the stomach into the small intestine along with the rest of the nutrients and other substances in a meal (chyme). Once in the small intestine, the partially digested proteins (and any fats accompanying them) trigger the release of the hormone cholecystokinin (CCK) from the walls of the small intestine. CCK, in turn, travels through the bloodstream to the pancreas, where it causes the pancreas to release protein-splitting enzymes, such as **trypsin.** These digestive enzymes further divide the chains of amino acids into segments of two to three amino acids and some individual amino acids. Eventually, this mixture is digested into amino acids, using other enzymes from the lining of the small intestine and enzymes present in the absorptive cells themselves.

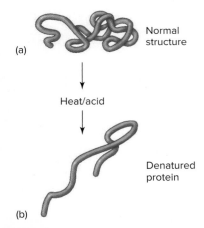

(a) Normal structure

Heat/acid

(b) Denatured protein

FIGURE 6-11 ▲ Denaturation. (a) Protein showing typical coiled state. (b) Protein is partly uncoiled by heat or acid. This uncoiling can reduce biological activity and allow digestive enzymes to act on peptide bonds.

pepsin A protein-digesting enzyme produced by the stomach.

trypsin A protein-digesting enzyme secreted by the pancreas to act in the small intestine.

Protein Digestion and Absorption

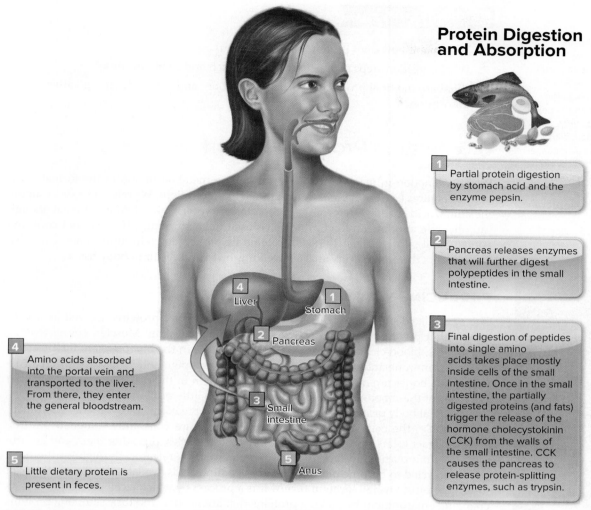

1. Partial protein digestion by stomach acid and the enzyme pepsin.

2. Pancreas releases enzymes that will further digest polypeptides in the small intestine.

3. Final digestion of peptides into single amino acids takes place mostly inside cells of the small intestine. Once in the small intestine, the partially digested proteins (and fats) trigger the release of the hormone cholecystokinin (CCK) from the walls of the small intestine. CCK causes the pancreas to release protein-splitting enzymes, such as trypsin.

4. Amino acids absorbed into the portal vein and transported to the liver. From there, they enter the general bloodstream.

5. Little dietary protein is present in feces.

Liver

Stomach

Pancreas

Small intestine

Anus

FIGURE 6-12 ▲ A summary of protein digestion and absorption. Enzymatic protein digestion begins in the stomach and ends in the absorptive cells of the small intestine, where any remaining short groupings of amino acids are broken down into single amino acids. Stomach acid and enzymes contribute to protein digestion. Absorption from the intestinal lumen into the absorptive cells requires energy input.

ABSORPTION

The short chains of amino acids and any individual amino acids in the small intestine are taken up by active transport into the absorptive cells lining the small intestine. Any remaining peptide bonds are broken inside intestinal cells to yield individual amino acids. They are water soluble, so the amino acids travel to the liver via the portal vein, which drains absorbed nutrients from the intestinal tract (see Fig. 6-12). In the liver, individual amino acids can undergo several modifications, depending on the needs of various body tissues. Individual amino acids may be (1) combined into the proteins needed by specific cells; (2) broken down for energy needs; (3) released into the bloodstream; or (4) converted into nonessential amino acids, glucose, or fat. With excess protein intake, amino acids are converted into fat as a last resort.

Except during infancy, it is uncommon for intact proteins to be absorbed from the digestive tract. In infants up to 4 to 5 months of age, the gastrointestinal tract is somewhat permeable to small proteins, so some whole proteins can be absorbed. Because proteins from some foods (e.g., cow's milk and egg whites) may predispose an infant to food allergies, experts recommend waiting until an infant reaches 4 to 6 months of age to introduce solid foods[10] (see Chapter 15 for details).

Gluten Sensitivity

Recall from the discussion of celiac disease and the gluten-free diet in Chapter 3 that gluten is a type of protein found in wheat, rye, and barley. Small peptides that arise from partial gluten digestion can be absorbed into the cells lining the small intestine and cause an inflammatory reaction in people with a genetic predisposition for celiac disease. Celiac disease is not a food allergy but an autoimmune response. Strict dietary avoidance of food products containing wheat, rye, and barley is the only proven way to manage the disease.[11] You will learn more about food allergies in Section 15.7.

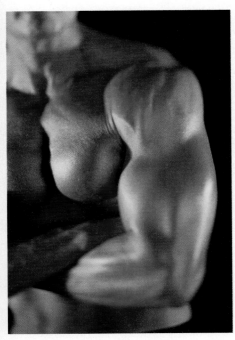

▲ Protein contributes to the structure and function of muscle. ©Ingram Publishing

protein turnover The process by which cells break down old proteins and resynthesize new proteins. In this way, the cell will have the proteins it needs to function at that time.

capillary bed Network of one-cell-thick vessels that create a junction between arterial and venous circulation. It is here that gas and nutrient exchange occurs between body cells and the blood.

extracellular space The space outside cells; contains one-third of body fluid.

edema The buildup of excess fluid in extracellular spaces.

☑ **CONCEPT CHECK 6.4**

1. Where and how does protein digestion begin?
2. What digestion steps take place in the stomach and small intestine?
3. What are the final products of protein digestion, and where do they go after absorption?

6.5 Putting Proteins to Work in the Body

Proteins function in many crucial ways in human metabolism and in the formation of body structures (see the Protein Concept Map in this section). We rely on foods to supply the amino acids needed to form these proteins; however, only when we also eat enough carbohydrate and fat can food proteins be used most efficiently. If we do not consume enough total calories to meet needs, proteins are broken down to supply energy to cells. This renders the amino acids unavailable for growth and repair of body tissues.

PRODUCING VITAL BODY STRUCTURES

The amino acid pool in a cell can be used to form body proteins, as well as a variety of other possible compounds. Every cell contains protein. Muscles, connective tissue, mucus, blood-clotting factors, transport proteins in the bloodstream, lipoproteins, enzymes, immune antibodies, some hormones, visual pigments, and the support structure inside bones are made of protein. Excess protein in the diet does not enhance the synthesis of these body components, but eating too little protein can prevent it.

Most vital body proteins are in a constant state of breakdown, rebuilding, and repair. For example, the cells of the intestinal tract lining are constantly sloughed off. The digestive tract treats sloughed cells just like food particles, digesting them and absorbing their amino acids. In fact, most of the amino acids released throughout the body can be recycled to become part of the pool of amino acids available for the synthesis of future proteins. Overall, **protein turnover** is a process by which a cell can respond to its changing environment by making proteins that are needed and disassembling proteins that are not needed.

During a 24-hour period, an adult turns over (makes and degrades) about 250 grams of protein, recycling many of the amino acids. Relative to the 65 to 100 grams of protein typically consumed by adults in North America, recycled amino acids make an important contribution to total protein metabolism. If a person's diet is low in protein for a long period, the processes of rebuilding and repairing body proteins will slow down. Over time, skeletal muscles, blood proteins, and vital organs such as the heart and liver will decrease in size or volume. Only the brain resists protein breakdown.

MAINTAINING FLUID BALANCE

Blood proteins help maintain body fluid balance. Normal blood pressure in the arteries forces blood into capillary beds. The blood fluid then moves from the **capillary beds** into the spaces between nearby cells (**extracellular spaces**) to provide nutrients to those cells (Fig. 6-13). Proteins in the bloodstream are too large, however, to move out of the capillary beds into the tissues. The presence of these proteins in the capillary beds attracts the proper amount of fluid back to the bloodstream, partially counteracting the force of blood pressure.

With an inadequate consumption of protein, the concentration of proteins in the bloodstream drops below normal. Excessive fluid then builds up in the surrounding tissues because the counteracting force produced by the smaller amount of blood proteins is too weak to pull enough of the fluid back from the tissues into the bloodstream. As fluids accumulate in the tissues, the tissues swell, causing **edema.** Because edema may be a symptom of other medical problems, an important step in diagnosing the cause is

Arterial end of a capillary bed

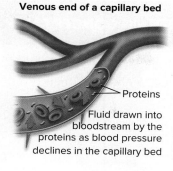

Fluid forced into tissue spaces by blood pressure generated by pumping action of heart

Blood cells

(a)

Venous end of a capillary bed

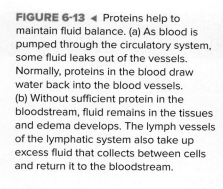

Proteins

Fluid drawn into bloodstream by the proteins as blood pressure declines in the capillary bed

FIGURE 6-13 ◄ Proteins help to maintain fluid balance. (a) As blood is pumped through the circulatory system, some fluid leaks out of the vessels. Normally, proteins in the blood draw water back into the blood vessels. (b) Without sufficient protein in the bloodstream, fluid remains in the tissues and edema develops. The lymph vessels of the lymphatic system also take up excess fluid that collects between cells and return it to the bloodstream.

Normal tissue

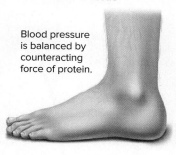

Blood pressure is balanced by counteracting force of protein.

Swollen tissue (edema)

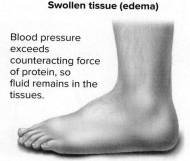

Blood pressure exceeds counteracting force of protein, so fluid remains in the tissues.

(b)

to measure the concentration of blood proteins. The lymphatic system also helps maintain fluid balance by collecting excess fluid and substances, including proteins, from tissues and depositing them in the bloodstream.

CONTRIBUTING TO ACID–BASE BALANCE

Proteins help regulate acid–base balance in the blood. Proteins located in cell membranes pump chemical ions in and out of cells. The ion concentration that results from the pumping action, among other factors, keeps the blood slightly alkaline. In addition, some blood proteins are especially good **buffers** in the bloodstream. Buffers are compounds that maintain acid–base conditions within a narrow range.

buffer Compounds that cause a solution to resist changes in acid–base conditions.

FORMING HORMONES AND ENZYMES

Many hormones, our internal body messengers, are proteins and therefore require amino acids for synthesis. Some hormones, such as the thyroid hormones, are made from only one type of amino acid, tyrosine. Insulin, on the other hand, is a hormone composed of 51 amino acids. Almost all enzymes are proteins or have a protein component.

CONTRIBUTING TO IMMUNE FUNCTION

Proteins are a key component of cells within the immune system. Consider, for example, antibodies, which are proteins produced by one type of white blood cell. These antibodies can bind to foreign proteins in the bloodstream—an important step in removing invaders from the body. Without sufficient dietary protein, the immune system lacks the materials needed to function properly. For example, a low-protein status can turn an infection such as measles into a fatal disease for a malnourished child.

Neurotransmitters, released by nerve endings, are often derivatives of amino acids. This is true for dopamine and norepinephrine (both synthesized from the amino acid tyrosine) and serotonin (synthesized from the amino acid tryptophan). Most neurotransmitters are the size of a single amino acid.

FORMING GLUCOSE

In Chapter 4, you learned that a fairly constant concentration of glucose must be maintained in the blood to supply energy for the brain, red blood cells, and nervous tissue. At rest, the brain uses about 19% of the body's energy requirements, and it gets most of that energy from glucose. If you do not consume enough carbohydrate to supply the

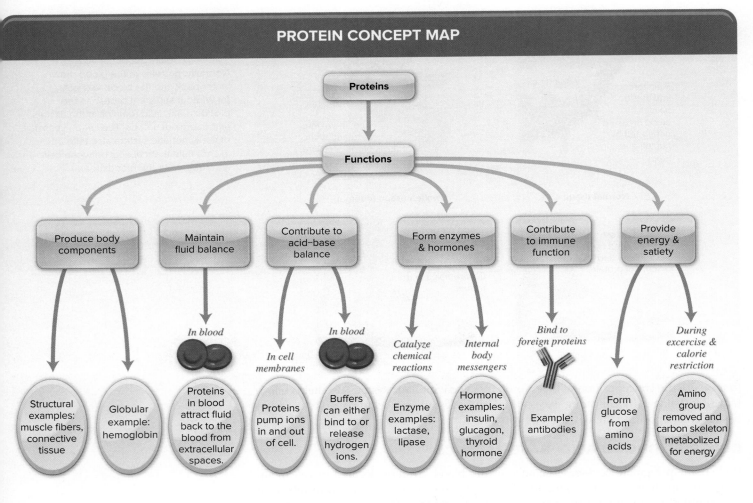

PROTEIN CONCEPT MAP

Proteins

Functions

| Produce body components | Maintain fluid balance | Contribute to acid–base balance | Form enzymes & hormones | Contribute to immune function | Provide energy & satiety |

In blood

In cell membranes

In blood

Catalyze chemical reactions

Internal body messengers

Bind to foreign proteins

During excercise & calorie restriction

Structural examples: muscle fibers, connective tissue

Globular example: hemoglobin

Proteins in blood attract fluid back to the blood from extracellular spaces.

Proteins pump ions in and out of cell.

Buffers can either bind to or release hydrogen ions.

Enzyme examples: lactase, lipase

Hormone examples: insulin, glucagon, thyroid hormone

Example: antibodies

Form glucose from amino acids

Amino group removed and carbon skeleton metabolized for energy

glucose, your liver (and kidneys, to a lesser extent) will be forced to make glucose from amino acids present in body tissues (Fig. 6-14).

Making some glucose from amino acids is normal. For example, when you skip breakfast and have not eaten since 7:00 P.M. the preceding evening, glucose must be manufactured. In an extreme situation, however, such as in starvation, amino acids from muscle tissue are regularly converted into glucose, which wastes muscle tissue and can produce edema.

PROVIDING ENERGY

Proteins supply little energy for a person at a healthy weight. Two situations in which a person does use protein to meet energy needs are during prolonged exercise and during calorie restriction, as with a weight-loss diet. In these cases, the amino group ($-NH_2$) from the amino acid is removed, and the remaining carbon skeleton is metabolized for energy needs (see Fig. 6-14). When the carbon skeletons of amino acids are metabolized to produce glucose or fat, ammonia (NH_3) is a resulting waste product. The ammonia is converted into **urea** and excreted in the urine. Under most conditions, cells primarily use fats and carbohydrates for energy needs. Although proteins contain the same amount of calories (on average, 4 kcal per gram) as carbohydrates, proteins are a costly source of calories, considering the amount of processing the liver and kidneys must perform to use this calorie source.

CONTRIBUTING TO SATIETY

Compared to the other macronutrients, proteins provide the highest feeling of **satiety** after a meal. Thus, including some protein with each meal helps control overall food

The vitamin niacin can be made from the amino acid tryptophan, illustrating another role of proteins.

urea Nitrogenous waste product of protein metabolism; major source of nitrogen in the urine,

$$\begin{array}{c} O \\ \parallel \\ NH_2{-}C{-}NH_2 \end{array}$$

chemically

satiety A state in which there is no longer a desire to eat; a feeling of satisfaction.

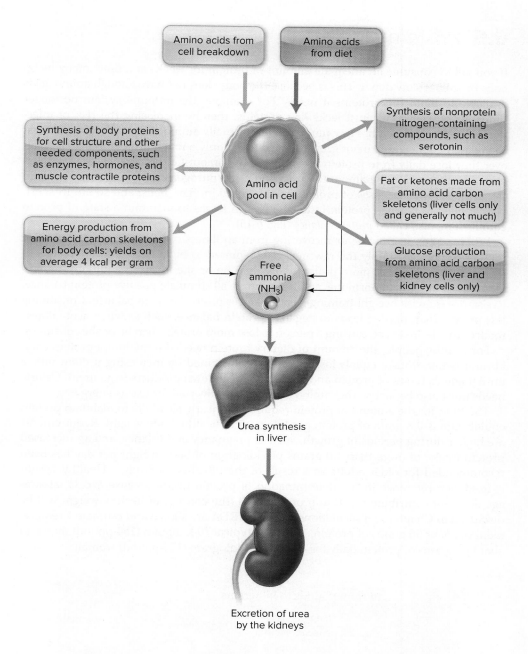

Amino acids from cell breakdown

Amino acids from diet

Synthesis of nonprotein nitrogen-containing compounds, such as serotonin

Synthesis of body proteins for cell structure and other needed components, such as enzymes, hormones, and muscle contractile proteins

Amino acid pool in cell

Fat or ketones made from amino acid carbon skeletons (liver cells only and generally not much)

Energy production from amino acid carbon skeletons for body cells: yields on average 4 kcal per gram

Free ammonia (NH₃)

Glucose production from amino acid carbon skeletons (liver and kidney cells only)

Urea synthesis in liver

Excretion of urea by the kidneys

FIGURE 6-14 ◄ Amino acid metabolism. The amino acid **pool** in a cell can be used to form body proteins, as well as a variety of other possible products. When the **carbon skeletons** of amino acids are metabolized to produce glucose or fat, ammonia (NH_3) is a resulting waste product. The ammonia is converted into urea and excreted in the urine.

pool The amount of a nutrient stored within the body that can be mobilized when needed.

carbon skeleton Amino acid structure that remains after the amino group (—NH_2) has been removed.

intake. Many experts warn against skimping on protein when trying to reduce energy intake to lose weight. Meeting protein needs is still important, and exceeding needs somewhat may provide an additional benefit when dieting to lose weight. Several effective weight-loss diets include a percentage of calories from protein at the upper end of the Acceptable Macronutrient Distribution Range of 10% to 35% for protein (see Appendix G). In general, these diets are appropriate if otherwise nutritionally sound, especially with regard to being moderate in fat and having enough fiber.

✓ CONCEPT CHECK 6.5

1. Which body constituents are mainly proteins?
2. What is the turnover rate of protein each day?
3. How is glucose produced from protein?

6.6 Protein Needs

If you fail to consume an adequate amount of protein for weeks at a time, many metabolic processes slow down. This is because the body does not have enough amino acids available to build the proteins it needs. For example, the immune system no longer functions efficiently when it lacks key proteins, thereby increasing the risk of infections, disease, and death. How much protein (actually amino acids) do we need to eat each day? People who are not growing need to eat only enough protein to match whatever they lose daily from protein breakdown. The amount of breakdown can be determined by measuring the amount of urea and other nitrogen-containing compounds in the urine, as well as losses of protein from feces, skin, hair, nails, and so on. In short, people need to balance protein intake with such losses to maintain a state of **protein equilibrium,** also called *protein balance* (Fig. 6-15).

When a body is growing or recovering from an illness or injury, it needs a **positive protein balance** to supply the raw materials required to build new tissues. To achieve this, a person must eat more protein daily than he or she loses. In addition, the hormones insulin, growth hormone, and testosterone all stimulate positive protein balance. Resistance exercise (weight training) also enhances positive protein balance. Consuming less protein than needed leads to **negative protein balance,** such as when acute illness reduces the desire to eat, causing a person to lose more protein than he or she consumes.

For healthy people, the amount of dietary protein needed to maintain protein equilibrium (where intake equals losses) can be determined by increasing protein intake until it equals losses of protein and its related breakdown products (e.g., urea). Calorie needs must also be met so that amino acids are not diverted for use as energy.

The RDA for the amount of protein required for nearly all adults to maintain protein equilibrium is 0.8 gram of protein per kilogram of healthy body weight. Requirements are higher during periods of growth, such as pregnancy and infancy, and an increased protein intake of more than 1.0 grams per kilogram of body weight per day has been recommended for older adults as a result of the PROT-AGE Study.[12] Healthy weight is used as a reference in the determination of protein needs because excess fat storage does not contribute much to protein needs (the concept of healthy weight will be discussed in Chapter 7). Calculations using this RDA are shown and estimate a requirement of about 56 grams of protein daily for a typical 70-kilogram (154-pound) man and about 46 grams of protein daily for a typical 57-kilogram (125-pound) woman.

protein equilibrium A state in which protein intake is equal to related protein losses; the person is said to be in protein balance.

positive protein balance A state in which protein intake exceeds related protein losses, as is needed during times of growth.

negative protein balance A state in which protein intake is less than related protein losses, such as often seen during acute illness.

The Dietary Guidelines for Americans recommend a variety of protein foods, including seafood, lean meats and poultry, eggs, legumes (beans and peas), nuts, seeds, and soy products. The following shifts are also recommended to increase variety in protein food choices and to make more nutrient-dense choices:

- Increase the amount and variety of seafood consumed by choosing seafood in place of some meat and poultry.
- Increase seafood intake, but the foods to be replaced depend on the individual's current intake from the other protein subgroups.
- Incorporate seafood as the protein foods choice in meals twice per week in place of meat, poultry, or eggs.
- Use legumes or nuts and seeds in mixed dishes instead of some meat or poultry.
- Shift to nutrient-dense options, including lean and lower sodium options, to improve the nutritional quality of protein food choices and support healthy eating patterns.
- Some individuals, especially teen boys and adult men, also need to reduce overall intake of protein foods by decreasing intakes of meats, poultry, and eggs and increasing amounts of vegetables or other underconsumed food groups.

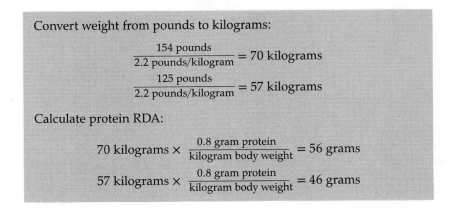

Convert weight from pounds to kilograms:

$$\frac{154 \text{ pounds}}{2.2 \text{ pounds/kilogram}} = 70 \text{ kilograms}$$

$$\frac{125 \text{ pounds}}{2.2 \text{ pounds/kilogram}} = 57 \text{ kilograms}$$

Calculate protein RDA:

$$70 \text{ kilograms} \times \frac{0.8 \text{ gram protein}}{\text{kilogram body weight}} = 56 \text{ grams}$$

$$57 \text{ kilograms} \times \frac{0.8 \text{ gram protein}}{\text{kilogram body weight}} = 46 \text{ grams}$$

The RDA for protein translates into about 10% of total calories. Many experts recommend up to 15% of total calories as protein to provide flexibility in diet planning and to allow for the variety of protein-rich foods typically consumed. The Dietary Guidelines encourage the consumption of protein-rich foods such as beans, nuts, seeds, fat-free milk, and seafood. The Food and Nutrition Board has set an upper range for protein intake at 35% of calories consumed. It is easy to meet these currently suggested daily

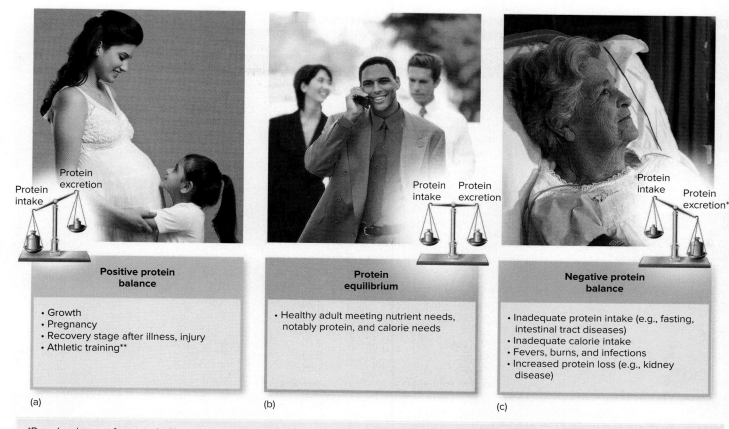

Protein
intake
Protein
excretion

Positive protein balance

- Growth
- Pregnancy
- Recovery stage after illness, injury
- Athletic training**

(a)

Protein
intake
Protein
excretion

Protein equilibrium

- Healthy adult meeting nutrient needs, notably protein, and calorie needs

(b)

Protein
intake
Protein
excretion*

Negative protein balance

- Inadequate protein intake (e.g., fasting, intestinal tract diseases)
- Inadequate calorie intake
- Fevers, burns, and infections
- Increased protein loss (e.g., kidney disease)

(c)

*Based on losses of urea and other nitrogen-containing compounds in the urine, as well as protein lost from feces, skin, hair, nails, and other minor routes.
**Only when additional lean body mass is being gained. Nevertheless, the athlete is probably already eating enough protein to support this extra protein synthesis; protein supplements are not needed.

FIGURE 6-15 ▲ Protein balance in practical terms: (a) positive protein balance, (b) protein equilibrium, and (c) negative protein balance. ©Sudipta Halder/Getty Images RF (left); ©Stockbyte/Punchstock Images (middle); ©Dynamic Graphics/JupiterImages (right)

protein needs, as given in Table 6-2. On a daily basis in North America, the typical man and woman consume about 100 and 65 grams of protein, respectively. Thus, most of us consume much more protein than the RDA recommends because we like many high-protein foods and can afford to buy them. Our bodies cannot store excess protein once it is consumed, so the excess amino acids are stripped of the nitrogen-containing amino group and may be turned into glucose or ketone bodies and contribute to a positive energy balance, which would be undesirable if weight loss is the goal (review Fig. 6-14).

Meal Protein Requirements Maintaining a more equal distribution of protein at each meal has recently been found important for the more optimal function of protein.[13] Many protein functions such as maintaining body composition and bone health and regulating glucose are sensitive to the concentration of amino acids in blood and cells after meals. Meal-based responses to dietary protein have been linked to amino acids acting as signals. The best characterized of these postmeal amino acid signals is that of leucine stimulating the synthesis of skeletal muscle.

Emerging research is pointing to the need to redistribute daily dietary protein for optimum health.[13] Studies have found that consuming at least 20 to 30 grams of protein at a given meal has positive effects on muscle protein synthesis, compared with spreading the same total amount of protein across multiple small meals. Researchers now recommend that adults consume at least 30 grams of protein at more than one meal in order to maintain healthy muscles and bones. Protein at breakfast is especially

TABLE 6-2 ■ Protein Content of Sample Menus Containing 1600 and 2000 kcal

Menu		1600 kcal		2000 kcal	
		Serving Size	Protein (g)	Serving Size	Protein (g)
Breakfast					
	Low-fat granola	⅔ cup	5	⅔ cup	5
	Blueberries	1 cup	1	1 cup	1
	Fat-free (skim) milk	1 cup	8.5	1 cup	8.5
	Coffee	1 cup	0	1 cup	0
Lunch					
	Broiled chicken breast	3 ounces	25	4 ounces	33
	Salad greens	3 cups	5	3 cups	5
	Baked taco shell strips	½ cup	2	½ cup	2
	Low-fat salad dressing	2 tbsp	0	2 tbsp	0
Dinner					
	Fat-free (skim) milk	1 cup	8.5	1 cup	8.5
	Brown rice	1 cup	5	2 cups	10
	Shrimp	4 large	5	6 large	7
	Mussels	4 medium	8	6 medium	12
	Clams	5 small	12	10 small	24
	Peas	¼ cup	2	½ cup	4
	Sweet red pepper	½ cup	0	½ cup	0
Snack					
	Muffin	1 small	4	1 small	4
	Swiss cheese	1 ounce	7.5	1 ounce	7.5
	Banana	½ small	0.5	½ small	0.5
	Total		101		132

©Image Source/Corbis (Breakfast); ©John A. Rizzo/Getty Images (Lunch); ©Kevin Sanchez/Cole Group/Getty Images (Dinner); ©John A. Rizzo/Getty Images (Snack)

critical to regulate appetite and daily food intake and to replenish body proteins after an overnight fast. Read more about this issue in What the Dietitian Chose at the end of this chapter.

Protein Needs for Older Adults The concept of meal requirements for protein has also been studied in older adults.[12] Research shows that the responses to dietary protein decline with advancing age or reduced physical activity. An increased daily protein intake of more than 1.0 grams per kilogram for older adults is recommended in the consensus position paper from the PROT-AGE Study Group, along with an emphasis on the need to focus on meal quantity and timing of protein as important factors in adult health.[12] Specific recommendations are for older adults to consume meals with greater than 20 grams of protein, including more than 2.2 grams of leucine, to optimize protein synthesis in skeletal muscle. Regarding activity, resistance exercise enhances the protein synthesis response, especially muscle growth, in older adults. Research indicates that with these increases in resistance exercise and protein intakes, older adults can achieve rates of muscle protein synthesis similar to young adults. In contrast, declining daily activity, including short-term bed rest due to hospitalization, illness, or injury, blunts the amino acid signaling response and results in a significant loss of lean tissue in both young and older adults.

ASK THE RDN Paleo Diet

Dear RDN: Is the Paleo Diet™ a healthy way to include a good amount of high-quality protein into my eating plan?

The Paleo Diet, also called the Stone Age or Caveman Diet, is based on what was eaten during the Paleolithic period. Acceptable foods, therefore, are ones that can be hunted, fished, or gathered. Meats include those that are grass fed and pasture raised or wild game such as venison. Wild-caught fish, poultry, eggs, vegetables, fruits, fungi, roots, and nuts are also part of the diet. Dairy products and grains are excluded based on the assumption that the human body has not adapted genetically to allow for the consumption of grains and dairy, and that these foods contribute to health problems such as overweight/obesity and heart disease. Legumes (beans and peanuts), potatoes, added salt, refined sugar, and processed oils are also excluded.

Desirable aspects of the Paleo Diet are that it is rich in high-quality proteins and produce, yet low in added sugar and sodium—all factors that can help keep blood sugar, blood pressure, and weight under control. This very strict diet, however, has inadequate research to support its proposed benefits; and it is nearly impossible to gather and consume foods in the manner they existed in prehistoric times. Most of the meat we eat today is domesticated rather than wild game. Available fruits and vegetables are also grown on farms rather than harvested from the wild. Paleo followers often modify the plan by eating wild-caught fish, grass-fed meat, and organic fruits and vegetables, but even this becomes a challenge given the expense, lack of variety, and need for extensive planning and supplementation.

In sum, the Paleo Diet typically exceeds recommendations for fat and protein intake yet falls short of carbohydrate needs. The elimination of whole grains, legumes, and dairy—foods that are rich in nutrients and fiber—is more likely to lead to nutrient deficiencies than to weight loss. The lack of dairy jeopardizes calcium and vitamin D status and necessitates the use of supplements. Some good attributes of the diet that you can incorporate into a healthy dietary pattern are to eat more lean protein and less refined carbohydrates (more whole grains) to promote weight loss and satiety; a wide variety of fruits and vegetables to obtain vitamins, minerals, fiber, and phytochemicals; and more foods that are local, seasonal, and minimally processed because they provide more nutrients and fiber than a highly processed version of the food.

Eating for today,

Anne M. Smith, PhD, RDN, LD (author)

Mental stress, physical labor, and recreational weekend sports activities do not require an increase in the protein RDA. For some highly trained athletes, such as those participating in endurance or strength training, protein consumption may need to exceed the RDA. Many North Americans, especially men, already consume that much protein. The effect of physical activity on protein requirements is covered in Sections 10.4 and 10.5.

AMINO ACID SUPPLEMENTS

Protein and amino acid supplements are used primarily by those trying to lose weight and by athletes hoping to build muscle. The branched-chain amino acids are especially popular with athletes looking to enhance their performance. Although the right amount of protein in the diet will aid athletic performance and help in weight control, consuming protein in the form of amino acid supplements cannot be considered safe. Because the body's gastrointestinal system is adapted to handle whole proteins as a dietary source of amino acids, individual amino acid supplements can overwhelm the absorptive mechanisms in the small intestine. Amino acid imbalances occur in the intestinal tract because groups of chemically similar amino acids compete for absorption sites in the absorptive cells. For example, an excess of lysine can impair absorption of arginine because they are absorbed by the same transporter. The amino acids methionine, cysteine, and histidine are most likely to cause toxicity when consumed in large amounts. Due to this potential for imbalances and toxicities, the best advice to ensure adequacy is to stick to whole foods as sources of amino acids rather than supplements. Amino acid supplements also have a disagreeable odor and flavor and are much more expensive than food protein. In Canada, the sale of individual amino acids to consumers is banned.

> ☑ **CONCEPT CHECK 6.6**
>
> 1. During what situations is the body in positive protein balance?
> 2. What is the RDA for protein for a 70-kilogram person?
> 3. How much protein does the average American consume?

protein-calorie malnutrition (PCM)
A condition resulting from regularly consuming insufficient amounts of calories and protein. The deficiency eventually results in body wasting, primarily of lean tissue, and an increased susceptibility to infections. Also known as *protein-energy malnutrition (PEM)*.

kwashiorkor A disease occurring primarily in young children who have an existing disease and consume a marginal amount of calories and insufficient protein in relation to needs. The child generally suffers from infections and exhibits edema, poor growth, weakness, and an increased susceptibility to further illness.

marasmus A disease resulting from consuming a grossly insufficient amount of protein and calories; one of the diseases classed as protein-calorie malnutrition. Victims have little or no fat stores, little muscle mass, and poor strength. Death from infections is common.

6.7 Protein-Calorie Malnutrition

Protein deficiency is rarely an isolated condition and usually accompanies a deficiency of calories and other nutrients resulting from insufficient food intake. In the developed world, alcoholism can lead to cases of protein deficiency because of the low protein content of alcoholic beverages that make up a high percent of calories. Protein and calorie malnutrition is a significant problem in hospitals worldwide, affecting patients from infancy through older adulthood. Malnutrition can be caused by the illnesses or injuries for which patients are admitted to the hospital and by the hospitalization itself.[14] In developing areas of the world, people often have diets low in calories and protein. This state of undernutrition stunts the growth of children and makes them more susceptible to disease throughout life. (Undernutrition is a main focus of Chapter 12.) People who consume too few of their calories as protein can eventually develop **protein-calorie malnutrition (PCM),** also referred to as *protein-energy malnutrition (PEM)* (Fig. 6-16). In its milder form, it is difficult to tell if a person with PCM is consuming too little calories or protein, or both. When an inadequate intake of nutrients, including protein, is combined with an existing disease, especially an infection, a form of malnutrition called **kwashiorkor** can develop. But if the nutrient deficiency—especially for calories—becomes severe, a deficiency disease called **marasmus** can result. Both conditions are

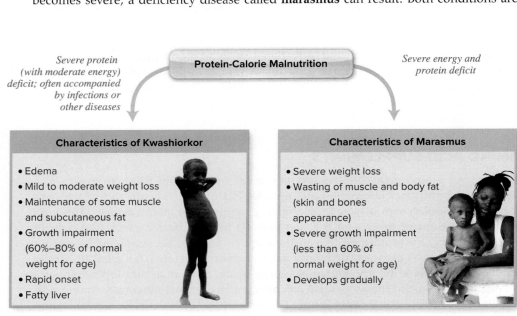

Severe protein (with moderate energy) deficit; often accompanied by infections or other diseases

Protein-Calorie Malnutrition

Severe energy and protein deficit

Characteristics of Kwashiorkor
- Edema
- Mild to moderate weight loss
- Maintenance of some muscle and subcutaneous fat
- Growth impairment (60%–80% of normal weight for age)
- Rapid onset
- Fatty liver

Characteristics of Marasmus
- Severe weight loss
- Wasting of muscle and body fat (skin and bones appearance)
- Severe growth impairment (less than 60% of normal weight for age)
- Develops gradually

FIGURE 6-16 ▲ Classification of undernutrition in children. (kwashiorkor): ©Christine Osborne Pictures/Alamy (left); ©Phanie/Alamy (right)

seen primarily in children but also may develop in adults, even in those hospitalized in North America. These two conditions form the tip of the iceberg with respect to states of undernutrition, and symptoms of these two conditions can even be present in the same person.

KWASHIORKOR

Kwashiorkor is a word from Ghana that means "the disease that the first child gets when the new child comes." Infants in developing areas of the world are usually breastfed from birth. Often by the time the child reaches 1 to 1.5 years of age, the mother is pregnant or has already given birth again, and the newborn infant gets preference for breastfeeding. The older child's diet then abruptly changes from nutritious human milk to starchy roots and **gruels,** which are low in protein compared to their calorie content. Additionally, the foods are usually high in bulky plant fibers, which are very filling and thus prevent the child from consuming enough food to meet calorie needs. Infections also raise calorie and protein needs. For these reasons, it is a challenge to meet the child's calorie needs, and his or her protein consumption is grossly inadequate, especially in view of the increased amount needed to combat infections. Many vitamin and mineral needs are also far from being fulfilled. Famine victims face similar problems.

gruels A thin mixture of grains or legumes in milk or water.

The major symptoms of kwashiorkor are apathy, diarrhea, listlessness, failure to grow and gain weight, and withdrawal from the environment. These symptoms complicate other diseases present. For example, a condition such as measles, a disease that normally makes a well-nourished child ill for only a week or so, can become severely debilitating and even fatal. Further symptoms of kwashiorkor are changes in hair color, potassium deficiency, flaky skin, fatty liver, reduced muscle mass, and massive edema in the abdomen and legs. The presence of edema in a child who has some subcutaneous fat (i.e., fat directly under the skin) is the hallmark of kwashiorkor (review Fig. 6-16). In addition, these children seldom move or cry. When you hold them, you feel the plumpness of edema, not muscle and fat tissue.

Many symptoms of kwashiorkor can be explained based on what we know about proteins. Proteins play important roles in fluid balance, lipoprotein transport, immune function, and production of tissues such as skin, cells lining the GI tract, and hair. Children with an insufficient protein intake do not grow or mature normally. If children with kwashiorkor are helped in time—that is, if infections are treated and the dietary pattern becomes plentiful in protein, calories, and other essential nutrients—then the disease process reverses. They begin to grow again and may even show no signs of their previous condition, except perhaps shortness of stature. Unfortunately, by the time many of these children reach a hospital or care center, they already have severe infections. Despite the best care, they still die. Or, if they survive, they return home only to become ill again.

MARASMUS

Marasmus (referred to as *protein-calorie malnutrition,* especially when experienced by older children and adults) typically occurs as an infant slowly starves to death. It is caused by diets containing minimal amounts of calories, as well as too little protein and other nutrients. The word *marasmus* means "to waste away," in Greek. Victims have a "skin-and-bones" appearance, with little or no subcutaneous fat (review Fig. 6-16). Marasmus commonly develops in infants who either are not breastfed or have stopped breastfeeding in the early months. When people are poor and sanitation is lacking, bottle feeding often leads to marasmus. Often the weaning formula used is improperly prepared because of unsafe water and because the parents cannot afford sufficient infant formula for the child's needs. If parents dilute the formula to provide more feedings, they will be providing only more water for the infant.

Marasmus in infants commonly occurs in the large cities of poverty-stricken countries. In cities, bottle feeding is often necessary because the infant is cared for by others

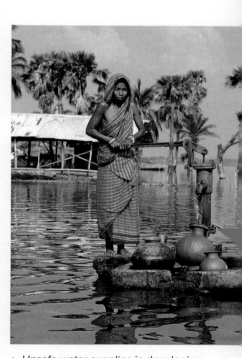

▲ Unsafe water supplies in developing countries contribute to the incidence of marasmus, particularly in bottle-fed infants. ©Digital Vision/PunchStock

preterm An infant born before 37 weeks of gestation; also referred to as *premature.*

when the mother is working or away from home. An infant with marasmus requires large amounts of calories and protein, similar to the needs of a **preterm** infant, and, unless the child receives them, full recovery from the disease may never occur. The majority of brain growth occurs between conception and the child's first birthday, with the brain growing at its highest rate after birth. If human milk or formula does not support brain growth during the first months of life, the brain may not grow to its full adult size, leading to diminished intellectual function. Both kwashiorkor and marasmus plague infants and children, causing mortality rates in developing countries to be often 10 to 20 times higher than in North America.

✓ CONCEPT CHECK 6.7

1. What are the characteristics of kwashiorkor and marasmus?
2. Why are bottle-fed infants at high risk for marasmus in poverty-stricken countries?

6.8 Nutrition and Your Health
Vegetarian and Plant-Based Dietary Patterns

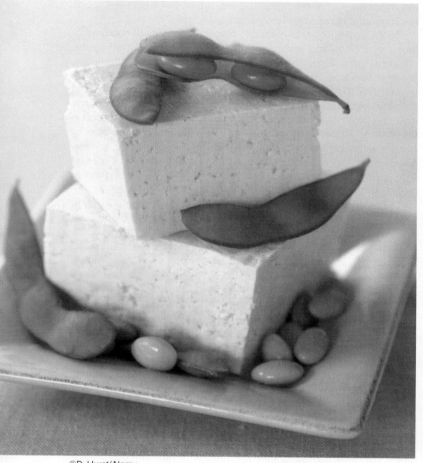

©D. Hurst/Alamy

There are many documented health benefits of following a vegetarian eating pattern. Studies show that death rates from some chronic diseases, such as certain forms of cardiovascular disease, hypertension, many forms of cancer, type 2 diabetes, and obesity, are lower for vegetarians than for nonvegetarians. Vegetarians often live longer, as shown in religious groups that practice vegetarianism. Other factors of healthful lifestyles, such as not smoking, abstaining from alcohol and drugs, and regular physical activity, are typical of vegetarians and probably partially account for the lower risks of chronic disease and longer lives seen in this population.

As you learned in Sections 2.2 and 2.3, the Dietary Guidelines for Americans and MyPlate emphasize a plant-based diet of whole grain breads and cereals, fruits, and vegetables. In addition, the American Institute for Cancer Research promotes "The New American Plate," which includes plant-based foods covering two-thirds (or more) of the plate and meat, fish, poultry, or low-fat dairy covering only one-third (or less) of the plate. Although these recommendations allow the inclusion of animal products, they are definitely more "vegetarian-like" than typical North American diets.

Vegetarianism has evolved over the centuries from a necessity into an option. A 2016 study from the Vegetarian Resource Group found 3.3% of U.S. adults (8 million people) to be vegetarian with only 3.7 million being strictly vegan.[15] Vegetarianism is popular among college students and campus dining services offer vegetarian options at every meal. According to the 2016 poll, 6% of young adults (18 to 34 years of age) are vegetarian or vegan. In contrast, only 2% of adults 65 years or older are vegetarian.

The growing popularity of vegetarian diets has prompted changes in the marketplace. Many restaurants offer vegetarian meals in response to the growing number of customers who want a vegetarian option when they eat out. Campus dining services offer vegetarian options at every meal.

As nutrition science has grown, new information has enabled the design of nutritionally adequate vegetarian diets. It is important for vegetarians to take advantage of this information because an eating pattern of only plant-based foods has the potential to promote various nutrient deficiencies and growth retardation in infants and children. People who choose a vegetarian eating pattern can meet their nutritional needs by following a few basic rules and knowledgeably planning their diets.

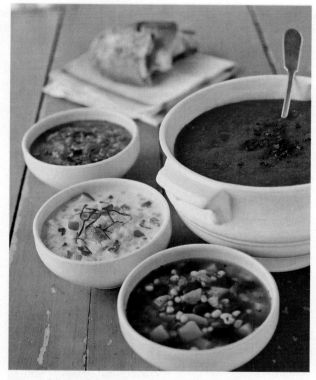

▲ Meatless Monday (www.meatlessmonday.com) is a nonprofit initiative that began in the United States in 2003 to reduce dietary saturated fat and is now worldwide, active in 44 countries. The Meatless Monday campaign recommends that we cut meat from our diet on Monday and thus encourages us to increase our consumption of fruits, vegetables, whole grains, and legumes. Ideally, this eating pattern will flow into other days of the week and translate into healthier eating habits. ©Jonelle Weaver/Getty Images

Why Do People Become Vegetarians?

People choose vegetarianism for a variety of reasons, including ethics, religion, economics, and health. Some believe that killing animals for food is unethical. Hindus and Trappist monks eat vegetarian meals as a practice of their religion. In North America, many Seventh Day Adventists base their practice of vegetarianism on Biblical texts and believe it is a more healthful way to live.

Some advocates of vegetarianism base their food preference upon the inefficient use of animals as a source of protein. In the United States, nearly 70% of the grain crop is used for animal feed, and globally 35% of the grain harvest is used to produce animal protein. Although animals that humans eat sometimes eat grasses that humans cannot digest, many also eat grains that humans can eat. According to the United Nations Environment Programme, it takes approximately 3 kilograms of grain to produce 1 kilogram of animal protein in cereal-fed animals.[2] An advantage of grass-fed livestock that eat from a pasture is that they convert grass into protein more efficiently than those raised on grains.

People might also practice vegetarianism because it limits saturated fat and cholesterol intake, while encouraging a high intake of complex carbohydrates; vitamins A, E, and C; carotenoids; magnesium; and fiber.

Good for Disease Prevention

Heart Health. Plant sources of proteins can positively impact heart health in several ways. First, the plant foods we eat contain no cholesterol nor *trans* fat and little saturated fat. As noted in Chapter 5, a vegan diet coupled with regular exercise and other lifestyle changes can lead to a reversal of atherosclerotic plaque in various arteries in the body. The major types of fat in plant foods are monounsaturated and polyunsaturated fats.

Beans and nuts contain soluble fiber, which binds to cholesterol in the small intestine and prevents it from being absorbed by the intestinal cells. Also, due to the activity of some phytochemicals, foods made from soybeans can lower production of cholesterol by the liver (by about 2% to 6%). Since 1999, the Food and Drug Administration (FDA) has allowed health claims for the cholesterol-lowering properties of soy foods, and the American Heart Association has recommended inclusion of some soy protein in the diets of people with high blood cholesterol. As noted in Chapter 2, to list a health claim for soy on the label, a food product must have at least 6.25 grams of soy protein and less than 3 grams of fat, 1 gram of saturated fat, and 20 milligrams of cholesterol per serving.

There are several other heart-protective compounds in plant foods. Some of the phytochemicals may help to prevent blood clots and relax the blood vessels. Nuts are an especially good source of nutrients implicated in heart health, including vitamin E, folate, magnesium, and copper. Frequent consumption of nuts (about 1 ounce of nuts five times per week) is associated with a decreased risk of cardiovascular disease. Recall from Chapter 2 that the FDA allows a provisional health claim on food labels to link nuts with a reduced risk of developing cardiovascular disease.

Cancer Prevention. The numerous phytochemicals in plant foods are also thought to aid in preventing cancers of the breast, prostate, and colon. Many of the proposed anticancer effects of foods containing plant protein are through antioxidant mechanisms (see the Newsworthy Nutrition in this section).[16,17] In 2012, the American Institute for Cancer Research added soy to its list and online tool *AICR's Foods That Fight Cancer.*[TM][17] This website summarizes the current and emerging evidence on soy and cancer risk, which indicates that for all cancers, human studies show soy foods do not increase risk and in some cases may even lower it. This is especially good news for breast cancer patients and survivors who need no longer worry about eating moderate amounts of soy

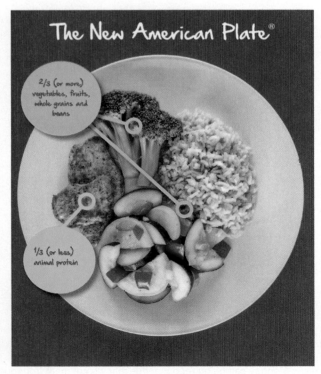

▲ "The New American Plate" published by the American Institute for Cancer Research was a forerunner of and embodies the same concepts as the MyPlate program.

Source: American Institute for Cancer Research.

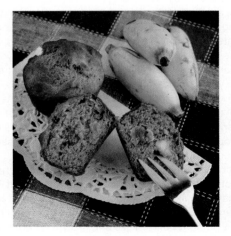

▲ Plant proteins, such as those in walnuts, can be incorporated into one's diet in numerous ways, such as adding them to banana nut muffins. ©YAY Media AS/Alamy

Newsworthy Nutrition

Vegetarian dietary patterns decrease risk of colorectal cancers

Because colorectal cancers are a leading cause of cancer deaths, it is of great interest to determine if eating patterns can decrease their risk. The hypothesis of this study presented an association between vegetarian dietary patterns and the incidence of cancers of the colon and rectum. The study design was a dietary assessment, using a validated quantitative food frequency questionnaire, of 77,659 Seventh-Day Adventist men and women for 7 years who were categorized into four vegetarian dietary patterns (vegan, lactoovovegetarian, pescovegetarian [a vegetarian who also eats aquatic animal protein], and semivegetarian) and a nonvegetarian dietary pattern. State cancer registries were used to identify cases of colorectal cancer. The results included 380 cases of colon cancer and 110 cases of rectal cancer during the 7.3-year follow-up of participants. As a group, vegetarians were 22% less likely to get colorectal cancers (19% for colon cancer; 29% for rectal cancer) than meat-eaters. When the risk was broken down by diet type, pescovegetarians had a 43% lower risk; vegans, 16%; lactoovovegetarians, 18%; and semivegetarians, 8% lower risk than meat-eaters. All of these effects were similar for men and women and for black and nonblack participants. These results support the hypothesis that vegetarian dietary patterns are associated with an overall lower incidence of colorectal cancers. Pescovegetarians had a much lower risk compared with nonvegetarians, suggesting that compounds in fish such as omega-3 fatty acids may play a protective role in the prevention of colorectal cancers.

Source: Orlich, MJ, et al. Vegetarian dietary patterns and the risk of colorectal cancer, *Journal of American Medical Association Internal Medicine* 175:767, 2015.

- Mix chopped walnuts into the batter of your banana bread to boost your intake of unsaturated fats.
- Eat soy nuts (oil-roasted soybeans) or edamame as a snack.
- Use peanut butter as your spread on bagels instead of butter or cream cheese.
- Make taco filling using a can of great northern beans heated with one-half packet of taco seasoning and chopped tomatoes.
- Use calcium-fortified soy milk, especially if you have lactose malabsorption or lactose intolerance.

FOOD PLANNING FOR VEGETARIANS

Of the estimated 3.3% of American adults who call themselves vegetarians, only about 1.5% are total vegetarians, or **vegans,** who eat only plant foods. **Fruitarians** primarily eat fruits, nuts, honey, and vegetable oils. This plan is not recommended because it can lead to nutrient deficiencies in people of all ages. **Lactovegetarians** and **ovovegetarians** are more liberal than vegans; they allow dairy and egg products, respectively, in their plant-based eating pattern. **Lactoovovegetarians** eat dairy products and eggs, as well as plant foods. These inclusions make food planning easier because the dairy and eggs are rich in some nutrients that are missing or minimal in plants, such as vitamin B-12 and calcium. The more variety in the diet, the easier it is to meet nutritional needs. A **pescovegetarian** diet, one that includes aquatic animal protein, has been associated with a lower risk of colon cancer (see the Newsworthy Nutrition in this section).[16] Anyone who goes meatless most of the time can call themselves a semivegetarian or a flexible vegetarian.

OPTIMIZING A VEGAN PLAN

Planning a vegan dietary pattern requires knowledge and creativity to yield high-quality protein and other key nutrients without animal

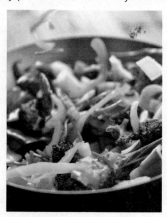

▲ Keep in mind that amino acids in vegetables are best used when a combination of sources is consumed. ©rez-art/iStockphoto/Getty Images

vegan A person who eats only plant foods.

fruitarian A person who primarily eats fruits, nuts, honey, and vegetable oils.

lactovegetarian A person who consumes plant products and dairy products.

ovovegetarian A person who consumes plant and egg products.

lactoovovegetarian A person who consumes plant products, dairy products, and eggs.

pescovegetarian A person who eats aquatic animal protein.

foods. Walnuts are another plant source of protein that have been recognized as an *AICR's Foods That Fight Cancer.*™[18]

Diabetes Control. Plants also may be particularly good sources of protein for people with diabetes or impaired glucose tolerance because the high fiber content of plant foods leads to a slower increase in blood glucose. Frequent nut consumption may reduce the risk of gallstones, obesity, and type 2 diabetes.

INCREASING PLANT PROTEINS IN YOUR DIET

The following are some suggestions for including plant proteins in your diet.

- Try a veggie burger instead of a hamburger. These are usually made from beans and come in a variety of delicious flavors. They are available in the frozen foods section of the grocery store, and many restaurants have added them to their menus.
- Sprinkle sunflower seeds or chopped almonds on top of your salad to add taste and texture.

TABLE 6-3 ■ **Food Plan for Vegetarians Based on MyPlate**

Food Group	MyPlate Servings		Key Nutrients Supplied‡
	Lactovegetarian*	Vegan†	
Grains	6–11	8–11	Protein, thiamin, niacin, folate, vitamin E, zinc, magnesium, iron, and fiber
Beans and other legumes	2–3	3	Protein, vitamin B-6, zinc, magnesium, and fiber
Nuts, seeds	2–3	3	Protein, vitamin E, and magnesium
Vegetables	3–5 (include 1 dark-green or leafy variety daily)	4–6 (include 1 dark-green or leafy variety daily)	Vitamin A, vitamin C, folate, vitamin K, potassium, and magnesium
Fruits	2–4	4	Vitamin A, vitamin C, and folate
Dairy Fortified soy milk	3 ——	—— 3	Protein, riboflavin, vitamin D, vitamin B-12, and calcium

*This plan contains about 75 grams of protein in 1650 kcal.

†This plan contains about 79 grams of protein in 1800 kcal.

‡One serving of vitamin- and mineral-enriched ready-to-eat breakfast cereal is recommended to meet possible nutrient gaps. Alternatively, a balanced multivitamin and mineral supplement can be used. Vegans also may benefit from the use of fortified soy milk to provide calcium, vitamin D, and vitamin B-12.

products.[18] In Section 6.3, you learned about complementary proteins, whereby the essential amino acids deficient in one protein source are supplied by those of another consumed at the same meal or the next (see Fig. 6-8). Many legumes are deficient in the essential amino acid methionine, whereas grains are limited in lysine. Eating a combination of legumes and grains, such as beans and rice, will supply the body with adequate amounts of all essential amino acids (see Fig. 6-8). As with any meal plan, variety is an especially important characteristic of a nutritious vegan dietary pattern. Table 6-3 lists vegetarian food plans, which emphasize grains, legumes, nuts, and seeds to help meet protein needs.

Aside from amino acids, low intakes of certain micronutrients can be a problem for the vegan. At the forefront of nutritional concerns are riboflavin, vitamin B-12, iron, zinc, iodine, calcium, and vitamin D. Although use of a balanced multivitamin and mineral supplement can help, the following dietary advice should be implemented.

Riboflavin can be obtained from green leafy vegetables, whole grains, yeast, and legumes—components of most vegan plans. Vitamin B-12 only occurs naturally in animal foods. Vegans can prevent a vitamin B-12 deficiency by finding a reliable source of this vitamin, such as fortified soybean milk, ready-to-eat breakfast cereals, and special nutritional yeast grown on media rich in vitamin B-12. Plants can contain soil or microbial contaminants that provide trace amounts of vitamin B-12, but these are negligible sources of the vitamin. Because the liver can store vitamin B-12 for about 4 years, it may take a long time for a vitamin B-12 deficiency to surface after removal of animal foods from the dietary pattern. If dietary B-12 inadequacy persists, deficiency can lead to anemia, nerve damage, and mental dysfunction. These deficiency consequences have been noted in the infants of vegetarian mothers whose breast milk was low in vitamin B-12.

For iron, the vegan can consume whole grains and ready-to-eat breakfast cereals, dried fruits and nuts, and legumes. The iron in these foods is not absorbed as well as iron in animal foods, but consuming these foods with a good source of vitamin C can enhance iron absorption. Cooking in iron pots and skillets can also add iron to food.

The vegan can find zinc in whole grains (especially ready-to-eat breakfast cereals), nuts, and legumes, but phytic acid and other substances in these foods limit zinc absorption. Breads are a good source of zinc because the leavening process (rising of the bread dough) reduces the influence of phytic acid. Iodized salt is a reliable source of iodine. It should be used instead of plain salt, both of which are found in U.S. supermarkets.

Of all nutrients, calcium and vitamin D are the most difficult to consume in sufficient quantities for vegans. Fortified foods including fortified soy milk, fortified orange juice, calcium-rich tofu (check the label), and certain ready-to-eat breakfast cereals and snacks are the vegan's best option for obtaining these nutrients. In addition to fortified foods, alternate sources of vitamin D include some mushroom varieties and regular sun exposure. Green leafy vegetables and nuts also contain calcium, but the mineral is either not well absorbed or not very plentiful from these sources. Dietary supplements are another option. Special diet planning is always required because even a multivitamin and mineral supplement will not supply enough calcium to meet the needs for bone health.

Consuming adequate quantities of omega-3 fatty acids is yet another nutritional concern for vegetarians, especially vegans. Fish and fish oils, abundant sources of these heart-healthy fats, are omitted from many types of vegetarian plans. Alternative plant sources of omega-3 fatty acids include canola oil, soybean oil, seaweed, microalgae, flax seeds, chia seeds, and walnuts.

Special Concerns for Infants and Children

Infants and children, notoriously picky eaters in the first place, are at highest risk for nutrient deficiencies as a result of improperly

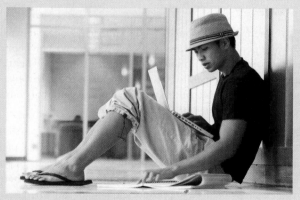

▲ Children can safely enjoy vegetarian and vegan diets as long as certain adjustments are made to meet their age-specific nutritional needs. ©Brand X Pictures/Getty Images

planned vegetarian and vegan dietary patterns. With the use of complementary proteins and good sources of the problem nutrients just discussed, the calorie and nutrient needs of vegetarian and vegan infants and children can be met.[18] The most common nutritional concerns for vegetarian and vegan infants and children are deficiencies of iron, vitamin B-12, vitamin D, and calcium.

Vegetarian and vegan plans tend to be high in bulky, high-fiber, low-calorie foods that cause a feeling of fullness. While this is a welcome advantage for most adults, children have small stomach capacity and relatively high nutrient needs, and thus may feel full before their calorie needs are met. The fiber content of a child's dietary pattern may need to be decreased by replacing high-fiber sources with some refined grain products, fruit juices, and peeled fruit. Other concentrated sources of calories for vegetarian and vegan children include fortified soy milk, nuts, dried fruits, and avocados.

CASE STUDY Planning a Vegetarian Dietary Pattern

Jordan is a freshman in college. He lives in a campus residence hall and teaches martial arts in the afternoon. He eats two or three meals a day at the residence hall cafeteria and snacks between meals. Jordan and his roommate both decided to become vegetarians because they recently read an article on a fitness website describing the health benefits of a vegetarian dietary pattern. Yesterday, Jordan's vegetarian plan consisted of a Danish pastry for breakfast and a tomato-rice dish (no meat) with pretzels and a diet soft drink for lunch. In the afternoon, after his martial arts class, he had a milkshake and two cookies. At dinnertime, he had a vegetarian sub sandwich consisting of lettuce, sprouts, tomatoes, cucumbers, and cheese, with two glasses of fruit punch. In the evening, he had a bowl of popcorn.

1. What type of health benefits can Jordan expect from following a well-planned vegetarian dietary pattern?
2. What is missing from Jordan's current dietary plan in terms of foods that should be emphasized in a vegetarian dietary pattern?
3. Which nutrients are missing in this current dietary plan?
4. Are there any food components in the current diet plan that should be minimized or avoided?
5. How could he improve his new dietary pattern at each meal and snack to meet his nutritional needs and avoid undesirable food components?

▲ Has Jordan planned a healthy and nutritious vegetarian dietary pattern? ©Purestock/SuperStock

Complete the Case Study. Responses to these questions can be provided by your instructor.

Summary (Numbers refer to numbered sections in the chapter.)

6.1 Amino acids, the building blocks of proteins, contain a very usable form of nitrogen for humans. Of the 20 common types of amino acids found in food, nine must be consumed in food (essential) and the rest can be synthesized by the body (nonessential).

6.2 Individual amino acids are bonded together to form proteins. The sequential order of amino acids determines the protein's ultimate shape and function. This order is directed by DNA in the cell nucleus. Diseases such as sickle cell anemia can occur if the amino acids are incorrect on a polypeptide chain. When the three-dimensional shape of a protein is unfolded—denatured—by treatment with heat, acid or alkaline solutions, or other processes, the protein also loses its biological activity.

6.3 Almost all animal products are nutrient-dense sources of protein. The high quality of these proteins means that they can be easily converted into body proteins. Rich plant sources of protein, such as beans, are also available.

High-quality (complete) protein foods contain ample amounts of all nine essential amino acids. Lower-quality (incomplete) protein foods lack sufficient amounts of one or more essential amino acids. This is typical of plant foods, especially cereal grains. Different types of plant foods eaten together often complement each other's amino acid deficits, thereby providing high-quality protein in the diet. Excessive intake of red meat, especially processed forms, has been linked to colon cancer and deaths caused by cardiovascular disease and cancer.

6.4 Protein digestion begins in the stomach, where stomach acid and pepsin break down proteins into shorter polypeptide chains of amino acids. In the small intestine, these polypeptide chains eventually separate into amino acids in the absorptive cells. The free amino acids then travel via the portal vein that connects to the liver. Some then enter the bloodstream.

6.5 Important body components—such as muscles, connective tissue, transport proteins in the bloodstream, visual pigments, enzymes, some hormones, and immune cells—are made of proteins. These proteins are in a state of constant turnover. The carbon chains of proteins may be used to produce glucose (or fat) when necessary.

6.6 The protein RDA for adults is 0.8 gram per kilogram of healthy body weight. This corresponds to 56 grams of protein daily for a 70-kilogram (154-pound) person and 46 grams per day for a 57-kilogram (125-pound) person. The North American diet generally supplies plenty of protein, with men consuming about 100 grams of protein daily and women consuming closer to 65 grams. These protein intakes are also of sufficient quality to support body functions. To maintain a state of protein balance, people need to balance protein intake with losses. A positive protein balance is needed to supply the raw materials required to build new tissues during growth or recovery from an illness or injury. To achieve this, a person must eat more protein daily than he or she loses. Consuming less protein than needed leads to negative protein balance, such as when acute illness reduces the desire to eat. Researchers now recommend that adults consume at least 30 grams of protein at each of three meals daily in order to maintain healthy muscles and bones.

Problems with high protein intakes primarily stem from eating patterns rich in animal products. A high-protein intake may overburden the kidneys by forcing them to excrete the extra nitrogen as urea. Due to this potential for imbalances and toxicities, the best practice to ensure adequacy is to stick to whole foods as sources of amino acids rather than supplements.

6.7 Undernutrition can lead to protein-calorie malnutrition in the form of kwashiorkor or marasmus. Kwashiorkor results primarily from an inadequate protein intake in comparison with body needs, which often increase with concurrent disease and infection. Kwashiorkor often occurs when a child is weaned from human milk and fed mostly starchy gruels. Marasmus results from extreme starvation—a negligible intake of both protein and calories. Marasmus commonly occurs during famine, especially in infants.

6.8 Vegetarian and other plant-based dietary patterns provide many health benefits, including lower risks of such chronic diseases as cardiovascular disease, diabetes, and certain cancers. The benefits associated with the plant-based diets appear to stem from the lower content of saturated fat and cholesterol and the higher amount of fiber, vitamins, minerals, and phytochemicals.

Check Your Knowledge (Answers are available at the end of this question set.)

1. The "instructions" for making proteins are located in the
   a. cell membrane.
   b. cell nucleus.
   c. cytoplasm.
   d. lysosome.

2. A nutrient that could easily be deficient in the diet of a vegan would be
   a. vitamin C.
   b. folic acid.
   c. calcium.
   d. carbohydrate.

3. An example of protein complementation used in vegetarian dietary planning would be the combination of
   a. cereal and milk.
   b. bacon and eggs.
   c. rice and beans.
   d. macaroni and cheese.

4. If an essential amino acid is unavailable for protein synthesis,
   a. then the cell will make the amino acid.
   b. then protein synthesis will stop.
   c. then the cell will continue to attach amino acids to the protein.
   d. then the partially completed protein will be stored for later completion.

5. An individual who eats only plant food is referred to as a
   a. planetarium.
   b. vegan.
   c. lactovegetarian.
   d. lactoovovegetarian.

6. Which of the following groups accounts for the differences among amino acids?
   a. Amine group
   b. Side chain
   c. Acid group
   d. Keto group

7. Absorption of amino acids primarily takes place in the
   a. stomach.
   b. liver.
   c. small intestine.
   d. large intestine.

8. Jack is not an athlete and weighs 176 pounds (80 kilograms). His daily protein requirement is _____ grams.
   a. 32
   b. 40
   c. 64
   d. 80

9. The basic building block of a protein is called a(n)
   a. fatty acid.
   b. monosaccharide.
   c. amino acid.
   d. gene.

10. Which of the following is true about protein intake of people in the United States?
   a. Most do not consume enough protein.
   b. Most consume the amount needed to balance losses.
   c. Athletes do not get enough protein without supplementation.
   d. Most consume more than is needed.

Answer Key: 1. b (LO 6.2), 2. c (LO 6.3), 3. c (LO 6.3), 4. b (LO 6.2), 5. b (LO 6.8), 6. b (LO 6.1), 7. c (LO 6.4), 8. c (LO 6.6), 9. c (LO 6.1), 10. d (LO 6.6)

Study Questions (Numbers refer to Learning Outcomes)

1. Discuss the relative importance of essential and nonessential amino acids in the diet. Why is it important for essential amino acids lost from the body to be replaced in the diet? **(LO 6.1)**

2. What is the role of cholecystokinin (CCK) in protein digestion? **(LO 6.4)**

3. What is a limiting amino acid? Explain why this concept is concern in a vegetarian diet. How can a vegetarian compensate for limiting amino acids in specific foods? **(LO 6.1)**

4. Briefly describe the organization of proteins. How can this organization be altered or damaged? What might be a result of damaged protein organization? **(LO 6.2)**

5. Describe four functions of proteins. Provide an example of how the structure of a protein relates to its function. **(LO 6.5)**

6. How are DNA and protein synthesis related? **(LO 6.2)**

7. What would be one health benefit of reducing high-protein intake(s) to RDA amounts for some people? **(LO 6.6)**

8. Which eight foods are the major sources of proteins that cause food allergies? **(LO 6.3)**

9. Outline the major differences between kwashiorkor and marasmus. **(LO 6.7)**

10. What are the possible long-term effects of an inadequate intake of dietary protein among children between the ages of 6 months and 4 years? **(LO 6.7)**

What the Dietitian Chose

Consuming adequate protein is important for muscle repair and synthesis, but it is not a good idea to take individual amino acid supplements. Your digestive tract is adapted to handle whole proteins: hydrochloric acid and enzymes break polypeptides into amino acids that can be absorbed by the cells of the small intestine. Taking large doses of one amino acid can impair the absorption and/or metabolism of other amino acids.

Studies have shown that consuming protein spread over multiple small meals throughout the day had less of an effect on muscle protein synthesis than eating the same total amount of protein in one or more large meals of at least 30 grams of protein. Whey protein, a by-product of cheese production from cow's milk, is considered to be a high-quality protein because it is easily digested and contains all of the essential amino acids. It is a source of the BCAAs valine, leucine, and isoleucine. BCAAs can be used for fuel by exercising muscles and are particularly important for synthesizing muscle tissue. The rationale is that whey protein supports muscle recovery and anabolism after exercise. Protein and amino acid supplements, however, are expensive and may be detrimental to health. Animal protein is often a source of excess total and saturated fat. Not only will this hinder efforts at weight loss, but it is detrimental to heart health. The unbalanced meal distribution of protein with more than 60% of daily protein consumed during a single evening meal and less than 15 g at breakfast is typical for many adults. Studies have now shown that protein distribution (and quantity of the amino acid leucine) is critical for optimum muscle protein synthesis.

Consuming at least 20 to 30 grams of protein at a given meal optimizes muscle protein growth. In addition, resistance exercise appears to increase the efficient use of the essential amino acids for muscle growth. It is safer and more economical to consume the high end of the recommended protein intake (35% of calories) well distributed over three meals and from a variety of lean sources of protein. This will pair best with a weight training program to optimize muscle growth.

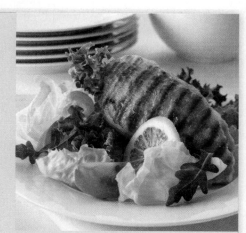
▲ This 4-ounce grilled chicken breast is an excellent choice, providing 38 grams of high-quality yet inexpensive lean protein. ©Ingram Publishing/SuperStock

Further Readings

1. Food and Agriculture Organization: *Dietary protein quality evaluation in human nutrition: Report of an FAO Expert Consultation.* FAO Food and Nutrition Paper 92, 2013. (Accessed January 21, 2017).

2. Sabate J and others: The environmental cost of protein food choices. *Public Health Nutr* 2015; 18:2067.

3. Dernini S and others: Med Diet 4.0: The Mediterranean diet with four sustainable benefits. *Public Health Nutr* 2016; 22:1.

4. Food and Agriculture Organization of the United Nations: *Dietary protein quality evaluation in human nutrition: Report of an FAO Expert Consultation.* FAO Food and Nutrition Paper 92, 2013.

5. Messina V: Nutritional and health benefits of dried beans. *Am J Clin Nutr* 2014; 100(suppl 1):437S.

6. Bouvard V and others: International Agency for Research on Cancer Monograph Working Group, et al. Carcinogenicity of consumption of red and processed meat. *Lancet Oncol* 2015; 16:1599.

7. Pan A and others: Red meat consumption and mortality: Results from two prospective cohort studies. *Arch Intern Med* 2012; 172:555.

8. Micha R and others: Red and processed meat consumption and risk of incident coronary heart disease, stroke, and diabetes mellitus: A systemic review and meta-analysis. *Circulation* 2010; 121:2271.

9. Haring B and others: Dietary protein sources and risk for incident chronic kidney disease: Results from the Atherosclerosis Risk in Communities (ARIC) Study. *J Ren Nutr* 2017 (in press). (Epub ahead of print; DOI: http://dx.doi.org/10.1053/j.jrn.2016.11.004).

10. Fleischer DM and others: Primary prevention of allergic disease through nutritional interventions. *J Allergy Clin Immunol: In Practice* 2013; 1:29.

11. Cooper CC: Gluten free and healthy. *Today's Dietitian* 2012; 14(5):24.

12. Bauer J and others: Evidence-based recommendations for optimal dietary protein intake in older people: A position paper from the PROT-AGE Study Group. *J Am Med Dir Assoc* 2013; 14:542.

13. Layman, DK and others: Defining meal requirements for protein to optimize metabolic roles of amino acids. *Am J Clin Nutr* 2015; 101(Suppl):1330S.

14. Barker LA and others: Hospital malnutrition: Prevalence, identification and impact on patients and the healthcare system. *Int J Environ Res Public Health* 2011; 8:514.

15. Stahler C: How often do Americans eat vegetarian meals? And how many adults in the U.S. are vegetarian? The Vegetarian Resource Group website. http://www.vrg.org/nutshell/Polls/2016_adults_veg.htm. (Accessed January 25, 2017).

16. Orlich MJ and others: Vegetarian dietary patterns and the risk of colorectal cancers. *J Amer Med Asso Intern Med* 2015; 175:767.

17. American Institute for Cancer Research: *AICR'S Foods That Fight Cancer™* http://www.aicr.org/foods-that-fight-cancer/ (Accessed January 25, 2017).

18. Academy of Nutrition and Dietetics: Position of the Academy of Nutrition and Dietetics: Vegetarian diets. *J Acad Nutr Diet* 2016; 116:1970.

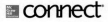 **To get the most out of your study, visit Connect where you will find NutritionCalc Plus, SmartBook®, and many other dynamic tools.**

Rate Your Plate

Protein and the Vegetarian

Alana weighs 110 pounds and is excited about all the health benefits that might accompany a vegetarian dietary pattern. However, she is concerned that she will not consume enough protein to meet her needs. She is also concerned about possible vitamin and mineral deficiencies. Use NutritionCalc Plus or a food composition table to calculate her protein intake and see if her concerns are valid.

	Protein (grams)
Breakfast Calcium-fortified orange juice, 1 cup Soy milk, 1 cup Fortified bran flakes, 1 cup Banana, medium	
Snack Calcium-enriched granola bar	
Lunch Garden burger, 4 ounces Whole wheat bun Mustard, 1 tbsp Soy cheese, 1 ounce Apple, medium Green leaf lettuce, 1 ½ cups Peanuts, 1 ounce Sunflower seeds, 1/4 cup Tomato slices, 2 Mushrooms, 3 Vinaigrette salad dressing, 2 tbsp Iced tea	
Dinner Kidney beans, 1/2 cup Brown rice, 3/4 cup Fortified margarine, 2 tbsp Mixed vegetables, 1/4 cup Hot tea	
Dessert Strawberries, 1/2 cup Angel food cake, 1 small slice Soy milk, 1/2 cup	
	Total Protein (grams) _____

Alana's dietary plan contained 2150 kcal, with _____ grams (you fill in) of protein (Is this plenty for her?), 360 grams of carbohydrate, 57 grams of total dietary fat (only 9 grams of which came from saturated fat), and 50 grams of fiber. Her vitamin and mineral intake with respect to those of concern to vegetarians—vitamin B-12, vitamin D, calcium, iron, and zinc—met her needs. How many grams of protein did Alana consume at each meal? Was her protein intake distributed evenly over her three main meals?

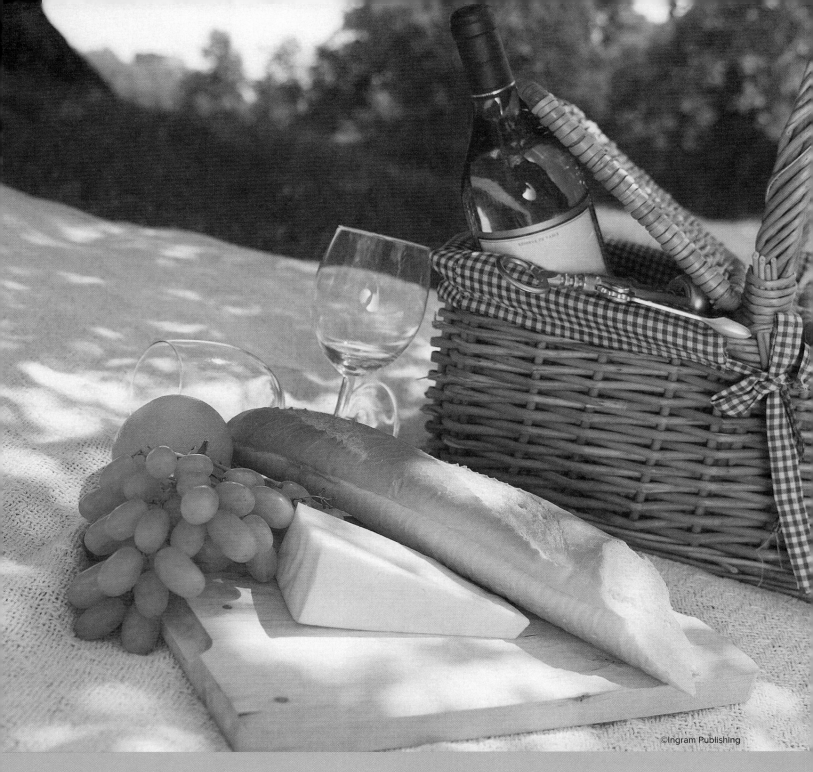

©Ingram Publishing

Student Learning Outcomes

Chapter 7 is designed to allow you to:

7.1 Describe energy balance and the various uses of energy by the body.

7.2 Compare methods to determine energy use by the body.

7.3 Discuss methods for assessing body composition and determining whether body weight and composition are healthy.

7.4 Explain obesity risk factors and related health consequences.

7.5 List and discuss characteristics of a sound weight-loss program.

7.6 Describe why reduced calorie intake is key to weight loss and maintenance.

7.7 Discuss why physical activity is a key component in weight loss and especially important for later weight maintenance.

Chapter 7
Energy Balance and Weight Control

In the last 25 years, there has been a dramatic increase in the percentage of individuals who are overweight or obese. Recall from Chapter 1 that the obesity epidemic remains a crisis not only in the United States but also globally among affluent people and in developing countries where Westernized dietary patterns (high saturated fat, refined sugars, and sodium) are increasing in popularity while more sedentary lifestyles are adopted. Excess body fat increases the likelihood of many health problems, such as cardiovascular disease, cancer, hypertension, stroke, bone and joint disorders, and type 2 diabetes, especially if a person performs minimal physical activity.

Currently, most diets fail before dieters reach a healthy weight range. Popular ("fad") diets are generally monotonous, highly restrictive, and short-lived. Many of these diets may even endanger some vulnerable populations, such as children, teenagers, pregnant women, and individuals with various health issues. A more logical approach is to change lifestyle behaviors. Focusing on altering dietary and physical activity patterns should include: (1) reducing calorie intake; (2) increasing physical activity; and (3) changing behaviors and patterns.[1]

A variety of organizations, including government agencies, the food industry, health professionals, and community groups, have begun to address the obesity epidemic in North America. It is expected that without a national effort to promote effective new approaches to maintaining healthy weight, the current trends will continue (Fig. 7-1).[2] This chapter will guide you into a deeper understanding of the causes, consequences, and potential treatments of overweight and obesity.

7.8   Describe how modifying lifestyle behaviors fits into a sound and sustainable weight-loss program.

7.9   Outline the pros and cons of various weight-loss methods for severe obesity.

7.10   Discuss the causes and treatment of underweight.

7.11   Evaluate popular weight-reduction methods, and determine which are safest and most successful.

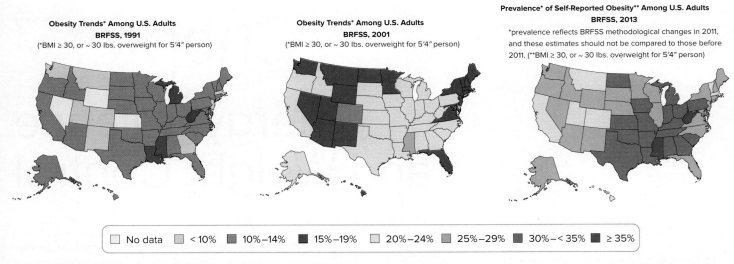

Obesity Trends* Among U.S. Adults
BRFSS, 1991
(*BMI ≥ 30, or ~ 30 lbs. overweight for 5′4″ person)

Obesity Trends* Among U.S. Adults
BRFSS, 2001
(*BMI ≥ 30, or ~ 30 lbs. overweight for 5′4″ person)

Prevalence* of Self-Reported Obesity Among U.S. Adults**
BRFSS, 2013
*prevalence reflects BRFSS methodological changes in 2011, and these estimates should not be compared to those before 2011. (**BMI ≥ 30, or ~ 30 lbs. overweight for 5′4″ person)

☐ No data   ☐ < 10%   ☐ 10%–14%   ☐ 15%–19%   ☐ 20%–24%   ☐ 25%–29%   ☐ 30%–< 35%   ☐ ≥ 35%

FIGURE 7-1 ▲ Obesity trends among U.S. adults: 1991, 2001, 2013.

Source: CDC Behavioral Risk Factor Surveillance System

7.1 Energy Balance

We begin this chapter with good and bad news. The good news is that if you obtain and maintain a healthy body weight, you increase your chances of living a long and healthy life. The bad news is that over 70% of all North American adults are overweight or obese, significantly more than in the 1980s. Of those, about 37% of adults and 17% of youth are obese (Fig. 7-2). There is a good chance that any of us could become part of those statistics if we do not pay attention to the prevention of significant weight gain in adulthood. Rapid weight gain (> 10 pounds) signals that a reevaluation of lifestyle is in order.

The prevalence and trends in obesity in the United States have been analyzed in several studies. One such study estimated the prevalence of adult obesity and severe obesity through the year 2030 using statistical modeling of Centers for Disease Control and Prevention (CDC) obesity data. The study estimated a 33% increase in obesity prevalence and a 130% increase in severe obesity

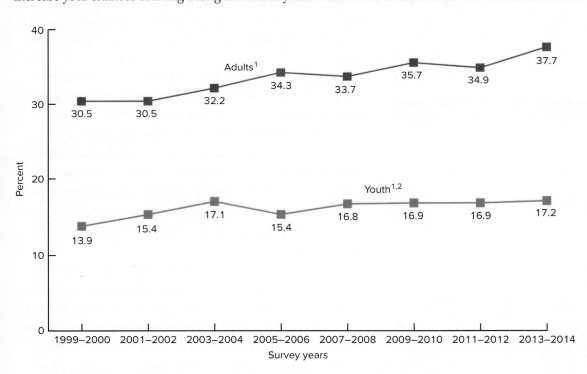

[1]Significant increasing linear trend from 1999–2000 through 2013–2014.

[2]Test for linear trend for 2003–2004 through 2013–2014 not significant ($p > 0.05$).

NOTE: All adult estimates are age-adjusted by the direct method to the 2000 U.S. census population using the age groups 20–39, 40–59, and 60 and over.

FIGURE 7-2 ▲ Trends in obesity prevalence among adults aged 20 and over (age-adjusted) and youth aged 2–19 years: United States, 1999–2000 through 2013–2014.[3]

Source: CDC/NCHS, National Health and Nutrition Examination Survey

prevalence over the next two decades, with 51% of the population projected to be obese by 2030. If obesity rates stop climbing and remain at current levels, the savings in medical expenditures over the next two decades would be over $549 billion.[4]

There is no quick cure for overweight or obesity, despite what many advertisements claim. The most reliable and successful weight loss comes from hard work and commitment. A combination of decreased calorie intake, increased physical activity, and behavior modification is considered to be the most reliable treatment for the overweight condition. And without a doubt, the *prevention* of the overweight condition in the first place is the most successful approach.

POSITIVE AND NEGATIVE ENERGY BALANCE

A healthy weight can result from paying more attention to the important concept of **energy balance** (Fig. 7-3). Think of energy balance as an equation consisting of energy input and energy output:

> Energy input   =   Energy output
> (calories from food intake)   (metabolism; digestion, absorption, and transport of nutrients; physical activity)

The balance of energy (or calories, measured in kilocalories) on the two sides of this equation can influence energy stores, especially the amount of triglyceride stored in adipose tissue. When energy input is greater than energy output, the result is **positive energy balance.** The excess calories consumed are stored in the body, which results in weight gain. There are some situations in which positive energy balance is normal and healthy. During pregnancy and lactation (breastfeeding), a surplus of calories supports the developing fetus. Infants and children also require a positive energy balance for normal growth and development during youth and puberty. In adults, however, even a small positive energy balance typically results in fat storage rather than muscle and bone and, over time, this can contribute to increased body fatness.

On the other hand, if energy input is less than energy output, there is a calorie deficit and **negative energy balance** results. A negative energy balance is necessary for successful weight loss. It is important to realize that when we lose weight, we typically lose some lean tissue in addition to adipose tissue.

The maintenance of energy balance while at an optimal weight substantially contributes to optimal health and well-being by minimizing the risk of developing many common health problems associated with increased body fat. Adulthood is often a time of subtle weight which can lead to obesity and a greater risk of disease if left unchecked. Aging does not directly cause weight gain; rather the problem stems from a pattern of excess energy intake coupled with limited physical activity and slower metabolism. Now, let us explore the factors that affect the energy balance equation.

ENERGY INTAKE

Energy needs are met by dietary intake, represented by the number of calories consumed each day. Determining the appropriate amount and type of food to meet our energy needs is a challenge for many of us. Our desire to consume food and the ability of our bodies to use it efficiently are survival mechanisms that have evolved with humans. The overabundance of energy-dense food and high-calorie beverages lead to overconsumption and excess stores of body fat. Given the cheap cost and wide availability of palatable food in vending machines, drive-through windows, social gatherings, and fast-food restaurants—combined with *supersized* portions—it is no wonder that the average adult is 10 pounds heavier than just 10 years ago.

The total annual cost attributable to obesity-related disease is about $200 billion in the United States. This is double what it was nearly a decade ago. At least half of this cost is supported by the taxpayers, who fund Medicare and Medicaid.

energy balance The state in which energy (calorie) intake, in the form of food and beverages, matches the energy expended, primarily through basal metabolism and physical activity.

positive energy balance The state in which energy intake is greater than energy expended, generally resulting in weight gain.

negative energy balance The state in which energy intake is less than energy expended, resulting in weight loss.

Weight Status Objectives from *Healthy People 2020*
- Increase by 10% the proportion of adults who are at a healthy weight.
  - Target for 2020:   33.9%
  - Baseline in 2005–2008:   30.8%
- Reduce by 10% the proportion of adults who are obese.
  - Target for 2020:   30.6%
  - Baseline in 2005–2008:   34.0%
- Reduce by 10% the proportion of children and adolescents, 2 to 19 years, who are considered obese.
  - Target for 2020:   14.6%
  - Baseline in 2005–2008:   16.2%
- Prevent inappropriate weight gain in youth and adults.

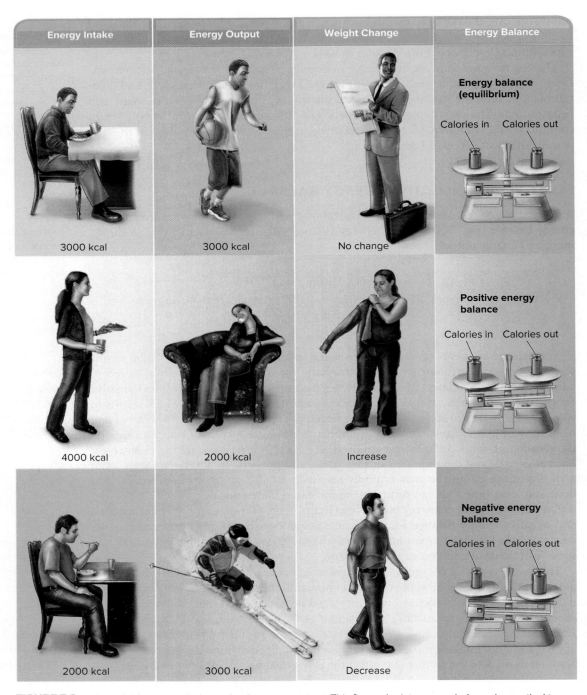

Energy Intake	Energy Output	Weight Change	Energy Balance
3000 kcal	3000 kcal	No change	**Energy balance (equilibrium)** Calories in Calories out
4000 kcal	2000 kcal	Increase	**Positive energy balance** Calories in Calories out
2000 kcal	3000 kcal	Decrease	**Negative energy balance** Calories in Calories out

FIGURE 7-3 ▲ A model for energy balance: Intake versus output. This figure depicts energy balance in practical terms.

bomb calorimeter An instrument used to determine the calorie content of a food.

The number of calories in a food is determined with an instrument called a **bomb calorimeter.** This calorie determination is shown in Figure 7-4. The bomb calorimeter measures the amount of calories (kilocalories) coming from carbohydrate, fat, protein, and alcohol. Recall that carbohydrates and proteins each yield 4 kcal per gram, fats yield 9 kcal per gram, and alcohol yields 7 kcal per gram. These calorie estimates have been adjusted for: (1) the body's ability to digest the food; and (2) substances in food, such as fibrous plant parts, that burn in the bomb calorimeter but are not absorbed by our bodies, so they do not provide calories to the human body. The figures are then rounded to whole numbers.

ENERGY OUTPUT

The body uses energy for three general purposes: (1) basal metabolism; (2) physical activity; and (3) digestion, absorption, and processing of ingested nutrients. A fourth minor form of energy output, known as adaptive thermogenesis, refers to energy expended during fidgeting or shivering when cold (Fig. 7-5).

Basal Metabolism. **Basal metabolism** is expressed as basal metabolic rate (BMR) and represents the minimal amount of calories expended in a fasting state to keep a resting, awake body alive in a warm, quiet environment. For a sedentary person, basal metabolism accounts for about 60% to 75% of total energy use by the body. Some of the processes that utilize energy include the beating of the heart, respiration by the lungs, and the activity required by other organs, such as the liver, brain, and kidney. It does not include energy used for physical activity or digestion, absorption, and processing of recently consumed nutrients. If the person is not fasting or completely rested, the term **resting metabolism** is used and expressed as resting metabolic rate (RMR). An individual's RMR is typically higher than his or her BMR.

To see how basal metabolism contributes to energy needs, consider a 130-pound woman. First, knowing that there are 2.2 pounds (lbs) for every kilogram (kg), convert her weight into metric units:

$$130 \text{ lb} \div 2.2 \text{ lb/kg} = 59 \text{ kg}$$

Then, using a rough estimate of BMR of 0.9 kcal per kilogram per hour for an average female (note 1 kcal per kilogram per hour is used for an average male), and calculate her BMR:

$$59 \text{ kg} \times 0.9 \text{ kcal/kg} = 53 \text{ kcal/hr}$$

Finally, use this hourly BMR to find her BMR for an entire day (24 hours):

$$53 \text{ kcal/hr} \times 24 \text{ hr} = 1272 \text{ kcal/day}$$

These calculations provide an estimate of basal metabolism, as it can vary as much as 25% to 30% among individuals.

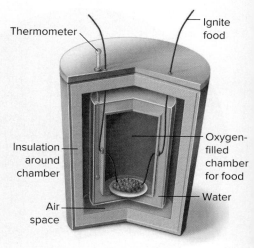

FIGURE 7-4 ▲ Bomb calorimeters measure calorie content by igniting and burning a dried portion of food. The burning food raises the temperature of the water surrounding the chamber holding the food. The increase in water temperature indicates the number of calories in the food because 1 kcal equals the amount of heat needed to raise the temperature of 1 kilogram of water by 1 degree Celsius.

basal metabolism The minimal amount of calories the body uses to support itself in a fasting state when resting and awake in a warm, quiet environment. It amounts to roughly 1 kcal per kilogram per hour for men and 0.9 kcal per kilogram per hour for women; these values are often referred to as *basal metabolic rate (BMR)*.

resting metabolism The amount of calories the body uses when the person has not eaten in 4 hours and is resting (e.g., 15 to 30 minutes) and awake in a warm, quiet environment. It is usually slightly higher (10%) than basal metabolism due to the less strict criteria for the test; often referred to as *resting metabolic rate (RMR)*.

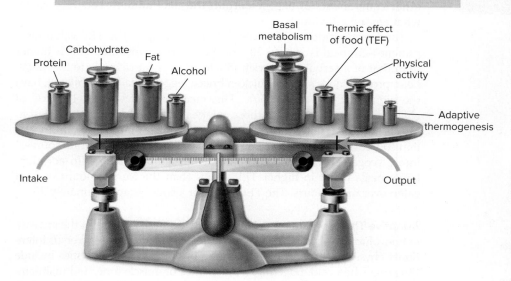

FIGURE 7-5 ▲ The components of energy intake and expenditure. This figure incorporates the major variables that influence energy balance. *Remember that alcohol is an additional source of energy.* The size of each weight on the scale represents the relative contribution of that component to energy balance.

CRITICAL THINKING

As she gets closer to age 30, a 28-year-old classmate of yours has been thinking about the process of aging. One of the things she fears most as she gets older is gaining weight. How would you suggest that she adjust her energy balance as she gets older?

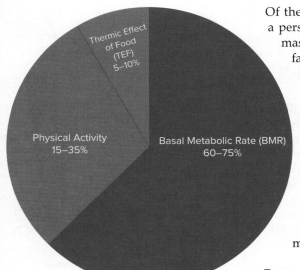

FIGURE 7-6 ▲ Contributions of BMR, activity, and TEF to energy output.

thermic effect of food (TEF) The increase in metabolism that occurs during the digestion, absorption, and metabolism of energy-yielding nutrients. This represents 5% to 10% of calories consumed.

adaptive thermogenesis This term refers to the ability of humans to regulate body temperature within narrow limits (thermoregulation). Two visible examples of thermogenesis are fidgeting and shivering when cold.

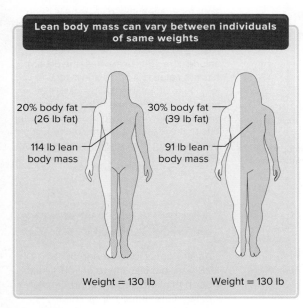

FIGURE 7-7 ▲ Lean body mass (LBM), the most important determinant of the basal metabolic rate, varies greatly between individuals. Persons of the same body weight can have different amounts of LBM and body fat and, therefore, have varying energy needs.

Of the factors affecting BMR listed in Figure 7-6, the amount of lean body mass a person has is the most important. Persons with higher amounts of lean body mass have a higher BMR because lean tissue is more metabolically active than fat. The lean tissue, therefore, requires more energy to support its activity. Although overweight and obese persons have an increased amount of body fat, they also typically have a high amount of lean body mass to support their weight and therefore a high BMR to go along with it (Fig. 7-7).

In contrast to factors that increase basal metabolism, a low calorie intake, such as an extreme diet regime, decreases basal metabolism by about 10% to 20% (about 150 to 300 kcal per day) as the body shifts into a conservation or starvation mode. In addition, the effects of aging also make weight maintenance a challenge. As lean body mass slowly and steadily decreases, basal metabolism declines 1% to 2% for each decade past the age of 30. However, because physical activity helps maintain lean body mass, remaining active as one ages helps to preserve a higher basal metabolism and, in turn, aids in weight control.

Energy for Physical Activity Physical activity increases energy expenditure above and beyond basal energy needs by as much as 15% to 35%. The calorie expenditure from physical activity varies widely among people. For example, climbing stairs rather than riding the elevator, walking rather than driving to class, and standing at a workstation rather than sitting for long periods all increase physical activity and, hence, energy use. The increasing incidence of obesity in North America is partially the result of our inactivity and sedentary lifestyles. Jobs demand less physical activity, and leisure time for many is often spent in front of a television or computer screen.

Thermic Effect of Food In addition to basal metabolism and physical activity, the body uses energy to digest food, and absorb and further process the nutrients recently consumed. Energy used for these tasks is referred to as the **thermic effect of food (TEF).** TEF is similar to a sales tax; it is like being charged about 5% to 10% for the total amount of calories you eat to cover the cost of processing that food. This "tax," equates to between 5 and 10 kcal extra for every 100 kcal needed for basal metabolism and physical activity. If your daily calorie intake was 3000 kcal, for example, TEF would account for 150 to 300 kcal. As with other components of energy output, the total amount can vary somewhat among individuals.

Food composition influences TEF. For example, the TEF value for a protein-rich meal is 20% to 30% of the calories consumed and is higher than that of a carbohydrate-rich (5% to 10%) or fat-rich (0% to 3%) meal. Lean protein foods such as chicken breast, egg whites, and whitefish have the highest TEF at almost 30%. This means that if you eat 100 kcal of chicken breast, almost 30 of those calories are burned off just to digest it. This is because it takes more energy to metabolize amino acids (from protein sources) into fat than to convert glucose (from carbohydrate sources) into glycogen or transfer absorbed fat into adipose stores. In addition, large meals result in higher TEF values than the same amount of food eaten over many hours. The TEF value for alcohol is approximately 20%.

Adaptive Thermogenesis **Adaptive thermogenesis** represents the increase in nonvoluntary physical activity triggered by reflex responses (versus intentional physical activity). Some examples of nonvoluntary activities include shivering when cold, fidgeting, maintenance of muscle tone, and maintaining body posture when not lying down. Some activities, such as eating, include both types of movement. Chewing is a voluntary movement, while the muscular contractions of the esophagus and intestine are not under conscious control.

The contribution of thermogenesis to overall calorie output is fairly small. The combination of BMR and TEF accounts for 70% to 85% of energy used by a sedentary person. The remaining 15% to 30% is used mostly for physical activity, with a small amount used for thermogenesis.

Brown adipose tissue is a specialized form of adipose tissue that is brown in color and participates in thermogenesis. The brown appearance results from its greater number of mitochondria. Brown fat contributes to thermogenesis by releasing some of the energy from energy-yielding nutrients into the environment as heat instead of producing ATP. Hibernating animals use brown adipose tissue to generate heat to withstand a long winter. In infants, brown adipose tissue is metabolically active and contributes as much as 5% of body weight and regulates heat to protect internal organs. Adults have very little brown adipose tissue, and its role in adulthood remains unknown.

While a person (130-pound woman) is resting, the percentage of total energy use and corresponding energy use by various organs are approximately:

Brain	19%	242 kcal/day
Skeletal muscle	18%	229 kcal/day
Liver	27%	343 kcal/day
Kidney	10%	127 kcal/day
Heart	7%	89 kcal/day
Other	19%	242 kcal/day
Total	100%	1272 kcal/day

✓ CONCEPT CHECK 7.1

1. What are the main components of energy balance?
2. How is the energy content of food determined and expressed?
3. What are the main purposes for which the body uses energy? Approximately how much does each component contribute to overall energy use by the body?

7.2 Determination of Energy Use by the Body

The amount of energy a body uses can be measured by both direct and indirect calorimetry or can be estimated based on height, weight, degree of physical activity, and age.

DIRECT AND INDIRECT CALORIMETRY

Direct calorimetry measures the amount of body heat released by a person. The individual is put into an insulated metabolic chamber, often the size of a very small bedroom, and over the course of 24 hours, body heat released raises the temperature of a layer of water surrounding the chamber. A calorie (kilocalorie), as you recall, is related to the amount of heat required to raise the temperature of water. By measuring the water temperature in the direct calorimeter before and after the body releases heat, the energy expended can be calculated. Direct calorimetry works because almost all the energy used by the body eventually leaves as heat. However, because of its expense and complexity, direct calorimetry is rarely used.

The most commonly used method of **indirect calorimetry** measures the respiratory gas exchange, which is the amount of oxygen a person consumes and the amount of carbon dioxide he or she expels (Fig. 7-8). A relationship exists between the body's use of energy and oxygen. For example, when metabolizing a typical mixed diet of the energy-yielding nutrients (carbohydrate, fat, or protein), the human body uses 1 liter of oxygen to yield about 4.85 kcal of energy.

Instruments to measure oxygen consumption for indirect calorimetry are widely used, relatively inexpensive, and portable. They can be mounted on carts (metabolic carts) or carried in a backpack while a person engages in physical activity to measure how many calories are burned during these activities. There are even portable instruments to estimate indirect calorimetry. Tables presenting energy costs of various forms

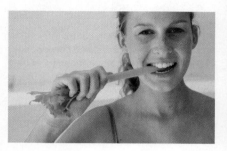

▲ A few foods, such as celery, have been hypothesized to use more calories for TEF than they contain, making them negative calorie foods. Despite its recurring popularity in fad diet plans, there is no scientific evidence supporting the idea that any food is calorically negative. Although these foods still yield some calories, they remain excellent choices to include in a weight-loss plan because they have such low energy density. ©Ingram Publishing

brown adipose tissue A specialized form of adipose (fat) tissue that produces large amounts of heat by metabolizing energy-yielding nutrients without synthesizing much useful energy for the body. The unused energy is released as heat.

direct calorimetry A method of determining a body's energy use by measuring heat released from the body. An insulated chamber is typically used.

indirect calorimetry A method to measure energy use by the body by measuring oxygen uptake and carbon dioxide output. Formulas are then used to convert this gas exchange value into energy use, estimating the proportion of energy nutrients that are being oxidized for energy in the fuel mix.

of exercises rely on information gained from indirect calorimetry studies. You will also see an estimation of calories burned during a workout on most exercise equipment and wearable fitness tracking devices. The accuracy of these values is discussed in Section 7.7.

ESTIMATES OF ENERGY NEEDS

As covered in Section 2.6, the Food and Nutrition Board has published a number of formulas to estimate energy needs, referred to as *Estimated Energy Requirements* (EER). Those for adults are shown below. As you calculate your own EER, remember to do multiplication and division before addition and subtraction! The calories used for basal metabolism are already factored into these formulas.

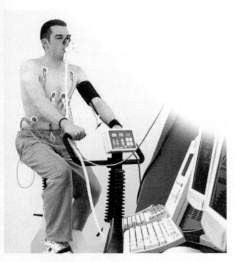

FIGURE 7-8 ▲ Indirect calorimetry measures oxygen intake and carbon dioxide output from respirations to predict energy expended during activities. ©Samuel Ashfield/ScienceSource

The variables in the formulas correspond to the following:

EER = Estimated Energy Requirement
AGE = age in years
PA = physical activity estimate (see following table)
WT = weight in kilograms (pounds divided by 2.2)
HT = height in meters (inches divided by 39.4)

Estimated Energy Requirement Calculation for Men 19 Years and Older:

$$EER = 662 - (9.53 \times AGE) + PA \times (15.91 \times WT + 539.6 \times HT)$$

Estimated Energy Requirement Calculation for Women 19 Years and Older:

$$EER = 354 - (6.91 \times AGE) + PA \times (9.36 \times WT + 726 \times HT)$$

Track Your Energy Needs

Use the forms in Appendix C to track your energy expenditure and estimate your energy needs. List all of your activities for a 24-hour period. Record the number of minutes spent in each activity to total 1440 minutes (24 hours in a day). Record the energy cost, in calories, for each activity, and multiply the energy cost by the minutes to obtain the energy expended for each activity. Total all the calorie values for your estimated energy expenditure for the day.

Physical Activity (PA) Estimates

Activity Level	PA (Men)	PA (Women)
Sedentary (e.g., no exercise)	1.00	1.00
Low activity (e.g., walks the equivalent of 2 miles per day at 3 to 4 mph)	1.11	1.12
Active (e.g., walks the equivalent of 7 miles per day at 3 to 4 mph)	1.25	1.27
Very active (e.g., walks the equivalent of 17 miles per day at 3 to 4 mph)	1.48	1.45

The following is a sample calculation for a man who is 25 years old, 5 feet 9 inches (1.75 meters), 154 pounds (70 kilograms), and has an active lifestyle. His EER is as follows:

$$EER = 662 - (9.53 \times 25) + 1.25 \times (15.91 \times 70 + 539.6 \times 1.75) = 2997 \text{ kcal}$$

The next equation is a sample calculation for a woman who is 25 years old, 5 feet 4 inches (1.62 meters), 120 pounds (54.5 kilograms), and has an active lifestyle. Her EER is as follows:

$$EER = 354 - (6.91 \times 25) + 1.27 \times (9.36 \times 54.5 + 726 \times 1.62) = 2323 \text{ kcal}$$

You have determined the man's EER to be about 3000 kcal and the woman's EER to be about 2300 kcal per day. Remember that this is only an estimate; many other factors, such as genetics and hormones, can also affect actual energy needs.

The www.ChooseMyPlate.gov website provides an interactive tool to estimate your calorie needs called MyPlate Checklist Calculator. Figure 7-9 shows the range of activity levels and calorie recommendations for age and gender groups.

✅ **CONCEPT CHECK 7.2**

1. What methods can be used to measure energy use by the body?
2. Estimated Energy Requirement (EER) can be calculated based on what five factors?

7.3 Assessing Healthy Body Weight

Numerous methods are used to establish what body weight should be, typically called *healthy weight*. Older terms, such as *ideal weight* and *desirable body weight,* are subjective and are no longer used in the literature. Several tables exist, generally based on weight-for-height criteria. When applied to a population, they provide adequate estimates of weight associated with health and longevity; however, they do not necessarily indicate the healthiest body weight for each individual. For example, athletes with more lean muscle mass but low fat mass will often have higher body weights (and BMI) than sedentary individuals.

Listening to the body's hunger cues, regularly eating a balanced and healthy dietary pattern, and remaining physically active are all positive behaviors that help one maintain a healthy weight over time. Healthy body weight is based upon both personal and individual factors. Body weight must be considered in terms of overall health, not a mathematical calculation. Under the guidance of a registered dietitian nutritionist or primary care provider, an individual can establish a *personal* healthy weight based on weight history, body fat distribution patterns, physical activity, dietary patterns, family history of obesity, and current health status.

Indications that your weight may be unhealthy include the following:
- Hypertension (high blood pressure)
- Elevated non-HDL cholesterol
- Family history of obesity or obesity-related diseases
- Pattern of upper-body (apple-shaped) android fat distribution
- Elevated blood glucose (hyperglycemia)

These criteria and current height/weight standards serve only as a rough guide. A healthy lifestyle may make a more important contribution to a person's health status than the number on the scale. Being fit and overweight are not necessarily mutually exclusive, and neither is *thin* synonymous with *healthy* if the person is not physically active.

BODY MASS INDEX

Currently, **body mass index (BMI)** is the most widely used weight-for-height standard because it is a noninvasive clinical measurement related to risk of disease for most individuals (Fig. 7-10).

$$\text{Body mass index} = \frac{\text{body weight (in kilograms)}}{\text{height}^2 \text{ (in meters)}}$$

An alternate method for calculating BMI is $\dfrac{\text{weight (pounds)} \times 703}{\text{height}^2 \text{ (inches)}}$

MyPlate Calorie Guidelines		
Children	**Sedentary** ⟶	**Active**
2–3 years	1000 ⟶	1400
Females	**Sedentary** ⟶	**Active**
4–8 years	1200 ⟶	1800
9–13	1400 ⟶	2200
14–18	1800 ⟶	2400
19–30	1800 ⟶	2400
31–50	1800 ⟶	2200
51+	1600 ⟶	2200
Males	**Sedentary** ⟶	**Active**
4–8 years	1200 ⟶	2000
9–13	1600 ⟶	2600
14–18	2000 ⟶	3200
19–30	2400 ⟶	3000
31–50	2200 ⟶	3000
51+	2000 ⟶	2800

FIGURE 7-9 ▲ MyPlate Calorie Guidelines for age and gender.

body mass index (BMI) Weight (in kilograms) divided by height (in meters) squared; a value of 25 and above indicates overweight and a value of 30 and above indicates obesity.

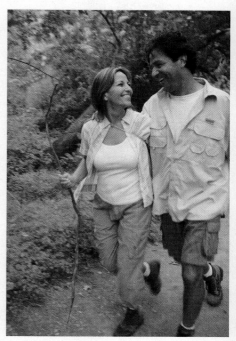

▲ Physical activity, such as walking, is an important component of energy expenditure. ©Ronnie Kaufman/Blend Images LLC

Women   Men

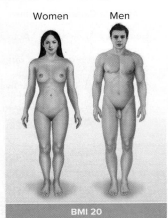

BMI 20

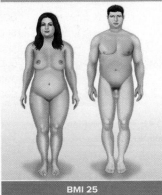

BMI 25

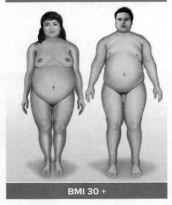

BMI 30 +

FIGURE 7-10 ▲ Estimates of body shapes at different BMI classifications.

underwater weighing
Also known as hydrostatic weighing or hydrodensitometry, this is a method of estimating total body fat by weighing the individual on a standard scale and then weighing him or her again once submerged in water. The difference between the two weights is used to estimate total body volume.

▶ A high BMI may not accurately reflect overweight or body fatness. Extra muscle mass can result in a false high BMI.
©McGraw-Hill Education/Jill Braaten, photographer

BMI weight classifications are shown below in Table 7-1. A healthy weight for height is defined by a BMI between 18.5 and 24.9. Obesity-related health risks increase when BMI is 25 or more. These are general cutoff values for the presence of overweight and obesity, respectively. Figure 7-11 lists the BMI for various heights and weights.

The concept of BMI is convenient to use because it is inexpensive, easy to obtain, and the values apply to both men and women (i.e., gender neutral). However, any weight-for-height standard remains a crude measure and does not consider body fatness. Keep in mind that a BMI of 25 to 29.9 is a marker of *overweight* (compared to a standard population) and not necessarily a marker of excessive body fatness. Many men (especially athletes) have a BMI greater than 25 because extra muscle mass weighs more. Also, very short adults (under 5 feet tall) may have a high BMI that may not necessarily reflect overweight or fatness. For this reason, BMI should be used only as a screening tool for overweight or obesity. Adult BMIs should not be applied to children, growing adolescents, frail older adults, pregnant and lactating women, and highly muscular individuals. Pregnant women and children have unique BMI standards that will be addressed later in the text.

TABLE 7-1 ■ **Body Mass Index Categories**

Category	BMI
Underweight	< 18.5
Healthy weight	18.5–24.9
Overweight	25–29.9
Obese	30–39.9
Severely (morbidly) obese	≥ 40

BMI is a useful measure of weight-for-height standards and estimated body fat.
Source: Adapted from World Health Organization 1995, 2000, and 2004.

ESTIMATING BODY FAT CONTENT AND DIAGNOSING OBESITY

If calorie intake exceeds calorie expenditure over time, overweight (and often obesity) is a likely result. Often, obesity-related health problems eventually follow (Table 7-2). As mentioned, BMI values can be used as a convenient clinical tool to screen for overweight (BMI ≥ 25), obesity (BMI ≥ 30), and morbid obesity (BMI ≥ 40) in individuals older than 20 years of age (Table 7-1). Medical experts, however, recommend that an individual's diagnosis of obesity should not be based primarily on body weight or BMI but rather on the total amount of fat in the body, the location of body fat, and the presence or absence of weight-related medical conditions.

Body fat varies widely among individuals. Good to acceptable amounts of body fat are about 11% to 20% for men and 16% to 30% for women. Men with over 25% body fat and women with over 35% body fat are considered obese. A higher range of body fat percentage for women is needed physiologically to maintain reproductive functions, including estrogen production.

To measure body fat content accurately, both body weight and body volume of the person are used to calculate body density. Body weight is easy to measure on a conventional scale. Of the typical methods used to estimate body volume, **underwater (hydrostatic) weighing** remains the most accurate. This technique determines body volume using the difference between conventional body weight and body weight measured while submerged under water, along with the relative densities of fat tissue and lean tissue, using a mathematical

TABLE 7-2 ■ Selected Health Problems Associated with Excess Body Fat

Health Problem	Likely Cause
Surgical complications	Increased anesthesia needs; greater risk of wound infections (decreased immune function)
Pulmonary disease and sleep disorders	Excess weight stressing the lungs and pharynx
Type 2 diabetes	Enlarged adipose (fat) cells poorly bind insulin and inadequately respond to insulin signals; reduced synthesis of factors that promote insulin action and increased synthesis of factors that counter insulin action
Hypertension	Increased miles of blood vessels found in the adipose tissue, increased blood volume, and increased resistance to blood flow related to hormones made by adipose cells
Cardiovascular disease (e.g., coronary heart disease and stroke)	Increased LDL cholesterol and triglycerides; reduced HDL cholesterol; increased synthesis of blood clotting and inflammatory factors by enlarged adipose cells; potential for altered heart rhythm
Bone and joint disorders (including gout)	Excess pressure placed on knees, ankles, and hip joints
Gallstones	Increased cholesterol content of bile
Skin disorders	Accumulation and trapping of moisture and microorganisms in tissue folds
Various cancers	Estrogen and other hormones contribute to tumor growth by adipose cells; increased hyperinsulinemia or insulin resistance; systemic inflammation associated with cancer risk; excess calorie intake may encourage tumor development (animal studies)
Shorter stature (in some forms of obesity)	Earlier onset of puberty
Pregnancy risks	More difficult delivery; increased birth defects and gestational diabetes; greater anesthesia needs
Reduced physical agility and increased risk of accidents and falls	Excess weight impairs physical movement and gait
Menstrual irregularities and infertility	Hormone imbalances; insulin resistance; increased oxidative stress
Vision problems	Higher rates of cataracts and other eye disorders
Premature death	Comorbidities and greater risk factors for numerous chronic diseases and complications
Infections	Reduced immune system activity
Liver damage and eventual failure	Excess fat accumulation in the liver (fatty liver)
Erectile dysfunction in men	Low-grade inflammation caused by reduced function of the cells lining the blood vessels and impaired blood circulation

The greater the degree of body fatness, the more likely and the more serious these health problems generally become. They are much more likely to appear in people who show an upper-body fat distribution pattern and/or are greater than twice their healthy body weight.

formula. This procedure requires that an individual be totally submerged in a tank of water, with a trained technician directing the procedure (Fig. 7-12). **Air displacement (Bod Pod)**® is another method of determining body volume. Body volume is quantified by measuring the space a person takes up inside a measurement chamber (Fig. 7-13).

air displacement A method for estimating body composition that makes use of the volume of space taken up by a body inside a small chamber (Bod Pod). This tool is also known as air displacement plethysmography.

$$\text{Body density} = \frac{\text{body weight}}{\text{body volume}}$$

$$\text{\% body fat} = (495 \div \text{body density}) - 450$$

Skinfold thickness measurements are also a common anthropometric method to estimate total body fat content, although there are some limits to its accuracy. Clinicians use calipers to measure the fat layer directly under the skin at multiple sites and then plug these values into a mathematical formula (Fig. 7-14).

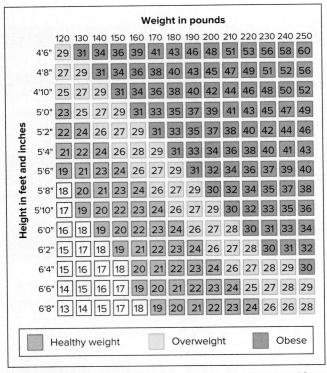

Weight in pounds

	120	130	140	150	160	170	180	190	200	210	220	230	240	250
4'6"	29	31	34	36	39	41	43	46	48	51	53	56	58	60
4'8"	27	29	31	34	36	38	40	43	45	47	49	51	52	56
4'10"	25	27	29	31	34	36	38	40	42	44	46	48	50	52
5'0"	23	25	27	29	31	33	35	37	39	41	43	45	47	49
5'2"	22	24	26	27	29	31	33	35	37	38	40	42	44	46
5'4"	21	22	24	26	28	29	31	33	34	36	38	40	41	43
5'6"	19	21	23	24	26	27	29	31	32	34	36	37	39	40
5'8"	18	20	21	23	24	26	27	29	30	32	34	35	37	38
5'10"	17	19	20	22	23	24	26	27	29	30	32	33	35	36
6'0"	16	18	19	20	22	23	24	26	27	28	30	31	33	34
6'2"	15	17	18	19	21	22	23	24	26	27	28	30	31	32
6'4"	15	16	17	18	20	21	22	23	24	26	27	28	29	30
6'6"	14	15	16	17	19	20	21	22	23	24	25	27	28	29
6'8"	13	14	15	17	18	19	20	21	22	23	24	26	26	28

Height in feet and inches

☐ Healthy weight   ☐ Overweight   ☐ Obese

Developed by the National Center for Health Statistics in collaboration with the National Center for Chronic Disease Prevention and Health Promotion

FIGURE 7-11 ▲ Convenient height/weight table based on BMI. A healthy weight for height generally falls within a BMI range of 18.5 to 24.9 kg/m² (shown in green).

bioelectrical impedance (BIA) The method to estimate total body fat that uses a low-energy electrical current. The more fat storage a person has, the more impedance (resistance) to electrical flow will be exhibited.

dual energy X-ray absorptiometry (DEXA) A scientific tool used to measure bone mineral density and body composition.

upper-body (android) obesity The type of obesity in which fat is stored primarily in the abdominal area; defined as a waist circumference more than 40 inches (102 centimeters) in men and more than 35 inches (88 centimeters) in women; closely associated with a high risk for cardiovascular disease, hypertension, and type 2 diabetes. Also known as visceral or central obesity.

The analysis of **bioelectrical impedance (BIA)** is also used to estimate body fat content. This procedure sends a painless, low-energy electrical current through the body to estimate body fat. This estimation is based on the assumption that adipose (fat) tissue resists electrical flow more than lean tissue because it has a lower electrolyte and water content. More adipose tissue has proportionately greater electrical resistance than lean tissue. Within a few seconds, bioelectrical impedance analyzers convert body electrical resistance into an approximate estimate of total body fat, as long as hydration is adequate in the person being measured. Dehydration skews these results (Fig. 7-15). Body composition monitors, better known as body fat calculators, which use bioelectric impedance, are now available for home use. These machines are similar in shape and use to bathroom scales, but their main purpose is to measure body fat. An electrical current passes easily through conductive foot pads and/or handheld electrodes. These in-home devices will hopefully encourage individuals to be less concerned with what they weigh than whether their weight comes from fat or muscle.

A more advanced determination of body fat content can be made using **dual energy X-ray absorptiometry (DEXA).** DEXA is considered the most accurate way to determine body fat, but the equipment is expensive and not widely available. This x-ray system allows the clinician to separate body weight into separate components: fat, fat-free soft tissue, and bone mineral. Additional software can determine body fat distribution. The typical whole-body scan requires about 10 to 25 minutes, and the dose of radiation is less than a chest X ray. An assessment of bone mineral density and the risk of osteoporosis can also be made using DEXA (Fig. 7-16).

There are other methods of assessing body composition, but those detailed here are the most commonly used in health clinics, fitness centers, and research. In the hands of a trained clinician, these assessments provide valuable information about body fat beyond simple measures of height and weight.

USING BODY FAT DISTRIBUTION TO FURTHER EVALUATE OBESITY

In addition to the amount of fat we store, the location of that body fat is an important predictor of health risks. Some people store fat in upper-body areas, whereas others store fat lower on the body. **Upper-body (android) obesity,** characterized by a large abdomen or waist, is more often called *abdominal, visceral,* or *central* obesity and is related to insulin resistance and fatty liver leading to obesity-related chronic diseases such as cancer, type 2 diabetes, high blood lipids, and heart disease. Because men typically develop upper-body obesity, it is also known as *android* obesity. While other adipose cells empty fat into general blood circulation, the fat released from abdominal adipose cells goes directly to the liver, by way of the portal vein. This influx of fat interferes with the liver's ability to use insulin and negatively affects lipoprotein metabolism by the liver. These upper-body adipose cells are not just storage depots; they are metabolically active cells that release many hormones and other peptides, called adipokines, involved in long-term energy regulation. When they fill with excess fat, the cells become dysfunctional, resulting in inflammation, insulin resistance, and other adverse health conditions leading to chronic disease.

High blood testosterone levels encourage upper-body obesity, as does excessive alcohol intake, and smoking. This pattern of fat storage is commonly known as the *apple shape* (large abdomen and small buttocks and thighs). Upper-body obesity is assessed by measuring the circumference of the abdomen at the waist. A waist circumference

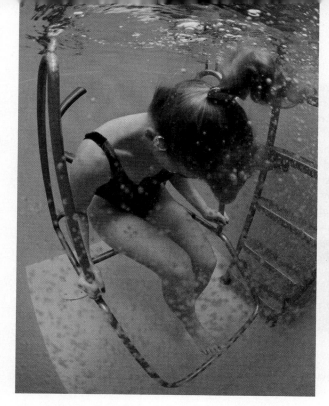

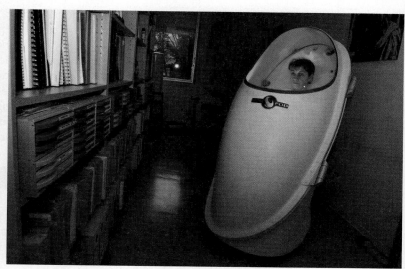

FIGURE 7-13 ▲ Bod Pod.® This device determines body volume based on the volume of displaced air, measured as a person sits in a sealed chamber.

FIGURE 7-12 ▲ Underwater (hydrostatic) weighing. In this technique, the subject exhales as much air as possible and then holds his or her breath and bends at the waist to become totally submerged. Once submerged, the underwater weight is recorded. Using this value, body volume can be calculated.

FIGURE 7-14 ▼ Skinfold measurements. With proper technique and calibrated equipment, skinfold measurements taken at various sites around the body can be used to predict body fat content in about 10 minutes. Measurements are made at several locations, including the triceps (pictured here).

Caliper

Fat

Triceps brachii muscle

Skin

Bone

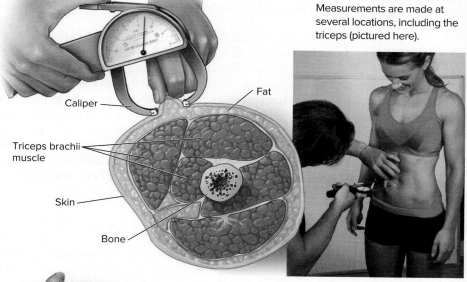

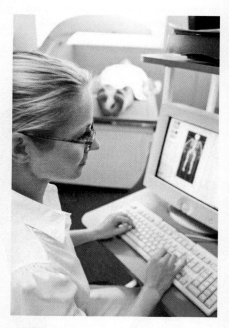

FIGURE 7-16 ▲ Dual energy X-ray absorptiometry (DEXA). This method measures body fat by passing small doses of radiation through the body. The radiation reacts differently with fat, lean tissue, or bone, allowing these components to be quantified. The scanner arm moves from head to toe and in doing so can determine body fat and bone density. DEXA is currently considered the most accurate method for determining body composition (as long as the person can fit under the arm of the instrument). The radiation dose is minimal.

FIGURE 7-15 ◄ Bioelectrical impedance estimates total body fat in less than 5 minutes and is based on the principle that body fat resists the flow of electricity, since it is low in water and electrolytes. The degree of resistance to electrical flow is used to estimate body fatness. This handheld device (along with home scales using foot pads) sends an electrical current through the body and gives a percentage of body fat when it has completed its process.

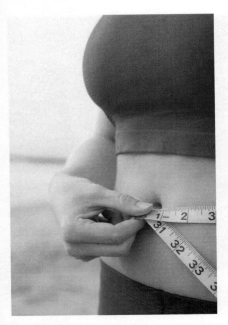

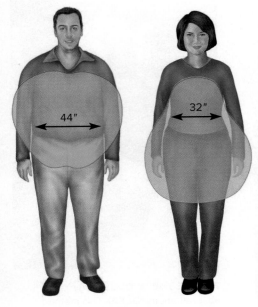

Upper-body fat distribution (android: apple shape)

Lower-body fat distribution (gynoid: pear shape)

FIGURE 7-17 ▲ Body fat stored primarily in the upper body (android) brings higher risks of obesity-related diseases than lower-body (gynoid) obesity. Here, the woman's waist circumference of 32 inches and the man's waist circumference of 44 inches indicate that the man has upper-body obesity but the woman does not, based on the waist circumference measures of 35 inches for women and 40 inches for men.

more than 40 inches (102 centimeters) in men and more than 35 inches (88 centimeters) in women indicates risk for upper-body obesity (Fig. 7-17). If BMI is also 25 or more, health risks are significantly increased.

Estrogen and progesterone encourage **lower-body (gynoid) obesity**—the typical female pattern. The small abdomen and much larger buttocks and thighs give a *pear shape* appearance. Fat deposited in the lower body is not mobilized as easily as android fat cells and often resists being released. After menopause, blood estrogen levels fall, encouraging greater upper-body fat distribution and raising the risk of chronic disease dramatically for postmenopausal females.

✓ CONCEPT CHECK 7.3

1. How is body mass index (BMI) determined?
2. What are the BMI, body fat percentage, and waist circumference values for men and women that are associated with increased risk of health problems related to being overweight?
3. What are five methods by which body fat content can be estimated?
4. Obesity leads to an increased risk of which diseases?

7.4 Why Some People Are Obese—Nature Versus Nurture

The energy imbalance that promotes obesity stems from cultural, economic, and social factors.[4] Many studies of obesity attribute the increasing trends to the growth of the global food system, including advancements in energy-dense food processing, marketing, and the widespread availability of more affordable energy-dense foods.

Both genetic (nature) and environmental (nurture) can increase the risk for obesity (Table 7-3). The location of fat storage is strongly influenced by genetics. For example, research studies have found that offspring born to obese mothers are at heightened risk of obesity later in life. Consider the possibility that obesity is nurture allowing nature to express itself. Some obese people begin life with a slower basal metabolism, maintain a sedentary lifestyle, and consume highly refined, calorie-dense diets. These people are nurtured into gaining weight, promoting their natural genetic predisposition toward obesity. Even with a genetic tendency toward obesity, individuals can attain a healthier body weight by engaging in positive lifestyle behaviors with increased physical activity and decreased calorie consumption.

HOW DOES NATURE CONTRIBUTE TO OBESITY?

Studies in pairs of **identical twins** provide insight into the contribution of nature (genetics) relative to obesity. Even when identical twins are raised apart, they tend to show similar weight gain patterns, both in overall weight and body fat distribution.

It appears that nurture (environment), which includes dietary patterns and lifestyle behaviors, varies slightly between twins raised apart. Nurture appears to have less to do with obesity than nature. A child with no obese parent has approximately a 10% chance of becoming obese. When a child has one obese parent, that risk increases to 40%, and with two obese parents, it soars to 80%. Our genes play a role in our metabolic rate, fuel use, and differences in brain chemistry—all of which ultimately affect body weight.

We also inherit specific body types. Tall, thin people appear to have an inherently easier time maintaining healthy body weight. This is probably because BMR increases as body surface increases; therefore, taller people use more calories than shorter people, even at rest.

TABLE 7-3 ■ **What Encourages Excess Body Fat Stores and Obesity?**

Factor	How Fat Storage Is Affected
Age	Excess body fat is more common in adults and middle-age individuals due to loss of lean body mass and reduction in physical activity.
Menopause	Hormonal changes result in increased abdominal fat deposition.
Gender	Females have more fat mass than males due to less lean body mass and reduced surface area (height).
Energy balance	Over time, dietary patterns consistent with positive energy balance promote storage of excess body fat.
Dietary patterns	Excess calorie intake from saturated fat, alcohol, and calorie-dense foods and beverages contribute to obesity.
Physical activity patterns	Sedentary behavior promotes positive energy balance and body fat storage.
Basal metabolism	A low BMR due to factors such as genetics, thyroid problems, or energy restriction is linked to weight gain.
Thermic effect of food	Some obese individuals metabolize nutrients more efficiently and thus expend fewer calories for digestion and absorption.
Increased hunger sensations	Some individuals appear to have blunted satiety, which may alter brain signals involved in food reward pathways.
Ratio of fat to lean tissue	A high ratio of fat mass to lean body mass is correlated with weight gain.
Fat uptake by adipose tissue	Fat storage efficiency is high in some obese individuals and may even increase with weight loss.
Social and behavioral factors	Obesity is associated with socioeconomic status; familial conditions; social networks; binge eating; intakes of of inexpensive, "supersized" high saturated fat food; sedentary lifestyles; increased screen time; smoking cessation; excessive alcohol intake; and frequency of meals eaten away from home.
Genetic predisposition	Genetic factors may affect metabolism, energy expenditure, deposition of adipose tissue or lean tissue, satiety, and the relative proportion of fuels used by the body.
Ethnicity	In some groups, higher body weight is socially acceptable, which may promote overeating.
Certain medications	Changes in hunger/appetite can be a side effect of many medications.
Childbearing	A pattern of weight gain during the childbearing years can occur to support fetus. Fat stored during pregnancy to support lactation may not be fully lost in women who do not breastfeed.
Region of residence	Regional environmental and lifestyle differences, such as calorie-laden diets and sedentary lifestyles, especially in the South and Midwest, are associated with higher rates of obesity.

Humans have inherited a so-called "thrifty" metabolism that enables us to store fat readily. In early human history, our genes adapted to an environment where food was sometimes scarce; thus, a metabolism that efficiently stored fat would have been a safeguard against starvation in times of famine. Now, with a constant overabundance of food, we require wise food choices and regular physical activity to maintain energy balance. Depending on genetic traits we inherit from our parents, some of us are more prone to weight gain in the modern food environment than others.

Does the Body Have a Set-Point for Weight? The **set-point** theory of weight maintenance proposes that humans have a genetically predetermined body weight or body fat content, which the body closely regulates. Several physiological changes that occur during calorie reduction and weight loss support this theory. For example, research suggests that the **hypothalamus** monitors the amount of body fat in humans and tries to keep that amount constant over time. The release and circulation of the hormone **leptin,** from adipose cells, promotes a satiety and a sense of fullness, thus reducing appetite. As adipose cells increase in size and number, overall production of leptin increases,

lower-body (gynoid) obesity The type of obesity in which fat storage is primarily located in the buttocks and thigh area. Also known as gynoid or gynecoid obesity.

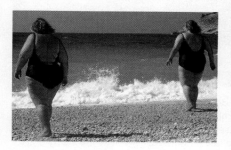

▲ Studies in identical twins give us insight into the genetic contribution to obesity.
©Ingram Publishing/SuperStock

identical twins Two offspring that develop from a single ovum and sperm and, consequently, have the same genetic makeup.

set-point Theory of weight status that refers to the close regulation of body weight. It is not known what cells control this set-point or how it functions in weight regulation. There is evidence, however, that complex mechanisms exist that help regulate weight.

hypothalamus A region at the base of the brain that contains cells that play a role in the regulation of energy intake, respiration, body temperature, satiety, and other body functions.

leptin A hormone made by adipose tissue in proportion to total fat stores in the body that influences long-term regulation of fat mass. Leptin also influences appetite and the release of insulin.

which should suppress appetite. If fat mass is reduced, leptin levels are reduced, so appetite should be increased. This system, however, is not foolproof. Research has shown that overweight persons have large amounts of leptin coming from the excess body fat, but their brains seem to be *leptin resistant* and are not receiving the signal to stop eating.

Thyroid hormone levels change in relation to body fatness, too. When calorie intake is reduced, the blood concentration of thyroid hormones falls, which slows BMR. Also, the calorie cost of weight-bearing activity decreases, so that an activity that burned 100 kcal before weight loss may only burn 80 kcal after weight loss. Furthermore, as weight loss occurs, the body becomes more efficient at storing fat by increasing the activity of the enzyme lipoprotein lipase, which permits fat entry into cells. All of these changes protect the body from losing weight.

If a person overeats, in the short term, BMR tends to increase. This causes some resistance to weight gain. In the long run, however, resistance to weight gain is much less than resistance to weight loss. When a person gains weight and stays at a stable weight for some time, the body tends to establish energy balance at a new set point.

Opponents of the set-point theory argue that weight does not remain constant throughout adulthood: the average person gains weight slowly through old age. Also, if an individual is placed in a different social, emotional, or physical environment, weight can be altered and maintained at a markedly higher or lower point. These arguments suggest that humans, rather than having a set-point determined by genetics or the number of adipose cells, settle into a particular stable weight based on their circumstances, often regarded as a "settling point."

A nondiet acceptance program, called Health At Every Size,® embraces the following core principles. See www.sizediversityandhealth.org for more information.

- Accepting and respecting the diversity of body shapes and sizes;
- Recognizing that health and well-being are multidimensional and that they include physical, social, spiritual, occupational, emotional, and intellectual aspects;
- Promoting all aspects of health and well-being for people of all sizes;
- Promoting eating in a manner that balances individual nutritional needs, hunger, satiety, appetite, and pleasure; and
- Promoting individually appropriate, enjoyable, life-enhancing physical activity, rather than exercise that is focused on a goal of weight loss.

DOES NURTURE PLAY A ROLE?

Environmental factors, such as consuming an energy-dense dietary pattern and failing to meet physical activity guidelines, literally shape us. This seems reasonable when we consider that our gene pool has not significantly changed in the past 25 years, whereas the ranks of obese people have grown to epidemic proportions over the last 25 years.

Some would argue that body weight similarities between family members stem more from learned behaviors than genetic similarities. Even couples, who have no genetic link, may behave similarly toward food and eventually assume similar degrees of leanness or fatness. Adult obesity in women is often correlated with childhood obesity. In addition, relative inactivity and periods of stress or boredom, as well as excess weight gain during pregnancy, contribute to female obesity. These patterns suggest both social and genetic interactions contribute to body weight. Male obesity, however, is not strongly linked to childhood obesity and, instead, tends to appear after age 30. This powerful and prevalent pattern suggests a primary role of nurture in obesity, with less genetic influence.

Is poverty associated with obesity? Ironically, in developed nations, the answer is *yes.* North Americans of lower socioeconomic status, especially single mothers, are more likely to be obese than those of higher socioeconomic status. Several social and behavioral factors promote fat storage and support the link between socioeconomic

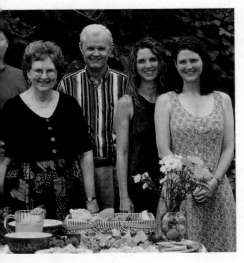

▲ Body weight is influenced by many factors related to both nature and nurture. We resemble our parents because of the genes we have inherited, as well as the lifestyle habits, including diet, that we have learned from them. ©Jack Hollingsworth/Getty Images

status and obesity. These factors may include lower socioeconomic status, overweight friends and family, a cultural/ethnic group that prefers higher body weight, a lifestyle that discourages healthy meals and adequate exercise, easy availability of inexpensive high-calorie food, limited access to fresh fruits and vegetables, excessive screen time, lack of adequate sleep, emotional stress, meals frequently eaten away from home, and smoking cessation. Weight gain associated with cessation of smoking has been shown to be a result of increased calorie consumption, with 96% of the weight gain as fat.

ASK THE RDN   Detox Diets

Dear RDN: I put on 10 pounds last year, and I can't seem to shed the extra weight. Can a detox diet help?

There is little consensus about the definition of a detoxification diet, but in general, such plans are meant to assist the body's natural mechanisms to get rid of harmful toxins that arise from metabolism and from our environment. When you look at the advocates of detox diets, it should raise a red flag that its praises are sung primarily by celebrities, tabloid magazines, and TV talk-show hosts who claim that detox diets cause weight loss, improve energy, and reduce risk of chronic diseases.

We are exposed to toxins every day. Some are produced by the body—such as the ammonia that arises from metabolism of amino acids. Many more are present in the foods we eat, the water we drink, and the air we breathe. Fortunately, the human body has several natural detoxification systems that convert harmful substances into water-soluble compounds that can be excreted via urine, sweat, bile, or feces.

Scientific evidence shows that the body's detoxification pathways are effective without any extra intervention. Popular culture detox diets have become a fad that features extreme, uninformed, and nutritionally inadequate dietary practices. One of the most harmful regimens instructs dieters to subsist on a liquid diet of lemon juice, maple syrup, water, and cayenne pepper for a week or more. Some plans rely on herbal laxatives to purge the colon of waste materials. Others involve consuming up to 8 cups per day of juice made from organic fruits and vegetables. Such plans, while they may boost certain nutrients and phytochemicals, are extremely low in calories and protein.

Currently, there is no clinical evidence to support the benefits of these detox diets. Side effects such as fatigue, headaches, or decreased mental acuity are signs of low blood sugar. Taken to an extreme, prolonged fasts and nutritionally inadequate diets can lead to chemical imbalances, which could affect heart function.

In summary, an overly restrictive diet is difficult to maintain and may end up decreasing lean mass and basal metabolic rate. Sustained weight loss requires a lifestyle change, not a quick fix! If weight loss is your goal, moderate calorie restriction combined with physical activity will support gradual and sustainable weight loss. B vitamins, antioxidant nutrients, phytochemicals (e.g., flavonoids), dietary fiber, and plenty of fluid are what the body requires to detoxify and flush harmful compounds. The best prescription to support your body's detoxification pathways is to consume a dietary pattern rich in fruits, vegetables, and whole grains, and to emphasize plant sources of protein every day—not just for a few days a year.

Pure and simple,

Angela Collene, MS, RDN, LD (author)

CONCEPT CHECK 7.4

1. Explain how body weight is influenced by nature (genetics).
2. What role does nurture (environment) play in determining body weight?

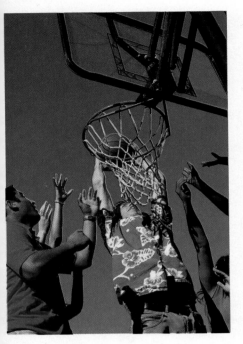

▲ Student life is often full of physical activity. This is not necessarily true when a person begins working full-time; hence, weight gain is highly possible. ©SW Productions/Getty Images

7.5 Treatment of Overweight and Obesity

Treatment of overweight and obesity should be long term and similar to that for any chronic disease. Treatments require sustainable lifestyle changes, rather than quick fixes promoted by many popular *fad* diets. We often view a *diet* as something one attempts temporarily, only to resume prior (typically poor) behaviors once satisfactory results have been achieved. This is a primary reason so many people regain lost weight. Instead, an emphasis on healthy, active living with acceptable dietary patterns and behaviors will promote weight loss and sustained weight maintenance. Maintenance of a healthy weight requires lifelong changes in behaviors, not short-term and rapid weight loss as seen in so-called crash diets.

LOSING BODY FAT

One pound of weight loss includes adipose tissue plus supporting lean tissues and fluids, and represents approximately 3300 kcal per pound (about 7.2 kcal per gram). Because there are approximately 3500 kcal in 1 pound of fat, the past 50 years of weight-loss advice has centered on the notion that a deficit of approximately 500 kcal per day is required to lose 1 pound of fat tissue per week. This fairly simple *3500-kcal rule*, however, may be an inaccurate predictor of weight change, resulting in unrealistic expectations. Over the years, energy balance research has shown that weight loss occurs more gradually than would be predicted by the 3500-kcal rule because of several factors, including the loss of muscle along with fat during weight loss. Experts have developed new weight-loss prediction formulas that estimate a much slower and realistic pattern of weight loss. Researchers emphasize that weight change is not linear. Rather, it occurs most rapidly during the first year after a change in energy balance and tapers off over the next 2 years. In addition, changes in energy intake and physical activity must be strictly maintained over time. Research has also shown that individuals have a tendency to overestimate their self-reported physical activity levels and underestimate their dietary intakes.

A web-based *body weight simulator* can help predict expected weight loss over time. The Body Weight Planner, which can be found at http://bwsimulator.niddk.nih.gov, projects weight loss over time based on an individual's height, weight, age, current calorie intake, calorie reduction, and activity level. As always, guidelines emphasize that the daily calorie deficit can come from decreased calorie intake, increased physical activity, or ideally, a combination of both.

WHAT TO LOOK FOR IN A SOUND WEIGHT-LOSS PLAN

Individuals can develop a weight-management plan by seeking advice from a health professional such as a registered dietitian nutritionist (RDN). Interactive tools such as www.ChooseMyPlate.gov can also aid in weight loss and maintenance. Overall, a sound weight-loss program should include the components listed in Figure 7-18.

A one-sided approach that focuses only on restricting calories is a difficult plan of action. Instead, adding physical activity and an appropriate behavioral component will contribute to success in weight loss and eventual weight maintenance (Fig. 7-19). The Dietary Guidelines for Americans recommendations focus on healthier dietary patterns translating to reduced discretionary calorie intake and meeting physical activity recommendations.

WEIGHT LOSS IN PERSPECTIVE

Three principles point to the importance of preventing obesity. Public health strategies to address the current obesity problem must speak to all age groups. There is a particular need to focus on children and adolescents because patterns of excess weight and

---

The Dietary Guidelines for Americans provide the following recommendations related to "Consume a healthy eating pattern that accounts for all foods and beverages within an appropriate calorie level."

- Choose a healthy eating pattern at an appropriate calorie level to help achieve and maintain a healthy body weight, support nutrient adequacy, and reduce the risk of chronic disease.

- To meet nutrient needs within calorie limits, choose a variety of nutrient-dense foods across and within all food groups in recommended amounts.

- Consume an eating pattern low in added sugars, saturated fats, and sodium.

- Choose nutrient-dense foods and beverages across and within all food groups in place of less healthy choices.

- Aim to achieve and maintain a healthy body weight. The relationship between diet and physical activity contributes to calorie balance and managing body weight.

Source: 2015–2020 Dietary Guidelines for Americans

RATE OF WEIGHT LOSS

☐ Encourages slow and steady weight loss, rather than rapid weight loss

☐ Sets goal of no more than 1 to 2 pounds of weight loss per week

☐ Includes a period of weight maintenance for a few months after 10% of body weight is lost

☐ Evaluates need for further weight loss before more weight loss begins

FLEXIBILITY

☐ Supports participation in normal activities (e.g., dining out, attending parties)

☐ Adapts the plan to individual habits and tastes

DIETARY PATTERN

☐ Meets nutrient needs (with low-calorie intake)

☐ Includes common foods, with no foods being promoted as magical or special

☐ Uses MyPlate or a comparable food guide as a pattern for food choices

BEHAVIOR CHANGE

☐ Promotes reasonable changes that can be maintained

☐ Encourages social support

☐ Includes plans for relapse, so that one does not quit after a setback

☐ Promotes changes that control problem eating behaviors

☐ Promotes self-monitoring practices such as keeping food diaries and setting goals

OVERALL HEALTH

☐ Requires screening by a physician for people with existing health problems, those over 40 (men) to 50 (women) years of age who plan to increase physical activity substantially, and those who plan to lose weight rapidly

☐ Encourages regular physical activity, sufficient sleep, stress reduction, and other healthy changes in lifestyle

☐ Addresses underlying psychological weight issues, such as depression or marital stress

FIGURE 7-18 ▲ Characteristics of a sound weight-loss plan. Use this checklist to evaluate any weight-loss plan before putting it into practice.

sedentary lifestyles developed during youth may form the basis for a lifetime of weight-related conditions and increased mortality. In the adult population, attention should be directed toward weight management and maintenance by encouraging healthy dietary patterns and increasing physical activity.

1. **Decrease calorie intake** by approximately 500 kcal per day to allow for slow and steady weight loss.
2. **Increase physical activity** to the equivalent of more than 150 minutes of moderate-intensity aerobic activity each week.
3. **Make positive behavior changes** to sustain lifestyle modifications promoting health.

FIGURE 7-19 ▶ Weight-loss triad. The key to weight loss and maintenance can be thought of as a triad, which consists of three interrelated components: (1) controlling calorie intake, (2) performing regular physical activity, and (3) engaging in positive behaviors. Without one component of the triad, weight loss and later maintenance becomes highly unlikely. ©Sam Edwards/age fotostock (top); ©Purestock/SuperStock (right); ©chrisgramly/Getty Images (left)

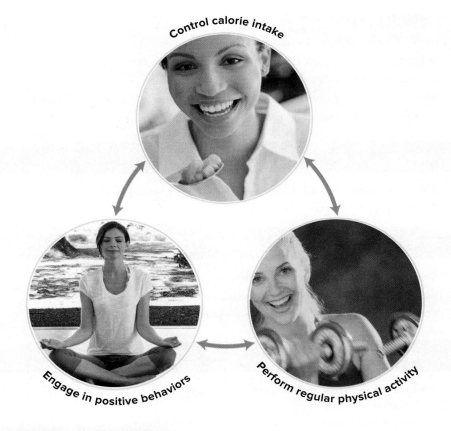

Control calorie intake

Engage in positive behaviors

Perform regular physical activity

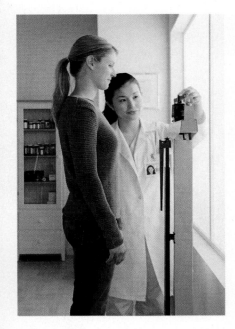

▲ Slow, steady weight loss is one of the characteristics of a sound weight-loss program. ©Image Source/age fotostock

ASK THE RDN   Biggest Loser Eating Plan

Dear RDN: *I'm a fan of* The Biggest Loser *TV show and see they have a diet and exercise plan. After reading all about the perils of fad diets in this chapter, I want to be sure this program is safe. Can you help?*

Sure! *The Biggest Loser* program has a popular diet and exercise plan. The first *Biggest Loser* book, released in 2005, has been expanded to include a *30-Day Jump Start* edition, *6 Weeks to a Healthier You,* and *The Biggest Loser: The Weight Loss Program to Transform Your Body, Health and Life* (released in 2013). In addition, there is now an online 6-week express program, "Biggest Loser Club," which costs approximately $20 per month.

Overall, the *Biggest Loser* plan is based on sound nutrition and physical activity principles, but it does require some effort and discipline. This program is based on eating small, frequent meals of nutrient-dense and high-fiber foods. It follows the *Biggest Loser's* 4-3-2-1 Pyramid: four servings of fruits and vegetables, three servings of lean protein, two servings of whole grains, and 200 kcal of "extras." This plan also recommends drinking six to eight glasses of water per day, limiting sodium and saturated fats, and avoiding caffeine.

Limitations: Although supplements are not recommended, some of the meal plans may fall below 1200 kcal per day and require a supplement. If you select the more interactive online version (Biggest Loser Club), there is a fee to participate.

Strengths: This plan focuses on both diet and physical activity, which are essential components for long-term weight management. All food groups are well represented, and the foods may be purchased at any grocery store. Vegetarian, vegan, and gluten-free options are all possible within this plan. The online version includes additional support, recipes, videos, and tracking tools.

In sum, choosing dietary and physical activity patterns that closely align with evidence-based recommendations is always the goal! The combination of diet and physical activity has been shown to improve success in long-term weight loss and maintenance.

Eat well, exercise, and prosper,

Colleen Spees, PhD, RDN, LD, FAND (author)

FARM to FORK Stone Fruits

Stone fruits, such as peaches, nectarines, apricots, cherries, and plums are soft-fleshed fruits with a hard (*stone*) seed. These fruits can contribute to a sound weight management plan while providing key nutrients.

Grow

- The best time to plant stone fruit trees is in winter, when they are dormant. They prefer cold winters and warm, dry summers to produce flowers and fruit.
- Dwarf or semidwarf fruit trees allow those with small yards to grow stone fruits. Most trees produce their first viable crops after 3 to 4 years.
- Harvest stone fruits, such as peaches, at a U-pick orchard for fruit picked at the height of ripeness.

Shop

- While the most flavorful stone fruits are locally grown and harvested when ripe, shipped fruits are often harvested prior to ripening and exposed to cold temperatures, resulting in mealy, leathery, and dry fruit.
- Choose fruit that is dent-free and without bruises. Ripe stone fruit has a slight give when gently pressed between your palms.
- Select peaches and nectarines by their background color, not their blush. White-fleshed peaches and nectarines are higher in antioxidants than the yellow varieties, and the less common red flesh, or *blood peaches*, are the most nutritious.
- Apricots are one of the most nutritious stone fruits; deep orange and red dried apricots pack the most nutrients.
- Dark skins and flesh of plums have more anthocyanins. Dried plums (also known as *prunes*) are highly nutritious and rich in both soluble and insoluble fibers and have a reputation for relieving constipation.
- When selecting cherries, look for bright green and flexible stems. Darker cherries contain higher levels of anthocyanins and can reduce inflammation.

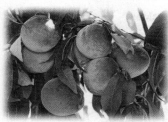

©iStockphoto/Getty Images

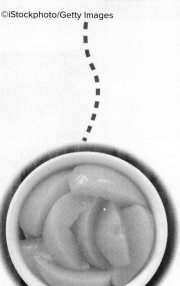

©FotografiaBasica/Getty Images

Store

- Freezing preserves more antioxidants than canning when storing stone fruits. To retain the highest levels of nutrients and prevent browning, slice the fruit and sprinkle with lemon juice and sugar.
- If you must store cherries, do so in a microperforated plastic bag (with pin-size holes to allow moisture to escape) in the crisper drawer to allow gas exchange and decrease oxidation.

Prep

- Dried plums (prunes) are an excellent source of antioxidants and have been linked to everything from reduced inflammation to bone health. To stew prunes, cover with water in a saucepan, bring to a boil, then reduce heat to simmer for 20 minutes. Add a sprinkle of sugar or slice of lemon for flavor.
- Eating the skin will provide the most fiber and nutrients. To de-fuzz stone fruits, wipe gently with a clean cloth.
- If frozen, thaw stone fruits in the microwave to retain the most antioxidants.

Source: Robinson J. "Stone Fruits: Time for a Flavor Revival," in *Eating on the Wild Side*. New York: Little, Brown and Company, 2013.

✔ CONCEPT CHECK 7.5

1. What are the characteristics of an appropriate weight-loss program?
2. What are the Dietary Guidelines related to "Choose a healthy eating pattern at an appropriate calorie level to help achieve and maintain a healthy body weight, support nutrient adequacy, and reduce the risk of chronic disease"?

> For interactive dietary and physical activity tools, see SuperTracker and Daily Food Plan at www.ChooseMyPlate.gov.

7.6 Control of Calorie Intake Is Essential for Weight Management

Per day, the average woman requires approximately 1800 to 2400 kcal and the average male requires 2200 to 3000 kcal. A goal of losing 1 pound or so of stored fat per week may require limiting calorie intake by 500 kcals per week to 1200 kcal per day for women and 1500 kcal per day for men. Although the number of calories allowed could be higher for physically active people, reducing calorie intake is typically necessary in

Nutrition Facts

7.5 servings per container

Serving size	2/3 cup (65g)

Amount per serving

Calories 134

	% Daily Value*
Total Fat 3g	**5%**
Saturated Fat 1.5g	**9%**
Trans Fat 0g	
Cholesterol 0mg	**3%**
Sodium 42mg	**2%**
Total Carbohydrate 23g	**8%**
Dietary Fiber 0g	**0%**
Total Sugars 18g	
Includes 12g Added Sugars	**24%**
Protein 4g	
Vitamin D 0.1mcg	1%
Calcium 80mg	8%
Iron 0mg	0%
Potassium 204mg	6%

* The % Daily Value (DV) tells you how much a nutrient in a serving of food contributes to a daily diet. 2,000 calories a day is used for general nutrition advice.

Nutrition Facts

7.5 servings per container

Serving size	2/3 cup (106g)

Amount per serving

Calories 362

	% Daily Value*
Total Fat 23g	**35%**
Saturated Fat 15g	**75%**
Trans Fat 0g	
Cholesterol 160mg	**53%**
Sodium 114mg	**5%**
Total Carbohydrate 27g	**9%**
Dietary Fiber 0g	**0%**
Total Sugars 20g	
Includes 16g Added Sugars	**32%**
Protein 7g	
Vitamin D 0.2mcg	2%
Calcium 112mg	11%
Iron 0mg	0%
Potassium 175mg	5%

FIGURE 7-20 ▲ Reading labels helps you choose foods with fewer calories. Which of these frozen desserts is the best choice, per ½-cup serving, for a person on a weight-loss diet? The percent Daily Values are based on a 2000-kcal diet. Read more about these dessert choices in What the Dietitian Chose.

Newsworthy Nutrition

Plant-Based Dietary Pattern Promotes Healthy Body Weight

The hypothesis of this study was that a plant-based diet would promote healthier body weights. The study design included over 146,000 participants from the Nurses' Health Study (NHS), Health Professionals Follow-Up Study (HPFS), and Nurses' Health Study II (NHS II) were assessed for the effect of diet quality over time on body weight. Healthy diet quality scores were correlated with greater intakes of fruits and vegetables, whole grains, and nuts. The results showed that subjects who had greater adherence to a plant-based dietary pattern, especially younger women or overweight individuals, gained significantly less weight over a 4-year period. The results of this study underscore the importance of healthy dietary patterns in promoting healthy body weight.

Source: Fung TT, et al. "Long-term change in diet quality is associated with body weight change in men and women." *Journal of Nutrition* 145:1850, 2015.

our increasingly sedentary society. Keep in mind that any calorie reduction will promote the loss of some lean mass along with fat tissue. With regard to consuming fewer calories, some experts suggest consuming less saturated fat; others suggest consuming less added sugars; others recommend consuming excessive protein. At this time, a primarily plant-based, high-fiber dietary pattern has proven the most successful in long-term studies. A recent report (see Newsworthy Nutrition) confirms that the kinds of food we eat have a large effect on weight gain over the years.[5] Finding what works for you is a process of trial and error. The notion that any type of diet promotes significantly greater calorie use by the body remains unfounded.

Portion control is another challenge that influences our calorie intake and requires a change in our approach to eating. The concept of energy density can help dieters choose more nutrient-rich foods with fewer calories per gram. With this technique, we can fill our plates with larger portions of low-energy-density foods, which are low in calories but high in volume. These low-energy-density foods enable us to eat fewer calories without eating less volume and help us feel full and satisfied while we are losing weight. Fruits and vegetables are great examples of low-energy-density foods. The Volumetrics Diet is based on this energy-density approach to eating.[6] This diet is based on the theory that people typically eat the same amount, or volume, of food each day. Since foods vary in terms of energy and nutrient density, the volumetrics approach promotes consuming more nutrient-rich, lower-calorie foods that provide fewer calories in the same amount of volume. Foods that have low density (low in calories but high volume) promote satiety. Fruits and vegetables are good examples of foods that fit into this plan.

One way to monitor calorie intake at the start of a weight-loss program is by reading labels. Label reading is critical because many foods are more energy dense than people realize (Fig. 7-20). Another method is to write down everything you eat and drink for 24 hours (Appendix C) and then calculate calorie intake by using your diet-analysis software.

With knowledge of current calorie intake, future food choices can be adjusted as needed. People often underestimate portion sizes when recording food intake, so measuring cups and a food scale can help.

Table 7-4 shows how to start reducing calorie intake. As you should realize, it is best to consider healthy eating a lifestyle change, rather than a fad diet or rapid weight-loss plan. Also, liquids deserve attention because liquid calories do not stimulate satiety mechanisms to the same extent as solid foods. The best bet is water and limiting any sugar-sweetened beverages.

TABLE 7-4 ▪ Saving Calories: Ideas for Getting Started

Save This Much	By Choosing This	Instead of This
45 kcal	1 cup 1% milk	1 cup whole milk
50 kcal	12 oz light beer	12 oz regular beer
60 kcal	1 cup cornflakes cereal	1 cup sugar-coated flakes cereal
65 kcal	½ cup boiled potatoes	½ cup fried potatoes
135 kcal	1 cup plain popcorn	1 oz potato chips
140 kcal	3 oz lean beef	3 oz marbled beef
140 kcal	1 cup raw vegetables	½ cup potato salad
150 kcal	2 tbsp low-calorie salad dressing	2 tbsp regular salad dressing
150 kcal	1 English muffin	1 Danish pastry
150 kcal	6 oz wine cooler made with sparkling water	6 oz gin and tonic
150 kcal	12 oz sugar-free soft drink	12 oz regular soft drink
175 kcal	½ broiled chicken	½ batter-fried chicken
185 kcal	1 slice angel food cake	1 slice white cake with icing
210 kcal	3 oz lean roast beef	½ cup beef stroganoff
310 kcal	1 apple	1 slice apple pie

CONTROLLING HUNGER

A challenge to most weight-loss programs is to regulate hunger while eating less and exercising more. Separating true hunger from habit or emotional eating is the first step toward controlling the hunger that can sabotage eating patterns. Hormones and your nervous system tell you when you are hungry. The hormone ghrelin in your blood, along with an empty stomach, signals the brain that you are hungry. Likewise, nerves in the stomach signal the brain when you are full, but it can take up to 20 minutes for these satiety signals to reach the brain. The goal is to be hungry at mealtime but not so ravenous that you are tempted to binge. Eat slowly and stop eating when you are comfortably full. If hunger strikes between meals, determine if you are feeling true hunger; if you are, then choose a small, high-fiber snack to hold you over until the next meal. Drinking a glass of water can also help decrease hunger pangs between meals. Including lean protein (nuts, low-fat dairy, soy protein, or lean meat, fish, or chicken) in meals and snacks will also keep hunger at bay. Eating high-volume foods that are rich in water and fiber will provide bulk with fewer calories, fill your stomach, and send satiety signals to the brain. Becoming aware of what you eat will go a long way to controlling hunger and overall calorie intake. When you slow down, you will not only enjoy each mouthful but also give your stomach time to signal your brain that you are full.

CONQUERING THE WEIGHT-LOSS PLATEAU

It is important for anyone on a weight-loss program to know that healthy weight loss is slow and sometimes erratic, and it is normal to reach a weight-loss plateau. After losing weight for weeks, suddenly weight refuses to budge. Fortunately, there are some strategies to overcome these plateaus and start obtaining results again. There are several reasons why weight loss may stall. During the first part of a weight-loss program, individuals are typically losing fluid in addition to fat, causing a weight loss larger than the expected 1 to 2 pounds per week. Because a healthy weight-loss program is designed to cause fat loss rather than loss of muscle or fluid, your weight loss will begin to slow after the first week or so. Also the level of calorie deprivation needed to lose weight is hard to maintain, and you may begin to eat a few more calories. This *calorie creep* can contribute to the weight-loss plateau and eventually lead to weight gain. When this happens, it is important to go back to tracking your calories by logging what you eat and drink and weighing yourself frequently. Another possible reason for the weight-loss plateau is that your metabolism is adjusting to your lower calorie intake. In this case, it may be time to reduce your calories somewhat and drink plenty of water. Your metabolism may also be adapting to your physical activity routine. Varying the intensity of your workout routine, therefore, will help your muscles burn more calories and can help get you past the weight plateau. Strength training, along with the calorie-burning cardio exercises, is important to build muscle mass, which ultimately uses more calories for metabolism.

✓ CONCEPT CHECK 7.6

1. How are hormones involved in hunger control?
2. What are "calorie creep" and the weight-loss plateau, and how can they lead to weight gain?

7.7 Regular Physical Activity Promotes Weight Loss and Maintenance of a Healthy Weight

Regular physical activity is important for everyone, especially those trying to lose weight or maintain a lower body weight. Calorie burning is enhanced both during and after physical activity. Therefore, activity greatly complements a reduction in calorie intake for weight loss. Many of us rarely do more than sit, stand, and sleep. More calories are used during physical activity than at rest. Expending only 100 to 500 extra calories per day above and beyond normal daily activity, while controlling calorie intake, can lead to a steady and sustained weight loss. Furthermore, physical activity has many other benefits, including a boost for overall self-esteem and quality of life. A Key Recommendation from the Dietary Guidelines is to meet physical activity guidelines and reduce time spent in sedentary behaviors. Although some adults may need a higher level of physical activity than others, it is recommended that adults perform a minimum of 150 minutes of moderate-intensity aerobic activity each week to achieve and maintain a healthy body weight. Some individuals may need more than the equivalent of 300 minutes per week.

Adding any of the activities in Table 7-5 to one's lifestyle can increase calorie expenditure, promote health, and reduce body fat over time. Physical activity should be enjoyable so it becomes part of a healthy pattern of living. Although the goal is to achieve 150 minutes per week of activity, everything counts! If you can't squeeze in 30 minutes a day, try shorter bouts of activity in 5-to-10 minute intervals. Some resistance (strength-training) exercises should also be incorporated into your routine to increase and retain lean body mass and, in turn, fat use (see Section 14.2). As lean muscle mass increases, so will one's BMR. Keep in mind that aerobic activity, including brisk walking, jogging, or cycling, burns more fat than resistance activity. An added benefit of including exercise in a weight-reduction program is maintenance of bone health. In sum, any type of physical activity is better than no activity at all.

Unfortunately, opportunities to expend calories in our daily lives are diminishing as technology systematically eliminates almost every reason to move our muscles. The easiest way to increase physical activity is to make it an enjoyable part of a daily routine. To start, one might pack a pair of athletic shoes and walk around the block after school or work every day. Other ideas are avoiding elevators in favor of stairs and parking the car farther away from your destination.

Pedometers or wearable fitness trackers are relatively inexpensive devices that monitor activity and steps. A recommended goal for activity is to take at least 10,000 steps per day; typically, we take about half that many or less. A pedometer tracks

Calorie Estimation on Exercise Machines

The control panel of your fitness machine will typically display your time, speed, distance covered, and calories burned. Time, speed, and distance are generally accurate values, but calories burned is a rough estimate based on the weight you enter before you start your workout. The calories burned are estimates that are not completely accurate because they do not consider factors other than weight, such as body fat percentage, fitness level, form, and running efficiency.

Treadmills and other cardio machines have been shown to overestimate calories burned by up to 20%. A heart rate monitor or fitness tracker is usually more accurate at estimating the number of calories you burn during a workout than are calorie estimators on stationery fitness machines.

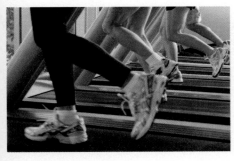

▲ Physical activity complements any weight-loss or maintenance plan. ©Zefa/Alamy RF

steps and often distance. Fitness trackers (like Fitbit® and Jawbone)® are wearable devices that often track steps, distance, active minutes, sleep patterns, and calorie expenditures throughout the day. Fitness trackers calculate calories by measuring heart rate, sweat rate, or heat loss and production. Like pedometers, these devices can motivate users to engage in more activity and reinforce positive behaviors.

TABLE 7-5 ■ Approximate Calorie Costs of Various Activities and Specific Calorie Costs Projected for a 150-Pound (68-Kilogram) Person

Activity	Kcal per kg per hour	Total kcal per hour
Aerobics—heavy	8.0	544
Aerobics—light	3.0	204
Basketball—vigorous	10.0	680
Calisthenics—light	4.0	272
Cleaning	3.6	243
Cooking	2.8	190
Cycling (13 mph)	9.7	659
Cycling (5.5 mph)	3.0	204
Dressing/showering	1.6	106
Driving	1.7	117
Eating (sitting)	1.4	93
Golf (using power cart)	3.6	244
Ice skating (10 mph)	5.8	394
Jogging—medium	9.0	612
Jogging—slow	7.0	476
Jogging (10 mph)	13.2	897
Lying down	1.3	89
Rowing machine (moderate)	7.0	478
Swimming (0.25 mph)	4.4	299
Tennis	6.1	414
Walking (3.75 mph)	4.4	299
Weight lifting—heavy	9.0	612
Weight lifting—light	4.0	272
Writing (sitting)	1.7	118

The values above refer to total energy expenditure, including that needed to perform the physical activity, plus that needed for basal metabolism, the thermic effect of food, and thermogenesis. You can find the calorie costs of additional activities using the Physical Activity Calorie Counter at http://www.acefitness.org/acefit/tools-and-calculators/.

✓ CONCEPT CHECK 7.7

1. What should individuals remember about physical activity as part of their weight-loss plan?

7.8 Behavioral Strategies for Weight Management

Setting realistic goals should be the first step toward successful weight loss and management. Realistic weight-loss goals will keep you more focused and motivated, and help to guarantee success. A successful weight-loss program requires transitioning to a healthier lifestyle. The most helpful goals will focus on changes to your behavior, such as engaging in physical activity 150 minutes per week, drinking plenty of water, or eating five servings of fruits and vegetables a day, rather than reaching for a certain weight. Making lifestyle changes means identifying the behaviors and barriers that led to weight gain in the first place. Controlling calorie intake means addressing those barriers and modifying *problem* behaviors. Only you can decide what behaviors may be preventing weight management and calorie control. What triggers you to start (or stop) eating? What factors influence your food choices?

The Dietary Guidelines identify ways to empower people to make healthy *shifts* in their dietary patterns to encourage weight management:

- Consume more fruits and vegetables.
- Make half of all grains consumed be whole grains.
- Consume more dairy products in nutrient-dense forms.
- Increase variety in protein food choices and make more nutrient-dense choices.
- Shift from solid fats to oils.
- Replace high-calorie, high-sodium intakes with more nutrient-dense options:
  - Reduce added sugar consumption to less than 10% of calories per day.
  - Reduce saturated fat intake to less than 10% of calories per day.
  - Reduce sodium intake to less than 2300 milligrams per day.
- Consume no-sugar-added beverages.
- Reduce portion sizes of nonnutrient-dense foods and beverages.
- Meet the physical activity guidelines.

EATING MINDFULLY OR MINDLESSLY—OR WHATEVER WORKS!

As emphasized throughout this chapter, becoming aware of your eating patterns will ultimately help you obtain and maintain a healthy weight. The concept of *mindful eating* has become increasingly popular. Mindful eating refers to being consciously aware of the

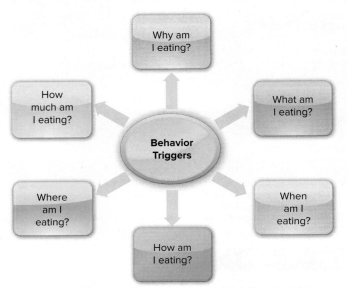

▲ This figure captures the questions you can ask to help you identify and define your unique behavior triggers.

entire eating experience, from food preparation to consumption, including recognizing and respecting everything in between (hunger cues, satiety, flavor, taste, texture, etc.).

If the thought of mindful eating is a bit too overwhelming, give mindless eating a try. Mindless eating focuses on making the healthier choice the easier choice. The average person makes 250 food-related decisions every day. Many of us overeat in response to a constant barrage of triggers in our environment—social networks, sights, sounds, smells, schedules, and other prompts throughout our day. The concept of *nudging* involves implementing subtle changes in your environment to promote positive behavior change.[7] Try a few of these nudges to start:

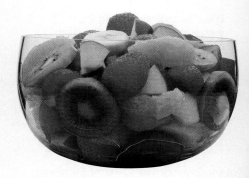

▲ Fruit is a great snack—high in nutrients and low in calories. ©Dennis Gray/Cole Group/ Getty Images RF

- Cover those cookies! When individuals leave desserts visible out on the counter, they tend to weigh about 10 pounds more than their hidden-dessert counterparts.
- Change up your colors! Research has shown that when the color of your plate matches the color of your food (think mashed potatoes on a cream-colored plate), subjects consume up to 30% more food.
- Pretty, pretty fruit bowl. Keeping produce visible on the counter is a reminder to snack healthy. Families that keep a fruit bowl on their counters weigh 8 pounds less than those that don't.
- Shift from 12-inch plates to 10-inch plates and reduce your caloric intake by 22% (see image below).

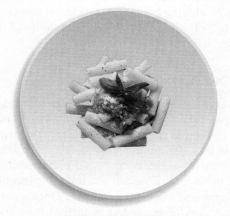 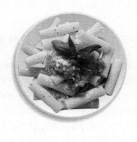

large dinner plate   **medium dinner plate**

▲ The dinner plate on the left is larger and makes the serving size of the food appear smaller. The dinner plate on the right is smaller and makes the serving size of the food appear much larger. This visual illusion tricks our minds into feeling satisfied more quickly when using smaller plates. This optical illusion was first documented in 1865 and termed the *Delboeuf effect.* ©FoodCollection

When changing behaviors, there is no one-size-fits-all approach. Experiment with different approaches and find what works for you!

OTHER BEHAVIORAL STRATEGIES

Chain-breaking, stimulus control, cognitive restructuring, contingency management, and self-monitoring are behavior modification strategies used by clinicians that help put problem behaviors in perspective and organize the intervention into manageable steps. **Chain-breaking** separates behaviors that tend to occur together (e.g., overindulging on potato chips while watching television). Although these activities do not have to occur together, they often do. Individuals need to identify and break these chain reactions.

chain-breaking Breaking the link between two or more behaviors that encourage overeating, such as snacking while watching television.

stimulus control Altering the environment to minimize the stimuli for eating such as, removing foods from sight by storing them in kitchen cabinets.

cognitive restructuring Changing one's frame of mind regarding eating; for example, instead of using a difficult day as an excuse to overeat, a person would substitute other pleasures for rewards, such as a relaxing walk with a friend.

contingency management Forming a plan of action to respond to a situation in which overeating is likely, such as when snacks are within arm's reach at a party.

self-monitoring Tracking foods eaten and conditions affecting eating; actions are usually recorded in a diary, along with location, time, and state of mind. This is a tool to help people understand more about their eating habits.

Stimulus control puts us in charge of temptations. Options include covering tempting food with foil, removing energy-dense snacks from the kitchen counter, and avoiding bringing home especially tempting items. Provide a positive stimulus by keeping healthier snacks available to satisfy hunger and appetite.

Cognitive restructuring changes our frame of mind. For example, after a hard day, avoid using alcohol or comfort foods as quick relief for stress. Instead, plan for healthful, relaxing activities for stress reduction. Find a positive outlet such as taking a walk or catching up with a good friend.

Labeling some foods as "off limits" sets up an internal struggle to resist the urge to eat that food. This hopeless battle can make us feel deprived, and we eventually lose the fight. Managing food choices with the principle of moderation is best. If a favorite food becomes troublesome, place it off limits temporarily, until it can be enjoyed in moderation.

Contingency management prepares one for situations that may trigger overeating (e.g., when snacks are served at a party) or hinder physical activity (e.g., rain).

Self-monitoring can reveal problem eating behaviors—such as unconscious overeating—that may lead to weight gain. Records of dietary and physical activity behaviors can encourage new habits that will counteract unwanted behaviors. Obesity experts note this is a key behavioral tool to use in any weight-loss program. Several of these monitoring tools are available online and as apps for smartphones and other mobile devices.[8]

Overall, it's important to address specific barriers to success such as snacking, compulsive eating, and mealtime overeating. Modifying behaviors is a critical component of weight reduction and maintenance (Table 7-6). Without it, it is difficult to make lifelong lifestyle changes needed to achieve weight-control goals.

RELAPSE PREVENTION IS IMPORTANT

Preventing *relapse* is thought to be the hardest part of weight control—even harder than losing weight. Successful weight managers plan for lapses, do not overreact, and take charge immediately. Change responses include changing your internal language from "I ate that cookie; I'm a failure" to "I ate that cookie, but I did well to stop after only one!" When individuals lapse from their plan, newly learned food habits should steer them back on track. Without a strong behavioral program for **relapse prevention** in place, a lapse frequently turns into a relapse and a potential collapse. Once a pattern of poor food choices begins, individuals may feel failure and stray farther from the plan. As the relapse lengthens, the entire plan collapses and falls short of the weight-loss goal. Losing weight is difficult. Overall, maintenance of weight loss is fostered by the *3 Ms*: motivation, movement, and monitoring.

relapse prevention A series of strategies used to help prevent and cope with weight-control lapses, such as recognizing high-risk situations and deciding beforehand on appropriate responses.

SOCIAL SUPPORT AIDS BEHAVIORAL CHANGE

Healthy social support and networking are helpful in weight control. Family and friends can provide praise and encouragement. Unfortunately, your social network can also sabotage your efforts, so be aware of whom you can trust for support. A registered dietitian nutritionist (RDN) or other trained interventionist can keep you accountable and help you navigate difficult situations. Long-term contact with a professional can be helpful for later weight maintenance. Groups of individuals attempting to lose weight or maintain losses can also provide empathetic support.

SOCIETAL EFFORTS TO REDUCE OBESITY

The incidence of obesity in the United States is now considered an *epidemic*. An epidemic is a public health problem, and such problems call for collective action. In fact, improvement in the health of our nation requires an approach that includes many sectors. Partnerships, programs, and policies that support healthy eating and active living must be coordinated.

Food and Activity Tracking

Here are some websites where you can download apps and record your food and physical activity for free:

- www.myfitnesspal.com/
- www.supertracker.usda.gov/
- www.loseit.com
- www.livestrong.com
- www.sparkpeople.com

TABLE 7-6 ■ Behavioral Tactics for Weight Loss

Shopping
1. Shop for food after eating so you are not hungry.
2. Shop from a list or use a shopping app.
3. Limit purchases of irresistible "problem" foods.
4. Shop for fresh foods around the perimeter of the store first.
5. Avoid highly processed, ready-to-eat foods.
6. Put off food shopping until absolutely necessary.

Planning
1. Plan meals in advance; keep healthy foods washed and prepared.
2. Substitute periods of physical activity for snacking.
3. Eat meals and snacks at scheduled times; don't skip meals.
4. Drink plenty of water throughout the day.

Activities
1. Store food out of sight to discourage impulsive eating.
2. Eat all food in a designated "dining" area; avoid buffet-type meals.
3. Keep serving dishes off the table, especially dishes of sauces and gravies.
4. Use smaller dishes and utensils.

Holidays and Parties
1. Drink fewer alcoholic beverages; alternate water with alcohol.
2. Eat a low-calorie snack before parties.
3. Plan eating behavior before parties.
4. Practice polite ways to decline food.
5. Don't get discouraged by an occasional setback.

Eating Behavior
1. Put the fork down between bites; chew thoroughly and slowly before taking the next bite.
2. Leave some food on the plate.
3. Pause in the middle of the meal and evaluate satiety (feeling of fullness) signals.
4. Do nothing else while eating (e.g., reading, texting, watching television).

Rewards
1. Plan specific rewards for positive behavior (behavioral contracts); allow for a small treat on exercise days.
2. Solicit help from family and friends; engage in exercise and healthy cooking together.
3. Use self-monitoring records (diet, physical activity, body weight) as basis for rewards. Many tracking apps are available.

Self-Monitoring
1. Note the time and place of eating.
2. List the type and amount of food and beverages consumed.
3. Record who is present and how you feel.
4. Use the dietary intake diary to identify problem areas.
5. Use online or mobile apps to track your progress, including your new nutrition and health goals and habits.

Cognitive Restructuring
1. Avoid setting unreasonable goals; focus on small and manageable steps.
2. Focus on long-term progress, not occasional setbacks.
3. Avoid imperatives such as *always* and *never.*
4. Counter negative thoughts with positive restatements.

Portion Control
1. Make healthy substitutions, such as small fries instead of large fries or add cucumbers instead of croutons to salads.
2. Think small. Order the entrée and share it with another person. Order a cup of soup instead of a bowl or an appetizer in place of an entrée.
3. Use a take-home box. Ask your server to pack half the entrée in a take-home box before bringing it to the table.

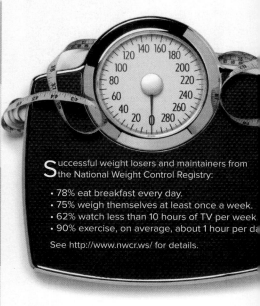

Successful weight losers and maintainers from the National Weight Control Registry:
- 78% eat breakfast every day.
- 75% weigh themselves at least once a week.
- 62% watch less than 10 hours of TV per week
- 90% exercise, on average, about 1 hour per da

See http://www.nwcr.ws/ for details.

©DNY59/Getty Images RF

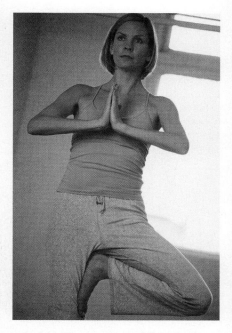

▲ Individuals who successfully maintain their weight loss employ a variety of strategies, such as physical activity or meditation, to cope with the stresses and challenges of changing problem behaviors.
©Royalty-Free/Corbis

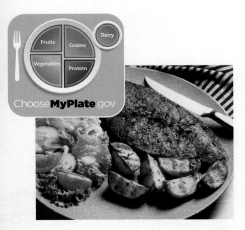

▲ Large portions of food, such as this steak, provide us with many opportunities to overeat. It takes much perseverance to eat sensibly. How do the portion sizes shown here compare to those recommended by MyPlate? Source: ChooseMyPlate.gov; ©Ernie Friedlander/Cole Group/Getty Images RF

The Dietary Guidelines Strategies for Action include:

1. Identifying and addressing successful approaches for change.
2. Improving knowledge of what constitutes healthy eating and physical activity patterns.
3. Enhancing access to adequate amounts of healthy, safe, and affordable food choices.
4. Promoting change in social and cultural norms and values to embrace, support, and maintain healthy eating and physical activity behaviors.

Public, private, and nonprofit organizations have begun to work together to address and reverse this public health crisis. For example, the U.S. Food and Drug Administration (FDA) has brought together leaders from industry, government, academia, and the public health community to seek solutions to the obesity epidemic by making changes in foods eaten outside the home (restaurant and carry-out foods). These groups collaborate and made recommendations to support the consumer's ability to manage calorie intake. Recommendations include *social marketing* programs that promote healthy eating and active living.

✓ CONCEPT CHECK 7.8

1. What behavioral techniques are helpful in changing problem eating behaviors to improve weight-loss success?
2. How does mindful and mindless eating help control hunger?

7.9 Professional Help for Weight Loss

The first professional to seek for advice about a weight-loss program is a primary care provider. This professional is equipped to assess overall health and current weight status by examining health parameters such as blood pressure, blood lipids, and blood glucose that can be altered because of excess weight. Your clinician may then recommend a registered dietitian nutritionist for a specific behavioral weight-loss plan and answers to nutrition-related questions. RDNs are uniquely qualified to help design a weight-loss plan because they understand both food composition and the psychological importance of food. Sports dietitians and exercise physiologists can provide advice about programs to improve physical activity. The expense for such professional interventions is tax deductible in the United States in some cases (consult a tax advisor) and often covered by health insurance plans if prescribed by a primary care provider or covered by a student wellness plan.

Many communities have a variety of weight-loss organizations. These include self-help groups, such as Weight Watchers,® which offer social support and education. Other programs, such as Jenny Craig® and Physicians' Weight Loss Center,® are less desirable for the average person because they require expensive food purchases and don't encourage healthy food preparation. Often, the leaders are not credentialed dietitians or other trained professionals. These programs tend to be expensive because of their requirements for intense counseling or mandatory diet foods and supplements. The diet programs that require product purchases promote weight cycling, sometimes called *yo-yo dieting*, and ultimately result in rebound weight gain at a higher body fat level. In addition, the Federal Trade Commission has charged these and other commercial diet programs with misleading consumers through unsubstantiated weight-loss claims and deceptive testimonials.

MEDICATIONS FOR WEIGHT LOSS

Candidates for medications to treat obesity, also called anti-obesity drugs or *diet pills*, include those with a BMI ≥ 30 or BMI ≥ 27 with at least one obesity-associated comorbid condition (e.g., type 2 diabetes, cardiovascular disease, hypertension) and who are motivated to lose weight. For specific populations, medication, also known as pharmacotherapy, may be considered to supplement lifestyle interventions to help achieve targeted weight loss and health goals. Drug therapy alone has not been found to be successful for long-term weight maintenance. Success with medications has been shown only in those who also modify their behavior, decrease calorie intake, and increase physical activity. For a drug to be considered effective in treating obesity, it must pass FDA guidelines and prove to be relatively safe (Table 7-7).

One class of medication approved by the FDA for weight loss is orlistat (Xenical).® This medication reduces fat digestion by about 30% by inhibiting lipase enzyme action in the small intestine (Fig. 7-21). This cuts absorption of dietary fat by one-third for about 2 hours when taken along with a meal containing fat. This malabsorbed fat is deposited in the feces. Fat intake has to be controlled, however, because large amounts of fat in the feces cause numerous side effects, such as diarrhea, gas, bloating, and oily discharge. The malabsorbed fat also carries fat-soluble vitamins (vitamins A, D, E, K) into the feces, so the person taking orlistat must take a multivitamin and mineral supplement at bedtime. In this way, any micronutrients not absorbed during the day can be replaced. A low-dose form of orlistat (Alli)® is now available over the counter without a prescription.

Other approved weight-loss medications work in various ways to curb appetite. Table 7-7 has a summary of the most common FDA-approved medications. Sometimes, physicians may prescribe medications that are not approved for weight loss but have weight loss as a side effect. Such an application is termed *off-label*. Over-the-counter medications and supplements are widely marketed as miracle cures for obesity, but in some cases, they do

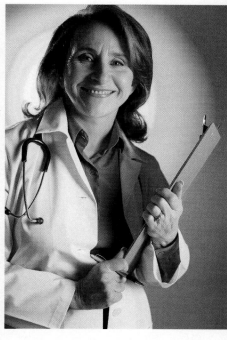

▲ All weight-loss programs should begin with a visit to your primary care provider.
©Dynamic Graphics/JupiterImages RF

TABLE 7-7 ■ **Medications Approved for Obesity Treatment**

Medication	Approval	Action	Possible Side Effects
Lorcaserin (Belviq)®	Adults	Acts on serotonin brain receptors Thought to promote satiety	Headaches, dizziness, fatigue, nausea, dry mouth, cough, and constipation Should not be taken with selective serotonin reuptake inhibitors and monoamine oxidase inhibitors
Orlistat (Xenical® by prescription or alli® over-the-counter)	Xenical – over age 12; Alli® – adults	Blocks fat absorption	Stomach pain, gas, diarrhea, leaky oily stools Rare cases of severe liver injury; should not take with cyclosporine
Phentermine-topiramate (Qsymia,® Fastin,® Lonamin)®	Adults	Combination of appetite suppressor and migraine/seizure medication	Tingling of hands and feet, dizziness, taste alterations, trouble sleeping, constipation, and dry mouth Do not use if pregnant or planning to become pregnant
Liraglutide (Saxenda)®	Adults	Slows gastric emptying and enhances satiety	Long-term effects remain unknown.
Others: phentermine benzphetamine diethylpropion phendimetrazine	Adults	Alter brain chemicals to promote appetite suppression. Approved by the FDA for use up to 12 weeks	Dry mouth, difficulty sleeping, dizziness, headache, feeling nervous, upset stomach, diarrhea, constipation, and feeling restless

Sources: http://www.fda.gov/ohrms/dockets/ac/04/briefing/2004-4068B1_05_Approved-Drugs.htm, and http://www.todaysdietitian.com/newarchives/060114p44.shtml

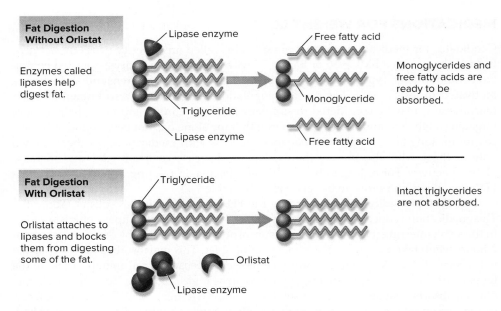

FIGURE 7-21 ▲ Orlistat is a weight-loss drug that works in the digestive system to block digestion and subsequent absorption of about one-third of the fat in the food we eat. A low-dose form of this drug (alli)® is now available without a prescription.

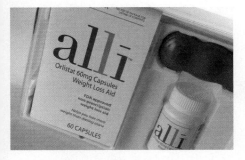

▲ alli® (orlistat) is an over-the-counter weight-loss drug that blocks fat digestion and absorption. ©McGraw-Hill Education/Jill Braaten, photographer

very-low-calorie diet (VLCD) This diet allows a person fewer than 800 calories per day, often in liquid form. Of this, 120 to 480 calories are typically from carbohydrate, and the rest are mostly from high-quality protein.

more harm than good. Today more than ever, let the buyer beware concerning any purported weight-loss aid not prescribed by a primary care provider.

Although prescription medications can aid weight loss in some instances, they do not replace the need for reducing calorie intake, modifying *problem* behaviors, and increasing physical activity, both during and after therapy. Often, any weight loss during drug treatment can be attributed mostly to the individual's hard work at balancing calorie intake with calorie output.

TREATMENT OF SEVERE OBESITY

Severe (morbid) obesity, having a BMI ≥ 40 or weighing at least 100 pounds over healthy body weight (or twice one's healthy body weight), often requires professional treatment. Because of the serious health implications of severe obesity, drastic measures may be necessary. Such treatments are recommended only when traditional diets and medications fail. Drastic weight-loss procedures are not without side effects, both physical and psychological, making careful monitoring by a primary care provider a necessity.

Very-Low-Calorie Diets If more traditional diets have failed, treating severe obesity with a **very-low-calorie diet (VLCD)** is possible, especially if the person has obesity-related diseases that are not well controlled (e.g., hypertension, type 2 diabetes). Some clinicians believe that people with body weight greater than 30% above their healthy weight are appropriate candidates. A VLCD is dangerous because of its rapid weight loss and potential for severe health complications, including heart problems and gallstones. Often providing fewer than 800 kcal per day, all VLCD programs should be administered under strict medical supervision, as careful monitoring by a trained clinician is crucial throughout this very restrictive form of weight loss.

Optifast® and other VLCD meal replacements are commercial programs. In general, these diets allow a person to consume only 400 to 800 kcal per day, often in liquid form. These diets were previously known as protein-sparing modified fasts. Of this amount, approximately 30 to 120 grams (120 to 480 kcal) are carbohydrates. The rest are from high-quality protein in the amount of 70 to 100 grams per day (280 to 400 kcal).

This low carbohydrate intake may cause *ketosis*, an acidic state caused by inadequate glucose for fuel, which may decrease hunger. The main reasons for weight loss, however, are the minimal energy consumption and restricted food choices. About 2 to 4 pounds can be lost per week, primarily water and lean body mass losses. When physical activity and resistance training augment this diet, a greater loss of adipose tissue occurs.

Weight regain remains a likely scenario, especially without a behavioral and physical activity component. If behavioral therapy and physical activity supplement a long-term support program, maintenance of the weight loss is more likely but still difficult. Any program under consideration should include a detailed maintenance plan. Today, anti-obesity medications may also be included in this phase of the program.

Intermittent Fasting The dietary practice known as *intermittent fasting*, where one cycles days of so-called normal eating with a day or days of eating little to nothing, is gaining popularity. Despite evidence that intermittent fasting can promote weight loss in some individuals, most dietitians and clinicians remain skeptical of this approach for any length of time. More specific information on intermittent fasting, binge eating, and other weight-loss methods can be found in Chapter 11 (Ask the RDN).

AspireAssist® The FDA has recently approved an obesity treatment device that uses a surgically placed tube to drain a portion of the stomach contents after every meal. AspireAssist® is only intended for obese adults (BMI ≥ 35) who have failed to achieve and maintain weight loss through nonsurgical weight-loss therapy.

The device is inserted in the stomach surgically and connected to a disk-shaped port valve outside the body, flush against the abdomen. Approximately 20 to 30 minutes after a meal, the patient attaches tubing to the port valve and drains the contents. Once the valve is opened, it takes approximately 5 to 10 minutes to drain food matter through the tube and into the toilet. The device removes approximately 30 percent of the calories consumed.

Ongoing medical visits are necessary to monitor device use and weight loss, and to provide education and training. The device also contains a safety feature that tracks the number of drain cycles and stops after 115 cycles (~5 to 6 weeks of therapy). This ensures the patient will return for frequent medical visits. Side effects include occasional indigestion, nausea, vomiting, constipation, and diarrhea.

Bariatric Surgery **Bariatrics** is the medical specialty focusing on the treatment of obesity. Bariatric surgery is only considered for people with severe obesity (BMI ≥ 40 or BMI ≥ 35 with obesity-related comorbid conditions) and includes surgery aimed at promoting weight loss. Figure 7-22 provides details about common bariatric procedures.

bariatrics The medical specialty focusing on the treatment of obesity.

The risks of bariatric surgery are serious and include death and both early and late postoperative complications, such as bleeding, blood clots, hernias, electrolyte imbalances, and severe infections. Risk of death from these demanding and complex surgeries can be as high as 2%. These risks depend on many factors related to the surgeon and facility, the patient, and the procedure. The procedures that are simply restrictive (e.g., adjustable gastric banding and sleeve gastrectomy) do not cause malabsorption and rarely affect bowel function. However, for those procedures that induce malabsorption (e.g., Roux-en-Y gastric bypass), nutrient deficiencies are of greater concern if the person is not adequately treated in the years following the surgery. Anemia and bone loss might then be the result.

Bariatric surgery is costly and may not be covered by medical insurance. The average cost for gastric bypass procedures is $18,000 to $35,000 and for adjustable gastric banding is $17,000 to $30,000. In addition, follow-up surgery is often needed after weight loss to correct stretched skin, previously filled with fat. Furthermore, the surgery necessitates major lifestyle changes, such as the need to plan frequent, small meals. Therefore, the dieter who has chosen this drastic approach to weight loss faces months of difficult adjustments.

Types of Bariatric Surgery

Gastric Bypass

This procedure, also called Roux-en-Y gastric bypass, creates a small pouch that significantly limits the amount the stomach can comfortably hold. The stomach continues to make digestive juices, so this permits the digestive juices to flow to the small intestine. Because food now bypasses a portion of the small intestine, fewer calories and nutrients are absorbed.

BENEFITS: Greater weight loss than gastric band with no foreign objects used in the procedure.

LIMITATIONS: Increased risk of surgery-related issues with longer recovery. This procedure is difficult to reverse and nutrient deficiencies may occur.

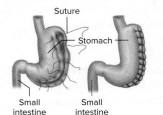

Before surgery   **After surgery**

1. Staples divide the stomach.

Stomach
Flow of food
Stomach and duodenum bypassed
Pouch
Duodenum
Jejunum
Small intestine
Jejunum

2. Part of the small intestine, called the jejunum, is connected to the pouch.

Laparoscopic Adjustable Gastric Banding

This procedure involves placing an inflatable band around the top portion of the stomach. This limits the space available for food and increases satiety. LAGB is often recommended for people who have tried other weight-loss plans without long-term success.

BENEFITS: The surgical procedure is rapid (30–60 minutes) and can be reversed. This surgery has the lowest risk of vitamin and mineral deficits.

LIMITATIONS: Results in less weight loss than other surgeries. The surgical procedure is challenging and requires multiple steps. In addition, the band may slip, so frequent follow-up is required.

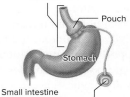

This procedure divides stomach into two sections. This creates a small pouch with a narrow opening that goes into the larger section of the stomach.

Pouch
Stomach
Small intestine
Port is used to adjust the gastric band after surgery.

Gastric Plication

This is a restrictive procedure that shrinks the size of the stomach by suturing large folds in the stomach's lining. This reduces the stomach volume by approximately 80%, and increases satiety. The procedure typically takes between 40 minutes and 2 hours to complete.

BENEFITS: Increased weight loss over gastric band with no change in the intestines. This procedure has a relatively rapid recovery period.

LIMITATIONS: This procedure cannot be reversed, and there is an increased risk of acid reflux. As with most bariatric procedures, vitamin and mineral deficiencies are a serious concern.

Suture
Stomach
Small intestine
Small intestine

Vertical Sleeve Gastrectomy

In this bariatric procedure, 80% to 85% of the stomach is removed to create a smaller stomach pouch. This limits the amount of food consumed and increases satiety. Vertical sleeve gastrectomy has most often been done on people who are too heavy to safely have other types of weight-loss surgery.

BENEFITS: This is a rapid surgical procedure, taking 30–60 minutes, that is safer than other procedures.

LIMITATIONS: This procedure cannot be reversed. Weight loss is typically slower than with other bariatric procedures.

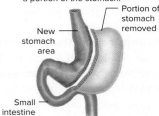

1. Using a video monitor to guide the instruments, surgeon removes a portion of the stomach.

Portion of stomach removed
New stomach area
Small intestine

2. The remaining portion of the stomach is closed using staples.

Ileal Transposition

The metabolic procedure is often used for overweight individuals with type 2 diabetes. The technique relocates the distal part of the small intestine to the proximal part of the small intestine. This is a longer operation than other procedures (3–3.5 hours) and requires more advanced equipment, longer hospital stays, and higher costs than other commonly used, simpler procedures.

BENEFITS: Results in greater glycemic control than other procedures; considered key to managing the twin epidemics of obesity and diabetes.

LIMITATIONS: As with all invasive procedures, surgical complications are possible.

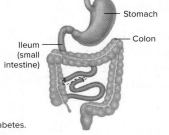

Stomach
Colon
Ileum (small intestine)

FIGURE 7-22 ▲ Bariatric surgery promotes weight loss by altering the digestive track anatomy, limiting the volume of food that can be consumed and digested. These surgical procedures are appropriate for everyone and candidates must be screened carefully. In addition, many of the procedures are relatively new and research on long-term effects remain unknown. The American Society for Bariatric Surgery has a certification for qualified surgeons.

Despite potential adverse effects, the benefits of bariatric surgery for those who are eligible usually outweigh the risks. In terms of long-term weight-loss success, bariatric surgeries have the best results of any intervention. An increasing number of youth are turning to bariatric surgery to treat obesity. Table 7-8 details the pros and cons of the most common bariatric procedures for children. Weight-loss statistics vary by surgical method, but on average, about 75% of people with severe obesity eventually lose and keep off 50% or more of excess body weight. In addition, many patients experience significant improvements in blood sugar, cholesterol, and blood pressure. By no means is bariatric surgery a quick and easy fix for obesity, but with a serious commitment to permanent lifestyle changes and long-term follow-up with a health professional, these procedures can positively impact both quality and quantity of life.

Liposuction *Spot reducing* by using diet and physical activity is not possible. Problem local fat deposits can be reduced in size, however, using suction liposuction, or lipectomy. This invasive procedure involves surgical removal of fat. A pencil-thin tube is inserted into an incision in the skin, and the fat tissue, often in the buttocks and thigh area,

TABLE 7-8 ■ **Bariatric Surgeries Performed on Youth**

	Adjustable Gastric Banding	Gastric Bypass
Strengths	Low rate of complications and quicker recovery	Most frequent bariatric procedure in youth
	Intestine not altered so vitamin deficiencies are rare	High success rate
Limitations	Weight loss not as rapid	Longer recovery due to intestinal trauma
	May require replacement surgery after time	Irreversible procedure
Possible Side Effects	Infection, bleeding, band slippage or erosion, stomach pouch enlargement, stoma blockage	Infection, bleeding, blood clots, bowel obstruction, "leaky" abdomen

is suctioned out through a tube and discarded. This invasive procedure involves risks, such as infection, permanent depressions in the skin, nerve damage, and blood clots, which can lead to kidney failure and sometimes death. The procedure is designed to help a person lose about 4 to 8 pounds per treatment. The costs vary greatly and depend upon site and clinician, but the average cost is approximately $3000 per procedure.

✓ CONCEPT CHECK 7.9

1. What are the surgical options for morbidly obese people who have failed to lose weight with other weight-loss strategies?

2. How restrictive is a very-low-calorie diet plan? Why is monitoring by a qualified health professional important?

7.10 Treatment of Underweight

Underweight is defined by a BMI < 18.5 and can be caused by a variety of factors, such as cancer, infectious disease (e.g., tuberculosis), digestive tract disorders (e.g., chronic inflammatory bowel disease), and excessive dieting or physical activity. Genetic factors may also lead to a higher RMR, a slight body frame, or both. Health problems associated with underweight include the loss of menstrual function (*amenorrhea*), low bone mass, complications with pregnancy and surgery, and slow recovery after illness. Significant underweight is also associated with increased death rates, especially when combined with smoking. We frequently hear about the risks of obesity but seldom of underweight. In our culture, being underweight is much more socially acceptable than being overweight or obese.

Sometimes being underweight requires medical intervention. A thorough physical exam should be obtained first to rule out hormonal imbalances, depression, cancer, infectious disease, digestive tract disorders, excessive physical activity, and other hidden diseases such as a serious eating disorder (see Chapter 15 for a detailed discussion of eating disorders).

The causes of underweight are not altogether different from the causes of obesity. Internal and external satiety-signal irregularities, the rate of metabolism, genetic factors, and psychological traits can all contribute to underweight.

In growing children, the high demand for calories to support physical activity and growth can cause underweight. During growth spurts, active children and adolescents may not take the time to consume enough calories to support their needs. Moreover, gaining

underweight A BMI below 18.5. The cutoff is less precise than for obesity BMI classifications because this condition has been less studied.

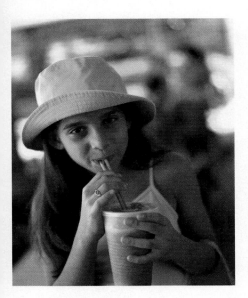

▲ Underweight people should increase their consumption of calorie-dense foods, such as smoothies, that are also loaded with nutrients and often calorie-dense.
©Dynamic Graphics Group/Creatas/Alamy RF

weight can be a formidable task for an underweight person. An extra 500 kcal per day may be required to gain weight, and this can prove challenging for active children. Individuals attempting to gain weight may need to increase portion sizes and include frequent snacks.

When underweight requires a specific intervention, one approach for treating adults is to gradually increase their consumption of calorie-dense foods, especially those high in vegetable fats. Nuts and granola can be good calorie sources with low saturated fat content. Dried fruits and bananas are good fruit choices. Underweight people should replace sugar-free drinks with good calorie sources, such as 100% fruit juices and nutrient-rich smoothies.

Encouraging a regular meal and snack schedule also aids in weight gain and maintenance. Sometimes underweight individuals have experienced stress at work or have been too busy to eat. Making regular meals a priority may not only help them attain an appropriate weight but also help with digestive disorders, such as constipation, sometimes associated with irregular eating times.

GAINING WEIGHT AS MUSCLE, NOT FAT

A combination of high-quality nutrition and strength training is needed to gain weight as muscle. Strength training slows muscle loss that comes with dieting and aging, increases the strength of your muscles and connective tissues, and increases bone density. When weight is lost, up to a quarter of the loss may come from muscle mass, which can slow basal metabolism. Strength training helps protect against lean body mass losses and rebuilds any muscle lost by dieting—or prevents it from being lost in the first place. The best bet when starting a strength-training program is to seek individualized counseling from a qualified sports dietitian or certified fitness trainer who can address personal goals and limitations and can help with alignment and execution of each exercise.

There are several things to consider when designing dietary patterns to accompany training. During a workout, it is normal for the body to break down some muscles due to the stress placed on them. Once you're finished strength training, you want to repair and build muscle again. It is very important to get proper nutrients into the body after a workout to promote recovery and muscle building. Immediately before and again after strength training, a serving of high-quality protein should be consumed to optimize performance and build lean muscle mass. It is also important to have some carbohydrate along with protein to increase the protein absorption, replete glycogen stores, and provide future fuel for workouts. Chocolate milk has shown to be a great source of protein, carbohydrate, and fluid immediately post-activity. Although a quick protein bar or shake is great when you're at the gym, it should not be the only source of protein. During meals, lean protein sources such as tuna, lean chicken, soy, and beans are the most appropriate. Those who work out but eat nothing but food high in saturated fat and calories will gain fat in addition to any muscle gains. To gain lean muscle mass, one needs a balanced diet rich in protein and carbohydrates, including plenty of fruits, vegetables, and whole grains. The number of calories you require each day varies greatly and will depend on your weight, activity level, age, and muscle mass. If you are working out 3 days a week, you can eat about 15 kcal per pound of body weight. If you work out 5 days a week, you can increase that calorie count to 20 kcal per pound.

✓ CONCEPT CHECK 7.10

1. How is underweight defined, and what are some of its primary causes?
2. What are the components necessary to gain weight as muscle and not as fat?

Popular Diets—Cause for Concern

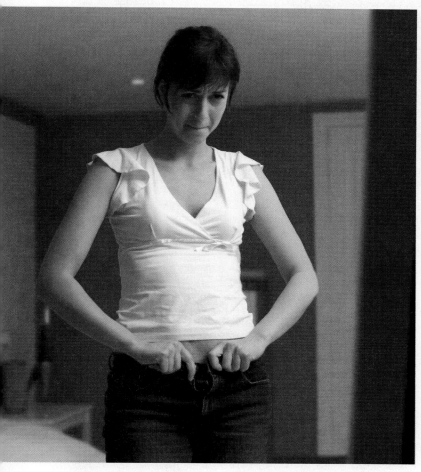

©BananaStock/PunchStock

Many overweight people try to help themselves by using the latest popular (also called *fad*) diets. But, as you will see, most of these fad diets do not help, and some can actually harm those who follow them. Research has shown that early dieting and unhealthful weight-control practices in adolescents can lead to an increased risk of weight gain, overweight, and eating disorders.

At the request of the U.S. Department of Agriculture (USDA), researchers were convened to evaluate weight-loss diets. They came to this conclusion: forget these fad diets when it comes to dieting. Most of the popular diets are nutritionally inadequate and include certain foods that people would not normally choose to consume in large amounts. The experts stated that eating less of one's favorite foods and becoming more physically active can be much more effective when trying to implement a weight-loss strategy. People need a plan they can live with in the long run so that a healthy weight becomes permanent. The goal should be weight management over a lifetime, not immediate weight loss. Every popular diet leads to some immediate weight loss simply because daily intake is monitored and monotonous food choices

are typically part of the plan. Overall, a healthy dietary pattern coupled with regular physical activity is recommended for weight loss.

People on diets often fall within a healthy BMI of 18.5 to 25. Rather than worrying about weight loss, these individuals should focus on a healthy lifestyle that allows for weight maintenance. Incorporating necessary lifestyle changes, especially regular physical activity, and learning to accept one's individual body characteristics should be the overriding goals.

The dieting mania can be viewed as mostly a social problem, stemming from unrealistic weight expectations (especially for women) and lack of appreciation for the natural variety in body shape and size. Not every woman can or should look like a fashion model, nor can every man look like a Greek god, but all of us can strive for good health and, if physically possible, an active lifestyle.

The size-acceptance nondiet movement, "Health at Every Size," has attempted to shift the paradigm away from the use of "popular" weight-loss diets. Goals of the movement are all independent of body weight and include improvement of self-image, normalization of eating behavior, and increase in physical activity. The best weight-loss plans of 2016 are listed in Table 7-9.

How to Recognize a Fad Diet

The criteria for evaluating weight-loss programs with regard to their safety and effectiveness were discussed in Section 7.5. In contrast, unreliable fad diets typically share some common characteristics:

1. They promote rapid weight loss. This is the primary temptation that attracts the dieter. As mentioned, this initial weight loss primarily results from water loss and lean muscle mass depletion.
2. They often limit food selections and dictate specific rituals, such as eating only fruit for breakfast or cabbage soup every day.
3. They use testimonials from famous people and tie the diet to well-known cities, such as Beverly Hills or South Beach.
4. They bill themselves as cure-alls. These diets claim to work for everyone, whatever the type of obesity or the person's genetic or environmental makeup.
5. They often recommend expensive supplements or meals.
6. No attempts are made to change eating habits permanently. Dieters follow the diet until the desired weight is reached and then revert to old behaviors; they are told, for example, to eat rice for a month, lose weight, and then return to old habits.
7. They are generally critical of and skeptical about the scientific community. The lack of a quick fix from medical and dietetic professionals has led some of the public to seek advice from those who appear to have the answer.
8. They claim that there is no need to exercise.

Probably the cruelest characteristic of these diets is that they essentially guarantee failure for the dieter. Fad diets are not designed for permanent weight loss. Habits are not changed, and the food selection is so limited that the person cannot follow the

TABLE 7-9 ■ Best Weight-Loss Plans 2016

Diet Plan	Rank	Score (out of 5)	Concept
DASH Diet	1	4.2	Focuses on a healthy eating pattern as key to deflating high blood pressure with additional benefits as well (weight loss)
Mediterranean Diet	2	4.1	Promotes an active lifestyle, weight control, and a diet low in red meat, sugar, and saturated fat and high in produce, nuts, and other healthful foods
MIND Diet	3	4.0	Takes two proven diets (DASH and Mediterranean) and zeroes in on the foods in each that specifically affect brain health
Flexitarian Diet	4 (tie)	3.9	Based on a flexible vegetarian approach that promotes a plant-based diet most of the time with room for occasional animal proteins
Mayo Clinic	4 (tie)	3.9	Focuses on recalibrating eating habits to break negative behaviors and replace them with positive behaviors

A panel of experts evaluated popular diets and ranked them. To be highly ranked, a plan must be easy to follow, nutritious, safe, effective for weight loss and protective against chronic disease. The government-endorsed Dietary Approaches to Stop Hypertension (DASH) diet took the top spot, while the Mediterranean diet came in second.

Source: *U.S. News and World Report,* 2016 (http://health.usnews.com/best-diet/dash-diet)

diet in the long run. Although dieters assume that they have lost fat, they have lost mainly muscle mass and body fluids. As soon as they begin eating normally again, much of the lost tissue is replaced as fat mass. In a matter of weeks or months, most of the lost weight is back. The dieter appears to have failed, when actually the *diet* has failed. The gain and loss cycle is called weight cycling or *yo-yo* dieting. This whole scenario can add more blame and guilt, challenging the self-worth of the dieter. It can also come with some health costs, such as increased upper-body fat deposition. If someone needs help losing weight, consult a nutrition expert, such as a registered dietitian nutritionist. It is unfortunate that current trends suggest that people are spending more time and money on *quick fixes* than on such professional help.

Types of Popular Diets

HIGH-PROTEIN, LOW-CARBOHYDRATE APPROACHES

High-protein, low-carbohydrate diets are a popular approach to losing weight. These diets typically recommend at least 30% to 50% of their total calories from protein and drastically restrict carbohydrate. Low-carbohydrate intake leads to less glycogen synthesis and therefore less water in the body (about 3 grams of water are stored per gram of glycogen). As discussed in Chapter 4, a very-low-carbohydrate intake also forces the liver to produce needed glucose. The source of carbons for this glucose is mostly proteins from tissues such as muscle, resulting in loss of protein tissue, which is about 72% water. Essential ions, such as potassium, are also lost in the urine. In the initial stages of a low-carbohydrate diet, losses of glycogen stores, lean tissue, and water cause rapid

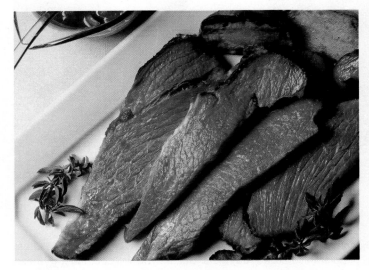

▲ In time, the very-low-carbohydrate, high-protein diets typically leave a person fatigued and wanting more variety in meals, and so the diets are abandoned. Dropout rates are high on these diets.
©Ernie Friedlander/Cole Group/Getty Images RF

weight loss. When a normal diet is resumed, the protein tissue is rebuilt and the weight is regained.

In addition, restricting carbohydrate causes your body to burn fat instead of carbohydrate for fuel. In theory, this burning of excess fat stores makes sense for weight loss. Remember, however, that when we burn fat without carbohydrate, it causes the body to go into the metabolic state called ketosis. This disruption in the body's acid–base balance has the short-term benefit of making you feel less hungry, yet long-term ketosis can become dangerous when ketones build up. High levels of ketones lead to dehydration and alterations in the chemical balance of your blood.

For most dieters, a low-carb plan is such a major change from normal habits that it is very difficult to maintain. However, research indicates that low-carbohydrate diets may be an effective alternative to low-fat diets for some people.[8] The most popular diet using a low-carbohydrate approach is Dr. Atkins' New Diet Revolution. More moderate approaches are found in the various Zone diets (40% of calorie intake as carbohydrate), Sugar Busters Diet, and the South Beach Diet.

CARBOHYDRATE-FOCUSED DIETS

Several recent diets do not restrict carbohydrates but rather emphasize the *good* carbohydrates in place of the *bad* or *harmful* ones. These diets recommend eating plenty of fruits, vegetables, and whole grains, and cutting out simple sugars and processed or refined grains. In theory, these foods will cause a slow, steady rise and fall in blood sugar after a meal, which may help control hunger.

LOW-FAT APPROACHES

Very-low-fat diets contain approximately 5% to 10% of calories as fat and are often very high in carbohydrates. If followed consistently, these approaches lead to weight loss and may be helpful for reducing heart disease risks; however, they are difficult to follow. People are quickly bored with this type of diet because they cannot eat many of their favorite foods. These dieters eat primarily plant-based foods (grains, fruits, and vegetables), which many people cannot maintain for very long. Eventually, the person wants some foods higher in fat or protein. Furthermore, such diets may have too much carbohydrate for some people who have a family history of diabetes.[9]

NOVELTY DIETS

A variety of diets are built on gimmicks. Some novelty diets emphasize one food or food group and exclude almost all others. A rice diet was designed in the 1940s to lower blood pressure; now it has resurfaced as a weight-loss diet. The first phase consists of eating only rice and fruit. On the Beverly Hills Diet, you eat mostly fruit. The Paleo Diet is designed to mimic the diets of cavemen and includes meats, seafood, vegetables, fruits, and nuts.

The Military Diet promises an *emergency* weight loss of up to 10 pounds without strenuous exercise or medications. Foods allowed include apples, bananas, meat, peanut butter, eggs, green beans, vanilla ice cream, water, coffee, and stevia. On the four off-days, any foods are allowed as long as total calories are 1500 or fewer.

Over 30 years ago, the Health Management Resources (HMR) program was launched. The diet requires food purchases including entrees, low-calorie shakes, and nutrition bars. The plan also allows fruits and vegetables to help keep the dieter satisfied. The typical dieter consumes a minimum of three shakes per day, two HMR entrées (provided to client), and five 1-cup servings of fruits and vegetables. Although a low-calorie plan will result in weight loss, it doesn't teach clients lifelong behavior skills. This can result in weight gain once they go off the diet.

The 10-Day Green Smoothie Cleanse claims that dieting won't remove bodily toxins, so detoxification should be completed. This cleanse promotes three smoothies, snacks, and water or detox tea each day for 10 days. Smoothies are made from raw vegetables along with fruits. Cleansing plans are often dangerously low in calories (< 1000 kcal), which often results in nutrient deficiencies. Side effects include fatigue, dizziness, and nausea. Advocates of cleanses fail to understand that the liver and kidneys serve as our body's detoxification organs.

Other popular diet plans include the Bulletproof Diet, Whole30, and a variety of fasting or intermittent eating regimens. Note that the Academy of Nutrition and Dietetics provides reviews of a variety of fad diet plans at www.eatright.org/resources/health/weight-loss/fad-diets.

MEAL REPLACEMENTS

Meal replacements come in many forms, including beverages or formulas, frozen or shelf-stable entrees, and meal or snack bars. Most meal replacements are fortified with vitamins and minerals and are appropriate to replace one or two regular meals or snacks per day. Although they are not a *magic bullet* for weight loss, they have been shown to help some people lose weight. Advantages of these convenient products are that they provide portion- and calorie-controlled foods that can serve as a visual education on appropriate portion sizes. A disadvantage is that when dieters rely on foods selected and prepared by someone else, they do not learn behaviors necessary to select and prepare healthy foods on their own.

QUACKERY IS CHARACTERISTIC OF MANY POPULAR DIETS

Many popular diets fall under the category of *quackery*—people taking advantage of others. They usually involve a product or service that costs a considerable amount of money. Often, those offering the product or service don't realize that they are promoting quackery because they were victims themselves. For example, they tried the product and, by pure coincidence, felt it worked for them, so they promote it to all their friends and relatives.

Numerous other gimmicks for weight loss have come and gone and are likely to resurface. If in the future an important aid for weight loss is discovered, you can feel confident that major journals, such as the *Journal of the Academy of Nutrition and Dietetics, Journal of the American Medical Association,* or *New England Journal of Medicine,* will report it. Quackwatch.com is an online resource for consumers to help identify quackery.

CASE STUDY Choosing a Weight-Loss Program

Joe has a hectic schedule. During the day, he works full time at a warehouse distribution center filling orders. At night, three times a week, he attends class at the local community college in pursuit of computer certification. On weekends, he likes to watch sports on television, spend time with family and friends, and study. Joe has little time to exercise or think about what he eats—that is, convenience rules. He stops for coffee and a pastry on his way to work, has a burger or pizza for lunch at a fast-food restaurant, and for dinner picks up fried chicken or fish at the drive-through on his way to class. Unfortunately, over the past few years, Joe's weight has been climbing. He is 5 feet, 10 inches tall and weighs 200 pounds. Lately, he has frequently been short of breath during his shift at work. Watching a game on television a few nights ago, he saw an infomercial for a weight-loss supplement that promises to increase his energy level and allow him to continue to eat large portions of tasty foods but not gain weight. A famous actor supports the claim that this product allows one to eat at will and not gain weight. This claim is tempting to Joe.

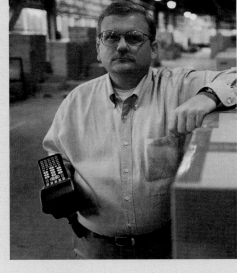

▲ What changes can Joe make in his daily routine and diet to prevent weight gain?
©Ryan McVay/Getty Images RF

1. Has Joe been experiencing positive or negative energy balance over the past few years? What is his current BMI?
2. What aspects of Joe's lifestyle (other than diet) are causing this effect on his energy balance?
3. What changes could Joe make to his diet and physical activity patterns that would promote weight loss or maintenance?
4. Why should Joe be skeptical of the claims he heard about the weight-loss product in the infomercial?
5. Referring back to the characteristics of unreliable diets, what advice can you offer Joe for evaluating weight-loss programs?

Complete the Case Study. Responses to these questions can be provided by your instructor.

Summary (Numbers refer to numbered sections in the chapter.)

7.1 Energy balance considers energy intake and energy output. Negative energy balance occurs when energy output surpasses energy intake, resulting in weight loss. Positive energy balance occurs when calorie intake is greater than output, resulting in weight gain.

Basal metabolism, the thermic effect of food, physical activity, and adaptive thermogenesis account for total energy use by the body. Basal metabolism, which represents the minimum amount of calories required to keep the resting, awake body alive, is primarily affected by lean body mass, surface area, and thyroid hormone concentrations. Physical activity is energy use above that expended at rest. The thermic effect of food describes the increase in metabolism that facilitates digestion, absorption, and processing of the nutrients recently consumed. Adaptive thermogenesis includes nonvoluntary activities, such as shivering and fidgeting, that increase energy use and may counter extra calories from overeating. In a sedentary person, about 70% to 85% of energy use is accounted for by basal metabolism and the thermic effect of food.

7.2 Energy use by the body can be measured as heat given off by direct calorimetry or as oxygen used by indirect calorimetry. A person's Estimated Energy Requirement can be calculated based on the following factors: gender, height, weight, age, and amount of physical activity.

7.3 A body mass index (weight in kilograms ÷ height^2 in meters) of 18.5 to 24.9 is one measure of healthy weight. A healthy weight is best determined in conjunction with a thorough health evaluation by a clinician or dietitian. A body mass index of 25 to 29.9 represents overweight. Obesity is defined as a body mass index of 30 or move or a total body fat percentage over 25% (men) or 35% (women).

Fat distribution greatly determines health risks associated with obesity. Upper-body fat storage (android), as measured by a waist circumference greater than 40 inches (102 centimeters) for men or 35 inches (88 centimeters) for women, typically results in higher risks of hypertension, cardiovascular disease, and type 2 diabetes than lower-body fat storage (gynoid).

7.4 Both genetic (nature) and environmental (nurture) factors can increase the risk of obesity. The set-point theory proposes that we have a genetically predetermined body weight or body fat content, which the body strives to regulates.

7.5 A sound weight-loss program should meet the individual's nutritional needs by emphasizing a wide variety of low-calorie, high-fiber foods; adapts to one's lifestyle; consists of readily obtainable foods; strives to change poor eating behaviors; stresses regular physical activity; and stipulates the supervision by a clinician if weight is to be lost rapidly, if the person is obese (body mass index over 40), or if the individual is over the age of 40 (men) or 50 (women) and plans to perform substantially greater physical activity than recommended.

7.6 Appropriate weight loss consists of a caloric deficit of 500 kcal per day from reduced calorie intake, increased physical activity, or a combination of both. This should results in approximately 1 pound of weight loss per week initially. Weight change is not linear; it occurs most rapidly during the first year after a change in energy balance but tapers off over the next 2 years if changes in energy intake and physical activity are strictly maintained over time.

7.7 Physical activity as part of a weight-loss program should be focused on duration rather than intensity. The recommendations promote 150 minutes of physical activity per week. Ideally, about 60 minutes of moderate-intensity physical activity should be part of each day to prevent adult weight gain.

7.8 Behavior changes are a vital part of a weight-loss program because individuals may have many habits that discourage successful weight loss and maintenance. Specific behavior modification techniques, such as stimulus control and self-monitoring, can be used to help change problem behavior.

7.9 Medications to blunt appetite can aid weight loss. Orlistat (Xenical) reduces fat absorption from a meal when taken with the meal. Weight-loss drugs are reserved for those who are obese or have weight-related problems, and they must be administered under close physician supervision.

The treatment of severe obesity may include very-low-calorie diets containing 400 to 800 kcal per day or bariatric surgery to reduce stomach volume to approximately 30 milliliters (1 ounce). Both of these measures should be reserved for people who have failed at more conservative approaches to weight loss. They also require close medical supervision.

7.10 Underweight can be caused by a variety of factors, such as excessive physical activity and genetics. Sometimes being underweight requires medical attention. A primary care provider should be consulted first to rule out underlying health issues. The underweight person may need to increase portion sizes, learn to incorporate calorie-dense foods frequently, and drink fluids between meals. In addition, encouraging a regular meal and snack schedule aids in both weight gain and weight maintenance.

7.11 Many overweight people try popular fad diets that most often are not helpful and may actually be harmful. Unreliable diets typically share some common characteristics, including promoting quick weight loss, limiting food selections, using personal testimonials as proof, and requiring no physical activity.

Check Your Knowledge (Answers are available at the end of this question set.)

1. An energy deficit of 500 kcal per day would result in a total weight loss of about 1 pound over a _____ period.
   a. 1-week
   b. 1-month
   c. 1-year
   d. 3-year

2. Thermic effect of food represents the energy cost of
   a. chewing food.
   b. peristalsis.
   c. basal metabolism.
   d. digesting, absorbing, and packaging nutrients.

3. A well-designed weight-loss diet should
   a. increase physical activity.
   b. alter problem behaviors.
   c. reduce energy intake.
   d. include all of the above.

4. All of the following factors are associated with a higher basal metabolic rate *except*
   a. stress.
   b. low calorie intake.
   c. fever.
   d. pregnancy.

5. The intent of bariatric surgery is to
   a. reduce stomach volume.
   b. slow transit time.
   c. surgically remove adipose tissue.
   d. prevent snacking.

6. Basal metabolism
   a. represents about 30% of total energy expenditure.
   b. is energy used to maintain heartbeat, respiration, other basic functions, and physical activities.
   c. represents about 60% to 75% of total calories used by the body during a day.
   d. includes energy to digest food.

7. It is recommended that adults should do the equivalent of _____ minutes of moderate-intensity aerobic activity each week for weight loss and to achieve and maintain a healthy body weight.
   a. 30
   b. 90
   c. 150
   d. 300

8. Probably the most important contributing factor for obesity rates today in the United States is
   a. food advertising.
   b. snacking practices.
   c. inactivity.
   d. eating processed food.

9. The major goal for weight reduction in the treatment of obesity is the loss of
   a. weight.
   b. body fat.
   c. body water.
   d. body protein.

10. For most adults, the greatest portion of their energy expenditure is for
    a. physical activity.
    b. sleeping.
    c. basal metabolism.
    d. the thermic effect of food.

10. c (LO 7.1)
5. a (LO 7.10), 6. c (LO 7.1), 7. c (LO 7.8), 8. c (LO 7.5), 9. b (LO 7.6),
Answer Key: 1. b (LO 7.6), 2. d (LO 7.2), 3. d (LO 7.6), 4. b (LO 7.1),

Study Questions (Numbers refer to Learning Outcomes)

1. Explain how nurture and nature can contribute to the development of obesity. What are the two most convincing pieces of evidence that both genetic and environmental factors play significant roles in the development of obesity? **(LO 7.4)**

2. How does energy imbalance, including the role of physical activity, lead to weight gain and obesity? **(LO 7.1)**

3. Define how a healthy weight may be determined. **(LO 7.3)**

4. Describe a practical tool to define obesity in a clinical setting. **(LO 7.3)**

5. List three health issues that are related to obesity and the mechanism or reason that each condition occurs. **(LO 7.3)**

6. List three key characteristics of a sound weight-loss program. **(LO 7.5)**

7. Why is the claim for quick, effortless weight loss by any method always misleading? **(LO 7.5)**

8. List examples of positive behaviors that can lead to weight management. **(LO 7.8)**

9. Why should obesity treatment be viewed as a lifelong commitment rather than a short diet or episode of weight loss? **(LO 7.5)**

10. What steps are important to remember when an underweight person wants to gain muscle but not fat? **(LO 7.10)**

What the Dietitian Chose

In this case, the dietitian starts with the Nutrition Facts panel (label) on the package when making a dessert choice. Research has shown that reading labels plays a role in decreasing obesity, especially in women, who were found to be more likely to read nutrition labels.[10] Regular varieties of ice cream contain at least 10% milk fat by weight and are therefore a source of saturated fat and cholesterol. The milk fat gives the product the smooth, creamy texture for which ice cream is famous. You can see that the regular ice cream has 240 kcal, 13 grams fat, 8 grams saturated fat, and 87 mg cholesterol. The sugar content is 25 grams; some of this comes from natural milk sugar (lactose), and some sugar is added for flavor.

Premium ice cream varieties, such as those you would find in an ice cream shop, may have up to 300 kcal, 18 grams fat, and 30 grams sugar per ½-cup serving! That's equivalent to 4 teaspoons of butter and 7 teaspoons of sugar. Such decadent treats can be enjoyed in moderation but are best reserved for special occasions.

Reduced-fat, low-fat, light, or fat-free varieties of ice cream have less than 10% milk fat. This can be accomplished by starting with lower-fat milk, using gelatin instead of eggs, using fat replacers, incorporating more air into the product (e.g., "churned"), or any combination thereof. "Reduced fat" means the product has at least 25% less fat than the original product. "Low fat" sets the standard at 3 grams of fat or less per ½-cup serving.

"Light" ice cream has at least 50% less fat than the original product. "Fat free" signifies 0.5 gram of fat or less per ½-cup serving. The brand shown here is "light": it contains lower fat and sugar than the regular ice cream. It has 145 kcal, 4 grams fat, 2.5 grams saturated fat, 13 milligrams cholesterol, and 19 grams sugar per serving. For weight-management purposes, this saves you 95 kcal, 9 grams of fat, and 6 grams of sugar per serving compared to regular ice cream. Reducing the fat content of ice cream might also reduce the creamy texture, but for most reduced-fat, low-fat, and light products, the change is barely noticeable.

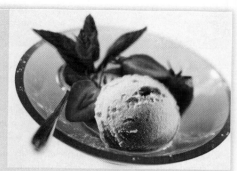

©Ingram Publishing/SuperStock

Frozen yogurt is not always a lower-calorie option than ice cream. It does not have to comply with the same 10% milk fat standard as ice cream does, so there may be a wide range of fat and sugar contents. This brand of frozen yogurt has 240 kcal, 4 grams fat, 1.3 grams saturated fat, and 64 milligrams cholesterol. The product is marketed as "low fat"—and it does only contain 4 grams of fat per ½-cup serving—but there are still 23 grams of sugar. This is a great example of how low fat does not necessarily mean low calorie.

Serving size is the most important part of the Nutrition Facts panel when it comes to calorie control. No matter how low the calorie, fat, and sugar contents are, if you consume multiple servings of any product, you are likely to take in too many calories. Likewise, you can control your calorie intake by choosing a smaller portion of premium ice cream.

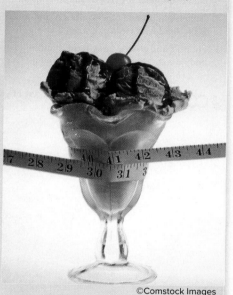

©Comstock Images

Nutrition Facts

Kroger Private Selection—Country Made Vanilla Ice Cream

Serving Size:			2/3 cup

Calories — **240**

Total Fat	13 g	Total Carbs	25 g
Saturated	8 g	Dietary Fiber	0 g
Trans	0 g	Total Sugars 25g	
Polyunsaturated	0 g	Includes 19g	
Monounsaturated	0 g	Added Sugars	38%
Cholesterol	87 mg	Protein	8 g
		Sodium	60 mg

Vitamin D 0.2mcg	2%	Iron 0.4mg	2%
Calcium 100mg	10%	Potassium 175mg	4%

The % Daily Value (DV) tells you how much a nutrient in a serving of food contributes to a daily diet. 2,000 calories a day is used for general nutrition advice.

Nutrition Facts

Kroger Deluxe—Vanilla Bean Light Ice Cream

Serving Size:			2/3 cup

Calories — **145**

Total Fat	4 g	Total Carbs	23 g
Saturated	2.5 g	Dietary Fiber	0 g
Trans	0 g	Total Sugars 19g	
Polyunsaturated	0 g	Includes 12g	
Monounsaturated	0 g	Added Sugars	24%
Cholesterol	13 mg	Protein	4 g
		Sodium	67 mg

Vitamin D 0.1mcg	1%	Iron 0mg	0%
Calcium 100mg	10%	Potassium 211mg	4%

The % Daily Value (DV) tells you how much a nutrient in a serving of food contributes to a daily diet. 2,000 calories a day is used for general nutrition advice.

Nutrition Facts

Häagen-Dazs—Yogurt Frozen Low Fat Vanilla

Serving Size:			2/3 cup

Calories — **240**

Total Fat	4 g	Total Carbs	40 g
Saturated	1.3 g	Dietary Fiber	0 g
Trans	0 g	Total Sugars 30g	
Polyunsaturated	0 g	Includes 23g	
Monounsaturated	0 g	Added Sugars	46%
Cholesterol	64 mg	Protein	12 g
		Sodium	60 mg

Vitamin D 0.2mcg	2%	Iron 0mg	0%
Calcium 200mg	20%	Potassium 180mg	4%

The % Daily Value (DV) tells you how much a nutrient in a serving of food contributes to a daily diet. 2,000 calories a day is used for general nutrition advice.

Further Readings

1. Academy of Nutrition and Dietetics: Position of the Academy of Nutrition and Dietetics: Total diet approach to healthy eating. *J Acad Nutri Diet* 2014; 113:307.

2. Centers for Disease Control and Prevention. *Overweight and obesity.* Updated September 1, 2016. https://www.cdc.gov/obesity/data/prevalence-maps.html. (Accessed January 4, 2016).

3. Ogden CL, and others: Prevalence of obesity among adults and youth: United States, 2011–2014. NCHS data brief, no. 219. Hyattsville, MD: National Center for Health Statistics. 2015.

4. Finkelstein EA and others: Obesity and severe obesity forecasts through 2030. *Am J Prev Med* 2012; 42(6):563.

5. Fung TT and others: Long-term change in diet quality is associated with body weight change in men and women. *J Nutri* 2015; 145:1850.

6. Rolls B and Hermann M: *The Ultimate Volumetrics Diet: Smart, Simple, Science-Based Strategies for Losing Weight and Keeping It Off.* New York: Harper Collins, 2012.

7. Wansink B: *Slim by Design.* New York: HarperCollins, 2014.

8. Dyczkowski CT and Seher CL: Smartphone apps for heart-healthy living—clients can track diet and exercise habits at their fingertips. *Today's Dietitian* 2012; 14(8):18.

9. Bazzano LA and others: Effects of low-carbohydrate and low-fat diets: A randomized trial. *Ann Intern Med* 2014; 161(5):309.

10. Loureiro ML and others: The effects of nutritional labels on obesity. *Agricultural Economics* 2012; 43:333.

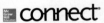 **connect** To get the most out of your study, visit Connect where you will find NutritionCalc Plus, SmartBook®, and many other dynamic tools.

Rate Your Plate

A Close Look at Your Weight Status

Determine the following two indices of your body status: body mass index and waist circumference.

Body Mass Index (BMI)

Record your weight in pounds: _____ pounds

Divide your weight in pounds by 2.2 to determine your weight in kilograms: _____ kilograms

Record your height in inches: _____ inches

Divide your height in inches by 39.4 to determine your height in meters: _____ meters

Calculate your BMI using the following formula:

BMI = weight (kilograms)/height^2 (meters)

BMI = _____ kg/ _____ m^2 = _____

Waist Circumference

Use a tape measure to measure the circumference of your waist (just above the hip bone with your stomach relaxed; see http://www.cdc.gov/healthyweight/assessing/). Circumference of waist (umbilicus) = _____ inches

Interpretation

1. BMI is greater than 25, health risks from obesity often begin. It is especially advisable to consider weight loss if your BMI exceeds 30. Does yours exceed 25 (or 30)?

    Yes _____ No _____

2. When a person has a BMI greater than 25 and a waist circumference of more than 40 inches (102 centimeters) in men or 35 inches (88 centimeters) in women, there is an increased risk of cardiovascular disease, hypertension, and type 2 diabetes. Does your waist circumference exceed the standard for your gender?

    Yes _____ No _____

3. Do you feel you need to pursue a program of weight loss?

    Yes _____ No _____

Application

From what you have learned in Chapter 7, list three specific actions you can take to move toward (or maintain) a healthy weight.

_____

_____

_____

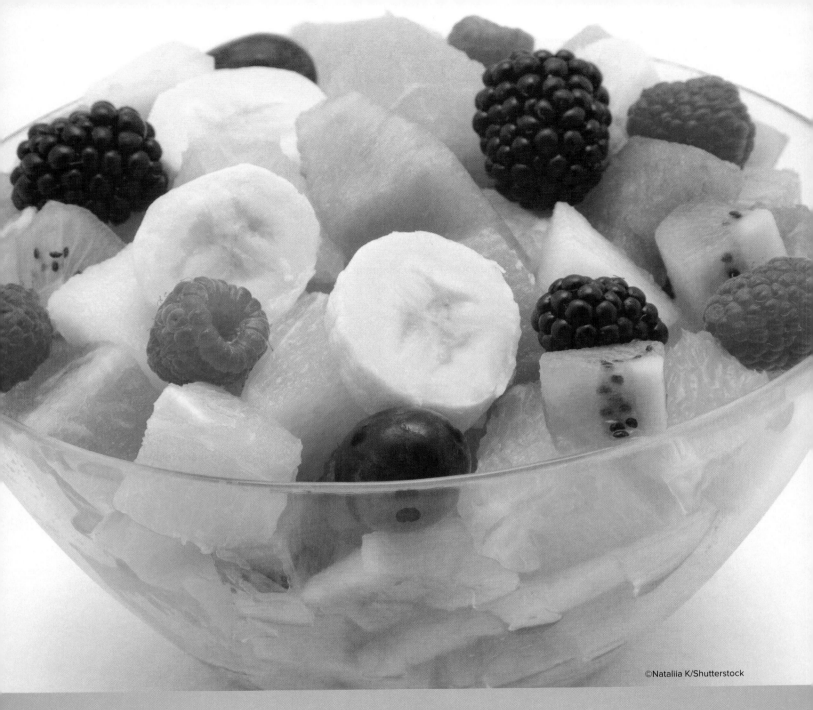

©Nataliia K/Shutterstock

Student Learning Outcomes

Chapter 8 is designed to allow you to:

8.1 Describe the general characteristics of the fat-soluble and water-soluble groups of vitamins, the general process of vitamin absorption and storage, the dangers of vitamin deficiency and toxicity, and the preservation of vitamins in foods. Explain several health benefits of phytochemicals and identify main sources of phytochemicals.

8.2 Describe the functions of vitamin A and carotenoids in vision, growth, development, reproduction, and cancer prevention, as well as the signs and symptoms of deficiency and toxicity, and understand its dietary requirements and how to get enough vitamin A in the diet and avoid too much from dietary supplements.

8.3 Explain the functions and sources of vitamin D, including its synthesis by the action of ultraviolet radiation; understand its dietary requirements; and describe the signs and symptoms of vitamin D deficiency and toxicity.

8.4 Summarize the functions of vitamin E, understand its dietary requirements, and describe its food sources and deficiency and toxicity symptoms.

8.5 Describe the role of vitamin K in blood clotting and the signs and symptoms of deficiency and toxicity, understand its dietary requirements, and identify its food sources.

8.6 Describe the characteristics of the water-soluble vitamins and the roles of the B vitamins in energy metabolism.

8.7 Describe the functions of thiamin in carbohydrate metabolism, and list its sources, dietary requirements, and deficiency symptoms.

Chapter 8
Vitamins

Although the vitamins are essential nutrients, the amount of vitamins we need to prevent deficiency is quite small. Some people believe that consuming vitamins far in excess of their needs provides them with extra energy, protection from disease, and prolonged youth. They seem to think that if a little is good, then more must be better. More than half of the U.S. adult population have taken vitamin and/or mineral supplements on a regular basis, some at unsafe levels.

Vitamins are naturally found in plants and animals. Plants synthesize all the vitamins they need and are a healthy source of vitamins for animals. Animals vary in their ability to synthesize vitamins. For example, guinea pigs and humans are two of the few organisms unable to make their own supply of vitamin C.

Every major public health authority recommends that we increase our intake of fruits and vegetables. Which vitamins are especially found in fruits and vegetables? What are some other health-related attributes of plant-based foods in general? Which chronic diseases are associated with a poor intake of fruits and vegetables? Should we take a daily vitamin supplement if we do not include fruits and vegetables in our diet? This chapter provides some answers.

8.8 Describe the functions of riboflavin in energy metabolism and understand the dietary requirements and sources of riboflavin that will prevent deficiency symptoms.

8.9 Describe the functions of niacin in energy metabolism and list its sources, dietary requirements, and deficiency and toxicity symptoms.

8.10 Describe the functions of vitamin B-6 in amino acid metabolism and understand how to get enough vitamin B-6 in the diet to avoid a deficiency and prevent toxicity from dietary supplements.

8.11 Describe the functions of pantothenic acid and biotin in energy metabolism, understand their dietary requirements, and list their food sources and deficiency signs and symptoms.

8.12 Summarize the functions of folate in cell metabolism, understand the dietary requirements needed to prevent megaloblastic anemia, and identify its food sources.

8.13 Understand the process of vitamin B-12 absorption and its role in folate metabolism, identify the dietary requirements for vitamin B-12 needed to avoid deficiency, and identify its food sources.

8.14 Describe the functions of vitamin C as well as its dietary requirements, sources, and deficiency and toxicity signs and symptoms.

8.15 Understand the functions and sources of choline and other vitamin-like substances.

8.16 Evaluate the use of dietary supplements with respect to their potential benefits and hazards to the body.

8.17 Describe how calorie and fat intakes contribute to cancer risk and understand the role other food constituents play in inhibiting cancer.

vitamin An essential organic (carbon-containing) compound needed in small amounts in the diet to help regulate and support chemical reactions and processes in the body.

fat-soluble vitamins Vitamins that dissolve in fat and some chemical compounds but not readily in water. These vitamins are A, D, E, and K.

water-soluble vitamins Vitamins that dissolve in water. These vitamins are the B vitamins and vitamin C.

scurvy The vitamin C–deficiency disease characterized by weakness, fatigue, slow wound healing, bone pain, fractures, sore and bleeding gums, diarrhea, and pinpoint hemorrhages on the skin.

rickets A disease characterized by poor mineralization of newly synthesized bones because of low calcium content. Arising in infants and children, this deficiency is caused by insufficient amounts of vitamin D in the body.

8.1 Vitamins: Vital Dietary Components

By definition, **vitamins** are essential organic (carbon-containing) substances needed in small amounts in the diet for normal function, growth, and maintenance of the body. All humans require the same essential vitamins, but the amount required can vary depending on age, gender, and presence of illness. Although vitamin requirements are very small, each vitamin is essential for one or more functions in the body (Fig. 8-1). Vitamins can be divided into two broad classes based on solubility: vitamins A, D, E, and K are **fat-soluble vitamins,** whereas the B vitamins and vitamin C are **water-soluble vitamins.** The B vitamins include thiamin, riboflavin, niacin, pantothenic acid, biotin, vitamin B-6, folate, and vitamin B-12. Choline is a vitamin-like nutrient but is not technically classified as a vitamin.

Vitamins are essential in human diets because they cannot be synthesized in the human body or produced in sufficient amounts. Notable exceptions to having a strict dietary need for a vitamin are vitamin A, which we can synthesize from certain pigments in plants; vitamin D, synthesized in the body if the skin is exposed to adequate sunlight; niacin, synthesized from the amino acid tryptophan; and vitamin K and biotin, synthesized to some extent by the bacteria in the intestinal tract.

To be classified as a vitamin, a compound must meet the following criteria: (1) the body is unable to synthesize enough of the compound to maintain health and (2) absence of the compound from the diet for a defined period produces deficiency symptoms that, if caught in time, are quickly reversed when the compound is reintroduced. A compound does not qualify as a vitamin merely because the body cannot make it. Evidence must suggest that health declines when the substance is not consumed.

As scientists began to identify various vitamins, related deficiency diseases such as **scurvy** (vitamin C) and **rickets** (vitamin D) were dramatically cured. For the most part, as the vitamins were discovered, they were named alphabetically: A, B, C, D, E, and so on. Later, many substances originally classified as vitamins were found not to be essential for humans and were removed from the list. Other vitamins, thought at first to be only one chemical, turned out to be several chemicals, so the alphabetical names had to be broken down by numbers (B-6, B-12, and so on).

In addition to their use in correcting deficiency diseases, a few vitamins have also proved useful in treating several nondeficiency diseases. These medical applications require administration of **megadoses,** amounts well above typical human needs for the vitamins. For example, megadoses of a form of niacin are used as part of blood cholesterol-lowering treatment for those in need. Still, any claimed benefits from use of vitamin supplements, especially intakes in excess of the Upper Level (if established), should be viewed critically because unproved claims are common. Remember, whenever you take a supplement at high doses, you are taking it at a pharmacological dose—that of a drug. Expect side effects as you would from any drug.

Vitamins isolated from foods or synthesized in the laboratory (*synthetic*) are the same chemical compounds and work equally well in the body. Contrary to claims on social media and in health food stores,

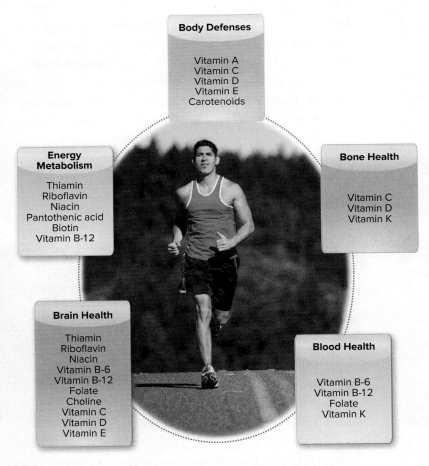

Body Defenses

Vitamin A
Vitamin C
Vitamin D
Vitamin E
Carotenoids

Energy Metabolism

Thiamin
Riboflavin
Niacin
Pantothenic acid
Biotin
Vitamin B-12

Bone Health

Vitamin C
Vitamin D
Vitamin K

Brain Health

Thiamin
Riboflavin
Niacin
Vitamin B-6
Vitamin B-12
Folate
Choline
Vitamin C
Vitamin D
Vitamin E

Blood Health

Vitamin B-6
Vitamin B-12
Folate
Vitamin K

FIGURE 8-1 ▲ Vitamins contribute to many functions in the body.
©John Lund/Getty Images

natural vitamins isolated from foods are, with few exceptions, no different than those labeled *synthetic*. Of note, the natural form of vitamin E is much more potent than the synthetic form. In contrast, synthetic folic acid, the form of the vitamin added to ready-to-eat breakfast cereals and flour, is 1.7 times more potent than the natural vitamin form.[1]

ABSORPTION AND STORAGE OF VITAMINS IN THE BODY

The fat-soluble vitamins (A, D, E, and K) are absorbed with dietary fat. These vitamins then travel with dietary fats as part of chylomicrons through the bloodstream to reach body cells. Special carriers in the bloodstream help distribute some of these vitamins. Fat-soluble vitamins are stored mostly in the liver and fatty tissues.

When fat absorption is efficient, about 40% to 90% of the fat-soluble vitamins are absorbed. Anything that interferes with normal digestion and absorption of fats, however, also interferes with fat-soluble vitamin absorption. For example, people with cystic fibrosis, a disease that often hampers fat absorption, may develop deficiencies of fat-soluble vitamins. Some medications, such as the weight-loss drug orlistat (Alli),® discussed in Chapter 7, also interfere with fat absorption. Unabsorbed fat carries these vitamins to the large intestine, and they are excreted in the feces. People with fat-malabsorption conditions are especially susceptible to vitamin K deficiency because body stores of vitamin K are lower than those of the other fat-soluble vitamins. Vitamin supplements, taken under a primary care provider's guidance, are part of the treatment for preventing a vitamin deficiency associated with fat malabsorption. Finally, people who use mineral oil as a laxative risk fat-soluble vitamin deficiencies. Fat-soluble vitamins dissolve in the mineral oil, but the intestine does not absorb mineral oil. Hence, the fat-soluble vitamins are eliminated with the mineral oil in the feces.

Water-soluble vitamins are handled much differently than fat-soluble vitamins. After being ingested, the B vitamins from food are first broken down from their active **coenzyme** forms into free vitamins in the stomach and small intestine. The vitamins are then absorbed, primarily in the small intestine. Typically, about 50% to 90% of the water-soluble vitamins in the diet are absorbed, which means they have relatively high **bioavailability.** Water-soluble vitamins are transported to the liver via the hepatic portal vein and are distributed to body tissues. Once inside cells, the active coenzyme forms are resynthesized. Although some supplement manufacturers sell vitamins in their coenzyme forms, there is no benefit in consuming the coenzyme forms, as these are broken down during digestion and activated inside cells as needed.

Excretion of vitamins varies primarily on their solubility. Except for vitamin K, fat-soluble vitamins are not readily excreted from the body. Hence, toxicity can be an issue. Water-soluble vitamins are excreted based on **tissue saturation,** the degree to which the tissue vitamin stores are full. Tissue storage capacity is limited. As the tissues become saturated, the rate of excretion via the kidney increases sharply, preventing potential toxicity. Unlike other water-soluble vitamins, B-6 and B-12 are stored in the liver and not easily excreted in the urine.

In light of the limits of tissue saturation for many water-soluble vitamins, these vitamins should be consumed in the diet daily. However, an occasional lapse in the intake of water-soluble vitamins causes no harm. Symptoms of a vitamin deficiency occur only when that vitamin is lacking in the diet and the body stores are essentially exhausted. For example, for an average person, the diet must be devoid of thiamin for 10 to 14 days or lacking in vitamin C for 20 to 40 days before the first symptoms of deficiencies of these vitamins appear.

VITAMIN TOXICITY

For most water-soluble vitamins, when you consume more than the RDA or AI, the kidneys efficiently filter the excess from the blood and excrete these compounds in urine. Notable exceptions are vitamin B-6 and vitamin B-12, which are stored in the liver. Although they are water-soluble, these two B vitamins may accumulate to toxic levels.

megadose Intake of a nutrient well beyond estimates of needs to prevent a deficiency or what would be found in a balanced diet; 2 to 10 times above human needs is typically a starting point for such a dosage.

coenzyme A compound (e.g., water-soluble vitamin) that combines with an inactive enzyme to form a catalytically active form. In this manner, coenzymes aid in enzyme function.

bioavailability The degree to which an ingested nutrient is digested and absorbed and thus is available to the body.

tissue saturation The limited storage capacity of water-soluble vitamins in the tissues.

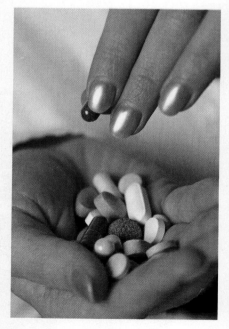

▲ Vitamins are not likely to be toxic unless taken in large amounts as supplements.
©liquidlibrary/PictureQuest

In contrast to the water-soluble vitamins, fat-soluble vitamins are not readily excreted, so some can easily accumulate in the body and cause toxic effects. Although a toxic effect from an excessive intake of any vitamin is theoretically possible, toxicity of the fat-soluble vitamin A is the most frequently observed. Vitamin A causes toxicity at intakes as little as 2 times the RDA. Vitamin E and the water-soluble vitamins niacin, vitamin B-6, and vitamin C can also cause toxic effects but only when consumed in very large amounts (15 to 100 times human needs). Overall, vitamins are unlikely to cause toxic effects unless taken in supplement (pill) form.

Some people believe that consuming vitamins far in excess of their needs provides them with extra energy, protection from disease, and prolonged youth. They seem to think that if a little is good, then more must be better. A *one-a-day* type of multivitamin and mineral supplement usually contains less than two times the Daily Values of its components, so daily use of these products is unlikely to cause toxic effects. However, consuming multiple pills, especially single-dose supplements such as vitamin A, can cause problems. See Section 8.16 to learn more about appropriate uses of dietary supplements.

PRESERVATION OF VITAMINS IN FOODS

Good sources of vitamins can be found in all food groups, especially fruits and vegetables (Fig. 8-2). However, storage time and environmental factors can affect vitamin content of foods. Fully ripe food contains more vitamins, but substantial amounts of vitamins can be lost from the time a fruit or vegetable is harvested until it is eaten. Therefore, it is best to eat fresh produce as soon as possible after harvest. Food cooperatives, **community-supported agriculture (CSA),** and farmers' markets are great sources of freshly harvested fruits and vegetables. The water-soluble vitamins, particularly thiamin, vitamin C, and folate, can be destroyed with improper storage and excessive cooking. Heat, light, exposure to the air, cooking in water, and alkalinity are factors that can destroy vitamins.

There are several steps you can take to preserve nutrients when you are purchasing, storing, and preparing fruits and vegetables (Table 8-1). Frozen vegetables and fruits are often as nutrient-rich as freshly harvested ones because fruits and vegetables are typically frozen immediately after harvesting. As part of the freezing process, vegetables are quickly blanched in boiling water. Blanching destroys the enzymes that would otherwise degrade the vitamins over time. If produce will not be eaten within a few days of harvest, freezing is the best preservation method to retain nutrients.

community-supported agriculture (CSA) Farms that are supported by a community of growers and consumers who provide mutual support and share the risks and benefits of food production, usually including a system of weekly delivery or pickup of vegetables and fruit, and sometimes dairy products and meat.

FIGURE 8-2 ▶ Certain food groups on MyPlate are especially rich sources of various vitamins and choline. Each may be also found in other MyPlate groups but in lower amounts. In addition to those vitamins listed here, pantothenic acid is present in moderate amounts in many groups, and vitamin E is abundant in plant oils.

Source: United States Department of Agriculture, ChooseMyPlate.Gov

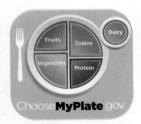

MyPlate:
Sources of Vitamins
and Choline

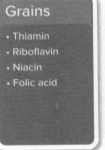

Grains
- Thiamin
- Riboflavin
- Niacin
- Folic acid

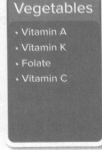

Vegetables
- Vitamin A
- Vitamin K
- Folate
- Vitamin C

Fruits
- Vitamin A
- Vitamin C

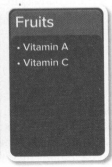

Dairy
- Vitamin D
- Riboflavin
- Vitamin B-12
- Choline

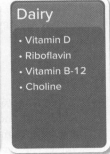

Protein
- Thiamin
- Riboflavin
- Niacin
- Biotin
- Vitamin B-6
- Vitamin B-12
- Choline

TABLE 8-1 ■ **Tips for Preserving Vitamins in Fruits and Vegetables**

Preservation Methods	Reason
Keep fruits and vegetables cool until eaten.	Enzymes in produce begin to degrade vitamins once it is harvested. Chilling slows down this process.
Refrigerate fruits and vegetables (except bananas, onions, potatoes, and tomatoes) in the vegetables drawer.	Nutrients keep best at temperatures near freezing, at high humidity, and away from air.
Trim, peel, and cut fruits and vegetables minimally and just prior to eating.	Oxygen breaks down vitamins faster when more of the food surface is exposed. Whenever possible, cook fruits and vegetables in their skins.
Microwave, steam, or stir-fry vegetables.	More nutrients are retained when there is minimal contact with water.
Minimize cooking time.	Prolonged cooking (slow simmering) and reheating reduce vitamin content.
Avoid adding fats to vegetables during cooking if you plan to discard the liquid.	Fat-soluble vitamins will be lost in discarded fat. If you want to add fats, do so after vegetables are fully cooked and drained.
Avoid adding baking soda to vegetables to enhance the green color.	Alkalinity destroys vitamin D, thiamin, and other vitamins.
Store canned and frozen fruits and vegetables carefully.	To protect canned foods, store them in a cool, dry location. To protect frozen foods, store them at 0°F (−32°C) or colder. Eat within 12 months.

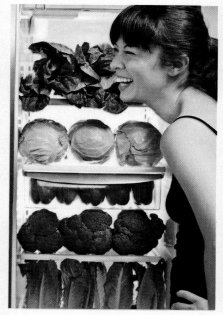

▲ It is time for a healthy snack! Store most fresh produce in the refrigerator to preserve vitamin content and reduce spoilage. ©Jill Giardino/Getty Images

PHYTOCHEMICALS

In addition to the approximately 45 essential nutrients, there are thousands of other compounds in food. For many years, a great deal of nutrition research concentrated on gaining knowledge about carbohydrates, lipids, proteins, vitamins, and minerals. Now, there is growing interest about the potential health benefits of other substances found in food. Foods that are sources of the chemicals that provide health benefits beyond being essential dietary nutrients are termed **functional foods.** Oatmeal is an example of a functional food as it contains soluble fiber that can lower cholesterol levels. Other foods are modified to improve health benefits. For example, some orange juice is fortified with calcium for bone health. Functional foods can be placed into two categories: (1) **zoochemicals,** health-promoting compounds found in animal food; and (2) phytochemicals, health-promoting compounds found in plant foods (*phyto* means "plant" in Greek). Phytochemicals are responsible for the unique colors, flavors, and odors observed in plants. For plants, phytochemicals serve as an environmental protective mechanism to help plants survive the elements (UV exposure, insects, and other predators). Interestingly, these chemicals improve human health when dietary patterns high in plant foods are consumed. In addition to the carotenoids discussed in Section 8.2, some of the phytochemicals being studied include allicin, phytosterols, isothiocyanates, lignans, stanols, ellagic acid, flavonoids, saponins, glucosinolates, polyphenols, phytoestrogens, sulphides, lectins, and many more. Examples of foods that are rich sources of phytochemicals include fruits, vegetables, whole grains, legumes, beans, herbs, spices, nuts, and seeds.

Over 4000 compounds have been identified in a single black raspberry, and over 600 carotenoids are found in plants. The full extent of these health benefits are just beginning to be elucidated. We do know that phytochemicals cannot be synthesized in the

functional foods Foods that have health benefits beyond basic nutrition.

zoochemicals Chemicals found in animal products that have health-protective actions.

body, so we must obtain them from food; however, they are not considered essential nutrients because a deficiency disease is not observed when they are removed from the diet. Thus, even though you may see the word *phytonutrient* in some sources, *phytochemical* remains the most accurate term.

Phytochemical Functions Although the study of the metabolic actions of phytochemicals is relatively new, numerous mechanistic protective health benefits of these plant-based foods have been noted, beyond those conferred by their vitamin and mineral contents:

- Stimulate the immune system
- Reduce inflammation
- Prevent DNA damage and aid in DNA repair
- Reduce oxidative damage to cells
- Regulate intracellular signaling of hormones and gene expression
- Activate insulin receptors
- Inhibit the initiation and proliferation of cancer, and stimulate spontaneous cell death
- Alter the absorption, production, and metabolism of cholesterol
- Mimic or inhibit hormones and enzymes
- Decrease the formation of blood clots

Phytochemical Recommendations There are no specific dietary recommendations for the amount of phytochemicals that should be consumed, except that they should be consumed as food. At present, we know that phytochemicals have protective functions with minimal side effects when consumed naturally in a variety of foods. Therefore, it is wise to eat a wide variety of whole plant foods to obtain the optimum amount of macronutrients, vitamins, minerals, fiber, and phytochemicals. A combination of different plant foods will also increase the antioxidant capacity of the total diet, and there is no doubt that we need to consume a greater variety and quantity of antioxidant-rich foods.

✓ CONCEPT CHECK 8.1

1. In a previous chapter, you learned that coenzyme Q (CoQ) is an organic compound that is required for the electron transport chain and has some antioxidant functions. This compound is synthesized within cells, and under most circumstances, the body synthesizes enough CoQ to meet its needs. Is CoQ a vitamin? Why or why not?

2. What is a megadose? Are there any negative consequences of consuming megadoses of vitamins? Are there any situations in which megadoses of vitamins are useful?

3. List at least three differences between fat-soluble and water-soluble vitamins.

4. List three ways to preserve vitamin content when storing, preparing, or cooking foods.

5. Give one example of a functional food.

6. Which food group has the richest supply of phytochemicals?

8.2 Vitamin A (Retinoids) and Carotenoids

Vitamin A was the first fat-soluble vitamin to be recognized as an important component of food essential for human health. Almost all (90%) of vitamin A is stored in the liver; the remaining 10% is in adipose tissue, kidneys, and the lungs. Either a deficiency or toxicity can cause severe problems, and there is a narrow range of optimal intakes between these two states.

Vitamin A is in a group of compounds known as **retinoids.** There are three active forms of vitamin A: **retinol, retinal,** and **retinoic acid.** These are often called preformed vitamin A. They exist only in animal products. When retinol is stored, it is esterified (joined to a fatty acid) and becomes **retinyl.** In supplements, you will often find vitamin A listed as retinyl acetate or retinyl palmitate.

Besides the retinoids, which come from animal sources, many foods of plant origin contain carotenoids, some of which can be converted into vitamin A in the body. **Carotenoids** are not essential nutrients; they are categorized as phytochemicals. Although hundreds carotenoids have been identified, just three can be converted to retinol in the body: alpha carotene, beta-carotene, and beta-cryptoxanthin. Because these carotenoids can be turned into vitamin A, they are termed **provitamin A.** Of these three, only beta-carotene serves as a significant source of vitamin A. Neither the absorption of carotenoids nor the conversion of the provitamin A carotenoids into vitamin A is an efficient process. Other carotenoids that may play a role in human health but are not vitamin A precursors include lycopene, zeaxanthin, and lutein.

FUNCTIONS OF VITAMIN A AND CAROTENOIDS

Health of Epithelial Cells and Immune Function Vitamin A maintains the health of epithelial cells, which line internal and external surfaces of the lungs, intestines, stomach, vagina, urinary tract, and bladder, as well as those of the eyes and skin. Retinoic acid is required for immature epithelial cells to develop into mature, functional epithelial cells. Without vitamin A, mucous-forming cells, such as those in the intestines and lungs, deteriorate and lose function. For the eye, this can lead to blindness. *Hyperkeratosis*, also a result of vitamin A deficiency, is a condition in which skin cells produce too much keratin, blocking the hair follicles and causing *gooseflesh* or *toadskin* appearance. The excessive keratin in these skin cells causes the skin to be hard and dry.

The epithelial tissues serve as important barriers to infection. Vitamin A also supports the activity of certain immune system cells, specifically, the T-lymphocytes, or T-cells. Vitamin A–deficient humans have an increased infection rate, but when they are supplemented with vitamin A, the immune response improves.

Vision The link between vitamin A and night vision has been known since ancient Egyptians used juice extracted from liver to cure **night blindness.** Vitamin A performs important functions in light-dark vision and, to a lesser extent, color vision. Light entering the back of the eye reaches a lining called the **retina.** The retina consists of rods, cones, and nerve cells. Rods detect black and white, and are responsible for night vision. Cones are responsible for color vision. Rods and cones require vitamin A for normal function. One form of vitamin A (retinal) allows certain cells in the eye to adjust to dim light (such as after seeing the headlights of an oncoming car; Fig. 8-3). Without sufficient dietary vitamin A, the cells in the eye cannot quickly readjust to dim light, causing night blindness.

If vitamin A deficiency progresses, the cells that line the cornea of the eye (the clear window of the eye) lose the ability to produce mucus. The eye then becomes dry. This disease is called **xerophthalmia,** which means dry eye. Eventually, dirt particles scratch the dry surface of the eye, leading to blindness. Xerophthalmia can progress to the stage where there is an accumulation of dead cells and secretions on the surface of the eye. This condition is called *Bitot's spots* (Fig. 8-4).

Vitamin A deficiency is the leading cause of blindness worldwide. North Americans are at low risk because typical American diets contain plentiful sources of preformed vitamin A, such as eggs and fortified milk. However, poor vitamin A intakes, low-fat intakes that do not allow for sufficient vitamin A absorption, and low stores of vitamin A lessen the ability of children to meet high needs during periods of rapid growth. Worldwide, about one-third of children suffer from vitamin A deficiency. Hundreds of thousands of children in developing nations, especially Southeast Asia and Sub-Saharan

retinoids Chemical forms of preformed vitamin A; one source is animal foods.

retinol Alcohol form of vitamin A.

retinal Aldehyde form of vitamin A.

retinoic acid Acid form of vitamin A.

retinyl Storage form of vitamin A.

carotenoids Precursors of vitamin A found in plant foods.

provitamin A A substance that can be converted into vitamin A.

night blindness Vitamin A–deficiency disorder that results in loss of the ability to see under low-light conditions.

retina A light-sensitive lining in the back of the eye. It contains retinal.

xerophthalmia Hardening of the cornea and drying of the surface of the eye, which can result in blindness.

FIGURE 8-3 ▶ Vitamin A functions to maintain vision. Light enters the eye through the cornea and lens, and then hits the retina. The light reacts with vitamin A–containing rhodopsin, which is stored in the rod cells of the retina. Rod cells allow us to see black-and-white images. When light reacts with rhodopsin, retinal is cleaved from rhodopsin (bleaching), a process that stimulates an electrical impulse to the brain. A new molecule of vitamin A then combines with opsin to regenerate rhodopsin. The yellow background indicates the bleaching events that occur in the light; the gray background indicates the regenerative events that can occur in either light or dark conditions.

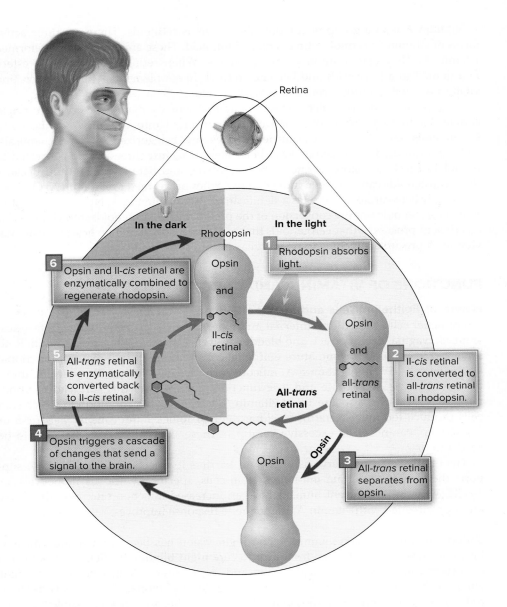

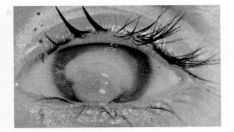

FIGURE 8-4 ▲ Vitamin A deficiency eventually leads to blindness. Bitot's spots are most common in developing countries. Courtesy of Dr. Alfred Sommer

Africa, become blind each year because of vitamin A deficiency. Some of these children ultimately die from infections. Worldwide, attempts to reduce this problem have included promoting breastfeeding, providing megadoses of vitamin A, and fortifying sugar, margarine, and monosodium glutamate with vitamin A. These food vehicles are used because they are commonly consumed by inhabitants of less-developed nations. This effort has proven effective in some countries.

Among pregnant women, night blindness is a marker of vitamin A deficiency that will likely lead to pregnancy-related deaths, malnutrition, anemia, or infant mortality. Screening and supplementing populations of pregnant women can be effective in treating and preventing this serious public health issue.

Some carotenoids are also important for vision. The macula (also known as the macula lutea, meaning *yellow spot*) is in the central area of the retina and is responsible for the most detailed central vision. It contains the carotenoids lutein and zeaxanthin in high enough concentrations to impart a yellow color. Age-related macular degeneration the leading cause of blindness among older adults in North America, occurs because of changes in this macular area of the retina (Fig. 8-5). In one study of older adults, the higher the total number of carotenoids (beta-carotene, lutein, and zeaxanthin) consumed in the diet, the lower the risk for age-related macular degeneration. The richest sources of lutein and zeaxanthin are green leafy vegetables (Table 8-2).

These carotenoids may also decrease the risk of cataracts in the eyes. Research studies point toward the actual fruit and vegetables with their high carotenoid content as contributing to reduced risk for eye disorders. Consuming just carotenoids as supplements for this purpose is not recommended. Multi-vitamin and mineral supplements formulated for older adults (e.g., Centrum Silver)™ are being marketed as a source of lutein. Consumers must be aware that studies on carotenoids are generally conducted with food rather than supplements.

Cardiovascular Disease Prevention Carotenoids may play a role in preventing cardiovascular disease in persons at high risk. This may be linked to carotenoids' ability to inhibit the oxidation of low-density lipoproteins (LDLs). Until definitive studies are complete, many scientists recommend that we consume a total of at least five servings of a combination of fruits and vegetables per day as part of an overall effort to reduce the risk of cardiovascular disease. Other phytochemicals, including flavonoids, phenolic acids, and phytoestrogens, may have a more significant effect in cardiovascular disease prevention than carotenoids. Until we have more answers, focus on consuming a diet rich in phytochemicals from whole foods.

Growth, Development, and Reproduction Vitamin A participates in the processes of growth, development, and reproduction in several ways. At the genetic level, vitamin A binds to receptors on DNA to increase synthesis of a variety of proteins. Some of these proteins are required for growth. During early fetal growth, vitamin A functions in the differentiation and maturation of cells, which ultimately form tissues and organs. Vitamin A–deficient children experience stunted growth. For bones to grow and elongate, old bone must be remodeled (broken down) so that new bone can be formed. Vitamin A assists with breakdown and formation of healthy bone tissue. Adequate intake of vitamin A is also needed for reproduction; it aids in sperm production (associated with its epithelial role) and in a normal reproductive cycle for women.

Cancer Prevention Vitamin A and carotenoids have potential benefits but also potential dangers where cancer prevention is concerned. It plays a role in cellular differentiation and embryonic development. Numerous studies have found that diets rich in provitamin A carotenoids are associated with a lower risk of skin, lung, bladder, and breast cancers. Still, because of the potential for toxicity, unsupervised use of megadose vitamin A or carotenoid supplements to reduce cancer risk is not advised and can be potentially dangerous.

Population studies show that regular consumption of foods rich in carotenoids decreases the risk of several types of cancer, including cancers of the lung, skin, oral cavity, and prostate gland. In particular, the dietary carotenoid lycopene (the red pigment found in tomatoes, watermelon, pink grapefruit, and guava) seems to protect against prostate cancer—one of the most common cancers among North American men. Some food companies have even marketed their tomato products as important sources of lycopene. The role of carotenoids in cancer prevention is thought to be a by-product of their antioxidant activity.

While dietary carotenoid intake appears to be protective against some cancer, such as the those of the **prostate gland,** supplementation with carotenoids has not proven beneficial. Although research continues, most researchers are convinced that beta-carotene supplementation offers no protection against cancer. Overall, the best advice is to rely on whole plant sources of both the retinoids and carotenoids to promote optimal health.

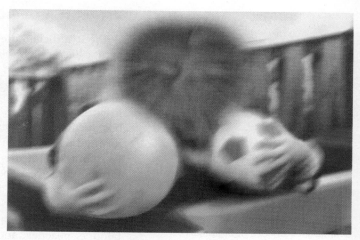

FIGURE 8-5 ▲ The blurry center of the image simulates the vision of a person with macular degeneration. ©National Eye Institute

TABLE 8-2 ■ **Vegetables Rich in Lutein and Zeaxanthin**

Vegetables (serving size)	Lutein and Zeaxanthin (mg)
Kale (1 cup cooked)	23.8
Spinach (1 cup cooked)	20.4
Swiss chard (1 cup cooked)	19.2
Collard greens (1 cup cooked)	14.6
Spinach (2 cups raw)	7.4
Peas (1 cup cooked)	3.8
Broccoli (1 cup cooked)	2.4
Romaine lettuce (2 cups raw)	2.2
Brussels sprouts (1 cup cooked)	2.0
Zucchini (1 cup cooked)	2.0

Vitamin A

RDA

    Men: 900 micrograms RAE

    Women: 700 micrograms RAE

DV: 900 micrograms RAE

UL: 3000 micrograms RAE

prostate gland A solid, chestnut-shaped organ surrounding the first part of the urinary tract in the male. The prostate gland secretes substances into the semen.

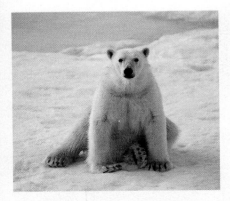

▲ Inuits long knew and explorers soon learned to avoid eating the liver of polar bears. Just 4 ounces (120 grams) of polar bear liver will deliver a toxic dose of vitamin A that is almost 140 times the RDA! ©Digital Vision/Getty Images RF

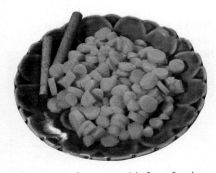

▲ Provitamin A carotenoids from foods (not supplements) are the safest way to meet your vitamin A needs. A serving of these carrots would be an excellent addition to the vegetable section of MyPlate. Cooking food sources of carotenoids actually makes them more bioavailable. ©CDC/James Gathany

international unit (IU) A crude measure of vitamin activity, often based on the growth rate of animals in response to the vitamin. Today IUs have largely been replaced by more precise milligram or microgram measures.

fetus The developing human life-form from 8 weeks after conception until birth.

VITAMIN A DEFICIENCY

Without sufficient dietary vitamin A, the cells in the eye cannot quickly readjust to dim light, causing night blindness.

GETTING ENOUGH VITAMIN A AND CAROTENOIDS

Preformed vitamin A (e.g., retinol, retinal, and retinoic acid) is found in liver, fish, fish oils, fortified milk, butter, yogurt, and eggs (Fig. 8-6). Margarine and spreads are also fortified with vitamin A.

About 70% of the vitamin A in the typical North American diet comes from preformed vitamin A sources, whereas provitamin A (carotenoids) dominates in the diet among poor people in other parts of the world. The provitamin A carotenoids are mainly found in dark green and yellow-orange vegetables and some fruits. Carrots, spinach and other leafy greens, winter squash, sweet potatoes, broccoli, mangoes, cantaloupe, peaches, and apricots are examples of such sources. Beta-carotene accounts for some of the orange color of carrots. Green vegetables also contain provitamin A. The yellow-orange beta-carotene is masked by dark-green chlorophyll pigments. Green, leafy vegetables, such as spinach and kale, have high concentrations of lutein and zeaxanthin. Tomato products contain significant amounts of lycopene. Cooking food and consuming food with small amounts of healthy fat improve the bioavailability of carotenoids. In raw fruits and vegetables, carotenoids are bound to proteins. Cooking disrupts this protein bond and frees the carotenoid for better absorption, and fat increases bioavailability.

The RDA for vitamin A is expressed in retinol activity equivalents (RAE). These RAE units consider the activity of both preformed vitamin A and the carotenoids that are synthesized into vitamin A in humans. There is no separate DRI for beta-carotene or any of the other carotenoids. The total RAE value for a food is calculated by adding the concentration of preformed vitamin A to the amount of provitamin A carotenoids in the food that will be converted into vitamin A.

You may have noticed that the RDA for vitamin A is given in micrograms, whereas the vitamin A content on Nutrition Facts labels is given in **international units (IU).** Legally, supplement manufacturers still must provide amounts of vitamin A in IU, which is a measure of the biological activity of a nutrient rather than its absolute quantity (see next page for conversion factors).

The diets of North American adults typically contain adequate vitamin A. Most adults in North America have liver reserves of vitamin A 3 to 5 times higher than needed for good health. Thus, the use of vitamin A supplements by most people is unnecessary. Populations in North America that may be at risk for vitamin A deficiency include those with low produce intakes (e.g., some children, older adults, and food insecure individuals); people with alcoholism or liver disease; or people with severe fat malabsorption.

AVOIDING TOO MUCH VITAMIN A AND CAROTENOIDS

Intakes in excess of the UL for vitamin A are linked to birth defects and liver toxicity. Other possible side effects include an increased risk of hip fracture and poor pregnancy outcomes.

During the early months of pregnancy, a high intake of preformed vitamin A is especially dangerous because it may cause fetal malformations and spontaneous abortions. This is because vitamin A binds to DNA and thus influences cell development. The Food and Drug Administration (FDA) recommends that women of childbearing age limit their overall intake of preformed vitamin A from diet plus supplements to a total of about 100% of the Daily Value. It is also important to limit consumption of rich food sources, such as liver. These precautions also apply to women who may possibly become pregnant; vitamin A is stored in the body for long periods, so women who ingest large amounts during the months before pregnancy place their **fetus** at risk.

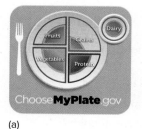

FIGURE 8-6 ▼ Food sources of vitamin A and carotenoids. (a) The fill of the background color (none, 1/3, 2/3, or completely covered) within each food group on MyPlate indicates the average nutrient density for vitamin A and provitamin A carotenoids in that group. (b) The bar graph shows the vitamin A content of several foods from each food group compared to the RDA for adult males and females. Overall, the fruits and vegetables groups provide many rich sources of carotenoids, whereas fortified dairy products and certain choices in the protein group are good sources of preformed vitamin A. The grains group also contains some foods that are nutrient dense because they are fortified with vitamin A.

Source: Nutrition data from USDA National Nutrient Database for Standard Reference, Release 26

(a)

(b)

Food Item and Amount	Vitamin A (micrograms RAE)*	% RDA for Adult Males (900 micrograms RAE)	% RDA for Adult Females (700 micrograms RAE)
Cream of Wheat,® Cooked, ½ cup	280	31%	40%
Kellogg's Raisin Bran® cereal, 1 cup	228	25%	33%
Corn muffin, 1 medium	59	7%	8%
Sweet potato, baked, 1 large	1730	192%	247%
Spinach, cooked, 1 cup	943	105%	135%
Kale, cooked, 1 cup	885	98%	126%
Cantaloupe, 1 cup	300	33%	43%
Apricots, dried, ½ cup	117	13%	17%
Mango, 1 cup	90	10%	13%
Milk, fat-free, 1 cup	150	17%	21%
Soy milk (fortified), 1 cup	134	15%	19%
Cheese, cheddar, 1.5 ounces	113	13%	16%
Beef liver, pan-fried, 3 ounces	6273	697%	896%
Tuna, bluefin, broiled, 3 ounces	643	71%	92%
Egg, hard-boiled, 1 large	74	8%	11%
Butter, 1 teaspoon	34	4%	5%
Margarine, 1 teaspoon	0	0%	0%
Olive oil, 1 teaspoon	0	0%	0%

(Food groups left margin: Grains, Vegetables, Fruits, Dairy, Protein, Fats & Oils)

* Retinol activity equivalents.

In contrast, ingesting large amounts of vitamin A–yielding carotenoids does not appear to cause toxic effects. A high carotenoid concentration in the blood (called *hypercarotenemia*) can occur if someone routinely consumes large amounts of carrots or takes pills containing beta-carotene (more than 30 milligrams daily) or if infants eat an excessive amount of squash. The skin turns yellow-orange, particularly the palms of the hands and soles of the feet. It differs from jaundice, a sign of liver failure. In jaundice, the yellow discoloration extends to the sclera (whites) of the eye, whereas in hypercarotenemia, it does not. Hypercarotenemia does not appear to cause harm and disappears when carotenoid intake decreases. Dietary carotenoids do not produce toxic effects because: (1) their rate of conversion into vitamin A is relatively slow and regulated; and (2) the efficiency of carotenoid absorption from the small intestine decreases markedly as oral intake increases.

1 RAE =
- 1 microgram of retinol (or retinal or retinoic acid: all the same)
- 12 micrograms of β-carotene from food or supplements
- 24 micrograms of other carotenoids from food

Converting IU to RAE
- IU ÷ 3.3 if the supplement is preformed vitamin A (such as retinyl acetate)
- IU ÷ 6.6 if the supplement is carotenoids (usually β-carotene)

Medicine Cabinet

Two derivatives of vitamin A are used to treat moderate to severe acne. Tretinoin (Retin-A)® is used topically (applied to the skin), and isotretinoin (Roaccutane)® is taken orally. These drugs appear to work by altering genes expressed by the skin cells. However, taking vitamin A supplements or making a paste from supplements and applying it to your skin will have no effect on acne. In fact, high doses of vitamin A can induce toxic symptoms, including birth defects. Isotretinoin's label clearly advises against the use of the medication during pregnancy, and its use is strictly monitored by the FDA. In order for women to receive this medication, they must have two negative pregnancy tests; sign a patient information/consent form; agree to use two effective forms of birth control; register, along with their primary care providers and pharmacists, with iPLEDGE (https://www.ipledgeprogram.com/); and agree to follow all instructions of the program.

©Peter Dazeley/Photographer's Choice/Getty Images

7-dehydrocholesterol Precursor of vitamin D found in the skin.

vitamin D₃ (cholecalciferol) Previtamin form found naturally in some animal sources, including fish and egg yolks.

25-hydroxyvitamin D₃ (calcidiol or calcifediol) Form found in blood. Sometimes shortened to 25(OH)D₃.

1,25-dihydroxyvitamin D₃ (calcitriol) Biologically active form of vitamin D.

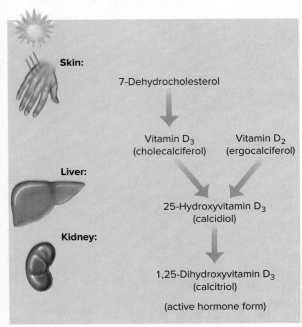

FIGURE 8-7 ▲ A precursor to vitamin D is synthesized when skin is exposed to sunlight. Previtamin D must be further modified by the liver and kidney for maximal activity.

✓ **CONCEPT CHECK 8.2**

1. What are the names of two carotenoids known to have antioxidant functions?
2. How are the carotenoids related to vitamin A?
3. What are the consequences of vitamin A deficiency?
4. What are some rich food sources of carotenoids?

8.3 Vitamin D (Calciferol or Calcitriol)

Vitamin D is a fat-soluble vitamin with two unique qualities. First, vitamin D is the only nutrient that is also a hormone. A hormone is a compound manufactured by one organ or tissue in the body that enters the bloodstream and has a physiological effect on another organ or tissue. The cells that participate in the synthesis of the active vitamin D hormone (skin, liver, and kidney) are different from the cells that respond to vitamin D (e.g., bone and intestine); therefore, vitamin D is a hormone.

Second, vitamin D is the only nutrient that can be produced in the skin upon exposure to ultraviolet light. The human production of vitamin D begins when the ultraviolet B (UVB) rays of the sun convert a cholesterol precursor of vitamin D **(7-dehydrocholesterol)** found in the skin into an inactive form of **vitamin D₃ (cholecalciferol)**. As illustrated in Figure 8-7, this compound must be activated to **25-hydroxyvitamin D₃ (calcidiol)** in the liver and to **1,25-dihydroxyvitamin D₃ (calcitriol)** in the kidney before it can function as the vitamin D hormone.

Our ability to absorb UVB rays and synthesize vitamin D is affected by many factors. Dark skin pigmentation, geographic latitude, time of day, season of the year, weather conditions, and amount of body surface covered with clothing or sunscreen affect the skin's exposure to UVB rays and therefore vitamin D synthesis. Something as simple as complete cloud cover or severe pollution can reduce UVB rays by about 50%. In addition, UVB rays will not penetrate glass. Aging reduces our ability to synthesize vitamin D—as much as 70% by age 70! Sunlight exposure of the hands, face, and arms for about 15 minutes daily will support adequate vitamin D synthesis for most healthy children and young adults. However, older adults and individuals with dark skin pigmentation require about 3 to 5 times this amount of sun exposure to synthesize an equivalent amount of vitamin D. Table 8-3 summarizes the various factors that can inhibit vitamin D synthesis, absorption, and activation.

FUNCTIONS OF VITAMIN D

Blood Calcium Regulation The main function of vitamin D (calcitriol) is to maintain the normal range of calcium and phosphorus in the blood. Together with the hormones parathyroid hormone (PTH) and calcitonin, vitamin D closely maintains blood calcium within a narrow range. This tight regulation of blood calcium ensures that an appropriate amount of calcium is available to all cells. Vitamin D regulates blood calcium in three ways: (1) it influences the absorption of calcium and phosphorus from the small intestine; (2) it works in combination with PTH and calcitonin, to regulate calcium excretion via the kidney; and (3) it affects the deposition or withdrawal of minerals from the bones (Fig. 8-8).

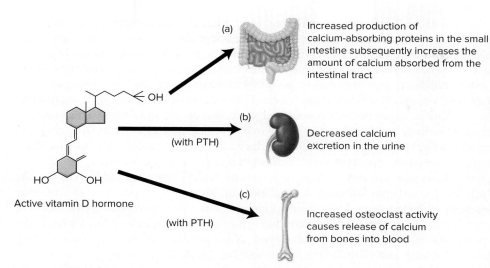

(a) Increased production of calcium-absorbing proteins in the small intestine subsequently increases the amount of calcium absorbed from the intestinal tract

(b) (with PTH) Decreased calcium excretion in the urine

Active vitamin D hormone

(c) (with PTH) Increased osteoclast activity causes release of calcium from bones into blood

FIGURE 8-8 ▲ Vitamin D regulates blood calcium. When blood levels of calcium begin to drop from the normal range, PTH stimulates the synthesis of the most active form of vitamin D (calcitriol) by the kidney. Calcitriol acts at three different sites to increase blood calcium: (a) small intestine; (b) kidney; and (c) bone. When blood calcium levels increase above the normal range, PTH release is inhibited and calcitonin is released, which has the opposite effects of PTH.

Gene Expression and Cell Growth It is now accepted that the biological effects of vitamin D extend far beyond its roles in calcium regulation and bone health. Vitamin D is involved in gene expression and cell growth; it binds to and subsequently affects cells of the immune system, brain and nervous system, parathyroid gland, pancreas, skin, muscles, and reproductive organs. In fact, vitamin D is considered one of the most potent regulators of cell growth, capable of influencing normal development of some cells (e.g., skin, colon, prostate, and breast), in turn reducing cancer risk in these sites.[2] Besides its role in influencing cancer risk, evidence suggests that vitamin D has a role in the prevention of several other chronic diseases, such as cardiovascular disease, diabetes, and hypertension.

VITAMIN D DEFICIENCY

When vitamin D levels are adequate, about 30% to 40% of dietary calcium is absorbed by the small intestine. If blood levels of vitamin D are low, the small intestine is able to absorb only about 10% to 15% of calcium from the diet, which is not enough to maintain the calcium requirements for bone health and other functions. Without adequate levels of vitamin D in the blood, calcium absorption from the small intestine decreases. Subsequently, calcium and phosphorus deposition during bone synthesis is reduced, resulting in weak bones that do not develop properly. Vitamin D deficiency can be traced to poor dietary intake, poor absorption (e.g., fat malabsorption in children with cystic fibrosis), altered metabolism (e.g., liver or kidney disease), or inadequate sun exposure. Studies have shown that vitamin D deficiency can be a problem in individuals with dark skin and the elderly. Vitamin D deficiency is a concern among young infants who are not receiving: (1) vitamin D supplementation; (2) sufficient exposure to sunlight; or (3) fortified food (e.g., cereal and dairy products).

Vitamin D deficiency can occur at any time, but when it occurs during infancy and early childhood, the resulting disease is known as *rickets*. The skeletal abnormalities of rickets include bowed legs, thick wrists and ankles, curvature of the spine, a pigeon chest (chest protrudes above the sternum), skull malformations, and pelvic deformities (Fig. 8-9). Studies show that vitamin D deficiency is prevalent among children and adolescents in the Unites States. It was estimated that 9% of children (7.6 million) in the U.S. were vitamin D deficient in 2009.[3] For the prevention of rickets, infants should be provided supplemental vitamin D (under a primary care provider's guidance). Keep in mind, however, that supplements need to be used carefully to avoid vitamin D toxicity in the infant.[3]

TABLE 8-3 ■ Factors That Impair Vitamin D Status

Inadequate sun exposure • Northern latitudes • Excess clothing (e.g., robes/veils) • Air pollution (i.e., smog) • Sunscreen with SPF > 8 • Excessive time spent indoors
Age
Dark skin pigmentation
Inadequate dietary intake
Fat malabsorption • Liver disease • Cystic fibrosis • Weight-loss medications
Obesity
Liver diseases
Kidney diseases

The pigment that imparts color to skin, melanin, is a potent natural sunscreen. Anthropologists believe that dark skin is protective against UVB rays because it is found in populations that have lived near the equator for many generations.

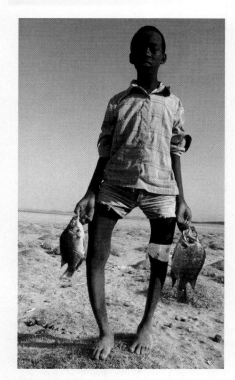

FIGURE 8-9 ▲ Vitamin D deficiency causes rickets, in which the bones and teeth do not develop normally.
©Jeff Rotman/Alamy

osteomalacia Adult form of rickets. The bones have low mineral density and subsequently are at risk for fracture.

vitamin D$_2$ (ergocalciferol) Form of vitamin D found in nonanimal sources, such as in some mushrooms.

Vitamin D

RDA: 15 micrograms (600 IU)
DV: 10 micrograms (400 IU)
UL: 100 micrograms (4000 IU)

Many tanning machines produce ultraviolet light of the appropriate wavelength to cause vitamin D synthesis in the skin. Relying on tanning machines, however, is not recommended by the FDA and the American Academy of Dermatology because of the potential health hazards (burns, damage to eyes, and skin cancer) associated with this practice.

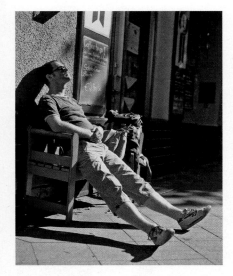

▲ Solar radiation (UVB rays) on the skin is the most reliable way to maintain vitamin D status and provides about 80% to 100% of the vitamin D humans use. In the absence of adequate sun exposure, the body must rely on dietary sources of vitamin D to meet needs. To get the vitamin D value of 10 to 15 minutes' exposure to sunlight, you would have to eat 30 servings of fortified cereal or 30 cups of fortified orange juice. ©Royalty-free/Corbis

Osteomalacia, which means soft bone, is an adult disease comparable to rickets. It can result from inadequate calcium intake, inefficient calcium absorption in the intestine, or poor conservation of calcium by the kidneys. It occurs most commonly in people with kidney, stomach, gallbladder, or intestinal disease (especially when most of the intestine has been removed) and in people with cirrhosis of the liver. These diseases affect both vitamin D activation and calcium absorption, leading to a decrease in bone mineral density. Bones become porous and weak, and break easily. Research shows that treatment with 10 to 20 micrograms (400 to 800 IU) per day of vitamin D, in conjunction with adequate dietary calcium, can reduce fracture risk among older adults. Thus, vitamin D is just as important as calcium when it comes to bone health.

Individuals who are most at risk of a vitamin D deficiency are older than the age of 60, live in northern latitudes, have dark skin, are rarely outdoors or always wear sunscreen while outdoors, have chronic kidney disease, take medications that interfere with vitamin D absorption, have a condition that prevents fat absorption, or have had part of their stomach or intestine removed. A combination of sun exposure, dietary vitamin D intake, and vitamin D supplementation can prevent deficiency.

GETTING ENOUGH VITAMIN D

There are two forms of vitamin D: vitamin D$_2$ and vitamin D$_3$. **Vitamin D$_2$ (ergocalciferol)** is a synthetic product derived from the irradiation of plant sterols (ergosterol) and is used in some supplements. Vitamin D$_3$ (cholecalciferol)—the form synthesized in the human body—is more commonly used in supplements and fortified foods. Both forms of vitamin D must be modified by chemical reactions that occur in the kidney and liver (Fig. 8-7) before they can be active in the body.

Sunlight is the best source of vitamin D. Unlike with supplements, you will never receive a toxic dose. With just 10 to 15 minutes of exposure of the arms and legs to sunlight, it is estimated that we synthesize roughly 3000 IU of vitamin D. To some extent, vitamin D synthesized on sunny days can be stored "for a rainy day" in the liver and adipose cells. However, most people now limit sun exposure to decrease their risk of skin cancer. Unless you live in a year-round sunny climate and find yourself outside most days between 10 A.M. and 3 P.M., you are not meeting your vitamin D needs from sun exposure alone. Therefore, people residing in northern climates and with limited sun exposure in general should find alternative (whole food) sources, especially in the winter months (Fig. 8-10). Overall, anyone who does not receive enough direct exposure to sunshine to synthesize an adequate amount of vitamin D must have a dietary source of the vitamin.

Dietary sources of vitamin D are limited, with very few foods being naturally high in vitamin D (Fig. 8-11). Fatty fish are considered the richest natural sources of vitamin D. Wild-caught salmon tops the list with around 600 to 1000 IU of vitamin D in a 3.5-ounce serving. Farmed salmon contains less at between 100 to 250 IU per 3.5-ounce serving. Tuna is a bit farther down the list with 6 ounces of canned light tuna providing about 300 IU. Eggs are another natural source with 1 large egg yolk delivering 41 IU. Although butter, liver, and a few brands of margarine contain some vitamin D, large servings must be eaten to obtain an appreciable amount of the vitamin; therefore, these foods are not considered significant sources.

Fortified foods and supplements are effective ways to add vitamin D to your diet. Use of vitamin D–fortified milk, which began in the 1930s, effectively wiped out rickets in the United States. Because vitamin D is a fat-soluble vitamin, there is slightly more in a cup of whole milk (124 IU) compared to 1% (120 IU) or nonfat (115 IU). Ready-to-eat breakfast cereals are also fortified with vitamin D and other vitamins and minerals. A few provide up to 100 IU per 1-cup serving, but most offer closer to 40 IU per serving. You will almost double your intake of vitamin D if you add milk on top of your fortified cereal. Some brands of orange juice are now fortified with vitamin D (about 140 IU of vitamin D per 1-cup serving). You can count on foods fortified with vitamin D containing not much more than 100 IU per serving because U.S. government regulations cap the added amount at that level.

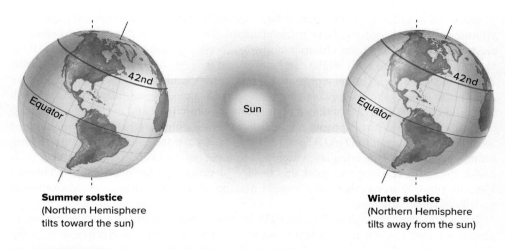

FIGURE 8-10 ◄ Seasonal variations to sunlight intensity. If you live north of 42° N latitude, the angle of the winter sun is such that the sun's rays must pass through more of the atmosphere than at other times of the year. As a result, skin forms less pro-hormone vitamin D in the winter. The 42nd parallel crosses North America at the northern border of California on the West Coast and Boston on the East Coast. In the far north (e.g., Alaska), this effect can last up to 6 months. Living below the 34th parallel (i.e., south of Los Angeles to Columbia, South Carolina), 10 minutes of UVB exposure per day is adequate to meet vitamin D needs year-round.

Summer solstice
(Northern Hemisphere tilts toward the sun)

Winter solstice
(Northern Hemisphere tilts away from the sun)

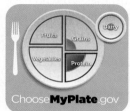

FIGURE 8-11 ◄ Food sources of vitamin D. (a) The fill of the background color (none, 1/3, 2/3, or completely covered) within each food group on MyPlate indicates the average nutrient density for vitamin D in that group. (b) The bar graph shows the vitamin D content of several foods compared to the RDA for adult males and females. Overall, the richest sources of vitamin D are fish, fortified dairy products, and fortified breakfast cereals. The vegetables group is not included in the bar graph because, aside from a select variety of mushrooms, vegetables are not a source of vitamin D.

Source: Nutrition data from USDA National Nutrient Database for Standard Reference, Release 26

(a)

(b)

	Food Item and Amount	Vitamin D (micrograms)	% RDA for Adult Males and Females (15 micrograms)
Grains	Total® Raisin Bran cereal, 1 cup	2.5	17%
Grains	Cheerios® cereal, 1 cup	1.0	7%
Grains	White bread, 1 slice	0.0	0%
Fruits	Orange juice (fortified), 1 cup	2.5	17%
Fruits	Blackberries, 1 cup	0.0	0%
Fruits	Kiwi, 1 cup	0.0	0%
Dairy	Milk, whole, 1 cup	3.2	21%
Dairy	Milk, fat-free, 1 cup	2.9	19%
Dairy	Almond milk, sweetened, 1 cup	2.4	16%
Protein	Salmon, baked, 3 ounces	11.0	73%
Protein	Egg, hard-boiled, 1 large	1.1	7%
Protein	Cod, baked, 3 ounces	1.0	7%
Fats & Oils	Margarine (fortified), 1 teaspoon	0.5	3%
Fats & Oils	Butter, 1 teaspoon	0.1	1%
Fats & Oils	Olive oil, 1 teaspoon	0.0	0.0

It takes some planning to meet daily vitamin D requirements from food sources. If you work indoors, live in a northern location, have a family history of skin cancer, and are not eating wild salmon every day, you may need a supplement. In supplements and fortified foods, vitamin D is available as vitamin D_2 and vitamin D_3; recent research shows that vitamin D_3 is most effective at raising blood levels of vitamin D and reducing fracture risk.

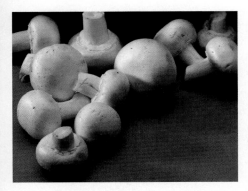

▲ The newest addition to foods naturally high in vitamin D is mushrooms. Mushrooms are the only vegetable to contain *ergosterol*, the precursor of vitamin D. Similar to humans, mushrooms also have the ability to make vitamin D when exposed to ultraviolet light. Although mushrooms are typically grown in the dark and do not contain the vitamin, some brands are now grown in ultraviolet light to stimulate vitamin D production. A vitamin D–rich portobello mushroom that provides 400 IUs of vitamin D per 3-ounce serving (about 1 cup of diced mushrooms) is already available in stores. ©Purestock/SuperStock

The Dietary Guidelines for Americans recommend that most individuals should choose more foods that provide vitamin D, which is a nutrient of public health concern in American diets.

During times of growth (i.e., from infancy through adolescence), consuming adequate vitamin D supports optimal bone mineralization. The American Academy of Pediatrics recommends that all infants, children, and adolescents consume a minimum of 400 IU of vitamin D daily. Until such intake can be obtained from whole foods, vitamin D supplementation is endorsed (under a primary care provider's guidance). This recommendation includes all infants (exclusively breastfed, partially breastfed, or formula-fed). As you will learn in Chapter 15, breast milk is a poor source of vitamin D, and exclusively breastfed infants with limited sun exposure are at risk for developing rickets. Even though infant formula contains vitamin D (60 IU per 100 kcal), the total intake of formula among young infants may not provide adequate vitamin D to meet needs. Evidence from clinical trials and historical precedence support this dosage of vitamin D for infants and children.[4] Keep in mind, however, that supplements need to be used carefully to avoid vitamin D toxicity in the infant.

For adults over the age of 70, the RDA increases because of the reduced ability to absorb vitamin D from the intestine and the decreased ability to synthesize it in the skin. A number of experts suggest older adults, especially those over age 70 who have limited sun exposure or dark skin, receive about 1000 IU (25 micrograms) from a combination of vitamin D–fortified foods and a multivitamin and mineral supplement, with an individual supplement of vitamin D added, if needed.[5]

Other population groups that have difficulty meeting vitamin D needs include vegans and people with milk allergies or lactose intolerance. Vitamin D supplements or vitamin D–fortified soy milk or fruit juices are options for people who do not consume dairy products.

AVOIDING TOO MUCH VITAMIN D

Too much vitamin D taken regularly can create serious health consequences in infants and children. Due to the role of vitamin D in calcium absorption, excretion, and release of calcium from bone, supplementation with high doses of vitamin D can cause calcium levels in the blood to increase above the normal range. The UL is based on the risk of overabsorption of calcium and eventual calcium deposits in the kidneys and other organs. Calcium deposits in organs can cause metabolic disturbances and cell death. Toxicity symptoms also include weakness, loss of appetite, diarrhea, vomiting, mental confusion, and increased urine output. Please note that vitamin D toxicity does not result from excessive exposure to the sun because the body regulates the amount of vitamin D made in the skin (i.e., as exposure to sunlight increases, vitamin D synthesis efficiency decreases).

✓ CONCEPT CHECK 8.3

1. Why is vitamin D sometimes not considered an *essential* nutrient?
2. How is vitamin D activated in the body?
3. How does vitamin D work to maintain blood calcium levels?
4. What are some rich food sources of vitamin D?
5. Can vitamin D be toxic?

8.4 Vitamin E (Tocopherols)

In the 1920s, a fat-soluble compound was found to be essential for fertility in rats. This compound was named tocopherol from the Greek words *tokos,* meaning "birth," and *phero,* meaning "to bring forth." Later, this essential nutrient was named vitamin E. Vitamin E is a family of four tocopherols and four tocotrienols called alpha, beta, gamma, and delta. They differ in that tocopherols have a saturated side chain, whereas the tocotrienols have an unsaturated side chain. Tocotrienols have not been as extensively

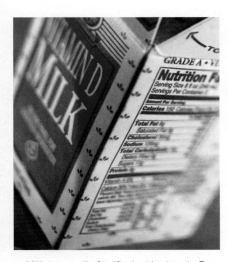

▲ Milk is usually fortified with vitamin D as well as vitamin A. Note that the DV for vitamin D is lower than the RDA for adults. ©Royalty Free/Corbis

studied as tocopherols, but recent research explores their potential roles in prevention of cancer, diabetes, and cardiovascular diseases. Of these eight forms of vitamin E, alpha (α)-tocopherol is the most biologically active and the most potent.

FUNCTIONS OF VITAMIN E

Antioxidant The principal function of vitamin E in humans is as an antioxidant. Vitamin E is a fat-soluble vitamin found primarily in adipose tissue and in the lipid bilayers of cell membranes (Fig. 8-12). Many of the lipids within these membranes are polyunsaturated fatty acids (PUFA), which are particularly susceptible to oxidative attack by free radicals. The formation of free radicals may destabilize the cell membrane, which may ultimately alter the ability of the cell to function properly. Vitamin E can donate electrons or hydrogen to free radicals found in membranes, thereby making them more stable. The antioxidant function of vitamin E appears to be critical in cells continually exposed to high levels of oxygen, particularly red blood cells and the cells lining the lungs.

Increasing vitamin E intake has been suggested as a way to prevent several chronic diseases that are linked to oxidative damage. For example, oxidized LDL cholesterol is a major component of the plaque that develops in arteries, which leads to atherosclerosis. Vitamin E is thought to attenuate the development of atherogenic plaque due to its ability to prevent or reduce the formation of oxidized LDL cholesterol.[6] In addition, oxidative damage to proteins in the eye leads to the development of cataracts. Oxidized proteins combine and precipitate in the lens, causing cloudiness and decreasing visual acuity. Insufficient consumption of antioxidants from foods increases one's risk of these diseases.

Experts do not know whether supplementation with megadoses of vitamin E can confer any significant protection against diseases linked to oxidative damage. The consensus among the scientific community is that the established benefits of lifestyle choices have a far greater effect than any proposed benefits of antioxidant supplementation. The position of scientific research organizations (e.g., American Heart Association, U.S. Preventive Services Task Force) is that it is premature to recommend vitamin E supplements to the general population, based on current knowledge and the failure of large clinical trials to show any consistent benefit. This conclusion is in agreement with the latest report on vitamin E by the Food and Nutrition Board of the National Academy of Sciences. In addition, the FDA has denied the request of the dietary supplement industry to make a health claim that vitamin E supplements reduce the risk of cardiovascular disease or cancer.

Other Roles of Vitamin E Although vitamin E is essential for fertility in many animal species, it does not appear to serve this role in humans. It is, however, important for the formation of muscles and the central nervous system in early human development. Vitamin E has been shown to improve vitamin A absorption if the dietary intake of vitamin A is low. It also functions in the metabolism of iron within cells, and it helps maintain nervous tissue and immune function.

VITAMIN E DEFICIENCY

Specific population groups are especially susceptible to developing marginal vitamin E status. Preterm infants tend to have low vitamin E stores because this vitamin is transferred from mother to baby during the late stages of pregnancy. Hence, the potential for oxidative damage, which could cause the cell membranes of red blood cells to break (hemolysis), is of particular concern for preterm infants. The rapid growth of preterm infants, coupled with the high oxygen needs of their immature lungs, greatly increases the stress on red blood cells. Special vitamin E–fortified formulas and supplements designed

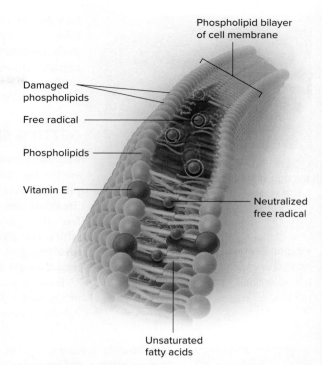

Phospholipid bilayer of cell membrane

Damaged phospholipids

Free radical

Phospholipids

Vitamin E

Neutralized free radical

Unsaturated fatty acids

FIGURE 8-12 ▲ Fat-soluble vitamin E can insert itself into cell membranes, where it helps stop free-radical chain reactions. If not interrupted, these reactions cause extensive oxidative damage to cells and, ultimately, cell death.

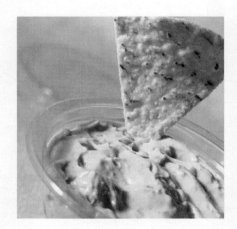

▲ The avocado in guacamole and the sunflower oil in the tortilla chip are good sources of vitamin E. ©Banana Stock/Punchstock

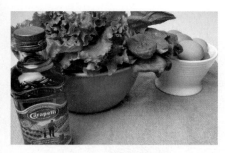

▲ Olive oil, leafy greens such as spinach, and egg yolks are sources of vitamin E.
©McGraw-Hill Education/Jill Braaten, photographer

Vitamin E
RDA: 15 milligrams
DV: 30 milligrams
UL: 1000 milligrams

for preterm infants compensate for this lack of vitamin E. Smokers are another group at high risk for vitamin E deficiency, as smoking readily destroys vitamin E in the lungs. One study showed that megadosing will not correct this vitamin E destruction by smokers. It remains unknown if any adjustment in vitamin E requirements is needed in those who smoke or are routinely exposed to smoke. Others at risk of vitamin E deficiency include adults on very low-fat diets (< 15% total fat) or those with fat-malabsorption disorders.

GETTING ENOUGH VITAMIN E

Because vitamin E is only synthesized by plants, plant products (especially the oils) are the best sources. In the North American diet, nearly two-thirds of vitamin E is supplied by salad oils, margarines, spreads (low-fat margarine), and shortening (Fig. 8-13). Breakfast cereals fortified with vitamin E are good sources, but other than wheat germ, few other grain products provide much vitamin E. Milling of grains removes the germ, which contains the oils (mostly PUFAs) and vitamin E. By removing the germ, the resulting grain product has less chance of spoiling (i.e., rancidity of the PUFAs) and thus a longer shelf life. Other good sources of vitamin E are nuts and seeds.

Because plant oils contain mostly unsaturated fatty acids, the relatively high amount of vitamin E in plant oils naturally protects these unsaturated lipids from oxidation. Animal products (meat, dairy, and eggs) and fish oils, on the other hand, contain almost

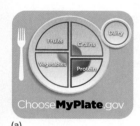

(a)

FIGURE 8-13 ◄ Food sources of vitamin E. (a) The fill of the background color (none, 1/3, 2/3, or completely covered) within each food group on MyPlate indicates the average nutrient density for vitamin E in that group. (b) The bar graph shows the vitamin E content of several foods compared to the RDA for adult males and females. Overall, the richest sources of vitamin E are nuts, seeds, plant oils, and fortified breakfast cereals. The dairy group is not pictured in the bar graph because, except for plant-based dairy alternatives, foods in this group yield no vitamin E.

Source: Nutrition data from USDA National Nutrient Database for Standard Reference, Release 26

(b)

	Food Item and Amount	Vitamin E (milligrams)	Vitamin E (IU)	% RDA for Adult Males and Females (15 milligrams)
Grains	Total® Raisin Bran cereal, 1 cup	13.5	20.1	90%
Grains	Whole wheat bread, 1 slice	0.9	1.3	6%
Grains	Quinoa, cooked, ½ cup	0.6	0.9	4%
Vegetables	Spinach, cooked, 1 cup	3.7	5.5	25%
Vegetables	Asparagus, cooked, 1 cup	2.7	4.0	18%
Vegetables	Sweet potato, baked, 1 cup	1.4	2.1	9%
Fruits	Blackberries, 1 cup	1.7	2.5	11%
Fruits	Mango, 1 cup	1.5	2.2	10%
Fruits	Olives, 5 large	0.7	1.0	5%
Protein	Sunflower seeds, dry roasted, 1 ounce	7.4	11.0	49%
Protein	Shrimp, cooked, 3 ounces	1.9	2.8	12%
Protein	Egg, hard-boiled, 1 large	0.5	0.8	3%
Fats & Oils	Sunflower oil, 1 teaspoon	1.9	2.8	12%
Fats & Oils	Salad dressing, Italian, 2 tablespoons	0.6	1.0	4%
Fats & Oils	Butter, 1 teaspoon	0.1	0.2	1%

no vitamin E (Fig. 8-13). Vitamin E is susceptible to destruction by oxygen, metals, light, and heat, especially when oil is repeatedly reused in deep-fat frying; thus, the vitamin E content of a food depends on how it is harvested, processed, stored, and cooked.

The RDA of vitamin E for adults is 15 milligrams per day of alpha-tocopherol, the most active, natural form of vitamin E (d isomer). This amount equals 22.4 milligrams of the less active, synthetic source (dl isomer). Typically, North American adults consume about two-thirds of the RDA for vitamin E from food sources. The Daily Value used on food and supplement labels is 30 milligrams.

As with vitamin A, the vitamin E content of dietary supplements is given in international units rather than simple metric measurements. International units reflect the different biological activity of natural vitamin E compared with synthetic preparations of vitamin E. Supplements may contain any of the variety of chemical forms and stereoisomers of vitamin E. Typical synthetic preparations of vitamin E contain a mixture of equal parts of d and l stereoisomers, only half of which are biologically active. Therefore, a supplement containing synthetic vitamin E has lower biological activity (i.e., lower IU) than the same quantity of natural vitamin E. The more expensive natural vitamin E supplements contain only the biologically active d-form. See the margin for conversion factors used to calculate the vitamin E content of dietary supplements.

AVOIDING TOO MUCH VITAMIN E

Unlike other fat-soluble vitamins, vitamin E is not as readily stored in the liver. It is stored in adipose tissue throughout the body. The UL for vitamin E is 1000 milligrams per day of supplemental alpha-tocopherol. Excessive intake of vitamin E can interfere with vitamin K's role in the clotting mechanism, leading to hemorrhage. The risk of insufficient blood clotting is especially high if vitamin E is taken in conjunction with anticoagulant medications (e.g., Coumadin or heavy aspirin use). Always be cautious about using dietary supplements. In addition to the significant risk of drug interference and prolonged bleeding, vitamin E supplements can produce nausea, gastrointestinal distress, and diarrhea.

> ✓ **CONCEPT CHECK 8.4**
>
> 1. How does vitamin E work to prevent oxidative damage?
> 2. What are some rich food sources of vitamin E?
> 3. Why are preterm infants, smokers, and people with fat-malabsorption disorders particularly susceptible to oxidative damage to cell membranes?
> 4. What are the possible results of vitamin E toxicity?

8.5 Vitamin K (Quinone)

A family of compounds known collectively as vitamin K is found in plants, plant oils, fish oils, and animal products. Vitamin K is also synthesized by bacteria in the human colon, which normally fulfills approximately 10% of human requirements. Vitamin K has three forms: (1) phylloquinone, the most abundant form of vitamin K, synthesized by green plants; (2) menaquinone, synthesized by gut bacteria; and (3) menadione, the synthetic form found in supplements. Interestingly, the synthetic menadione form of vitamin K is twice as biologically available as the other two!

FUNCTIONS OF VITAMIN K

Vitamin K serves as a cofactor in chemical reactions that add CO_2 molecules to various proteins, thus enabling these proteins to bind calcium. This is the biochemical basis for vitamin K's role in the life-and-death process of blood clotting. In the clotting cascade

---

Calculating Vitamin E Content of Dietary Supplements

To find milligrams of *natural* vitamin E (d-alpha-tocopherol), multiply IU by 0.67. Conversely, to calculate IU from milligrams, multiply milligrams by 1.49.

Example: The RDA for vitamin E is 15 milligrams per day. This is equal to how many IU of natural vitamin E?

15 mg × 1.49 IU/mg = 22.35 IU

To find milligrams of *synthetic* vitamin E (dl-alpha-tocopherol), multiply IU by 0.45. Conversely, to calculate IU from milligrams, multiply milligrams by 2.22.

Example: If a vitamin E supplement contains 400 IU of dl-alpha-tocopherol, then how many milligrams of vitamin E does it contain?

400 IU × 0.45 mg/IU = 180 mg

Vitamin K

AI
    Men: 120 micrograms
    Women: 90 micrograms
DV: 80 micrograms
UL: None

Medicine Cabinet

People who are prone to develop blood clots may take anticoagulants or *blood thinners*. One example is Plavix (clopidogrel), which works by inhibiting the activity of platelets. Another commonly prescribed anticoagulant is Coumadin (warfarin). This medication inhibits vitamin K-dependent coagulation factors. When taking Coumadin or similar drugs, it is important to keep vitamin K intake consistent from day to day.[7]

©Peter Dazeley/Photographer's Choice/Getty Images

FIGURE 8-14 ▼ Vitamin K works to activate clotting factors, which are then able to bind to calcium. The binding of calcium to clotting factors is necessary for clot formation. ©Science Photo Library/Getty Images RF

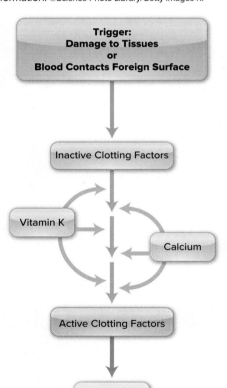

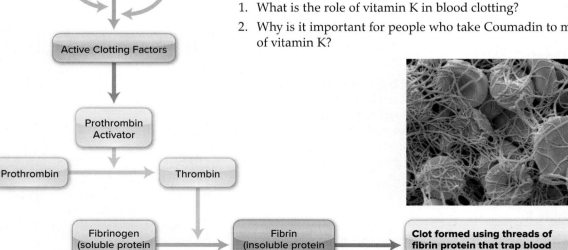

(Fig. 8-14), vitamin K imparts calcium-binding ability to seven different proteins, eventually leading to the conversion of soluble fibrinogen into insoluble fibrin (i.e., the clot). The "K" stands for *koagulation* in the language spoken by the Danish researchers who first noted the relationship between vitamin K and blood clotting.

Besides its role in blood clotting, vitamin K is also important for bone health. Three calcium-binding proteins (e.g., osteocalcin) in the bone depend upon vitamin K for their function in bone mineralization.

VITAMIN K DEFICIENCY

At birth, a newborn has a *sterile gut*—an intestinal tract with an insufficient amount of bacteria. Thus, the newborn cannot produce enough vitamin K to allow for effective blood clotting if the infant is injured or needs surgery. Therefore, vitamin K is routinely administered by injection shortly after birth. In adults, deficiencies of vitamin K have occurred when a person takes antibiotics for an extended time. Chronic antibiotic use destroys the bacteria that normally produce some of the vitamin K that is absorbed and used by the body. Vitamin K deficiency may also occur when fat absorption is limited.

GETTING ENOUGH VITAMIN K

Major food sources of the phylloquinone form of vitamin K are green, leafy vegetables, broccoli, asparagus, and peas (Fig. 8-15). The menaquinone form of vitamin K is found in some meats, eggs, and dairy products, and is the form synthesized by bacteria. Compared to that of plant sources, the nutrient density of vitamin K in foods of animal origin is rather low. Vitamin K is resistant to cooking losses.

As with other fat-soluble vitamins, absorption of vitamin K requires dietary fat and adequate liver and pancreatic secretions. Unlike other fat-soluble vitamins, though, not much vitamin K is stored in the body, and excesses can be excreted via urine. Thus, a deficiency could develop rather quickly if dietary intake of this nutrient is poor, which can be a problem among older adults whose diets lack vegetables. However, because vitamin K is fairly widespread in foods and some can be synthesized by bacteria in the colon, deficiencies of this vitamin rarely occur. No reports of toxicity have been published.

Table 8-4 reviews what we have covered so far regarding the fat-soluble vitamins.

✓ CONCEPT CHECK 8.5

1. What is the role of vitamin K in blood clotting?
2. Why is it important for people who take Coumadin to monitor their dietary intake of vitamin K?

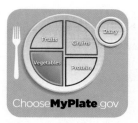

FIGURE 8-15 ◄ Food sources of vitamin K. (a) The fill of the background color (none, 1/3, 2/3, or completely covered) within each food group on MyPlate indicates the average nutrient density for vitamin K in that group. (b) The bar graph shows the vitamin K content of several foods compared to the AI for adult males and females. Overall, the richest sources of vitamin K are green, leafy vegetables. The grains group is not shown in the bar graph because grains provide very little vitamin K.

Source: Nutrition data from USDA National Nutrient Database for Standard Reference, Release 26; and Elder SJ and others: Vitamin K contents of meat, dairy, and fast food in the U.S. diet. *Journal of Agricultural and Food Chemistry* 54: 463, 2006

(a)

(b)

	Food Item and Amount	Vitamin K (micrograms)	% AI for Adult Males (120 micrograms)	% AI for Adult Females (90 micrograms)
Vegetables	Spinach, cooked, 1 cup	889	741%	987%
	Broccoli, cooked, 1 cup	220	183%	244%
	Brussels sprouts, cooked, 1 cup	219	183%	243%
Fruits	Rhubarb, cooked, 1 cup	51	42%	56%
	Blueberries, 1 cup	29	24%	32%
	Pomegranates, 1 cup arils	29	24%	32%
Dairy	Cheese, cheddar, 1.5 ounces	6*	5%	7%
	Soy milk, 1 cup	4	3%	4%
	Milk 2%, 1 cup	1*	1%	1%
Protein	Tofu, firm, cooked, 1 cup	6*	5%	7%
	Egg, hard-boiled, 1 large	4*	3%	4%
	Beef liver, pan-fried, 3 ounces	3	3%	4%
Fats & Oils	Soybean oil, 1 teaspoon	8	7%	9%
	Margarine, 1 teaspoon	4	4%	5%
	Butter, 1 teaspoon	0	0%	0%

* Value includes phylloquinone and menaquinone.

TABLE 8-4 ■ **Summary of the Fat-Soluble Vitamins**

Vitamin	Major Functions	RDA or AI	Dietary Sources	Deficiency Symptoms	Toxicity Symptoms
Vitamin A (preformed and provitamin A)	• Required for normal vision • Gene expression • Growth, development, reproduction • Embryonic development • Immune function • Cancer prevention	*Men:* 900 micrograms RAE (3000 IU preformed vitamin A) *Women:* 700 micrograms RAE (2300 IU preformed vitamin A)	• Liver • Fortified dairy • Fish, fish oils • Darkly colored fruits and leafy vegetables • Fortified milk • Eggs	• Night blindness • Xerophthalmia • Inadequate growth • Dry skin • Inadequate immune function	• Birth defects • Bone pain and fractures • Liver toxicity • Nervous system disorders • Nausea and vomiting UL = 3000 micrograms (10,000 IU) of preformed vitamin A

(continued)

TABLE 8-4 ■ Summary of the Fat-Soluble Vitamins (*continued*)

Vitamin	Major Functions	RDA or AI	Dietary Sources	Deficiency Symptoms	Toxicity Symptoms
Vitamin D (calciferol)	• Maintain serum calcium and phosphorus concentrations • Bone health • Gene expression and cell growth	15 micrograms (600 IU)	• Fish liver oils • Flesh of fatty fish • Egg yolk • Fortified dairy • Fortified cereals	• Rickets in children • Osteomalacia in adults • Delayed growth • Reduced immunity	• Hypercalcemia • Decreased renal function and hypercalciuria • Kidney failure • Cardiovascular system failure • Calcification of soft tissues UL = 100 micrograms (4000 IU)
Vitamin E	• Antioxidant • Prevents breakdown of vitamin A and unsaturated fatty acids	15 milligrams alpha-tocopherol (22 IU natural form, 33 IU synthetic form)	• Vegetable oils • Unprocessed cereal grains • Nuts • Fruits • Vegetables • Fortified cereals	• Hemolysis of red blood cells • Nerve damage • Anemia	• Hemorrhagic toxicity UL = 1000 milligrams (1100 IU synthetic form, 1500 IU natural form)
Vitamin K	• Coenzyme during the synthesis of proteins involved in blood clotting and bone metabolism	*Men:* 120 milligrams *Women:* 90 milligrams	• Green leafy vegetables • Liver • Plant oils and margarine	• Hemorrhage • Fractures	• Disruption of anticlotting medications No UL

Abbreviations: RDA = Recommended Dietary Allowance; AI = adequate intake; RAE = retinol activity equivalents; IU = international units; UL = Upper Intake Level

8.6 The Water-Soluble Vitamins and Choline

Regular consumption of good sources of the water-soluble vitamins is important. Most water-soluble vitamins are readily excreted from the body with any excess generally ending up in the urine or stool and very little being stored. They dissolve in water, so large amounts of these vitamins can be lost during food processing and preparation. As emphasized earlier in this chapter, vitamin content is best preserved by light cooking methods, such as stir-frying, steaming, and microwaving (Table 8-1).

The B vitamins are thiamin, riboflavin, niacin, pantothenic acid, biotin, vitamin B-6, folate, and vitamin B-12. Choline is a related nutrient that has vitamin-like characteristics but currently is not classified as a vitamin. Vitamin C is also a water-soluble vitamin.

The B vitamins often occur together in the same foods, so a lack of one B vitamin may mean other B vitamins are also low in a diet. The B vitamins function as coenzymes, small molecules that interact with enzymes to enable the enzymes to function. In essence, the coenzymes contribute to enzyme activity (Fig. 8-16).

As coenzymes, the B vitamins play many key roles in metabolism. The metabolic pathways used by carbohydrates, fats, and amino acids all require input from B vitamins. Because of their role in energy metabolism, needs for many B vitamins increase somewhat as energy expenditure increases. Still, this is not a major concern because this increase in energy expenditure is usually accompanied by a corresponding increase in food intake, which contributes more B vitamins to a diet. Many B vitamins are interdependent because they participate in the same processes (Fig. 8-17). B vitamin–deficiency symptoms typically occur in the brain and nervous system, skin, and gastrointestinal (GI) tract. Cells in these tissues are metabolically active, and those in the skin and GI tract are also constantly being replaced.

ASK THE RDN   Raw Food Diet Plan

Dear RDN: *My roommate follows a raw food diet and claims that cooking foods destroys key nutrients and makes foods toxic. Is this true?*

This highly restrictive diet includes consuming uncooked, unprocessed, mostly organic fruits, vegetables, and spouted grains. Some may consume unpasteurized dairy products and raw eggs, meat, and fish. Advocates of this diet believe that heat destroys key nutrients and enzymes that are necessary to fight disease. Although some phytochemicals and nutrients are more bioavailable in raw form, there are many plant-based foods (e.g., tomatoes) that actually become more digestible once exposed to heat. In addition, many uncooked and unpasteurized products are sources of foodborne pathogens. Food poisoning is of particular concern for pregnant women, young children, older adults, immunocompromised individuals, and those with chronic disease.

Limitations: This diet is extremely difficult to maintain, especially when dining out, because of its many restrictions. Complete exclusion of food groups (e.g., dairy and meat) may lead to nutrient deficiencies, so supplements (e.g., iron, calcium, and vitamin B-12) may be necessary. Also, the cost and limited availability of organic foods may be prohibitive.

Strengths: This plan is compatible with vegetarian, vegan, and gluten-free dietary patterns. Raw food adopters often lose or maintain weight, given most of the foods allowed are low in calories and fat.

In sum, a plant-based dietary pattern is recommended for Americans; however, there is no evidence to support the nutritionally inadequate, extreme, and potentially harmful raw food practices.

Warm regards,

Colleen Spees, PhD, RDN, LD, FAND (author)

After being ingested, the B vitamins are first broken down from their active coenzyme forms into free vitamins in the stomach and small intestine. The vitamins are then absorbed, primarily in the small intestine. Typically, about 50% to 90% of the B vitamins in the diet are absorbed, which means that they have relatively high bioavailability. Once inside cells, the active coenzyme forms are resynthesized. There is no need to consume the coenzyme forms themselves. Some vitamins are sold in their coenzyme forms, but these are broken down during digestion, and we activate them when needed.

B VITAMIN INTAKES OF NORTH AMERICANS

The nutritional health of most North Americans with regard to the B vitamins is good. Typical diets contain plentiful and varied natural sources of these vitamins. In addition, many common foods, such as ready-to-eat breakfast cereals, are fortified with one or more of the B vitamins. In some developing countries, however, deficiencies of the B vitamins are more common, and the resulting deficiency diseases pose significant health problems. Global nutritional deficiencies will be discussed in more detail in Chapter 12.

Because B vitamins are water soluble, very little is stored and excess ends up in the urine or stool. About 10% to 25% of these vitamins are lost from food during food processing and preparation because they dissolve in water. Light cooking methods, such as stir-frying, steaming, and microwaving, best preserve vitamin content (Table 8-1).

Despite the adequate B vitamin status of North Americans, marginal deficiencies of these vitamins may occur in some cases, especially among older adults who consume small amounts of food and in people with inadequate dietary patterns. In the short run, a marginal deficiency likely leads only to fatigue or other unspecified physical effects. Although the long-term effects of such marginal deficiencies are yet unknown, increased risks of cardiovascular disease, cancer, and cataracts of the eye are suspected. With rare

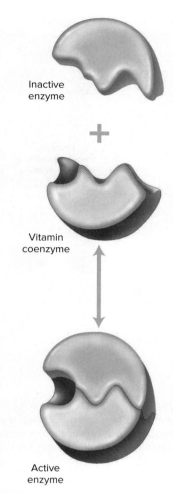

Inactive enzyme

+

Vitamin coenzyme

Active enzyme

FIGURE 8-16 ▲ Coenzymes, such as those formed from B vitamins, aid in the function of various enzymes. Without the coenzyme, the enzyme cannot function properly, and deficiency symptoms associated with the missing vitamin eventually appear. Health-food stores sell the coenzyme forms of some vitamins. These more expensive forms of vitamins are unnecessary. The body makes all the coenzymes it needs from vitamin precursors.

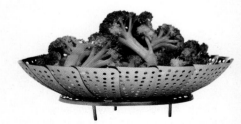

▲ Rapid cooking of vegetables in minimal fluids aids in preserving vitamin content. Steaming is one effective method.
©C Squared Studios/Getty Images

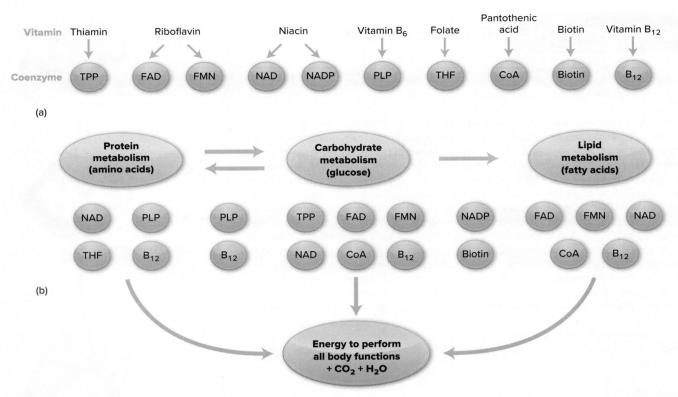

FIGURE 8-17 ▲ B vitamins are essential components of many coenzymes involved in energy metabolism. (a) The B vitamins and their coenzymes (shown as their commonly used abbreviation): TPP, thiamin pyrophosphate; FAD, flavin adenine dinucleotide; FMN, flavin mononucleotide; NAD, nicotinamide adenine dinucleotide; NADP, nicotinamide adenine dinucleotide phosphate; PLP, pyridoxal phosphate; CoA, coenzyme A. (b) The coenzymes are shown associated with the metabolic pathways for which they are essential.

exceptions, healthy adults do not develop the more serious B vitamin–deficiency diseases from dietary inadequacy alone. The main exceptions are people with alcoholism. The combination of extremely unbalanced diets and alcohol-induced alterations of vitamin absorption and metabolism creates significant risks for serious nutrient deficiencies among people with alcoholism.

B VITAMINS IN GRAINS

The production of refined grains, such as white flour from wheat, leads to the loss of B vitamins as well as other vitamins and minerals. In milling grains to make refined products, seeds are crushed and the germ, bran, and husk layers are discarded, leaving just the starch-containing endosperm in the refined grains. This starch is used to make white flour, bread, and cereal products. Unfortunately, many nutrients are lost along with the discarded germ, bran, and husk materials. To counteract these losses, in the United States, bread and cereal products made from milled grains are enriched with four B vitamins (thiamin, riboflavin, niacin, and folic acid) and with the mineral iron.

Food enrichment was initiated by federal legislation in the 1930s to help combat nutrient deficiencies such as pellagra (niacin deficiency) and iron-deficiency **anemia.** Federal regulations added folate to the list of nutrients required to be added to refined grain products in 1998. Not all nutrients lost in milling are added back through enrichment; these products remain lower in vitamins E and B-6, potassium, magnesium, fiber, and other nutrients than the whole grains. This lower nutrient density is why dietitians and the Dietary Guidelines advocate daily consumption of whole grain products, such as whole wheat bread and brown rice, rather than refined grain products (Fig. 8-18).

anemia A decreased oxygen-carrying capacity of the blood. This can be caused by many factors, such as iron deficiency or blood loss.

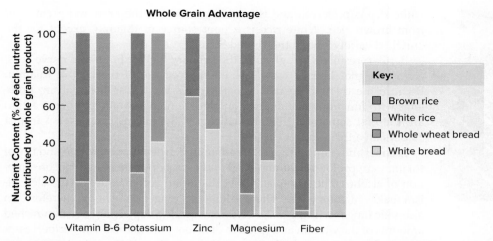

FIGURE 8-18 ▲ Compare the relative nutrient contents of refined versus whole grains. Nutrients are expressed as a percentage of the nutrient contribution of the whole grain product.

✓ CONCEPT CHECK 8.6

1. What are the coenzymes associated with each of the B vitamins involved in energy metabolism?
2. What body organs or tissues are most likely to show symptoms if there is a deficiency of B vitamins?
3. Why are B vitamins lost when foods are cooked in water?
4. What group of people is at very high risk of deficiency of B vitamins?
5. What happens during the refining of grains that causes a decrease in nutrient density?
6. What is added during the "enrichment" of grain products, and why is it important?

8.7 Thiamin (Vitamin B-1)

FUNCTIONS OF THIAMIN

Thiamin was the first water-soluble vitamin to be discovered. One of its primary functions is to help release energy from carbohydrate. Its coenzyme form, thiamin pyrophosphate (TPP), participates in reactions in which carbon dioxide (CO_2) is released. Such reactions are particularly important in the body's ATP-producing energy pathways, which involve the breakdown of carbohydrates and certain amino acids (Fig. 8-17). Thiamin also functions in chemical reactions that make RNA, DNA, and neurotransmitters.

THIAMIN DEFICIENCY

The thiamin-deficiency disease is called **beriberi,** a word that means "I can't, I can't" in the Sri Lankan language of Sinhalese. This disease was described long before thiamin was discovered to be a vitamin in 1910. The symptoms include weakness, loss of appetite, irritability, nervous tingling throughout the body, poor arm and leg coordination, and deep muscle pain in the calves. A person with beriberi often develops an enlarged heart and sometimes severe edema.

Beriberi is seen in areas where rice is a staple and polished (white) rice is consumed rather than brown (whole grain) rice. In most parts of the world, even poor countries,

beriberi The thiamin-deficiency disorder characterized by muscle weakness, loss of appetite, nerve degeneration, and sometimes edema.

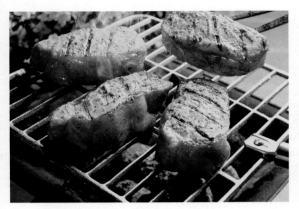

▲ Pork is an excellent source of thiamin.
©D. Fischer and P. Lyons/Cole Group/Getty Images

white rice is preferred and is made by removing the bran and germ layer from brown rice. White rice is a poor source of thiamin, except for the enriched variety sold in the United States.

Beriberi results when glucose, the primary fuel for brain and nerve cells, cannot be metabolized to release energy because of the lack of thiamin. Because the thiamin coenzyme participates in glucose metabolism, problems with functions that depend on glucose such as brain and nerve action are the first signs of a thiamin deficiency. Symptoms can develop in just 10 days on a thiamin-free diet.

Alcohol abuse increases risk for thiamin deficiency. Absorption and use of thiamin are profoundly diminished and excretion is increased by consumption of alcohol. The low-quality diet that often accompanies severe alcoholism makes matters worse. There is limited storage in the body; therefore, an alcoholic binge lasting 1 to 2 weeks may quickly deplete already diminished amounts of the vitamin and result in deficiency symptoms. The beriberi associated with alcoholism is also called Wernicke-Korsakoff syndrome.

GETTING ENOUGH THIAMIN

Average daily intakes of thiamin for men exceed the DV by 50% or more and for women exceed by about 26%. Adults with low incomes and older people may have difficulty meeting their needs for thiamin. Potential contributors to thiamin deficiency are diets dominated by highly processed and unenriched foods, sugar, and fat; and heavy alcohol intake combined with a inadequate diet. Oral thiamin supplements are typically nontoxic because thiamin is rapidly lost in the urine. Thus, no UL has been set for thiamin.

Major sources of thiamin include pork products, whole grains (wheat germ), ready-to-eat breakfast cereals, enriched grains and flour, green beans, milk, orange juice, organ meats, peanuts, dried beans, and seeds (Fig. 8-19). When considering the sections of MyPlate, the protein and grains groups contain the most foods that are nutrient-dense sources of thiamin.

Thiamin

RDA

Men: 1.2 milligrams

Women: 1.1 milligrams

DV: 1.5 milligrams

UL: none

> ✓ CONCEPT CHECK 8.7

1. How is thiamin involved in energy metabolism?
2. What body organs or tissues are most likely to show symptoms if there is a deficiency of thiamin?
3. What group of people is at very high risk of deficiency of thiamin?
4. What are some excellent sources of thiamin?

8.8 Riboflavin (Vitamin B-2)

FUNCTIONS OF RIBOFLAVIN

Riboflavin derives its name from its yellow color (*flavus* means "yellow" in Latin). The coenzyme forms of riboflavin, flavin dinucleotide (FAD) and flavin mononucleotide (FMN), participate in many energy-yielding metabolic pathways, such as the breakdown of fatty acids (Fig. 8-17). Some metabolism of vitamins and minerals also requires riboflavin. Indirectly, riboflavin also has an antioxidant role in the body through its support of the enzyme glutathione peroxidase.

RIBOFLAVIN DEFICIENCY

Symptoms associated with riboflavin deficiency **(ariboflavinosis)** include inflammation of the mouth and tongue, dermatitis, cracking of tissue around the corners of the mouth

Riboflavin

RDA

Men: 1.3 milligrams

Women: 1.1 milligrams

DV: 1.7 milligrams

UL: None

ariboflavinosis Riboflavin-deficiency disease resulting in irritation of the skin, mouth, and throat; usually accompanied by low overall intakes of calories and protein.

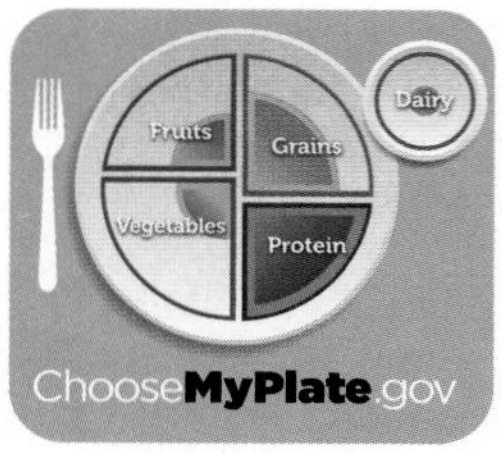

FIGURE 8-19 ◄ Food sources of thiamin. (a) The fill of the background color (none, 1/3, 2/3, or completely covered) within each food group on MyPlate indicates the average nutrient density for thiamin in that group. (b) The bar graph shows the thiamin content of several foods in each food group compared to the RDA for adult males and females. Overall, the richest sources of thiamin are meats (especially pork), whole grains, and fortified breakfast cereals.

Source: Nutrition data from USDA National Nutrient Database for Standard Reference, Release 26

(a)

(b)

Food Item and Amount	Thiamin (milligrams)	% RDA for Adult Males (1.2 milligrams)	% RDA for Adult Females (1.1 milligrams)
Grains Cheerios® cereal, 1 cup	0.4	31%	34%
Wheat germ, 2 tablespoons	0.3	25%	27%
Flour tortilla, 8″	0.2	17%	18%
Vegetables Green peas, cooked, 1 cup	0.4	35%	38%
Acorn squash, cooked, 1 cup	0.3	29%	31%
Corn, cooked, 1 cup	0.1	12%	13%
Fruits Orange juice, fresh, 1 cup	0.2	17%	18%
Raisins, ½ cup	0.1	6%	7%
Watermelon, 1 cup	0.1	4%	5%
Dairy Yogurt, plain, nonfat, 1 cup	0.1	10%	11%
Milk, fat-free, 1 cup	0.1	9%	10%
Soy milk, 1 cup	0.1	6%	6%
Protein Ham, canned, 3 ounces	0.8	68%	74%
Kidney beans, cooked, ½ cup	0.1	12%	13%
Chicken breast, roasted, 3 ounces	0.1	5%	5%

(called **cheilosis**), various eye disorders, sensitivity to the sun, and confusion (Fig. 8-20). Such symptoms develop after approximately 2 months on a riboflavin-poor diet. Riboflavin deficiency typically would occur jointly with deficiencies of niacin, thiamin, and vitamin B-6 because these nutrients often occur in the same foods.

GETTING ENOUGH RIBOFLAVIN

On average, daily intakes of riboflavin are above the RDA. As with thiamin, people with alcoholism risk riboflavin deficiency because they eat nutrient-poor diets. No specific symptoms indicate that riboflavin taken in megadoses is toxic, so no UL has been set. Riboflavin supplementation, including the riboflavin found in multivitamin supplements or in a heavily fortified breakfast cereal, can cause the urine to become bright yellow.

The grains, dairy, and protein groups of MyPlate contain the most nutrient-dense sources of riboflavin (Fig. 8-21). Major sources of riboflavin are ready-to-eat breakfast cereals, milk and milk products, enriched grains, meat, and eggs. Vegetables such as asparagus, broccoli, and various greens (e.g., spinach) are also good sources. Riboflavin is a relatively stable water-soluble vitamin; however, it is destroyed by light. Milk is sold in paper or opaque plastic containers rather than clear glass to protect the riboflavin. In

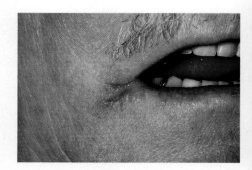

FIGURE 8-20 ▲ Angular cheilitis, also called cheilosis or angular stomatitis, is result of a riboflavin deficiency. It causes painful cracks at the corners of the mouth. Angular cheilitis can be caused by other medical conditions; thus, further evaluation is required before diagnosing a nutrient deficiency. ©Dr. P. Marazzi

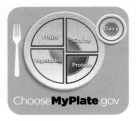

FIGURE 8-21 ◄ Food sources of riboflavin. (a) The fill of the background color (none, 1/3, 2/3, or completely covered) within each food group on MyPlate indicates the average nutrient density for riboflavin in that group. (b) The bar graph shows the riboflavin content of several foods in each food group compared to the RDA for adult males and females. Overall, the richest sources of riboflavin are meats (especially liver), dairy products, and fortified breakfast cereals. Fruits (not shown) are not particularly good sources of riboflavin.

Source: Nutrition data from USDA National Nutrient Database for Standard Reference, Release 26

(a)

(b)

	Food Item and Amount	Riboflavin (milligrams)	% RDA for Adult Males (1.3 milligrams)	% RDA for Adult Females (1.1 milligrams)
Grains	Kellogg's All Bran® cereal, 1 cup	0.8	62%	73%
Grains	Egg noodles, cooked, ½ cup	0.1	8%	9%
Grains	Bread, white, 1 slice	0.1	8%	9%
Vegetables	Mushrooms, raw, 5 medium	0.4	31%	36%
Vegetables	Spinach, cooked, 1 cup	0.4	31%	36%
Vegetables	Asparagus, cooked, 1 cup	0.3	23%	27%
Dairy	Yogurt, plain, nonfat, 1 cup	0.5	38%	45%
Dairy	Milk, fat-free, 1 cup	0.4	31%	36%
Dairy	Cheese, feta, 1.5 ounces	0.4	31%	36%
Protein	Beef liver, pan-fried, 3 ounces	2.8	215%	255%
Protein	Egg, hard-boiled, 1 large	0.3	23%	27%
Protein	Black beans, cooked, ½ cup	0.1	4%	5%

cheilosis Inflammation of the skin at one or both corners of the mouth; may be a nonspecific symptom of a nutrient deficiency or just opportunistic infection; also called *angular cheilitis*.

the United States, many meet the riboflavin recommendation by consuming three servings of dairy products each day.

☑ **CONCEPT CHECK 8.8**

1. How is riboflavin involved in energy metabolism?
2. What body organs or tissues are most likely to show symptoms if there is a deficiency of riboflavin?
3. What types of foods are the best sources of riboflavin?

8.9 Niacin (Vitamin B-3)

FUNCTIONS OF NIACIN

Niacin functions in the body as one of two related compounds: nicotinic acid and nicotinamide. The coenzyme forms of niacin function in many cellular metabolic pathways. When you are generating energy (ATP) by burning carbohydrate and fat, a niacin coenzyme, nicotinamide adenine dinucleotide (NAD) or nicotinamide adenine dinucleotide phosphate (NADP), is used. Anabolic pathways in the cell—those that make new compounds—also often use a niacin coenzyme. This is especially true for fatty-acid synthesis (Fig. 8-17).

Nicotinic acid has been promoted as a natural method to lower blood lipids including LDL cholesterol; however, due to potential adverse side effects, its use is discouraged.

NIACIN DEFICIENCY

Because niacin coenzymes function in over 200 enzymatic reactions, niacin deficiency causes widespread problems in the body. Early symptoms include poor appetite, weight loss, and weakness. The distinct group of niacin-deficiency symptoms is known as **pellagra,** which means rough or painful skin (Fig. 8-22). The symptoms of the disease are **dementia,** diarrhea, and dermatitis (especially on areas of skin exposed to the sun). Left untreated, death often results.

Pellagra is the only dietary deficiency disease ever to reach epidemic proportions in the United States. It became a major problem in the southeastern United States in the late 1800s and persisted until the 1930s, when standards of living and diets improved. Pellagra was particularly prevalent in populations that consumed corn as a major part of their diet. Niacin in corn is bound by a protein that inhibits its absorption, making it less bioavailable. Soaking corn in an alkaline solution, such as lime water (water with calcium hydroxide), releases bound niacin and renders it more bioavailable. Hispanic people traditionally soak corn in lime water before making tortillas. This treatment is one of the reasons why the Hispanic population rarely experienced pellagra. Today, pellagra is rare in Western societies but can be seen in the developing world.

GETTING ENOUGH NIACIN

Besides the preformed niacin found in foods, we can synthesize niacin from the amino acid tryptophan. In this manner, we synthesize about 50% of the niacin required each day. This reaction requires two other vitamins (riboflavin and vitamin B-6) to function as coenzymes in this chemical conversion. The adult RDA of niacin is expressed as *niacin equivalents* (NE) to account for niacin received intact from the diet, as well as that synthesized from tryptophan: 60 milligrams of tryptophan in a diet yield about 1 milligram of niacin. The DV used on food and supplement labels is 20 milligrams.

Intakes of niacin by adults are about double the RDA, not including the contribution from tryptophan. Tables of food composition values ignore tryptophan contributions. The best food sources of niacin are found in the protein group on MyPlate (Fig. 8-23).

Niacin

RDA

  Men: 16 milligrams

  Women: 14 milligrams

DV: 20 milligrams

UL: 35 milligrams (nicotinic acid form)

pellagra Niacin-deficiency disease characterized by dementia, diarrhea, and dermatitis, and possibly leading to death.

dementia A general loss or decrease in mental function.

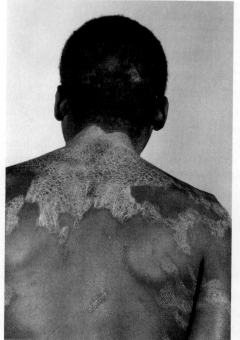

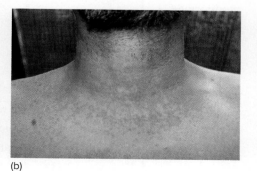

FIGURE 8-22 ◄ The dermatitis of pellagra. (a) Dermatitis on both sides (bilateral) of the body is a typical symptom of pellagra. Sun exposure worsens the condition. (b) The rough skin around the neck is referred to as Casal's necklace. (a): ©Dr M.A. Ansary/Science Source; (b): ©Gary Corbett/age fotostock/Alamy

(a)

(b)

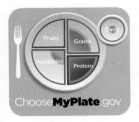

ChooseMyPlate.gov

FIGURE 8-23 ◄ Food sources of niacin. (a) The fill of the background color (none, 1/3, 2/3, or completely covered) within each food group on MyPlate indicates the average nutrient density for niacin in that group. (b) The bar graph shows the niacin content of several foods compared to the RDA for adult males and females. Overall, the richest sources of niacin are foods in the protein group and fortified breakfast cereals. Foods in the dairy group (not shown) contain very little niacin, but the tryptophan in dairy foods can be converted into niacin.

Source: Nutrition data from USDA National Nutrient Database for Standard Reference, Release 26

(a)

(b)

	Food Item and Amount	Niacin (milligrams)	% RDA for Adult Males (16 milligrams)	% RDA for Adult Females (14 milligrams)
Grains	Total® Raisin Bran cereal, 1 cup	20	125%	143%
Grains	Tortilla, flour, 8″	1.8	11%	13%
Grains	Bread, whole wheat, 1 slice	1.4	9%	10%
Vegetables	Raw mushrooms, 5	4.7	29%	34%
Vegetables	Potato, 1	2.1	13%	15%
Vegetables	Asparagus, cooked, 1 cup	2.0	13%	14%
Fruits	Orange juice, fresh, 1 cup	1.0	6%	7%
Fruits	Banana, 1 medium	0.8	5%	6%
Fruits	Blueberries, 1 cup	0.6	4%	4%
Protein	Tuna, yellow fin, grilled, 3 ounces	18.8	118%	134%
Protein	Chicken breast, roasted, 3 ounces	11.8	74%	84%
Protein	Peanut butter, 2 tablespoons	4.2	26%	30%

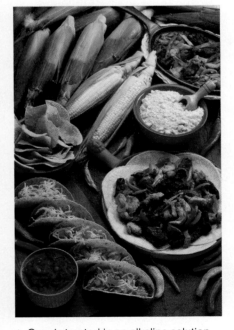

▲ Corn is treated in an alkaline solution to release protein-bound niacin so it can be available in corn products such as tortillas, taco shells, tortilla chips, and corn flour. Source: Scott Bauer/USDA

Major sources of niacin are tuna, poultry, peanuts, fish, ready-to-eat cereals, beef, and asparagus. Coffee and tea also contribute some niacin to the diet. Niacin is heat stable, thus little is lost in cooking.

AVOIDING TOO MUCH NIACIN

The UL for niacin pertains only to the nicotinic acid form (found in supplements). Side effects of niacin toxicity include headache; itching; and increased blood flow to the skin because of blood vessel dilation or flushing in various parts of the body. These symptoms are especially seen when intakes are above 100 milligrams per day. In the long run, GI tract and liver damage are possible, so any use of megadoses, including large doses recommended for treatment for cardiovascular disease, requires close medical monitoring.

✓ CONCEPT CHECK 8.9

1. How is niacin involved in energy metabolism?
2. What are the three distinct signs of a niacin deficiency?
3. What are some excellent sources of niacin?
4. What is the relationship between tryptophan and niacin?

8.10 Vitamin B-6 (Pyridoxine)

This vitamin is known by its number, rather than its general name. Vitamin B-6 is a family of three structurally similar compounds. All can be converted into the active vitamin B-6 coenzyme, pyridoxal phosphate (PLP).

FUNCTIONS OF VITAMIN B-6

The coenzymes of vitamin B-6 are needed for the activity of numerous enzymes involved in carbohydrate, protein, and lipid metabolism. One of the primary functions is as a coenzyme in over 100 chemical reactions that involve the metabolism of amino acids and protein (see Fig. 8-17). The B-6 coenzyme, PLP, participates in reactions that allow the synthesis of nonessential (dispensable) amino acids by helping to split the nitrogen group ($-NH_2$) from an amino acid and making it available to another amino acid.[8]

Vitamin B-6 also plays a role in **homocysteine** metabolism. Among the other important functions of vitamin B-6 are synthesis of neurotransmitters such as serotonin and gamma aminobutyric acid; conversion of tryptophan to niacin; breakdown of stored glycogen to glucose; and synthesis of white blood cells and the heme portion of **hemoglobin.**

homocysteine An amino acid that arises from the metabolism of methionine. Vitamin B-6, folate, vitamin B-12, and choline are required for its metabolism. Elevated levels are associated with an increased risk of cardiovascular disease.

hemoglobin The iron-containing part of the red blood cell that carries oxygen to the cells and carbon dioxide away from the cells. The heme iron portion is also responsible for the red color of blood.

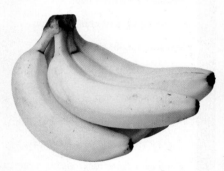

▲ Bananas are a plant source of vitamin B-6. ©lynx/iconotec.com/Glow Images

VITAMIN B-6 DEFICIENCY

Because of the role of vitamin B-6 in hemoglobin synthesis, a deficiency in vitamin B-6 would affect multiple body systems, including the cardiovascular, immune, and nervous systems, as well as overall energy metabolism. Vitamin B-6 deficiency also results in widespread symptoms, including depression, vomiting, skin disorders, irritation of the nerves, anemia, and impaired immune response.

People with alcoholism are susceptible to a vitamin B-6 deficiency. A metabolite formed in alcohol metabolism can displace the coenzyme form of B-6, increasing its tendency to be destroyed. In addition, alcohol decreases the absorption of vitamin B-6 and decreases the synthesis of its coenzyme form. Cirrhosis and hepatitis (both can accompany alcoholism) also destroy healthy liver tissue. Thus, a cirrhotic liver cannot adequately metabolize vitamin B-6 or synthesize its coenzyme form.

GETTING ENOUGH VITAMIN B-6

With their ample consumption of animal products, North Americans have an average daily consumption of vitamin B-6 that is greater than the RDA. There is some research to indicate that athletes may need slightly more vitamin B-6 than sedentary adults. The athlete's body processes large quantities of glycogen and protein, and the metabolism of these compounds requires vitamin B-6. However, unless athletes restrict their food intake, they are likely to consume plenty of this B vitamin.

Major sources of vitamin B-6 are animal products and fortified ready-to-eat breakfast cereals (Fig. 8-24). Other sources are vegetables and fruits such as potatoes, spinach, bananas, and cantaloupes. Overall, the protein group of MyPlate offers most of the food sources of vitamin B-6, and animal sources and fortified grain products are the most reliable because the vitamin B-6 they contain is more absorbable than that in plant foods. Vitamin B-6 is rather unstable; heating and freezing can easily destroy it.

AVOIDING TOO MUCH VITAMIN B-6

The UL for vitamin B-6 (see margin) is based on the risk of developing nerve damage. Studies have shown that intakes of 2 to 6 grams of vitamin B-6 per day for 2 or more months can lead to irreversible nerve damage. Symptoms of vitamin B-6 toxicity include walking difficulties, and hand and foot tingling and numbness. Some nerve damage in

Vitamin B-6

RDA
　Men: 1.3 milligrams
　Women: 1.3 milligrams
DV: 2 milligrams
UL: 100 milligrams

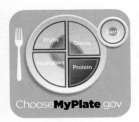

ChooseMyPlate.gov

(a)

FIGURE 8-24 ◄ Food sources of vitamin B-6. (a) The fill of the background color (none, 1/3, 2/3, or completely covered) within each food group on MyPlate indicates the average nutrient density for vitamin B-6 in that group. (b) The bar graph shows the vitamin B-6 content of several foods compared to the RDA for adult males and females. Overall, the richest and most bioavailable sources of vitamin B-6 are animal sources of protein and fortified breakfast cereals. However, dairy foods (not shown) are not a particularly good source of vitamin B-6.

Source: Nutrition data from USDA National Nutrient Database for Standard Reference, Release 26

(b)

Food Item and Amount	Vitamin B-6 (milligrams)	% RDA for Adult Males and Females (1.3 milligrams)
Special K® cereal, 1 cup	2.0	154%
Kellogg's® Eggo® waffles, home-style, 2 each	0.4	31%
Brown rice, cooked, ½ cup	0.1	3%
Potato, baked with skin, 1 medium	0.5	10%
Spinach, cooked, 1 cup	0.4	9%
Butternut squash, cooked, 1 cup	0.3	5%
Banana, 1 medium	0.4	8%
Raisins, ½ cup	0.1	3%
Watermelon, 1 cup	0.1	1%
Beef liver, pan-fried, 3 ounces	0.8	16%
Turkey breast, roasted, 3 ounces	0.7	14%
Sunflower seeds, dry roasted, 1 ounce	0.2	5%

©Ivary Inc./Alamy

individual sensory neurons is probably reversible, but damage to the ganglia (where many nerve fibers converge) appears to be permanent. With 500-milligram tablets of vitamin B-6 available in health-food stores, taking a toxic dose is easy.[8]

✔ CONCEPT CHECK 8.10

1. What is the role of vitamin B-6 in energy metabolism and other body functions?
2. What are the primary sources of vitamin B-6?
3. Are vitamin B-6 supplements safe?

8.11 Pantothenic Acid (Vitamin B-5) and Biotin (Vitamin B-7)

PANTOTHENIC ACID

Pantothenic acid is required for the synthesis of coenzyme A (CoA), a coenzyme in chemical reactions that allow the release of energy from carbohydrates, lipids, and protein. It also activates fatty acids so they can yield energy (Fig. 8-17) and is used in the initial steps of fatty-acid synthesis. Pantothenic acid is so widespread in foods that a nutritional deficiency among healthy people who eat varied diets is unlikely. *Pantothen* means "from every side" in Greek.

Pantothenic Acid Deficiency A deficiency of pantothenic acid might occur in alcoholism, along with a nutrient deficient diet. However, the symptoms would probably be

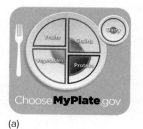

(a)

FIGURE 8-25 ◄ Food sources of pantothenic acid. (a) The fill of the background color (none, 1/3, 2/3, or completely covered) within each food group on MyPlate indicates the average nutrient density for pantothenic acid in that group. (b) The bar graph shows the pantothenic acid content of several foods in each food group compared to the AI for adult males and females. Overall, fortified foods and foods rich in protein are the best sources of pantothenic acid.

Source: Nutrition data from USDA National Nutrient Database for Standard Reference, Release 26

(b)

	Food Item and Amount	Pantothenic Acid (milligrams)	% AI for Adult Males and Females (5 milligrams)
Grains	Whole Grain Total® cereal, 1 cup	10.0	200%
Grains	Brown rice, cooked, ½ cup	0.4	8%
Grains	White bread, 1 slice	0.1	2%
Vegetables	Mushrooms, raw, 5 medium	1.3	26%
Vegetables	Acorn squash, cooked, 1 cup	1.0	20%
Vegetables	Broccoli, cooked, 1 cup	1.0	20%
Fruits	Orange juice, fresh, 1 cup	0.5	10%
Fruits	Blueberries, 1 cup	0.2	4%
Fruits	Apple, Fuji, 1 medium	0.1	2%
Dairy	Yogurt, plain, nonfat, 1 cup	1.6	32%
Dairy	Milk, fat-free, 1 cup	0.9	18%
Dairy	Soy milk, 1 cup	0.3	6%
Protein	Power bar, 1 each	10.8	216%
Protein	Beef liver, pan-fried, 3 ounces	5.6	112%
Protein	Sunflower seeds, dry roasted, ¼ cup	2.6	52%

hidden among deficiencies of thiamin, riboflavin, vitamin B-6, and folate, so the pantothenic acid deficiency might be unrecognizable.

Getting Enough Pantothenic Acid The AI set for pantothenic acid is 5 milligrams per day for adults. Average consumption is well in excess of this amount. The DV on food and supplement labels is 10 milligrams. Rich sources of pantothenic acid are sunflower seeds, mushrooms, peanuts, and eggs (Fig. 8-25). Other rich sources are meat, milk, and many vegetables. No toxicity is known for pantothenic acid, so no UL has been set.

BIOTIN

In its coenzyme form, biotin aids in dozens of chemical reactions. Biotin assists in the addition of CO_2 to other compounds, a reaction critical in synthesizing glucose and fatty acids, as well as breaking down certain amino acids.

Biotin Deficiency Symptoms of biotin deficiency include a scaly inflammation of the skin, changes in the tongue and lips, decreased appetite, nausea, vomiting, a form of anemia, depression, muscle pain and weakness, and poor growth.

Getting Enough Biotin Foods rich in protein, such as egg yolks, peanuts, and cheese, are good sources of biotin (Fig. 8-26). The biotin content of food is typically not measured and therefore often not available in food composition tables or nutrient databases.

Pantothenic Acid
AI: 5 milligrams
DV: 10 milligrams
UL: none set

Biotin
AI: 30 micrograms
DV: 300 micrograms
UL: none set

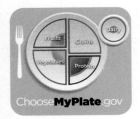

ChooseMyPlate.gov

(a)

FIGURE 8-26 ◀ Food sources of biotin. (a) The fill of the background color (none, 1/3, 2/3, or completely covered) within each food group on MyPlate indicates the average nutrient density for biotin in that group. (b) The bar graph shows the biotin content of several foods compared to the AI for adult males and females. Overall, foods rich in protein are the best sources of biotin. Grains (even fortified varieties) contain very little biotin, so they are not shown in the bar graph.

Source: Nutrition data from Staggs CG, et al. "Determination of the biotin content of select foods using accurate and sensitive HPLC/avidin binding," *J Food Compost Anal* 2004;17:767–776

(b)

	Food Item and Amount	Biotin (micrograms)	% AI for Adult Males and Females (30 micrograms)
Vegetables	Sweet potato, baked, 1 cup	2.9	10%
	Mushrooms, canned, ½ cup	1.7	6%
	Carrots, cooked, 1 cup	0.9	3%
Fruits	Strawberries, 1 cup	2.3	8%
	Orange juice, from concentrate, 1 cup	1.0	3%
	Raisins, ½ cup	0.3	1%
Dairy	Cheese, American, 2 ounces	1.7	6%
	Cheese, cheddar, 1.5 ounces	0.6	2%
	Milk, nonfat, 1 cup	0.3	1%
Protein	Beef liver, pan-fried, 3 ounces	35.0	106%
	Egg, hard-boiled, 1 large	10.0	33%
	Peanuts, dry roasted, 1 ounce	4.9	16%

Because intestinal bacteria synthesize some biotin that you can absorb, a biotin deficiency is unlikely. Scientists are not sure how much of the bacteria-synthesized biotin in our intestines is absorbed, so we still need to consume some in our diet. If bacterial synthesis in the intestines is not sufficient, as in people who are missing a large part of the colon or who take antibiotics for many months, special attention must be paid to meeting biotin needs.

Biotin's bioavailability varies significantly among foods based on the food's biotin-protein complex. In raw egg whites, biotin is bound to avidin, which inhibits absorption of the vitamin. Consuming many raw egg whites can eventually lead to biotin-deficiency disease. Cooking, however, denatures the protein avidin in eggs so it cannot bind biotin. In addition to food safety concerns, this is an important reason to avoid consuming raw eggs.

Our food supply is thought to provide 40 to 60 micrograms per person per day. The DV used on food and supplement labels is 10 times the AI; the DV for biotin was set years before the vitamin had an AI level set and is based on outdated recommendations. However, biotin is relatively nontoxic. Large doses (up to 1 milligram per day) have been given over an extended period without harmful side effects to children who exhibit defects in biotin metabolism. Thus, no UL for biotin has been set.

✓ CONCEPT CHECK 8.11

1. What is the role of pantothenic acid in energy metabolism?
2. What are some rich sources of pantothenic acid?
3. What is the role of biotin in energy metabolism?
4. What are the signs and symptoms of biotin deficiency?
5. What are the best sources of biotin?
6. Why does consumption of raw eggs lead to biotin deficiency?

8.12 Folate (Vitamin B-9)

The term *folate* is used to describe a variety of forms of this B vitamin found in foods and in the body. Folic acid is the synthetic form added to fortified foods and present in supplements.

FUNCTIONS OF FOLATE

A key role of the folate coenzyme is to supply or accept single carbon compounds. In this role, folate coenzymes help form DNA and metabolize amino acids and their derivatives, such as homocysteine. Folate works along with vitamins B-6 and B-12 to metabolize homocysteine. Folate also functions in the formation of neurotransmitters in the brain. Meeting folate needs can improve the depressed state in some cases of mental illness.

Research is underway on the link between folate and cancer protection. Because folate aids in DNA synthesis, adequate folate status is important to maintain DNA integrity, including the control of certain cancer-promoting genes. Meeting the RDA for folate may be one way to reduce cancer risk.

FOLATE DEFICIENCY

One major result of a folate deficiency is that in the early phases of red blood cell synthesis, immature cells cannot divide because they cannot form new DNA. The cells grow progressively larger because they can still synthesize enough protein and other cell parts to make new cells. When the time comes for the cells to divide, the amount of DNA is insufficient to form two nuclei. The cells then remain in a large immature form, known as a **megaloblast** (Fig. 8-27).

Few mature red blood cells arrive in the bloodstream because the bone marrow of a folate-deficient person produces mostly immature megaloblast cells. When fewer mature red blood cells are present, the blood's capacity to carry oxygen decreases, causing a condition known as **megaloblastic anemia** (also called *macrocytic* or large-cell anemia).

Clinicians focus on red blood cells as an indicator of folate status because they are easy to collect and examine. Folate deficiency, however, disrupts cell division throughout the entire body. Other symptoms of folate deficiency are inflammation of the tongue, diarrhea, poor growth, mental confusion, depression, and problems in nerve function.

Maternal folate deficiency (along with a genetic abnormality related to folate metabolism) has been linked to the development of **neural tube defects** in the fetus. These defects include **spina bifida** (spinal cord or spinal fluid bulge through the back) and **anencephaly** (absence of a brain). Adequate folate status is crucial for all women of childbearing age because the neural tube closes within the first 28 days of pregnancy, a time when many women are not even aware that they are pregnant.

Older people may be at risk for folate deficiency due to a combination of inadequate folate intake and decreased absorption. Perhaps these people fail to consume sufficient amounts of fruits and vegetables because of inadequate access to food or physical problems, such as poor dental health. In addition, folate deficiencies often occur with alcoholism, mostly due to poor intake and absorption. Symptoms of a folate-related anemia can alert a primary care provider to the possibility of alcoholism.

GETTING ENOUGH FOLATE

Folate's name is derived from the Latin word *folium,* which means "foliage" or "leaves." Quite predictably, the richest sources of folate are green, leafy vegetables. In addition, other vegetables, orange juice, dried beans, and organ meats are excellent sources of folate (Fig. 8-28). Fortified ready-to-eat breakfast cereals, bread, and milk are important sources of folic acid for many adults.

megaloblast A large, immature red blood cell that results from the inability of the cell to divide normally (*megalo* = large; *blast* = primitive or immature).

megaloblastic (macrocytic) anemia Anemia characterized by the presence of abnormally large red blood cells.

neural tube defect A defect in the formation of the neural tube occurring during early fetal development. This type of defect results in various nervous system disorders, such as spina bifida. Folate deficiency in the pregnant woman increases the risk that the fetus will develop this disorder.

spina bifida Birth defect resulting from improper closure of the neural tube during embryonic development. The spinal cord or fluid may bulge outside the spinal column.

anencephaly Birth defect characterized by the absence of some or all of the brain and skull.

FIGURE 8-27 ▶ Macrocytic (megaloblastic) anemia occurs when red blood cells are unable to divide, leaving large, immature red blood cells. Either a folate or vitamin B-12 deficiency may cause this condition. Measurements of blood concentrations of both vitamins are taken to help determine the cause of the anemia.

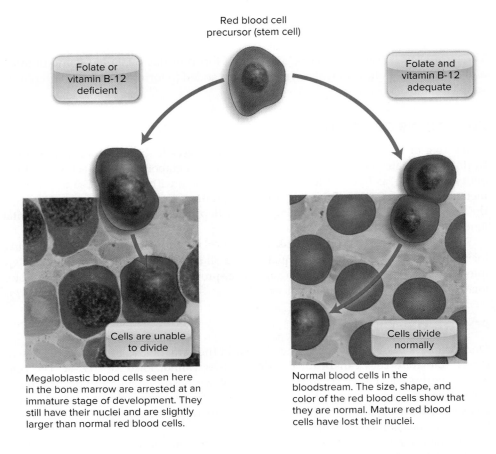

Red blood cell precursor (stem cell)

Folate or vitamin B-12 deficient

Folate and vitamin B-12 adequate

Cells are unable to divide

Cells divide normally

Megaloblastic blood cells seen here in the bone marrow are arrested at an immature stage of development. They still have their nuclei and are slightly larger than normal red blood cells.

Normal blood cells in the bloodstream. The size, shape, and color of the red blood cells show that they are normal. Mature red blood cells have lost their nuclei.

Folate

RDA: 400 micrograms

DV: 400 micrograms

UL: 1000 micrograms (synthetic only)

Dietary Folate Equivalents

1 DFE = 1 microgram folate from food

= 0.6 microgram folic acid from food

= 0.5 microgram folic acid from a supplement on an empty stomach

Folate is susceptible to destruction by heat and oxygen. The vitamin C present in some food sources of folate, such as orange juice, helps to reduce folate destruction, but food processing and preparation destroy 50% to 90% of the folate in food. This underscores the importance of regularly eating fresh fruits and raw or lightly cooked vegetables.

Folate recommendations for all but women of childbearing age are based on dietary folate equivalents (DFE). Synthetic folic acid, found in supplements and fortified foods, is more bioavailable than the folate that naturally occurs in food. The DFE unit considers these differences in bioavailability (see margin).

Pregnant women need extra folate (a total of 600 micrograms DFE) to accommodate the increased rates of cell division and DNA synthesis in their bodies and in the developing fetus. A healthy diet can supply this much. Still, prenatal care often includes a specially formulated multivitamin and mineral supplement enriched with folic acid to meet the higher RDA during pregnancy.

Prior to 1998, average daily folate intakes in the United States were approximately 320 micrograms for men and 220 micrograms for women. In 1998, the FDA mandated the fortification of grain products with folate with the aim of reducing birth defects of the spine. With this mandate, average intakes have increased by about 200 micrograms per day. Factors other than folate deficiency (e.g., genetics and environment) play a role in the development of neural tube defects, but studies have shown that fortification of grain products with folic acid has decreased the rates of neural tube defects in infants by an estimated 15% to 30% in the United States and up to 50% in other countries with higher background rates of neural tube defects.[9]

The mandated folic acid enrichment of grains has also been accompanied by a noticeable decline in cardiovascular risk, especially risk for stroke, owing to a drop in blood homocysteine levels among U.S. adults. Supplements of folic acid, B-12, and B-6 have been promoted to help lower homocysteine and decrease cardiac and stroke risks. This is only likely to be effective for individuals who start out with elevated homocysteine

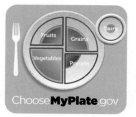

FIGURE 8-28 ◄ Food sources of folate. (a) The fill of the background color (none, 1/3, 2/3, or completely covered) within each food group on MyPlate indicates the average nutrient density for folate in that group. (b) The bar graph shows the folate content of several foods in each food group compared to the RDA for adult males and females. Overall, the richest sources of folate are green, leafy vegetables and fortified grains.

Source: Nutrition data from USDA National Nutrient Database for Standard Reference, Release 26

(a)

(b)

	Food Item and Amount	Folate (micrograms DFE)	% RDA for Adult Males and Females (400 micrograms DFE)
Grains	Cheerios® cereal, 1 cup	336	84%
Grains	Wheat germ, 2 tablespoons	150	38%
Grains	Flour tortilla, 8″	98	25%
Vegetables	Asparagus, cooked, 1 cup	268	67%
Vegetables	Spinach, cooked, 1 cup	263	66%
Vegetables	Broccoli, cooked, 1 cup	168	42%
Fruits	Orange juice, fresh, 1 cup	74	19%
Fruits	Cantaloupe, 1 cup	37	9%
Fruits	Strawberries, raw, 1 cup	36	9%
Dairy	Yogurt, plain, 1 cup	29	7%
Dairy	Cottage cheese, low-fat, 1 cup	23	6%
Dairy	Soy milk, 1 cup	22	6%
Protein	Beef liver, pan-fried, 3 ounces	211	53%
Protein	Lentils, cooked, ½ cup	179	45%
Protein	Sunflower seeds, dry roasted, ¼ cup	76	19%

levels. Taking pharmacological doses of folate is not likely to benefit people who have blood homocysteine levels in the normal range. In addition, some research indicates that too much folic acid could promote tumor development. Thus, even though folic acid fortification has been a public health success story for prevention of neural tube defects, there are concerns about the appropriate dose for the entire population.[9]

AVOIDING TOO MUCH FOLATE

The UL for folate only refers to folic acid. This is because folate, the natural form in food, has limited absorption. Large doses of folic acid can hide the signs of vitamin B-12 deficiency and therefore complicate its diagnosis. Specifically, regular consumption of large amounts of folate can prevent the appearance of an early warning sign of vitamin B-12 deficiency: enlarged red blood cell size. For this reason, FDA limits the amount of folic acid in supplements (for nonpregnant adults) to 400 micrograms.

✓ **CONCEPT CHECK 8.12**

1. Explain why macrocytic (megaloblastic) anemia occurs.
2. Why do daily folate needs increase from 400 to 600 micrograms for pregnant women?

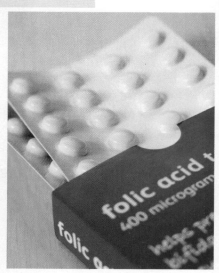

▲ An objective of *Healthy People 2020* is to increase by 10% the proportion of women of childbearing potential who take supplements containing folic acid prior to pregnancy. ©Banana Stock/Punchstock

8.13 Vitamin B-12 (Cobalamin or Cyanocobalamin)

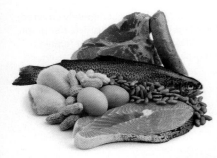

▲ With age, absorption of vitamin B-12 from food becomes less efficient, usually owing to the decreases in stomach acid production. ©Alamy RF

R-proteins Proteins produced by the salivary glands that bind to free vitamin B-12 in the stomach and protect it from stomach acid.

intrinsic factor A protein-like compound produced by the stomach that enhances vitamin B-12 absorption in the ileum.

Vitamin B-12 is quite unique among the water-soluble vitamins. It is the only vitamin that contains a mineral as part of its structure. Its structure is the largest of all the vitamins. Unlike most water-soluble vitamins, B-12 can be stored to a significant extent in the liver, so it takes many months on a diet devoid of vitamin B-12 for a deficiency to surface. Vitamin B-12 is only naturally found in foods of animal origin. Finally, the means by which the body absorbs vitamin B-12 is complex; a problem at any one of several steps could impair absorption and lead to deficiency. To illustrate the multistep process by which vitamin B-12 is absorbed, we will trace the path of a meal containing vitamin B-12 through the digestive tract (Fig. 8-29).

In food, much of the vitamin B-12 is bound to protein and therefore cannot be absorbed. When food enters the mouth, **R-proteins** are secreted by the salivary glands. The bolus of food, including the R-proteins, travels down the esophagus to the stomach. Acid and enzymes present in the stomach release vitamin B-12 from food proteins, and the free vitamin B-12 then binds to R-protein. While food is in the stomach, the stomach cells release a protein-like compound called the **intrinsic factor.** When the chyme reaches the duodenum, pancreatic enzymes release vitamin B-12 from R-proteins. The

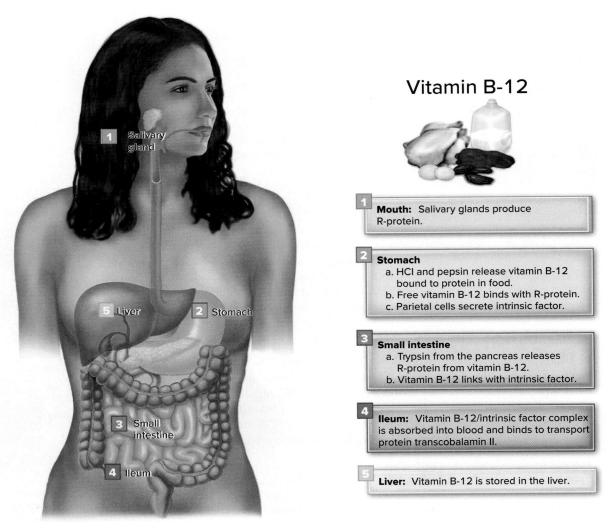

Vitamin B-12

1 Mouth: Salivary glands produce R-protein.

2 Stomach
a. HCl and pepsin release vitamin B-12 bound to protein in food.
b. Free vitamin B-12 binds with R-protein.
c. Parietal cells secrete intrinsic factor.

3 Small intestine
a. Trypsin from the pancreas releases R-protein from vitamin B-12.
b. Vitamin B-12 links with intrinsic factor.

4 Ileum: Vitamin B-12/intrinsic factor complex is absorbed into blood and binds to transport protein transcobalamin II.

5 Liver: Vitamin B-12 is stored in the liver.

FIGURE 8-29 ▲ The absorption of vitamin B-12 requires several compounds produced in the mouth, stomach, and small intestine. Defects arising in the stomach or small intestine can interfere with absorption and result in vitamin B-12 deficiency.

free vitamin B-12 then combines with intrinsic factor. The vitamin B-12–intrinsic factor complex travels the length of the small intestine to the ileum, where vitamin B-12 is finally absorbed.

If any of these steps fails or is altered, absorption can drop to 1% to 2%. In these cases, the person usually takes monthly injections of vitamin B-12, uses nasal gels of the vitamin to bypass the need for absorption, or takes megadoses of a supplemental form (300 times the RDA). In this latter case, the vitamin B-12 absorption defect is overcome by providing enough of the vitamin via simple diffusion across the intestinal tract.

About 95% of cases of vitamin B-12 deficiencies in healthy people result from defective absorption, rather than from inadequate dietary intakes. This is especially true for older people. As we age, stomach acid production declines, and our stomachs have a decreased ability to synthesize the intrinsic factor needed for vitamin B-12 absorption.

FUNCTIONS OF VITAMIN B-12

Vitamin B-12 participates in a variety of cellular processes. The most important function is folate metabolism. Vitamin B-12 is required to convert folate coenzymes into the active forms needed for metabolic reactions, such as DNA synthesis. Without vitamin B-12, reactions that require certain active forms of folate do not take place in the cell. Thus, a deficiency of vitamin B-12 can result in symptoms of a folate deficiency, including elevated homocysteine levels and macrocytic anemia.

Another vital function of vitamin B-12 is maintaining the myelin sheath that insulates neurons. Initial neurological symptoms of vitamin B-12 deficiencies include irregular muscular actions and impaired reflexes. Eventual destruction of the myelin sheath causes paralysis and, perhaps, even death. In the past, vitamin B-12 deficiencies eventually led to death, mainly due to the destruction of nerves.

VITAMIN B-12 DEFICIENCY

The fatal consequences of vitamin B-12 deficiency can be observed in a disease known as **pernicious anemia.** The word *pernicious* means "leading to death." Indeed, before the discovery that consuming large doses of raw liver—a rich source of vitamin B-12—could be used to treat this particular disease, many people did die from it. Pernicious anemia is characterized by macrocytic anemia (with all the usual signs of anemia), sore mouth, depression, back pain, apathy, and severe nerve degeneration that can lead to tingling in the extremities, weakness, paralysis, and, eventually, death from heart failure.

People with pernicious anemia usually do not lack vitamin B-12 in their diets. Instead, they suffer from an autoimmune disease that destroys the stomach cells that produce gastric acid and intrinsic factor. The resulting malabsorption of vitamin B-12 is responsible for all the symptoms of the disease. Because we are able to store some vitamin B-12, symptoms of nerve destruction do not develop for years. Unfortunately, substantial nerve destruction often occurs before clinical signs of deficiency, such as anemia, are detected. The nerve destruction is irreversible.

Pernicious anemia, which affects about 2% of older adults, is the most common cause of vitamin B-12 malabsorption. Other causes are age-related atrophy of the acid-producing cells of the stomach and bacterial overgrowth in the small intestine. When acid production is low, bacteria normally present in the large intestine may colonize the small intestine and compete with our intestinal cells for vitamin B-12 absorption. Certain medications also impair vitamin B-12 absorption (see Medicine Cabinet in margin).

Inadequate intake of vitamin B-12 is rarely responsible for deficiency, but it can occur. Vegan diets supply little vitamin B-12 unless they include vitamin B-12–enriched food (e.g., soy milk) or supplements. Infants breastfed by vegetarian mothers are at risk for vitamin B-12 deficiency accompanied by anemia and long-term nervous system problems, such as diminished brain growth, degeneration of the spinal cord, and poor intellectual development. The problems may have their origins during pregnancy if

pernicious anemia The anemia that results from a lack of vitamin B-12 absorption; it is *pernicious* because of associated nerve degeneration that can result in eventual paralysis and death.

Medicine Cabinet

Some medications may limit vitamin B-12 absorption. Antacids or other medications used to inhibit acid secretions will increase the pH within the stomach, thereby limiting release of B-12 from protein. People who have ulcers or reflux may take these drugs. Metformin, a popular medication for controlling diabetes, may reduce B-12 absorption. With any of these medications, you should check with your primary care provider to see if supplemental B-12 is recommended.

©Peter Dazeley/Photographer's Choice/Getty Images

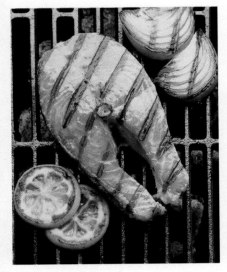

▲ Salmon, rainbow trout, and other types of seafood are excellent sources of B-12.
©Michael Lamotte/Cole Group/Getty Images

Newsworthy Nutrition

Folic Acid and Vitamin B-12 May Prevent Cognitive Decline

The hypothesis of this study was that B vitamins could prevent cognitive decline in a cohort of older adults with depression. The study design was a secondary data analysis of a randomized controlled trial that enrolled over 900 older adults (aged 60 to 74 years). Participants were given either a placebo or a dietary supplement containing 400 micrograms of folic acid and 100 micrograms of vitamin B-12 for 24 months. The results revealed that subjects who received long-term folic acid and vitamin B-12 performed better on tests of cognitive function. The authors concluded that supplementation with some B vitamins may help older adults with depression maintain cognitive functioning as they age.

Source: Walker JG and others: Oral folic acid and vitamin B-12 supplementation to prevent cognitive decline in community-dwelling older adults with depressive symptoms—the Beyond Ageing Project: A randomized controlled trial. *American Journal of Clinical Nutrition* 95:194, 2012.

the mother is deficient in vitamin B-12. Certainly, achieving an adequate vitamin B-12 intake is a key goal for vegans.

GETTING ENOUGH VITAMIN B-12

Vitamin B-12 compounds are originally synthesized by bacteria, fungi, and other lower organisms, then become incorporated into animal tissues when animals consume them. Organ meats (e.g., liver, kidneys, and heart) are especially rich sources of vitamin B-12. Other major sources of vitamin B-12 include meat, seafood, fortified breakfast cereals, milk, and eggs (Fig. 8-30). Adults over age 50 are encouraged to seek a synthetic vitamin B-12 source to increase absolute absorption, which can be limited due to both reduced intrinsic factor and stomach acid output. Synthetic vitamin B-12 is not food-bound, so it does

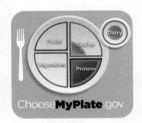

FIGURE 8-30 ◄ Food sources of vitamin B-12. (a) The fill of the background color (none, 1/3, 2/3, or completely covered) within each food group on MyPlate indicates the average nutrient density for vitamin B-12 in that group. (b) The bar graph shows the vitamin B-12 content of several foods compared to the RDA for adult males and females. Overall, foods of animal origin and fortified grains are the richest sources of vitamin B-12. Except for fortified grains, foods of plant origin (not shown) do not contain vitamin B-12.

Source: Nutrition data from USDA National Nutrient Database for Standard Reference, Release 26

(a)

(b)

	Food Item and Amount	Vitamin B-12 (micrograms)	% RDA for Adult Males and Females (2.4 micrograms)
Grains	Cheerios® cereal, 1 cup	1.9	79%
Grains	Egg noodles, cooked, ½ cup	0	0%
Grains	Quinoa, cooked, ½ cup	0	0%
Dairy	Soy milk (fortified), 1 cup	2.1	86%
Dairy	Yogurt, plain, nonfat, 1 cup	1.5	63%
Dairy	Milk, fat-free, 1 cup	1.2	50%
Protein	Claims, baked, 3 ounces	84.1	3504%
Protein	Beef liver, pan-fried, 3 ounces	67.3	2804%
Protein	Kidney beans, cooked, ½ cup	0	0%

not need stomach acid to release it from foods. It will be more readily absorbed than the form found in food.[10] Fortified breakfast cereals and dietary supplements are two possible synthetic sources.

On average, adults consume two times the RDA or more. This high intake provides the average meat-eating person with 2 to 3 years' storage of vitamin B-12 in the liver. A person would have to consume a diet essentially free of vitamin B-12 for approximately 20 years before exhibiting nerve destruction caused by a dietary deficiency. Pernicious anemia develops more rapidly because of the reduced ability to reabsorb vitamin B-12 excreted into the GI tract during digestion, coupled with reduced absorption of dietary sources. Still, vegans, who eat no animal products, should find a reliable source of vitamin B-12, such as fortified soy or rice milk, ready-to-eat breakfast cereals, and a form of yeast grown on media rich in vitamin B-12. Use of a multivitamin and mineral supplement containing vitamin B-12 is another option. Vitamin B-12 supplements are essentially nontoxic, so no UL has been set.

> **Vitamin B-12**
> RDA: 2.4 micrograms
> DV: 6 micrograms
> UL: None

✓ CONCEPT CHECK 8.13

1. Explain the role of specific factors required for vitamin B-12 absorption.
2. Which two nutrient deficiencies could be responsible for macrocytic anemia?
3. Identify two population groups that are at risk for vitamin B-12 deficiency. Explain why these people are at risk.

8.14 Vitamin C (Ascorbic Acid)

FUNCTIONS OF VITAMIN C

Formation of Body Proteins The best understood function of vitamin C (also known as *ascorbic acid* or *ascorbate*) is its role in the synthesis of collagen. This protein is highly concentrated in connective tissue, bone, teeth, tendons, and blood vessels. The important function of vitamin C in the formation of connective tissue is exemplified in the early symptoms of a deficiency: pinpoint hemorrhages under the skin (Fig. 8-31), bleeding gums, and joint pain. Vitamin C is very important for wound healing; it strengthens structural tissues by increasing the cross-connections between amino acids found in collagen.

Formation of Other Compounds Vitamin C has a specific function in the synthesis of numerous other compounds in the body. It is required for the synthesis of carnitine, a compound that transports fatty acids into the mitochondria. In addition, it takes part in the formation of two neurotransmitters, serotonin, and norepinephrine.

Antioxidant Vitamin C also has a more general function as an antioxidant because it can readily accept and donate electrons. These antioxidant properties have been postulated to reduce the formation of cancer-causing nitrosamines in the stomach. Vitamin C also aids in the reactivation of vitamin E after it has donated an electron to a free radical. Population studies suggest that the antioxidant properties of vitamin C may be effective in the prevention of certain cancers (esophagus, mouth, and stomach) and cataracts. The extent to which vitamin C functions in the reduction of specific diseases is debatable based on the scientific studies to date.

Absorption of Iron Vitamin C enhances iron absorption by keeping iron in its most absorbable form, especially as the mineral travels through the alkaline environment of the small intestine. Consuming 75 milligrams or more of vitamin C at a meal significantly increases absorption of the iron consumed at that meal. Increasing intake of vitamin C–rich foods is beneficial for those with poor iron status or for those who choose to limit iron-rich food sources. Iron-deficiency anemia is common in the United States and is the number–one nutritional deficiency worldwide.

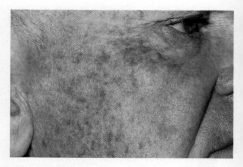

FIGURE 8-31 ▲ Pinpoint hemorrhages of the skin—an early symptom of scurvy. The spots on the skin are caused by slight bleeding. The person may experience poor wound healing. These are signs of defective collagen synthesis.
©Dr P. Marazzi/Science Source

Immune Function Last, but certainly not least, vitamin C is vital for the proper function of the immune system. Not only does vitamin C protect the immune cells from being degraded by the powerful oxidant reactions they use to kill pathogens, but it also promotes the proliferation of white blood cells. Can taking vitamin C fend off the common cold? Numerous well-designed, double-blind studies have failed to show that vitamin C prevents colds. Nevertheless, vitamin C does appear to reduce the duration of symptoms by a day or so and to lessen the severity of the symptoms. The key to success is to start the supplement as soon as symptoms appear. Once the cold has taken hold, it is too late!

VITAMIN C DEFICIENCY

On long sea voyages before the mid-eighteenth century, half or more of sailing crews died due to scurvy, the vitamin C–deficiency disease. The symptoms of scurvy, which include bleeding gums, tooth loss, bruising, and scaly skin, illustrate the important function of vitamin C in the formation of connective tissue. Without vitamin C, the skin and blood vessels weaken and wounds will not heal. In 1740, the Englishman Dr. James Lind first showed that citrus fruits—two oranges and one lemon a day—could prevent the development of scurvy. Fifty years after Lind's discovery, daily rations for British sailors included limes (thus their nickname, *limeys*). Even after this discovery, scurvy continued to affect many people as thousands died during the American Civil War owing to inadequate intake of vitamin C.

GETTING ENOUGH VITAMIN C

Fresh, ripe fruits and vegetables are loaded with vitamin C. Besides the foods listed in Figure 8-32, other citrus fruits, papayas, broccoli, cauliflower, and many types of peppers pack a lot of vitamin C into a low-calorie package. Ready-to-eat breakfast cereals, potatoes, and fortified fruit drinks are also good sources of vitamin C. The 5 to 9 servings of fruit and vegetables suggested by MyPlate's Daily Checklist can easily provide enough

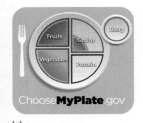

FIGURE 8-32 ◄ Food sources of vitamin C. (a) The fill of the background color (none, 1/3, 2/3, or completely covered) within each food group on MyPlate indicates the average nutrient density for vitamin C in that group. (b) The bar graph shows the vitamin C content of several foods compared to the RDA for adult males and females. Overall, fruits and vegetables are the richest sources of vitamin C. Foods in the dairy and protein groups (not shown) are poor sources of vitamin C.

Source: Nutrition data from USDA National Nutrient Database for Standard Reference, Release 26

(a)

(b)

	Food Item and Amount	Vitamin C (milligrams)	% RDA for Adult Males (90 milligrams)	% RDA for Adult Females (75 milligrams)
Grains	Whole Grain Total® cereal, 1 cup	60	67%	80%
	Tortellini with cheese filling, ½ cup	0	0%	0%
	Brown rice, cooked, ½ cup	0	0%	0%
Vegetables	Red peppers, raw, 1 cup	190	211%	253%
	Brussels sprouts, cooked, 1 cup	97	108%	129%
	Spinach, raw, 2 cups	17	19%	23%
Fruits	Strawberries, 1 cup	89	99%	119%
	Orange, 1 medium	83	92%	111%
	Grapefruit juice, canned, 1 cup	72	80%	96%

FARM to FORK Crucifers

Cruciferous vegetables are cool-weather vegetables with flowers that have four petals that resemble a cross. The most common crucifers include broccoli, cauliflower, cabbage, bok choy, Brussels sprouts, and green leafy vegetables such as kale and arugula. Ounce for ounce, crucifers have it all—vitamins, minerals, fiber, and an abundance of disease-fighting phytochemicals.

Grow
- The freshest and most nutrient dense crucifers always come straight from the garden. Sadly, up to 80% of nutrients are lost in the transport from farm to fork.
- For crucifer container gardening, estimate 1 broccoli plant per 5 gallons of soil (see https://ofbf.org/2008/06/05/vegetable-container-gardens/).
- Most crucifers require full sun and moist, fertile soil that's slightly acidic. Broccoli can germinate in soil with temperatures as low as 40°F, but check online for growing recommendations in your region.

Shop
- At the store, look for broccoli with dark green crowns, tight bud heads, and moist and firm stems. Avoid yellowing and dry produce that is not kept chilled.
- Intact heads of broccoli are not only more nutritious but less expensive than precut florets.

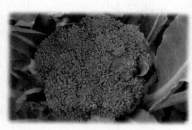

©Mary-Jon Ludy, Bowling Green State University, Garden of Hope images

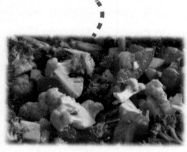

©Mary-Jon Ludy, Bowling Green State University, Garden of Hope images

Store
- To preserve the abundance of nutrients, antioxidants, and phytochemicals in crucifers, keep them cool and eat within days of harvest.
- If storing for any period, place in a plastic bag with about 20 pinprick holes (*micro-perforated* bag) in the crisper drawer.
- Prior to freezing broccoli, it is essential to *blanch* the produce to deactivate its enzymes (see http://ohioline.osu.edu/factsheet/HYG-5333).

Prep
- In most cases, the leaves or flower buds of crucifers are eaten, but there are a few where either the roots or seeds are also eaten.
- Compounds known as glucosinolates are responsible for much of the bitterness and the health benefits offered by these amazing plants.
- Cooking and preservation expose crucifers to heat, oxygen, and light—all significantly decreasing nutrient and phytochemical content. Lower temperatures as well as drier and shorter cooking times reduce losses.
- Steaming for less than 5 minutes or sautéing with a small amount of extra virgin olive oil is recommended.

Source: Robinson J. "Incredible Crucifers: Tame their bitterness and reap the rewards," In *Eating on the Wild Side: The Missing Link to Optimum Health*. New York: Little, Brown and Company, 2013.

---

vitamin C to meet the RDA. The brighter the fruit or vegetable, the higher it tends to be in vitamin C. For example, while a green bell pepper has 96 milligrams of vitamin C, a red bell pepper provides 152 milligrams of vitamin C. Keep in mind, however, that vitamin C is rapidly lost in processing and cooking as it is unstable in the presence of heat, iron, copper, or oxygen and is water soluble. Boiling fruits and vegetables can destroy much of the vitamin C or cause it to leach out of the food. Extended time on grocery store shelves or on your countertop at home will also decrease vitamin C content. Thus, you should consume fresh fruits and vegetables as soon after harvest as possible.

The adult RDA of vitamin C is 75 milligrams for women and 90 milligrams for men per day. The Daily Value used on food and supplement labels is 60 milligrams. Tobacco users need to add an extra 35 milligrams per day to the RDA. The toxic by-products of cigarette smoke and the oxidizing agents found in tobacco products increase the need for the antioxidant action of vitamin C. Average daily consumption of vitamin C in the United States is in the range of 70 to 100 milligrams, and at this level of intake, absorption efficiency is about 80% to 90%.

AVOIDING TOO MUCH VITAMIN C

The Upper Level (UL) of vitamin C is 2000 milligrams. Note that when vitamin C is consumed in large doses, the amount in excess of daily needs mostly ends up in the feces or urine. The kidneys start rapidly excreting vitamin C when intakes exceed 100 milligrams per day. As the amount ingested increases, absorption efficiency decreases precipitously—to approximately 50% with intake of 1000 milligrams per day and to 20% with intakes of

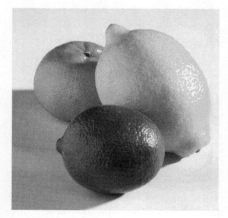

▲ Citrus fruits are good sources of vitamin C. ©Purestock/SuperStock

Vitamin C

RDA

  Men: 90 milligrams

  Women: 75 milligrams

DV: 60 milligrams

UL: 2000 milligrams

6000 milligrams daily. Regular consumption of more than 2000 milligrams per day may cause stomach inflammation and diarrhea. Even 1000-milligram supplement pills can cause some nausea and GI distress. A recent study found that men who said they took a vitamin C supplement regularly were at higher risk of developing kidney stones; therefore, ingesting large amounts of vitamin C supplements is discouraged in people predisposed to kidney stones. Because vitamin C enhances the absorption of iron, vitamin C supplements are also not recommended for those who overabsorb iron or have excessive iron stores. High doses of vitamin C may interfere with medical tests for diabetes or blood in the feces. If you take vitamin C supplements at any dose, be sure to inform your primary care provider. Primary care providers may misdiagnose conditions if they do not realize the influence of large doses of vitamin on your medical test results.

✓ CONCEPT CHECK 8.14

1. How does vitamin C function as an antioxidant and regenerate vitamin E?
2. How do the signs of vitamin C deficiency relate to the many roles of the vitamin discussed in this chapter?
3. Why are fresh foods the best sources of vitamin C?

8.15 Choline and Other Vitamin-Like Compounds

The dietary component choline is the latest addition to the list of essential nutrients. In 1998, the National Academy of Medicine recognized choline as an essential nutrient. When the Dietary Reference Intakes were released in 2000, only limited research on the dietary requirements for choline existed. One study of male volunteers showed decreased choline stores and liver damage when they were fed choline-deficient intravenous nutrition solutions. Based on this human study, plus laboratory animal studies, choline has been deemed essential and *vitamin-like*, but it is not yet classified as a vitamin.

FUNCTIONS OF CHOLINE

Despite its lack of vitamin status, choline is needed by all cells and plays several important roles in the body.

Cell Membrane Structure Choline is a precursor for several phospholipids. Phosphatidylcholine (also known as *lecithin*) accounts for about half of the phospholipids in cell membranes. Recall from Chapter 5 that phospholipids contribute to the flexibility of cell membranes and allow for the presence of both water- and fat-soluble compounds in cell membranes. With its role in cell membrane structure, choline is important for the health of every cell and particularly for the health of brain tissue, where it is present in high levels.

Single-Carbon Metabolism Choline is a precursor for betaine, a compound that participates in many chemical reactions that involve the transfer of single-carbon groups in metabolism. Important examples of metabolic pathways that involve the transfer of single-carbon groups include the synthesis of neurotransmitters, modifications of DNA during embryonic development, and the metabolism of homocysteine. As you learned earlier in this chapter, high levels of homocysteine in the blood are related to increased risk of heart disease. Betaine and the B vitamin folate both donate single-carbon groups to convert homocysteine into another compound, thus reducing levels of homocysteine in the blood.

Research points to a role of adequate choline for the prevention of birth defects.[11] Choline's purported role in prevention of birth defects is similar to that of folate. Both folate and choline are involved in the formation of DNA during embryonic development. As you will read in Chapter 14, problems with DNA formation lead to birth defects. Indeed, animal studies show that maternal choline supplementation during critical stages of embryonic development can improve learning and memory in the offspring. In humans,

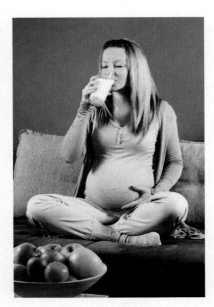

▲ Choline is important for proper development of the fetal brain. Milk and other dairy products supply some choline. ©InesBazdar/Shutterstock

as well, studies show that babies born to women with low choline intakes have four times higher rates of birth defects than babies born to women with high choline intakes.

Nerve Function and Brain Development Choline is part of acetylcholine, a neurotransmitter associated with attention, learning, memory, muscle control, and many other functions. Sphingomyelin, a choline-containing phospholipid, is part of the myelin sheath that insulates nerve cells. As mentioned, brain tissue is particularly high in choline. During pregnancy, the concentration of choline in amniotic fluid is high, supplying choline to the developing brain of the fetus. Animal studies demonstrate that choline deficiencies during pregnancy lead to poor brain development, learning ability, and memory. The AI for choline is increased during pregnancy and breastfeeding to assist in proper brain development. Choline also may be useful for preventing or treating neurological disorders such as Alzheimer's disease.

Lipid Transport As part of phospholipids, choline is a component of lipoproteins, which carry lipids through the blood. Choline deficiencies in animals and humans lead to decreased production of lipid transport proteins, such as very low density lipoproteins (VLDL). The inability of the liver to export fat to the rest of the body leads to the buildup of fat in the liver. A small amount of fat in the liver is normal, but excess fat leads to scarring of the liver tissue and eventual dysfunction. Fatty liver is a common cause of cirrhosis.

The roles of choline in lipid transport and homocysteine metabolism have implicated the nutrient in the prevention of cardiovascular disease. However, research has also raised some concerns about possible negative effects of choline on cardiovascular disease risk. Recent findings have shown that metabolism of dietary phosphatidylcholine, from foods such as eggs, by the intestinal microbiota produces an atherosclerosis-promoting compound that has been associated with an increased risk of major adverse cardiovascular events.[11]

GETTING ENOUGH CHOLINE

Choline is widely distributed in foods (Fig. 8-33). Soybeans, egg yolks, beef, cauliflower, almonds, and peanuts are good sources. In addition to natural food sources, lecithin is often added to food products as an emulsifier during processing, so many other foods are sources of choline.

Choline can exist in foods as free choline or as part of other compounds, such as phospholipids. Pancreatic enzymes break down some of the phospholipid forms prior to absorption. Free choline is water soluble and can be absorbed from the small intestine into portal circulation for transport to the liver. Choline that is part of phospholipids, on the other hand, is fat soluble and gets absorbed into the lymphatic system.

To some extent, choline also can be synthesized in the body by a process that involves other nutrients, such as folate and the amino acid methionine. If the body must synthesize choline to meet its needs, functional deficiencies of folate could result.

Eggs (with yolks) are by far the most nutrient-dense source of choline. One whole egg supplies about ¼ of the daily choline needs in a 70-kcal package. Choline researchers suggest that an average of one egg per day would assist in achieving the AI for choline while still supplying less than the 300 milligram per day for cholesterol.

An AI has been set for adults (see margins), but it is unknown whether a dietary supply is essential for infants or children. As already noted, some choline can be synthesized in the body, but recent research indicates that synthesis by the body is not sufficient to meet the body's needs for choline. Nutrition surveys show that fewer than 10% of Americans meet the AI for choline. In addition, the AIs do not reflect wide genetic variation in individual choline requirements. Research suggests that at least half the population has genetic variations that increase dietary requirements for nutrients that serve in single-carbon metabolism, including choline and folate. Thus, even meeting the AI may not provide enough choline to support the body's needs for some people.

The AI for choline increases during pregnancy (to 450 milligrams per day) and breastfeeding (to 550 milligrams per day) to support the brain development of the fetus or infant. Prenatal vitamins do not contain choline. Therefore, consumption of rich dietary sources of choline, such as eggs, is important for pregnant and breastfeeding women.

Choline
AI
  Men: 550 milligrams
  Women: 425 milligrams
DV: not established
UL: 3.5 grams

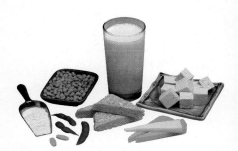

▲ Dairy products, soy, almonds, and peanuts are natural sources of choline.
©C Squared Studios/Getty Images

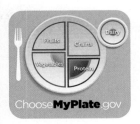

(a)

FIGURE 8-33 ◄ Food sources of choline. (a) The fill of the background color (none, 1/3, 2/3, or completely covered) within each food group on MyPlate indicates the average nutrient density for choline in that group. (b) The bar graph shows the choline content of several foods compared to the RDA for adult males and females. Overall, foods that are rich sources of protein are good sources of choline. Grains and fruits are not included in the bar graph because, in general, these are poor sources of choline.

Source: Nutrition data from USDA National Nutrient Database for Standard Reference, Release 26

(b)

	Food Item and Amount	Choline (milligrams)	% AI for Adult Males (550 milligrams)	% AI for Adult Females (425 milligrams)
Vegetables	Swiss chard, cooked, 1 cup	50	9%	12%
Vegetables	Cauliflower, cooked, 1 cup	49	9%	12%
Vegetables	Mushrooms, shiitake, 4 each	30	5%	7%
Dairy	Milk, fat-free, 1 cup	38	7%	9%
Dairy	Yogurt, plain, nonfat, 1 cup	37	7%	9%
Dairy	Cottage cheese, low-fat, ½ cup	18	3%	4%
Protein	Beef liver, pan-fried, 3 ounces	339	62%	78%
Protein	Egg, hard-boiled, 1 large	147	27%	35%
Protein	Cod, baked, 3 ounces	71	13%	17%

AVOIDING TOO MUCH CHOLINE

The choline UL for adults is set at 3.5 grams per day. Routinely exceeding the UL will result in a fishy body odor and low blood pressure.

OTHER VITAMIN-LIKE COMPOUNDS

A variety of vitamin-like compounds are found in the body. These include the following:

- Carnitine, needed to transport fatty acids into cell mitochondria
- Inositol, part of cell membranes
- Taurine, part of bile acids
- Lipoic acid, which participates in carbohydrate metabolism and acts as an antioxidant

These vitamin-like compounds can be synthesized by cells using common building blocks, such as amino acids and glucose. Our diets are also a source. In disease states or periods of active growth, the synthesis of vitamin-like compounds may not meet needs, so dietary intake can be crucial. The needs for vitamin-like compounds in certain groups of individuals, such as for preterm infants, are being investigated. Although promoted and sold by health-food stores, these vitamin-like compounds need not be included in the diet of the average healthy adult.

Table 8-5 summarizes much of what we know about the water-soluble vitamins. Now that you have studied the vitamins, review MyPlate and note how each food group can make an important vitamin contribution (Fig. 8-2).

✓ CONCEPT CHECK 8.15

1. Describe three functions of choline in the human body.

2. List three ways to incorporate more choline into the diet.

3. Is it necessary to take dietary supplements of vitamin-like compounds, such as carnitine and taurine? Why or why not?

TABLE 8-5 ■ **Summary of the Water-Soluble Vitamins and Choline**

Vitamin	Major Functions	RDA or AI	Dietary Sources*	Deficiency Symptoms	Toxicity Symptoms
Thiamin	• Coenzyme in metabolism of carbohydrates and branched-chain amino acids	*Men:* 1.2 milligrams *Women:* 1.1 milligrams	• Enriched, fortified, or whole grains • Ready-to-eat cereals • Pork	• Beriberi resulting in nervous system dysfunction	• Unknown No UL
Riboflavin†	• Coenzyme in numerous redox reactions	*Men:* 1.3 milligrams *Women:* 1.1 milligrams	• Organ meats • Milk • Bread products and fortified cereals	• Inflammation of the mouth and tongue • Eye disorders	• Unknown No UL
Niacin	• Coenzyme in many biological reduction and oxidation reactions required for energy metabolism	*Men:* 16 milligrams (NE) *Women:* 14 milligrams (NE)	• Meat, fish, poultry • Enriched and whole grains • Fortified ready-to-eat cereals	Pellagra: • Diarrhea • Dermatitis • Dementia • Death	• Flushing and itchy skin • GI distress UL = 35 milligrams
Pantothenic acid	• Coenzyme in fatty acid metabolism	5 milligrams	• Organ meats • Poultry • Beef • Potatoes • Broccoli • Whole grains • Tomato products • Yeast • Egg yolk	No natural deficiency disease or symptoms	• Unknown No UL
Biotin	• Coenzyme in synthesis of fat, glycogen, and amino acids	30 micrograms	• Liver • Small amounts in fruits and meats	• Dermatitis • Tongue soreness • Anemia • Depression	• Unknown No UL
Vitamin B-6†	• Coenzyme for amino acid metabolism • Neurotransmitter synthesis • Red blood cell synthesis	*Men (up to 50 years):* 1.3 milligrams *Women (up to 50 years):* 1.3 milligrams	• Fortified cereals • Organ meats • Fortified soy-based meat substitutes	• Anemia • Convulsions • Nausea • Dermatitis • Depression	• Sensory neuropathy UL = 100 milligrams
Folate (folic acid)†	• Coenzyme in nucleic and amino acid metabolism • Red blood cell synthesis	400 micrograms (DFE)	• Enriched cereal grains • Dark leafy vegetables • Enriched and whole grains • Fortified ready-to-eat cereals	• Megaloblastic anemia • Neural tube birth defects • Diarrhea • Depression • Fatigue	• Masks vitamin B-12 deficiency UL = 1000 micrograms synthetic folic acid (exclusive of food folate)
Vitamin B-12†	• Coenzyme in nucleic acid metabolism • Red blood cell synthesis	2.4 micrograms Older adults and vegans may need fortified foods or supplements	• Fortified cereals • Meat • Fish • Poultry	• Megaloblastic anemia • Nerve damage • Fatigue	• Unknown No UL

(continued)

TABLE 8-5 ■ (*continued*)

Vitamin	Major Functions	RDA or AI	Dietary Sources*	Deficiency Symptoms	Toxicity Symptoms
Vitamin C (ascorbic acid)	• Connective tissue synthesis • Hormone and neurotransmitter synthesis • Antioxidant • Immune function • Improves nonheme iron absorption	*Men:* 90 milligrams *Women:* 75 milligrams Smokers should add 35 milligrams	• Citrus fruits • Potatoes • Brussels sprouts • Cauliflower • Broccoli • Spinach • Strawberries	• Scurvy • Poor wound healing • Pinpoint hemorrhages • Bleeding gums • Fatigue • Infections • Bruises	• GI disturbances • Kidney stones • Excess iron absorption UL = 2 grams
Choline†	• Neurotransmitter and phospholipid synthesis	*Men:* 550 milligrams *Women:* 425 milligrams	• Milk • Liver • Eggs • Peanuts	No natural deficiency	• Fishy body odor • Sweating • Hypotension • Hepatotoxicity UL = 3.5 grams per day, based on development of fishy body odor and reduced blood pressure

Abbreviations: RDA =Recommended Dietary Allowance; AI = adequate intake; RAE = retinol activity equivalents; IU = international units; UL = Upper Intake Level; NE = niacin equivalents; DFE = dietary folate equivalents; UL = Upper Intake Level

*Fortified ready-to-eat breakfast cereals are good sources for most of these vitamins and a common source of B vitamins for many of us.

†These nutrients also participate in homocysteine metabolism; meeting the RDA or AI may reduce the risk of developing cardiovascular disease.

8.16 Dietary Supplements— Who Needs Them?

The phrase *multivitamin* and *mineral supplement* has been mentioned many times so far in this textbook. Often, these and other supplements are marketed as cures for anything and everything. This cure-all approach is promoted by the supplement industry and countless health-food stores, pharmacies, and supermarkets.

According to the Dietary Supplement Health and Education Act of 1994 (DSHEA), a supplement in the United States is a product intended to supplement the diet that bears or contains one or more of the following ingredients:

- A vitamin
- A mineral
- An herb or another botanical
- An amino acid
- A dietary substance to supplement the diet, which could be an extract or a combination of the first four ingredients in this list

The definition is broad and covers a wide variety of nutritional substances. The use of dietary supplements is a common practice among North Americans and generates about $35 billion annually for the industry in the United States (Fig. 8-34). Supplements can be sold without proof that they are safe and effective. Unless the FDA has evidence that a supplement is inherently dangerous or marketed with an illegal claim, it will not regulate such products closely. The vitamin folate is an exception. The FDA has limited resources to police supplement manufacturers and has to act against these manufacturers one at a time. Thus, we cannot rely on the FDA to protect us from vitamin and mineral supplement overuse and misuse. We bear that responsibility ourselves, with the help of professional advice from a primary care provider or registered dietitian nutritionist.

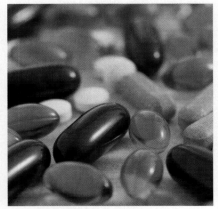

©Nancy R. Cohen/Getty Images

FIGURE 8-34 ▼ The dietary supplement industry is a growing multibillion-dollar business in the United States.

Sales in $ Billions

36
30
24
18
12
6

2000 2001 2002 2003 2004 2005 2006 2007 2008 2009 2010 2011 2012 2013 2014 2015 2016

The supplement makers can make broad claims about their products under the *structure or function* provision of the law. The products, however, cannot claim to prevent, treat, or cure a disease. Menopause in women and aging are not diseases per se, so products alleging to treat symptoms of these conditions can be marketed without FDA approval. For example, a product that claims to treat hot flashes arising during menopause can be sold without any evidence to prove that the product works, but a product that claims to decrease the risk of cardiovascular disease by reducing blood cholesterol must have results from scientific studies that justify the claim.

Why do people take supplements? Frequently given reasons include:

- Maintain overall health
- Fill nutrient gaps in the diet
- Reduce susceptibility to health conditions (e.g., colds)
- Reduce stress
- Increase "energy"
- Prevent disease (cancer, osteoporosis, etc.)

CRITICAL THINKING

Believing that supplements provide the nutrition her body needs, Janice regularly takes numerous supplements while paying relatively little attention to daily food choices. How would you explain to her that this practice may lead to health problems?

Newsworthy Nutrition

Increased Emergency Department Visits for Dietary Supplement Users

Intake of dietary supplements, including herbals, vitamins, and mineral supplements, continues to increase in the United States, yet few studies have investigated safety of these products. The aim of this study was to evaluate adverse events directly related to dietary supplement intake that resulted in emergency department visits. Surveillance data were collected from 63 nationally representative emergency departments from 2004 to 2013. Over 23,000 emergency department visits per year were attributed to adverse events related to dietary supplement intake, resulting in 2154 hospitalizations annually. Of emergency department visits, 28% related to supplement use involving young adults (ages 20 to 34). After excluding dietary supplement intake by unsupervised children, 66% of supplement-related emergency department visits involved herbal or complementary nutritional products and 32% involved micronutrients. Herbals and complementary nutritional products for weight loss and enhanced energy were prevalent. These products resulted in complaints of heart palpitations, chest pain, or tachycardia. In light of the fact that the dietary supplement industry is not well regulated, supplement users must be extremely cautious and stay well informed of the potential health risks.

Source: Geller, A, et al. "Emergency department visits for adverse events related to dietary supplements," *New England Journal of Medicine* 15:373, 2015.

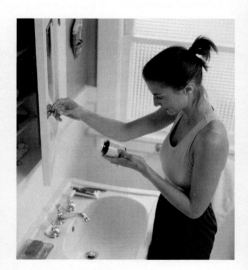

▲ Long-term intake of just three times the Daily Value for some fat-soluble vitamins—particularly preformed vitamin A—can cause toxic effects. Know what you are taking if you use supplements. ©Ryan McVay/Getty Images

Top Five Dietary Supplements in 2016:
1. Multivitamins
2. Vitamin D
3. Calcium
4. Vitamin C
5. Vitamin B/B Complex

Source: Council for Responsible Nutrition

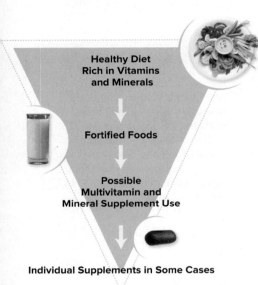

FIGURE 8-35 ▲ Supplement savvy—an approach to the use of nutrient supplements. Emphasizing a healthy dietary pattern rich in vitamins and minerals is always the first option.

A few websites to help you evaluate ongoing claims and evaluate safety of supplements are:
- www.acsh.org
- www.quackwatch.com
- www.ncahf.org
- ods.od.nih.gov
- www.eatright.org
- www.usp.org/dietary-supplements/overview

These sites are maintained by groups or individuals committed to providing reasoned and authoritative nutrition and health advice to consumers.

SHOULD YOU TAKE A SUPPLEMENT?

Multivitamin and mineral supplements (MVMs) are popularly regarded as a simple back-up plan or an insurance policy, even for people who consciously try to consume a balanced diet. Users aim to prevent nutrient deficiencies or chronic diseases by filling any gaps between dietary intake and nutrient needs. However, evidence to support the widespread use of MVMs is mixed. While there is little risk of harm from consuming a balanced MVM that supplies no more than 100% of the Daily Value for the nutrients it contains, most studies indicate no discernible advantage. The National Institutes of Health, in its *State-of-the-Science Report*, concluded that the present evidence is insufficient to recommend either for or against the use of MVMs by Americans to prevent chronic disease.[12]

Do specific vitamin or mineral supplements provide any benefit? Only a few studies of vitamin and mineral supplements demonstrate beneficial effects for the prevention of deficiencies or chronic diseases. For example, postmenopausal women may benefit from taking calcium and vitamin D supplements to increase bone mineral density and decrease fracture risk. Table 8-6 outlines the population groups that are most likely to benefit from taking dietary supplements.

While there may be moderate benefits of consuming dietary supplements, uninformed use of supplements can be risky. Indeed, most cases of nutrient toxicity are a result of supplement use. High doses of one nutrient can affect absorption or metabolism of other nutrients. For example, excessive zinc intake can inhibit copper absorption, and large amounts of folate can mask signs and symptoms of a vitamin B-12 deficiency. In addition, some supplements can interfere with medications. For instance, high intakes of vitamin K or vitamin E alter the action of anticlotting medications, vitamin B-6 can offset the action of L-dopa (used in treating Parkinson's disease), and large doses of vitamin C might interfere with certain cancer therapy regimens.

For most Americans, finding ways to incorporate the recommended servings of fruits, vegetables, and whole grains into the diet is the safest and healthiest way to ensure nutrient adequacy.[13] Many of the health-promoting effects of foods cannot be found in a bottle. Recall the discussions of phytochemicals in Chapter 1 and the benefits of fiber in Chapter 4. Few or no phytochemicals or fiber are present in most supplements. Multivitamin and mineral supplements also contain little calcium to keep the pill size small. Furthermore, the oxide forms of magnesium, zinc, and copper used in many supplements are not as well absorbed as forms found in foods. Overall, supplement use cannot fix an inadequate dietary pattern in all respects.

As illustrated in Figure 8-35, when it comes to improving nutrient intake, emphasize foods before considering dietary supplements. First, you should assess your current dietary patterns. MyPlate is a tool consumers can use to plan a healthy dietary pattern (see Chapter 2). If nutrient gaps still remain, identify food sources that can help. For example, fortified, ready-to-eat breakfast cereals supply a variety of micronutrients, including vitamin E, folic acid, vitamin B-6, and highly absorbable forms of vitamin B-12. Other fortified foods, such as calcium-fortified orange juice, can also be helpful. Be mindful of portion sizes of highly fortified foods, however, as multiple servings could lead to excessive intakes of some nutrients, such as vitamin A, iron, and synthetic folic acid. Lastly, if supplement use is desired, educate yourself and discuss it with your primary care provider or registered dietitian nutritionist.

WHICH SUPPLEMENT SHOULD YOU CHOOSE?

If you decide to take a multivitamin and mineral supplement, start by choosing a nationally recognized brand (from a supermarket or pharmacy) that contains about 100% of the Daily Values for the nutrients present. A multivitamin and mineral supplement should generally be taken with or just after meals to maximize absorption. Make sure also that intake from the total of this supplement, any other supplements used, and highly fortified foods (such as ready-to-eat breakfast cereals) provides no more than the

TABLE 8-6 ■ **Who Is Most Likely to Benefit from Dietary Supplements?**

Type of Supplement	Who May Benefit
Multivitamin/mineral supplement	• People on restrictive diets (< 1200 kcal per day), vegans, vegetarians • People with unbalanced or inadequate diets (e.g., in cases of food insecurity or *picky* eaters) • People with malabsorptive diseases • People who take medications that interfere with nutrient absorption or metabolism • Older adults (over 50 years of age) • Pregnant women or those of childbearing age
Various B vitamins	• People who abuse alcohol
Folic acid	• Women of childbearing age (especially during pregnancy and breastfeeding)
Vitamin B-12	• Older adults • Strict vegans
Vitamin C	• People who smoke
Vitamin D	• People with limited milk intake (due to allergies or lactose intolerance) • People with limited exposure to sunlight (e.g., all infants, many African-Americans, and some older adults) • Strict vegans
Vitamin E	• People who follow diets low in fat (especially low in plant oils)
Vitamin K	• Newborns (given by injection shortly after birth)
Calcium	• Strict vegans • Older adults with bone loss
Fluoride	• Some older infants and children (as directed by a dentist)
Iron	• Women with excessive bleeding during menstruation • Women who are pregnant • Strict vegans
Zinc	• Strict vegans

Upper Level for each vitamin and mineral. This is especially important with regard to preformed vitamin A intake. Two exceptions are: (1) both men and older women should make sure any product used is low in iron or iron-free to avoid possible iron overload (see Chapter 9 for details); and (2) somewhat exceeding the Upper Level for vitamin D is likely a safe practice for adults. Read the labels carefully to be sure of what is being taken (Fig. 8-36). Because research on a variety of nutrient supplements has revealed a lack of product quality, the FDA now requires supplement makers to test the identity, purity, strength, and composition of all their products. As an extra protection, select supplements that bear the logo of the United States Pharmacopeial Convention (USP). The USP is an independent, nonprofit group of scientists that reviews products for strength, quality, purity, packaging, labeling, speed of dissolution, and shelf-stability. The USP designation on a supplement label indicates that the product has been evaluated and meets professionally accepted standards of supplement quality.

Another consideration in choosing a supplement is avoiding superfluous ingredients, such as para-aminobenzoic acid (PABA), hesperidin complex, inositol, bee pollen, and lecithins. These are not needed in our diets. They are especially common in expensive supplements sold in health-food stores and online. In addition, use of l-tryptophan and high doses of beta-carotene or fish oils is discouraged.

✓ **CONCEPT CHECK 8.16**

1. Name four types of ingredients that are classified as dietary supplements by the Dietary Supplement Health and Education Act.
2. Identify three potential risks from use of dietary supplements.
3. Describe three situations in which use of dietary supplements is necessary.

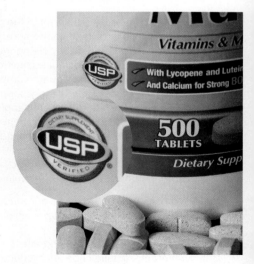

▲ If you must take vitamins, look for the USP symbol on your vitamin or mineral supplement to ensure quality and safety. ©McGraw-Hill Education/Jill Braaten, photographer

FIGURE 8-36 ▶ Nutrient supplements display a nutrition label different from that of foods. This Supplement Facts label must list the ingredient(s), amount(s) per serving, serving size, suggested use, and % Daily Value if one has been established. In addition, this label includes structure/function claims, which are not mandatory elements of the supplement label. When structure/function claims are made, however, the label also must include the FDA warning that these claims have not been evaluated by the agency.

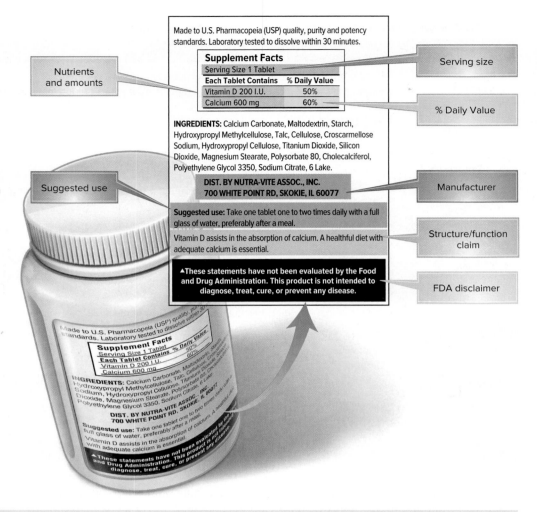

Nutrients and amounts

Suggested use

Made to U.S. Pharmacopeia (USP) quality, purity and potency standards. Laboratory tested to dissolve within 30 minutes.

Supplement Facts

Serving Size 1 Tablet

Each Tablet Contains	% Daily Value
Vitamin D 200 I.U.	50%
Calcium 600 mg	60%

INGREDIENTS: Calcium Carbonate, Maltodextrin, Starch, Hydroxypropyl Methylcellulose, Talc, Cellulose, Croscarmellose Sodium, Hydroxypropyl Cellulose, Titanium Dioxide, Silicon Dioxide, Magnesium Stearate, Polysorbate 80, Cholecalciferol, Polyethylene Glycol 3350, Sodium Citrate, 6 Lake.

DIST. BY NUTRA-VITE ASSOC., INC.
700 WHITE POINT RD, SKOKIE, IL 60077

Suggested use: Take one tablet one to two times daily with a full glass of water, preferably after a meal.

Vitamin D assists in the absorption of calcium. A healthful diet with adequate calcium is essential.

▲These statements have not been evaluated by the Food and Drug Administration. This product is not intended to diagnose, treat, cure, or prevent any disease.

Serving size

% Daily Value

Manufacturer

Structure/function claim

FDA disclaimer

CASE STUDY — Getting the Most Nutrition from Your Food

In the dietary supplements aisle of the grocery store, the choices are endless—and expensive. Julie, a college sophomore, just read the Academy of Nutrition and Dietetics' position paper on nutrient supplementation for her class. She learned that dietary supplements, such as a balanced multivitamin and mineral supplement, can be a good back-up plan to ensure adequate nutrition, but the jury is still out when it comes to demonstrating a benefit of dietary supplements for long-term health. The majority of Americans regularly take nutrient supplements, but it is usually the people who already consume a healthy diet who take them. Getting more than the recommended amount of a nutrient does not confer additional health benefits. In fact, too much of some vitamins and minerals can lead to toxicity.

Julie decides she would rather focus on getting her nutrients from whole foods. How can she get the most vitamins and minerals out of the foods she eats?

1. What factors can damage or reduce vitamins in food?
2. To maximize vitamin content, what should Julie keep in mind as she selects fresh produce for purchase?
3. How does food processing affect vitamin and mineral content? Does it make a difference if Julie chooses products with whole grains or refined grains?
4. When storing fruits and vegetables in her apartment, what steps can Julie take to minimize nutrient losses?
5. Which cooking methods are best for preserving vitamin content?

Complete the Case Study. Responses to these questions can be provided by your instructor.

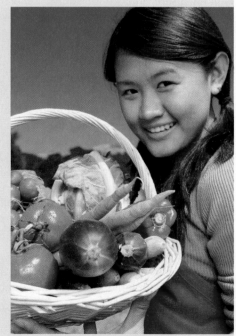

©Tanya Constantine/Blend Images LLC

8.17 Nutrition and Your Health

Nutrition and Cancer

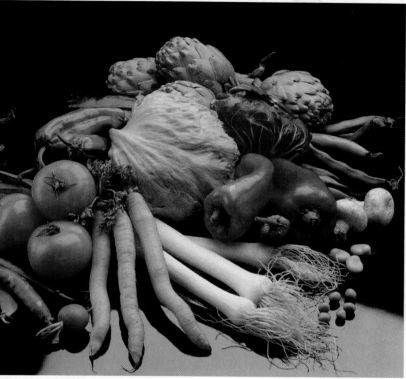

©Pixtal

Cancer is the second leading cause of death for North American adults. It is estimated that more than 1620 people die each day of cancer in the United States, accounting for one in four deaths. Cancer-related medical expenses exceed $88 billion each year and are projected to reach $158 billion by 2020. The top four cancers, causing approximately 50% of cancer deaths are lung, colorectal, breast, and prostate.

Cancer is many complex diseases; each differs in the types of cells affected and, in some cases, in the factors contributing to cancer development and progression (Fig. 8-37). For example, the environmental and genetic factors leading to skin cancer often differ from those leading to breast cancer. Similarly, the treatments for the different types of cancer must also vary.

Cancer Progression

The initiation of cancer occurs when a DNA mutation occurs in a cell. Promotion and progression of cancer occurs when mutated cells multiply and proliferate uncontrollably. Without prompt and effective treatment, cancer continues to grow and spread. Most cancers take the form of tumors, although not all tumors are cancers. A **tumor** is spontaneous new tissue growth that appears to serve no physiological purpose. It can be either **benign,** such as a wart, or **malignant,** such as most lung cancers. The terms *malignant tumor* and *malignant neoplasm* are synonymous with cancer.

Whereas benign (noncancerous) tumors are dangerous if their presence interferes with normal bodily functions, malignant

(cancerous) tumors invade surrounding structures, including blood vessels, the lymph system, and nervous tissue. Cancer can spread, or **metastasize,** to distant sites via the blood and lymphatic circulation, thereby producing invasive tumors in almost any part of the body. Cancer metastasis is much more difficult to treat as each new cancer takes on distinct characteristics in response to its new environment. The fact that uncontrolled cancers spread explains why early detection and targeted treatment are critical. Cancers that are often diagnosed in the early stages, mainly due to widespread screening programs, are those in the colon, breast, and cervix.

Early Detection of Cancer

The CAUTION acronym listed below is a useful aid for remembering many early warning signs for cancer. Unexplained weight loss can be an additional symptom that should not be ignored.

- **C**hange in bowel or bladder habits
- **A** sore that does not heal
- **U**nusual bleeding or discharge
- **T**hickening or lump in the breast or elsewhere
- **I**ndigestion or difficulty in swallowing
- **O**bvious change in a wart or mole
- **N**agging cough or hoarseness

Routine screenings are important for early detection of cancer. The American Cancer Society and others publishes current cancer screening guidelines based upon expert recommendations and research. Families with genetic predispositions to cancer should consult their primary care provider to discuss enhanced surveillance.

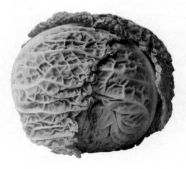
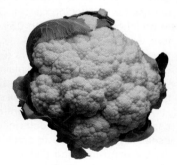

▲ Cruciferous vegetables such as cabbage and cauliflower are rich in cancer-preventing phytochemicals. ©C Squared Studios/Getty Images

tumor Mass of cells; may be cancerous (malignant) or noncancerous (benign).

benign Noncancerous; tumors that do not spread.

malignant Malicious; in reference to a tumor, the property of spreading locally and to distant sites.

metastasize The spreading of disease from one part of the body to another, even to parts of the body that are remote from the site of the original tumor. Cancer cells can spread via blood vessels, the lymphatic system, or direct growth of the tumor.

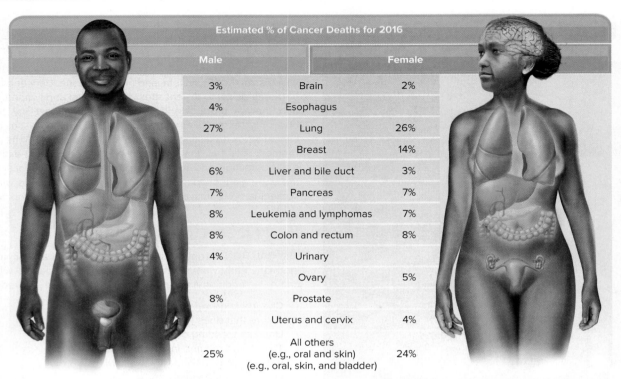

Estimated % of Cancer Deaths for 2016		
Male		Female
3%	Brain	2%
4%	Esophagus	
27%	Lung	26%
	Breast	14%
6%	Liver and bile duct	3%
7%	Pancreas	7%
8%	Leukemia and lymphomas	7%
8%	Colon and rectum	8%
4%	Urinary	
	Ovary	5%
8%	Prostate	
	Uterus and cervix	4%
25%	All others (e.g., oral and skin) (e.g., oral, skin, and bladder)	24%

FIGURE 8-37 ▲ Cancer is many diseases. Numerous types of cells and organs are its target. About one-third of all cancers arise from smoking (primarily lung cancer). Source: American Cancer Society, Inc., Surveillance Research, 2016

Factors That Influence the Development of Cancer

Genetics, environment, and lifestyle are potent forces that influence the risk for developing cancer. Of cancers, 5% to 10% are thought to be inherited and 90% to 95% are related to environmental factors. Genetic predispositions to cancer are most prevalent in colon, breast, and prostate cancers (Fig. 8-37). Modifiable lifestyle and environmental exposures explain the huge variation in cancer rates from country to country. Excessive body fatness and dietary patterns account for over half of all environmentally related cancers.

Although we have little control over our genetic risk factors for cancer, we have tremendous influence over our lifestyle behaviors, especially with regard to smoking, alcohol intake, physical activity, UV exposure, and dietary patterns. Indeed, over one-third of all cancers in North America are due to tobacco use. About half of the cancers of the mouth, pharynx, and larynx are associated with heavy use of alcohol. The combined use of both alcohol and tobacco increases cancer risks even higher than either alone.

A Closer Look at the Influence of Diet on Cancer

Some food constituents may contribute to cancer development, whereas others have a protective effect (Table 8-7). Next, the association between body fat/calorie intake and cancer risk is presented, followed by a list of food constituents that may reduce the risk for cancer.[15]

Body Fatness Linked to Cancer Risk

An estimated one of every three cancer deaths in the United States is linked to excess body fat, poor nutrition, and inadequate physical activity. Of these, body weight appears to have the greatest impact on cancer risk. Excess body weight alone contributes to one of five cancer-related deaths. This includes cancer of the breast, colon and rectum, esophagus, kidney, pancreas, gallbladder, liver, cervix, ovary, and **endometrium;** non-Hodgkin's lymphoma; multiple myeloma; and aggressive prostate cancer.

There are several ways excess body fat can influence cancer risk. Adipose tissue secretes hormones, such as estrogen and insulin, that promote the development of cancer. Other proteins are secreted as well that regulate hormonal actions. Also, chronic and systemic inflammation and oxidative stress often typical among overweight and obese individuals contribute to carcinogenesis.

A strong link exists between cancer risk and excess calories in the diet. In animal experiments, restricting total calorie intake to about 70% of usual intake results in about a 40% reduction in tumor development, regardless of the macronutrient composition of the diet. Currently, calorie restriction appears to be the most effective technique for preventing cancer in laboratory animals.

endometrium The membrane that lines the inside of the uterus. It increases in thickness during the menstrual cycle until ovulation occurs. The surface layers are shed during menstruation if conception does not take place.

TABLE 8-7 ■ Food Constituents Associated with Cancer

Constituent	Dietary Sources	Action
Protective when consumed in recommended ranges*		
Vitamin A	Liver, fortified milk, fruits, vegetables	Encourages normal cell development.
Vitamin D	Fortified milk, fatty fish	Increases production of a protein that suppresses cell growth.
Vitamin E	Whole grains, vegetable oils, green leafy vegetables	Prevents formation of nitrosamines; antioxidant.
Vitamin C	Fruits, vegetables	Can block conversion of nitrites and nitrates to potent carcinogens; antioxidant.
Folate	Fruits, vegetables, whole grains	Encourages normal cell development; reduces the risk of colon cancer.
Selenium	Meats, whole grains	Part of antioxidant system that inhibits tumor growth and kills cancer cells.
Carotenoids, such as lycopene	Fruits, vegetables	Antioxidant-like properties; possibly influences cell metabolism.
Flavonoids, indoles, phenols, and other phytochemicals	Vegetables, especially cabbage, cauliflower, broccoli, Brussels sprouts, garlic, onions, tea	May reduce cancer in the stomach and other organs.
Calcium	Milk products, green vegetables	Slows cell division in the colon and binds bile acids and free fatty acids, thus reducing colon cancer risk.
Omega-3 fatty acids	Cold-water fish, such as salmon and tuna	May inhibit tumor growth.
Soy products	Tofu, soy milk, tempeh, soy nuts	Phytic acid possibly binds carcinogens in the intestinal tract; genistein component possibly reduces growth and metastasis of malignant cells.
Conjugated linoleic acid	Milk products, meats	May inhibit tumor development and act as an antioxidant.
Fiber-rich foods	Fruits, vegetables, whole grain breads and cereals, beans, nuts	Colon and rectal cancer risk may be decreased by accelerating intestinal transit or binding carcinogens such that they are excreted.
Possibly carcinogenic		
Excessive calorie intake	All macronutrients can contribute.	Excess fat mass leading to obesity; increased synthesis of estrogen and other sex hormones, which may increase the risk for some cancer; resulting excess insulin output from creation of an insulin-resistant state is also implicated.
Saturated fats	Meats, high-fat milk and milk products, animal fats, and vegetable oils	The strongest evidence is for excessive saturated and polyunsaturated fat intake; saturated fat is linked to an increased risk of prostate cancer.
High glycemic load carbohydrates	Cookies, cakes, sugared soft drinks, candy	Insulin surges associated with these foods may increase tumor growth, such as in the colon.
Alcohol	Beer, wine, liquor	Contributes to cancers of the throat, liver, bladder, breast, and colon (especially if the person does not consume enough folate).
Nitrites, nitrates	Cured meats, especially ham, bacon, and sausages	Under very high temperatures will bind to amino acid derivatives to form nitrosamines, potent carcinogens.
Multiring compounds: aflatoxin	Formed when mold is present on peanuts or grains.	May alter DNA structure and inhibit its ability to properly respond to physiologic controls; aflatoxin in particular is linked to liver cancer.
Benzo(a)pyrene and other heterocyclic amines	Charcoal-broiled foods, especially meats	Linked to stomach and colon cancer; to limit this risk, trim fat from meat before cooking, cut barbecuing time by partially cooking meat (such as in a microwave oven) prior to grilling, and don't consume blackened parts.

*Many of the actions listed for these possibly protective agents are speculative and have been verified only by experimental animal studies. The best evidence supports obtaining these nutrients and other food constituents from foods. The U.S. Preventive Services Task Force supports this statement, noting there is no clear evidence that nutrient supplements provide the same benefits.

Unfortunately, it is difficult for humans to reduce dietary calories to 70% of usual intake. While the data obtained from animal studies are interesting, understand that severe calorie restrictions are not feasible and sustainable for most individuals. In addition, once cancer is present, calorie restriction may no longer be helpful.

Cancer-Fighting Foods

Many nutrients and plant compounds exhibit anticancer properties. These include antioxidants and phytochemicals (Table 8-7). The antioxidant activity of vitamins C and E helps to prevent the formation of **nitrosamines** in the GI tract, thus reducing carcinogen exposure. Vitamin E also helps protect unsaturated fatty acids from damage by free radicals. Overall, carotenoids, vitamin E, vitamin C, and selenium from whole foods function as or contribute to antioxidant protection for the body. Some of these protective systems prevent DNA mutations by electron-seeking compounds, the main factor promoting cancer initiation.

Research shows that fruits and vegetables protect against a range of cancers. As well as containing key vitamins and minerals, which strengthen our immune system, they are good sources of biologically active phytochemicals. Foods containing fiber are also linked to a reduced risk of cancer. Fiber is thought to speed up *gut transit time*, or the length of time it takes food to move through the digestive system. It has been suggested that an adequate intake of vitamin D may prevent the risk for some forms of cancer. Vitamin D can "turn on" (express) or "turn off" (silence) a host of genes that regulate cell growth and inflammation. The exact role of vitamin D relative to carcinogenesis continues to be an active area of research.

Although no single food or food component can fully protect you against cancer, evidence clearly shows that dietary patterns that are rich in a variety of plant foods—vegetables, fruits, whole grains, beans—help to reduce the risk for many cancers. MyPlate is aimed at cancer and disease prevention. It is likely that consumption of a wide variety of plant-based foods and adequate physical activity result in a "cocktail" effect that, together, are more potent and protective than either in isolation.[14]

Evidence-Based Recommendations for Cancer Prevention

Given the devastating toll of cancer treatment and lack of a definitive cure, efforts at prevention are of prime importance. Several health organizations have issued their own sets of diet and lifestyle guidelines for cancer prevention and survivorship. Here, we present the recommendations of the American Institute for Cancer Research, which are consistent with the recommendations of other cancer organizations.

AMERICAN INSTITUTE FOR CANCER RESEARCH RECOMMENDATIONS FOR CANCER PREVENTION

1. *Be as lean as possible without becoming underweight.* Maintaining a healthy body weight is one of the most important things you can do to reduce your risk of cancer. Aim to be at the lower end of the healthy BMI range.

nitrosamine A carcinogen formed from nitrates and breakdown products of amino acids; can lead to stomach cancer.

2. *Be physically active for at least 30 minutes every day.* Physical activity in any form helps to lower cancer risk. Aim to build more activity, such as brisk walking, into your daily routine. Limit sedentary habits such as excessive screen time.
3. *Avoid sugary drinks. Limit consumption of energy-dense foods.* Choosing healthy foods and drinks instead of those that are high in refined carbohydrates and often in added sugar and fat can help us avoid overweight and obesity and thereby reduce cancer risk.
4. *Eat more of a variety of vegetables, fruits, whole grains, and legumes.* For good health, base all of your meals on plant foods. When preparing a meal, aim to fill at least two-thirds of your plate with vegetables, fruits, whole grains, and beans.
5. *Limit consumption of red meats and avoid processed meats.* Red meat refers to beef, pork, and lamb—foods such as hamburgers, steaks, pork chops, and roast lamb. The term *processed meat* refers to meats preserved by smoking, curing, or salting or by the addition of preservatives. Examples include ham, bacon, pastrami, salami, hot dogs, and sausages. To reduce risk, limit intake to no more than 18 ounces per week.
6. *If consumed at all, limit alcoholic drinks to two (men) or one (women) per day.* For cancer prevention, it is best to avoid alcohol completely, but alcohol does afford some protection against cardiovascular disease.
7. *Limit consumption of salty foods and foods processed with salt.* Consuming too much salt can be harmful to our health, increasing the risk of stomach cancer as well as hypertension.
8. *Don't use supplements to protect against cancer.* To reduce your risk of cancer, choose a balanced dietary pattern rich in a variety of whole foods rather than supplements.
9. *It is best for mothers to breastfeed exclusively for up to 6 months and then add other liquids and foods.* Breastfeeding reduces the risk of breast and other reproductive cancers for the mother and lowers the risk of future obesity in the infant.
10. *After treatment, cancer survivors should follow the recommendations for cancer prevention.* Anyone diagnosed with cancer should receive specialized nutritional advice from a registered dietitian nutritionist or clinician. Once active treatment is complete, aim to adhere to the cancer-prevention recommendations.

And always remember . . . Do not smoke or chew tobacco.

Nutrition Concerns During Active Cancer Treatment

Diet and lifestyle changes can exert a powerful influence on the risk for developing cancer, but it is important to note that they are no substitute for preventive screening and appropriate medical care. Once cancer has developed, diet and lifestyle changes will not be adequate to prevent cancer growth or metastasis. Nutrition concerns during active cancer treatment (chemotherapy, radiation, surgery) vary depending on the site and stage of the cancer, but the overall goals of nutrition therapy are to minimize weight fluctuations and prevent nutrient deficiencies.

Weight loss, particularly loss of muscle mass, is a major concern during cancer treatment because malnutrition can interrupt treatment regimens and impede recovery. Common effects of cancer and/or cancer treatments include fatigue, mouth sores, dry mouth, taste abnormalities, nausea, and diarrhea—all of which can lead to inadequate food intake.

During active treatment, the most appropriate food choices are those that the cancer patient craves and can tolerate. Although food choices vary widely based on each patient's individual symptoms, cool, nonacidic liquids and soft, mildly flavored foods are generally well accepted. Small, frequent meals and foods with high nutrient and calorie density should be emphasized to meet calorie and protein needs. Often, liquid nutritional supplements are needed. Because many cancer patients are immunocompromised as a result of their treatment, safe food handling practices are extremely important.

To learn more about cancer, review these sources of credible cancer information on the Internet:

American Cancer Society: www.cancer.org:

National Cancer Institute: www.cancer.gov:

American Institute for Cancer Research: www.aicr.org:

Abramson Cancer Center's Oncolink: www.oncolink.org:

Harvard School of Public Health's Disease Risk Index: www.diseaserisk index.harvard.edu

Summary (Numbers refer to numbered sections in the chapter.)

8.1 Vitamins are organic substances required in small amounts in the diet for growth, function, and body maintenance. These can be categorized as fat soluble (vitamins A, D, E, and K) or water soluble (B vitamins and vitamin C). Vitamins cannot be synthesized by the body in adequate amounts to support health, and absence of a vitamin from the diet leads to the development of a deficiency disease. Fat-soluble vitamins require dietary fat for absorption and are carried by lipoproteins in the blood. Vitamin toxicity is most likely to occur from megadoses of fat-soluble vitamins because they are readily stored in the body. Intakes of water-soluble vitamins that exceed the storage ability of tissues are typically excreted in urine. Some vitamins are susceptible to destruction by light, heat, air, or alkalinity, or may be lost from foods in cooking water or fats. Functional foods, such as oatmeal, provide health benefits beyond basic nutrition. Functional foods often contain large amounts of plant-derived compounds known as phytochemicals. These nonessential compounds are what provides plants with their unique color, odor, and flavor. Human consumption is linked to numerous protective health benefits.

8.2 Vitamin A maintains the health of epithelial tissues and is responsible for the function of mucous-secreting cells. Vitamin A is found in meats, fortified dairy products, fish, eggs, and a variety of red, orange, or leafy green vegetables. Carotenoids are phytochemicals that can be converted into vitamin A in the body. Three forms of carotenoids can yield vitamin A in humans: beta-carotene, alpha-carotene, and beta-cryptoxanthin. Although carotenoids are not essential nutrients, some have health-promoting qualities for humans. In addition to their contribution to vitamin A intake, carotenoids are powerful antioxidants. The antioxidant abilities of several carotenoids are linked to prevention of macular degeneration, cataracts, cardiovascular disease, and cancer. Carotenoids are plentiful in dark-green and orange vegetables.

8.3 Vitamin D is both a hormone and a vitamin. Human skin synthesizes it using sunshine and a cholesterol-like substance. If we do not spend enough time in the sun, foods such as fish and fortified milk can supply the vitamin. The active hormone form of vitamin D helps regulate blood calcium in part by increasing calcium absorption from the intestine. Infants and children who do not get enough vitamin D may develop rickets, and adults with inadequate amounts in the body develop osteomalacia. Older people and infants often need a supplemental source. Toxicity may lead to calcification of soft tissue, weakness, and gastrointestinal disturbances.

8.4 Vitamin E functions primarily as an antioxidant and is found in plant oils. By donating electrons to electron-seeking, free-radical (oxidizing) compounds, it neutralizes them. This effect shields cell membranes and red blood cells from breakdown. Claims are made about the curative powers of vitamin E, but more information is needed before megadose vitamin E recommendations for healthy adults can be made with certainty. The Upper Level is set at about 50 times adult needs.

8.5 Vitamin K is essential for blood clotting and imparts calcium-binding ability to various proteins, including those in bone. Some vitamin K absorbed each day comes from bacterial synthesis in the intestine, but most comes from foods, primarily green, leafy vegetables.

8.6 The B vitamins yield no energy directly, but they contribute to energy-yielding chemical reactions in the body by virtue of their coenzyme functions. B vitamins are highly bioavailable. North American diets are typically adequate in B vitamins except in cases of food insecurity, metabolic disorders, or alcoholism. Whole grains are more nutrient-dense sources of B vitamins (as well as other nutrients) than refined grains. Several B vitamins function as coenzymes in energy metabolism.

8.7 Thiamin's coenzyme form is involved in the metabolism of carbohydrates and proteins as well as the synthesis of RNA, DNA, and neurotransmitters. Rich food sources of thiamin include pork, enriched or fortified grain products, and milk. Beriberi, the thiamin-deficiency disease, leads to muscle weakness and nerve damage. Thiamin toxicity is unknown, and no UL has been set.

8.8 The coenzymes of riboflavin participate in the catabolism of fatty acids, metabolism of other vitamins and minerals, and antioxidant activity of glutathione peroxidase. Dairy products, enriched and fortified grain products, meat, and eggs are rich food sources of riboflavin. Symptoms of ariboflavinosis include glossitis and angular cheilitis. There is no evidence of toxicity with high doses of riboflavin; no UL has been set.

8.9 Niacin's coenzymes function in many synthetic reactions, especially fatty-acid synthesis. Rich food sources include seafood, poultry, meats, peanuts, and enriched or fortified grains. Pellagra, the disease of niacin deficiency, results in dermatitis, diarrhea, dementia, and, eventually, death. Megadoses of niacin have been used to lower blood lipids, but they cause side effects, such as flushing of the skin.

8.10 Vitamin B-6 coenzymes activate many enzymes of carbohydrate, lipid, and, especially, protein metabolism. They also help synthesize neurotransmitters and participate in homocysteine metabolism. Rich food sources include animal products and enriched or fortified grain products, as well as some fruits and vegetables. A deficiency of vitamin B-6 leads to headaches, depression, gastrointestinal symptoms, skin disorders, nerve problems, anemia, and impaired immunity. Vitamin B-6 toxicity can result in nerve damage.

8.11 Pantothenic acid functions as a coenzyme in reactions that yield energy from carbohydrates, lipids, and protein, as well as fatty-acid synthesis. It is widely distributed among foods, with sunflower seeds, mushrooms, peanuts, and eggs among the richest sources. A deficiency of pantothenic acid is unlikely, but symptoms would be similar to those seen with deficiencies of other B vitamins. There is no known toxicity and no UL for pantothenic acid. Biotin's coenzyme form aids in reactions that synthesize glucose and fatty acids and in the metabolism of amino acids. Egg yolks, peanuts, and cheese provide dietary biotin, but this vitamin is also synthesized by bacteria in the intestines. Consuming raw egg whites may lead to a biotin deficiency because avidin in egg whites binds biotin and reduces its bioavailability. Biotin deficiency can lead to inflammation of the skin and mouth, gastrointestinal symptoms, muscle pain and weakness, poor growth, and anemia. No UL has been set for biotin as no toxicity has ever been observed.

8.12 Folate plays an important role in DNA synthesis and homocysteine metabolism. Symptoms of a deficiency include generally poor cell division in various areas of the body, megaloblastic anemia, tongue inflammation, diarrhea, and poor growth. Pregnancy puts high demands for folate on the body; deficiency during the first month of pregnancy can result in neural tube defects in offspring. A deficiency can also occur in people with alcoholism. Food sources are leafy vegetables, organ meats, and orange juice.

8.13 Vitamin B-12 is needed to metabolize folate and homocysteine, and to maintain the insulation surrounding nerves. Absorption of vitamin B-12 is a complex process that requires a salivary protein, adequate stomach acid production, and an intrinsic factor produced by the stomach. A deficiency, which results in anemia and nerve degeneration, most likely results from poor absorption of vitamin B-12 rather than poor dietary intake. Pernicious anemia is one condition that can impair vitamin B-12 absorption. Vitamin B-12 is found in foods of animal origin, fortified foods, and supplements.

8.14 Vitamin C is a potent antioxidant and functions in the synthesis of collagen, carnitine, and neurotransmitters. A vitamin C deficiency results in scurvy, evidenced by pinpoint hemorrhages in the skin, bleeding gums, and joint pain. Vitamin C also modestly enhances iron absorption. Fresh fruits and vegetables, especially citrus fruits, are good sources. A great amount of vitamin C is lost in storage and cooking; therefore, the diet should emphasize fresh or minimally cooked fruits and vegetables. Deficiencies can occur in people with alcoholism and those whose diets lack sufficient fruits and vegetables. Smoking increases the possibility of vitamin C deficiency. The Upper Level is set at about 20 times adult needs.

8.15 Choline is an essential nutrient but has not yet been classified as a vitamin. As a component of phospholipids, it is important for cell membrane structure, myelination of nerves, and lipid transport. Like folate, choline plays a role in single-carbon metabolism, which has implications for prevention of birth defects, cancer, and heart disease. Egg yolks, meats, dairy products, soybeans, and nuts are good food sources of choline.

8.16 To meet nutrient needs and prevent chronic disease, foods should be emphasized, but dietary supplements can be useful in some circumstances. For example, women of childbearing age, older adults, vegans, and people with malabsorptive diseases are most likely to benefit from dietary supplements. Consumers should educate themselves about possible benefits and risks.

8.17 Given the toll of cancer treatment and lack of a definitive cure, efforts at prevention are key. A variety of dietary changes will reduce your risk for cancer. Start by making sure that your diet is moderate in calorie and fat content and that you consume many fruits and vegetables, whole grain breads and cereals, beans, some fish, and low-fat or fat-free milk products. In addition, remain physically active; avoid obesity; consume alcohol in moderation (if at all); and limit intake of animal fat and salt-cured, smoked, and nitrate-cured foods.

Check Your Knowledge (Answers to the following questions are below)

1. Vitamins are classified as
   a. organic and inorganic.
   b. fat soluble and water soluble.
   c. essential and nonessential.
   d. elements and compounds.

2. A vitamin synthesized by bacteria in the intestine is
   a. A.
   b. D.
   c. E.
   d. K.

3. A deficiency of vitamin A can lead to the disease called
   a. xerophthalmia.
   b. osteomalacia.
   c. scurvy.
   d. pellagra.

4. Vitamin D is called the sunshine vitamin because
   a. it is available in orange juice.
   b. exposure to sunlight converts a precursor into vitamin D.
   c. it can be destroyed by exposure to sunlight.
   d. it is an ingredient in sunscreen.

5. Vitamin E functions as
   a. a coenzyme.
   b. a hormone.
   c. an antioxidant.
   d. a peroxide.

6. Bowed legs, an enlarged and misshapen head, and enlarged knee joints in children are all symptoms of
   a. rickets.
   b. xerophthalmia.
   c. osteoporosis.
   d. vitamin D toxicity.

7. A deficient intake of _____ has been shown to increase the risk of having a baby with a neural tube defect such as spina bifida.
   a. vitamin A
   b. vitamin C
   c. vitamin E
   d. folate

8. Vitamin C is necessary for the production of
   a. stomach acid.
   b. collagen.
   c. insulin.
   d. clotting factors.

9. B vitamins, including thiamin, riboflavin, and niacin, are called the "energy" vitamins because they
   a. can be broken down to provide energy.
   b. are ingredients in energy drinks such as Powerade.
   c. are part of coenzymes needed for release of energy from carbohydrates, fats, and proteins.
   d. are needed in large amounts by competitive athletes.

10. Noodles, spaghetti, and bread are made from wheat flour that is enriched with all of the following nutrients except
    a. vitamin B-6.
    b. thiamin.
    c. niacin.
    d. riboflavin.

11. Which of the B vitamins is sensitive to and can be degraded by light?
    a. Riboflavin
    b. Niacin
    c. Thiamin
    d. Pantothenic acid

12. Niacin can be synthesized in the body from the amino acid
    a. tyrosine.
    b. tryptophan.
    c. phenylalanine.
    d. glutamine.

13. Avidin, a component of raw egg whites, may decrease the absorption of
    a. biotin.
    b. thiamin.
    c. iron.
    d. riboflavin.

14. Choline is an important component of
    a. cholesterol.
    b. an antioxidant.
    c. a phospholipid.
    d. proteins.

15. Which of the following meals is most compatible with American Institute for Cancer Research guidelines for cancer prevention?
    a. Flame-broiled chicken breast, baked potato, and mixed vegetables
    b. Poached salmon, steamed broccoli, and corn on the cob
    c. Baked ham, sweet potato casserole, and spinach salad
    d. Cheese pizza and bread sticks with marinara sauce

Answer Key: 1. b (LO 8.1), 2. d (LO 8.5), 3. a (LO 8.2), 4. b (LO 8.3), 5. c (LO 8.4), 6. a (LO 8.3), 7. d (LO 8.12), 8. b (LO 8.14), 9. c (LO 8.6), 10. a (LO 8.6), 11. a (LO 8.8), 12. b (LO 8.9), 13. a (LO 8.11), 14. c (LO 8.15), 15. b (LO 8.17)

Study Questions (Numbers refer to Learning Outcomes)

1. Why is the risk of toxicity greater with the fat-soluble vitamins A and D than with water-soluble vitamins in general? **(LO 8.1)**

2. Diets rich in phytochemicals have been associated with which protective health benefits? **(LO 8.1)**

3. How would you determine which fruits and vegetables displayed in the produce section of your supermarket are likely to provide plenty of carotenoids? **(LO 8.2)**

4. What is the primary function of the vitamin D hormone? Which groups of people likely need to supplement their diets with vitamin D, and on what do you base your answer? **(LO 8.3)**

5. Describe how vitamin E functions as an antioxidant. **(LO 8.4)**

6. Milling (refining) grains removes which vitamins and minerals? Which of these are replaced during processing? **(LO 8.6)**

7. What are the best food sources for thiamin? **(LO 8.7)**

8. What are the signs of a riboflavin deficiency? **(LO 8.8)**

9. Describe the three signs of the niacin deficiency pellagra. **(LO 8.9)**

10. Describe how the RDA, DV, and UL for vitamin B-6 should be used in everyday life. **(LO 8.10)**

11. How is pantothenic acid involved in energy metabolism? **(LO 8.11)**

12. Why does the consumption of raw eggs lead to a biotin deficiency? **(LO 8.11)**

13. Why does FDA limit the amount of folate that may be included in supplements and fortified foods? **(LO 8.12)**

14. Is it necessary for North Americans to consume a great excess of vitamin C to avoid the possibility of a deficiency? Do vitamin C intakes well above the RDA have any negative consequences? **(LO 8.14)**

15. Why is choline not considered a vitamin? **(LO 8.15)**

What the Dietitian Chose

Who does not occasionally yearn for more energy? In our fast-paced society, it is not surprising that energy supplements are the fastest-growing segment of the supplement industry. Products marketed as energy boosters typically contain at least 100% of the DV of the B vitamins that are involved in energy metabolism. As you learned in Chapter 8, the B vitamins function as coenzymes in chemical reactions that yield usable energy from carbohydrates, fats, and protein. However, taking B vitamins *alone* will not give you any energy. To obtain energy, you must also take in adequate calories. Furthermore, supplemental B vitamins will only enhance energy metabolism if they compensate for a pre-existing deficiency. If your current B vitamin status is adequate, you will not gain any extra energy. How is your current B vitamin status? How much, if any, should you take? Are there other ingredients that can help to boost your energy level? Let us take a closer look at our options.

The 5-Hour Energy shot catches your eye because it promises a quick, convenient boost of energy with fewer calories (it is artificially sweetened) than full-size energy drinks. This product provides 188% of the DV of niacin, 2353% of the DV for vitamin B-6, and 20,833% of the DV for vitamin B-12! In addition, 5-Hour Energy contains a proprietary *energy blend*, which includes several stimulant ingredients (e.g., caffeine and citicholine) and amino acids that are purported to enhance physical and mental performance.

Do you need that much niacin, vitamin B-6, and vitamin B-12? If your current B vitamin status is adequate, taking these B vitamins will offer no boost of energy. On the other hand, if your usual intake of B vitamins is poor, this product could optimize your B vitamin status and thereby enhance energy metabolism. Beyond your body's needs, however, excess water-soluble vitamins will be excreted in urine. In addition, the

B vitamins are highly interdependent. Consuming unbalanced quantities of B vitamins could prevent them from working together properly in energy-yielding metabolic processes. Recognize that the high dose of niacin in this product has been known to cause uncomfortable symptoms of flushing in sensitive individuals.

Experts agree that caffeine provides most of the kick from an energy shot. Presently, energy shot makers are not required to disclose their products' caffeine content on the supplement facts label, but on its website, 5-Hour Energy volunteers that each shot contains around 200 milligrams of caffeine. You should be cautious if using energy shots alongside coffee or other caffeinated drinks. Excess caffeine can cause nervousness, trouble sleeping, nausea, vomiting, rapid heartbeats, and higher blood pressure. The mix of other ingredients in energy shots, such as the taurine, tyrosine, and phenylalanine in 5-Hour Energy, are cause for concern; there is currently not enough research on how they react together.

Finally, note that 5-Hour Energy provides no energy! The metabolic reactions that involve the coenzyme form of these B vitamins require some carbohydrates, fats, or proteins to generate energy. Therefore, even though this small shot has as much caffeine as a 12-ounce cup of coffee and 20 times the Daily Value of vitamin B-6, it still does not have the necessary source of sustained energy: calories.

Leaving behind the proprietary energy blend of the energy shot, let us take a look at a B-complex. The product label for Nature Made® B-Complex with Vitamin C claims that it *"helps convert food into energy."* The supplement facts panel reveals that it contains a variable amount of nutrients related to the recommended Daily Values. As with the 5-Hour Energy Shot, the B vitamins in this supplement can assist the chemical reactions that generate energy but only in the presence of adequate carbohydrates, fats, and/or proteins. The B-complex will not enhance energy levels in a person who already has adequate B vitamin status. The quantities of B vitamins in this product exceed human needs; much of it will be excreted. Unless there is a specific medical need, it is not necessary to supplement with more than 100% of the DV for any nutrient. Bluntly stated, you will be flushing your hard-earned cash down the toilet!

These megadoses of B vitamins are not necessary, but what if you would like a simple backup plan for days when your dietary intake is less than adequate? In this case, a balanced multivitamin-mineral supplement providing no more than 100% of the DV for nutrients is a prudent idea. The Centrum® product shown here claims to support energy and metabolism by providing B vitamins and iron (see Chapter 9), plus it contains a full array of essential vitamins and minerals needed for other aspects of overall health. With this product, you can meet (but not exceed) your needs for nutrients involved in energy metabolism. Keep in mind, for the majority of the healthy population, studies show that there is no overall benefit of taking multivitamin-mineral supplements.[14] Such products are most valuable for people who do not meet their nutrient requirements from food sources.

Although a deficiency of B vitamins theoretically can affect your energy levels, typical American diets supply ample B vitamins. Good animal sources are fish, poultry, meat, eggs, and dairy products. Leafy green vegetables, lentils, beans, peas, and whole grains are rich plant sources of B vitamins. Recall that grain products are enriched with thiamin, niacin, riboflavin, and folate. Fortified breakfast cereals are especially rich sources of B vitamins and many other micronutrients. If you consume a diet consistent with the Dietary Guidelines, you will likely meet your daily needs for B vitamins.

Try to gain perspective on some other factors that may be draining you of energy. Lack of sleep is a likely culprit for busy college students who try to balance school, work, and a social life. Besides B vitamin status, other common dietary causes for fatigue include inadequate calories and poor iron status. High levels of stress and a sedentary lifestyle could also leave you feeling tired. To boost energy levels naturally:

- Eat several small meals throughout the day rather than three large ones.
- Avoid large amounts of sugar and saturated fat.
- Do not skip meals, especially breakfast.
- Take a quick physical activity break, such as a short walk.
- Exercise regularly.
- Reduce stress.
- Get 7 to 9 hours sleep each night.

Nature Made® B-Complex w/Vitamin C

Supplement Facts

Serving Size 1 Caplet
Serving Per Container 100

	Amount Per Serving	% Daily Value
Vitamin C	300 mg	333%
Thiamin	15 mg	1250%
Riboflavin	10.2 mg	785%
Niacin	50 mg	313%
Vitamin B$_6$	5 mg	294%
Pantothenic Acid	10 mg	200%

5-Hour Energy Shot®

Supplement Facts

Serving Size 1.93 fl. oz.
Serving Per Container 1

	Amount Per Serving	% Daily Value
Niacin	30 mg	188%
Vitamin B$_6$	40 mg	2353%
Folic Acid	400 mcg	100%
Vitamin B$_{12}$	500 mcg	20833%
Sodium	18 mg	<1%

Other ingredients: Taurine, Glucuronic acid, Malic Acid, N-Acetyl L-Tyrosine, L-Phenylalanine, Caffeine, Citicholine

Centrum® Adult Multivitamin and Mineral Supplement

Supplement Facts

Serving Size 1 Tablet
Serving Per Container 100

	Amount Per Serving	% Daily Value
Vitamin A	1060 mcg	118%
Vitamin C	60 mg	67%
Vitamin D	10 mcg	50%
Vitamin E	30 mg	200%
Vitamin K	25 mcg	31%
Thiamin	1.5 mg	100%
Riboflavin	1.7 mg	100%
Niacin	20 mg	100%
Vitamin B$_6$	2 mg	100%
Folate	400 mcg	100%
Vitamin B$_{12}$	6 mcg	100%
Biotin	30 mcg	10%
Pantothenic Acid	10 mg	100%
Calcium	200 mg	20%
Iron	18 mg	100%
Phosphorus	20 mg	2%
Iodine	150 mcg	100%
Magnesium	50 mg	13%
Zinc	11 mg	73%
Selenium	55 mcg	79%

Further Readings

1. Fulgoni VL III and others: Foods, fortificants, and supplements: Where do Americans get their nutrients? *J Nutri* 2011; 141:1847.

2. Webb D: Vitamin D and cancer—evidence suggests this vital nutrient may cut risk. *Today's Dietitian* 2012; 14(10):58.

3. Keller M: Vitamin D deficiency in children. *Today's Dietitian* 2012; 14(12):26.

4. Wagner CL and others: Prevention of rickets and vitamin D deficiency in infants, children, and adolescents. *Pediatrics* 2008; 122(5):1142.

5. Office of Dietary Supplements, National Institutes of Health: *Dietary supplement fact sheet: Vitamin D.* Updated February 11, 2016. http://ods .od.nih.gov/factsheets/vitamind

6. Fortmann SP and others: Vitamin and mineral supplements in the primary prevention of cardiovascular disease and cancer: An updated systematic evidence review for the US Preventive Services Task Force. *Ann Intern Med* 2013; 159.12.

7. National Institutes of Health Clinical Center's Drug-Nutrient Interaction Task Force: *Important information to know when you are taking: Coumadin and vitamin K.* Updated September 5, 2012. http://www.cc.nih.gov/ccc/patient_education/drug_nutrient/coumadin1.pdf

8. Office of Dietary Supplements, National Institutes of Health: *Dietary supplement fact sheet: Vitamin B-6 fact sheet.* Updated September 15, 2011. http://ods.od.nih.gov/factsheets/vitaminb6

9. Krider KS, and others: Folic acid food fortification—its history, effect, concerns and future. *Nutrients* 2011; (3):370.

10. Office of Dietary Supplements, National Institutes of Health: *Dietary supplement fact sheet: Vitamin B-12 fact sheet.* Updated February 11, 2016. http://ods.od.nih.gov/factsheets/vitaminb12

11. Linus Pauling Institute: Oregon State University, Micronutrient: Information Center. *Choline.* Updated 2017. http://lpi.oregonstate.edu/mic/other-nutrients/choline#neural-tube-defects-prevention

12. Office of Dietary Supplements, National Institutes of Health: *Dietary supplements: What you need to know.* Updated June 17, 2011. https://ods.od.nih.gov/HealthInformation/DS_WhatYouNeedToKnow.aspx

13. ADA Reports: Position of the American Dietetic Association: Nutrient supplementation. *J Am Diet Assoc* 2009; 109:2073.

14. Kushi LH and others: American Cancer Society guidelines on nutrition and physical activity for cancer prevention: Reducing the risk of cancer with healthy food choices and physical activity. *CA Cancer J Clin* 2012; 62:30.

connect To get the most out of your study, visit Connect where you will find NutritionCalc Plus, SmartBook®, and many other dynamic tools.

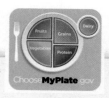

Rate Your Plate

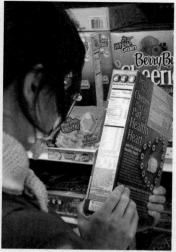

©McGraw-Hill Education/Andrew Resek, photographer

Throughout this book, you see breakfast cereals described as enriched, fortified, cold, or ready to eat. What do these terms mean?

The cereal you pour out of the box, add milk to, and enjoy is called ready-to-eat or cold cereal. Any addition of nutrients to a food product is called fortification. In the United States, the FDA strictly defines enrichment, which is a special type of fortification of refined grain products. Per pound of flour, all refined grains must contain at least 2.9 milligrams of thiamin, 1.8 milligrams of riboflavin, 24 milligrams of niacin, 0.7 milligrams of folic acid, and 20 milligrams of iron. Enrichment replaces some (but not all) of the nutrients lost during the milling of grains.

You can tell if a product is fortified by reading the Nutrition Facts Panel. See for yourself in the following table. **Cereal A** has been enriched to levels mandated by the FDA. **Cereal B,** the enriched or fortified choice, contains 100% of the DV for select vitamins and minerals, especially the B vitamins and iron. While all refined grain products are enriched with thiamin, riboflavin, niacin, folic acid, and iron, many food manufacturers choose to fortify their products with additional nutrients. In this book, when we refer to fortified breakfast cereals, we are referring to this latter group of food products.

Nutrient	Cereal A (1 ounce) % DV	Cereal B (1 ounce) % DV	Your Favorite Cereal % DV	Nutrient	Cereal A (1 ounce) % DV	Cereal B (1 ounce) % DV	Your Favorite Cereal % DV
Vitamin A	25	15		Niacin	25	100	
Vitamin C	25	100		Vitamin B-6	25	100	
Calcium	0	0		Folic acid	25	100	
Iron	50	100		Pantothenic acid	—*	100	
Vitamin D	10	10		Phosphorus	4	4	
Vitamin E	25	100		Magnesium	—*	4	
Thiamin	25	100		Zinc	—*	100	
Riboflavin	25	100					

*Information not provided on label.

Locate a nutrition facts panel for one of your favorite breakfast cereals. In the blank spaces in the table, record the % DV for each nutrient provided by one serving. If some data are missing, fill in the blanks with an asterisk. Based on your observations, answer the following questions.

1. Is your favorite cereal fortified? How can you tell?

   _____

   _____

2. Examine the calorie, saturated fat, and sugar content listed on your Nutrition Facts panel. How does the cereal compare to the recommendations of the Dietary Guidelines for Americans and other health authorities to limit calories, saturated fat, and added sugars?

   _____

   _____

3. Which special population groups can especially benefit from daily use of a fortified breakfast cereal?

   _____

   _____

4. What could you eat with your breakfast cereal to build a meal that resembles MyPlate?

   _____

   _____

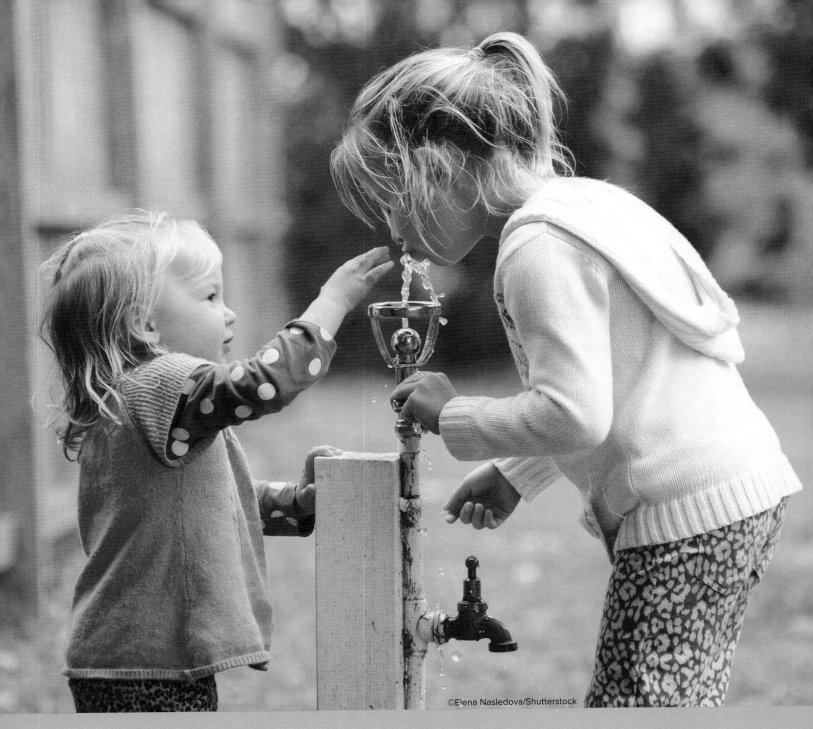

©Elena Nasledova/Shutterstock

Student Learning Outcomes

Chapter 9 is designed to allow you to:

9.1 Understand the functions of water in the body, the regulation of fluid balance, and the health consequences of fluid imbalance; list recommended intakes and sources of water.

9.2 Describe the general characteristics of the major and trace minerals, mineral absorption and storage, the dangers of mineral toxicities, and ways to preserve minerals in foods.

9.3 Describe the roles of sodium in controlling fluid balance, acid–base balance, and nerve impulse transmission and list its dietary sources and requirements, as well as the dangers of exceeding sodium recommendations.

9.4 List the functions, dietary sources, and requirements of potassium, as well as the dangers of getting too much potassium.

9.5 List the functions of chloride, as well as its dietary sources and requirements.

9.6 List the dietary sources and requirements of calcium, and describe its role in bone growth, maintenance and repair, as well as the process of osteoporosis development and prevention.

9.7 Describe the functions, dietary requirements, and sources of phosphorus, as well as the benefit of avoiding too much phosphorus.

9.8 List magnesium functions and sources, as well as the dangers of magnesium toxicity from nonfood sources.

Chapter 9
Water and Minerals

What Would You Choose?

Water is the best choice for everyday hydration: it quenches thirst without calories. There are currently many "water" choices available. Do you need water that contains vitamins and minerals? What's the difference between spring water and mineral water? Is bottled water safer to drink than tap water? As you peruse store shelves, which is the healthiest choice to take along to the student recreation center for your workout?

a Reusable bottle filled with tap water

b Aquafina® Pure Water

c S. Pellegrino® Mineral Water

d Vitaminwater®

Think about your choice as you read this chapter, then see What the Dietitian Chose at the end of the chapter.

Water (H_2O)—the most abundant molecule in the human body and the most versatile medium for a variety of chemical reactions—constitutes the major portion of the human body. Without water, biological processes necessary to life would cease in a matter of days. We must replenish water regularly because the body does not store it *per se*. Fluids must be consumed daily to replenish what is lost through respiration (lungs), perspiration (skin), and excretion (urine and feces). We recognize this constant demand for water as thirst, but the body has several intricate mechanisms to ensure fluid conservation. Maintenance of fluid balance relies on strict control of levels of dissolved minerals inside and outside the cells. These dissolved minerals—sodium, chloride, potassium, and phosphorus—are called electrolytes. Not only do they regulate the distribution of water throughout the body, they are also involved in maintenance of acid–base balance and in the conduction of nerve impulses. In this chapter, you will learn about the importance of water and how the electrolytes work together to regulate fluid balance, acid–base balance, and nerve function.

Like water, many minerals are vital to health. They are considered inorganic because they are typically not bonded to carbon atoms. In addition to water balance, minerals are key participants in body metabolism, muscle movement, body growth, and other wide-ranging processes (Fig. 9-1). We also know that some mineral deficiencies can cause severe health problems.

9.9 Describe the functions of iron in the maintenance of blood health, and list its sources, dietary requirements, and deficiency and toxicity problems.

9.10 Describe the functions of zinc, including its role in immune function, as well as its food sources, dietary requirements, and signs and symptoms of deficiency and toxicity.

9.11 Summarize the functions of selenium, and describe its dietary requirements, food sources, and symptoms of deficiency, as well as the dangers of toxicity from supplements.

9.12 Describe the functions of iodine in thyroid metabolism, and list its sources, dietary requirements, and problems of deficiency and toxicity.

9.13 Describe the functions of copper and its potential for toxicity, and list its sources, dietary requirements, and conditions that can lead to a deficiency.

9.14 Describe the role of fluoride in tooth development and bone health, and list its primary sources, as well as recommendations for use and problems of toxicity.

9.15 Describe the functions of chromium in glucose metabolism, and list its sources, dietary requirements, and deficiency symptoms.

9.16 Describe the functions of manganese and molybdenum, and understand how to get enough from dietary sources.

9.17 Describe factors that can contribute to the development of hypertension.

FIGURE 9-1 ▶ Water and minerals are involved in many processes in the body.
©Sam Edwards/age fotostock

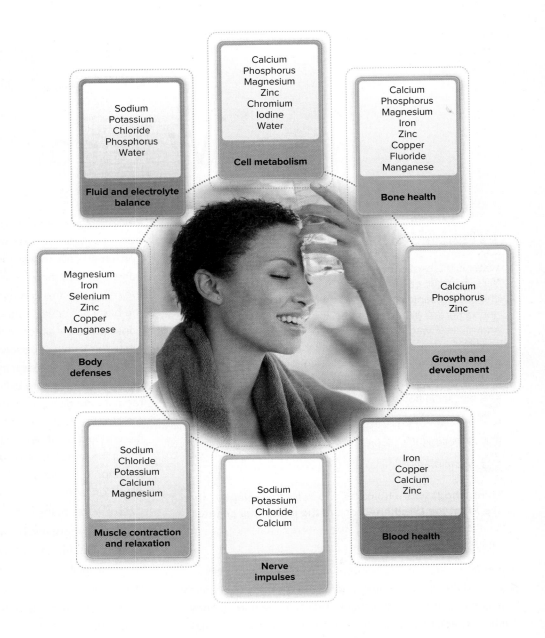

Sodium
Potassium
Chloride
Phosphorus
Water

Fluid and electrolyte balance

Calcium
Phosphorus
Magnesium
Zinc
Chromium
Iodine
Water

Cell metabolism

Calcium
Phosphorus
Magnesium
Iron
Zinc
Copper
Fluoride
Manganese

Bone health

Magnesium
Iron
Selenium
Zinc
Copper
Manganese

Body defenses

Calcium
Phosphorus
Zinc

Growth and development

Sodium
Chloride
Potassium
Calcium
Magnesium

Muscle contraction and relaxation

Sodium
Potassium
Chloride
Calcium

Nerve impulses

Iron
Copper
Calcium
Zinc

Blood health

WHERE'S THE WATER?

The percentage of water varies tremendously between tissues. For example, muscle is 73% water, adipose tissue is 10% to 20% water, and bone contains approximately 20% water. As the fat content of the body increases, the percentage of lean decreases, and subsequently, the percentage of body water decreases. When body composition measurements are performed on extremely lean athletes, the percentage of body water will be around 70%.

solvent A liquid substance in which other substances dissolve.

9.1 Water

Life as we know it could not exist without water. Every cell, tissue, and organ contains some water. Overall, water comprises 50% to 70% of the human body (Fig. 9-2). Indeed, water is essential for life. While humans can live for several weeks without food, we cannot survive for more than a few days without water. The simple H_2O molecule has some amazing properties: it is a versatile solvent, a heat sink, and a lubricant (Fig. 9-3). As detailed in the next few sections, these properties make water uniquely suited to carry out a number of essential roles in the human body.

WATER IS THE UNIVERSAL SOLVENT

Water is often called the "universal **solvent**" because so many different solutes can be dissolved in it. This property of water makes it (1) an ideal transport vehicle for nutrients and wastes and (2) a medium for many chemical reactions of human metabolism.

Water Transports Nutrients and Wastes. The majority of the nutrients we consume—carbohydrates, proteins, minerals, and many vitamins—are water soluble. Lipids, although they are not soluble in water, can be surrounded by a layer of water-soluble protein so that they can be dispersed throughout the water-based environment within and around cells and tissues (recall Chapter 5). As the primary component of blood and lymph, water acts to transport nutrients to all the cells of the body.

The metabolism of nutrients generates some waste products, most of which can dissolve in water and exit the body as part of urine. For example, when proteins are broken down as fuel, the nitrogen portion of amino acids cannot be used for energy production. Recall from Chapter 6 that the liver converts these nitrogenous waste products into urea. In addition, when we consume more than we need of some nutrients, such as sodium, the excess can be dissolved in water and excreted in urine. Typical urine output is about 1 liter per day, depending mostly on our intakes of fluid, protein, and sodium.

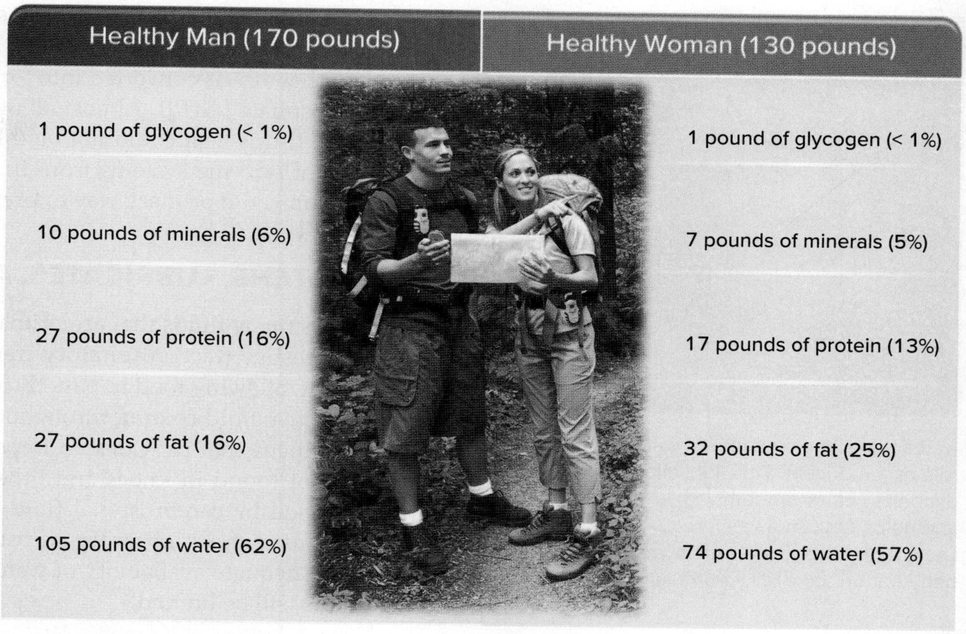

Healthy Man (170 pounds)	Healthy Woman (130 pounds)
1 pound of glycogen (< 1%)	1 pound of glycogen (< 1%)
10 pounds of minerals (6%)	7 pounds of minerals (5%)
27 pounds of protein (16%)	17 pounds of protein (13%)
27 pounds of fat (16%)	32 pounds of fat (25%)
105 pounds of water (62%)	74 pounds of water (57%)

FIGURE 9-2 ▲ Although the percentages vary for men and women, the main constituent of the body is water. ©Digital Vision/Getty Images

Water Is a Medium for Chemical Reactions. Because so many compounds dissolve in water, it provides a medium in which chemical reactions take place in the body. Furthermore, water itself (H_2O) is an important participant in many chemical reactions. When carbohydrates, lipids, and proteins are metabolized as sources of energy, water is one of the by-products. In fact, this **metabolic water** (1 cup or more per day) contributes to the maintenance of fluid balance in the body.

metabolic water Water formed as a by-product of carbohydrate, lipid, and protein metabolism.

WATER CONTRIBUTES TO BODY TEMPERATURE REGULATION

Water temperature changes slowly because water has a great ability to hold heat. It takes much more energy to heat water than it does to heat air. Water molecules are polar (charged), so they are attracted to each other. This attractive force is strong, and energy is required to separate the water molecules as water is heated. Because the human body is 50% to 70% water (see Fig. 9-2), it takes a lot of energy to change body temperature.

When overheated, the body secretes fluids in the form of perspiration, which evaporates through skin pores. As water evaporates from the skin, heat energy is released. So, as perspiration evaporates, heat energy is removed from the skin, cooling the body in the process (Fig. 9-4). In response to an increased body temperature, blood vessels in the skin become larger, allowing greater water loss through perspiration. Each quart (approximately 1 liter or 2 pounds) of perspiration that evaporates represents approximately 600 kilocalories of energy lost from the skin and surrounding tissues.

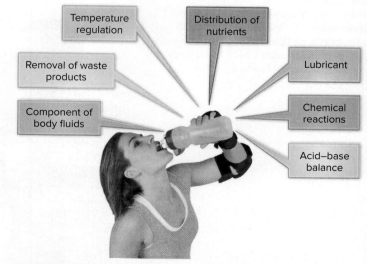

FIGURE 9-3 ▲ Water has many essential functions in the body.
©Ingram Publishing/Fotosearch

When carbohydrates, lipids, and proteins are used by cells in the body, energy is released in the form of heat. About 60% of the chemical energy in food is turned into body heat; the other 40% is converted into forms of energy that cells can use (principally adenosine triphosphate [ATP]). Almost all of that energy eventually leaves the body in the form of heat. If this heat could not be dissipated, the body temperature would rise enough to prevent enzyme systems from functioning efficiently, ultimately leading to death. Perspiration is the primary way to prevent this rise in body temperature.

WATER MOISTENS, LUBRICATES, AND CUSHIONS

The body secretes many fluids that are primarily water. Water-based secretions are produced by the digestive tract, respiratory tract, urogenital tract, eyes, and skin. Saliva acts as a lubricant, allowing food to pass through the esophagus to the stomach. Mucus provides a protective fluid coating throughout the digestive tract. The lungs are coated with a layer of mucus that provides an important immunologic function. Water helps form the lubricant found in knees and other joints of the body. The spinal cord and brain are cushioned by cerebrospinal fluid. Water is also the basis of amniotic fluid, which functions as a shock absorber surrounding the growing fetus in the mother's womb. Without adequate availability of water, the ability of the body to produce these critical secretions will be limited.

THE WATER BALANCING ACT

You have just learned about the many functions of water in the human body. Despite its critical importance for human survival, however, water is not stored in the body. It is continually lost through respiration (lungs), perspiration (skin), and excretion (urine and feces). Through mechanisms that monitor blood pressure and the concentration of solutes in body fluids, the nervous, endocrine, digestive, and urinary systems work elegantly together to maintain fluid balance and support life.

Water Intake. The Adequate Intake (AI) for *total* water is 2.7 liters (11 cups) for adult women and 3.7 liters (15 cups) for adult men. This amount is based primarily on average water intake from fluids and foods. For *fluid* alone, this corresponds to about 2.2 liters (9 cups) for women and about 3 liters (13 cups) for men.

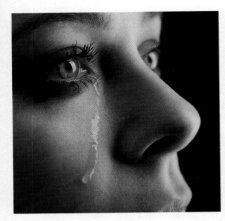

▲ Tears are one example of water's role as a lubricant. This fluid allows the eyeball to move smoothly in its socket and helps to flush away foreign particles. Lack of tear production is a symptom of dehydration. ©Danil Chepko/123RF

Should you feed a fever? Fever is an increase in body temperature caused by an immune response. When you have a fever, you do need more energy. For every increase of 1°F (0.5°C) in internal temperature above normal, your basal metabolic rate (BMR) increases by 7%. Although BMR is elevated for a person with a fever, physical activity will likely be lower than normal, which lowers overall energy needs. Thus, having a fever is not a reason to overeat.

FIGURE 9-4 ▶ Body temperature is reduced when heat is transported from the body through the bloodstream to the surface of the skin. As perspiration evaporates from the surface of the skin, heat is dissipated. This cools the blood, which circulates back to the body, reducing body temperature.

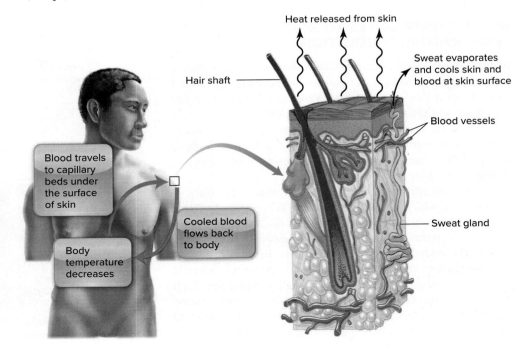

Heat released from skin

Hair shaft

Sweat evaporates and cools skin and blood at skin surface

Blood vessels

Sweat gland

Blood travels to capillary beds under the surface of skin

Cooled blood flows back to body

Body temperature decreases

Fluid intake—including water, fruit juice, coffee, tea, soft drinks, milk, and even alcoholic beverages—makes the biggest contribution to our total water needs. For the woman in Figure 9-5, fluid intake adds up to about 9 cups. In addition, nearly all foods contain water. Many fruits and vegetables are more than 80% water, and many meats contain at least 50% water (Fig. 9-6). In Figure 9-5, water from foods supplies another 2 cups. As mentioned previously, the body produces 250 to 350 milliliters (1 to 1½ cups) of water each day as a by-product of the chemical reactions used to metabolize energy. For the woman in Figure 9-5, metabolic water amounts to 1.25 cups. However, the amount of metabolic water produced can double in physically active people.

Water Output. Usually, urinary excretion of water accounts for the greatest source of output. The daily amount of urine produced may vary based on intake of fluids, protein, and sodium, but average urinary water loss per day is approximately 1650 milliliters (7 ½ cups). Removal of waste products requires at least 500 milliliters (2 cups) of urine production per day. Urine output consistently below this level is often a sign of chronic dehydration due to low fluid intake.

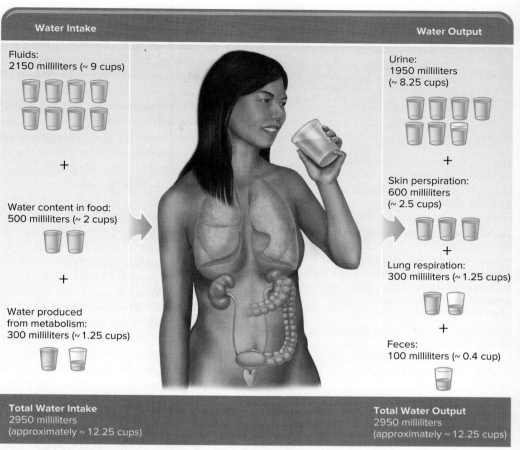

FIGURE 9-5 ▲ Estimate of water balance—intake versus output—in a woman. We primarily maintain body fluids at an optimum amount by adjusting water output to intake. As you can see with this woman, most water comes from the liquids we consume. Some comes from the moisture in foods, and the remainder is manufactured during metabolism. Water output includes that lost via urine, skin, lungs, and feces.

Water is lost through the skin in the form of perspiration. On days of low physical activity, these losses amount to about 1 liter. Under hot, humid conditions or with strenuous physical activity, losses can be much greater than 1 liter per day. Some water is also lost from the lungs in the form of water vapor in exhaled air. Together with

MyPlate: Sources of Water

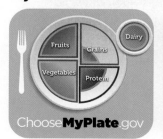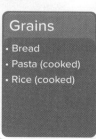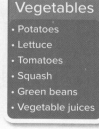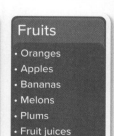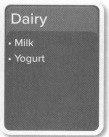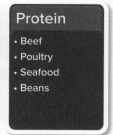

FIGURE 9-6 ▲ Sources of water from MyPlate. The fill of the background color (none, 1/3, 2/3, or completely covered) within each group on the plate indicates the average nutrient density for water in that group. Overall, the vegetables, fruits, dairy, and protein groups contain many foods that are nutrient-dense sources of water. Although not depicted on MyPlate, all beverages are nearly 100% water. Fats and oils, on the other hand, have almost no water.

Source: United States Department of Agriculture, ChooseMyPlate.gov

perspiration, the fluid lost through lung respiration is sometimes called "insensible" water loss because it is difficult to measure.

A relatively small amount of water is lost daily in the feces. About 8000 milliliters (34 cups) of water enter the digestive tract daily through secretions from the mouth, stomach, intestine, pancreas, and other organs, in addition to the variable amount of water ingested in the form of foods and fluids. When we consider the large amount of water used to lubricate the digestive tract, the loss of only 100 milliliters (½ cup) of water each day through the feces is remarkable. The small intestine absorbs most of this water, while the colon takes up a lesser but still important amount. The kidneys also greatly conserve water. They can reabsorb as much as 97% of the water filtered each day. The volumes of water intake and output shown in Figure 9-5 are estimates. Caffeine and alcohol intake, ambient temperature, humidity, altitude, and physical activity will influence water loss.

Fluid Conservation. The blood pressure and the concentration of solutes in the blood are closely monitored by receptors in the kidneys, blood vessels, and brain. Once the body registers a shortage of available water, it increases fluid conservation (Fig. 9-7). Hormones that participate in this process are **antidiuretic hormone (ADH), angiotensin,** and **aldosterone.** The pituitary gland, located in the brain, senses the concentration of solutes in the blood. When blood concentration of solutes is high, the pituitary gland releases ADH. The kidneys respond to ADH by reducing urine production and output. ADH also causes blood vessel constriction, which acts to raise blood pressure. Meanwhile, the kidneys possess receptors that monitor blood pressure. Low blood pressure triggers the release of an enzyme that activates angiotensin and, eventually, aldosterone, two hormones that signal the kidneys to retain more sodium and, in turn, more water via osmosis. As sodium and water are retained, blood pressure increases back to normal.

antidiuretic hormone A hormone secreted by the pituitary gland when blood concentration of solutes is high. It causes the kidneys to decrease water excretion, which increases blood volume.

angiotensin A hormone produced by the liver and activated by enzymes from the kidneys. It signals the adrenal glands to produce aldosterone and also directs the kidneys to conserve sodium (and therefore water). Both of these actions have the effect of increasing blood volume.

aldosterone A hormone produced by the adrenal glands when blood volume is low. It acts on the kidneys to conserve sodium (and therefore water) to increase blood volume.

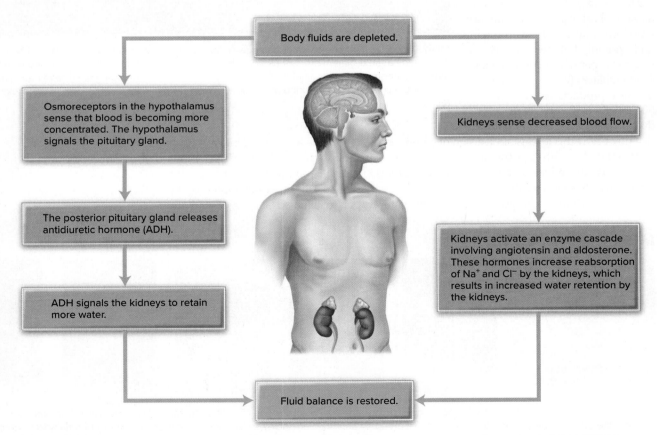

FIGURE 9-7 ▲ When body fluids are depleted, hormonal signals from the pituitary gland and the kidneys work together to increase fluid retention by the kidneys and thereby restore fluid balance.

Dehydration. Despite mechanisms that work to conserve water, fluid continues to be lost via the feces, skin, and lungs. Those losses must be replaced. In addition, there is a limit to how concentrated urine can become. Eventually, if fluid is not consumed, the body becomes dehydrated and suffers ill effects.

By the time a person loses 1% to 2% of body weight in fluids, he or she will be thirsty (Fig. 9-8). Even this small water deficit can cause one to feel tired and dizzy and to experience headaches. At a 4% loss of body weight, muscles lose significant strength and endurance, and central nervous system function is negatively affected (e.g., memory and reaction time are compromised, and one becomes impatient). By the time body weight is reduced by 10%, heat tolerance is decreased and weakness results. Ultimately, **dehydration** will lead to kidney failure, coma, and death.

Dehydration is a contributing factor to the development of heatstroke, a very serious condition. Performing strenuous physical activity in hot, humid conditions can lead to dehydration and the inability to control body temperature. Heart rate is increased and the skin becomes dry. Unassisted, the individual will become unconscious and die. Adequate fluid intake and, if possible, avoidance of physical activity in hot, humid conditions are the best steps to prevent heat illness.

Another potential consequence of inadequate fluid intake is kidney stones. When urine production is lower than about 500 milliliters per day, the kidneys are forced to form concentrated urine. Heavy ion concentration, in turn, increases the risk of kidney stone formation in susceptible people (generally men). Kidney stones form from minerals and other substances that have precipitated out of the urine and accumulate in the kidney.

The simplest way to determine if water intake is adequate is to observe the urine color (Fig. 9-9). If hydration is adequate, urine should be clear or pale yellow (like pale lemonade or the color of straw); concentrated urine is dark yellow (like apple juice). Urine color can be influenced by consuming supplements (especially some B vitamins), medications, and food. Lots of carrot juice, pumpkin, or winter squash can tint your urine orange. Too many fava beans or too much rhubarb will turn it dark brown. A

dehydration Inadequate intake of water to replace losses.

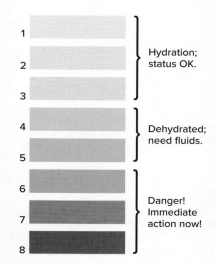

FIGURE 9-9 ▲ Monitoring the color of urine is a good gauge of hydration.

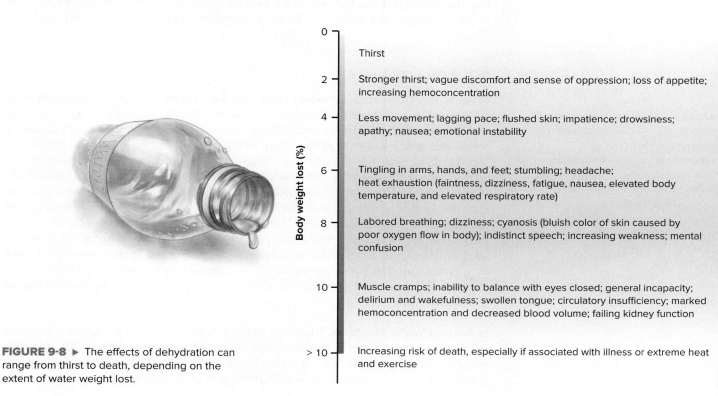

FIGURE 9-8 ▶ The effects of dehydration can range from thirst to death, depending on the extent of water weight lost.

reddish or pinkish urine results from eating too many beets or blackberries. A high intake of asparagus not only makes your urine smell funny but can also turn it a bit green.

Is Thirst a Good Indicator of Hydration Status? If you do not drink enough water, your body soon lets you know by signaling thirst. Your brain is communicating the need to drink. In most cases, drinking fluids in response to the thirst sensation will result in adequate hydration. However, the thirst mechanism can lag behind actual water loss during prolonged exercise and illness. The thirst sensation decreases with age, as well. Sick children, especially those with fever, vomiting, diarrhea, and increased perspiration, and older persons often need to be reminded to drink plenty of fluids.

As you will learn in Chapter 10, athletes need to monitor fluid status. They should weigh themselves before and after training sessions to determine their rate of water loss and, thus, their water needs. The old saying, "A pint's a pound the world around" does not apply here. True, 1 pound of water is 1 pint (2 cups) of water. However, the body can absorb only about 60% of the water consumed. So athletes should drink about 50% more than what they lose through sweat in a workout. Their goal is to consume 2 to 3 cups of fluid for every pound lost.

Can a Person Consume Too Much Water? Even though the kidneys of a healthy person can process up to 15 liters of urine per day, it is possible to drink too much water. As water intake increases above what is needed, kidneys process the excess fluid and excrete dilute urine. If water intake far exceeds the kidneys' processing ability, overhydration and sodium dilution in the blood result. This condition is commonly known as **water intoxication,** or more accurately, **hyponatremia.** Water intoxication can happen to healthy people when they drink a great deal of water in a very short period of time. Endurance athletes exercising for prolonged times, drinking large volumes of water to replace sweat losses, are especially at risk. Rapid dilution of the blood causes tissues to swell. The heartbeat becomes irregular, allowing fluid to enter the lungs; the brain and nerves swell, causing severe headaches, confusion, seizure, and coma. Unless water is restricted and a concentrated salt solution administered under close medical monitoring, the person will die. For endurance athletes and those who labor outdoors for many hours per day, sports drinks can be used to replace electrolytes along with fluids (see Chapter 10).

SOURCES OF WATER

What Is the Difference Between Hard and Soft Water? Water can be classified as either hard or soft. **Hard water** contains relatively high levels of the minerals calcium and magnesium. In North America, 89% of homes have hard water. Naturally occurring **soft water,** which can be high in sodium, is found in the Pacific North and Northwest, New England, South Atlantic-Gulf, and Hawaii. Hard water can be converted into soft water through the use of a commercial water softener. As water travels through the water softener, calcium and magnesium exchange with sodium found in the water softener device. The water that exits the softener has a low calcium and magnesium content; however, the sodium content is increased. The additional intake of sodium from softened water (about 12.5 milligrams per cup) is small compared to typical American intakes of the mineral but could be undesirable for people restricting sodium intake due to **hypertension.** The additional intake of calcium and magnesium afforded by consuming hard water would be more beneficial than increasing sodium intake through the use of softened water.

Is Bottled Water Healthier than Tap Water? Bottled water is a popular alternative to tap water; the latest statistics show that Americans consume 30.8 gallons of bottled water per capita per year. Many people choose bottled water because they believe that it is less likely to be contaminated with pathogens or impurities than tap water. There

---

water intoxication Potentially fatal condition that occurs with a high intake of water, which results in severe dilution of the blood and other fluid compartments.

hyponatremia Dangerously low blood sodium level.

hard water Water that contains high levels of calcium, magnesium, and sometimes iron.

soft water Water that contains little or no calcium or magnesium. Soft water may contain sodium and other minerals.

hypertension High blood pressure. The pressure inside the blood vessels exceeds 140/90 millimeters of mercury.

are some differences in water treatment methods: rather than using chlorine to disinfect water, most bottled water is treated with ozone, which does not impart a flavor to the water. However, the standards for quality and contaminant levels are identical for bottled and tap water. The Environmental Protection Agency regulates and monitors public water supplies, whereas the Food and Drug Administration (FDA) regulates bottled water. Truth be told, much of the bottled water produced in the United States is actually processed municipal tap water.

Beyond the level of contaminants, there are some definite differences between bottled and tap water. As you'll learn in Section 9.14, a small amount of fluoride is added to many municipal water supplies to prevent dental caries. Very few bottled water manufacturers add the mineral fluoride to the water. People who drink primarily bottled water should include regular tap water throughout the day in order to receive the benefits of fluoride. Trips to the drinking fountain or making coffee or tea with tap water should suffice.

Another big difference between bottled water and tap water is the way it is delivered. Tap water travels through pipes into your home, but bottled water requires extra packaging and more costly methods of transport and storage. The large amount of plastic used to package the more than 9 billion gallons of bottled water consumed in America each year creates huge energy use, recycling, and solid waste disposal concerns.

Beyond its impact on the environment, the use of plastics may pose additional threats to human health. Drinking water from a freshly washed or newly opened bottle is fine. But plastic, like the food we eat, has a shelf life. Over time, the chemicals that make up plastic break down and can leach into the liquid inside the container. Temperature, age of the bottle, acidity of the contents, and type of plastic (recycling code) all make a difference. Age of the consumer makes a difference, too, as babies and young children are more susceptible to problems than adults. Table 9-1 lists several guidelines to ensure the safety of the bottled water you drink.

ELECTROLYTES REGULATE FLUID BALANCE

Each cell of the body is surrounded by a membrane that allows water to pass freely through it. Water found inside the cell membrane is part of the **intracellular fluid.** Intracellular fluid accounts for 63% of fluid in the body. The remaining body fluid is found outside of cells in one of two extracellular spaces: (1) the fluid portion of blood (plasma) and lymph, accounting for 7% of body fluid; or (2) the fluid between cells (interstitial), making up 30% of body fluid (Fig. 9-10).

Although water can freely travel into and out of cells across the cell membrane, the body controls the amount of water in the intracellular and extracellular compartments mainly by controlling ion concentrations. **Ions** are minerals that dissolve in water and are either positively (+) or negatively (−) charged. These charged ions allow the

Water that comes out of your refrigerator dispenser or through a filter on your faucet typically runs through a charcoal (carbon) filter. The carbon attracts compounds present in tap water to remove off flavors. Importantly, it does not remove fluoride, a mineral essential to help fight tooth decay.

To find a list of brands of bottled water that contain fluoride, check out the website of the International Bottled Water Association at **http://www.bottledwater .org/fluoride.**

Since the 1930s, BPA has been used to make clear plastic bottles. Unfortunately, this organic compound can leach into a bottle's contents when the plastic is exposed to acidic or hot conditions. BPA is considered an endocrine disrupter. At low doses, it can mimic the body's own hormones. Thus, there is concern about chronic exposure for infants and young children. BPA has been banned for use in Canada and many European countries. In the United States, the FDA has banned the use of BPA in the manufacture of baby bottles and sippy cups. Many manufacturers of reusable water bottles are switching to "BPA free" plastics.

intracellular fluid Fluid contained within a cell; it represents about two-thirds of body fluid.

ion A positively or negatively charged atom.

TABLE 9-1 ■ Guidelines for Safe Use of Water Bottles

1. For repeated use, choose stainless steel bottles.

2. If you choose plastic, look for recycling codes 2 and 4. When these types of plastics break down, they are the least harmful.[1]

3. Avoid bottles with recycling codes 3 and 7 unless they have "BPA free" embedded in the plastic. These hard plastics may contain bisphenyl A (BPA, see margin). If your plastic bottle contains BPA, avoid cleaning it with harsh (i.e., laboratory) detergents or filling it with acidic (e.g., lemonade and fruit juices) or hot beverages.[2]

4. Choose a reusable bottle with a wide mouth so you can easily clean it. Wash and soak it in a sanitizer, such as ¼ teaspoon (4 milliliters) bleach in 1 quart (1 liter) water.

5. When your plastic bottle becomes scratched or cracked, throw it away. Bacteria can grow inside.

6. Do not store your containers of water in a hot garage or in the back of your hot car. The heat quickly breaks down the plastic. If a bottle has been exposed to heat, pitch the water and recycle the bottle.

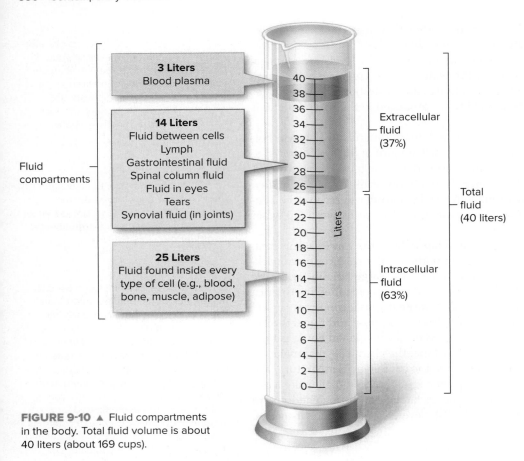

3 Liters
Blood plasma

14 Liters
Fluid between cells
Lymph
Gastrointestinal fluid
Spinal column fluid
Fluid in eyes
Tears
Synovial fluid (in joints)

25 Liters
Fluid found inside every
type of cell (e.g., blood,
bone, muscle, adipose)

Fluid
compartments

Extracellular
fluid
(37%)

Total
fluid
(40 liters)

Intracellular
fluid
(63%)

Liters

FIGURE 9-10 ▲ Fluid compartments
in the body. Total fluid volume is about
40 liters (about 169 cups).

electrolyte A mineral that separates into
positively or negatively charged ions
in water. They are able to transmit an
electrical current.

extracellular fluid Fluid found outside
the cells; it represents about one-third of
body fluid.

osmosis The passage of water through
a membrane from a less concentrated
compartment to a more concentrated
compartment.

isotonic Having equal concentration of
solutes.

hypertonic Having high concentration
of solutes.

hypotonic Having low concentration of
solutes.

transfer of electrical current, so they
are called **electrolytes.** Four electrolytes predominate: sodium (Na^+) and
chloride (Cl^-) are primarily found in
the **extracellular fluid,** and potassium (K^+) and phosphate (PO_4^-) are
the principal electrolytes in the intracellular fluid.

The term **osmosis** is used to
describe the passage of water through
a membrane from an area of lower
electrolyte concentration to an area
of higher electrolyte concentration.
Where ions move, water follows pas-
sively. Under normal conditions,
the concentration of electrolytes on
either side of the cell membrane is
controlled in such a way that the
intracellular fluid and extracellular fluid are **isotonic.** Thus, water
movement into and out of the cell is
in equilibrium (Fig. 9-11). However,
if the intracellular concentration
of electrolytes is greater than the
extracellular concentration—that is,
hypertonic—water will flow freely
into the cell. If too much water flows
in, the cell can burst, similar to filling a balloon with too much air. The
opposite can also occur. When the
intracellular concentration of electrolytes is relatively low or **hypotonic** compared to
the extracellular environment, water will exit the cell, leading to cell shrinkage.

The principle of osmosis is used by the digestive tract to absorb water from the colon.
Water from beverages, foods, and intestinal tract secretions makes the contents of the
intestinal tract high in water as it enters the colon from the small intestine. Cells that
line the colon lumen (inside the colon) actively absorb sodium. Water follows sodium,
causing a large amount of water to be absorbed from the colon. As a result, daily water
loss from feces is low—approximately 100 milliliters (0.5 cup).

During illness, when large volumes of fluid are lost through vomiting and diarrhea,
osmosis can lead to a life-threatening condition. Fluid losses from the gastrointestinal
tract result in an increased concentration of electrolytes in the extracellular space.
As intracellular water exits the cells in an attempt to dilute the extracellular fluid,
cells shrink and lose their ability to function normally. In the heart, this imbalance
can lead to a decreased ability of the heart to pump blood and, ultimately, to cardiac
failure. Infants and older adults are particularly susceptible to the effects of severe
dehydration.

✓ CONCEPT CHECK 9.1

1. Why is it significant that water is the "universal solvent"?
2. Describe how water regulates body temperature.
3. Provide two examples of water's role as a lubricant.
4. List the components of water intake and water output.
5. What is the AI for fluid intake for adult men? For adult women?

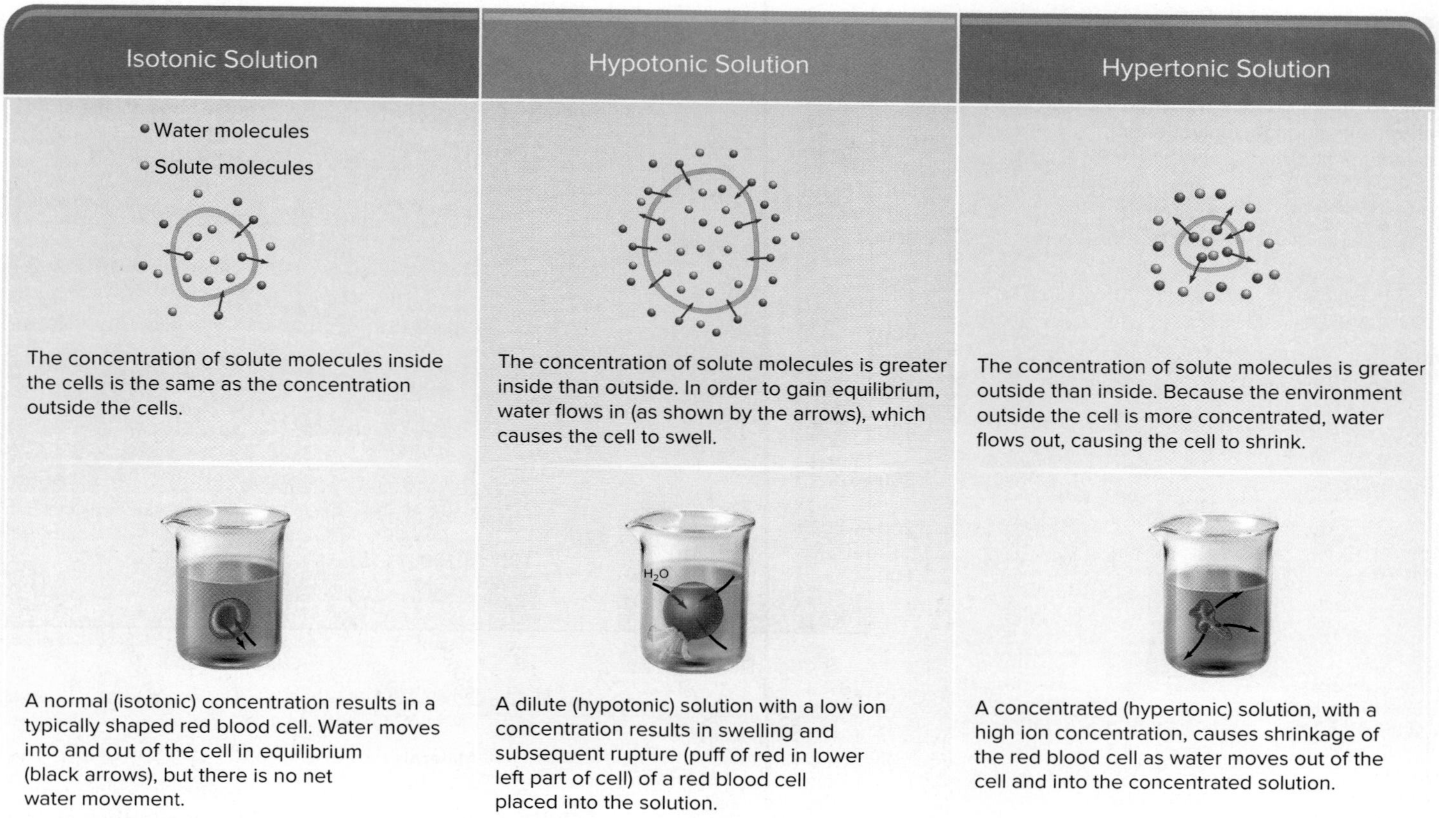

Isotonic Solution	Hypotonic Solution	Hypertonic Solution

• Water molecules
• Solute molecules

The concentration of solute molecules inside the cells is the same as the concentration outside the cells.

The concentration of solute molecules is greater inside than outside. In order to gain equilibrium, water flows in (as shown by the arrows), which causes the cell to swell.

The concentration of solute molecules is greater outside than inside. Because the environment outside the cell is more concentrated, water flows out, causing the cell to shrink.

A normal (isotonic) concentration results in a typically shaped red blood cell. Water moves into and out of the cell in equilibrium (black arrows), but there is no net water movement.

A dilute (hypotonic) solution with a low ion concentration results in swelling and subsequent rupture (puff of red in lower left part of cell) of a red blood cell placed into the solution.

A concentrated (hypertonic) solution, with a high ion concentration, causes shrinkage of the red blood cell as water moves out of the cell and into the concentrated solution.

FIGURE 9-11 ▲ Effects of various ion concentrations in a fluid on human cells. This shows the process of osmosis. Fluid is shifting into and out of the red blood cell in response to changing ion concentrations in the fluid surrounding the cells.

6. Examine Figure 9-7 and describe the hormonal regulation of water balance in your own words.

7. List two situations in which thirst is *not* a reliable indicator of fluid needs.

8. What is water intoxication?

9. Define *osmosis*.

9.2 Minerals: Essential Elements for Health

While vitamins are compounds consisting of many elements (e.g., carbon, oxygen, and hydrogen), **minerals** are individual chemical elements. They cannot be broken down further. The mineral content of foods is sometimes called "ash" because it is all that remains after the whole food has been destroyed by high temperatures or chemical degradation. In humans, minerals make up about 4% of adult body weight (Fig. 9-12). A mineral is essential for humans if a dietary inadequacy results in a physiological or structural abnormality and its addition to the diet prevents such illness or reinstates normal health. Sixteen minerals are known to be essential in the diet.

Minerals are categorized based on the amount we need per day. Recall from Chapter 1 that if we require greater than 100 milligrams (1/50 of a teaspoon) of a mineral per day, it is considered a **major mineral.** These include calcium, phosphorus, magnesium, sulfur, sodium, potassium, and chloride. **Trace minerals** are required at levels less than 100 milligrams per day. Nine essential trace minerals (iron, zinc, copper, iodide, selenium, molybdenum, fluoride, manganese, and chromium) have been identified for humans.

mineral Element used in the body to promote chemical reactions and form body structures.

major mineral Vital to health, a mineral required in the diet in amounts greater than 100 milligrams per day.

trace mineral Vital to health, a mineral required in the diet in amounts less than 100 milligrams per day.

FIGURE 9-12 ▶ Approximate amounts of various minerals present in the average human body. Other trace minerals of nutritional importance not listed include chromium, fluoride, molybdenum, selenium, and zinc.

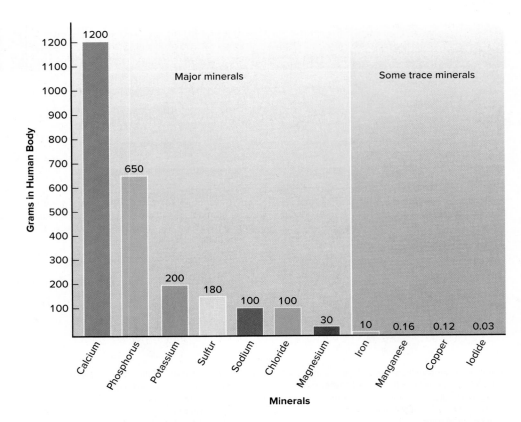

Sulfur is unique among the major minerals because it has no known dietary requirement. Proteins supply all the sulfur we need. It is found in many important compounds in the body, such as some amino acids (e.g., methionine) and vitamins (e.g., biotin and thiamin). Sulfur helps to maintain acid–base balance in the body and is an important part of the liver's drug-detoxifying pathways.

ultratrace mineral A mineral present in the human diet in trace amounts but that has not been shown to be essential to human health.

phytic acid (phytate) A constituent of plant fibers that binds positive ions to its multiple phosphate groups.

oxalic acid (oxalate) An organic acid found in spinach, rhubarb, and sweet potatoes that can depress the absorption of certain minerals present in the food, such as calcium.

Information about trace minerals is perhaps the most rapidly expanding area of knowledge in nutrition. With the exceptions of iron and iodine, the importance of trace minerals to humans has been recognized only within the last 50 years or so. Although we need 100 milligrams or less of each trace mineral daily, they are as essential to good health as are major minerals.

In some cases, discovering the importance of a trace mineral reads like a detective story, and the evidence is still unfolding. In 1961, researchers linked dwarfism in Middle Eastern villagers to a zinc deficiency. Other scientists recognized that a rare form of heart disease in an isolated area of China was linked to a selenium deficiency. In North America, some trace mineral deficiencies were first observed in the late 1960s and early 1970s, when the minerals were not added to synthetic formulas used for intravenous feeding.

It is difficult to define precisely our trace mineral needs because we need only minute amounts. Highly sophisticated technology is required to measure such small amounts in both food and body tissues.

There are several additional trace minerals (sometimes called **ultratrace minerals**) found in the human body, but many of them have no known requirements. These include arsenic, boron, nickel, silicon, and vanadium.

ABSORPTION AND STORAGE OF MINERALS IN THE BODY

Foods offer us a plentiful supply of many minerals, but the ability of our bodies to absorb and use them varies. The bioavailability of minerals depends on many factors, including many nonmineral components of foods. Age, gender, genetic variables, nutritional status, and diet will affect mineral absorption and bioavailability. Numerous prescription drugs also adversely affect mineral absorption. The mineral content listed in a food composition table is a starting point for estimating the contribution the food will make to our mineral needs.

Components of fiber, such as **phytic acid (phytate)** and **oxalic acid (oxalate),** can limit absorption of some minerals by binding to them. Spinach, for example, contains plenty of calcium, but only about 5% (compared to the average 25% bioavailability of calcium from foods) of it can be absorbed because of the high concentration of oxalic acid in spinach, which binds calcium. High-fiber diets—particularly those in excess of current recommendations of 25 (adult women) to 38 grams (adult men) of fiber per day—can decrease the absorption of iron, zinc, and possibly other minerals.

Many minerals, such as magnesium, calcium, iron, and copper, are of similar sizes and electrical charges (+2 charge). Having similar sizes and the same electrical charge causes these minerals to compete with each other for absorption; therefore, an excess of one mineral decreases the absorption and metabolism of other minerals. For example, a large intake of zinc decreases copper absorption. This becomes an issue with the use of individual mineral supplements, which should be avoided unless a dietary deficiency or medical condition specifically warrants it. Food sources pose little risk for these mineral interactions, giving us another reason to emphasize foods in meeting nutrient needs.

Several beneficial vitamin-mineral interactions occur during nutrient absorption and metabolism. When consumed in conjunction with vitamin C, absorption of certain forms of iron—such as that in plant products—improves. The active form of the vitamin D hormone improves calcium absorption. Many vitamins require specific minerals to act as components in their structure and as cofactors for their function. For example, without magnesium or manganese, the thiamin coenzyme cannot function efficiently.

The average North American diet derives minerals from both plant and animal sources. Overall, minerals from animal products are better absorbed than those from plants because binders such as fiber are not present to hinder absorption. Also, the mineral content of plants greatly depends on mineral concentrations of the soil in which they are grown. Vegans must be aware of the potentially poor mineral content of some plant foods and choose some concentrated sources of minerals. Soil conditions have less of an influence on the mineral content of animal products because livestock usually consume a variety of plant products grown from soils of differing mineral contents.

Like vitamins, the majority of the minerals are absorbed in the small intestine. Minor amounts may be absorbed in the stomach, and some sodium and potassium are absorbed in the large intestine. After minerals are absorbed, some travel freely in the bloodstream, but many are carried by specific transport proteins to their sites of action or storage. Calcium is one example of a mineral that can travel as an ion in the blood or bound to a blood protein called albumin. Iron, on the other hand, has damaging effects in its unbound form, so it is transported bound to proteins, such as transferrin.

Minerals are stored in various tissues throughout the body. Some minerals must remain in the bloodstream to maintain fluid balance and supply body functions. Others, such as calcium, phosphorus, magnesium, and fluoride, are stored mainly in bones. Iron, copper, zinc, and many trace minerals are stored in the liver. Still others are stored in muscle tissue, organs, or glands.

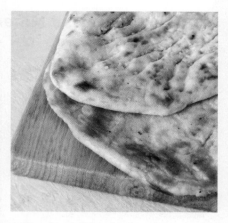

▲ The zinc deficiencies found among some Middle Eastern populations are attributed partly to their consumption of unleavened breads, resulting in low bioavailability of dietary zinc. If grains are leavened with yeast, as they are in bread making, enzymes produced by the yeast can break some of the bonds between phytic acid and minerals. This increases mineral absorption. ©Robyn Mackenzie/Shutterstock

CRITICAL THINKING

Gwen follows a vegetarian diet. What factors in foods of plant origin may limit the bioavailability of minerals, such as calcium and zinc, in her diet?

MINERAL TOXICITIES

Excessive mineral intake, especially of trace minerals such as iron and copper, can have toxic results. For many trace minerals, the gap between just enough and too much is small. Taking minerals in supplement form poses the biggest threat for mineral toxicity, whereas food sources are unlikely culprits. Mineral supplements exceeding current standards for mineral needs—especially those that supply more than 100% of the Daily Values on supplement labels—should be taken only under a primary care provider's supervision. The Daily Values for minerals are typically greater than our current standards (e.g., Recommended Dietary Allowances [RDA]). Without close monitoring, doses of minerals should not exceed any Upper Level set on a long-term basis.

The potential for toxicity is not the only reason to be cautious about the use of mineral supplements. Harmful interactions with other nutrients are possible as well as contamination of mineral supplements—with lead, for example. Use of brands approved by the United States Pharmacopeial Convention (USP) lessens this risk (see Chapter 8).

MyPlate: Sources of Minerals

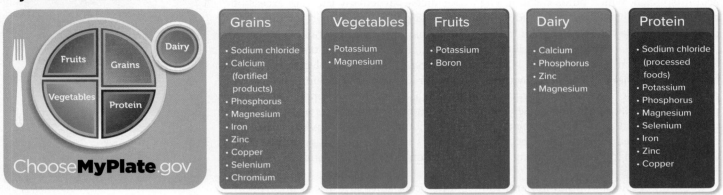

Grains	Vegetables	Fruits	Dairy	Protein
• Sodium chloride • Calcium (fortified products) • Phosphorus • Magnesium • Iron • Zinc • Copper • Selenium • Chromium	• Potassium • Magnesium	• Potassium • Boron	• Calcium • Phosphorus • Zinc • Magnesium	• Sodium chloride (processed foods) • Potassium • Phosphorus • Magnesium • Selenium • Iron • Zinc • Copper

ChooseMyPlate.gov

FIGURE 9-13 ▲ Certain groups of MyPlate are especially rich sources of various minerals. This is true for the minerals listed. Each mineral may also be found in other groups but in lower amounts. Other trace minerals are also present in moderate amounts in many groups. With regard to the grains group, whole grain varieties are the richest sources of most trace minerals listed.

Source: ChooseMyPlate.gov

PRESERVATION OF MINERALS IN FOODS

bioavailability The degree to which a consumed nutrient is absorbed and used by the body.

Minerals are found in plant and animal foods (Fig. 9-13), but as you previously read, the **bioavailability** of minerals varies widely. Minerals are not typically lost from animal sources during processing, storage, or cooking; but for plant sources, significant amounts may be lost during food processing. When grains are refined, the final products have lost the majority of their vitamin E, many B vitamins, and trace minerals. The more refined a plant food, as in the case of white flour, the lower its mineral content. During the enrichment of refined grain products, iron is the only mineral added, whereas the selenium, zinc, copper, and other minerals lost during refinement are not replaced. Following the recommendation of the 2015–2020 *Dietary Guidelines for Americans* to "make half your grains whole" will effectively improve the mineral content of a eating pattern.

✓ CONCEPT CHECK 9.2

1. Define *bioavailability*.
2. Are ultratrace minerals essential for humans? List three examples of ultratrace minerals.
3. Should people take individual mineral supplements? Why or why not?
4. Where are minerals stored in the body?

9.3 Sodium

Sodium (Na) is best known as one of the elements in common table salt. Salt is nutritionally important and once highly valued chemical compound! Historically, salt was treasured because it enabled people to preserve foods. Salt was traded and used as a form of payment. In fact, the word *salary* comes from the Latin *salarium,* which is linked to the use of salt to pay Roman soldiers. Salt is 40% sodium and 60% chloride by weight. (The chemical symbol Na represents the Latin term *natrium.*) One teaspoon of salt contains 2400 milligrams of sodium. What was once difficult to find, however, is now abundant in our food supply. Indeed, nearly all Americans exceed dietary requirements for sodium by so much that reducing sodium in our diets is the focus of major public health campaigns.

FUNCTIONS OF SODIUM

Nearly all the sodium we consume is absorbed by the digestive tract. When sodium chloride (NaCl) is dissolved in water, the chemical bond holding the two atoms together breaks and the charged ions Na^+ and Cl^- are released. These electrolytes, as well as others, attract water. The concentration of intracellular and extracellular water is controlled by the concentration of the electrolytes. Fluid balance is maintained by moving or actively pumping sodium ions where more water is needed. Sodium ions also function in nerve impulse conduction and absorption of some nutrients (e.g., glucose).

Although sodium consumption varies tremendously from day to day, even meal to meal (unless strictly controlled for health reasons), our blood levels vary only slightly. The kidneys function as a filter. If blood sodium is low, as blood flows through the kidney, sodium is secreted back into the blood, resulting in a decreased urine output. Conversely, if our blood sodium levels are too high, the sodium is filtered out by the kidneys and excreted into the urine. When this excess sodium is removed, water follows, resulting in greater urine output. Without drinking extra water, dehydration can result. Fortunately, high-sodium (salty) foods make us thirsty and drive us to drink more fluids.

SODIUM DEFICIENCY

A low sodium intake, coupled with excessive perspiration and persistent vomiting or diarrhea, has the ability to deplete the body of sodium. This state can lead to muscle cramps, nausea, vomiting, dizziness, and later shock and coma. The likelihood of this occurring is low because the kidney is very efficient at conserving sodium under conditions of low-sodium status.

When excessive perspiration leads to weight loss that exceeds 2% to 3% of total body weight (or about 5 to 6 pounds), sodium losses should raise concern. Even then, merely salting food or selecting some salty foods such as soup or crackers is sufficient to restore body sodium for most people. Athletes who perspire for hours during endurance activities need to consume electrolyte-replacement drinks during exercise to avoid depletion of sodium, which can lead to hyponatremia. Perspiration contains about two-thirds the sodium concentration found in blood or about 1 gram of sodium per liter.

GETTING ENOUGH SODIUM

About 77% of the sodium we consume is added in the form of salt during food manufacturing and food preparation at restaurants. Sodium added while cooking or at the table at home provides about 11% of our intake, and naturally occurring sodium in foods provides the remaining 12% (Fig. 9-14). Most unprocessed foods are relatively low in sodium; milk is one exception (about 120 milligrams per cup).

The more processed and restaurant food consumed, the higher one's sodium intake. Conversely, the more home-cooked meals prepared, the more control a person has over sodium in the diet. Major contributors of sodium in the adult diet are white bread and rolls; hot dogs and lunch meat; cheese; soups; and foods with tomato sauce—partly because these foods are consumed so often. Other foods that can be major contributors to sodium intake include French fries, pretzels, potato chips, sauces, and gravies.

If we ate only unprocessed foods and added no salt, we would consume about 500 milligrams of sodium per day. The AI for sodium is 1500 milligrams for adults through age 50. The recommendation is lower for older adults (see margin). If we compare 500 milligrams of sodium from an eating pattern of unprocessed foods with

Is sea salt a healthier choice than common table salt? Sea salt is made by evaporating seawater. It is minimally processed, which gives it a coarser texture, and it may contain traces of magnesium, calcium, and potassium. In contrast, table salt is typically mined from the earth and processed into fine grains. Many consumers prefer the taste and texture of sea salt over table salt, but when it comes to heart health, there is no significant difference in sodium or chloride content. Furthermore, as you will learn in Section 9.12, most of the table salt sold in North America is fortified with iodide, an essential nutrient for thyroid function. Next time you purchase salt, compare the labels of several products to assess any nutritional differences for yourself.

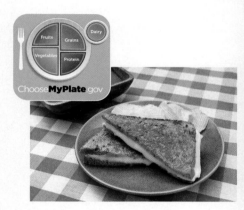

▲ How does this meal of a grilled cheese sandwich, chips, and tomato soup compare to MyPlate? How could you reduce the sodium content of this meal?
©Matthew Antonino/123RF

Sodium
AI
  9–50 years: 1500 milligrams
  51–70 years: 1300 milligrams
  > 70 years: 1200 milligrams
DV: 2400 milligrams
UL: 2300 milligrams

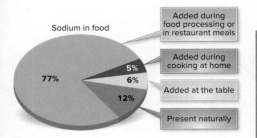

Sodium in food

Added during food processing or in restaurant meals — 5%

Added during cooking at home — 6%

Added at the table — 12%

Present naturally — 77%

FIGURE 9-14 ▲ Salt arrives in the American diet largely as a result of food processing.

Newsworthy Nutrition

No evidence for extreme sodium restrictions for older adults

The relationship between dietary sodium and health outcomes in older adults remains unclear. The aim of this study was to examine the association between sodium intake and the incidence of cardiovascular disease (CVD), heart failure (HF), and death in older adults. Data was obtained from 2642 older adults, aged 71 to 80 years, participating in a 10-year study beginning in 1997–1998. A food frequency questionnaire was used to assess dietary sodium intake at baseline. Participants were categorized according to sodium intake: < 1500 mg/d (291 participants [11.0%]), 1500 to 2300 mg/d (779 participants [29.5%]), and > 2300 mg/d (1572 participants [59.5%]). During the 10-year study, 881 participants died, 572 developed CVD, and 398 developed HF. Sodium intake was not associated with 10-year mortality or risk of CVD or HF. Adjusting for caloric intake and body mass index did not affect the results. There were no consistent interactions with sex, race, or hypertensive status observed for any outcome. In conclusion, sodium intake in adults aged 71 to 80 was neither associated with 10-year mortality nor incidence of CVD or HF. The authors emphasize the need for additional rigorous studies before recommending any further restrictions of sodium intake beyond the current UL of 2300 mg/d for adults.

Source: Kalogeropoulos AP and others: Dietary sodium content, mortality, and risk for cardiovascular events in older adults: The Health, Aging, and Body Composition (Health ABC) Study. *Journal of the American Medical Association Intern Med.* 175(3):410–419, 2015.

the 2300 to 4700 milligrams or more typically consumed by adults, it is clear that food processing, dining out, and salt added while cooking are the major contributors to sodium intake. When dietary sodium must be restricted, attention to food labels is valuable to monitor sodium intake.

Most people can adapt to wide variations in dietary sodium intakes; today's sodium intake is found in tomorrow's urine. However, approximately 10% to 15% of adults are *sodium sensitive;* that is, sodium intake has a direct effect on their blood pressure. As their sodium intake increases, so does their blood pressure. Among these people, lower-sodium diets (about 2000 milligrams daily) often decrease blood pressure. Groups that appear to be especially affected are African-Americans, Asian Americans, and people who have diabetes and/or are overweight (see the Nutrition and Your Health section on minerals and hypertension at the end of the chapter). Lifestyle factors such as being overweight and inactive are the major contributors to the development of hypertension.

Although current research suggests no association between sodium intake and risk of cardiovascular disease, heart failure, or death (see the Newsworthy Nutrition above), the medical community still recommends adults should reduce salt and sodium consumption to limit the risk of developing hypertension later in life. Read more about the American Heart Association's recommendation to "break up with salt" at https://sodiumbreakup.heart.org. It is also a good idea to have your blood pressure checked regularly. If you are diagnosed with hypertension, you should reduce sodium intake as you follow a comprehensive plan to treat this disease. Reducing sodium intake may also help maintain a healthy calcium status, as sodium intake greater than about 2000 milligrams per day may increase urinary calcium loss along with the sodium excreted. The effect of this increased urinary calcium loss on bone health is controversial.

Adopting a reduced-salt eating pattern is a significant lifestyle change for most people because many typical food choices will have to be limited (Fig. 9-15). At first, foods may taste bland, but eventually, you will perceive more flavor as the taste receptors in the tongue become more sensitive to the salt content of foods. It takes 6 to 8 weeks to retrain your taste buds to sense sodium at a lower level. Slowly reducing sodium intake by substituting lemon juice, herbs, and spices will allow you to become accustomed to an eating pattern that contains minimal amounts of salt. Many cookbooks and online sources offer excellent recipes for flavorful dishes.

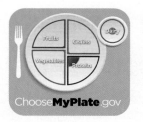

FIGURE 9-15 ◄ Food sources of sodium. (a) The fill of the background color (none, 1/3, 2/3, or completely covered) within each food group on MyPlate indicates the average nutrient density for sodium for *natural, unprocessed foods* in that group. (b) The bar graph shows the sodium content of several natural and processed foods from each food group compared to the AI for adult males and females. Overall, the dairy group is the only food group that provides much sodium in its natural form. Food processing adds significant sodium to foods such as canned vegetables and cured meats.

Source: Nutrition data from USDA National Nutrient Database for Standard Reference, Release 26

(a)

(b)

	Food Item and Amount	Sodium (milligrams)	% AI for Adult Males and Females (1500 milligrams)
Grains	Chicken noodle soup, canned, 1 cup	870	58%
Grains	Kellogg's Corn Flakes,® 1 cup	200	13%
Grains	Whole wheat bread, 1 slice	146	10%
Vegetables	Tomatoes, stewed (canned), 1 cup	564	38%
Vegetables	Green beans, cooked (from canned), 1 cup	461	31%
Vegetables	Green beans, cooked (from frozen), 1 cup	3	0%
Fruits	Olives, green, bottled, 5 medium	210	14%
Fruits	Cantaloupe, 1 cup	25	2%
Fruits	Fruit cocktail, 1 cup	9	1%
Dairy	Cottage cheese, low-fat, 1 cup	746	50%
Dairy	Cheddar cheese, 1.5 ounces	264	18%
Dairy	Milk, nonfat, 1 cup	103	7%
Protein	Pepperoni pizza, 2 slices	1538	103%
Protein	Ham steak, cooked, 3 ounces	1079	72%
Protein	Chicken breast, roasted, 3 ounces	64	4%

AVOIDING TOO MUCH SODIUM

The Upper Level (UL) for sodium for adults is 2300 milligrams (2.3 grams), approximately 1 teaspoon. Intakes exceeding this amount typically increase blood pressure. Recent research also links excessive sodium consumption to overweight and obesity. As salt intake increases, fluid intake also increases; if calorie-laden beverages are chosen, weight gain may ensue.[3] About 95% of North American adults have sodium intakes that exceed that UL. It must be noted that the Daily Value (DV) of 2400 milligrams exceeds the UL for sodium. A healthier goal is to aim for the AI of 1500 milligrams.

✓ CONCEPT CHECK 9.3

1. List three food sources of sodium in your diet.
2. Which organ regulates the amount of sodium in your blood?
3. Define *sodium sensitivity.*
4. List three specific changes you could make to your eating pattern to decrease your sodium intake.

The *Dietary Guidelines for Americans* recommend less than 2300 milligrams of sodium (approximately 1 teaspoon of salt) per day for those 14 years and older. This is the UL set by the National Academy of Medicine for individuals in this age group. The following strategies are recommended to shift food choices to reduce sodium intake:

- Use the Nutrition Facts label to compare sodium content of foods and choose the product with less sodium.
- Buy low-sodium, reduced-sodium, or no-salt-added versions of products.
- Choose fresh, frozen (no sauce or seasoning), or no-salt-added canned vegetables and fresh poultry, seafood, pork, and lean meat, rather than processed meat and poultry.
- Eat at home more often.
- Cook foods from scratch to control the sodium content of dishes.
- Limit sauces, mixes, and "instant" products, including flavored rice, instant noodles, and ready-made pasta.
- Flavor foods with herbs and spices instead of salt.

ASK THE RDN   Pass the Salt?

Dear RDN: As a college student, do I need to be concerned about the amount of salt in my diet, or are the limits just for older adults with high blood pressure?

Since the 1970s, Americans have been told to limit their salt, more specifically sodium, intakes to control blood pressure. For most Americans, this is a tough rule to follow because of our preference for salty foods. To complicate matters, the scientific community continues to debate this issue as the research presents conflicting evidence. Experts do agree that consuming too much salt may be harmful, especially for individuals with high blood pressure. Scientists disagree, however, on the definition of "too much" salt. The *Dietary Guidelines* define too much as > 2300 milligrams of sodium per day, the amount in 1 teaspoon of salt. This guideline was confirmed in a recent review by the National Academy of Medicine (formerly Institute of Medicine)[4] that determined the evidence linking sodium intake and blood pressure to be compelling. The American Heart Association recommends 1500 milligrams per day for those over 50 and for all African-Americans,[5] but the National Academy of Medicine found insufficient data to support such tight limits. Adding to the confusion, several new studies[6] failed to conclusively link dietary sodium intake with health outcomes such as heart disease and stroke.

Remember that sodium is the culprit in salt but is an essential nutrient that affects every body system, including the cardiovascular system. Indeed, too little sodium may pose serious health risks. The typical American, however, consumes over 3500 milligrams of sodium per day!

Current evidence links excessive sodium intake with high blood pressure. Most Americans, including college-age students, should reduce sodium intakes to < 2300 milligrams per day. To begin reducing overall sodium consumption, read food labels carefully and select foods low in sodium (140 milligrams or less per serving), consume more whole foods and fewer highly processed foods, cook at home, and ask for low-sodium options in restaurants. Deli meats and cheeses are very high in sodium. The sodium in breads, pizza, crackers, and snack foods adds up quickly because we typically eat so much of them. Also, reducing sodium while at the same time eating foods rich in potassium, such as fruits and vegetables, might achieve greater health benefits than reducing sodium alone. In sum, choosing fewer highly processed foods and preparing most of your meals at home will result in a healthy, yet achievable, sodium intake.

With just a dash of salt,

Anne M. Smith, PhD, RDN, LD (author)

9.4 Potassium

FUNCTIONS OF POTASSIUM

Potassium (K) performs many of the same functions as sodium, such as water balance and nerve impulse transmission. (The chemical symbol K represents the Latin term *kalium.*) All membranes contain an energy-dependent pump that can transfer sodium from inside to outside the cell. When sodium (Na^+) is actively pumped out of the cell, potassium (K^+) enters the cell in an attempt to balance the loss of the positively charged sodium ions. That makes potassium the principal positively charged ion inside cells. Intracellular fluids contain 95% of the potassium in the body. Higher potassium intake is associated with *lower* rather than higher blood pressure values.

POTASSIUM DEFICIENCY

Low blood potassium, also known as *hypokalemia,* is a life-threatening problem. Symptoms often include a loss of appetite, muscle cramps, confusion, and constipation. Eventually, the heart beats irregularly, decreasing its capacity to pump blood.

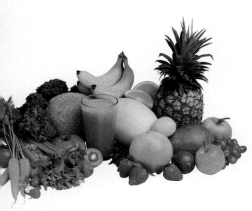

▲ Fruits and vegetables are rich sources of potassium. ©C Squared Studios/Getty Images

Hypokalemia can result from continually deficient food intake, but it is most commonly seen with chronic diarrhea or vomiting, or as a side effect of medications, including laxatives and some diuretics (see the Medicine Cabinet in this section). Vulnerable populations include people with certain eating disorders (see Chapter 11) or alcohol use disorders (see Chapter 16). Other populations at increased risk for potassium deficiency include people on very low-calorie diets and athletes who exercise for prolonged periods. These people should compensate for potentially low body potassium by consuming potassium-rich foods.

GETTING ENOUGH POTASSIUM

Unprocessed foods are rich sources of potassium, including fruits, vegetables, milk, whole grains, dried beans, and meats (Fig. 9-16). Here is an easy guide: the more processed your food, the higher it is in sodium and the lower it is in potassium. Major contributors of potassium to the adult diet include milk, potatoes, beef, coffee, tomatoes, and orange juice.

Medicine Cabinet

Some people take **diuretics** to lower their blood pressure. Diuretics cause the kidneys to excrete more urine but at the same time may increase urinary excretion of minerals. This is nutritionally relevant for regulation of blood levels of potassium, magnesium, and zinc. People who take potassium-wasting diuretics need to carefully monitor their dietary intake of this mineral. Increased intake of fruits and vegetables or potassium chloride supplements are prescribed by primary care providers.

Examples:

Hydrochlorothiazide (Microzide)

Furosemide (Lasix)

©Peter Dazeley/Photographer's Choice/Getty Images

diuretic A substance that increases urinary fluid excretion.

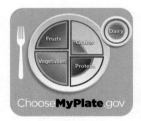

FIGURE 9-16 ◄ Food sources of potassium. (a) The fill of the background color (none, 1/3, 2/3, or completely covered) within each food group on MyPlate indicates the average nutrient density for potassium in that group. (b) The bar graph shows the potassium content of several foods in each food group compared to the AI for adult males and females. Overall, the richest sources of potassium are unprocessed foods of plant origin, such as fruits, vegetables, and beans.

Source: Nutrition data from USDA National Nutrient Database for Standard Reference, Release 26

(a)

(b)

	Food Item and Amount	Potassium (milligrams)	% AI for Adult Males and Females (4700 milligrams)
Grains	Raisin bran cereal, 1 cup	352	7%
Grains	Quinoa, cooked, ½ cup	159	3%
Grains	White bread, 1 slice	29	1%
Vegetables	Swiss chard, cooked, 1 cup	961	20%
Vegetables	Potato, baked (with skin), 1 medium	926	20%
Vegetables	Acorn squash, cooked, 1 cup	896	19%
Fruits	Orange juice, fresh, 1 cup	496	11%
Fruits	Cantaloupe, 1 cup	426	9%
Fruits	Banana, 1 medium	422	9%
Dairy	Yogurt, plain, nonfat, 1 cup	625	13%
Dairy	Milk, fat-free, 1 cup	382	8%
Dairy	Soy milk, 1 cup	296	6%
Protein	Kidney beans, cooked, ½ cup	358	8%
Protein	Sirloin steak, grilled, 3 ounces	286	6%
Protein	Pistachios, dry roasted, 1 ounce	285	6%

Potassium
AI: 4700 milligrams
DV: 3500 milligrams
UL: none

Approximately 90% of the potassium consumed is absorbed, but eating patterns are more likely to be lower in potassium than sodium because we add salt to our food, not potassium. In fact, North Americans typically consume only 2000 to 3000 milligrams of potassium per day, much less than the AI (see margin). Thus, many of us need to increase potassium intake, preferably by increasing fruit and vegetable intake.

AVOIDING TOO MUCH POTASSIUM

If the kidneys function normally, potassium from dietary sources will not lead to toxicity. Thus, no Upper Level for potassium has been set. When the kidneys function poorly, potassium builds in the blood, inhibiting heart function and leading to a slowed heartbeat. If left untreated, the heart eventually stops beating, resulting in a cardiac arrest and death. Therefore, in cases of kidney failure or kidney disease, close monitoring of blood levels of potassium and potassium intake becomes critical.

> ✓ **CONCEPT CHECK 9.4**
>
> 1. List two functions of potassium in the body.
> 2. How is potassium intake related to blood pressure?
> 3. List three specific changes you could make to your eating pattern to increase your potassium intake.

9.5 Chloride

FUNCTIONS OF CHLORIDE

Chloride (Cl^-) is a negative ion found primarily in the extracellular fluid. Along with sodium and potassium, chloride helps to regulate fluid balance in the body. In fact, chloride itself may be partially responsible for increases in blood pressure that accompany high-salt diets.

Chloride ions are also a component of the acid produced in the stomach (hydrochloric acid) and are important for overall maintenance of acid–base balance in the body. This electrolyte is used during immune responses as white blood cells attack foreign cells. In addition, nervous system function relies on the presence of chloride.

CHLORIDE DEFICIENCY

Low levels of chloride in the blood can lead to a disturbance of the body's acid–base balance. A chloride deficiency is unlikely, however, because our dietary salt intake is so high. Frequent and lengthy bouts of vomiting, if coupled with a nutrient-poor diet, can contribute to a deficiency because stomach secretions contain a lot of chloride. Therefore, individuals with bulimia or severe cases of gastroenteritis are at risk for chloride deficiency. In addition, low chloride levels could occur as a side effect of some medications, such as diuretics or laxatives.

GETTING ENOUGH CHLORIDE

When it comes to sources of chloride, it is important to make the distinction between the chloride ion, which is vital for body functions, and chlorine (Cl_2), which is a poisonous gas. *Chlorine* is used to disinfect municipal water supplies. A small amount of chlorine may remain in tap water, but the substance evaporates quickly. Municipal and well water usually contains some *chloride* (leached from the earth) as well, but water does not represent a significant source of chloride in the diet.

A few fruits and vegetables, such as seaweed, celery, tomatoes, and olives, are naturally good sources of chloride. Most of our dietary chloride, however, comes from salt

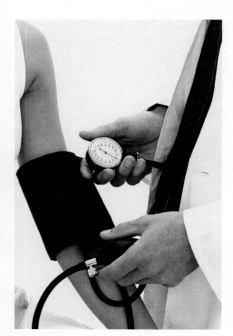

▲ Chloride is likely part of the blood-pressure-raising property of sodium chloride (salt). ©Stockdisc/PunchStock

added to foods. Salt is 60% chloride by weight, so knowing a food's salt content allows for a close prediction of its chloride content.

Like sodium, nearly all the chloride consumed is efficiently absorbed. The AI for chloride (see margin) is based on the 40:60 ratio of sodium to chloride in salt (1500 milligrams of sodium: 2300 milligrams of chloride). If the average adult consumes about 9 grams of salt daily, that yields 5.4 grams (5400 milligrams) of chloride. The principal route of excretion is the kidneys, although some chloride is lost in perspiration.

AVOIDING TOO MUCH CHLORIDE

The average adult typically consumes an excess of this mineral. Because chloride has a role in raising blood pressure, it is important that aging adults consciously control salt intake to decrease risk of developing hypertension. Learning at a young age to select foods lower in sodium chloride is the best way to start.

> **Chloride**
> AI: 2300 milligrams
> DV: 3400 milligrams
> UL: 3600 milligrams

✓ CONCEPT CHECK 9.5

1. List two functions of chloride in the body.
2. How is chloride intake related to blood pressure?

9.6 Calcium

FUNCTIONS OF CALCIUM

Bone Growth, Maintenance, and Repair Calcium (Ca) represents 40% of all the minerals present in the body and equals about 2.5 pounds (1200 grams) in the average person. All cells require calcium to function; however, more than 99% of the calcium in the body is used for growth, development, and maintenance of bones. Calcium is the main component of **hydroxyapatite,** the crystalline compound responsible for the structure and hardness of bone.

Muscle and Nerve Function Less than 1% of calcium is found in blood, but this circulating calcium is critical to supply the needs of cells other than bone cells. Forming and maintaining bone are calcium's major roles in the body, but it is critical for other processes as well. Muscle contraction is activated by calcium release and the flow of calcium along the surface of the muscle cell. In nerve transmission, calcium assists in the release of neurotransmitters and permits the flow of ions in and out of nerve cells.

Additional Functions and Health Benefits Calcium helps regulate cellular metabolism by influencing the activities of various enzymes and hormonal responses. Calcium also functions in the maintenance of cell membrane integrity, normal blood pressure, regulation of glucose concentration, and **cellular differentiation.** Calcium is also essential for blood clotting (see Section 8.5). It is the tight regulation of the concentration of calcium in the blood that keeps these processes going, even if a person fails to consume enough dietary calcium from day to day. There is some evidence that calcium has a role in preventing breast and colon cancer. Overall, the benefits of a diet providing adequate calcium extend far beyond bone health.

hydroxyapatite crystalline compound containing calcium, phosphorus, and sometimes fluoride, also known as bone mineral.

cellular differentiation The process of a less specialized cell becoming a more specialized type such as stem cells in the bone marrow becoming red and white blood cells.

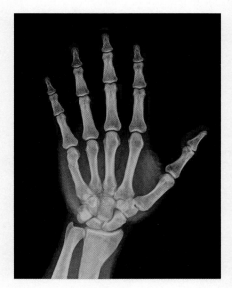

▲ Ninety-nine percent of calcium in the body is in bones. ©kravka/Shutterstock

CALCIUM DEFICIENCY

The body tightly regulates blood calcium concentration within a narrow range, regardless of dietary intake. If dietary calcium intake is inadequate and blood calcium concentration begins to decrease, three hormonally controlled actions are stimulated to reestablish calcium blood levels: (1) bones release calcium, (2) intestines absorb more calcium, and (3) the kidneys retain more calcium in the blood. (Recall the role of vitamin D

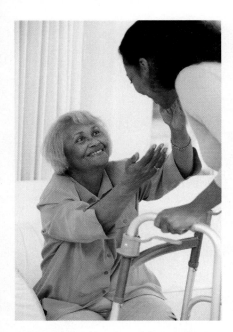

▲ Osteoporosis leads to millions of bone fractures each year, including debilitating fractures of the hip and spine. These fractures frequently result in the need for assistance with activities of daily living, as we see with this woman who needs a walker to help her navigate. ©Rolf Bruderer/Blend Images LLC

tetany A body condition marked by sharp contraction of muscles and failure to relax afterward; usually caused by abnormal calcium metabolism.

osteoporosis The presence of a stress-induced fracture or a T-score of −2.5 or lower. The bones are porous and fragile due to low mineral density.

osteopenia A bone disease defined by low mineral density.

type 1 osteoporosis Porous trabecular bone characterized by rapid bone demineralization following menopause.

in blood calcium regulation, discussed in Chapter 8.) Because of this tight hormonal regulation, poor dietary intake of calcium is not likely to result in low blood calcium. Rather, kidney diseases, hormonal abnormalities, or medications are the likely culprits. If blood calcium does fall below a critical point, muscles cannot relax after contraction and nerve function is disrupted. The result is a condition called **tetany,** in which muscles become stiff or twitch involuntarily.

You can see that the skeleton does more than simply provide the framework for the body; it also functions as a bank from which calcium can be added or withdrawn. Only about 1% of the calcium in bone is available at any time for this purpose. Over time, however, bone loss due to inadequate calcium intake and/or absorption may occur, though slowly. Clinical symptoms of the calcium loss from bones show after many years. By not meeting calcium needs, some people, especially women, are setting the stage for osteoporosis and future bone fractures.

Osteoporosis. *Healthy People 2020* identified the prevention of the bone disease **osteoporosis** as one of its major focus areas. In 2014, the National Osteoporosis Foundation reported that 54 million U.S. adults age 50 and older, more than one-half of the total U.S. adult population, is affected by osteoporosis and low bone mass.[7] Of those affected, 10.2 million currently have osteoporosis and another 43.4 million have low bone mass. Of those with osteoporosis, it is estimated that 7.7 million are non-Hispanic white, 0.5 million are non-Hispanic black, and 0.6 million are Mexican American. The numbers of adults over 50 with osteoporosis or low bone mass are increasing and expected to reach 64.4 million by 2020 and 71.2 million by 2030.

Osteoporosis continues to lead to approximately 2 million bone fractures per year in the United States, including nearly 300,000 broken hips. The health care costs associated with these fractures are projected to reach more than $25 billion by the year 2025, with the most rapid increases among minority populations.[8] The personal cost of a hip fracture surpasses any financial cost. Hip fractures are regarded as devastating. They result in loss of mobility and need for long-term care. Women experience 80% of hip fractures, and the average age at which a hip fracture occurs is 80 years.[9] Only 40% of people with hip fractures regain their earlier level of independence. More specifically, it is estimated that a year after fracturing a hip, 90% of those who needed no assistance climbing stairs before the fracture will not be able to climb five stairs; 66% will need help to get on or off a toilet; 50% will not be able to raise themselves from a chair; 31% will need assistance to get out of bed; and 20% will not be able to put on a pair of pants by themselves.

Hip fracture is associated with significant mortality. It is estimated that 20% to 30% of the 300,000 Americans 65 or older who fracture a hip each year will die within 12 months. Results from the national Fracture Intervention Trial showed a six times greater risk of mortality associated with a hip fracture among postmenopausal women with low bone mass. Other types of fractures or even fear of fracture due to osteoporosis can affect quality of life. Vertebral fractures, especially if there are several of them, cause significant pain, reduced lung function, loss of height, and a curved spine. Movement can be restricted and gait altered, increasing the risk and fear of falls and/or more fractures.

Women tend to lose 1% to 3% of their bone mass each year after menopause. Men also lose bone mass as they age, but the loss is more gradual. When the bone-demineralization activities of bone-resorbing cells exceed the bone-building activities of bone-building cells, bone mass declines. This is a normal part of aging and does not always lead to unhealthy bones. However, if bone mass is low when this process begins, even moderate bone demineralization can lead to a condition called **osteopenia.** As more bone is lost, the entire matrix of the bone tissue also begins to break down. When this occurs, osteoporosis is likely to result. About 25% of women older than age 50 develop or have osteoporosis. Among people older than age 80, osteoporosis becomes the rule, not the exception. To young adults, it may sound benign to have osteoporosis. To older adults, the diagnosis presents the reality of life permanently changed.

There are two types of osteoporosis. **Type 1 osteoporosis,** also called postmenopausal osteoporosis, typically occurs in women between 50 and 60 years of age. This type of osteoporosis is directly linked to decreased estrogen concentrations that occur at menopause. Type 1 osteoporosis most dramatically affects **trabecular bone,** as this type of bone undergoes faster remodeling than cortical bone (Fig. 9-17). A woman can lose 20% to 30% of trabecular bone and 5% to 10% of **cortical bone** between ages 50 and 60, unless intervention occurs (Fig. 9-18).

Trabecular bone has more bone-building and bone-resorbing cells than cortical bone. The bone-building cells require estrogen for maximal activity. After menopause, the rate of bone synthesis declines, whereas the rate of bone resorption remains high, leading to net bone loss. Minerals are released but not reincorporated into bone, leaving weak areas and open spaces within the bone matrix. The bones at greatest risk for osteoporotic fractures are the trabecular-rich bones of the pelvis (7% of fractures), vertebrae of the spine (27%) (Fig. 9-19), and portions of long bones such as the wrist (19%).

Type 2 osteoporosis tends to be diagnosed later in life (70 to 75 years of age). Type 2 osteoporosis is a result of breakdown of both cortical and trabecular bone. It is due to a combination of dietary and age-related factors; low dietary intake of bone-building nutrients compounds the problems associated with decreased ability to absorb or metabolize nutrients.

People with either form of osteoporosis can lose significant height and experience severe pain, especially in the vertebrae. A woman may lose an inch or more in height as the bone is demineralized (Fig. 9-19). Both men and women can develop a curvature in the upper spine called **kyphosis** or dowager's hump (see Fig. 9-19). Kyphosis is a major concern because the bending of the spine may decrease the volume of the chest cavity, resulting in difficulty breathing, abdominal pain, decreased appetite, and premature satiety. As already discussed, osteoporotic bone is also more susceptible to fracture following a fall.

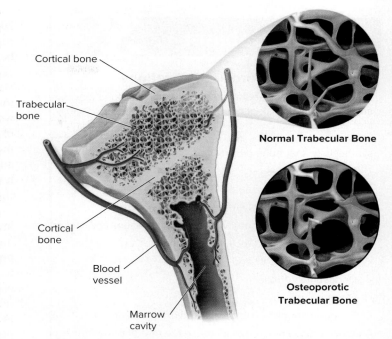

FIGURE 9-17 ▲ Cortical and trabecular bone. Cortical bone forms the shafts of bones and their outer mineral covering. Trabecular bone supports the outer shell of cortical bone in various bones of the body. Note how the osteoporotic bone has much less trabecular bone. This leads to a more fragile bone and is not reversible to any major extent with current therapies.

trabecular bone The less dense, more open structure bone found in the inner layer of bones.

cortical bone The compact or dense bone found on the outer surfaces of bone.

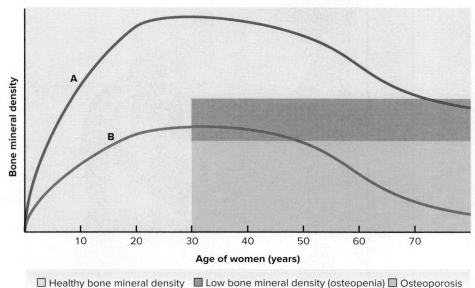

• **Woman A** had developed a high peak bone mass by age 30. Her bone loss was slow and steady between ages 30 and 50 and sped up somewhat after age 50 because of the effects of menopause. At age 75, the woman had a healthy bone mineral density value and did not show evidence of osteoporosis.

• **Woman B** with low peak bone mass experienced the same rate of bone loss as Woman A. By age 50, she already had low bone mineral density and by age 70, kyphosis and spinal fractures had occurred.

☐ Healthy bone mineral density ◼ Low bone mineral density (osteopenia) ☐ Osteoporosis

FIGURE 9-18 ▲ The relationship between peak bone mass and the ultimate risk of developing osteoporosis and related bone fractures.
Source: Based on data from R. Burge, "Incidence and economic burden of osteoporosisrelated fractures in the United States, 2005–2025," *Journal of Bone and Mineral Research,* 2007; 22:465.

Medicine Cabinet

Types of Osteoporosis Medications

Antiresorptive medications are used to prevent bone loss and decrease the risk of bone fractures. They slow bone loss that occurs during the breakdown phase of the remodeling cycle. These medicines slow bone loss without affecting bone synthesis so that bone density can increase.

- Bisphosphonates
  - Alendronate (Fosamax® and Fosamax Plus D)®
  - Ibandronate (Boniva)®
  - Risedronate (Actonel,® Actonel® with Calcium, and Atelvia)™
  - Zoledronic acid (Reclast)®
- Calcitonin (Fortical® and Miacalcin)®
- Denosumab (Prolia)®
- Estrogen therapy
- Estrogen agonists/antagonists (Raloxifene: Evista)®

Anabolic drugs are used to increase the rate of bone formation and decrease the risk of fractures.

- Teriparatide (Forteo)® is currently the only osteoporosis medicine approved by the FDA that rebuilds bone.

©Peter Dazeley/Photographer's Choice/Getty Images

According to the National Osteoporosis Foundation 2014 guidelines,[10] all men and women diagnosed with osteoporosis should first be counseled on risk factor reduction. Daily habits of calcium and vitamin D consumption as well as exercise should be stressed. Clear guidelines are provided to physicians for patients to be considered for pharmacological (drug) intervention. These drugs are indicated for postmenopausal women and men over 50 who meet specific standards for level of risk of future fracture as well as medical history.[10] Current medication options for men and women are **bisphosphonates** and **parathyroid hormone.** Women may also use calcium and hormone replacement therapy (see the Medicine Cabinet in this section for a list of osteoporosis medications).

The incidence of osteoporosis increases as a person ages. Its importance as a personal and public health problem is intensifying as the U.S. population ages. It appears, however, that a large percentage of the cases of osteoporosis can be prevented. The key to prevention is to build dense bones during the first 30 years of life and then limit the amount of bone loss in adulthood (Fig. 9-19). People with higher peak bone mass have more calcium to lose before bones become weak and fracture easily. A higher peak bone mass is also the reason males experience osteoporosis less often than females do; they have more bone mass to lose.

Bone Health Assessment. Today, we have tools that can quantitate bone mass and bone density, and, subsequently, the likelihood of a person's developing bone disease. The most

FIGURE 9-19 ▶ Normal and osteoporotic woman. Osteoporotic bones have less substance, so osteoporosis generally leads to loss of height, distorted body shape, fractures, and possibly loss of teeth. Monitoring changes in adult height is one way to detect early evidence of osteoporosis. Kyphosis, or curvature of the upper spine, results from demineralization of the vertebrae. This can lead to both physical and emotional pain. Kyphosis occurs in both men and women.

type 2 osteoporosis Porous trabecular and cortical bone observed in men and women after the age of 70.

kyphosis Abnormally increased bending of the spine.

bisphosphonates Drugs that bind minerals and prevent osteoclast breakdown of bone. Examples are alendronate (Fosamax) and risedronate (Actonel).

parathyroid hormone (PTH) A hormone made by the parathyroid gland that increases synthesis of the active form of vitamin D. This hormone works with vitamin D to increase blood levels of calcium.

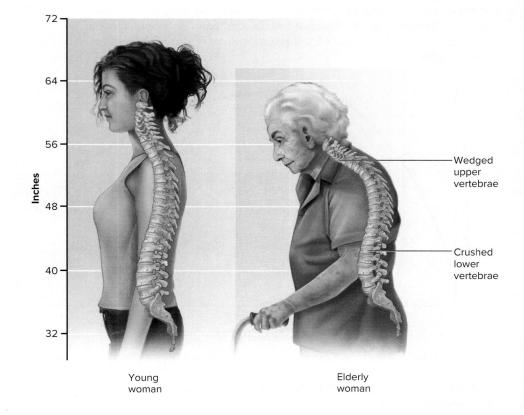

Young woman

Elderly woman

Wedged upper vertebrae

Crushed lower vertebrae

CASE STUDY Worried About Grandma

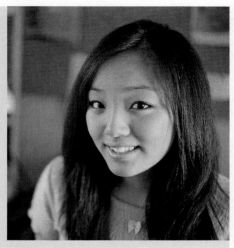

©Dennis Wise/Getty Images

Grace, a 23-year-old woman of Korean descent, is in her final year of nursing school in Boston. She also works 20 hours per week at a local pharmacy. Grace is worried about a phone call she just received from her mom. While out on her walk yesterday, Grandmother Kyon fell and broke her hip. The doctor diagnosed Grandmother Kyon with osteoporosis, and the family is worried about the long recovery ahead. As a nursing student, Grace knows how devastating a hip fracture can be. She also knows that osteoporosis can run in families. Grace resolves to do whatever she can to learn about osteoporosis and strengthen her bones now.

She starts by doing an online search for a website that can help her determine if she is at high risk for osteoporosis. The New York State Department of Health Osteoporosis Education Prevention Program, **www.health.ny.gov/diseases/conditions/osteoporosis/index.htm**, offers a list of risk factors for osteoporosis. For herself, Grace sees a few risk factors that she cannot change, but there are a few that are glaringly obvious. She uses this website to "bone up" on ways to promote her bone health while she is still young.

Grace discovers she is probably pretty low in vitamin D intake. She also does not have much free time for exercise. She cooks traditional Korean dishes for half of her meals but eats fast food or sandwiches for the rest. Daily, she takes a multivitamin/mineral pill plus one calcium carbonate pill. She generally takes them when she brushes her teeth at night before bed. On weekends, she gets out with friends and has a glass or two of wine. Grace does not smoke.

1. Go to the URL that Grace visited and click on the link for Risk Factors for Osteoporosis. What risk factors do you see for Grace? What additional questions would you ask Grace to assess her risk for osteoporosis?
2. Grace went to the section "Keeping Your Bones and Teeth Strong for Life" to determine key actions she can take to strengthen her bones now. Which ones does she already do? Which lifestyle actions could Grace integrate into her daily life right now?
3. What are the environmental conditions that inhibit Grace from adequately synthesizing vitamin D? How can she overcome some of them?
4. What are some calcium and vitamin D sources in traditional Korean dishes?
5. Give Grace some tips to increase her calcium and vitamin D intake at fast-food restaurants without significantly increasing costs or calories.
6. Would you recommend any changes to her supplement regimen?

Complete the Case Study. Responses to these questions can be provided by your instructor.

accurate test for assessing bone density is the central **dual energy X-ray absorptiometry (DEXA)** measurement of the hip and spine. The central DEXA procedure is simple, painless, safe, noninvasive, and generally takes less than 15 minutes. The hip and spine are measured because these sites are commonly affected by osteoporosis and are likely to result in more serious injuries. The ability of the bone to block the path of a low-level X ray is used as a measure of bone mineral density. A very low dose of radiation is used for the DEXA—about one-tenth of the exposure from a chest X ray.

From the DEXA measurement of bone density, a T-score is generated, which compares the observed bone density to that of a person at peak bone mass (e.g., age 30). The T-score is interpreted as shown in Figure 9-20.

The National Osteoporosis Foundation 2014 recommendations call for DEXA testing for the following groups of people:

- All women age 65 and older and men age 70 and older;
- Younger postmenopausal women and men (ages 50 to 69) who have risk factors;
- Women going through perimenopause (transitioning into menopause) who have low body weight, have prior low-trauma fracture, or take high-risk medications, such as steroids;
- Adults with fracture after age 50;
- Adults with a health condition for which they take steroids for a prolonged period (e.g., rheumatoid arthritis, Crohn's disease, asthma);
- Anyone being considered for medication for osteoporosis or receiving therapy for osteoporosis.

dual energy x-ray absorptiometry (DEXA) A scientific tool used to measure bone mineral density and body composition.

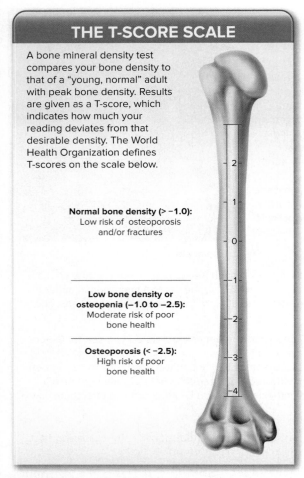

THE T-SCORE SCALE

A bone mineral density test compares your bone density to that of a "young, normal" adult with peak bone density. Results are given as a T-score, which indicates how much your reading deviates from that desirable density. The World Health Organization defines T-scores on the scale below.

Normal bone density (> –1.0):
Low risk of osteoporosis and/or fractures

Low bone density or osteopenia (–1.0 to –2.5):
Moderate risk of poor bone health

Osteoporosis (< –2.5):
High risk of poor bone health

FIGURE 9-20 ▲ The classification for diagnosing osteoporosis is used by the World Health Organization. A T-score of –1.0 or higher is normal; a T-score from –1.0 to –2.5 indicates low bone mass and is known as osteopenia, and a T-score less than –2.5 indicates osteoporosis. Severe osteoporosis is diagnosed with a T-score of less than –2.5 and a personal history of fragility fracture.

TABLE 9-2 ■ **Biological Factors Associated with Bone Status**

Biological Factors	Effect on Bone Status
Sex	Women have lower bone mass and density than men.
Age	Bone loss occurs after age 30.
Ethnicity	Individuals of Caucasian or Asian heritage are at greater risk for poor bone health than individuals of African descent.
Frame size	People with "small bones" have a lower bone mass.
Estrogen	Women at menopause and beyond should consider use of current medical therapies to reduce bone loss linked to the fall in estrogen output.

Whether or not you have had your bone mineral density tested, you can also use the online Fracture Risk Assessment Tool (FRAX) to estimate your risk of fracture. You can calculate your FRAX score at **http://www .shef.ac.uk/FRAX.** The National Osteoporosis Foundation Guide recommends that physicians consider prescribing medication if your risk of a hip fracture is at least 3% over the next 10 years. The incidence of osteoporosis is far less in many other countries than in the United States. In reviewing Tables 9-2 and 9-3, you can see that the contributions for the greater incidence in the United States are mainly related to diet and other lifestyle behaviors. That means that osteoporosis can largely be prevented.

GETTING ENOUGH CALCIUM

Calcium requires an acidic environment in the gastrointestinal tract to be absorbed efficiently. Absorption occurs primarily in the upper part of the small intestine. This area tends to remain somewhat acidic because it receives the acidic stomach contents. In the first section of the small intestine, secretions from the pancreas begin to increase the pH of the small intestine, and the pH becomes neutral to slightly basic, causing calcium absorption to decrease. Efficient calcium absorption in the upper small intestine also depends on the presence of the active form of vitamin D (review Chapter 8). Adults absorb about 30% of the calcium in the foods eaten, but during times when the body needs extra calcium, such as in infancy and pregnancy, absorption increases to as high as 60%. Aging negatively influences the absorption efficiency of calcium; due to decreased acid secretion in the stomach and lower synthesis, absorption, and activation of vitamin D, people over age 40 have a harder time meeting their needs for calcium.

The Recommended Dietary Allowance for calcium is 1000 milligrams per day for adults through 50 years of age. For women older than age 50 and for both men and women over age 70, the RDA increases to 1200 milligrams per day. The RDA is based on the amount of calcium needed each day to offset calcium losses in urine, feces, and other routes. The RDA for young people ages 9 to 18 (1300 milligrams per day) includes an additional amount to allow for increases in bone mass during growth and development.

The calcium intakes of many Americans fall short of meeting the RDA. During late childhood and adolescence—a critical time for accretion of bone mass—many youngsters are choosing sugar- and caffeine-laden beverages instead of milk or dairy alternatives. This calcium deficit sets the stage for osteoporosis later in life. Into adulthood, average daily calcium intakes are approximately 800 milligrams for women and 1000 milligrams for men. Approximately half of adult women in the United States consume less than 60% of the recommended intake of calcium. Some of this is due to their perception that dairy products are high in calories (although many reduced-fat dairy products are available). A growing number of Americans are choosing a plant-based eating pattern, including a vegan diet, which eliminates dairy products. Other adults simply lose their taste for milk as they age. In addition, lactose intolerance becomes more prevalent as people age.

Calcium is found in both plant and animal foods. Overall, dairy products provide about 75% of the calcium in North American eating patterns. In fact, fat-free milk is the most nutrient-dense (milligrams per kcal) source of this bone-building nutrient. Calcium tends to be highly bioavailable from dairy products because they contain vitamin D and lactose, which enhance calcium absorption. An exception is cottage cheese; much of its calcium is bound and unavailable for absorption.

TABLE 9-3 ■ **Modifiable Lifestyle Factors Associated with Bone Status**

Lifestyle Factors	Call to Action
Adequate diet containing an appropriate amount of nutrients	• Follow MyPlate with special emphasis on adequate amounts of fruits, vegetables, and low-fat and fat-free dairy products. • Consider use of fortified foods (or supplements) to make up for specific nutrient shortfalls, such as vitamin D and calcium.
Healthy body weight	• Maintain a healthy body weight (BMI of 18.5–24.9) to support bone health.
Normal menses	• During childbearing years, seek medical advice if menses cease (such as in cases of anorexia nervosa or extreme athletic training). • Women at menopause and beyond should consider use of current medical therapies to reduce bone loss linked to the fall in estrogen output.
Weight-bearing physical activity	• Perform weight-bearing activity as this contributes to bone maintenance, whereas bed rest and a sedentary lifestyle lead to bone loss. Strength training, especially upper body, is helpful to bone maintenance.
Smoking	• Smoking lowers estrogen synthesis in women. Cessation is advised. Passive exposure is a risk.
Medications	• Some medications (e.g., thyroid hormone, cortisol, and diuretics) stimulate urinary calcium excretion. • Some medications (e.g., alcohol, diuretics, and cancer medications) stimulate urinary excretion of magnesium.
Excessive intake of protein, phosphorus, sodium, caffeine, wheat bran, or alcohol	• Moderate intake of these dietary constituents is recommended. Problems primarily arise when excessive intakes of these nutrients are combined with inadequate calcium consumption. • Excessive soft drink consumption is especially discouraged.
Inadequate UV-B exposure	• If sunlight exposure is limited (<10–15 minutes per day without sunscreen), focus on food or supplements to meet current RDA for vitamin D.

Bread, rolls, crackers, and foods made with milk products also make a significant contribution to North Americans' calcium intake. Chia seeds, flaxseeds, and sesame seeds, as well as quinoa, also are rich sources. Other sources are leafy greens (such as kale), almonds, some legumes, sardines, and canned salmon (Fig. 9-21).

Through the production of more products fortified with calcium, food and beverage companies are responding to consumers' desire to increase consumption of calcium. Calcium-fortified foods such as orange juice, breakfast cereals, breakfast bars, waffles, and soy products provide considerable amounts of calcium. In fact, an 8-ounce glass of calcium-fortified orange juice can provide up to 350 milligrams of calcium, whereas a serving of milk has 300. Another source of calcium is soybean curd (tofu) if it is made with calcium (check the label). It is easy to assess the calcium content of foods because it is among those nutrients that are required to be listed on the Nutrition Facts panel on food labels. The revised Nutrition Facts label now lists the amount of calcium and vitamin D in a serving as well as the percent of the DV. The DV for calcium used for food and supplement labels is 1000 milligrams.

To estimate your calcium intake, use the rule of 300s. Count 300 milligrams for the calcium provided by foods scattered throughout the diet. Add another 300 milligrams to that for every cup of milk or yogurt or 1.5 ounces of cheese. If you eat a lot of tofu, almonds, or sardines, or drink calcium-fortified beverages, use Figure 9-21 or diet-analysis software such as NutritionCalc Plus in Connect to get a more accurate calculation of calcium intake.

Keep in mind, however, that many factors can influence the bioavailability of calcium. Calcium absorption can be reduced by the presence of oxalates, tannins, and phytic acid. These compounds chelate (chemically bind) calcium in the digestive tract. Oxalates are found in sweet potatoes, collard greens, spinach, and rhubarb. It is estimated that a person would have to consume over eight servings (8 cups) of spinach to absorb the same amount of calcium present in one serving (1 cup) of milk! Oxalates bind only the calcium in the food they are in; oxalate-containing foods do not affect the calcium availability from other foods. This does not hold true for phytates or tannins. Tea and some legumes

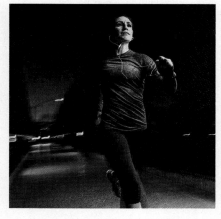

▲ Weight-bearing exercise such as walking or running is associated with increased bone density. Female athletes, however, must maintain an adequate energy intake to maintain estrogen levels, which stimulate bone formation. ©Image Source/Corey Jenkins

Calcium
RDA: 1000 milligrams
DV: 1000 milligrams
UL: 2500 milligrams

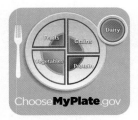

FIGURE 9-21 ◄ Food sources of calcium. (a) The fill of the background color (none, 1/3, 2/3, or completely covered) within each food group on MyPlate indicates the average nutrient density for calcium in that group. (b) The bar graph shows the calcium content of several foods in each food group compared to the RDA for adult males and females. Overall, the richest sources of calcium are dairy foods (and dairy alternatives), legumes, green leafy vegetables, and fortified foods.

Source: Nutrition data from USDA National Nutrient Database for Standard Reference, Release 26

(a)

(b)

	Food Item and Amount	Calcium (milligrams)	% RDA for Adult Males and Females (1000 milligrams)
Grains	Total Raisin Bran cereal, 1 cup	1000	100%
Grains	English muffin, whole wheat, 1 each	175	18%
Grains	Pancake, 4"	83	8%
Vegetables	Spinach, cooked, 1 cup	245	25%
Vegetables	Butternut squash, cooked, 1 cup	84	8%
Vegetables	Broccoli, cooked, 1 cup	62	6%
Fruits	Orange juice (fortified), 1 cup	349	35%
Fruits	Figs, dried, ½ cup	121	12%
Fruits	Raisins, ½ cup	36	4%
Dairy	Yogurt, plain, nonfat, 1 cup	488	49%
Dairy	Milk, fat-free, 1 cup	299	30%
Dairy	Soy milk, (fortified), 1 cup	299	30%
Protein	Tofu (with calcium sulfate), 3 ounces	574	57%
Protein	Salmon, canned with bones, 3 ounces	203	20%
Protein	Almonds, dry roasted, 1 ounce	76	8%

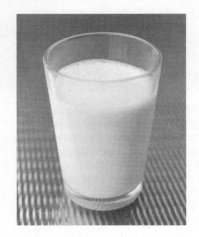

▲ Many milk alternatives are available including soy milk, almond milk, and rice milk. Not all milk substitutes have the same nutritional profiles as cow's milk. It is very important to know what nutrients you are looking for and to read labels carefully to compare products. ©Jonelle Weaver/Getty Images

are rich sources of tannins. Phytates are found in whole grains, raw beans, and nuts. Diets high in dietary fiber reduce mineral absorption. With this in mind, vegans should take extra care to include good sources of calcium in their diets. Read the Ask the RDN in this section for information on the negative effect of caffeine on calcium absorption.

Dairy Alternatives. There are many reasons why you may choose to avoid dairy products. These include following a vegan diet or just trying to avoid the antibiotics and hormones that may be used in the dairy industry. Or you may need to avoid dairy products because you have an allergy to milk protein or intolerance to lactose. If you do not eat dairy products, it is critical that you know how to make healthy food substitutions to get the nutrients you need, especially those related to bone health.[11] Many dairy alternatives are available in the grocery store today. These products look, feel, and taste like typical dairy foods but are not made from the milk of animals. Most of the milk alternatives are healthy and delicious, but not exact nutritional replicas of cow's milk (Table 9-4). *Soy milk* contains the highest quantity of protein of all the dairy alternatives with 6 to 10 grams per cup and also the best quality in that it contains all of the essential amino acids. It also has about the same proportion of protein (3.5%), fat (2%), and carbohydrate (3%) as cow's milk. It contains omega-3 fatty acids, fiber, magnesium, and manganese, and most brands are fortified with calcium, riboflavin, and vitamins A, D, and B-12. Most brands contain 450 milligrams of calcium (45% DV). Soy milk is a popular product for vegans because it is plant-based and for people with lactose intolerance

TABLE 9-4 ■ How Nondairy Milk Beverages Compare to the Nutrient Content of Cow's Milk

Nutrients per 1-Cup Serving	Whole Milk	Soy Milk	Rice Milk	Almond Milk	Coconut Milk	Coconut Milk Beverage	Flax Milk	Cashew Milk
Calories	149	90	120	40–60	552	70	50	60
Total Fat (grams)	7.7	3.5	2.5	3	57	4.5	2.5	2.5
Protein (grams)	8	6	1	1	5	0	0	<1
Calcium (% Daily Value)	28	45	30	20	4	10	30	45
Vitamin D (% Daily Value)	30	45	25	45	0	45	25	45

because it does not contain lactose. *Rice milk* is naturally sweeter than cow's milk, much higher in carbohydrates (24 grams per cup), and has significantly less protein (1 gram per cup) and no lactose. Most brands are fortified with calcium, iron, riboflavin, and vitamins A, D, and B-12 and contain about 300 milligrams of calcium per cup (30% DV).

Almond milk naturally contains a significant amount of calcium and vitamin D and is an excellent source of the antioxidant vitamin E. A cup of almond milk contains about 200 mg of calcium (20% DV), 100 IU of vitamin D (25% DV), and 10 mg of vitamin E (50% DV). Almond milk is much lower in calories than cow's milk and contains very little protein (1 gram per cup), carbohydrate (2 grams per cup), fat (3 grams per cup), and fiber (1 gram per cup). Because almond milk is low in fat and calories and contains some essential vitamins and minerals, it can be used as a milk substitute for those who would like to lose weight. Many find the taste of almond milk more acceptable compared to other dairy substitutes.

Coconut milk has a high oil content and therefore is much higher in calories, fat, and saturated fat than other milks and milk substitutes. A 1-cup serving of canned coconut milk contains 445 calories and 48 grams of fat, of which 43 grams are saturated fat. It contains very little calcium or vitamin D but does contain about 40% DV of iron. There are also coconut milk beverages available that compare closely to soy, rice, and almond milks. These beverages are a mixture of coconut cream and water, and per cup have only 5 grams of fat, 1 gram of protein, 80 calories, and 450 milligrams of calcium (45% DV).

Flax milk is cold-pressed flax oil mixed with filtered water. One cup has 50 calories, 1200 mg of omega-3s, and 30% DV of calcium but no protein. Flax milks are typically fortified with vitamin A (10%), vitamin D (25%), vitamin B-12 (25%), and calcium (30%).

Cashew milk is the most recent addition to the plant-based beverages industry. Although it has only 60 calories per cup and no saturated fat or cholesterol, it is creamier than skim milk and has nearly twice the calcium of cow's milk.

In summary, many dairy alternatives are available. Not all of these substitutes, however, have the same nutritional profiles as the original milk-based product. Thus, it is very important to know what nutrients you are looking for and then to read labels carefully to compare products.

Calcium Supplementation. There has been much debate over the effectiveness of calcium and vitamin D supplementation for maintaining bone health. Although achieving the RDAs for calcium and vitamin D through dietary modifications has been found to improve bone mineral density and reduce rate of fractures, use of supplements to meet RDAs may actually impair skeletal health and worsen cardiovascular health. Recent studies have ignited controversy over the potential health risks of consuming large amounts of these nutrients, especially for older adults. One of these studies found that a dietary intake of calcium near the current recommendations was not related to higher bone mineral density of the hip or lumbar spine compared with lower intakes of calcium in elderly men and women in the United States. In addition, calcium intake beyond the RDA for elderly women and men, usually achieved by calcium supplements, did not provide any

Many factors *enhance* calcium absorption, including:

- High need (e.g., during growth, pregnancy, lactation)
- Increased blood levels of parathyroid hormone and vitamin D
- The presence of lactose in the diet
- Decreased flow rate (motility) of digestive contents through the intestine
- Acidic environment of the stomach

Many factors *inhibit* calcium absorption, including:

- Large amounts of phytic acid and fiber from grains (if fiber intake exceeds 30 grams per day)
- Oxalates found in specific foods—but only calcium in the food itself; they do not inhibit calcium absorption from other foods.
- Great excess of phosphorus, magnesium, sodium, and zinc in the diet if calcium intake is very low
- Tannins (polyphenols) in tea and some legumes (e.g., soy)
- A vitamin D deficiency
- Diarrhea
- Old age
- Some medications (anticonvulsants, cortisone, antacids)

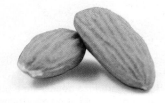

▲ Almonds are a natural source of calcium. One ounce contains 80 milligrams.
©Ingram Publishing/SuperStock

Dairy-Free Shopping Guide: Things to Consider

- Replacing dairy milk with a plant-milk alternative can be part of a plant-based eating plan.
- Look for the unsweetened varieties available in most product lines.
- Choose plant-based milks that are fortified with vitamin D and calcium.
- Remember that most plant-based milks have negligible protein. Only soy milk is similar to dairy milk in terms of protein. Be aware that almond milk that is extremely low in protein is becoming popular in coffee shops as a dairy-free creamer.
- Look for a dairy alternative with a short ingredient list (e.g., nuts, water, salt, and spices). Some dairy-free milks are full of additives, including stabilizers and thickening agents such as sugar, gums, inulin, and carrageenan.

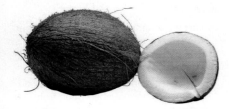

▲ Freshly pressed coconut milk is loaded with calories because of its high fat content and contains very little calcium and vitamin D. Coconut milk beverages sold alongside cow's milk have been altered to reduce fat content and increase bone-building nutrients. ©Author's Image/Glow Images

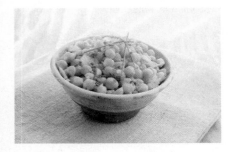

▲ Chickpeas (garbanzo beans) are a good plant source of calcium at 80 milligrams per cup. A cup of hummus made from chickpeas provides 93.5 milligrams of calcium. ©L. Mouton/PhotoAlto

ASK THE RDN — Coffee, Colas, and Bone Health

Dear RDN: I look forward to the caffeine boost I get from a cup of coffee in the morning and late afternoon, and I enjoy a diet cola with lunch. Could the caffeine in these drinks be damaging my bones and leading to osteoporosis?

Coffee and colas are major sources of caffeine. An 8-ounce cup of coffee usually contains at least 95 milligrams of caffeine, and a 12-ounce cola typically has about 30 milligrams. High intakes of caffeine are known to decrease intestinal calcium absorption and simultaneously increase the amount of calcium excreted in the urine, suggesting that excessive use of caffeine can eventually contribute to bone loss. Research has confirmed that consuming 330 milligrams or more of caffeine daily (the amount found in about four cups of coffee) increases the risk of brittle or broken bones. The evidence shows both coffee and colas having effects on bone density that could contribute to osteoporosis. It is interesting that these associations appear only in women and are not linked to the consumption of black tea, which also contains caffeine. In fact, older women who drink tea have been shown to have greater bone density than women who do not drink tea at all. While the tannins in tea are known to reduce the absorption of calcium, studies have suggested that phytochemicals in tea, such as flavonoids, may provide a protective effect against bone loss due to their estrogen-like properties.

In addition to caffeine, regular and diet colas also contain phosphoric acid that can affect bones. Phosphorus is widespread in our food supply, both naturally and as an additive. The abundance of phosphorus in our food raises some concern that we may actually be getting too much of a good thing. Getting more phosphorus is generally considered safe in people with healthy kidney function who consume adequate calcium. However, high phosphorus intakes are a concern when they are combined with a low calcium intake, which creates an imbalance in the calcium-to-phosphorus ratio that can contribute to bone loss. This situation is more common when you regularly substitute soft drinks for milk.

The bottom line is that you can enjoy coffee and cola as long as you get enough calcium to meet your body's needs and make up for any caffeine-induced calcium losses. Be sure and include calcium-rich foods in your dietary pattern and consult your primary care provider or dietitian to discuss calcium supplementation if your intake falls short of the recommendations. Most importantly, make sure that your coffee and colas are not replacing milk and calcium-fortified juice consumption that promotes bone health. Practice moderation with your caffeine consumption to prevent caffeine from interfering with calcium absorption and excretion. Less than two cans of cola per day is advised, and keep your coffee habit to no more than three (8-ounce) cups a day. Adding fat-free milk to your coffee can help offset any losses.

Start your day with café au lait,

Anne M. Smith, PhD, RDN, LD (author)

benefit for hip or lumbar spine bone mineral density in older adults.[12] Other large studies, including the large Women's Health Initiative trial, have also shown a small but statistically significant increase in the rate of heart attacks among older adults taking calcium supplements with or without vitamin D.[13] Although the observed relationships between calcium supplements and heart attack risk are small, the regular use of calcium supplements by so many older adults could translate into a large public health problem.

On the positive side, a more recent report from the Women's Health Initiative study indicates that long-term use of a daily calcium and vitamin D supplement that is close to the RDA results in a substantial reduction in the risk of hip fracture among postmenopausal women. These authors also reported that the level of calcium and vitamin D supplementation did not result in an increase in other chronic diseases, including heart disease. The more positive effects of supplementation appear to happen when the level of total calcium and vitamin D intake is kept very close to the RDA (see the Newsworthy Nutrition in this section). Therefore, taking 1000 milligrams of calcium carbonate or calcium citrate daily as a supplement in divided doses (about 500 milligrams per tablet) is probably safe in many instances.

So which is better: calcium from food or supplements? The National Osteoporosis Foundation continues to encourage all individuals to consume the recommended amounts of calcium and vitamin D to protect bone health. Experts agree that we should strive to meet our calcium and vitamin D needs from foods first and that more research is needed to better comprehend the benefits and risks associated with calcium and vitamin D supplementation. Modification of eating habits to include foods that are good sources of calcium is a better plan of action and appears to be the safest means to prevent osteoporosis without jeopardizing heart health. In addition to this important mineral, foods that contain calcium also supply other vitamins, minerals, phytochemicals, and fats needed to support health. Problems associated with excessive consumption of calcium, such as constipation, are not likely when foods are the primary sources of calcium.

In an effort to provide guidance for the public, the U.S. Preventive Services Task Force reviewed current research studies on the use of vitamin D and calcium supplements to prevent fractures and issued recommendations in its *Vitamin D and Calcium Supplementation to Prevent Fractures* report in February 2013. The recommendations apply to adult men and women who live at home. They do not apply to those living in assisted living or skilled nursing facilities or who have been diagnosed with osteoporosis or vitamin D deficiency. The Task Force conclusions are listed in the margin and are based on what is known about the potential benefits and harms of using these supplements.

Keeping in mind the recommendations just discussed, increasing calcium intake through the use of a calcium supplement is beneficial if you have a milk allergy; do not like milk; are ovovegetarian, vegan, or lactose intolerant; or cannot incorporate enough calcium-containing foods into your eating pattern.[14] Always look for a supplement with added vitamin D, as it enhances calcium uptake. This additional vitamin D typically does not add to the cost of the supplement. Table 9-5 compares the two most common forms of calcium supplements. Calcium carbonate should be taken with meals because it requires an acid environment in the stomach to dissolve and maximize calcium absorption. Calcium citrate is indicated for people who cannot remember to take

Vitamin D and Calcium Supplementation to Prevent Fractures
Task Force Conclusions:

(1) There is not enough evidence to determine whether vitamin D and calcium supplements can prevent fractures in men and in women who have not yet gone through menopause.

(2) There is not enough evidence to determine whether vitamin D and calcium supplements with greater than 400 IU of vitamin D and greater than 1000 mg of calcium can prevent fractures in noninstitutionalized postmenopausal women.

(3) There is enough evidence to recommend against daily supplementation with 400 IU or less of vitamin D and 1000 milligrams or less of calcium for the primary prevention of fractures in noninstitutionalized postmenopausal women because lower doses of vitamin D and calcium supplements do not prevent fractures in older women and may increase the risk of kidney stones.

The full Task Force statement can be viewed at https://www.uspreventiveservicestaskforce .org/Page/Document/UpdateSummaryFinal/ vitamin-d-and-calcium-to-prevent-fractures-preventive-medication.

Newsworthy Nutrition

Calcium supplements decrease risk of hip fracture in women

The Women's Health Initiative clinical trial randomly assigned 36,282 postmenopausal women in the United States to a placebo or 1000 milligram supplement of calcium carbonate plus 400 IU of vitamin D daily for 7.0 years. The hypothesis of this study was that calcium plus vitamin D supplementation would reduce hip fracture. This study also examined the health benefits and risks of calcium and vitamin D supplementation on total fractures, cardiovascular disease, cancer, and total mortality. Women in both groups were also allowed to take personal calcium and vitamin D supplements during the study, which was accounted for during the analysis of the data. Regarding bone health, the women who took the assigned calcium and vitamin D supplement but took no personal calcium supplements had a 75% lower risk of hip fracture than women who got the placebo and took no personal calcium supplements. The results also showed that women assigned to take calcium and vitamin D had no higher risk of heart disease, heart attacks, stroke, colorectal cancer, or total mortality. The supplement group did have a 17% increased risk of kidney stones. The authors concluded that long-term use of calcium and vitamin D appears to confer a substantial reduction in the risk of hip fracture among postmenopausal women. Because the risk reduction was significant only in women not taking any additional calcium supplements, it is recommended that women strive to consume the RDA for calcium (1200 milligrams per day) and vitamin D (600 IU/per day up to age 70 and 800 IU per day over 70) from food and supplements combined.

Source: Prentice, RL. "Health risks and benefits from calcium and vitamin D supplementation: Women's Health Initiative clinical trial and cohort study." *Osteoporosis International*, 24, 2, 2013, 567. Springer-Verlag London LTD.

TABLE 9-5 ■ Calcium Supplement Comparisons

	Calcium carbonate	Calcium citrate
Calcium content	40%	21%
Forms	Tablets, chewable tablets, soft chews	Pills (can be quite large), liquid (sometimes easier to tolerate)
Cost	Least expensive, most common form	Most expensive
Bioavailability and meal timing	Needs acid environment in stomach, so take with acid food or with meals	Best absorbed; does not need acid environment to be absorbed

calcium carbonate with meals and for those who have low-acid stomach conditions, such as people who take acid-reducing medications for ulcers or reflux, or have had surgery for obesity reduction.

Calcium supplements have side effects, including gas, bloating, or constipation. Distributing small-dose supplements throughout the day, taking it with meals, or even changing the brand of supplement may alleviate some problems. Intake of calcium from supplements and/or food above 500 milligrams at any one time significantly reduces the percent absorbed.

With calcium supplements, interactions with other minerals are a concern. There is evidence that calcium supplements may decrease zinc, iron, and other mineral absorption. An effect of calcium supplementation on iron absorption is possible; however, this appears to be small over the long term. To be safe, people using a calcium supplement on a regular basis should notify their primary care provider of the practice. Calcium supplements can also interfere with the body's ability to absorb certain antibiotics. Be sure to consult with your pharmacist about timing of your supplement, medications, and meals.

Tablet or liquid calcium supplements with the United States Pharmacopeia (USP) symbol are considered the safest. The FDA has cautioned the public on the use of calcium supplements from dolomite, bone meal, coral, or oyster shell because of the potential for unhealthy levels of environmental contaminants.

AVOIDING TOO MUCH CALCIUM

The Upper Level (UL) for calcium intake is 2500 milligrams per day for young adults, based on the observation that greater intakes increase the risk for some forms of kidney stones. Excessive calcium intakes by some people can also cause high blood and urinary calcium concentrations, irritability, headache, kidney failure, soft tissue calcification, and decreased absorption of other minerals, as noted previously.

✓ CONCEPT CHECK 9.6

1. What percent of calcium in the body is found in bone and teeth?
2. What are the two types of osteoporosis, and how do they differ?
3. What type of bone is most affected by osteoporosis?
4. Why is the achievement of peak bone mass as a young adult so important in preventing osteoporosis?
5. What are some current treatments for osteoporosis?
6. What is the most accurate test for bone density, and how is it done?
7. According to the National Osteoporosis Foundation, who should have their bone density checked?
8. Beyond its role in bone health, what are some other critical functions of calcium?
9. What role does vitamin D play in calcium metabolism?
10. What factors reduce calcium absorption?

9.7 Phosphorus

FUNCTIONS OF PHOSPHORUS

Phosphorus (P) is the second most abundant mineral in the body. Approximately 85% of phosphorus is found as a component of hydroxyapatite crystals that provide the functional component of bone and teeth. The remaining 15% of phosphorus is in the soft tissues, blood, and extracellular fluid. Phosphorus is part of DNA and RNA, the genetic material present in every cell. Therefore, phosphorus is critical for cellular replication and growth because DNA and RNA are responsible for mitosis and protein synthesis. Phosphorus is also a primary component of adenosine triphosphate (ATP), the energy molecule that fuels body functions. Phosphorus is essential for the activation and deactivation of many enzymes, and many of the B vitamins are functional only when a phosphate group is attached.

A major class of lipids contains phosphorus: phospholipids are the principal structural component of cell membranes, making up approximately 60% of membranes. These phospholipid membranes regulate the transport of nutrients and waste products into and out of cells. Phosphorus also serves as a buffer to maintain blood pH. Lastly, phosphorus (in the form of the phosphate ion) is the principal negatively charged ion in intracellular fluid and thus is essential for maintenance of fluid balance.

PHOSPHORUS DEFICIENCY

As a general rule, deficiencies of phosphorus are unlikely in healthy adults because it is so widespread in food and efficiently absorbed. If intakes of phosphorus are inadequate, the kidney compensates by increasing the reabsorption of phosphorus to prevent blood phosphorus levels from decreasing. Dietary phosphorus deficiency usually occurs only in cases of near-total starvation, including anorexia nervosa. Some health conditions such as diabetes and alcoholism, as well as medications such as antacids and diuretics, can cause phosphorus levels in the body to fall. Marginal phosphorus status can be found in preterm infants, vegans, older people with nutrient-poor eating patterns, and people with long-term bouts of diarrhea, as occurs in Crohn's disease and celiac disease. A small percentage of older women undergoing osteoporosis treatment have been shown to be at high risk for phosphorus deficiency because phosphorus intake is low and phosphorus absorption is inhibited by calcium supplements. Symptoms of phosphorus deficiency include loss of appetite, anemia, muscle weakness, bone pain, fragile bones, increased susceptibility to infection, numbness and tingling of the extremities, difficulty walking, and irregular breathing.[15]

GETTING ENOUGH PHOSPHORUS

In contrast to calcium, phosphorus is naturally abundant in many foods. Milk, cheese, meat, and bread provide most of the phosphorus in the adult diet. Nuts, fish, breakfast cereals, bran, and eggs are also good sources (Fig. 9-22). About 20% to 30% of dietary phosphorus comes from food additives, especially in baked goods, cheeses, processed meats, and many soft drinks (about 75 milligrams per 12 ounces). As a food additive, phosphorus is considered a GRAS (generally recognized as safe) substance, and its function is to increase water binding and taste. Phosphoric acid, which gives a tangy, sour taste, will also significantly lower the pH of a food or beverage (pH of a soft drink is less than 3). Absorption of phosphorus is generally high, ranging from 55% to 80%. Phosphorus absorption from grains, however, is reduced because of the high phytic acid content. Vitamin D enhances phosphorus absorption.

The RDA for phosphorus is 700 milligrams for adult men and women (see margin). The recommendation is higher (1250 milligrams per day) for young people ages 9 to 18 to support growth and development. Average daily adult consumption is about 1000 to 1600 milligrams.

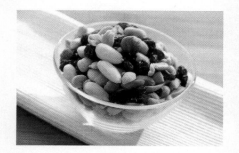

▲ Trail mix is rich in phosphorus.
©imagebroker/Alamy

Phosphorus
RDA: 700 milligrams
DV: 1000 milligrams
UL: 4000 milligrams

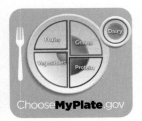

FIGURE 9-22 ◄ Food sources of phosphorus. (a) The fill of the background color (none, 1/3, 2/3, or completely covered) within each food group on MyPlate indicates the average nutrient density for phosphorus in that group. (b) The bar graph shows the phosphorus content of several foods compared to the RDA for adult males and females. Overall, the richest sources of phosphorus are dairy products and protein foods. Foods from the fruits group (not shown) are poor sources of phosphorus.

Source: Nutrition data from USDA National Nutrient Database for Standard Reference, Release 26

(a)

(b)

	Food Item and Amount	Phosphorus (milligrams)	% RDA for Adult Males and Females (700 milligrams)
Grains	Trail mix (with chocolate, nuts, seeds), ½ cup	283	40%
Grains	Raisin bran cereal, 1 cup	205	29%
Grains	Oatmeal, prepared with water, ½ cup	90	13%
Vegetables	Potato, baked (with skin), 1 medium	121	17%
Vegetables	Asparagus, cooked, 1 cup	97	14%
Vegetables	Mushrooms, white, raw, 1 cup	60	9%
Dairy	Yogurt, plain, nonfat, 1 cup	385	55%
Dairy	Milk, fat-free, 1 cup	247	35%
Dairy	Soy milk, 1 cup	104	15%
Protein	Salmon, baked, 3 ounces	218	31%
Protein	Great northern beans, cooked, ½ cup	146	21%
Protein	Almonds, dry roasted, 1 ounce	134	19%

AVOIDING TOO MUCH PHOSPHORUS

The UL for phosphorus intake is 3 to 4 grams per day. Intakes greater than this can result in mineralization of soft tissues. Phosphorus levels in the blood are regulated primarily by the kidneys, and these organs are particularly sensitive to phosphorus toxicity. High intakes can lead to serious problems in people with certain kidney diseases. In addition, a high phosphorus intake coupled with a low calcium intake can cause a chronic imbalance in the calcium-to-phosphorus ratio in the diet and contribute to bone loss. This situation most likely arises when the RDA for calcium is not met, as can occur in adolescents and adults who regularly substitute soft drinks for milk or otherwise underconsume calcium.

✓ CONCEPT CHECK 9.7

1. What are the key functions of phosphorus beyond bone health?
2. Is phosphorus deficiency very common, or is the RDA met by most North Americans?
3. What are the primary food sources of phosphorus?
4. What are the risks of excess intake of phosphorus?
5. What effect does vitamin D have on phosphorus absorption?

9.8 Magnesium

FUNCTIONS OF MAGNESIUM

Magnesium (Mg) is important for nerve and heart function and aids in many enzyme reactions. Magnesium is similar to calcium and phosphorus in that most of the magnesium in the body is found in bones. Bone contains 60% of the body's magnesium, where it serves a structural role to help provide rigidity and acts as a storage site drawn upon by other tissues when dietary intake is inadequate to meet the body's needs. Another notable function of magnesium as it relates to bone health is that magnesium is required for the synthesis of vitamin D in the liver. Magnesium functions to relax muscles after contraction. It promotes resistance to tooth decay by stabilizing calcium in tooth enamel. Over 300 enzymes use magnesium, and many energy-yielding compounds in cells require magnesium to function properly (e.g., ATP). Magnesium plays a critical role in the synthesis of DNA and protein.

Other possible benefits of magnesium in relation to cardiovascular disease include decreasing blood pressure by dilating arteries and preventing heart abnormalities. The results of a recent review of 40 studies of magnesium and risk of disease found that increasing dietary magnesium provided health benefits, including a reduced risk of stroke, heart failure, diabetes, and all-cause mortality.[16] People with cardiovascular disease should closely monitor magnesium intake, especially because they are often on medications such as diuretics that reduce magnesium status. An eating pattern rich in food sources of magnesium and calcium is associated with lower risk of type 2 diabetes in some populations.

MAGNESIUM DEFICIENCY

In humans, low blood magnesium causes an irregular heartbeat, sometimes accompanied by weakness, muscle pain, disorientation, and seizures. In terms of bone health, low magnesium disrupts the hormonal regulation of blood calcium by parathyroid hormone and affects the activity of vitamin D. You might expect that magnesium deficiency would result in diminished bone mass, but to date, this has only been observed in animals. (There is some evidence, however, that magnesium supplementation may improve bone density in postmenopausal women.)

Magnesium deficiency develops very slowly. Not only is the mineral present in foods of both plant and animal origin, but the kidneys also are very efficient at retaining magnesium. Thus, it is uncommon for healthy people to suffer a clinically relevant magnesium deficiency due to dietary inadequacy alone. Poor magnesium status is most commonly found among people with abnormal kidney function, whether as a result of kidney disease or as a side effect of certain diuretics. Alcohol use disorders also can increase the risk of deficiency because dietary intake may be poor and because alcohol increases magnesium excretion in the urine. The disorientation and weakness associated with alcohol use disorders closely resemble the behavior of people with low blood magnesium. In addition, people with malabsorptive diseases (e.g., Crohn's disease), heavy perspiration, or prolonged bouts of diarrhea or vomiting are susceptible to low blood levels of magnesium.

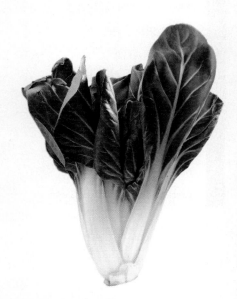

▲ Because magnesium is found in the chlorophyll of plants, it is in good supply in green leafy vegetables such as Swiss chard. ©lynx/iconotec.com/Glow Images

GETTING ENOUGH MAGNESIUM

Magnesium is found in the plant pigment chlorophyll, so rich sources for magnesium are plant products, such as spinach, whole grains (such as wheat bran), beans, nuts, seeds, and broccoli (Fig. 9-23). Animal products (e.g., milk and meats) and chocolate supply some magnesium, although not as much as foods of plant origin. Two other sources of magnesium are hard tap water, which contains a high mineral content, and coffee (espresso, not brewed).

The adult RDA for magnesium (see margin) is based on the amount needed to offset daily losses. Adult men consume on average 320 milligrams daily, whereas women

Magnesium

RDA

    Adult men: 400 milligrams

    Adult women: 310 milligrams

DV: 400 milligrams

UL: 350 milligrams (nonfood sources only)

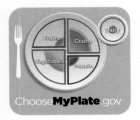

FIGURE 9-23 ◀ Food sources of magnesium. (a) The fill of the background color (none, 1/3, 2/3, or completely covered) within each food group on MyPlate indicates the average nutrient density for magnesium in that group. (b) The bar graph shows the magnesium content of several foods in each food group compared to the RDA for adult males and females. Overall, the richest sources of magnesium are vegetables and whole grains.

Source: Nutrition data from USDA National Nutrient Database for Standard Reference, Release 26

(a)

(b)

	Food Item and Amount	Magnesium (milligrams)	% RDA for Adult Males (400 milligrams)	% RDA for Adult Females (310 milligrams)
Grains	Raisin bran cereal, 1 cup	72	18%	23%
Grains	Whole wheat bread, 1 slice	24	6%	8%
Grains	White bread, 1 slice	7	2%	2%
Vegetables	Spinach, cooked, 1 cup	157	39%	51%
Vegetables	Okra, cooked, 1 cup	58	15%	19%
Vegetables	Sweet potato, baked, 1 cup	54	14%	17%
Fruits	Banana, 1 medium	32	8%	10%
Fruits	Blackberries, 1 cup	29	7%	9%
Fruits	Pineapple, 1 cup	20	5%	6%
Dairy	Yogurt, plain, nonfat, 1 cup	47	12%	15%
Dairy	Soy milk, 1 cup	36	9%	12%
Dairy	Milk, fat-free, 1 cup	27	7%	9%
Protein	Peanut butter, 2 tablespoons	49	12%	16%
Protein	Navy beans, cooked, ½ cup	48	12%	15%
Protein	Chicken breast, roasted, 3 ounces	25	6%	8%

consume closer to 220 milligrams daily, suggesting that many of us should improve our intakes of magnesium-rich foods, such as whole grain breads and cereals. The refined grain products that dominate the diets of many North Americans are poor sources of this mineral, as refining reduces the magnesium content by as much as 80%. This low value also reflects poor intake of green and other brightly colored vegetables. If dietary intake of magnesium is inadequate, a balanced multivitamin and mineral supplement containing approximately 100 milligrams of magnesium can help close the gap between intake and needs. Nutrient-nutrient interactions can reduce magnesium absorption. Diets very high in phosphorus or fiber (phytate) limit intestinal absorption, as do diets too low in protein.

AVOIDING TOO MUCH MAGNESIUM

The UL for magnesium intake is 350 milligrams per day, based on the risk of developing diarrhea. This guideline refers only to nonfood sources such as antacids, laxatives, or supplements.[14] Food sources are not known to cause toxicity. Magnesium toxicity especially occurs in people who have kidney failure or who overuse over-the-counter medications that contain magnesium, such as certain antacids and laxatives (e.g., milk of magnesia). Older people are at particular risk, as kidney function may be compromised.

Table 9-6 summarizes much of what we have covered regarding the major minerals.

TABLE 9-6 ■ **Summary of the Major Minerals**

Mineral	Major Functions	RDA or AI	Dietary Sources	Deficiency Symptoms	Toxicity Symptoms
Sodium	• Maintains fluid volume outside of cells and thus normal cell function	*Age 19–50 years:* 1500 milligrams *Age 51–70 years:* 1300 milligrams	• Processed foods to which sodium chloride (salt) has been added • Salted meats, nuts, cold cuts • Margarine, butter • Salt added to foods in cooking or at the table	• Muscle cramps	• Hypertension • Increased risk of cardiovascular disease and stroke UL = 2300 milligrams
Potassium	• Maintains fluid volume • Acts to blunt the rise of blood pressure in response to excess sodium intake • Decreases markers of bone turnover and recurrence of kidney stones	4700 milligrams	• Fruits • Vegetables • Dried peas • Dairy products • Meats • Nuts	• Irregular heartbeat • Loss of appetite • Muscle cramps	• None documented from food alone • Supplements or salt substitutes can result in hyperkalemia and possibly sudden death in susceptible individuals. No UL
Chloride	• With sodium, maintains fluid volume outside of cells and thus normal cell function	2300 milligrams	• Foods to which sodium chloride (salt) has been added	• Convulsions in infants	• In concert with sodium, results in hypertension UL = 3600 milligrams
Calcium	• Blood clotting • Muscle contraction • Nerve transmission • Bone and tooth formation	*Age 9–18 years:* 1300 milligrams *Age >18 years:* 1000–1200 milligrams	• Dairy • Corn tortillas • Calcium-set tofu • Chinese cabbage • Kale • Broccoli • Fortified foods and beverages	• Increased risk of osteoporosis	• Kidney stones • Hypercalcemia • Hypercalciuria • Prostate cancer • Constipation • Soft tissue calcification UL = 2500 milligrams
Phosphorus	• Maintenance of pH • Storage and transfer of energy • Nucleotide synthesis	*Age 9–18 years:* 1250 milligrams *Age >18 years:* 700 milligrams	• Dairy products • Soft drinks • Peas • Meat • Nuts • Eggs • Some cereals and breads	• Possibility of poor bone maintenance	• Metastatic calcification • Skeletal porosity • Interference with calcium absorption UL = 4 grams
Magnesium	• Cofactor for enzyme systems and vitamin D activation • Reduces tooth decay	*Men: 400– 420 milligrams* *Women: 310– 320 milligrams*	• Green leafy vegetables • Beans and peas • Nuts • Meat • Peanut butter • Milk	• Weakness • Muscle pain • Irregular heartbeat • Seizures	• Osmotic diarrhea UL = 350 milligrams (nonfood sources only)
Sulfur	• Part of vitamins and amino acids • Aids in drug detoxification • Acid–base balance	None established	• Protein foods • Dried fruit • Soy flour • Fruit juices • Coconut milk • Red and white wine • Bread • Meats that are high in sulfur amino acids	• None observed	• Osmotic diarrhea where water supply has high levels No UL

Abbreviation: UL = Upper Intake Level; RDA = Recommended Dietary Allowance; AI = adequate intake

1. What are the key functions of magnesium other than bone health?
2. What are the primary food sources of magnesium?
3. Who is at greatest risk of developing a magnesium deficiency?
4. When is magnesium toxicity most likely to occur?

9.9 Iron

Iron (Fe) is the trace mineral present in the largest amount in the body (Fig. 9-12). Although the importance of dietary iron has been recognized for many years, iron deficiency is the most common nutrient deficiency worldwide. About 30% of the world's population is anemic, with half of these cases caused by iron deficiency. Iron is the only nutrient for which young women have a greater RDA than do adult men.

FUNCTIONS OF IRON

Iron is part of the hemoglobin in red blood cells and myoglobin in muscle cells. Hemoglobin molecules in red blood cells transport oxygen (O_2) from the lungs to cells and then transport carbon dioxide (CO_2) from cells to the lungs for excretion. In addition, iron is used as part of many enzymes, some proteins, and compounds that cells use in energy production. Iron also is needed for brain and immune function, drug detoxification in the liver, and synthesis of collagen for bone health.

IRON DEFICIENCY

When neither the diet nor body stores can supply the iron needed for hemoglobin synthesis, the concentration of hemoglobin in red blood cells decreases. The percentage of blood made up of red blood cells **(hematocrit)** as well as the hemoglobin concentration are used to assess iron status. Other measures of iron status include the concentration of iron and iron-containing proteins in blood (serum iron, **ferritin,** or **transferrin**).

When hematocrit and hemoglobin fall, an iron deficiency is suspected. In severe deficiency, hemoglobin and hematocrit fall so low that the amount of oxygen carried in the bloodstream is decreased. This condition is called iron-deficiency anemia.

Iron deficiency can be categorized into three stages:

- **Stage 1:** Iron stores become depleted, but no physiological impairment is observed.
- **Stage 2:** The amount of iron in transferrin is depleted; some physiological impairment occurs. Heme production is decreased, and activities of enzymes that require iron as a cofactor are limited.
- **Stage 3 (iron-deficiency anemia):** Red blood cells are small (microcytic), pale (hypochromic), and reduced in number; oxygen-carrying capacity of red blood cells declines.

Clinical symptoms of iron-deficiency anemia are associated with the lack of oxygen getting to the tissues. One experiences pale skin, fatigue upon exertion, poor temperature regulation (always cold, especially toes and fingers), loss of appetite, and apathy. Poor iron stores may decrease learning ability, attention span, work performance, and immune status even before a person is anemic. Children with chronic anemia have abnormal cognitive development.

It is important to note that many more North Americans have an iron deficiency without anemia (stages 1 or 2) than have iron-deficiency anemia (stage 3). Their blood hemoglobin values are still normal, but they have no stores to draw from in times of pregnancy or illness, and basic functioning may be marginally impaired. That could

hematocrit The percentage of blood made up of red blood cells.

ferritin A protein that stores iron and releases it in a controlled manner. Acts as a buffer against iron deficiency and iron overload.

transferrin Iron-binding protein; controls the level of free iron in blood.

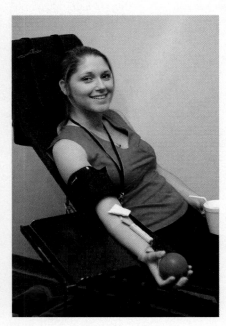

▲ Red blood cells contain about two-thirds of the body's total iron supply. Each time blood is donated, about 10% of total blood volume is sacrificed, which removes about 7% of the body's iron supply. Over the next few weeks, the red blood cells will be replaced, so healthy people can usually donate blood two to four times a year without harmful consequences. As a precaution, blood banks first screen potential donors' blood for the presence of anemia. ©David H. Lewis/Getty Images

mean anything from too little energy to perform everyday tasks in an efficient manner to difficulties staying mentally alert.

There are many conditions that lead to an anemic state; iron-deficiency anemia is the most prevalent nutrient deficiency worldwide. Probably about 10% of North Americans in high risk categories have iron-deficiency anemia. This appears most often in infancy, the preschool years, and at puberty for both males and females. Growth—with accompanying expansion of blood volume and muscle mass—increases iron needs, making it difficult to consume enough iron. Women are vulnerable to anemia during childbearing years due to menstrual blood loss. Anemia is also found in pregnant women because blood volume expands during pregnancy and extra iron is needed to synthesize red blood cells for the mother and the fetus. Iron-deficiency anemia in adult men is usually caused by blood loss from ulcers, colon cancer, or hemorrhoids. Athletes can have increased iron requirements due to increased blood loss in feces and urine and chronic lysis of red blood cells in the feet due to the trauma of running.

To cure iron-deficiency anemia, a person needs to take iron supplements.[17] A primary care provider should also find the cause so that the anemia does not reoccur. Changes in the dietary pattern may *prevent* iron-deficiency anemia, but supplemental iron is the only reliable *cure* once it has developed. Supplements must be taken for 3 to 6 months or perhaps longer. Hemoglobin levels respond quickly to dietary changes and supplementation, but stopping supplements too soon means that iron stores (blood, bone marrow, etc.) will not be replenished. Remember, it takes longer than 1 month to become anemic, so it will take longer than 1 month to cure it.

ABSORPTION AND DISTRIBUTION OF IRON

Overall, iron absorption depends on the following factors: (1) the person's iron status, (2) its form in food, (3) the acidity of the GI tract, and (4) other dietary components consumed with iron-containing foods. Controlling iron levels in the body is important because there is a narrow gap between just enough and too much iron. As you've learned, too little iron can impair oxygen transport. To prevent deficiency, the human body highly conserves iron. Except for bleeding associated with menstruation, injury, or childbirth, body loss of iron is minimal. Approximately 90% is recovered and reused every day. On the other hand, too much iron in the body is also extremely damaging. It can accumulate in organs and promote oxidative damage. To avoid toxicity, iron absorption from the small intestine is tightly regulated.

The most important factor influencing iron absorption is body need. Iron needs are increased during pregnancy and growth. At high altitudes, the lower oxygen concentration of the air causes an increase in the hemoglobin concentration of blood and thus an increase in iron needs.

The principal mechanism to regulate iron content in the body is tight control of absorption. High doses of iron can still be toxic, but absorption is carefully regulated under most conditions. In general, healthy people with adequate iron stores absorb between 5% and 15% of dietary iron, which is quite low compared to other nutrients. When iron stores are inadequate or needs are high due to growth or pregnancy, the main protein that carries iron (transferrin) more readily binds iron, shifting it from intestinal cells into the bloodstream. Absorption efficiency in times of need can be as high as 50%. On the other hand, if iron stores are adequate and the iron-binding protein in the blood is fully saturated with iron, absorption from the intestinal cells is minimal—as low as 2%. The iron remains in the intestinal cells, and it will be excreted in the feces when those intestinal cells slough off, which occurs every 5 to 6 days.

Another major influence on iron absorption is the form of iron in the food. **Heme iron,** derived from hemoglobin and **myoglobin,** comprises 40% of the iron in meat, fish, and poultry (MFP). Absorption of heme iron ranges from about 15% to 35%. Almost nothing affects its absorption. **Nonheme iron,** on the other hand, is subject to many conditions that can either enhance or inhibit its absorption, which ranges from 2% to 8%. Table 9-7 summarizes dietary factors that affect bioavailability of nonheme iron.

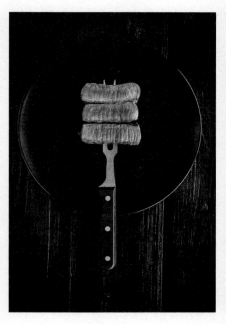

▲ Red meat is a major source of iron in the North American diet. Heme iron, which makes up about 40% of the iron in foods of animal origin, is better absorbed than nonheme iron. ©Mikhaylovskiy/Shutterstock

heme iron Iron provided from animal tissues in the form of hemoglobin and myoglobin. Approximately 40% of the iron in meat, fish, and poultry is heme iron; it is readily absorbed.

myoglobin Iron-containing protein that binds oxygen in muscle tissue.

nonheme iron Iron provided from plant sources, supplements, and animal tissues other than in the forms of hemoglobin and myoglobin. Nonheme iron is less efficiently absorbed than heme iron; absorption is closely dependent on body needs.

Iron

RDA

  Men: 8 milligrams

  Women: 18 milligrams (8 milligrams after menopause)

DV: 18 milligrams

UL: 45 milligrams

The iron added to foods and in most dietary supplements is nonheme iron.

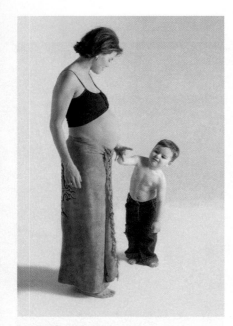

▲ During both pregnancy and childhood, demands for iron are high. Young children and women of reproductive age are at risk for iron-deficiency anemia. ©Ingram Publishing/AGE Fotostock

TABLE 9-7 ■ Dietary Iron Enhancers and Inhibitors

Nonheme Enhancers	Nonheme Inhibitors

• Vitamin C
  • Add marinara sauce to your spaghetti noodles.
• MFP (meat, fish, poultry) meat protein
  • Add some tuna to your snack of crackers.
	• Tannins (found in tea)
	  • Can lower absorption up to 60%, so drink tea between meals. Does not apply to herbal "tea," which contains no tea leaves.
	• Oxalates (spinach, rhubarb, and chard)
	• Phytates (whole grains, bran, and soybean)
	• Megadoses of zinc, calcium, or copper

Nonheme iron makes up 60% of iron in MFP and 100% of the iron found in dairy, eggs, fruit, vegetables, grains, fortified foods, and supplements. Because most of our dietary iron is nonheme iron, our overall dietary iron absorption is 5% to 15%.

Acidity also affects iron absorption: an acidic environment solubilizes iron and keeps it in a form that can be readily absorbed. Therefore, any medication or health condition that lowers acid production of the stomach can decrease iron absorption. For example, acid-reducing medications that people take to control heartburn or ulcers can impair iron absorption. Also, as people age, gastric acid secretion may decline. This puts older adults at risk for iron-deficiency anemia.

Lastly, other micronutrients affect iron absorption and availability. Megadoses of zinc or calcium compete with iron for absorption in the small intestine. In contrast, adequate copper is important for iron metabolism, and vitamin C is a powerful enhancer of iron absorption. Doses of 75 milligrams of vitamin C can increase nonheme absorption by 4%—a lot for nonheme. If you want to get the most iron out of your dietary supplement, take it with a glass of orange juice.

GETTING ENOUGH IRON

Animal sources contain approximately 40% heme iron, the most bioavailable form. The major iron sources in the adult eating pattern are ready-to-eat breakfast cereals, beans, and animal products (Fig. 9-24). Iron is added to flour during the enrichment process. Other iron sources are peas and legumes, but the absorption of nonheme iron found in these products is relatively low. Milk and eggs are poor sources of iron. A common cause of iron-deficiency anemia in children is high consumption of milk coupled with insufficient meat intake. Vegans are particularly susceptible to iron-deficiency anemia because of their lack of dietary heme iron.

The adult RDA is based on a 10% absorption rate to cover average losses of about 0.8 milligrams per day. For women of reproductive age, menstrual losses are an average of about 1 gram of additional iron per day. Thus, iron is the only nutrient for which women have higher requirements than men. Most women do not consume the recommended 18 milligrams of iron daily. The average daily amount consumed by women is closer to 13 milligrams, while in men, it is about 18 milligrams per day. Women of reproductive age can close this gap between average daily intakes and needs by seeking out iron-fortified foods, such as ready-to-eat breakfast cereals that contain at least 50% of the DV. Use of a balanced multivitamin and mineral supplement containing up to 100% of the DV for iron is another option. Consuming more than that much iron is not advised unless recommended by a primary care provider.

AVOIDING TOO MUCH IRON

The UL for iron is 45 milligrams per day. Higher amounts can lead to stomach irritation. Although iron overload is not as common as iron deficiency, the consequences can be dire. Even a large single dose of 60 milligrams of iron can be life threatening to

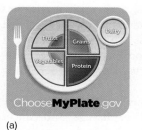

FIGURE 9-24 ◀ Food sources of iron. (a) The fill of the background color (none, 1/3, 2/3, or completely covered) within each food group on MyPlate indicates the average nutrient density for iron in that group. (b) The bar graph shows the iron content of several foods in each food group compared to the RDA for adult males and females. Overall, the richest sources of iron are meats, legumes, and fortified grain products.

Source: Nutrition data from USDA National Nutrient Database for Standard Reference, Release 26

(a)

(b)

	Food Item and Amount	Iron (milligrams)	% RDA for Adult Males (8 milligrams)	% RDA for Adult Females (18 milligrams)
Grains	Frosted mini wheats, 24 biscuits	17.6	220%	98%
Grains	Flour tortilla, 8″	1.0	13%	6%
Grains	Whole wheat bread, 1 slice	0.8	10%	4%
Vegetables	Spinach, cooked, 1 cup	6.4	80%	36%
Vegetables	Parsley, raw, 1 cup	3.7	47%	21%
Vegetables	Potato, baked (with skin), 1 medium	1.9	23%	10%
Fruits	Prune juice, 1 cup	3.0	38%	17%
Fruits	Raisins, ½ cup	1.6	19%	9%
Fruits	Orange, navel, 1 medium	0.2	2%	1%
Dairy	Soy milk, 1 cup	1.0	13%	6%
Dairy	Feta cheese, 1.5 ounces	0.3	4%	2%
Dairy	Milk, fat-free, 1 cup	0.1	1%	0%
Protein	Oysters, steamed, 3 ounces*	7.8	98%	44%
Protein	Kidney beans, cooked, ½ cup	2.0	25%	11%
Protein	Sirloin steak, grilled, 3 ounces*	1.5	18%	8%

*Contains heme iron

a 1 year old. Children are frequently victims of iron poisoning (acute toxicity) because supplements, which look a lot like candy, may be easily accessible on kitchen tables and from cabinets. The FDA requires that all iron supplements carry a warning about toxicity. Furthermore, supplements with 30 milligrams of iron or more per tablet must be individually wrapped.

Iron toxicity accompanies the genetic disease, hereditary **hemochromatosis.** The disease is associated with a substantial increase in iron absorption from both food and supplements. The harshest effects are seen in iron-storing organs such as the liver and heart. Some iron is deposited in the pancreas and muscles. Blood levels of iron remain high too, which increases the likelihood of infections and may promote cardiovascular disease.

Development of hereditary hemochromatosis requires that a person carry two defective copies of a particular gene. People with one defective gene and one normal gene (i.e., carriers) may also absorb too much dietary iron but not to the same extent as those with two defective genes. About 5% to 10% of North Americans of Northern European descent are carriers of hemochromatosis. Approximately 1 in 250 North Americans has both hemochromatosis genes. These numbers are high, considering that many primary care providers regard hemochromatosis as a rare disease and therefore do not routinely test for it.

hemochromatosis A disorder of iron metabolism characterized by increased iron absorption and deposition in the liver and heart. This eventually poisons the cells in those organs.

Anyone who has a blood relative (including uncles, aunts, and cousins) who has hemochromatosis or is a carrier should be screened for iron overload. At your next visit to a primary care provider, ask for a transferrin saturation test to assess iron stores. A ferritin test may also be added to assess your stores. Hemochromatosis can go undetected until a person is in his or her 50s or 60s, so some experts recommend screening for anyone over the age of 20.

If the disease goes untreated, iron accumulates and serious health problems may result: darkening of skin, arthritis, heart disease, diabetes, liver disease, and cancer (colon). Even with iron overload, the person may have anemia due to damage to the bone marrow or liver. Treatment of hemochromatosis is relatively easy, but it must be monitored consistently. **Therapeutic phlebotomy** to remove excess iron is essential. One must be very careful about the diet. Few sources of heme iron should be eaten, and supplements with iron or vitamin C should be avoided. Highly fortified breakfast cereals must also be avoided.

therapeutic phlebotomy Periodic blood removal, as a blood donation, for the purpose of ridding the body of excess iron.

✔ CONCEPT CHECK 9.9

1. List three symptoms of iron deficiency. How do these symptoms relate to the roles of iron in the body?
2. What are heme and nonheme iron? What can you do to enhance your absorption of nonheme iron?
3. What is hemochromatosis?

9.10 Zinc

Zinc (Zn) deficiency was first recognized in the early 1960s in Egypt and Iran, where it was linked to growth retardation and poor sexual development (Fig. 9-25). Even though the zinc content of the diets of people in these areas was fairly high, absorption of the mineral was limited by the phytic acid in unleavened bread. Parasite infestation and the practice of eating clay and other parts of soil also contributed to the severe zinc deficiency.

FUNCTIONS OF ZINC

Approximately 200 enzymes require zinc as a cofactor for activity. Adequate zinc intake is necessary to support many physiological functions:

- DNA synthesis and function
- Protein metabolism, wound healing, and growth
- Development of bones and reproductive organs
- Storage, release, and function of insulin
- Cell membrane structure and function
- Component of superoxide dismutase, an enzyme that aids in the prevention of oxidative damage to cells (zinc, therefore, has an indirect antioxidant function)
- White blood cell formation

It is important to note that although zinc is important for immune function, intakes in excess of the RDA do not provide any extra benefit for immune function. In fact, chronic excessive intakes of zinc can actually depress immune function. Zinc supplementation may be useful to slow the progression of macular degeneration of the eye and reduce the risk for developing certain forms of cancer.

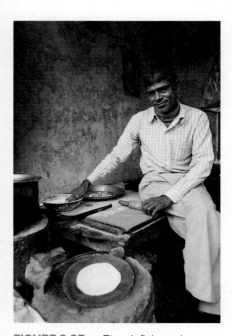

FIGURE 9-25 ▲ Zinc deficiency has been associated with the consumption of unleavened bread in Middle Eastern countries because the phytic acid in this bread inhibits the absorption of zinc.
©hadynyah/Getty Images

ZINC DEFICIENCY

Symptoms of adult zinc deficiency include an acnelike rash, diarrhea, lack of appetite, delayed wound healing, impaired immunity, reduced sense of taste (metallic-like) and smell, and hair loss. In children and adolescents with zinc deficiency, growth, sexual development, and learning ability may also be hampered.

GETTING ENOUGH ZINC

Protein-rich diets, especially those that include many animal sources of protein, are high in zinc. The average North American consumes 10 to 14 milligrams of zinc per day, about 80% of which is provided by meat, fish, poultry, fortified cereal, and dairy products (Fig. 9-26). There are no indications of moderate or severe zinc deficiencies in an otherwise healthy adult population. It is likely, however, that some North Americans—especially some poor children, vegans, and older people with alcohol use disorders—have marginal zinc status. These and other people who show deterioration in taste sensation, recurring infections, poor growth, or depressed wound healing should have their zinc status checked.

Overall, about 40% of dietary zinc is absorbed. Absorption efficiency depends on the body's need for zinc and the form of the mineral in foods. When zinc status is poor, absorption of the mineral increases. The zinc found in animal foods is better absorbed than that found in plants. Worldwide, however, most people rely on unfortified cereal grains (low in zinc) as their source of protein, calories, and zinc. Phytic acid in plant foods binds to zinc and limits its availability. Adding yeast to grains (leavening) breaks

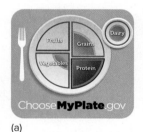

FIGURE 9-26 ◀ Food sources of zinc. (a) The fill of the background color (none, 1/3, 2/3, or completely covered) within each food group on MyPlate indicates the average nutrient density for zinc in that group. (b) The bar graph shows the zinc content of several foods compared to the RDA for adult males and females. Overall, the richest sources of zinc are in the protein group. Foods in the fruits group (not shown) provide very little zinc.

Source: Nutrition data from USDA National Nutrient Database for Standard Reference, Release 26

(a)

(b)

	Food Item and Amount	Zinc (milligrams)	% RDA for Adult Males (11 milligrams)	% RDA for Adult Females (8 milligrams)
Grains	White rice, enriched, ½ cup	1.1	10%	14%
Grains	Quinoa, cooked, ½ cup	1.0	9%	13%
Grains	Special K® cereal, 1 cup	0.4	4%	5%
Vegetables	Asparagus, cooked, 1 cup	1.1	10%	14%
Vegetables	Zucchini, cooked, 1 cup	0.6	5%	7%
Vegetables	Spinach, raw, 2 cups	0.3	3%	4%
Dairy	Mozzarella cheese, part skim, 1.5 ounces	1.2	11%	15%
Dairy	Milk, fat-free, 1 cup	1.0	9%	13%
Dairy	Soy milk, 1 cup	0.6	6%	8%
Protein	Oysters, steamed, 3 ounces	66.8	607%	835%
Protein	Beef pot roast, 3 ounces	7.9	71%	98%
Protein	Peanuts, dry roasted, 1 ounce	0.9	9%	12%

down phytic acid, increasing zinc bioavailability from leavened grain products. In populations that consume mainly unleavened bread, zinc deficiency can be a problem.

The form generally used in multivitamin and mineral supplements (zinc oxide) is not as well-absorbed as zinc found naturally in foods but still contributes to meeting zinc needs. High-dose calcium supplementation decreases zinc availability if taken too close to mealtime. Finally, zinc competes with copper and iron for absorption, and vice versa, when supplemental sources are consumed. Supplements with more than 100% of the Daily Value for individual minerals are not recommended without medical supervision.

AVOIDING TOO MUCH ZINC

Excessive zinc intake over time can lead to problems by interfering with copper metabolism. The interference with copper metabolism is the basis for setting the UL (see margin). Zinc toxicity can occur from zinc supplements and overconsumption of zinc-fortified foods. A person using megadose supplementation should be under close medical supervision and take a supplement containing copper (2 milligrams per day). Zinc intakes over 100 milligrams result in diarrhea, cramps, nausea, vomiting, and loss of appetite. Intakes consistently over 2000 milligrams per day can lead to depressed immune function and decreased high density lipoproteins.

Zinc
RDA:
  Men: 11 milligrams
  Women: 8 milligrams
DV: 15 milligrams
UL: 40 milligrams

CONCEPT CHECK 9.10

1. List three good sources of zinc.
2. What are the consequences of zinc deficiency?

9.11 Selenium

FUNCTIONS OF SELENIUM

Selenium (Se) is a trace mineral that exists in many readily absorbed chemical forms. Selenium's best-understood role is aiding the activity of one of the body's natural antioxidant enzymes, glutathione peroxidase. Glutathione peroxidase chemically converts potentially damaging peroxides (hydrogen peroxide, for example) into water. In functioning as part of our natural antioxidant enzyme system, selenium spares vitamin E and indirectly helps maintain cell-membrane integrity. Selenium is also a component of an enzyme essential for the activation of thyroid hormone.

SELENIUM DEFICIENCY

Selenium content of foods is strongly dependent on the selenium content of the soil where plants are raised or animals graze. Worldwide, only one region—Keshan County in China—has such low soil selenium levels that selenium deficiencies result. Such deficiencies were first reported by Chinese scientists in 1979. (Of note, communication and relations between the West and China were closed from 1949 until 1972. In the mid- and late 1970s, medical dialogue opened significantly.)

Selenium deficiency symptoms in humans include muscle pain and wasting, and a certain form of heart damage. Also, due to its role in thyroid hormone metabolism, selenium deficiency may impair thyroid function, thereby limiting growth. In China's Keshan County unless they receive selenium supplements, children and adults develop characteristic muscle and heart disorders associated with inadequate selenium intake.

Selenium
RDA: 55 micrograms
DV: 70 micrograms
UL: 400 micrograms

Low blood levels of selenium have been linked with an increased incidence of some forms of cancer, specifically prostate cancer. Although selenium could prove to have a role in prevention of cancers in those with low or marginal selenium stores, it is premature to recommend selenium supplementation for this purpose. Animal studies in this area are conflicting. Current studies examine the interaction of selenium and vitamin E on **gene expression** in some cancers.

gene expression Use of DNA information on a gene to produce a protein. Thought to be a major determinant of cell development.

GETTING ENOUGH SELENIUM

Fish, meat (especially organ meats), shellfish, and eggs are good animal sources of selenium (Fig. 9-27). Brazil nuts, and grains and seeds grown in soils containing selenium are good plant sources. Garlic and onions can be rich sources of selenium because they have the ability to accumulate it from soil, increasing their ability to protect against carcinogenesis. Read more about getting the most from garlic and onions in the Farm to Fork feature. Overall, the major selenium contributors to the adult dietary pattern are animal and grain products. Some geographic regions with low-selenium soil in North America include the Northeast, Pacific, Southwest, and coastal plain of the Southeast in the United States; and the north central and eastern regions in Canada. We eat a varied diet of foods supplied from many geographic areas, so it is unlikely that local areas with low soil selenium will mean inadequate selenium in our eating patterns.

The RDA for selenium is 55 micrograms per day for adults. This intake maximizes the activity of selenium-dependent enzymes. The Daily Value used on food and supplement labels is 70 micrograms. Adults meet the RDA, consuming on average 105 micrograms each day.

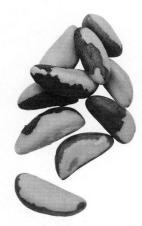

▲ Be careful with Brazil nuts. This portion of 10 nuts contains 960 micrograms of selenium, which exceeds the Upper Limit for selenium of 400 micrograms per day. ©4kodiak/Getty Images

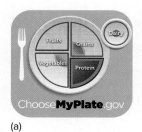

FIGURE 9-27 ◄ Food sources of selenium. (a) The fill of the background color (none, 1/3, 2/3, or completely covered) within each food group on MyPlate indicates the average nutrient density for selenium in that group. (b) The bar graph shows the selenium content of several foods compared to the RDA for adult males and females. Overall, the richest sources of selenium are found in the protein foods and grains groups. Foods from the fruits group (not shown) provide very little selenium.

Source: Nutrition data from USDA National Nutrient Database for Standard Reference, Release 26

(a)

(b)

Food Item and Amount	Selenium (micrograms)	% RDA for Adult Males and Females (55 micrograms)
Egg noodles, cooked, ½ cup	19	35%
Puffed wheat cereal, 1 cup	19	34%
White rice, cooked, ½ cup	7	13%
Mushrooms, crimini, raw, 1 cup	19	35%
Asparagus, cooked, 1 cup	11	20%
Spinach, cooked, 1 cup	3	5%
Swiss cheese, 1.5 ounces	8	14%
Milk, fat-free, 1 cup	8	14%
Soy milk, 1 cup	6	10%
Brazil nuts, 2 each	192	349%
Tuna, grilled, 3 ounces	92	167%
Oysters, steamed, 3 ounces	34	62%

AVOIDING TOO MUCH SELENIUM

High concentrations of selenium are rarely found in food, with the exception of Brazil nuts. Therefore, selenium toxicity has not been reported from eating food. Excessive selenium supplementation for an extended period has been shown to be toxic. The UL for selenium is 400 micrograms per day for adults. This is based on overt signs of selenium toxicity, such as hair loss, weakness, nausea, vomiting, and cirrhosis. Because Brazil nuts are such a concentrated source of selenium, it is recommended to avoid consuming them daily, thus preventing an inadvertent overload.

✓ CONCEPT CHECK 9.11

1. How does selenium play an antioxidant role?
2. What other functions does selenium play in the body?
3. What are the signs of a selenium deficiency?
4. What food groups are the best sources of selenium?
5. What are the signs of selenium toxicity?

FARM to FORK   Onions and Garlic

Onions and garlic, along with shallots, scallions, chives, and leeks, are part of the allium family. The alliums have long been associated with health and medicinal properties. The hot, pungent flavor of alliums comes from thiosulfinates, compounds that contain the mineral sulfur. Quercetin, the main phytonutrient in onions, and allicin, the active ingredient in garlic, have been shown to have antiviral and antibacterial properties, respectively.

Grow
- The most common garlic grown in America, the California silverskin, is very productive. Plant one clove and a new head grows with 16 cloves.
- Several varieties of onions are grown, including white, yellow, red, pearl, and the sweet onions, such as Vidalia.
- Farmers have cultivated larger and sweeter varieties of onions that are popular but have much lower health benefits.
- Green onions, or scallions, are one of the most nutritious alliums and are easy to grow even in small gardens.

Shop
- Buy garlic bulbs that are plump and tightly encased in their papery outer wrapping. If the outer skin is loose or frayed, the bulbs are likely to be dried or moldy.
- Purchase onions with their papery skin intact; this outer skin preserves the juiciness of the onion and protects it from mold and fungal infections.

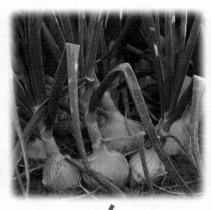
©Pixtal/age fotostock

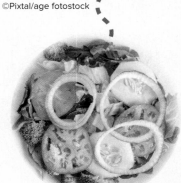
©McGraw-Hill Education

Store
- Garlic can be stored for 1 or 2 months but does become more pungent the longer it is stored.
- Store sweet onions and garlic on a shelf in the refrigerator to keep them freshest. Keep them out of the crisper drawer where the high humidity will cause them to sprout. Other onions can be stored in a net bag in a cool, dark location such as an unheated room or basement.

Prep
- Before cooking, garlic should be sliced, chopped, or minced, and then allowed to rest for 10 minutes. This will maximize the production of allicin before heat destroys the enzyme that creates it.
- Onions can be cooked as soon as you slice or chop them without losing any health benefits. In fact, all cooking methods, except boiling, have been shown to increase the quercetin content of onions. Cooking also makes the hottest onions mild and sweet.

Source: Robinson J. "Alliums: All things to all people." in *Eating on the Wild Side*. New York: Little, Brown and Company, 2013.

9.12 Iodine

FUNCTIONS OF IODINE

The thyroid gland actively accumulates and traps iodine (I) from the bloodstream to support thyroid hormone synthesis. Thyroid hormones are synthesized using iodine and the amino acid tyrosine. Because these hormones help regulate metabolic rate and promote growth and development throughout the body, iodine adequacy is important for overall energy metabolism.

IODINE DEFICIENCY

During World War I, a link was discovered between a deficiency of iodine and an enlarged thyroid gland, a condition called **goiter.** Men drafted into the military from areas such as the Great Lakes Region of the United States had a much higher rate of goiter than did men from other areas of the country. The soils in these areas have low iodine contents. In the 1920s, a researcher in Ohio found that low doses of iodine given to children over a 4-year period could prevent goiter. That finding led to the addition of iodine to salt beginning in the 1920s, the first time a nutrient was purposely added to food to prevent a disease.

Today, many nations, such as Canada, require iodine fortification of salt. In the United States, salt can be purchased either iodized or plain. Check for this on the label when you purchase salt. Some areas of Europe, such as northern Italy, have very low soil levels of iodine but have yet to adopt an iodine-fortification program. People in these areas, especially women, still suffer from goiter, as do people in areas of Latin America, the Indian subcontinent, Southeast Asia, and Africa. About 2 billion people worldwide are at risk of iodine deficiency, and approximately 800 million of these people have suffered the widespread effects of such a deficiency. Eradication of iodine deficiency is a goal of many health-related organizations worldwide.

If a person's iodine intake is insufficient, the thyroid gland enlarges as it attempts to take up more iodine from the bloodstream. This eventually leads to goiter. Simple goiter is a painless condition but, if uncorrected, can lead to pressure on the trachea (windpipe), which may cause difficulty in breathing. Although iodine can prevent goiter formation, it does not significantly shrink a goiter once it has formed. Surgical removal may be required in severe cases.

If a woman has an iodine-deficient diet during the early months of her pregnancy, the fetus suffers iodine deficiency because the mother's body uses up the available iodine. The infant then may be born with short length and develop intellectual delays. Collectively, the stunted growth and developmental delays that result are known as **congenital hypothyroidism** (formerly called cretinism). This deficiency disease appeared in North America before iodine fortification of table salt began. Today, congenital hypothyroidism still appears in Europe, Africa, Latin America, and Asia. Recent studies have shown a link between mild iodine deficiency during pregnancy and decreased IQ in offspring in the United Kingdom and Australia.[18,19] Marginal iodine status has been detected recently in women of childbearing years in the United States.

GETTING ENOUGH IODINE

The RDA for iodine (see margin) was set to support thyroid gland function. This is the same as the DV used on food and supplement labels. A half teaspoon of iodine-fortified salt (about 2 grams) supplies that amount. Most North American adults consume more iodine than the RDA—an estimated 190 to 300 micrograms daily, not including that from use of iodized salt at the table. The amount of iodine we consume adds up because dairies use it as a sterilizing agent, bakeries use it as a dough conditioner,

goiter An enlargement of the thyroid gland; this is often caused by insufficient iodide in the diet.

congenital hypothyroidism The stunting of body growth and poor development in the offspring that result from inadequate maternal intake of iodide during pregnancy that impairs thyroid hormone synthesis (formerly called cretinism).

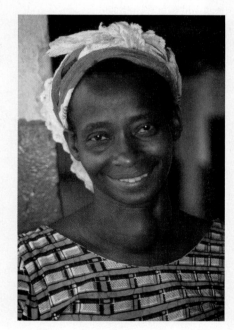

▲ This woman has an enlargement of the thyroid gland (also known as a goiter) caused by insufficient iodide in the diet. ©Scott Camazine/Science Source

Iodine
RDA: 150 micrograms
DV: 150 micrograms
UL: 1.1 milligrams

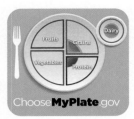

FIGURE 9-28 ◄ Food sources of iodine. (a) The fill of the background color (none, 1/3, 2/3, or completely covered) within each food group on MyPlate indicates the average nutrient density for iodine in that group. (b) The bar graph shows the iodine content of several foods compared to the RDA for adult males and females. Overall, the richest sources of iodine are iodized salt (added to foods in any group), seafood and seaweed, and dairy products. Fruits (not shown) and vegetables other than seaweed, are poor sources of iodine.

Source: Nutrition data from FDA/CFSAN Total Diet Study Statistics on Elements Results—2006–2008

(a)

(b)

	Food Item and Amount	Iodide (micrograms)	% RDA for Adult Males and Females (150 micrograms)
Grains	Iodized salt, ½ tsp	195	130%
Grains	White bread, 1 slice	29	19%
Grains	Corn muffin, 1 small	21	14%
Grains	Whole wheat bread, 1 slice	8	5%
Vegetables	Seaweed, whole or sheet, 1 g	16 to 2984	11% to 1989%
Vegetables	Lima beans, mature, boiled, ½ cup	8	5%
Vegetables	Green peas, frozen, boiled, ½ cup	3	2%
Dairy	Yogurt, plain, nonfat, 1 cup	106	71%
Dairy	Milk, fat-free, 1 cup	103	69%
Dairy	Cheese, cheddar, 1.5 ounces	22	15%
Protein	Pepperoni pizza, 1 slice	51	34%
Protein	Eggs, hard-boiled, 1 large	32	21%
Protein	Tuna, grilled, 3 ounces	13	9%

food producers use it as part of food colorants, and it is added to salt. There is concern, however, that vegans may not consume enough unless iodized salt is used. Iodized salt, dairy products, and grain products contain various forms of iodine (Fig. 9-28). Sea salt and kosher salt, however, are not typically iodized.

AVOIDING TOO MUCH IODINE

The UL for iodine is 1.1 milligrams per day. When high amounts of iodine are consumed, thyroid hormone synthesis is inhibited, as in a deficiency. This can appear in people who eat a lot of seaweed because some seaweeds contain as much as 1% iodine by weight. Total iodine intake then can add up to 60 to 130 times the RDA.

✓ CONCEPT CHECK 9.12

1. What is the role of iodide in thyroid metabolism?
2. What are the effects of iodide deficiency?
3. What is a goiter?
4. Is salt always a good source of iodide?

9.13 Copper

Copper (Cu) and iron are similar in terms of food sources, absorption, and functions. Copper is a component of blood. In the body, it is found in highest concentration in the liver, brain, heart, kidneys, and muscles. **Ceruloplasmin** is the name of the protein that carries most of the body's copper in the blood.

ceruloplasmin Copper-containing protein in the blood; functions in the transport of iron.

FUNCTIONS OF COPPER

Copper is a cofactor for many enzymes, including some involved in the body's antioxidant defenses. Copper serves as a cofactor for superoxide dismutase, an enzyme that defends the body against free-radical damage. Copper also has a role in the function of enzymes that create cross-links in connective tissue proteins, such as the collagen in bone. Another very important role of copper is as a cofactor in the last stage of energy metabolism, which converts the energy stored in carbohydrates, fats, and proteins into ATP.

Copper is important for blood health because one of its roles is making iron available for the formation of red blood cells. Copper is part of three different enzymes that assist in the transport of iron out of intestinal cells, through the blood, and to the bone marrow, where iron is incorporated into hemoglobin. Copper is also a cofactor for enzymes involved in blood clotting, immune system function, and blood lipoprotein metabolism. In addition, copper is needed for brain health through its role in enzymes involved in nerve myelination and neurotransmitter synthesis.

COPPER DEFICIENCY

Considering the myriad roles of copper discussed, it is not surprising that copper deficiency affects so many different body systems. Symptoms of copper deficiency include a form of anemia, low white blood cell count, bone loss, poor growth, and some forms of cardiovascular disease.

The groups most likely to develop copper deficiencies are preterm infants recovering from semistarvation on a milk-dominated dietary pattern (a poor source of copper) and people recovering from intestinal surgery. A copper deficiency can also result from overzealous supplementation of zinc, because zinc and copper compete with each other for absorption.

A genetic disease called **Menkes syndrome** decreases the amount of copper available to the brain and nervous system. Babies born with Menkes syndrome suffer from nervous system disorders, weak muscle tone, and delays in physical and cognitive development related to the lack of copper-containing enzymes that help to form nervous tissue and synthesize neurotransmitters. They usually do not live past the age of 3.

Menkes syndrome An inherited X-linked recessive pattern disorder that affects copper levels in the body.

GETTING ENOUGH COPPER

Rich sources of copper include liver, legumes, seeds, whole grain breads and cereals, and cocoa (Fig. 9-29). Milk and dairy products, fruit, and vegetables are generally poor sources of copper. Also, the form of copper typically found in multivitamin and mineral supplements (copper oxide) is not readily absorbed. It is best to rely on food sources to meet copper needs.

Copper absorption is highly variable, with higher intakes associated with lower absorption efficiency. Absorption takes place in the stomach and upper small intestine. Excess copper is not stored to a great extent, so when intake exceeds needs, the liver incorporates it into bile, which is excreted as part of the feces. Phytates, fiber, and excessive zinc and iron supplements may all interfere with copper absorption.

The copper status of adults appears to be good: the average adult intake is about 1 milligram for women and 1.6 milligrams for men per day. However, sensitive laboratory tests to determine copper status are lacking.

Copper
RDA: 900 micrograms
DV: 2 milligrams
UL: 10 milligrams

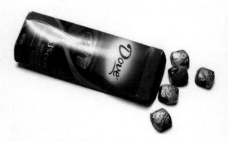

▲ Dark chocolate is a rich source of copper. These candies containing 53% cacao solids provide 1400 micrograms of copper, which is 72% of the Daily Value. ©McGraw-Hill Education/Mark Dierker, photographer

AVOIDING TOO MUCH COPPER

A single dose of copper greater than 10 milligrams can cause toxicity. Consequences of copper toxicity include GI distress, vomiting blood, tarry feces, and damage to the

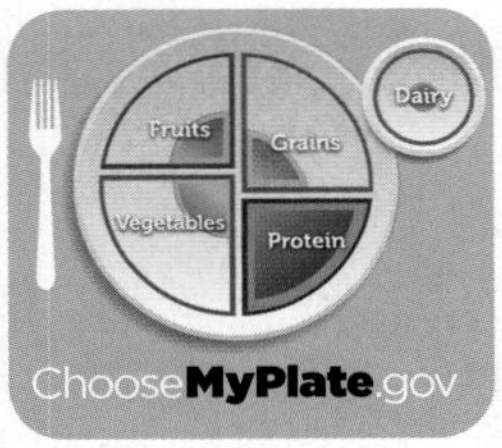

FIGURE 9-29 ◄ Food sources of copper. (a) The fill of the background color (none, 1/3, 2/3, or completely covered) within each food group on MyPlate indicates the average nutrient density for copper in that group. (b) The bar graph shows the copper content of several foods in each food group compared to the RDA for adult males and females. Overall, the richest sources of copper are found in the protein foods and grains groups.

Source: Nutrition data from USDA National Nutrient Database for Standard Reference, Release 26

(a)

(b)

	Food Item and Amount	Copper (micrograms)	% RDA for Adult Males and Females (900 micrograms)
Grains	Whole Grain Total cereal, 1 cup	140	16%
Grains	Whole wheat bread, 1 slice	73	8%
Grains	White rice, cooked, ½ cup	35	4%
Vegetables	Spinach, cooked, 1 cup	313	35%
Vegetables	Potato, baked (with skin) medium	185	21%
Vegetables	Butternut squash, cooked, 1 cup	133	15%
Fruits	Blackberries, fresh, 1 cup	238	26%
Fruits	Red seedless grapes, 1 cup	192	21%
Fruits	Orange juice, fresh, 1 cup	109	12%
Dairy	Soy milk, 1 cup	401	45%
Dairy	Cottage cheese, 1 cup	68	8%
Dairy	Milk, fat-free, 1 cup	32	4%
Protein	Beef liver, pan-fried, 3 ounces	11816	1313%
Protein	Walnuts, 1 ounce	386	43%
Protein	Kidney beans, cooked, ½ cup	191	21%

Wilson's disease A genetic disorder that results in accumulation of copper in the tissues; characterized by damage to the liver, nervous system, and other organs.

liver and kidneys. Toxicity cannot occur with food, only with supplements or excessive exposure to copper salts used in agriculture.

Wilson's disease is a genetic disease in which the liver cannot synthesize ceruloplasmin. In turn, copper accumulates in tissues, such as lungs and liver. People with Wilson's disease suffer damage to the liver and nervous system. A primary treatment for Wilson's disease is a vegan eating pattern, as fruits and vegetables are low in copper. Researchers are currently interested in how excess copper in the blood may influence the development of Alzheimer's disease and Parkinson's disease.

✓ CONCEPT CHECK 9.13

1. List three functions of copper.
2. Describe some interactions among iron, zinc, and copper in the body.
3. What changes to the dietary pattern will be required for a person with Wilson's disease?

9.14 Fluoride

The fluoride ion (F^-) is the form of this trace mineral essential for human health. Nearly all (about 95%) of the fluoride in the body is found in the teeth and skeleton. Dentists in the early 1900s noticed a lower rate of dental caries (cavities) in the southwestern United States. These areas contained high amounts of fluoride in the water. The amounts of fluoride were sometimes so high that small spots developed on the teeth (mottling). Even though mottled teeth were discolored, they contained few dental caries. Experiments in the early 1940s showed that fluoride in the water decreased the incidence of dental caries by 20% to 80% in children. Fluoridation of public water supplies in many parts of the United States has since been instituted.[20]

FUNCTIONS OF FLUORIDE

Fluoride functions in the following ways to prevent dental caries: (1) fluoride is incorporated into the tooth structure, causing it to be stronger and more resistant to acid degradation from bacteria found in plaque; (2) stimulation of remineralization of enamel and inhibition of tooth demineralization; and (3) antibacterial effect on acid-producing microorganisms found in plaque.

Fluoride has been shown to increase protein synthesis in the bone-building cells and subsequently have an effect on the production of new bone. The combination of calcium and fluoride supplementation has been investigated regarding increasing bone mass; however, to date, the studies have been inconclusive. Except for increased risk of dental caries, there is no fluoride-deficiency disease.

GETTING ENOUGH FLUORIDE

The list of foods that are good sources of fluoride is rather short: marine fish, clams, lobster, crab, shrimp, tea, and seaweed. Most of our fluoride actually comes from oral hygiene products and the water supply. Numerous products are available to apply fluoride to teeth topically. These include gels applied at a dentist's office or toothpaste and mouth rinses for everyday use. Fluoride is also available in supplement form, although use should be directed by a dentist or pediatrician. The most economical method of distributing fluoride is to add the mineral to the community's drinking water.

In a few areas of the world, the fluoride content of groundwater is naturally high, but most groundwater supplies contain low levels of fluoride. In the 1950s, after researchers established a connection between fluoride and rates of dental caries, communities in the United States began adding fluoride to the municipal water supply to achieve a fluoride level of 0.7 to 1.2 milligrams per liter. (The lower levels are for communities in hotter climates, where total water consumption is higher.) About two-thirds of North Americans currently consume fluoridated water; these policies are made by individual municipalities. Because most people now have ample access to oral hygiene products with fluoride, in 2011, the U.S. Department of Health and Human Services and the Environmental Protection Agency issued new recommendations to lower the level of water fluoridation to just 0.7 milligrams per liter.

The AI for fluoride for adults is 3.1 to 3.8 milligrams per day. This range of intake provides the benefit of resistance to dental caries without causing ill effects. As described above, typical fluoridated water contains about 1 milligram per liter, which works out to about 0.25 milligrams per cup. In communities without fluoridated water (e.g., those that rely on private well water), use of fluoride-containing oral hygiene products or dietary supplements is of heightened importance for combating dental decay. Note that fluoride is generally not added to bottled water. Frequent use of bottled water or a household reverse osmosis water purification system significantly restricts fluoride intake. A refrigerator or Brita® filter does not remove fluoride. When water fluoridation

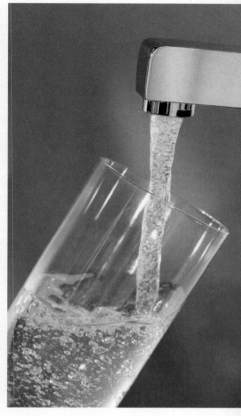

▲ *Healthy People 2020* objectives for the nation set a target goal of 79.6% of the population using piped water to have that water optimally fluoridated. As of 2014, the benefits of community water fluoridation reached nearly 74.7% of the U.S. population served by community water systems. ©amelaxa/Shutterstock

Fluoride	
AI:	3.1 to 3.8 milligrams
UL	
Young children:	1.3 to 2.2 milligrams
> 9 years:	10 milligrams

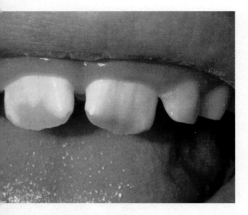

▲ Example of mottling (brown spots) in a tooth caused by overexposure to fluoride. ©Dr. P. Marazzi/Getty Images

fluorosis Discoloration of tooth enamel sometimes accompanied with pitting due to consuming a large amount of fluoride for an excessive period.

and fluoridated oral hygiene products are used in combination, the reductions in dental caries are additive.

AVOIDING TOO MUCH FLUORIDE

The UL for fluoride is set at 1.3 to 2.2 milligrams per day for young children and 10 milligrams per day for children over 9 years of age and adults, based on skeletal and tooth damage seen with higher doses. Children may swallow large amounts of fluoride toothpaste as part of daily tooth care and develop **fluorosis.** During tooth development (first decade of life), fluorosis permanently damages teeth. Fluorosis leads to stained and pitted teeth. Not swallowing toothpaste and limiting the amount used to "pea" size are the best ways to prevent this problem. In addition, children under 6 years should have tooth brushing supervised by an adult and should never use fluoride mouthwash. In adults, fluorosis is associated with hip fractures, weak or stiff joints, and chronic stomach inflammation.

There have been opponents to the fluoridation of public water supplies. Some people argue that water fluoridation standards were set at a time when much of the population did not have adequate access to fluoride-containing oral hygiene products and that addition of fluoride to the water supply is no longer necessary. Other critics claim that chronic exposure to fluoridated water is linked to a variety of health ailments affecting the skeletal, nervous, or endocrine systems. At this time, there is little scientific evidence to support claims that water fluoridation at current levels has adverse health effects other than dental fluorosis, but this is definitely an area for continued study. The updated recommendations for the level of water fluoridation aim to take advantage of the oral health benefits of fluoride while limiting unwanted health effects, including fluorosis.[21]

✓ CONCEPT CHECK 9.14

1. When is fluoride incorporated into teeth?
2. How does fluoride help to reduce the development of dental caries?
3. What are our primary sources of fluoride?
4. What are the risks of excessive fluoride intake?

9.15 Chromium (Cr)

FUNCTIONS OF CHROMIUM

Chromium enhances the function of insulin, so it is required for glucose uptake into cells. The mineral is involved in the metabolism of lipids and proteins as well, although the exact mechanisms are not known. Chromium supplements have been promoted for building muscle mass and for weight loss, but there is not much evidence to support these claims.

CHROMIUM DEFICIENCY

A chromium deficiency is characterized by impaired blood glucose control and elevated blood cholesterol and triglycerides. Low or marginal chromium intakes may contribute to an increased risk for developing type 2 diabetes, but opinions are mixed on the true degree of this effect. Chromium deficiency appears in people maintained on intravenous nutrition solutions not supplemented with chromium and in children with malnutrition. Marginal deficiencies may go undetected because sensitive measures of chromium status are not available.

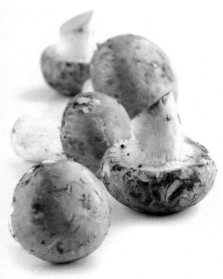

▲ Mushrooms are a good source of chromium. ©Ingram Publishing

GETTING ENOUGH CHROMIUM

Specific data regarding the chromium content of various foods are scant, and most food-composition tables do not include values for this trace mineral. Because of two major limits, we really cannot accurately determine the amount of chromium in food: (1) the content is significantly affected by agricultural and manufacturing processes; and (2) when foods are analyzed, they may be "contaminated" by the chromium in the instruments themselves. Meat, whole grain products, eggs, mushrooms, nuts, beer, and spices are relatively good sources of chromium. Brewer's yeast is also a very good source.

Chromium absorption is quite low: only 0.4% to 2.5% of the amount consumed. Absorption is enhanced by vitamin C and niacin. Any unabsorbed chromium is excreted in the feces. Once absorbed, it is stored in the liver, spleen, soft tissue, and bone, and excreted via urine. Certain conditions can enhance urinary excretion of chromium: diets high in simple sugars (more than 35% of total calories), significant infection, acute prolonged exercise, pregnancy and lactation, and major physical trauma. If chromium intakes are already low, these states potentially can lead to deficiency.

The Adequate Intake (AI) for chromium is 25 to 35 micrograms per day, based on the amount present in a balanced eating pattern. The DV used on food and supplement labels is 120 micrograms. Average adult intakes in North America are estimated at about 30 micrograms per day but could be somewhat higher.

No UL for chromium has been set because toxicity from food sources has not been observed. Chromium toxicity, however, has been reported in people exposed to industrial waste and in painters who use art supplies with high chromium content. Liver damage and lung cancer can result. Use of any supplement should normally not exceed the DV unless supervised by a primary care provider because of the risk of toxicity.

> **Chromium**
> AI
>   Men: 35 micrograms
>   Women: 25 micrograms
> DV: 120 micrograms
> UL: none

✓ CONCEPT CHECK 9.15

1. How is chromium involved in carbohydrate metabolism?
2. Why is it hard to know the chromium content of foods?
3. Which foods are considered the best sources of chromium?

9.16 Other Trace Minerals

MANGANESE (Mn)

The mineral manganese is easily confused with magnesium (Mg). Not only are their names similar, but they also often substitute for each other in metabolic processes. As a participant in energy metabolism, manganese is required as a cofactor for synthesis of glucose and metabolism of some amino acids. Manganese is also needed by some enzymes, especially superoxide dismutase used in free-radical metabolism. Manganese is also important in bone formation.

Manganese deficiency does not develop in humans unless the mineral is purposely removed from the diet. Animals on manganese-deficient diets suffer alterations in brain function, bone formation, and reproduction. If human dietary patterns were low in manganese, these symptoms would probably appear as well. As it happens, our need for manganese is very low, and our eating patterns tend to be adequate in this trace mineral.

The AI for manganese is 1.8 to 2.3 milligrams to offset daily losses. Average intakes fall within this range. The DV used on food and supplement labels is 2 milligrams. Good food sources of manganese are nuts, rice, oats, and other whole grains, beans, and leafy vegetables. Manganese is toxic at high doses. Supplements are not recommended because large doses can decrease absorption of other minerals. People with low iron stores must avoid manganese supplements or risk worsening anemia. The UL

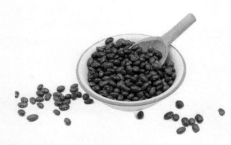
▲ Beans are sources of manganese and molybdenum. ©Pixtal/AGE Fotostock

> **Manganese**
> AI
>   Men: 2.3 milligrams
>   Women: 1.8 milligrams
> DV: 2 milligrams
> UL: 11 milligrams

is 11 milligrams per day. This value is based on the development of nerve damage. Miners who have inhaled dust fumes high in manganese experience symptoms that mimic Parkinson's disease, including cognitive and muscular dysfunction.

MOLYBDENUM (Mo)

Several human enzymes use molybdenum, including some involved in metabolism of amino acids that contain sulfur. No molybdenum deficiency has been reported in people who consume food and beverages orally. Deficiency symptoms have appeared in people maintained on intravenous nutrition devoid of this trace mineral. Symptoms include increased heart and respiratory rates, night blindness, mental confusion, edema, and weakness.

Good food sources of molybdenum include milk and dairy products, beans, whole grains, and nuts. The RDA for molybdenum is 45 micrograms to offset daily losses. The DV used on food and supplement labels is 75 micrograms. Our daily intakes average 76 micrograms (for women) and 109 micrograms (for men). The Upper Level for molybdenum is 2 milligrams per day. When consumed in high doses, molybdenum causes toxicity in laboratory animals, resulting in weight loss and decreased growth. Toxicity risk in humans is quite low.

Table 9-8 summarizes much of what we know about the trace minerals.

Molybdenum
RDA: 45 micrograms
DV: 75 micrograms
UL: 2 milligrams

✓ CONCEPT CHECK 9.16

1. What are the primary functions of manganese and molybdenum in metabolism of nutrients?
2. What are the good food sources of manganese and molybdenum?
3. Why is a deficiency of manganese or molybdenum possible when patients are fed intravenously?

TABLE 9-8 ■ **Summary of Key Trace Minerals**

Mineral	Major Functions	RDA or AI	Dietary Sources	Deficiency Symptoms	Toxicity Symptoms
Iron	• Component of hemoglobin and numerous enzymes • Immune function • Cognitive development	*Men:* 8 milligrams *Premenopausal women:* 18 milligrams	Nonheme plant sources: • Fruits • Vegetables • Fortified bread and grain products Heme animal sources: • Meat and poultry	• Fatigue • Microcytic hypochromic anemia	• GI distress UL = 45 milligrams
Zinc	• Component of multiple enzymes and proteins • Regulation of gene expression • Protein metabolism • Wound healing and growth	*Men:* 11 milligrams *Women:* 8 milligrams	• Fortified cereals • Red meats • Seafood	• Skin rash • Diarrhea • Decreased appetite and sense of taste • Hair loss • Poor growth and development • Poor wound healing	• Reduced copper status UL = 40 milligrams
Selenium	• Defense against oxidative stress • Regulation of thyroid hormone action • Reduction and oxidation status of vitamin C and other molecules	55 micrograms	• Organ meats • Seafood • Plants (depending on soil selenium content)	• Muscle pain • Weakness • Form of heart disease	• Hair and nail brittleness and loss UL = 400 micrograms

TABLE 9-8 ■ *(continued)*

Mineral	Major Functions	RDA or AI	Dietary Sources	Deficiency Symptoms	Toxicity Symptoms
Iodine	• Component of the thyroid hormones	150 micrograms	• Foods of marine origin • Processed foods • Iodized salt	• Goiter • Mental retardation • Congenital hypothyroidism: Poor growth in infancy when mother is iodine deficient during pregnancy	• Elevated thyroid stimulating hormone concentration UL = 1.1 milligrams
Copper	• Component of enzymes in iron metabolism • Collagen synthesis	900 micrograms	• Organ meats • Seafood • Nuts and seeds • Wheat bran cereals, whole grain products • Cocoa	• Anemia • Low white blood cell count • Poor growth	• GI distress • Liver damage UL = 8 to 10 milligrams
Fluoride	• Inhibits the initiation and progression of dental caries • Stimulates new bone formation	*Men:* 4 milligrams *Women:* 3 milligrams	• Fluoridated water • Fluoridated dental products • Tea • Marine fish	• Increased risk of dental caries	• Enamel and skeletal fluorosis UL = 10 milligrams
Chromium	• Helps to maintain normal blood glucose levels	*Men (up to 50 years):* 35 micrograms *Women (up to 50 years):* 25 micrograms	• Some cereals • Meats • Poultry • Fish • Beer	• High blood glucose after eating	• Chronic renal failure No UL
Manganese	• Involved in the formation of bone • Cofactor for enzymes involved in amino acid, cholesterol, and carbohydrate metabolism	*Men:* 2.3 milligrams *Women:* 1.8 milligrams	• Nuts • Legumes • Tea • Oats	• None observed in humans	• Elevated blood concentration and neurotoxicity UL = 11 milligrams
Molybdenum	• Cofactor for enzymes involved in catabolism of sulfur amino acids, purines, and pyridines	45 micrograms	• Legumes • Grain products • Nuts	• None observed in healthy humans	• Reproductive effects observed in animal studies UL = 2 milligrams

Abbreviation: RDA = Recommended Dietary Allowance; AI = adequate intake; UL = Upper Intake Level

9.17 Nutrition and Your Health

Minerals and Hypertension

©Picturenet/Blend Images LLC

In the United States, 78 million or an estimated one in five adults has hypertension. Over the age of 65, the number rises to one in every two adults. Only about half of cases are being treated. Blood pressure is expressed by two numbers. The higher number represents systolic blood pressure, the pressure in the arteries when the heart muscle is contracting and pumping blood into the arteries. Optimal systolic blood pressure is 120 mmHg or less. The second value is diastolic blood pressure, the artery pressure when the heart is relaxed. Optimal diastolic blood pressure is 80 mmHg or less. Elevations in both systolic and diastolic blood pressure are strong predictors of disease (Fig. 9-30).

Hypertension is defined as sustained systolic pressure exceeding 139 mmHg or diastolic blood pressure exceeding 89 mmHg. Most cases of hypertension (about 95%) have no clear-cut cause. Such cases are classified as **primary** or **essential hypertension.** Kidney disease, sleep-disordered breathing (sleep apnea), and other causes often lead to the other 5% of cases, classified as **secondary hypertension.**

primary hypertension Blood pressure of 140/90 mmHg or higher with no identified cause; also called *essential hypertension.*

secondary hypertension Blood pressure of 140/90 mmHg or higher as a result of disease (e.g., kidney dysfunction or sleep apnea) or drug use.

African-Americans and Asian Americans are more likely than Caucasians to develop hypertension and to do so earlier in life.

Unless blood pressure is periodically measured, the development of hypertension is easily overlooked. Because it usually does not cause symptoms, it is described as a silent disorder.

Why Control Blood Pressure?

Blood pressure needs to be controlled mainly to prevent cardiovascular disease, kidney disease, strokes and related declines in brain function, poor blood circulation in the legs, problems with vision, and sudden death. These conditions are much more likely to be found in individuals with hypertension than in people with normal blood pressure. Smoking and elevated blood lipoproteins make these diseases even more likely. Individuals with hypertension need to be diagnosed and treated as soon as possible, as the condition generally progresses to a more serious stage over time and even resists therapy if it persists for years. The benefits of controlling blood pressure were confirmed by the results of a recent randomized study of patients at high risk for cardiovascular events.[22] Decreasing the systolic blood pressure of these patients to less than 120 mmHg, as compared with less than 140 mmHg, resulted in lower rates of fatal and nonfatal major cardiovascular events and death from any cause.

Contributors to Hypertension

Because we do not know the cause of 95% of the cases of hypertension, we can identify only risk factors that contribute to its development. A family history of hypertension is a risk factor, especially if both parents have (or had) the problem. In addition, blood pressure can increase as a person ages. Some increase is caused by atherosclerosis. As plaque builds up in the arteries, the arteries

How High Is High?

If your systolic and diastolic pressures fall into different categories, your risk depends on the higher category.

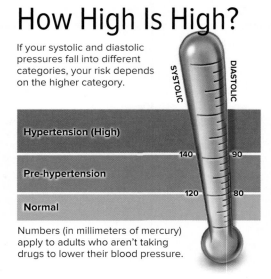

	SYSTOLIC	DIASTOLIC
Hypertension (High)	140	90
Pre-hypertension		
	120	80
Normal		

Numbers (in millimeters of mercury) apply to adults who aren't taking drugs to lower their blood pressure.

FIGURE 9-30 ▲ The cutoff for hypertension is 140/90 mmHg, but the risk of heart attacks and stroke precedes the rise in blood pressure.

become less flexible and cannot expand. When vessels remain rigid, blood pressure remains high. Eventually, the plaque begins to make the problem worse by decreasing the blood supply to the kidneys, which decreases their ability to control blood volume and, in turn, blood pressure.

Obesity Overweight people have a much greater risk of having hypertension than lean people. Overall, obesity is considered the number one lifestyle factor related to hypertension. This is especially the case in minority populations. Additional blood vessels develop to support excess tissue in overweight and obese individuals, and these extra miles of associated blood vessels increase work by the heart and also blood pressure. Hypertension is also linked to obesity when insulin-resistant adipose cells cause insulin levels to increase in the blood. This increased insulin level augments sodium retention in the body and accelerates atherosclerosis. In such cases, a weight loss of as little as 10 to 15 pounds often can help treat hypertension.

Inactivity Inactivity is considered the number two lifestyle factor related to hypertension. If an obese person can engage in regular physical activity (at least 5 days per week for 30 to 60 minutes) and lose weight, blood pressure often returns to normal.

Alcohol Third, excess alcohol intake is responsible for about 10% of all cases of hypertension, especially in middle-age males and among African-Americans in general. When hypertension is caused by excessive alcohol intake, it is usually reversible. A sensible alcohol intake for people with hypertension is two or fewer drinks per day for men and one or no drinks per day for women and all older adults.

Sodium In some people, particularly African-Americans and older overweight persons, blood pressure is especially sensitive to sodium. In these people, excess salt leads to fluid retention by the kidney and a corresponding increase in blood volume, resulting in increased blood pressure. It is not clear whether sodium or chloride is more responsible for the effect. Because most of our sodium comes in the form of salt, if one reduces sodium intake, chloride intake naturally falls. For the most part, a recommendation to consume less sodium is equivalent to a call for less salt in our dietary patterns. Only some North Americans are susceptible to increases in blood pressure from salt intake, so it is only the number four lifestyle factor related to hypertension. It is unfortunate that salt intake receives the major portion of public attention with regard to hypertension. Efforts to prevent hypertension should also focus on obesity, inactivity, and excessive consumption of alcohol.

Other Minerals and the DASH Diet

Minerals such as calcium, potassium, and magnesium also deserve attention when it comes to prevention and treatment of hypertension (see the Newsworthy Nutrition in this section). Studies show that a dietary pattern rich in these minerals and low in salt can decrease blood pressure within days of beginning this type of diet, especially among African-Americans. The response is even similar to that seen with commonly used medications. The diet is called the Dietary Approaches to Stop Hypertension (DASH) diet (Table 9-9). The diet is rich in calcium, potassium, and magnesium and low in

TABLE 9-9 ■ What Is the DASH Diet?
The DASH diet is low in fat and sodium and rich in fruits, vegetables, and low-fat dairy products. Here is the breakdown:

Per Day	Per Week
6–8 servings of grains and grain products	4–5 servings of nuts, seeds, or legumes
4–5 servings of fruit	5 servings of sweets and added sugars
4–5 servings of vegetables	
2–3 servings of low-fat or fat-free dairy products	
2 or fewer servings of meats, poultry, and fish	
2–3 servings of fats/oils	

salt. Both magnesium and calcium are important for healthy blood pressure because they help blood vessels relax. It takes a standard MyPlate Daily Food Plan; adds one to two extra vegetables and fruits servings; and emphasizes consumption of nuts, seeds, or legumes (beans) 4 to 5 days of the week. In DASH studies,

Newsworthy Nutrition

Slash sodium, but step up potassium to control blood pressure

Studies have linked high sodium and low potassium intakes to increased blood pressure. There is limited research, however, on the association of sodium-to-potassium intake ratio with blood pressure and hypertension. The hypothesis of this study was that the sodium-to-potassium ratio would be positively associated with blood pressure. Data on 10,563 participants in the 2005–2010 National Health and Nutrition Examination Survey (NHANES) were analyzed. Subjects were ≥ 20 years of age and were not taking antihypertensive medication or following a low-sodium diet. The average sodium intake (3569 mg/d), potassium intake (2745 mg/d), and sodium-to-potassium ratio (1.41) were all significantly associated with systolic blood pressure. For each 1000-mg/d increase in sodium intake, blood pressure increased by 1.04 mmHg, but for each 1000-mg/d increase in potassium intake, blood pressure decreased by 1.24 mmHg. Blood pressure also increased by 1.05 mmHg per 0.5-unit increase in sodium-to-potassium ratio. These results provide evidence that high sodium intakes combined with suboptimal potassium consumption are associated with hypertension.

Source: Zhang Z , et al. "Association between usual sodium and potassium intake and blood pressure and hypertension among U.S. adults: NHANES 2005–2010." *PLoS ONE* 8(10):e75289, 2013.

participants also consumed no more than 3 grams of sodium and no more than one to two alcoholic drinks per day. A DASH 2 diet trial tested three daily sodium intakes (3300 milligrams, 2400 milligrams, and 1500 milligrams). People showed a steady decline in blood pressure on the DASH diet as sodium intake declined. Overall, the DASH diet is seen as a total dietary approach to treating hypertension, with the many healthful practices of the dietary pattern being responsible for the fall in blood pressure. It is also impressive that a panel of health experts has named the DASH diet the best overall eating plan, ranking it first for the seventh year in a row on the *U.S. News & World Report's* 2017 Best Diets list.

Other studies also show a reduction in stroke risk among people who consume a diet rich in fruits, vegetables, and vitamin C (recall that fruits and vegetables are rich in vitamin C). Overall, a diet low in salt and rich in low-fat and fat-free dairy products, fruits, vegetables, whole grains, and some nuts can substantially reduce

hypertension and stroke risk in many people, especially those with hypertension.[23]

Medications to Treat Hypertension

There are a variety of high blood pressure medications otherwise known as antihypertensives. The different classes of these drugs are summarized in the Medicine Cabinet feature in this section. Diuretics, or "water pills," are one class that work to reduce blood volume (and therefore blood pressure) by increasing fluid output in the urine. Other medications act by slowing heart rate or by causing relaxation of the small muscles lining the blood vessels. A combination of two or more medications is commonly required to treat hypertension that does not respond to diet and lifestyle therapy.

Prevention of Hypertension

Many of the risk factors for hypertension and stroke are controllable, and appropriate lifestyle changes can reduce a person's risk (Fig. 9-31), depending on the severity of the hypertension. Experts also recommend that those with hypertension lower blood pressure through diet and lifestyle changes before resorting to blood pressure medications.

Medicine Cabinet

Diuretics are commonly prescribed to lower blood pressure. Diuretics cause the kidneys to excrete more urine but at the same time may increase urinary excretion of minerals and decrease blood levels of potassium, magnesium, and zinc. Those taking diuretics need to carefully monitor their dietary intake of these minerals, especially potassium, and increase intake of fruits and vegetables or potassium chloride supplements as prescribed by primary care providers.

Examples:

- Hydrochlorothiazide (Microzide)®
- Furosemide (Lasix)®

Beta-blockers decrease the heart's rate, as well as its workload and blood output.

Examples:

- Atenolol (Tenormin)®
- Metoprolol tartrate (Lopressor)®

ACE (angiotensin-converting enzyme) inhibitors cause the body to produce less **angiotensin,** which causes the blood vessels to relax and open up and thus lower blood pressure.

Examples:

- Benazepril hydrochloride (Lotensin)®
- Lisinopril (Prinivel,® Zestril)®

Source: American Heart Association: Types of blood pressure medications, http://www.heart.org.

©Peter Dazeley/Photographer's Choice/Getty Images

Advice	Details	Drop in Systolic Blood Pressure
Lose excess weight	For every 20 pounds you lose (if BMI > 25)	5 to 20 points
Adopt a DASH eating plan	Eat a lower-fat diet rich in vegetables, fruits, and low-fat dairy foods	8 to 14 points
Exercise daily	Get 30 minutes a day of aerobic activity (such as brisk walking)	4 to 9 points
Limit sodium	Eat no more than 2400 mg per day (1500 mg per day is better)	2 to 8 points
Limit alcohol	Have no more than 2 drinks per day for men, 1 drink per day for women (1 drink = 12 oz beer, 5 oz wine, or 1.5 oz 80-proof whiskey)	2 to 4 points

FIGURE 9-31 ▲ What works? If your blood pressure is high, here's how much lifestyle changes should lower it.

Source: The Seventh Report of the Joint National Committee on Prevention, Detection, Evaluation, and Treatment of High Blood Pressure (www.nhlbi.nih.gov/health-pro/guidelines/current/hypertension-jnc-7)

---

diuretic A substance that increases the volume of urine.

angiotensin A hormone produced by the liver and activated by enzymes from the kidneys. It signals the adrenal glands to produce aldosterone also and directs the kidneys to conserve sodium (and therefore water). Both of these actions have the effect of increasing blood volume.

Summary (Numbers refer to numbered sections in the chapter.)

9.1 Water constitutes 50% to 70% of the human body. Its unique chemical properties enable it to dissolve substances as well as serve as a medium for chemical reactions, temperature regulation, and lubrication. Water also helps regulate the acid–base balance in the body.

For adults, daily water needs are estimated at 9 cups (women) to 13 cups (men) per day; fluid intake contributes to meeting this need. Hormones participate in the process of fluid conservation. Receptors in the kidneys, blood vessels, and brain monitor blood pressure and solute concentration in the blood. Dehydration leads to kidney failure, coma, and death. The amount of water in the intracellular and extracellular compartments is controlled mainly by ion concentrations.

9.2 Minerals are categorized based on the amount we need per day. If we require greater than 100 milligrams of a mineral per day, it is considered a major mineral; otherwise it is considered a trace mineral. Many minerals are vital for sustaining life. For humans, animal products are the most bioavailable sources of most minerals. Supplements of minerals exceeding 100% of the Daily Values should be taken only under a primary care provider's supervision. Toxicity and nutrient interactions are especially likely if the Upper Level (when set) is exceeded on a long-term basis.

9.3 Sodium, the major positive ion found outside cells, is vital in fluid balance and nerve impulse transmission. The North American diet provides abundant sodium through processed foods and table salt. About 10% to 15% of the adult population, such as overweight people, is especially sodium-sensitive and at risk for developing hypertension from consuming excessive sodium.

9.4 Potassium, the major positive ion found inside cells, has a similar function to sodium. Milk, fruits, and vegetables are good sources. Low blood potassium, hypokalemia, is a life-threatening problem that is most commonly seen with chronic diarrhea or vomiting, or as a side effect of medications, including laxatives and some diuretics.

9.5 Chloride is the major negative ion found outside cells. It is important in digestion as part of stomach acid and in immune and nerve functions. Table salt supplies most of the chloride in our diets.

9.6 Calcium forms a part of bone structure and plays a role in blood clotting, muscle contraction, nerve transmission, and cell metabolism. Calcium absorption is enhanced by stomach acid and the active vitamin D hormone. Dairy products are important calcium sources, but many dairy alternatives such as soy or almond milk are available. Deficient calcium intake decreases bone mineralization, ultimately leading to osteopenia and osteoporosis. Women are particularly at risk for developing osteoporosis as they age. Numerous lifestyle and medical options can help reduce this risk, including an adequate intake of calcium and many other minerals.

9.7 Phosphorus aids enzyme function and forms part of key metabolic compounds, cell membranes, and bone. It is efficiently absorbed, and deficiencies are rare, although there is concern about possible poor intake by some older women. Good food sources are dairy products, bakery products, and meats.

9.8 Magnesium is a mineral found mostly in plant food sources. It is important for nerve and heart function and as an activator for many enzymes. Whole grain breads and cereals (bran portion), vegetables, nuts, seeds, milk, and meats are good food sources.

9.9 Iron absorption depends mainly on the form of iron present and the body's need for it. Heme iron from animal sources is better absorbed than the nonheme iron obtained primarily from plant sources. Consuming vitamin C or meat simultaneously with nonheme iron increases absorption. Iron operates mainly in synthesizing hemoglobin and myoglobin and in the action of the immune system. Women are at highest risk for developing iron deficiency, which decreases blood hemoglobin and hematocrit. When this condition is severe, iron-deficiency anemia develops. This decreases the amount of oxygen carried in the blood. Iron toxicity usually results from a genetic disorder called hemochromatosis. This disease causes overabsorption and accumulation of iron, which can result in severe liver and heart damage.

9.10 Zinc aids in the action of up to 200 enzymes important for growth, development, cell membrane structure and function, immune function, antioxidant protection, wound healing, and taste. A zinc deficiency results in poor growth, loss of appetite, reduced sense of taste and smell, hair loss, and a persistent rash. Zinc is best absorbed from animal sources. The richest sources of zinc are oysters, shrimp, crab, and beef. Good plant sources are whole grains, peanuts, and beans.

9.11 An important role of selenium is decreasing the action of free-radical (oxidizing) compounds. In this way, selenium acts along with vitamin E in providing antioxidant protection. Muscle pain, muscle wasting, and a form of heart damage may result from a selenium deficiency. Meats, eggs, fish, and shellfish are good animal sources of selenium. Good plant sources include grains and seeds.

9.12 Iodine forms part of the thyroid hormones. A lack of dietary iodine results in the development of an enlarged thyroid gland or goiter. Iodized salt is a major food source.

9.13 Copper is important for iron metabolism, cross-linking of connective tissue, and other functions, such as enzymes that provide antioxidant protection. A copper deficiency can result in a form of anemia. Copper is found mainly in liver, seafood, cocoa, legumes, and whole grains.

9.14 Fluoride as part of regular dietary intake or toothpaste use makes teeth resistant to dental caries. Most North Americans receive the bulk of their fluoride from fluoridated water and oral hygiene products.

9.15 Chromium aids in the action of the hormone insulin. Chromium deficiency results in impaired blood glucose control. Egg yolks, meats, and whole grains are good sources of chromium.

9.16 Manganese and molybdenum are used by various enzymes. One enzyme that uses manganese provides antioxidant protection. Clear deficiencies in otherwise healthy people are rarely seen for these nutrients. Human needs for other trace minerals are so low that deficiencies are uncommon.

9.17 Controlling weight and alcohol intake; exercising regularly; decreasing salt intake; and ensuring adequate potassium, magnesium, and calcium in the diet all can play a part in controlling high blood pressure.

Check Your Knowledge (Answers to the following questions are below.)

1. Dietary heme iron is derived from
   a. elemental iron in food.
   b. animal flesh.
   c. breakfast cereal.
   d. vegetables.

2. Chloride is
   a. a component of hydrochloric acid.
   b. an intracellular fluid ion.
   c. a positively charged ion.
   d. converted to chlorine in the intestinal tract.

3. Minerals involved in fluid balance are
   a. calcium and magnesium.
   b. copper and iron.
   c. calcium and phosphorus.
   d. sodium and potassium.

4. In a situation where there is an insufficient intake of dietary iodine, the thyroid-stimulating hormone promotes the enlargement of the thyroid gland. This condition is called
   a. Graves' disease.
   b. goiter.
   c. hyperparathyroidism.
   d. congenital hypothyroidism.

5. Ninety-nine percent of the calcium in the body is found in
   a. intracellular fluid.
   b. bones and teeth.
   c. nerve cells.
   d. the liver.

6. At the end of long bones, inside the spinal vertebrae, and inside the flat bones of the pelvis is a spongy type of bone known as _____ bone.
   a. cortical
   b. osteoporotic
   c. trabecular
   d. compact

7. Which compartment contains the greatest amount of body fluid?
   a. Intracellular
   b. Extracellular
   c. They contain the same amount.

8. The primary function of sodium is to maintain
   a. bone mineral content.
   b. hemoglobin concentration.
   c. immune function.
   d. fluid distribution.

9. Hypertension is defined as a blood pressure greater than
   a. 110/60.
   b. 120/65.
   c. 140/90.
   d. 190/80.

10. Which of the following individuals are most likely to develop osteoporosis?
    a. Premenopausal women athletes
    b. Women taking estrogen replacement therapy
    c. Slender, inactive women who smoke
    d. Women who eat a lot of high-fat dairy products

Answer Key: 1. b (LO 9.9), 2. a (LO 9.5), 3. d (LO 9.3), 4. b (LO 9.12), 5. b (LO 9.6), 6. c (LO 9.6), 7. a (LO 9.1), 8. d (LO 9.3), 9. c (LO 9.17), 10. c (LO 9.6)

Study Questions (Numbers refer to Learning Outcomes)

1. Approximately how much water do you need each day to stay healthy? Identify at least two situations that increase the need for water. Then list three sources of water in the average person's dietary pattern. **(LO 9.1)**

2. Identify four factors that influence the bioavailability of minerals from food. **(LO 9.2)**

3. What is the relationship between sodium and water balance, and how is that relationship monitored as well as maintained in the body? **(LO 9.3)**

4. List three sources of dietary calcium. Identify two factors that negatively influence the absorption of calcium. Identify two factors that positively influence the absorption of calcium. **(LO 9.6)**

5. Describe two methods that can be used to assess bone density. What demographic groups should have bone density measured? **(LO 9.6)**

6. List three roles of magnesium in the body. Identify two chronic diseases that may be affected by magnesium status. **(LO 9.8)**

7. Describe the symptoms of iron-deficiency anemia, and explain possible reasons they occur. **(LO 9.9)**

8. What is the relationship between iodine, the thyroid gland, and energy metabolism? **(LO 9.12)**

9. Describe the functions of fluoride in the body. List three sources of fluoride. **(LO 9.14)**

10. Explain the function of chromium in carbohydrate metabolism. **(LO 9.15)**

11. List three dietary strategies to lower blood pressure. **(LO 9.17)**

What the Dietitian Chose

Bottled water has become very popular. In 2015, each American consumed more than 36 gallons of bottled water, adding up to about 11.7 billion gallons for the nation. The public perception that bottled water is safer and healthier than tap water has stimulated the current bottle-toting habit. The truth is that bottled and tap water are both regulated: bottled water by the FDA and tap water by the Environmental Protection Agency (EPA). FDA requirements for bottled water mimic those of the EPA for water quality, but in neither does the water have to be contaminant-free.

Pure is an advertising term and means nothing about the quality of the water. Controversy over misleading advertising by major companies such as Pepsico and Coca-Cola that use public source water in their respective products, Aquafina and Dasani, has led to the printing of "Public Source Water" or "PSW" on labels.

Mineral water must contain consistent levels of natural elements from an underground source; no minerals may be added to the water. The precise mineral content varies by source, but some common minerals found in water include calcium, magnesium, potassium, sodium, sulfur, iron, fluoride, zinc, and some ultratrace minerals. The minerals impart some taste to the water but are typically a minor contributor to overall mineral intake.

There is no legal definition for "vitamin water." Manufacturers of vitamin water (i.e., soft-drink companies) usually use filtered or distilled water and add sweeteners (e.g., high-fructose corn syrup) and citric acid as flavoring agents, plus several vitamins (mostly vitamin C and an assortment of B vitamins). In 2010, the Coca-Cola Bottling Company was sued by the Center for Science in the Public Interest for false marketing of its popular vitaminwater® brand as "nutritious." These products are marketed as healthy because they contain added vitamins, but most of them also supply a surprising amount of sugar. Recall that the American Heart Association recommends that men and women get no more than 150 or 100 kcal per day, respectively, from added sugars. A 20-ounce bottle of vitaminwater® has 33 grams of sugar, providing 132 kcal from added sugar. This is

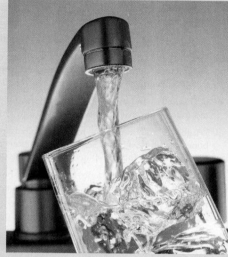
©Comstock Images

about half the sugar in a regular soft drink, but you can see how this can add up to excess. Furthermore, most North Americans consume adequate amounts of vitamin C and the B vitamins without the aid of these beverages.

Consumers should also be aware of FDA definitions for other types of bottled water.

- Artesian water must come from a confined aquifer.

- Springwater must flow naturally to the surface.

- Purified water is produced through an approved process such as distillation or reverse osmosis.

Relying on bottled water is an expensive habit, personally and environmentally. If you use bottled water to meet your recommended fluid needs, you will spend close to $1500 per year compared with about 50 cents for the same volume of tap water. On a larger scale, it is estimated that close to 90% of water bottles end up in the trash, clogging our landfills or being shipped to other countries for recycling. It is well known that America has some of the cleanest, safest tap water in the world. While following the recommendations to drink more water, hydrate with tap or home-filtered water in a reusable container.

Further Readings

1. Howard BC: What do recycling symbols on plastics mean? *The Daily Green.* November 2008. Available at: http://www.thedailygreen.com/green-homes/latest/recycling-symbols-plastics-460321 (Accessed February 5, 2017).

2. Food and Drug Administration: FDA continues to study BPA. *FDA Consumer Update.* March 2012. Available at: http://www.fda.gov/downloads/ForConsumers/ConsumerUpdates/UCM297971.pdf. (Accessed February 5, 2017).

3. Grimes CA and others: Dietary salt intake, sugar-sweetened beverage consumption, and obesity risk. *Pediatrics* 2013;131:14.

4. Institute of Medicine: *Sodium Intake in Populations: Assessment of Evidence.* Washington, DC: National Academies Press, 2013.

5. Cobb LK and others: Methodological issues in cohort studies that relate sodium intake to cardiovascular disease outcomes—A science advisory from the American Heart Association. *Circulation* 2014;129:1173.

6. O'Donnell M and others: Urinary sodium and potassium excretion, mortality, and cardiovascular events. *N Engl J Med* 2014;371:612.

7. Wright NC and others: The recent prevalence of osteoporosis and low bone mass in the United States based on bone mineral density at the femoral neck or lumbar spine. *J Bone Min Res* 2014;29:2520.

8. Burge R and others: Incidence and economic burden of osteoporosis related fractures in the United States, 2005–2025. *J Bone Min Res* 2007;22:465.

9. LeBlanc KE and others: Hip fracture: Diagnosis, treatment, and secondary prevention. *Am Fam Phys* 2014;89:945.

10. Cosman F and others: Clinician's guide to prevention and treatment of osteoporosis. *Osteoporis Int* 2014;25:2359.

11. Schaeffer J: What's new in the dairy-free aisle. *Today's Dietitian* 2013;17(2):30.

12. Anderson JJ and others: Calcium intakes and femoral and lumbar bone density of elderly U.S. men and women: National Health and Nutrition Examination Survey 2005–2006 analysis. *J Clin Endocrinol Metab* 2012;97:4531.

13. Bolland MJ and others: Calcium supplements with or without vitamin D and risk of cardiovascular events: Reanalysis of the Women's Health Initiative limited access dataset and meta-analysis. *BMJ* 2011;342:d2040.

14. Office of Dietary Supplements, National Institutes of Health: *Dietary Supplement Fact Sheet: Calcium.* Updated November 17, 2016. Available at: http://ods.od.nih.gov/factsheets/calcium, and *Dietary Supplement Fact Sheet: Magnesium.* Updated February 11, 2016. Available at: http://ods.od.nih.gov/factsheets/magnesium.

15. Linus Pauling Institute Micronutrient Information Center. *Phosphorus.* Updated June 2014. http://lpi.oregonstate.edu/mic/minerals/phosphorus (Accessed February 6, 2017).

16. Fang X and others: Dietary magnesium intake and the risk of cardiovascular disease, type 2 diabetes, and all-cause mortality: A dose-response meta-analysis of prospective cohort studies. *BMC Medicine* 2016;14:210.

17. Office of Dietary Supplements, National Institutes of Health: *Dietary supplement fact sheet: Iron.* Updated February 11, 2016. Available at: http://ods.od.nih.gov/factsheets/iron.

18. Bath SC and others: Effect of inadequate iodine status in UK pregnant women on cognitive outcomes in their children: Results from the Avon Longitudinal Study of Parents and Children (ALSPAC). *Lancet* 2013;382:331.

19. Hynes KL and others: Mild iodine deficiency during pregnancy is associated with reduced educational outcomes in the offspring: 9-year follow-up of the Gestational Iodine Cohort. *J Clin Endocrinol Metab* 2013;98:1954.

20. Rugg-Gunn AJ and Do L: Effectiveness of water fluoridation in caries prevention. *Community Dent Oral Epidemiol* 2012;240 (Suppl. 2):55.

21. Palmer CA and Gilbert JA: Position of the Academy of Nutrition and Dietetics: The impact of fluoride on health. *J Acad Nutr Dietet* 2012;112:1443.

22. SPRINT Research Group: A randomized trial of intensive versus standard blood-pressure control. *N Engl J Med* 2015;373:2103.

23. Aburto NJ and others: Effect of lower sodium intake on health: Systematic review and meta-analyses. *BMJ* 2013;346:f1326.

24. Popkin BM and others: A new proposed guidance system for beverage consumption in the United States. *Amer J Clin Nutr* 2006;83:529.

Rate Your Beverage Choices

Water is the key component in the guidelines that have been developed by the Beverage Guidance Panel (Table 9-10). These recommendations give guidance on the health and nutritional benefits as well as the risks of various beverage categories. The basis of the Beverage Guidance System is that fluids should not provide a significant amount of the energy nutrients in a healthy diet. More specifically, the system recommends that beverages provide less than 10% of total calories consumed for a 2200 kcal diet.[24]

TABLE 9-10 ■ The Beverage Guidance System

Level	Category*	Recommended Servings per Day
1	Water	50 fluid ounces (1.7 liters)
2	Tea or coffee, unsweetened	0 to 40 fluid ounces (0 to 1.4 liters)
3	Low-fat and skim milk and soy beverages	0 to 16 fluid ounces (0 to 0.5 liter)
4	Noncalorically sweetened beverages (diet drinks)	0 to 32 fluid ounces (0 to 1 liter)
5	Calorie beverages with some nutrients (100% fruit juices, alcoholic beverages, whole milk, and sports drinks)	0 to 8 fluid ounces 100% fruit juices (0 to 0.25 liter) 0 to 1 alcoholic drink for women 0 to 2 alcoholic drinks for men
6	Calorically sweetened beverages (regular soft drinks)	0 to 8 fluid ounces (0 to 0.25 liter)

*Categories established based on their possible health benefits or risks.

Source: Adapted from Popkin, et al. "A new proposed guidance system for beverage consumption in the United States." *American Journal of Clinical Nutrition* 83:529, 2006

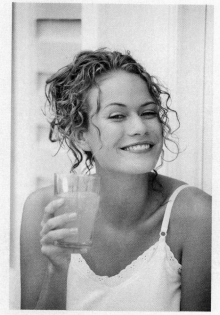
©Hoby Finn/Getty Images

1. Think of all the beverages you drank yesterday, from the time you woke up to the time you went to bed. Do your best to recall the types and amounts of your fluid intake in the space below.

   _____

   _____

   _____

   _____

2. Next to each beverage choice you listed for question 1, indicate its category from the Beverage Guidance System.

3. Did you come close to the recommendation to consume 50 fluid ounces (1.7 liters) of fluid in the form of water yesterday?

   _____

   _____

4. How many fluid ounces of your beverages fit into categories 2, 3, 4, 5, or 6? Did you exceed the recommended servings per day for these categories?

   _____

   _____

   _____

5. What changes could you make in your beverage choices to follow the Beverage Guidance System more closely? How does following the Beverage Guidance System contribute to good health?

   _____

   _____

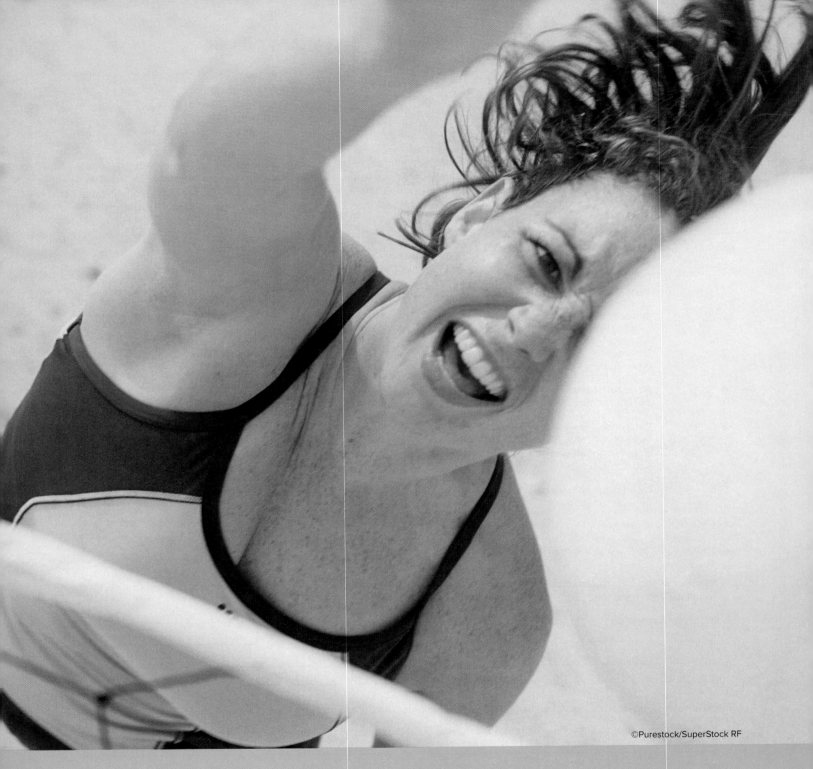

©Purestock/SuperStock RF

Student Learning Outcomes

Chapter 10 is designed to allow you to:

10.1 List five positive health-related outcomes of a physically active lifestyle.

10.2 List three key elements of a sound fitness regimen.

10.3 Describe the use of carbohydrates, fat, and protein to meet energy needs during different activities.

10.4 Differentiate between anaerobic and aerobic uses of glucose and identify advantages and disadvantages of each.

10.5 Explain how muscles and related organs adapt to an increase in physical activity.

10.6 Outline how to estimate an athlete's calorie needs and discuss the general principles for meeting overall nutrient requirements in the training diet.

10.7 Examine problems associated with dehydration and outline the importance of fluids during exercise.

Chapter 10
Nutrition: Fitness and Sports

You are gearing up to run your first half-marathon in a few weeks. From your long training runs, you know that physical and mental fatigue may set in a few miles before the finish. You've practiced great dietary patterns throughout training but have trouble eating during your runs. You want to try one of those sports nutrition products to help get you through the last few miles. What would you choose to take along during the race to help you make it to the finish line?

a Clif Shot® Turbo energy gel with 100 milligrams caffeine, 22 grams of carbohydrate, and electrolytes

b PowerBar ProteinPlus® energy bar with 23 grams of protein

c Powerade® sports drink with electrolytes, vitamins, and 14 grams of carbohydrate

d Essential Amino Energy™ drink with branched-chain amino acids

Think about your choice as you read this chapter, then see What the Dietitian Chose at the end of the chapter.

Are you a sedentary individual looking to start a personal fitness program? Do you participate in recreational sports, such as intramural volleyball? Or are you a competitive athlete who would like to take your performance to the next level? One thing is certain: at every level of fitness, sensible nutrition and physical activity complement each other in the pursuit of wellness.

Some individuals fall into the trap of thinking that participation in sports alleviates the need to pay close attention to eating habits. As you will learn in this chapter, adequate dietary patterns and hydration have a big impact on physical performance.

Most athletes are on the lookout for any advantage, whether real or perceived, that might enhance performance and give them the winning edge. For this reason, athletes are likely targets for nutrition quackery and misinformation. As you try to sort fact from fiction, be sure of this: long-term health promotion and maintenance should include adherence to evidence-based dietary and physical activity practices.

Overall, making informed choices about foods, beverages, and dietary supplements can optimize many aspects of physical performance, from preventing fatigue to gaining muscle to recovering from workouts. In this chapter, you will discover how physical activity benefits the entire body and how nutrition relates to physical performance. This information is important for the everyday, recreational athlete who exercises to manage weight or just to have fun. It is crucial, however, for elite athletes for whom a fraction of a second can make the difference between first and second place. A sports dietitian can assist in adapting the unique issues of individual athletes regarding overall health, nutrient requirements, performance goals, physique characteristics, barriers to success, and food preferences.

10.8 Understand how athletes can optimize performance by consuming foods and fluids before, during, and after exercise.

10.9 List several ergogenic aids and describe their effects, if any, on an athlete's performance.

10.1 An Introduction to Physical Fitness

Healthy People 2020 objectives focus on reducing the proportion of adults who engage in no leisure time physical activity and increasing the proportion of adults who meet the Physical Activity Guidelines for aerobic and muscle-strengthening physical activity.

physical activity Any movement of skeletal muscles that requires energy.

exercise Physical activities that are planned, repetitive, and intended to improve physical fitness.

physical fitness The ability to perform moderate to vigorous activity without undue fatigue.

Randi and Chandra used to chat over a cup of coffee after their 8:00 A.M. nutrition class, but now they meet at the student rec center for a workout. Terry listens to recorded nutrition lectures as he jogs around the track. Claudia takes the stairs instead of the elevator to her dorm room on the fourth floor. Marlie reviews her course notes while she works out on the recumbent bike. What do these students have in common? They each have found inventive ways to incorporate physical activity into their busy college schedules.

Without a doubt, the benefits of **physical activity** outweigh the risks for most Americans. The potential benefits of regular physical activity include improved heart health, sleep patterns, and body composition. Physical activity also can reduce stress and improve clinical parameters such as blood pressure, blood cholesterol, blood glucose regulation, and immune function. In addition, physical activity aids in weight control, both by raising resting energy expenditure and by increasing overall energy expenditure. In fact, as physical fitness improves, so does your ability to mobilize fat as a source of energy. See Figure 10-1 for a closer look at these and other benefits of a physically active lifestyle.[1]

It is important to note that physical activity and exercise are not synonymous. Physical activity refers to any movement of skeletal muscles that requires energy. It includes exercise, sports, as well as all the simple, unplanned activities of daily living, such as raking the yard, walking up and down the stairs, and carrying bags of groceries into the house. **Exercise** specifically refers to those physical activities that are planned, repetitive, and intended to improve **physical fitness.** Examples of exercise include walking, biking, swimming, participating in team sports, and running.

FIGURE 10-1 ▶ The benefits of regular, moderate physical activity and exercise.
©Rubberball Productions/Getty Images

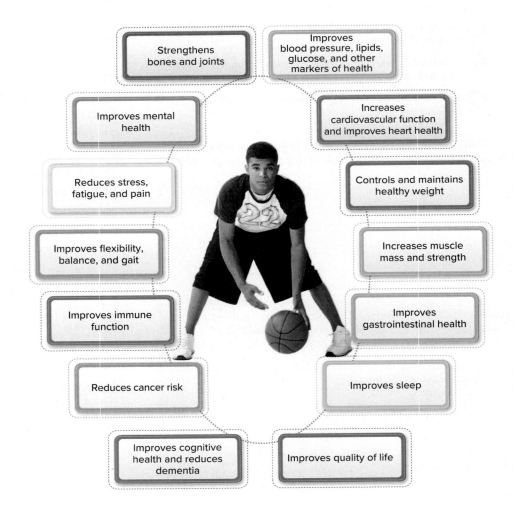

- Strengthens bones and joints
- Improves blood pressure, lipids, glucose, and other markers of health
- Improves mental health
- Increases cardiovascular function and improves heart health
- Reduces stress, fatigue, and pain
- Controls and maintains healthy weight
- Improves flexibility, balance, and gait
- Increases muscle mass and strength
- Improves immune function
- Improves gastrointestinal health
- Reduces cancer risk
- Improves sleep
- Improves cognitive health and reduces dementia
- Improves quality of life

The U.S. Department of Health and Human Services' (DHHS) Physical Activity Guidelines for Americans recommend that all adults should avoid inactivity.[2] Any physical activity is better than none, and adults who participate in any amount of physical activity gain some health benefits. The key Physical Activity Guidelines for adults include:

- For substantial health benefits, adults should do at least 150 minutes (2 1/2 hours) per week of **moderate-intensity,** or 75 minutes (1 1/4 hours) per week of **vigorous-intensity aerobic physical activity,** or an equivalent combination of moderate- and vigorous-intensity aerobic activity. Activity should be performed in episodes of at least 10 minutes, and preferably, it should be spread throughout the week.
- For additional and more extensive health benefits, adults should increase their physical activity to 300 minutes (5 hours) per week of moderate-intensity, or 150 minutes per week of vigorous-intensity aerobic physical activity, or an equivalent combination of moderate- and vigorous-intensity activity.
- Adults should also include **muscle-strengthening activities** that involve all major muscle groups on 2 or more days a week.

Complying with the Physical Activity Guidelines is the first step toward managing weight, reducing risks for chronic diseases, and improving physical fitness. Losing excess weight and maintaining weight loss will typically require more than 150 minutes of physical activity per week. Unfortunately, many North American adults lead sedentary lives. Only one in five American adults consistently achieves the level of physical activity set forth by the Physical Activity Guidelines.

moderate-intensity aerobic physical activity Aerobic activity that increases a person's heart rate and breathing to some extent (4–6 on RPE scale, Fig. 10-3). Examples include brisk walking, dancing, swimming, or bicycling on level terrain.

vigorous-intensity aerobic physical activity Aerobic activity that greatly increases a person's heart rate and breathing (7–8 on RPE scale, Fig. 10-3). Examples include jogging, singles tennis, swimming continuous laps, or bicycling uphill.

muscle-strengthening activity Physical activity that increases skeletal muscle strength, power, endurance, and mass. Examples include lifting weights, using weight machines, and calisthenics (e.g., push-ups).

✅ CONCEPT CHECK 10.1

1. Differentiate between physical activity and exercise.
2. How much physical activity is recommended by the Physical Activity Guidelines for Americans to reduce risks for chronic diseases?
3. List the five benefits of regular physical activity that are most important to you.

10.2 Achieving and Maintaining Physical Fitness

Much of the nutrition advice that appears later in this chapter focuses on enhancing the performance of highly competitive athletes; however, only a few students would describe themselves as elite athletes. Furthermore, in a health profession, most clients are at a beginner or intermediate level of fitness. Certainly, proper nutrition supports physical performance at all levels. Perhaps more importantly, nutrition and physical activity complement each other when it comes to improving health outcomes. This section outlines how to get started with a plan to achieve physical fitness.

ASSESS YOUR CURRENT LEVEL OF FITNESS

Start by assessing your current level of fitness. In some cases, it is beneficial to seek medical advice before getting started. Men aged 40 years or older and women aged 50 years or older, anyone who has been inactive for many years, or those who have an existing health problem should discuss their fitness goals with their primary care provider before increasing activity. Health problems that require medical evaluation before beginning an exercise program include obesity, cardiovascular disease (or family history), hypertension, diabetes (or family history), chest pains or shortness of breath, and arthritis. Even if you do not have preexisting medical problems, enlisting the aid of a sports dietitian or certified personal trainer can help you to determine a safe starting point and establish realistic goals.

SET A GOAL

For any behavior change, goal setting will enhance your success. Sports dietitians are trained professionals who can help you set reasonable physical activity goals based on your current level of fitness. For someone who has never exercised regularly, running a mile without stopping might be a worthwhile goal. An elite runner might strive to run that mile in under 4 minutes. Based on your long-term goal, also incorporate several smaller, short-term goals into your plan. Measurable, attainable, and realistic goals provide focus and motivation for any endeavor.

PLAN YOUR PROGRAM

What activities should you include in your physical activity program? Although your goal may focus on just one aspect of fitness, such as being able to bench-press your body weight, a balanced fitness program will include three key types of activities: aerobic exercise, strength training, and flexibility.

Many physical activity experts use the *FITT principle* to design a fitness program. FITT stands for *frequency, intensity, time,* and *type* of exercise. Frequency is the number of days per week you engage in a particular activity. Intensity is how hard you work when you exercise—that is, how much you increase your heart rate or how much resistance you use when you lift weights. Type (also called *mode*) is your choice of activity, such as walking or running. Table 10-1 summarizes the American College of Sports Medicine (ACSM) recommendations for planning a general fitness program.

Aerobic Exercise Enhances Heart and Lung Function As you learned earlier, *aerobic* means "with oxygen." Aerobic exercises use large muscle groups in a rhythmic fashion and aim to increase your heart rate. The ability to perform aerobic exercise depends on the health of your heart and lungs—the organ systems that provide oxygen to the cells of the body.

Aerobic activities usually form the backbone of a fitness program. Indeed, many of the benefits of fitness mentioned in Section 10.1 are direct effects of aerobic training. The ACSM recommends including at least 30 minutes per day of moderate-intensity aerobic activities on 5 days per week. Alternatively, less time spent in aerobic exercises of vigorous intensity can yield similar results. Walking, running, dancing, and biking are examples of aerobic activities.

TABLE 10-1 ■ **Elements of a Well-Rounded Fitness Program**

	Aerobic Fitness	Muscular Fitness	Flexibility
Frequency	5 days per week	2 to 3 days per week	2 to 3 days per week
Intensity	55% to 85% of MHR[a] or RPE[b] of 4 or higher (Fig. 10-3)	40% to 80% of 1 RM[c] (lower for endurance and higher for strength)	To the point of tension
Time	20 to 60 minutes per day	1 to 3 sets of 8 to 12 repetitions of 8 to 10 different exercises	2 to 4 repetitions of 8 to 10 different exercises, held for 15 to 30 seconds each
Type (examples)	Brisk walking, running, cycling, swimming, basketball, tennis, and soccer	Bench press, squat, biceps curl, and abdominal crunch	Hamstring stretch, shoulder reach, and side bend

[a] Maximal heart rate; [b] Rating of perceived exertion; [c] 1-repetition maximum

There are a few ways to determine the intensity of aerobic exercise. A popular and simple method is to use a percentage of your age-predicted *maximum heart rate* (MHR) (Fig. 10-2). To find your MHR, subtract your age from 220. For a 20-year-old person, MHR equals 200 beats per minute (220 − 20 (age) = 200 MRH).

At the initiation of an aerobic exercise program, aim for about 50% to 65% of MHR as a target heart rate for aerobic activity. Thus, (200 × 0.5) and (200 × 0.65) yield a target training zone of 100 to 130 beats per minute. As you progress and become more physically fit, you can work up to a higher heart rate. For an intermediate fitness enthusiast, 60% to 75% of MHR is recommended. For more experienced exercisers, 70% to 85% MHR is suitable.

Remember that heart rate is just an estimate of workout intensity. Medications, such as those for hypertension and other health conditions, may impact heart rate. If you have health concerns, a primary care provider can help to personalize your safe target heart rate zone.

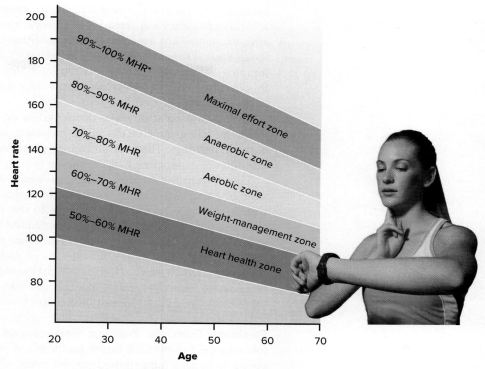

*MHR (maximum heart rate) = 220 − Age in years

FIGURE 10-2 ▲ Heart rate training chart. This chart shows the number of heart beats per minute that corresponds to various exercise intensities. ©Tetra Images/SuperStock RF

Another way of determining the intensity of exercise is the *Rating of Perceived Exertion (RPE) scale*. One version includes a range of 0 to 10, with each number corresponding to a subjective feeling of exertion. For example, the number 0 is "nothing at all" (e.g., sitting), and the number 10 is considered close to maximal effort or "very, very strong" (e.g., all-out sprint; Fig. 10-3).

When using the 10-point RPE scale, the goal is to aim for a minimum rating of 4, which corresponds to the beginning of "somewhat strong." This is the point at which you begin to obtain significant fitness results. If you are hovering around a RPE of 4 (somewhat strong perception of exersion), you should still be able to talk somewhat comfortably to a workout partner (sometimes called the *talk test*).

Measuring heart rate (pulse) is easy: stop and count your pulse for 10 seconds and then multiply that number by 6 to determine beats per minute. Most fitness equipment and some personal fitness devices now contain automatic heart rate monitors.

Muscular Fitness Encompasses Strength, Endurance, and Power Muscles can be trained in several ways. *Muscular strength* is the maximal force a muscle can exert against a load at one time (1-repetition maximum or 1 RM). For example, a strength-trained athlete may be able to dead-lift 400 pounds one time. *Muscular endurance* refers to the ability of the muscle to perform repeated, submaximal contractions over time without

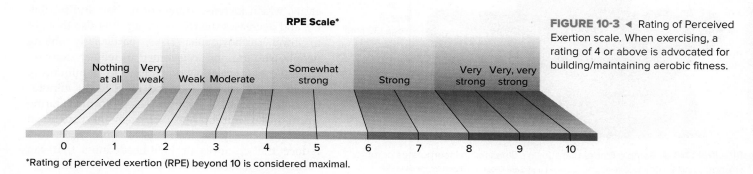

*Rating of perceived exertion (RPE) beyond 10 is considered maximal.

FIGURE 10-3 ◄ Rating of Perceived Exertion scale. When exercising, a rating of 4 or above is advocated for building/maintaining aerobic fitness.

becoming fatigued. An athlete training for muscular endurance may bench-press 80 to 100 pounds for several sets of 8 to 12 repetitions. Both muscular strength and endurance are important aspects of muscular fitness that relate to health for athletes of all levels. *Muscular power* combines strength with speed for explosive movements such as jumping or throwing. Power is a crucial aspect of muscular fitness for many athletes. Studies also show that developing muscular power can help to improve function and balance among older adults.

Overall, muscular fitness is developed by performing resistance exercises for all the major muscle groups of the body, including arms and shoulders, back, abdominals, buttock, and legs. This resistance may come from free weights (e.g., barbells), weight machines (e.g., leg press), or the weight of your own body (e.g., push-ups).

The Physical Activity Guidelines and ACSM recommend including muscle-strengthening activities in your fitness program on 2 to 3 nonconsecutive days per week (Fig. 10-4). Taking a day or more to rest between bouts of resistance exercise or alternating groups of muscles is recommended to allow time for muscles to recover and increase in size. Performing regular resistance exercises will help you become stronger and better able to handle the activities of daily living. It promotes increases in lean body mass, which assist efforts at weight management and control. Compared to aerobic exercise alone, resistance exercise can also provide further reductions in risks for cardiovascular diseases, osteoporosis, and type 2 diabetes.

Flexibility Exercises Enhance Balance and Stability *Flexibility* is an often overlooked aspect of physical health and tends to decline with age. Flexibility refers to the ability to move a joint through its full range of motion. Poor flexibility is often linked to chronic pain, especially in the lower back. Contrary to popular belief, research studies do not clearly support a role of flexibility exercises in preventing injury or muscle soreness from aerobic or strength-training activities. However, gains in flexibility can improve balance and stability, thereby reducing risks of falls and injuries, especially among older adults.

ACSM recommends performing flexibility exercises at least 2 to 3 days per week (Fig. 10-4). It is best to perform stretches when the muscles have already been warmed up—after a few minutes of light-intensity walking. Examples of flexibility exercises include hamstring stretch, side bends, and shoulder reach. Some forms of exercise, such as Pilates or tai chi, combine stretching with strength moves.

Warm-Up and Cool-Down Be sure to plan for adequate warm-up and cool-down periods as part of your physical activity routine. Begin by warming up with 5 to 10 minutes of low-intensity exercises, such as walking, slow jogging, or any low-intensity performance of the anticipated activity. This warms up your muscles so that muscle filaments slide over one another more easily, which increases range of motion and flexibility, and decreases the risk of injury. It is also thought to lower cardiovascular risks, particularly among people who are not accustomed to regular exercise. During cool-down, slow down for 5 to 10 minutes of low-intensity activity followed by 5 to 10 minutes of stretching. The same exercises performed during warm-up are appropriate. Although the cool-down does not actually prevent muscle soreness, it does reduce the dizziness or light-headedness that can occur with an abrupt end to a vigorous workout.

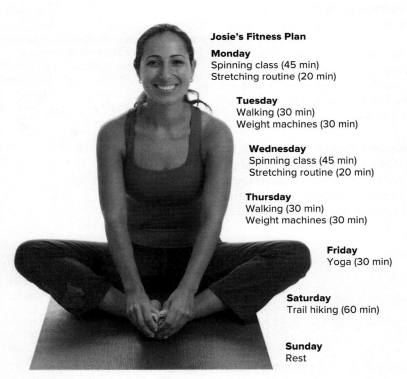

Josie's Fitness Plan

Monday
Spinning class (45 min)
Stretching routine (20 min)

Tuesday
Walking (30 min)
Weight machines (30 min)

Wednesday
Spinning class (45 min)
Stretching routine (20 min)

Thursday
Walking (30 min)
Weight machines (30 min)

Friday
Yoga (30 min)

Saturday
Trail hiking (60 min)

Sunday
Rest

FIGURE 10-4 ▲ Sample fitness plan. Josie's fitness plan incorporates aerobic, strength, and flexibility exercises. ©John Lund/Sam Diephuis/Blend Images LLC RF

Get Started For sedentary people who are otherwise healthy, gradual **progression** toward meeting the physical activity guidelines is recommended. During the first phase of a fitness program to promote health, you should begin to incorporate short periods of physical activity into your daily routine. This includes brisk walking, taking the stairs instead of the elevator, dancing, hiking, and other activities that cause you to "huff and puff" a bit. A sensible goal is a total of 30 minutes of this moderate type of physical activity on most (and preferably all) days of the week. If necessary, this can be broken up into increments lasting at least 10 minutes. If there is not much time for activity, you can obtain similar benefits from performing shorter sessions of increased intensity, such as running instead of walking or biking on hilly versus flat terrains.

Once you can perform physical activity for 30 minutes per day, turn your attention to more specific goals, such as increasing muscle mass and strength, to reap even more benefits.

progression Incremental increase in frequency, intensity, and time spent in each type of physical activity over several weeks or months.

> ### Stick with It!
>
> Even after all the effort of assessing baseline fitness, setting goals, and designing a program, it turns out that maintaining a physical activity program is the hardest part! To stick with an exercise program, experts recommend the following:
>
> - Start slowly and progress incrementally.
> - Vary your activities to keep it fresh; rotate indoor and outdoor activities.
> - Include friends and family members for additional motivation.
> - Frequently revisit both short- and long-term goals.
> - Set aside a specific time each day for exercise; set physical activity calendar appointments.
> - Reward yourself when achieving goals.
> - Forgive yourself for occasional setbacks; focus on the long-term benefits to your health.

✔ CONCEPT CHECK 10.2

1. Why is goal setting important for the success of a physical activity program?
2. What is the FITT principle? Demonstrate how you would use the FITT principle to make a plan for aerobic fitness.
3. Differentiate between muscular strength, muscular endurance, and muscular power.
4. List two evidence-supported benefits of flexibility exercises.
5. Provide three tips for a person who needs help maintaining a fitness program.

10.3 Energy Sources for Exercising Muscles

Like other cells, muscle cells cannot directly use the energy released from breaking down glucose or triglycerides. Muscle cells need a specific form of energy for contraction. Body cells must first convert food energy (i.e., calories) to **adenosine triphosphate (ATP).**

The chemical bonds between phosphates in ATP and related molecules are high-energy bonds. Using the energy obtained from food, cells make ATP from its breakdown product **adenosine diphosphate (ADP)** and a phosphate group (abbreviated P_i). Conversely, to release energy from ATP, cells partially break the compound down into ADP and P_i. The released energy is used for many cell functions (Fig. 10-5).

adenosine triphosphate (ATP) The main energy currency for cells. ATP energy is used to promote ion pumping, enzyme activity, and rapid muscular contraction.

adenosine diphosphate (ADP) A breakdown product of ATP. ADP is synthesized into ATP using energy from foodstuffs and a phosphate group (abbreviated P_i).

ANAEROBIC METABOLISM SUPPLIES ENERGY FOR SHORT BURSTS OF INTENSE ACTIVITY

Stored ATP Essentially, ATP is the immediate source of energy for body functions (Table 10-2). The primary goal in the use of any fuel, whether carbohydrate, fat, or protein, is to make ATP. A resting muscle cell contains only a small amount of ATP that can be used immediately. This amount of ATP could keep the muscle working maximally for only about 2 to 4 seconds if no resupply of ATP were possible. Fortunately, the cells have various mechanisms to resupply ATP. Overall, cells must constantly and repeatedly use and then reform ATP, using a variety of energy sources.

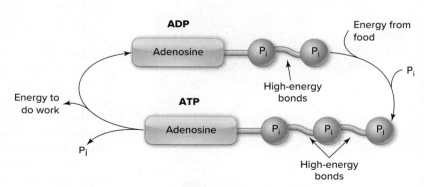

FIGURE 10-5 ▲ Food energy is stored in the chemical bonds between the phosphate groups in ATP. When a phosphate group is cleaved from ATP, energy to perform work is released. The product of the breakdown of ATP is adenosine diphosphate (ADP).

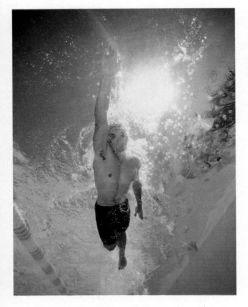

anaerobic Requiring no oxygen.
aerobic Requiring oxygen.

▲ Bursts of muscle activity, such as the 100-meter freestyle, use a variety of energy sources, including ATP, PCr, and glucose. ©Erik Isakson/Blend Images LLC RF

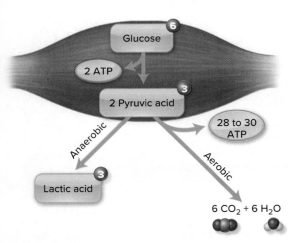

FIGURE 10-6 ▲ ATP yield from aerobic versus anaerobic glucose use. Encircled numbers indicate the number of carbons in each molecule.

TABLE 10-2 ■ **Energy Sources Used by Resting and Working Muscle Cells**

Energy Source*	When in Use	Activity
ATP	At all times	All types
Phosphocreatine (PCr)	All exercise initially; short bursts up to 10 seconds	Shot put, high jump, bench press
Carbohydrate **(anaerobic)**	High-intensity exercise, especially lasting 30 seconds to 2 minutes	200-yard (about 200-meter) sprint
Carbohydrate **(aerobic)**	Exercise lasting 2 minutes to several hours; the higher the intensity, the greater the use	Basketball, swimming, jogging, power walking
Fat (aerobic)	Exercise lasting more than a few minutes; greater amounts are used at lower intensities	Long-distance running or cycling; much of the fuel used in a 30-minute brisk walk is fat
Protein (aerobic)	Low amount used during all exercise; slightly more in endurance exercise, especially when carbohydrate fuel is depleted	Long-distance running

*At any given time, more than one source is used. The relative amount of use differs during various activities.

Phosphocreatine As soon as ATP stored in muscle cells begins to be used, another high-energy compound, **phosphocreatine (PCr),** is used to resupply ATP. An enzyme in the muscle cell is activated to split PCr into phosphate and **creatine.** This releases energy that can be used to reform ATP from its breakdown products. If no other source of energy for ATP resupply were available, PCr could probably maintain maximal muscle contractions for about 10 seconds.

The main advantage of PCr is that it can be activated instantly and can replenish ATP at rates fast enough to meet the energy demands of the fastest and most powerful actions, including jumping, lifting, throwing, and sprinting. The disadvantage of PCr is that not much of it is made and stored in the muscles. Strength-training athletes sometimes use creatine supplements in an effort to increase PCr in muscles (Section 10.6).

Anaerobic Glucose Breakdown Carbohydrates are an important fuel for muscles. The most useful form of carbohydrate fuel is the simple sugar glucose, available to all cells from the bloodstream. As you will recall, glucose is stored as glycogen in the liver and muscle cells. Blood glucose is maintained by the breakdown of liver glycogen. Breakdown of glycogen stored in a specific muscle also helps meet the carbohydrate demand of that muscle, but the actual amount of glycogen stored in muscle is limited (about 350 grams for all the muscles in the body, which would yield about 1400 kcal).

When oxygen supply in the muscle is limited (anaerobic conditions), glucose is broken down into a three-carbon compound called **pyruvic acid.** The pyruvic acid accumulates in the muscle and is then converted to **lactic acid.** Only about 5% of the total amount of ATP that could be formed from complete breakdown of glucose is released through this anaerobic process (Fig. 10-6).

The advantage of anaerobic glucose breakdown is, it is the fastest way to resupply ATP, other than PCr breakdown. It therefore provides most of the energy needed for events that require a quick burst of energy, ranging from about 30 seconds to 2 minutes. Examples of activities that primarily rely on anaerobic glucose breakdown include sprinting 400 meters or swimming 100 meters.

The two major disadvantages of the anaerobic process are: (1) the high rate of ATP production cannot be sustained for long periods; and (2) the rapid accumulation of lactic acid increases the acidity of the muscle. Normally, the pH of the muscle is about 7.1. Intense exercise that relies on anaerobic glucose breakdown can decrease the pH of muscle tissue to about 6.5. Acidity inhibits the activities of key enzymes in the muscle cells, slowing anaerobic ATP production and causing short-term fatigue. In addition, the acidity leads to a net potassium loss from muscle cells, which also contributes to fatigue. During exercise, you need to choose a sustainable pace according to the goals of the activity.

Before long, muscle cells release the accumulating lactic acid into the bloodstream. The liver (and the kidneys, to some extent) takes up the lactic acid and resynthesizes it into glucose. Glucose can then reenter the bloodstream, where it is available for cell uptake and breakdown. Individuals vary in their ability to clear lactic acid from the muscles and recycle it. Physical training may improve the ability of the body to remove and recycle lactic acid. Section 10.6 describes an ergogenic aid to neutralize lactic acid.

AEROBIC METABOLISM FUELS PROLONGED, LOWER-INTENSITY ACTIVITY

Carbohydrates If plenty of oxygen is available in the muscle (aerobic conditions), such as when the exercise is of low to moderate intensity, the bulk of the three-carbon pyruvic acid is shuttled to the mitochondria of the cell, where it is fully metabolized into carbon dioxide (CO_2) and water (H_2O) (Fig. 10-7). This aerobic breakdown of glucose yields approximately 95% of the ATP made from complete glucose metabolism (glucose $\rightarrow\rightarrow CO_2 + H_2O$).

phosphocreatine (PCr) A high-energy compound that can be used to reform ATP. It is used primarily during bursts of activity, such as lifting and jumping.

creatine An organic (i.e., carbon-containing) molecule in muscle cells that serves as part of a high-energy compound (termed *creatine phosphate* or *phosphocreatine*) capable of synthesizing ATP from ADP.

pyruvic acid A three-carbon compound formed during glucose metabolism; also called *pyruvate*.

lactic acid A three-carbon acid formed during anaerobic cell metabolism; a partial breakdown product of glucose; also called *lactate*.

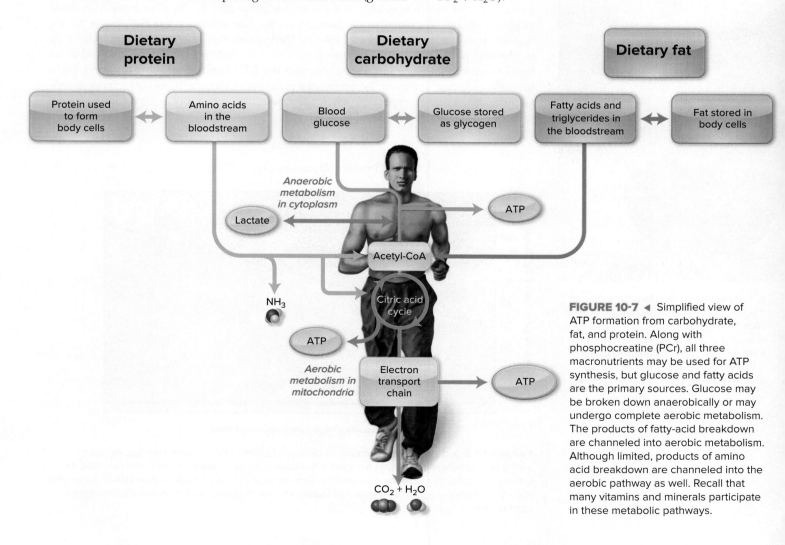

FIGURE 10-7 ◄ Simplified view of ATP formation from carbohydrate, fat, and protein. Along with phosphocreatine (PCr), all three macronutrients may be used for ATP synthesis, but glucose and fatty acids are the primary sources. Glucose may be broken down anaerobically or may undergo complete aerobic metabolism. The products of fatty-acid breakdown are channeled into aerobic metabolism. Although limited, products of amino acid breakdown are channeled into the aerobic pathway as well. Recall that many vitamins and minerals participate in these metabolic pathways.

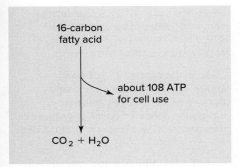

16-carbon
fatty acid

about 108 ATP
for cell use

$CO_2 + H_2O$

▲ ATP yield from aerobic fatty-acid utilization.

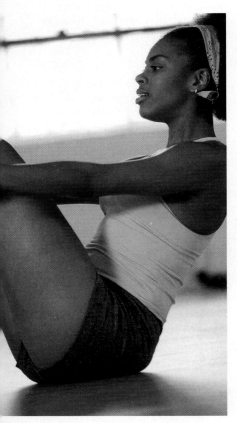

▲ Fatty acids are recruited from all over the body, not necessarily from fat stored near the active muscles. *This is why spot reducing does not work.* Exercise can tone the muscles near adipose tissue but does not preferentially use those stores. ©Comstock Images/Jupiterimages RF

Aerobic glucose breakdown supplies more ATP than the anaerobic process, but it releases the energy more slowly. This slower rate of aerobic energy supply can be sustained for hours. One reason is that the products are carbon dioxide and water, not lactic acid. Aerobic glucose breakdown makes a major energy contribution to activities that last anywhere from 2 minutes to several hours. Examples of such activities include jogging or distance swimming (Table 10-2).

Endurance athletes sometimes reach a point in an event at which extreme physical and mental fatigue sets in; it feels impossible to stand up, let alone continue competing. Long-distance runners call this phenomenon *hitting the wall,* and cyclists refer to it as *bonking.* This occurs because muscle glycogen has been depleted and blood glucose has begun to decline during exercise, leading to deterioration of both physical and mental function. As you will learn in Section 10.5, maximizing glycogen storage before exercise, supplying carbohydrates during activity, and replenishing glycogen stores between events can help athletes avoid the game-stopping effects of glycogen depletion.

Fat When fat stores in body tissues begin to be broken down for energy, each triglyceride first yields three fatty acids (*tri-*) and a glycerol molecule (*glyceride*). The majority of the stored energy is found in the fatty acids. During physical activity, fatty acids are released from various adipose tissue depots into the bloodstream and travel to the muscles, where they are taken into each cell and broken down aerobically to carbon dioxide and water. Some of the fat stored in muscles (intramuscular triglycerides) also is used, especially as activity increases from a low to a moderate pace.

Fat is an advantageous fuel for muscles: we generally have plenty of it stored, and it is a concentrated source of energy. For a given weight of fuel, fat supplies more than twice as much energy as carbohydrate does. However, the ability of muscles to use fat for fuel depends on the intensity of exercise. During intense, brief exercise, muscles may not be able to use much fat. The reason for this is that some of the steps involved in fat breakdown cannot occur fast enough to meet the ATP demands of short-duration, high-intensity exercise. However, fat becomes a progressively more important energy source as duration increases, especially when exercise remains at a low or moderate (aerobic) rate for more than 20 minutes (Fig. 10-8).

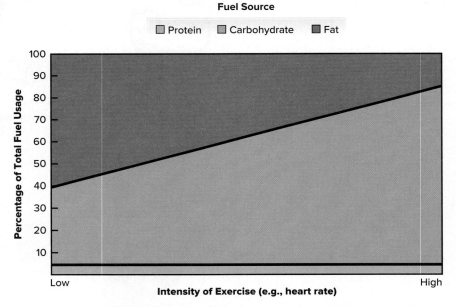

Fuel Source

☐ Protein ☐ Carbohydrate ■ Fat

FIGURE 10-8 ▲ Generalized relationship between fuel use and exercise intensity. At rest or during light activity, nearly equal amounts of carbohydrate and fat are used to generate ATP. As activity intensifies (e.g., sprinting), anaerobic processes supply quick fuel, so the relative proportion of carbohydrates used for fuel increases. Except during endurance exercise, very little protein is used for fuel.

For lengthy activities at a moderate pace (e.g., hiking) or even sitting at a desk for 8 hours a day, fat supplies about 70% to 90% of the energy required. Carbohydrate use is much less. As intensity increases, carbohydrate use goes up and fat use decreases. During a 5-mile run at a moderate pace, muscles use about a 50:50 ratio of fat to carbohydrate. In comparison, for a sprint, the contribution of fat to resupply ATP is minimal. To summarize, remember that the only fast-paced (anaerobic) fuel we eat is carbohydrate; slow and steady (aerobic) activity uses fat in addition to carbohydrate.

Protein Although amino acids derived from protein can be used to fuel muscles, their contribution is relatively small, compared with that of carbohydrate and fat. Most protein is reserved for building and repairing body tissues and for synthesizing important enzymes, hormones, and transporters. As a rough guide, only about 5% of the body's ATP comes from the metabolism of amino acids.

During endurance exercise, proteins can contribute importantly to energy needs, perhaps as much as 10%, especially as glycogen stores in the muscle are exhausted. Most of the energy supplied from protein comes from metabolism of the branched-chain amino acids: leucine, isoleucine, and valine. A healthy dietary pattern provides ample branched-chain amino acids to supply this amount of fuel; protein or amino acid supplements are rarely needed.

CAN PHYSICAL TRAINING AFFECT FUEL USE?

As people start exercising regularly (e.g., a minimum of 150 minutes per week of moderate-intensity aerobic activity), they experience a "training effect." Initially, these individuals might be able to exercise for 20 minutes before tiring. Months later, exercise can be extended to an hour before they become fatigued. The training effect results from changes in the ability of exercising cells to use food fuel to generate ATP.

Almost immediately after a person begins an exercise program, both aerobic and strength training improve the insulin sensitivity of cells. In other words, more glucose can be transported from the bloodstream into the cells, where it can be broken down either anaerobically or aerobically. Improved blood glucose management is an added benefit for preventing or treating metabolic syndrome or type 2 diabetes.

Endurance aerobic activities also increase the ability of muscles to store glycogen. This highly branched polymer of glucose can be broken down into individual glucose units when the energy needs of the cell are high or when blood glucose levels start to drop. Increasing glycogen storage will help to delay fatigue during prolonged exercise.

Fat is a concentrated source of calories; complete oxidation of a long-chain fatty acid yields about three times as much ATP as metabolism of glucose. Many endurance athletes attempt to train their muscles to more readily use fat for fuel and thereby conserve muscle glycogen. In Section 10.5, you will learn more about this technique, known as **fat adaptation.**

Protein use becomes more efficient with training, too. Endurance training increases the ability of muscle cells to use branched-chain amino acids for fuel during prolonged activity. However, the ability to use carbohydrates and fats for fuel is also increased; as long as the diet is adequate in carbohydrates and fat, most protein is spared for muscle synthesis and repair.

In addition, training increases the number of mitochondria within muscle cells. Recall that mitochondria are the powerhouses of the cells; this is where glucose and fat are broken down aerobically to generate ATP. With more mitochondria, muscle cells can use carbohydrates and fat more efficiently.

Overall, the cardiovascular and respiratory systems become more efficient at providing oxygen to the cells of the body. Plasma volume increases shortly after a training program is started, and red blood cell volume eventually increases as well. The heart pumps more blood with each contraction. Training also increases the number of capillaries in muscles, which increases oxygen supply to the muscles. Meanwhile, lung capacity increases, so more oxygen is available. The increased supply of oxygen translates into

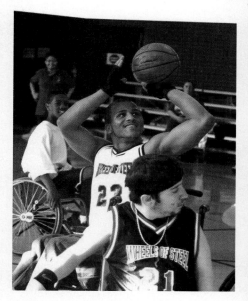

▲ The calories needed to perform come from carbohydrate, fat, and protein. The relative mix depends on many factors.
©Realistic Reflections RF

CRITICAL THINKING

Marty started going to the gym about 8 weeks ago. At first, he noticed that he began "huffing and puffing" about 7 minutes into his aerobic workout. Now, however, he can work out for about 25 minutes without tiring. What is a possible explanation for this ability to work out longer?

fat adaptation Manipulating the diet and physical training regimen so that muscles become more efficient at metabolizing fat as fuel during aerobic activity.

more efficient aerobic metabolism of carbohydrates and fats. Thus, lactic-acid production from anaerobic glucose metabolism decreases. Lactic acid contributes to short-term muscle fatigue, so the less lactic acid produced, the longer the exercise can be sustained.

Through all these adaptations, physical training improves the ability of cells to convert food energy into fuel for exercise.

✓ CONCEPT CHECK 10.3

1. Describe one process used to resupply ATP during a short, intense burst of activity, such as a 100-meter sprint.
2. How does the ATP yield of anaerobic breakdown of glucose compare to that of aerobic breakdown of glucose?
3. Why is fat a useful source of energy during exercise? Name three types of activity during which fat supplies 50% or more of fuel.
4. Is protein a useful source of energy during exercise? Why or why not?

10.4 Tailoring Nutrient Recommendations for Athletes

Athletic training and genetic makeup are two important determinants of athletic performance. Although a healthy dietary pattern can't substitute for either factor, it can help to enhance and maximize an athlete's potential. On the other hand, poor dietary patterns can seriously reduce performance.[3]

CALORIES

The daily calorie needs of athletes are highly individualized: genetics, hormones, age, sex, temperature, altitude, stress, physical health, medications, body size and composition, and training volume influence energy expenditure. A small, female gymnast may need only 1800 kcal daily to sustain her training regimen without losing body weight, whereas a large, muscular football player may need 4000 kcal per day. Because athletes are such a heterogeneous group, there is no perfect equation to estimate their daily calorie needs. Even for nonathletes, the *Estimated Energy Requirement* (EER) equation (Chapter 7) provides only a rough approximation. However, you can use the EER equation as a starting point and individualize recommendations based on trial and error.

An estimate of the calories required to sustain moderate activity is 5 to 8 kcal per minute. The calories required for sports training or competition, then, must be added to those used to carry on normal activities. For example, consider a 135-pound young woman who requires 2200 kcal per day to fuel her normal activities. If she starts teaching two 45-minute dance classes each day, she will need about 500 extra kcal (a total of 2700 kcal per day) to maintain her current body weight. If an athlete experiences daily fatigue, the first consideration should be whether he or she is consuming enough food. Up to six meals per day may be needed, including one before each workout.

How can we know if an athlete is getting enough calories? Consulting with a sports dietitian would help answer this question. Estimating daily intake from a food diary kept by the athlete is one way. Another option is to estimate the athlete's body fat percentage via body composition measures such as those detailed in Chapter 7 (e.g., bioelectrical impedance, skinfolds, etc.). Body fat should be the typical amount found for athletes in the specific sport practiced. The National Collegiate Athletic Association (NCAA) recommendations for healthy body fat ranges are 20% to 32% for females and 10% to 22% for males. The next step is to monitor body weight changes on a daily or weekly basis. If body weight starts to fall, calories should be increased; if weight rises and it is because of increases in body fat, the athlete should reduce calories or increase physical activity.

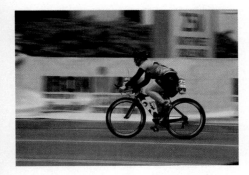

▲ Intense athletic training may require thousands of additional calories. This increased food intake should easily provide ample protein and other nutrients to support activity. ©Bernie McGroarty

Body mass index is not an appropriate surrogate for assessing body fat for athletes. Body composition assessments are preferred for determining body fatness. If assessments of body composition show that an athlete has too much body fat, the athlete should lower food intake by about 200 to 500 kcal per day, while maintaining a regular exercise program, until the desirable fat percentage is achieved. On the other hand, if an athlete needs to gain weight, increasing food intake by 500 to 700 kcal per day will eventually lead to the needed weight gain. A mix of carbohydrate, fat, and protein is advised. Continuing to exercise will ensure that weight gain is mostly in the form of lean tissue rather than stored fat.

Historically, athletes who competed in sports with weight classes (e.g., wrestlers, boxers) would try to lose weight before a competition. Being certified to compete in a lower weight class could help an athlete gain a mechanical advantage over an opponent of smaller stature. Many of the methods used to cut weight are unhealthy and dangerous. For example, an athlete could lose up to 22 pounds (10 kilograms) of body weight as water in 1 day by sitting in a sauna, exercising in a plastic sweat suit, or taking diuretic drugs, which speed water loss via the kidneys. As you learned, losing as little as 2% of body weight by dehydration can adversely affect physical and mental performance, especially in hot weather. A pattern of repeated weight loss or gain of more than 5% of body weight by dehydration carries risk of kidney dysfunction and heat-related illness. Death is also a possibility.

To discourage such unhealthy practices and prevent future deaths, the National Collegiate Athletic Association (NCAA) and many states have authorized physicians or athletic trainers to set safe weight and body fat content minimums (e.g., 7% or more of total body weight for male athletes and 12% or more for females) in weight-class sports. Under current guidelines, athletes are assigned to weight classes at the beginning of the season and are not allowed to *cut weight* to gain a competitive advantage. In addition, urine specific gravity is measured prior to events to check for hydration status. This practice deters athletes from dehydrating themselves before weigh-in. Weight gain in the days after a competition (reflecting regain of body water) can now be no greater than 2 pounds. If athletes, such as wrestlers, wish to compete in a lower-body weight class and have enough extra fat stores, they should begin a gradual, sustained reduction in calorie intake months before the competitive season starts.[4]

CARBOHYDRATES

Anyone who exercises vigorously, especially for more than 1 hour per day on a regular basis, needs to consume a diet that includes moderate to high amounts of carbohydrate. Numerous servings of varied grains, starchy vegetables, and fruits provide enough carbohydrate to maintain adequate liver and muscle glycogen stores.

Depletion of carbohydrate ranks just behind depletion of fluid and electrolytes as a major cause of fatigue. Optimal carbohydrate intake depends on the size of the athlete and the type of physical activity. Recall that your weight in pounds divided by 2.2 converts your weight into kilograms. For light or skill-based sports, 3 to 5 grams of carbohydrate per kilogram of body weight will suffice. For exercise of moderate intensity, consume 5 to 7 grams of carbohydrate per kilogram. Athletes who train for several hours per day may need up to 12 grams of carbohydrates per kilogram of body weight, which may be 600 grams per day (or more). Attention to carbohydrate intake is especially important when performing multiple training bouts in one day (e.g., two-a-day swim practices) or heavy training on successive days (e.g., cross-country running).

The *Choose Your Foods* system designed for people with diabetes is a useful tool for planning all types of diets, including high-carbohydrate diets for athletes (Appendix B). As noted, athletes should obtain at least 45% to 65% of their total energy needs from carbohydrate, especially if exercise duration is expected to exceed 2 hours and total caloric intake is about 3000 kcal per day or less. Diets providing 4000 to 5000 kcal per day can be as low as 50% carbohydrate, as these will still provide sufficient carbohydrate (e.g., 500 to 600 grams or so per day).

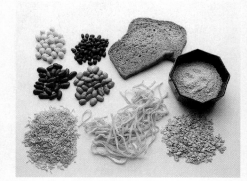

▲ Fruits, vegetables, and whole grains should form the foundation of the diet for athletes. ©Royalty-Free/Corbis

FARM to FORK | Citrus Fruit

Oranges, tangelos, grapefruit, lemons, and limes make up the glorious and sunny citrus fruit family. The most popular citrus is the navel orange, easily identified by its *belly button* on the blossom end of the fruit. Indeed, more than 11 million tons of oranges are grown in the United States each year. Yet few know that the most nutrient-dense part of citrus is the white inner membrane found just below the skin. Called the *pith*, this spongy substance contains the phytochemicals naringenin, hesperidin, and others that have known antioxidant, antibacterial, antiviral, anti-inflammatory, and anti-allergenic properties!

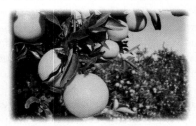

©Jason Patrick Ross/Shutterstock

Grow
- Most citrus is grown in California, Arizona, and Texas, while most orange juice and grapefruit is produced in Florida.
- To grow an indoor citrus tree, buy premixed potting soil formulated specifically for citrus trees. Most citrus trees require 8 to 12 hours of sunlight each day in a south-facing window.

Shop
- The first crop of U.S. oranges typically hits the supermarket shelves in October each year.

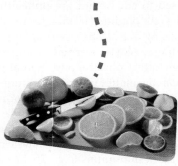

©lynx/iconotec.com/Glow Images

- When purchasing citrus, look for the largest fruits with the deepest colors; these have had more time to ripen on the tree.
- When purchasing orange juice, select juice concentrate to boost your flavonoids by 45%.

Store
- Citrus fruits do not ripen after they have been picked, so it is best to enjoy them soon after purchase.
- If you can't enjoy citrus within a few days of purchasing, refrigerate them. Do not place them in a plastic bag as this will increase moisture and mold.
- If you cannot eat your oranges with a few weeks, squeeze and make orange juice!

Prep
- Many recipes call for citrus peels or zest to add a splash of exotic flavor to favorite dishes.
- Sliced citrus makes a perfect addition to salads and adds an ample dose of phytochemicals to any meal.
- Citrus juice is also a component of many recipes and dressings.
- And let's not forget the simple pleasure of adding citrus slices to enhance the flavor of ice water.

Source: Robinson J. "Citrus Fruits: Beyond Vitamin C," in *Eating on the Wild Side*. New York: Little, Brown and Company, 2013.

Besides the total amount of carbohydrates, the *quality* of carbohydrates can certainly influence mental and physical performance, as well. Sports dietitians emphasize the difference between a high-carbohydrate meal and a high-carbohydrate/high-fat meal. Before endurance events, such as marathons or triathlons, some athletes seek to increase their carbohydrate reserves by eating foods such as potato chips, French fries, banana cream pie, and pastries. Although such foods provide carbohydrate, they also contain a lot of fat and are highly processed. Better high-fiber, high-carbohydrate dietary patterns are rich in whole grain pasta, brown rice, sweet potatoes, whole grain bread, fruit and 100% fruit juices, and various whole grain breakfast cereals. Be sure to check the Nutrition Facts panel for carbohydrate content (Table 10-3). Consuming a moderate (rather than high) amount of fiber during the final day of training is a good precaution to reduce the chances of bloating and intestinal gas during the next day's event. It is also essential to hydrate properly when consuming additional fiber.

FAT

A dietary pattern containing up to 35% of calories from fat is generally recommended for athletes. Rich sources of monounsaturated fat, such as canola oil, should be emphasized, and saturated fat and *trans* fat intake should be limited.

PROTEIN

For athletes, experts recommend protein intake within the range of 1.2 to 2.0 grams of protein per kilogram of body weight. This is considerably higher than the RDA of 0.8 gram per kilogram of body weight recommended by the Food and Nutrition Board for all adults. Sports dietitians contend that the RDAs have been set to prevent deficiency among the general population, not to optimize physical performance among athletes.[5]

▲ Fruits provide starches and natural sugars to maximize glycogen stores. ©Ingram Publishing/SuperStock RF

TABLE 10-3 ■ **Carbohydrate-Rich Foods**

Starches—One Serving = 15 Grams Carbohydrate (80 kcal)	
Dry breakfast cereal,* 1/2–3/4 cup	Baked potato, 1/4 large
Cooked breakfast cereal, 1/2 cup	Bagel, 1/4 (or 4 ounces)
Cooked rice, 1/3 cup	English muffin, 1/2
Cooked pasta, 1/3 cup	Bread, 1 slice
Baked beans, 1/3 cup	Pretzels, 3/4 ounce
Cooked corn, 1/2 cup	Saltine crackers, 6
Cooked dry beans, 1/2 cup	Pancake, 4-inch diameter, 1

Vegetables—One Serving = 5 Grams Carbohydrate (25 kcal)	
Cooked vegetables, 1/2 cup	Examples: carrots, green beans, broccoli,
Raw vegetables, 1 cup	cauliflower, spinach, tomatoes, and vegetable
Vegetable juice, 1/2 cup	juice

Fruits—One Serving = 15 Grams Carbohydrate (60 kcal)	
Canned fruit or berries, 1/2 cup	Grapes (small), 17
100% Fruit juice, 1/2 cup	Grapefruit, 1/2
Apple or orange, 1 small	Peach, 1
Banana, 1 small	Watermelon cubes, 1 1/4 cups

Milk—One Serving = 12 Grams Carbohydrate	
Milk, 1 cup	Soy milk, 1 cup
Plain low-fat yogurt, 2/3 cup	

Sweets—One Serving = 15 Grams Carbohydrate (variable calories)	
Cake, 2-inch square	Ice cream, 1/2 cup
Cookies, 2 small	Sherbet, 1/2 cup

*The carbohydrate content of dry cereal varies widely. Check the labels of the ones you choose and adjust the serving size accordingly.

Source: Modified from *Choose Your Foods: Food Lists for Diabetes* by the American Diabetes Association and Academy of Nutrition and Dietetics, 2014.

What are some reasons why athletes require more protein than sedentary adults?

- The overall calorie needs of athletes are increased to meet the demands of physical activity, so more amino acids will be metabolized as fuel. For endurance athletes, in particular, protein may provide up to 15% of overall energy needs.
- Athletes, most notably those involved in strength training, need additional amino acids for repair of damaged muscle tissue and synthesis of new muscle protein.
- Beyond their use as fuel or building blocks, certain amino acids also act as chemical signals that regulate protein synthesis and other metabolic processes.

The optimal protein intake for an athlete will vary based on the athlete's activity and level of fitness. Athletes who are just beginning a strength-training program are likely to need the most protein to supply the building blocks for synthesis of new muscle tissue. Once the desired muscle mass is achieved, daily protein intake need not exceed 1.2 grams per kilogram of body weight. Some strength-training athletes tend to aim for excessive protein intakes, sometimes as high as 3 or 4 grams of protein per kilogram of body weight. To date, there is little evidence that protein intake above 2.0 grams per kilogram of body weight will benefit the athlete. Protein intakes above this amount result in an increased use of amino acids for energy needs; no further increase in muscle protein synthesis is seen.

Is there an optimal dose of protein? Researchers suggest a dose of 20 to 25 grams of protein per meal is ideal to promote muscle synthesis.[6] Rather than simply focusing on total protein intake, athletes should consume foods that provide 20 to 25 grams of high-quality protein per meal spaced throughout the day.

Unless an athlete follows a low-calorie diet, the recommended range of 1.2 to 2.0 grams of protein per kilogram of body weight can be met by eating a variety of foods. To illustrate, a 117-pound (53-kilogram) woman performing moderate-intensity endurance activity can consume 58 grams of protein (53 × 1.1) during a single day by including 3 ounces of chicken (a chicken breast), 3 ounces of tuna, and two glasses of low-fat milk in her diet. Similarly, a 170-pound (77-kilogram) man who aims to gain muscle mass through strength training needs to consume only 6 ounces of chicken (a large chicken breast), 1/2 cup of cooked beans, a 6-ounce can of tuna, and three glasses of milk to achieve an intake of 154 grams of protein (77 × 2.0) in a day. For both athletes, these calculations do not include the protein present in grains or vegetables they will also eat. By simply meeting their calorie needs, many athletes consume more protein than is required.

Despite marketing claims, high-quality whole food proteins are superior to supplements for the maintenance, repair, and synthesis of skeletal muscle proteins. Studies have shown that the consumption of milk-based protein, especially after resistance exercise, is effective in increasing muscle strength and promotes positive in body composition. Although supplements are usually expensive and unnecessary, many athletes choose to use protein powders (e.g., whey, casein, or soy) to add additional protein to their diet. Whey protein is especially popular among strength-trained athletes. Whey protein is an easily digested, high-quality protein derived from cow's milk. It is particularly rich in leucine, an essential branched-chain amino acid that has been shown in some studies to stimulate gains in muscle mass during strength training.[6] Yet experts still recommend that individuals attempt to meet their protein needs via whole foods and plant-based proteins (nuts, legumes, seeds, dairy).

Consuming excessive amounts of protein has drawbacks. As noted in Section 6.7, it increases calcium loss somewhat in the urine. It also leads to increased urine production, which could increase dehydration. Excess animal protein also may lead to kidney stones in people with a history of this or other kidney problems. Last but not least, a dietary pattern that is so focused on animal protein may leave the athlete short on carbohydrates, leading to fatigue and poor athletic performance.

VITAMINS AND MINERALS

Compared to the needs of sedentary adults, vitamin and mineral needs are the same or slightly higher for athletes. At this time, there are not enough data to support separate DRIs specific to athletes for any of the micronutrients. Athletes usually have high calorie intakes, so they tend to consume plenty of vitamins and minerals. An exception is athletes consuming low-calorie diets (1200 kcal or less), as seen with some female athletes participating in events in which maintaining a low body weight is crucial. These diets may not meet B vitamin and other micronutrient needs. Vegan athletes may also be a concern. In these cases, consuming fortified foods, such as ready-to-eat breakfast cereals, or a balanced multivitamin and mineral supplement may be recommended. You can discuss options with a sports dietitian or your clinician. Vegetarian athletes are encouraged to consume generous amounts of fruits, vegetables, whole grains, and plant proteins (nuts, seeds, soy products, etc.) that contribute adequate fiber, phytochemicals, antioxidants, and other nutrients. Research remains inconclusive related to the influence on athletic performance from long-term vegetarianism.

B Vitamins Support Energy Metabolism and Red Blood Cell Health Recall that coenzyme forms of B vitamins facilitate chemical reactions that generate ATP from carbohydrates, proteins, and fats. Some B vitamins are involved in biosynthetic reactions, such as synthesis of glycogen from glucose, as well as reactions that metabolize amino acids. Compared to the metabolism of sedentary adults, the higher volume of energy metabolism of athletes will increase demands for these coenzymes. Although no separate DRIs have been set, athletes may need more than the current RDA for some B vitamins, such as riboflavin and vitamin B-6.

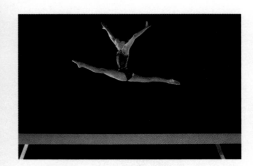

▲ Weight-restricted athletes should make sure they are consuming enough protein and other essential nutrients. ©Echo/Getty Images

ASK THE RDN   No-Meat Athlete

Dear RDN: For a variety of reasons, I am considering switching to a vegan diet. However, I am a sprinter on the college women's swimming and diving team, and I want to make sure that a vegan diet would not affect my athletic performance. Can a "no-meat athlete" compete?

A well-planned plant-based diet can absolutely support optimal athletic performance. From better weight management to reduced risk for chronic diseases, vegan diets offer many health benefits. However, some nutrient needs may be difficult to meet with a plant-based diet. These include protein, iron, calcium, and vitamin B-12.

Protein intakes of vegan athletes, especially young women, are often low. You may need more than the RDA for protein because first, you are an athlete, and second, the quality of plant proteins is lower than that of animal proteins. Protein recommendations for vegetarian and vegan athletes are 1.3 to 1.8 grams per kilogram of body weight. If you consume adequate calories, you can meet your protein needs without protein or amino acid supplements, but the *quality* of your protein matters. Be sure to consume a variety of plant proteins (legumes, grains, nuts) throughout the day to obtain all of the essential amino acids.

Iron delivers oxygen to exercising muscles and helps to convert food fuel into ATP—two processes that impact athletic performance. Iron needs can be difficult to meet even with omnivorous diets, so iron intake deserves special attention. Remember that plant (nonheme) sources of iron are not as well absorbed as animal (heme) sources, but foods with vitamin C can boost absorption of nonheme iron. Have your iron status checked periodically. If your iron stores are low, discuss options with your primary care provider or registered dietitian nutritionist.

Lean female athletes place themselves at risk for early osteoporosis if their diets are poor in calcium (and vitamin D). A vegan diet eliminates animal products, including dairy foods, which are excellent sources of these bone-building nutrients.

A deficiency of vitamin B-12 could also affect red blood cell health and possibly nerve function. Unlike iron and calcium, there are no plant-based alternatives for vitamin B-12. Use of fortified foods and/or dietary supplements will be crucial to meeting your vitamin B-12 needs.

One more concern is that this highly restrictive dietary change—even though it seems like a healthful choice—could promote disordered eating behaviors. Swimmers often hold themselves to unrealistic standards for lean physical appearance, but lower body fat does not automatically translate to better performance. As you move toward a plant-based diet, make sure that your overall energy intake is adequate to support your needs for competitive training. If your weight drops too low, it could significantly affect your athletic performance and long-term bone health.

Start slowly and follow these general recommendations: Begin your day with a bowl of fortified whole grain breakfast cereal. Check the label for brands of cereal that provide at least 20% of the DV for iron and vitamin B-12, such as Raisin Bran® (60% DV for iron, 40% DV for B-12) or Total® (100% DV for both iron and B-12). Top your cereal with almond milk (or a similar dairy alternative) that provides at least one-third of the DV for calcium. Also include calcium-fortified dairy alternatives as a substitute whenever you would have chosen dairy products. Enjoy a glass of calcium-fortified 100% orange juice with breakfast to enhance absorption of iron from your cereal. Throughout the day, be sure to choose plentiful and varied sources of plant proteins, including legumes, nuts, seeds, and whole grains. Try soy and quinoa, two versatile plant proteins that contain all essential amino acids. A dietary supplement, such as a one-a-day multivitamin and mineral supplement, could be a good backup plan to close any remaining nutrient gaps, especially for vitamin B-12. Lastly, monitor changes in your weight and performance. If your calorie intake is too low, consider incorporating more nuts, nut butters, avocados, and hummus into your meals and snacks, as these are energy-dense sources of healthy fats.

These are just a few basic ideas to help you remain healthy and compete at your highest level. To tailor your food intake to your specific needs, seek the expert advice of your team's registered dietitian nutritionist (RDN) at your university health center.

To your record-breaking success!

Angela Collene, MS, RDN, LD (author)

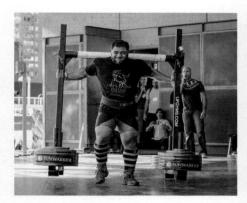

▲ Do strength-trained athletes need to ingest tuna, chicken, and lean beef at every meal to build muscle? Patrik Baboumian is a strongman competitor and former bodybuilder who follows a vegan diet. The plant-based protein sources that built his 250-pound physique include beans, peas, lentils, nuts, seeds, and protein shakes made with soy protein powder. Baboumian was a world record-holder for the log lift in his weight class and was named Germany's strongest man. ©David Cooper/Toronto Star via Getty Images

Furthermore, physical performance is highly dependent on the availability of oxygen to exercising muscles. Folate, vitamin B-6, and vitamin B-12 are involved in the formation of healthy red blood cells, which transport oxygen to all body tissues.

As you can imagine, an inadequate supply of B vitamins could impair an athlete's physical performance. Yet deficiencies of B vitamins are not very common. As athletes consume greater quantities of food to meet their increased calorie needs, they typically consume enough B vitamins from food sources to support energy metabolism and red blood cell health. Taking more than the RDA for B vitamins is not likely to enhance performance.

On the other hand, for a person who is deficient in one or more of the B vitamins, supplementation could improve athletic performance. At-risk populations include vegan or senior athletes (vitamin B-12), female athletes of childbearing age (folate), and any athlete who restricts dietary intake to control body weight (micronutrients). In these cases, fortified foods or a balanced multivitamin and mineral supplement may be beneficial to overall health and athletic performance.

Antioxidant Nutrients May Prevent Oxidative Damage Intense exercise leads to increased production of free radicals. The presence of some free radicals in muscle tissue is actually beneficial for muscle contraction and adaptation to exercise. However, excessive free radicals can lead to fatigue and cell damage.

Athletes' needs for antioxidants such as vitamin E and vitamin C may be somewhat greater because of the potential protection these nutrients provide. However, there is evidence that antioxidant systems in the body increase in activity as exercise training progresses. The use of large doses of antioxidants is not currently an accepted part of the dietary guidance for athletes. Experts suggest consuming a diet containing foods rich in antioxidants, such as fruits, vegetables, whole grains, and vegetable oils.[3]

Iron Deficiency Impairs Performance Iron is involved in red blood cell production, oxygen transport, and energy production, so a deficiency of this mineral can noticeably detract from optimal athletic performance. Some of the consequences of iron deficiency include weakness, fatigue, and decreased work capacity. The potential causes for iron deficiency in athletes vary.[3] As in the general population, female athletes are most susceptible to low iron status due to monthly menstrual losses. Special diets, such as low-calorie and vegan diets, are likely to be lower in iron. Distance runners should pay special attention to iron intake because their intense workouts may lead to gastrointestinal bleeding.

A less threatening concern is *sports anemia*. At the start of an endurance training regimen, plasma volume expands, but the synthesis of additional red blood cells is slower to increase. This results in a temporary dilution of the blood; even if iron stores are adequate, blood iron tests may appear low. Sports anemia is not detrimental to performance, but it is hard to differentiate between sports anemia and true anemia. If iron status is low and not replenished, iron-deficiency anemia can markedly impair endurance performance.

Although true iron-deficiency anemia (a depressed blood hemoglobin level) is not that common among athletes, some studies suggest that iron deficiency *without* anemia may have a negative impact on physical activity and performance. Recall that iron deficiency occurs long before anemia is detected clinically. As body stores of iron are depleted, body processes that use iron, such as energy-yielding reactions, are impaired.

It is a good idea for athletes (especially premenopausal women) to have their iron status checked at the beginning of a training season and at least once midseason. Current evidence suggests that as many as half of female athletes may be iron deficient. To identify iron deficiency without anemia among athletes, many experts advocate serum ferritin testing. Ferritin is an iron transport protein; low serum ferritin levels indicate low iron stores even before red blood cell health is affected.

Any blood test indicating low iron status—sports anemia or not—warrants follow-up. A primary care provider will need to determine the cause of iron depletion. Whatever the cause, once depleted, iron stores can take months to replenish. Dietary sources are

Recall that nutrients in dietary supplements should not exceed any Upper Levels set over the long term. As well, men should be cautious about any use of supplements containing iron.

Blood doping is the injection of red blood cells, naturally containing iron, to enhance aerobic capacity. This is an illegal and dangerous practice under Olympic guidelines.

typically not enough to correct iron-deficiency anemia; supplementation (under a primary care provider's supervision only) is required. Athletes must be especially careful to meet iron needs because preventing iron deficiency is a lot simpler than treating it.

Knowing that iron is required for red blood cell synthesis, athletes may be tempted to self-prescribe iron supplements in an attempt to boost the oxygen-carrying capacity of the blood. However, indiscriminate use of iron supplements for people with normal hemoglobin and serum ferritin levels is never advised.[7] Research does not support a benefit of iron supplementation on athletic performance for athletes with normal iron status. Furthermore, liver damage and increased rates of heart disease and some forms of cancer are possible consequences of iron toxicity. A safer alternative would be to have iron status checked periodically. In addition, monitor dietary patterns to become aware of usual iron intakes. If dietary iron intake is low, incorporate more food sources of heme iron and pair nonheme sources with vitamin C to enhance absorption. Avoid drinking tea or iced tea with meals since this may inhibit iron absorption. The decision to use an iron supplement is best left to a primary care provider.

Calcium Intake Is Important, Especially in Women Athletes, especially women trying to lose weight by restricting their intake of dairy products, can have marginal or low dietary intakes of calcium. This practice compromises optimal bone health. Of still greater concern are female athletes who have stopped menstruating because their arduous training and low body fat interferes with the normal secretion of reproductive hormones. Disturbing evidence shows that female athletes who do not menstruate regularly have bones far less dense than those of both nonathletes and female athletes who menstruate regularly. They are more likely to suffer **stress fractures** during training and will be susceptible to bone injuries throughout life. The negative impacts of low dietary calcium intake and irregular menses in female athletes outweigh the benefits of weight-bearing exercise on bone density. Increasing energy intake to restore body weight and body fat stores is important to correct hormonal imbalances and prevent further bone loss. This topic is discussed further in future chapters.

stress fracture A fracture that occurs from repeated jarring of a bone. Common sites include bones of the foot and shins.

Female athletes whose menstrual cycles become irregular should consult a primary care provider or sports dietitian to determine the cause. Decreasing the amount of training or increasing energy intake and body weight often restores regular menstrual cycles. If irregular menstrual cycles persist, severe bone loss (much of which is not reversible) and osteoporosis can result. Extra calcium in the diet does not necessarily compensate for these damaging effects of menstrual irregularities, but inadequate dietary calcium can make matters worse.

VITAMIN D

Recent studies have documented a relationship between vitamin D status and injury prevention, improved neuromuscular function, enhanced muscle size, decreased inflammation, and reduced risk of stress fractures. Athletes who live at latitudes above the 35th parallel or who predominately train indoors are at higher risk for vitamin D deficiency. Although vitamin D status is important for athletes and nonathletes alike, current data do not support vitamin D as an ergogenic aid. More data is needed to elucidate the role of vitamin D in athletics. Those who have a history of stress fractures, joint or overtraining injuries, or muscle pain and weakness should consult their primary care provider or sports dietitian.

FLUID

Fluid needs for an average adult are about 9 to 11 cups per day for women and 13 to 15 cups per day for men. Athletes generally need even more water to regulate body temperature. Heat production in contracting muscles can rise 15 to 20 times above that of resting muscles. Unless this heat is quickly dissipated, heat exhaustion, heat cramps, and potentially fatal heatstroke may ensue.

Fluid and electrolyte needs vary widely, based on differences in genetics, body mass, environmental conditions, level of training, and event duration. Because fluid needs are highly individualized and dynamic, it is difficult to make general recommendations for fluid replacement.[3] Rather, an athlete should consume enough fluid to prevent short-term (i.e., fluid-related) changes in body weight. The American College of Sports Medicine recommends losing *no more than 2%* of body weight during exercise, especially in hot weather. A football player wearing equipment in hot weather can lose this much within 30 minutes! However, it is important to remember this advice even when sweating can go unnoticed, such as when swimming or during the winter.

To determine fluid needs, the athlete should first calculate 2% of his or her body weight. Next, it is useful to know the body's hourly sweat rate, which can be calculated by comparing weight loss during exercise to the amount of fluid consumed during exercise. This will require some self-monitoring of pre- and post-workout weight and fluid intake during workouts. For reference, sweat rates during prolonged exercise can range from 3 to 8 cups (750 to 2000 milliliters) per hour. If weight change cannot be monitored, urine color is another measure of hydration status. Urine color should be no more yellow than lemonade.

Note that thirst is a late sign of dehydration. An athlete who drinks only when thirsty may take 48 hours to replenish fluid losses. After several days of training, an athlete relying only on thirst can build up a fluid debt that will impair performance. For healthy athletes, pale yellow urine is a good indicator that fluid needs are being met.

> The following fluid-replacement approach can meet an athlete's fluid needs in most cases.
> - Freely drink beverages (e.g., especially water) during the 24-hour period before an event, even if not particularly thirsty.
> - Drink 5 to 7 milliliters per kilogram of body weight (about 1.5 to 2 cups for a 150-pound male) of water at least 4 hours before exercise. This allows time for both adequate hydration and excretion of excess fluid.
> - During events lasting more than 30 minutes, athletes should consume fluid to prevent dehydration (losses of > 2% body weight). Recommendations for marathon runners suggest about 1.5 to 3.5 cups (400 to 800 milliliters) per hour to prevent dehydration. Football players wearing equipment for two-a-day practices during the heat of August may need even more than 800 milliliters per hour to prevent dehydration. The best plan is to determine individual rate of fluid losses during training and plan accordingly. In many cases, athletes, especially children and teenagers, need to be reminded to consume fluids during exercise.
> - Within 4 to 6 hours after exercise, about 2 to 3 cups of fluid should be consumed for every pound lost. It is important that weight be restored before the next exercise period. Skipping fluids before or during events will almost certainly impair performance.

Sports Drinks For sports that require less than 60 minutes of continuous exertion or when total weight loss is less than 5 to 6 pounds, the primary concern is replacing the water lost in sweat. When continuous exercise extends beyond 60 minutes, electrolyte (especially sodium) and carbohydrate replacement becomes increasingly important.

Use of sports drinks (Fig. 10-9) during long bouts of continuous exercise—especially in hot weather—offers several advantages for athletes:

- *Water* increases blood volume to allow for efficient cooling and transport of fuels and waste products to and from cells.
- *Carbohydrates* supply glucose to muscles as they become depleted of glycogen and also add flavor, which encourages athletes to drink.
- *Electrolytes* in sports drinks help to maintain blood volume, enhance the absorption of water and carbohydrate from the intestine, and stimulate thirst.

Overall, the decision to use a sports drink hinges primarily on the duration, type, and intensity of the activity. As the projected duration of continuous activity approaches 60 minutes or longer, the advantages of sports drinks over plain water emerge. However, athletes should experiment with sports drinks during practice, instead of trying them for the first time during competition. Also, both athletes and nonathletes should recognize that sports drinks can be a source of excess calories that may result in undesired weight gain (see Newsworthy Nutrition on the next page).

"Energy" Drinks The popularity of caffeine-containing energy drinks has surged in recent years. Some studies show that caffeine may improve athletic performance during endurance events (e.g., cycling) or sports that require a high level of mental alertness (e.g., archery). However, excessive caffeine consumption can lead to shakiness, nervousness, anxiety, nausea, irregular heart rate, elevated blood pressure, and insomnia. Chronic intakes of energy drinks can lead to fatigue and headaches. The high added sugar content also can lead to weight gain. In addition, the diuretic effect of caffeine may not support optimal hydration, particularly for athletes who are not accustomed to caffeine. Compare the caffeine and calorie contents of several top-selling energy drinks in Table 10-4.

Alcohol Excessive alcohol consumption, consistent with binge drinking patterns, is observed among some athletes, particularly in team sports. Besides the nonnutritive calorie load of alcohol (7 kcals/gram), alcohol has negative effects on performance and recovery from exercise. Research promoting alcohol consumption during sport is fraught with design flaws. A solid body of evidence cautions against consumption of significant amounts of alcohol before, during, or after exercise.

Heat-Related Illness As environmental temperature rises above 95°F (35°C), virtually all body heat is lost through the evaporation of sweat from the skin. As humidity rises, especially above 75%, evaporation slows and sweating is insufficient to cool the body. The result is rapid fatigue, increased work for the heart, and difficulty with prolonged exertion. Heat-related injuries—heat exhaustion, heat cramps, and heatstroke—can be deadly (Table 10-5). To decrease the risk of developing heat-related injuries, watch for rapid body-weight changes (2% or more of body weight), replace lost fluids, and avoid exercising under extremely hot, humid conditions.

Water Intoxication It is also possible for some athletes to drink so much water that they develop *water intoxication* (hyponatremia). Recall that hyponatremia (plasma sodium < 135 mmol/L) causes cardiovascular and neurological problems and can lead

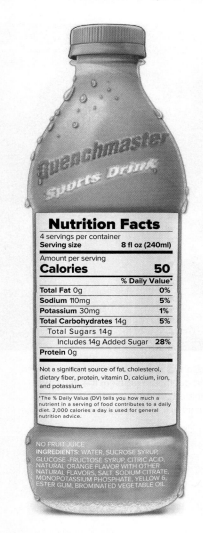

FIGURE 10-9 ▲ Sports drinks for fluid and electrolyte replacement typically contain a form of simple carbohydrate plus sodium and potassium. The various sugars in this product total 14 grams of carbohydrates per 1-cup (240-milliliter) serving. Sports drinks typically contain about 6% to 8% sugar. This provides ample glucose and other monosaccharides to fuel working muscles, and it is well tolerated. Drinks with a sugar content above 8% to 10%, such as soft drinks or fruit juices, may cause gastrointestinal distress, fail to empty from the stomach rapidly, and are not recommended.

TABLE 10-4 ■ **Caffeine, Calorie, and Sugar Content of Popular Energy Drinks**

Beverage	Container Size (fl oz)	Caffeine (mg)	Energy (kcal)	Sugars (g)
5-Hour Energy®	1.93	215*	4	0
Amp Energy®	16	142	220	58
Monster Energy®	16	160	200	54
NOS® PowerShot®	16	260	210	54
Red Bull®	8.4	80	110	27
Red Bull® Sugarfree	8.4	80	10	0
Rockstar®	16	160	280	62

*Determined by independent lab analysis reported by *Consumer Reports*, December 2012. Caffeine content is not specified by the manufacturer but rather as part of a total amount of "energy blend." The labels state that this product has approximately the same amount of caffeine as a strong cup of coffee (typical range: 80–175 milligrams).

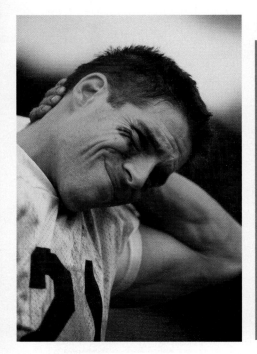

▲ Dehydration, which can lead to illness and death, is a problem that must be avoided during physical activity in hot, humid environments. ©Eyewire/Getty Images RF

Newsworthy Nutrition

Sports drinks cause weight gain among adolescents and young adults

Sales of sugar-sweetened soda pop continue to decline, yet sales of other sweetened beverages, such as sports drinks, are increasing. Although the value of sports drinks (e.g., Gatorade,® Powerade)® is well documented for replenishing fluids during continuous physical activity lasting more than 1 hour, the contribution of excess sugar intake to obesity remains a concern. The aim of this prospective study was to determine the associations between sports drinks and body mass index (BMI) gains among adolescents and young adults. Over 7500 U.S. youth, age 9 to 16, were followed from 2004 to 2011. Servings per day of beverages were assessed using a food frequency questionnaire. Intake of sports drinks predicted larger increases in BMI among all youth. In addition, boys who increased their intake over the 2- to 3-year interval gained significantly more weight than their peers during the same time interval. These results suggest that, although there is less sugar per ounce in sugar-sweetened sports drinks than in soda pop, sports beverages still contain sugar and calories that appear to promote increases in BMI for both adolescents and young adults.

Source: Field AE, et al. "Association of sports drinks with weight gain among adolescents and young adults," *Obesity* 22:2238, 2014.

to death. Symptoms of hyponatremia include bloating, puffiness, weight gain, nausea, vomiting, headache, confusion, delirium, seizures, respiratory distress, loss of consciousness, and possibly death, if left untreated.

TABLE 10-5 ■ **Heat-Related Illnesses**

Heat-Related Illness	Symptoms	Recommended Treatment
Heat exhaustion is the first stage of heat-related illness that occurs because of depletion of blood volume from fluid loss by the body.	• Profuse sweating • Headache • Dizziness • Nausea • Muscle weakness • Visual disturbances • Flushed skin • Hyperthermia • Heat cramps	• Move to cool environment. • Remove excess clothing. • Cool the skin with ice packs or cold water. • Replenish lost fluids and electrolytes.
Heat cramps are a frequent complication of heat exhaustion. They usually occur in people who have experienced large sweat losses from exercising for several hours in a hot environment and have consumed a large volume of water without replacing electrolytes.	• Painful skeletal muscle cramps • Involuntary muscle spasms	• Replenish lost fluids and electrolytes.
Heatstroke can occur when internal body temperature reaches 104°F. Sweating generally ceases if left untreated, and blood circulation is greatly reduced. Nervous system damage may ensue, and death results in 10% of cases.	• Hyperthermia • Hot, dry skin • Nausea • Confusion • Irritability • Poor coordination • Fainting • Seizures • Coma	• Cool the skin with ice packs or cold water. *SEEK PROFESSIONAL MEDICAL ATTENTION IMMEDIATELY.*

1. What does it mean to *cut weight* before a competition? How may this affect physical performance?

2. Greta, a point guard on the women's basketball team, complains of chronic fatigue. Describe three nutritional concerns you would investigate.

3. During one day of preseason training for football, David loses 7 pounds as a result of sweat losses. How much fluid should he drink to rehydrate after practice?

10.5 Specialized Advice for Endurance, Strength, and Power Athletes

In Section 10.4, you learned about ways in which nutrient needs can be universally affected by participation in sports. The definition of sports, however, is broad and each athlete is unique. Endurance athletes, who need to fuel activity that lasts several hours, should take a different approach to nutrition than strength and power athletes, who focus on gains in muscle mass. In this section, we present specific nutrition strategies for endurance, strength, and power athletes.

ENDURANCE ATHLETES: STRATEGIES TO DELAY OR PREVENT FATIGUE

The overarching goal for endurance athletes is to consume adequate carbohydrates and fluids. *Before* the event, endurance athletes should focus on maximizing muscle and liver glycogen stores, which will later be used to fuel muscles and maintain blood glucose. *During* an event, the goal is to prevent dehydration and glycogen depletion, as both of these conditions lead to fatigue and detract from physical performance. *After* an event, muscle glycogen stores need to be replenished, damaged muscle tissue must be repaired, and hydration should be restored.

Maximize Glycogen Stores Before the Event For athletes who compete in continuous, intense aerobic events lasting more than 90 minutes (or in shorter events taking place more than once within a 24-hour period), a **carbohydrate-loading** regimen can help to maximize the amount of energy stored in the form of muscle glycogen for the event. In one possible regimen, during the week prior to the event, the athlete gradually reduces the intensity and duration of exercise (*tapering*) while simultaneously increasing the percentage of total calories supplied by carbohydrates. Shorter carbohydrate-loading regimens (e.g., 1 or 2 days before an event) may also be effective.

For example, consider the carbohydrate-loading schedule of a 25-year-old man preparing for a marathon. His typical calorie needs are about 3500 kcal per day. Six days before competition, he completes a final, hard workout of 60 minutes. On that day, carbohydrates contribute 45% to 50% of his total calorie intake. As he goes through the rest of the week, the duration of his workouts decreases to 40 minutes and then to about 20 minutes by the end of the week. Meanwhile, he increases the amount of carbohydrate in his diet to reach 70% to 80% of total calorie intake as the week continues (Table 10-6).

carbohydrate-loading A process in which a high-carbohydrate diet is consumed for 6 days before an athletic event while tapering exercise duration in an attempt to increase muscle glycogen stores.

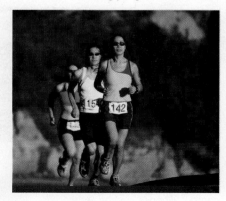

▲ Carbohydrate-loading is appropriate only for endurance activities such as a long-distance race. ©Corbis - All Rights Reserved RF

TABLE 10-6 ▪ Sample Carbohydrate-Loading Regimen

Days Before Competition	6	5	4	3	2	1
Exercise time (minutes)	60	40	40	20	20	Rest
Carbohydrate intake (grams)	450	450	450	600	600	600

Total calorie intake should decrease as exercise time decreases throughout the week. On the final day before competition, he rests while maintaining the high carbohydrate intake.

This carbohydrate-loading technique usually increases muscle glycogen stores by 50% to 90% over typical conditions (i.e., when dietary carbohydrate constitutes only about 50% of total calorie intake). A potential disadvantage of carbohydrate loading is that additional water (about 3 grams) is incorporated into the muscles along with each gram of glycogen. Although the additional water aids in maintaining hydration, for some individuals this additional water weight and related muscle stiffness detract from their sports performance.

Athletes considering a carbohydrate-loading regimen should test it out during training (and well before an important competition) to experience its effects on their performance. They can then determine whether it is worth the effort. Currently, expert advice is shifting away from such regimented carbohydrate loading in favor of supplying carbohydrates during the event (along with a consistent dietary pattern high in carbohydrate).

Even if an endurance athlete chooses not to practice a strict carbohydrate-loading regimen, a meal should be eaten 1 to 4 hours before an endurance event to top off muscle and liver glycogen stores, prevent hunger during the event, and provide extra fluid. A pre-event meal should consist primarily of carbohydrate, contain moderate fat or fiber, and include high-quality protein (Table 10-7). The longer the period before an event, the larger the meal can be, because there will be more time available for digestion. Anything consumed within 1 hour before an event should be blended or liquid to promote more rapid stomach emptying. Examples include diluted 100% juice, low-fat smoothies, and sports drinks.

Carbohydrate-rich food choices for a pre-event meal include spaghetti, muffins, bagels, pancakes with fresh fruit topping, oatmeal with fruit, a baked potato topped with a small amount of low-fat cheese, toasted bread with jam, bananas, or low-sugar breakfast cereals with reduced-fat milk. Liquid meal-replacement formulas, such as Carnation® Instant Breakfast, also can be used. Foods especially rich in fiber can be eaten the previous day to help empty the colon before an event, but they should not be

TABLE 10-7 ■ **Convenient High-Carbohydrate Pre-Event Meals**

Breakfast	
Cheerios,® ¾ cup	450 kcal
Reduced-fat milk, 1 cup	92 grams (82%) carbohydrate
Blueberry muffin, 1	482 kcal
Orange juice, 4 ounces	84 grams (68%) carbohydrate
or	
Low-fat fruit yogurt, 1 cup	
Plain bagel, ½	
Apple juice, 4 ounces	
Peanut butter (for bagel), 1 tbsp	
Lunch or Dinner	
Broiled chicken, 3 ounces	839 kcal
Rice, 1 ½ cups	120 grams (57%) carbohydrate
Steamed zucchini, 1 cup	
Low-fat chocolate milk, 1 cup	
Jello,® ½ cup	
or	
Spaghetti noodles, 2 cups	
Spaghetti sauce, 1 cup	761 kcal
Reduced-fat milk, 1 ½ cups	129 grams (66%) carbohydrate
Green beans, 1 cup	

With regard to the timing of pre-activity meals, a general guide is to allow 4 hours for a big meal (about 1200 kcal), 3 hours for a moderate meal (about 800 to 900 kcal), 2 hours for a light meal (about 400 to 600 kcal), and an hour or less for a snack (about 300 kcal).

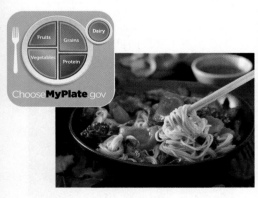

▲ Pre-event meals may require a higher proportion of grains than suggested by MyPlate to boost carbohydrate content. Choose starchy vegetables and grain-based snacks to help top off glycogen stores. Source: ChooseMyPlate.gov; ©cobraphotography/Shutterstock

eaten the night before or on the morning of the event. Avoid fatty or fried foods, such as sausage, bacon, sauces, and gravies. Some foods (e.g., dairy products) may cause gastrointestinal upset. Athletes should experiment with the size, timing, and composition of pre-event meals during training to determine what is best tolerated.

Emerging Research on Fat Adaptation Traditionally, high-carbohydrate diets have been the nutrition norm for endurance athletes. However, an alternative approach in training, known as *fat adaptation*, is becoming more popular among endurance athletes.

Of all the energy-yielding nutrients, carbohydrates are utilized most rapidly to fuel exercising muscles. When athletes consume a high-carbohydrate diet or practice carbohydrate loading before an endurance event, they ensure that muscle and liver glycogen will be available to muscles throughout the race. Even after carbohydrate loading, however, the total amount of energy available from muscle glycogen is limited to about 2500 kcal.

In comparison, the supply of energy from triglycerides stored in the muscle and adipose tissue is virtually limitless. Recall from Figure 10-7 that, depending on intensity, about half of the energy for endurance events comes from fat. The metabolism of fat for energy occurs more slowly, but it provides more than twice as many calories per gram as carbohydrates or protein.

With fat adaptation, rather than following a traditional high-carbohydrate diet (about 65% of calories from carbohydrates and only about 20% from fat) during the days leading up to an event, endurance athletes replace much of the carbohydrates with fat. For example, a high-fat training diet might consist of just 25% of calories from carbohydrate with a whopping 60% to 70% of calories from fat. The rationale is that high-carbohydrate diets, especially those with many simple sugars and refined grains, boost insulin secretion, which inhibits the breakdown of fat. By lowering carbohydrates and increasing the fat content of the diet, the cells will adapt to greater use of fat for fuel. If the athlete uses more fat for fuel during an endurance event, muscle glycogen might be spared, so that those stored carbohydrates would be available for a burst of speed at the end of the race.[8]

Research comparing the effects of high-carbohydrate or high-fat training diets on athletic performance has yielded mixed results. A possible explanation is that the muscles of *fat-adapted* athletes are able to break down more fat for fuel during exercise at low or moderate intensities, but the low carbohydrate intake depletes glycogen stores, so higher-intensity activity is impaired.

At this time, there is not enough research evidence to support a recommendation for high-fat diets for athletes. Evidence *does* clearly support a performance-enhancing effect of carbohydrate ingestion before and during physical activity.

Replenish Fuel During the Event We have already established the importance of consuming adequate fluids during endurance exercise. For continuous sporting events longer than 60 minutes, consumption of carbohydrate and electrolytes during activity can also improve athletic performance. Prolonged exercise depletes muscle glycogen stores and may transiently lower blood glucose, leading to physical and mental fatigue. One way to avoid *hitting the wall* is to maintain normal blood glucose concentrations by carbohydrate feedings during exercise. During short events (e.g., 30 minutes or so), carbohydrate intake during exercise is not as important because the muscles do not take up much blood glucose during short-term exercise, relying instead primarily on their glycogen stores for fuel.

A general guideline for endurance events is to consume 30 to 60 grams of carbohydrate per hour. A trend in sports nutrition is to use multiple sources of carbohydrates (e.g., glucose, fructose, and maltodextrin) with different routes and rates of absorption to maximize the supply of glucose to cells and lessen the risk of gastrointestinal distress.[8]

Some experts suggest that consuming protein with carbohydrate during exercise provides added benefit. In particular, branched-chain amino acids, which can be used for fuel, are thought to delay fatigue by supplying energy and altering the production of certain neurotransmitters.[5] This is an area of ongoing research, but there is not enough evidence at this time to support a clear recommendation for ingesting protein during exercise. Some products formulated for consumption during exercise do contain amino acids, so you can try various formulations to see what works best for you.

Compared to carbohydrates, fat is more slowly digested, absorbed, and metabolized. Thus, although fat serves as fuel during prolonged aerobic activity, consumption of fat during activity is unlikely to improve athletic performance and is likely to cause gastrointestinal distress.

Sports drinks are a good source of carbohydrate calories during continuous endurance events. Sports drinks, described in detail in the Section 10.3, usually contain about 14 grams of carbohydrate per 8-oz serving. They supply the necessary fluid, electrolytes, and carbohydrates to keep an athlete performing at his or her best in endurance or ultra-endurance events.

As an alternative to sports drinks, some athletes use carbohydrate gels or chews. Gels and chews are formulated with one or more sugars or starches to rapidly supply about 25 grams of carbohydrate per serving (Table 10-8). In addition, they provide electrolytes to replenish those lost in sweat. Some of these products also may contain certain amino acids, vitamins, caffeine (Section 10.6), or herbal ingredients. An advantage of gels compared to energy bars or sports drinks is they are convenient to carry.

Popular energy bars (e.g., PowerBar) typically provide about 180 to 250 kcal and anywhere from 2 to 45 grams of carbohydrate. The wide range of carbohydrate content in energy bars is due to a variety of marketing trends in the sports supplement industry. If a bar is chosen, look for one with about 40 grams of carbohydrate and no more than 10 grams of protein, 4 grams of fat, and 5 grams of fiber. The bars are fortified with vitamins and minerals in amounts ranging from about 25% to 100% of typical human needs. Remember that any carbohydrate-containing food must be accompanied by fluid to ensure adequate hydration. Outside of sporting events, some people use energy bars as a quick and convenient meal or snack. Keep in mind that energy bars contain a concentrated source of calories. Whole foods are always preferred for snacking.

Check the label on these products to gauge the amount of gel or bar that provides 30 to 60 grams of carbohydrate per hour. In addition, remember that any carbohydrate-containing food must be accompanied by fluid to ensure adequate hydration. At minimum, one serving of any of these products will cost at least $1, and some brands with all natural or organic ingredients cost as much as $5. Are sports drinks, energy bars, and gels worth the price? Critics suggest that these products are essentially the nutritional equivalent of a cup of low-fat yogurt and piece of fruit (Table 10-8). For an athlete on a tight budget, a small bag of graham crackers or jelly beans could just as easily provide a quick shot of glucose during a race. With a little bit of time and an Internet connection,

TABLE 10-8 ■ Energy and Macronutrient Content of Popular Energy Bars, Gels, and Chews

Energy Bars	Serving (oz)	Energy (kcal)	Carbohydrates (g)	Fiber (g)	Protein (g)	Fat (g)
Clif® Bar (chocolate chip)	2.4	250	45	4	10	5
Kashi® (chewy trail mix)	1.23	140	21	3	5	5
KIND® (peanut butter dark chocolate)	1.41	200	17	2.5	8	13
Luna® (nutz over chocolate)	1.69	200	24	3	9	8
PowerBar® (peanut butter)	2.13	230	44	2	9	4
Slim-Fast® (dark chocolate sea salt)	1.59	190	20	5	10	10
Energy Gels & Chews						
Clif Shot (vanilla)	1.1	100	24	0	0	0
GU™ Energy Gel (lemon sublime)	1.1	100	23	0	0	0
Jelly Belly Sport Beans® (berry)	1.0	100	24	0	0	0
PowerBar® Gel (strawberry banana)	1.44	110	27	0	0	0

Overall, choosing energy bars is preferable to choosing candy bars and packaged desserts. When used in athletic situations, these bars can be handy. Better yet, however, is to eat a variety of wholesome foods; these offer more health-protective compounds. This is also a much less expensive choice, especially for day-to-day snacking. An additional concern is that micronutrient toxicity might occur if numerous bars are eaten in a day, as many are highly fortified. Vitamin A and iron are two nutrients of special concern in this regard.

you can even find recipes to make your own sports drinks and energy bars at home for a fraction of the cost of name-brand products.

After Exercise, Replenish Glycogen and Fluid After prolonged aerobic exercise, muscle and liver glycogen stores will be depleted. An athlete's need to pay special attention to nutrition during recovery from exercise depends on the type of workout completed and the timing of the next workout. For example, multiple events in the same day will require rapid restoration of glycogen stores. However, if an athlete will be able to rest for 1 or 2 days before the next exercise session, immediate consumption of a post-workout meal is not as crucial.

To rapidly restore glycogen stores, carbohydrate-rich foods providing 0.8 to 1.5 grams of carbohydrate per kilogram body weight should be consumed within 30 minutes after continuous (endurance) exercise. Immediately after exercise is when glycogen synthesis is greatest because the muscles are insulin-sensitive at this point. This process should then be repeated every 2 hours for the next 4 to 6 hours. Foods such as fruit, fruit juice, bread, or a sports drink contribute to rapid restoration of glycogen stores.

Although carbohydrate intake is the most important factor for replenishing glycogen after endurance exercise, adding an appropriate amount of high-quality protein during recovery can be helpful for stimulating glycogen synthesis and repairing damaged muscle tissue. The current recommendation for protein after exercise is 0.4 grams of protein per kilogram body weight.

Fluid and electrolyte (i.e., sodium and potassium) intake is another essential component of recovery for an endurance athlete, especially if two workouts a day are performed or if the environment is hot and humid. Specialized recovery drinks containing carbohydrates, amino acids, and electrolytes are available, but if food and fluid intake is sufficient to restore weight loss, it generally will also supply enough electrolytes to meet needs during recovery from endurance activities. Low-fat chocolate milk is a great option to replenish the body!

STRENGTH AND POWER ATHLETES: STRATEGIES TO ENHANCE MUSCLE GAIN

Strength training—improving the maximal force that can be exerted by the muscle—should be part of any well-rounded physical activity program. Resistance exercises may utilize free weights, specialized weight machines, or one's own body weight. A workout typically includes 8 to 12 different exercises that target all the major muscle groups of the body. Most of the people you see lifting weights in the gym are probably performing several sets of 8 to 10 repetitions each, lifting about 50% of the maximum weight they could lift (1 RM). This type of workout improves muscular *endurance,* which is an important part of muscular fitness for overall health. However, to truly build muscular *strength,* athletes need to work against greater resistance (around 80% of 1 RM) over just a few repetitions (2 to 5 repetitions). For a few athletes, such as those who participate in weight-lifting or body-building competitions, muscular strength is the focus of training.

Muscular power combines strength with speed, improving the ability to apply force quickly. Examples of power sports include middle-distance running, gridiron football, rowing, and swimming. In reality, many sports and everyday activities involve muscular power: jumping for a rebound in basketball, delivering a roundhouse kick to an opponent in martial arts, or driving the ball down the fairway in a round of golf are examples of muscular power in sports.

For strength and power athletes, some sports nutrition alterations are warranted. First, calorie needs will be high due to the additional lean mass and high-volume training routines of these athletes. Recall that the primary types of fuel for strength and power moves are phosphocreatine (PCr) and carbohydrates for the brief bursts of activity, with fat providing energy during the resting stages. Very little protein is used as fuel during resistance exercises (Fig. 10-7). Second, there will be some extra emphasis on protein intake in the recovery phase.[9,10]

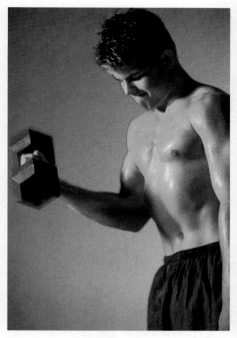

▲ A special nutrition issue that concerns strength-trained athletes is muscle dysmorphia, informally called *bigorexia.* In this disorder, individuals see themselves as being too thin, even though they are more muscular than average. People who suffer from muscle dysmorphia may practice disordered eating behaviors or use steroids to achieve high levels of muscularity. ©Ingram Publishing RF

Many power athletes utilize a training technique called **periodization,** in which physical stresses on the body change throughout the year:

- Early in the training season, athletes work on building aerobic endurance.
- After gains in aerobic capacity have been achieved, the focus shifts to building strength, power, and sport-specific skills.
- During the competitive season, daily workouts are scaled back, but activity is intense and of long duration on game days.
- In the off-season, athletes continue to work out to stay in shape, but the volume is certainly lower than it was in season.

Athletes taking part in periodized training will use the full spectrum of energy systems we have discussed. Nutrition recommendations should also be periodized to match such dynamic training plans.

periodization Cycling the volume, intensity, and activities of workouts throughout the training season.

Strength and power athletes tend to be extremely focused on consuming adequate protein to support muscle protein synthesis. Strength-training athletes in the early phases of training have the highest estimated protein needs of any athletes. Once desired muscle mass has been achieved, protein requirements for maintenance of muscular strength decrease slightly. Meeting these recommendations for protein intake optimizes muscle protein synthesis, but consuming more than the recommended range of protein intake does not appear to offer advantage and could be detrimental. Recall that excess amino acids are used as fuel or stored as fat; they do not directly translate into increased muscular strength.

Before and During Strength and Power Training, Focus on Calories, Carbohydrates, and Fluids Adequate hydration supports optimal athletic performance; strength and power athletes are no exception. Checking urine color or urine specific gravity is a good indication of fluid status. If the athlete is poorly hydrated before an event, water or a sports drink will be sufficient to restore hydration.

Similar to nutrition strategies for endurance athletes, adequate carbohydrate ingestion in the days leading up to and hours immediately before exercise has been shown to enhance performance for strength and power events, too. Athletes who perform many repetitions with moderate resistance will use more of their muscle glycogen stores than athletes who perform fewer repetitions with high resistance. Overall, research has shown that consuming 4 to 7 grams of carbohydrates per kilogram of body weight per day is appropriate for strength and power training. The optimal rate of carbohydrate ingestion before and during resistance activities has not yet been established, but some research indicates that 1 to 4 grams of carbohydrate per kilogram of body weight in a pre-event meal or beverage will enhance work capacity during resistance workouts.

In strength and power sports, many athletes also use creatine supplements to increase levels of phosphocreatine in muscles. Recall that phosphocreatine is used to resupply ATP during short, intense bursts of activity. When phosphocreatine stores are increased, muscle glycogen may be preserved.[9] Section 10.6 provides more information on creatine and other ergogenic aids.

Focus on achieving adequate hydration and maximizing muscle glycogen before activities because there may not be an opportunity to replenish fluids and carbohydrates during strength or power competitions. During extended training sessions, however, supplying fluids and carbohydrates will enhance both physical and mental performance.

While a few experts advocate ingesting protein before or during a resistance workout in an effort to promote muscle protein synthesis, the bulk of evidence points to emphasizing protein in the recovery meal.

For athletes (and adults in general), fat intake should fall into the range of 20% to 35% of overall calorie intake. Dietary analysis show that usual fat intake of resistance-trained athletes is slightly higher than recommended, probably because too many of their choices of protein-rich foods (e.g., meats and dairy products) are also rich sources of fat. If fat intake is above 35% of total calories, replacing the excess fat with carbohydrates would have a favorable effect on protein balance. This is because insulin, secreted in response to glucose in the blood, triggers uptake of amino acids by cells, which provides materials for protein synthesis within the cells.

After Strength and Power Activities, Consuming Carbohydrates and Protein Promotes Recovery Those first few hours after resistance exercise, according to many researchers, are the best time to provide carbohydrates and protein to replenish muscle glycogen and promote muscle repair and synthesis. Right after exercise, the cells are insulin sensitive, so they rapidly take up glucose from the blood and store it as glycogen. General ACSM guidelines are to consume 1.0 to 1.5 grams of carbohydrate per kilogram of body weight to restore muscle glycogen. To promote muscle protein synthesis along with glycogen restoration, many experts recommend intakes at the upper end of that range (e.g., 1.2 to 1.5 grams of carbohydrates per kilogram of body weight)

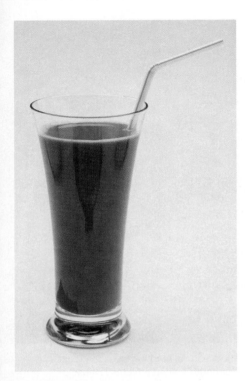

▲ Chocolate milk is the go-to recovery drink for many athletes. This 2-cup serving of low-fat chocolate milk is a tasty vehicle for 52 grams of carbohydrate and 16 grams of protein. ©Pixtal/SuperStock

TABLE 10-9 ■ Sample Recovery Meals

Option 1: 509 kcal, 71 grams carbohydrate, 33 grams protein, and 10 grams fat
Bagel, 1 regular
Deli turkey, 1 ounce
Mozzarella cheese, 1 ounce
Low-fat milk, 1 cup

Option 2: 533 kcal, 86 grams carbohydrate, 31 grams protein, and 8 grams fat
Low-fat flavored Greek yogurt, 16 ounces
Banana, 1 medium

Option 3: 380 kcal, 65 grams carbohydrate, 28 grams protein, and 1.5 grams fat
Gatorade Recover Post-Game Recovery Beverage, 1 (8 fluid ounce) carton
Gatorade Recover Protein Shake, 1 (11 fluid ounce) carton

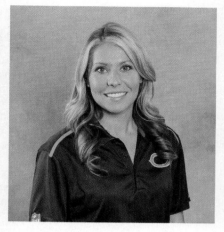

▲ Elite athletes are subject to all the same nutritional challenges as the general public: overreliance on convenience foods, abundance of nutrition misinformation, temptations to eat out of boredom or for emotional comfort. Furthermore, they must adapt to the seasonal demands of their sport and maintain exhausting training and travel schedules. In her role as a sports dietitian for the United States Olympic Committee, Jennifer Gibson, M.Sc., R.D.N, CSSD, carefully tailored nutrition recommendations for each of her athletes based on nutritional status, sport, season, position, and body composition goals. ©Jennifer Gibson

shortly after exercise.[9] The presence of certain amino acids further stimulates insulin secretion to enhance the uptake of glucose and synthesis of glycogen.

To promote gains in muscle mass, many experts recommend at least 15 to 25 grams of high-quality protein within the first 1 or 2 hours after exercise to maximize protein synthesis. Novice strength-training athletes who are seeking to gain muscle mass have the highest requirements for protein. With advanced training, the rate of protein turnover during exercise decreases. Therefore, well-trained strength athletes require less protein to repair and maintain muscles than their untrained counterparts. Some amino acids (e.g., leucine) may stimulate the metabolic pathways that lead to synthesis of muscle protein. The process of muscle protein synthesis not only requires amino acids as building blocks, of course, but also depends on carbohydrate as a source of energy.

Overall, recovery from resistance exercise requires a combination (3:1 ratio) of carbohydrates and high-quality protein. For a 154-pound (70-kilogram) athlete, this corresponds to about 70 grams of carbohydrate and 25 grams of protein in each 2-hour interval. Table 10-9 describes sample meals of this composition.

CONCLUDING REMARKS

Nutritional strategies have the potential to optimize athletic performance. Here, we have presented several generalized guidelines to plan nutritionally adequate diets that optimize energy stores, ensure hydration, and give athletes a competitive edge. We have stressed the importance of carbohydrates and fluids before, during, and after exercise, as well as protein for muscle recovery. Above all, recognize that each athlete is unique. Remember that genetics can impact nutrition requirements. Each type of exercise demands its own set of energy sources. Sports vary in training regimens, duration, and opportunities to acquire nourishment before, during, and between events. Even within a particular sport, each player's position has its own physical demands, which can alter nutritional needs.[11] Finally, personal taste preferences and gastrointestinal tolerance will dictate adherence to any nutrition plan. When working with athletes, start with your solid foundation of knowledge about nutrient needs, but be attentive to individual concerns, be adaptable, and always continue to learn.

✔ CONCEPT CHECK 10.5

1. Which nutrient(s) should be emphasized in a pre-event meal for an endurance athlete? Provide an example of a suitable pre-event meal for a long-distance cyclist.

2. What is carbohydrate loading? List three sports for which carbohydrate loading could enhance performance.

3. Why is a combination of carbohydrate and protein recommended for recovery after resistance exercise? When should a recovery meal be provided? Suggest a suitable recovery meal.

For more information on sports nutrition, check out the following websites:
Gatorade Sports Science Institute:
www.gssiweb.com
The Physician and Sportsmedicine:
http://www.tandfonline.com/toc/ipsm20/current
American College of Sports Medicine:
www.acsm.org
Centers for Disease Control and Prevention's Division of Nutrition, Physical Activity, and Obesity:
www.cdc.gov/nccdphp/dnpao
American Council on Exercise:
www.acefitness.org

CASE STUDY Planning a Training Diet

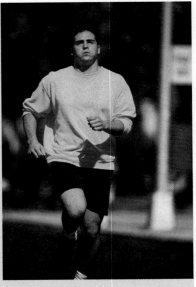

©Comstock Images RF

Michael is training for a 10K run coming up in 3 weeks. He has read a lot about sports nutrition and especially about the importance of eating a high-carbohydrate diet while in training. He also has been struggling to keep his weight in a range that he feels contributes to better speed and endurance. Consequently, he is also trying to eat as little fat as possible. Unfortunately, over the past week, his workouts in the afternoon have not met his expectations. His run times are slower, and he shows signs of fatigue after just 20 minutes into his training program.

   His breakfast yesterday was a large bagel with cream cheese and orange juice. For lunch, he had a small salad with fat-free dressing, a large plate of pasta with marinara sauce and broccoli, and a diet soft drink. For dinner, he had a small broiled chicken breast, a cup of rice, some carrots, and iced tea. Later, he snacked on fat-free pretzels.

1. Is a high-carbohydrate diet a good idea during Michael's training?
2. Are there any important components missing in Michael's diet? Are missing components contributing to his fatigue?
3. Describe some changes that should be made in Michael's diet, including specific foods that should be emphasized.
4. How should fluid needs be met during workouts?
5. Should Michael focus on fueling his body before, during, or after workouts?

Complete the Case Study. Responses to these questions can be provided by your instructor.

Ergogenic Aids and Athletic Performance

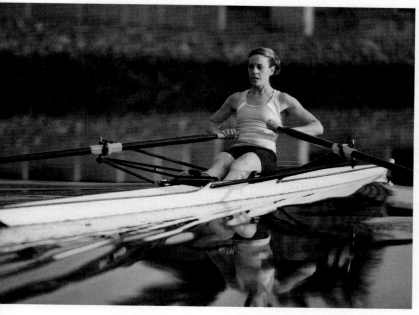

©Ty Milford/Aurora Open/Getty Images RF

TABLE 10-10 ■ Sample Ergogenic Aids

Substance/Practice	Purported Use
Beetroot juice	Enhance endurance performance by improving oxygen consumption
Beta-alanine	Increase muscle carnosine, a protein that neutralizes acidic compounds that contribute to muscle fatigue during high-intensity exercise
Caffeine	Increase vigilance and mental alertness; improve endurance performance; reduce perception of fatigue
Creatine	Increase lean mass; improve short-term intense exercise performance; aid muscle recovery
Sodium bicarbonate (baking soda)	Neutralize acidic compounds that contribute to muscle fatigue

Extreme diet manipulation to improve athletic performance is not a recent innovation. Today's athletes are as likely as their predecessors to experiment with any substance that promises a competitive advantage. In 2015, the U.S. sports nutrition supplement market reached $11 billion, accounting for 35% of the global market. Bee pollen, medium-chain triglycerides, chromium picolinate, carnitine, and ginseng are just some of the likely ineffective substances used by athletes in hopes of gaining an **ergogenic** edge.

Based on what is known at this time, today's athletes can benefit from scientific evidence documenting the ergogenic properties of a few dietary substances. These ergogenic aids include sufficient water and electrolytes, adequate carbohydrates, and a balanced and varied dietary pattern consistent with MyPlate. Protein and amino acid supplements are NOT needed as the vast majority of athletes can easily meet their protein needs from whole foods. In general, nutrient supplements should only be used to meet a specific dietary shortcoming, such as an inadequate iron intake. Beyond the proven benefits of the nutrition strategies presented in this chapter, Table 10-10 provides a short list of well-studied ergogenic aids.

Dietary supplements rumored to enhance athletic performance require careful evaluation and monitoring. Overall, there is little scientific evidence to support the effectiveness of many substances that are touted as performance-enhancing aids. Of these, many are useless, and some are dangerous enough to promote organ damage (Table 10-11). The liver and kidneys are particularly susceptible to damage because these organs help detoxify harmful compounds.[12]

ergogenic Work-producing. An ergogenic aid is a mechanical, nutritional, psychological, pharmacological, or physiological substance or treatment intended to directly improve exercise performance.

National Collegiate Athletic Association (NCAA) and Nutrition Supplements

The NCAA's Committee on Competitive Safeguards and Medical Aspects of Sports has developed lists of permissible and nonpermissible nutritional supplements for athletic departments to provide to student athletes. The NCAA has issued a warning advising students to discuss their use of *any* dietary supplement with their team medical staff to avoid unknowingly ingesting banned substances. Following are a few key examples:

Select Permissible Supplements

- Vitamins and minerals
- Energy bars (if no more than 30% protein)
- Electrolyte replacement drinks such as Gatorade® or Powerade®
- Calorie replacement drinks such as Ensure® or Boost®

Select Nonpermissible Supplements

- Amino acids (including amino acid chelates)
- CLA (conjugated linoleic acid)
- Chondroitin (unless for medical condition)
- Creatine/compounds containing creatine
- Ginkgo biloba
- Ginseng
- Glucosamine (unless for medical condition)
- Green tea
- Melatonin
- Protein powders
- St. John's wort
- Weight gainers

For a complete explanation of NCAA's rules regarding dietary supplements, see www.ncaa.org.

TABLE 10-11 ■ Dangerous, Banned, or Illegal Substances and Practices

Substance/Practice	Purported Use	Risks
Anabolic steroids (e.g., testosterone, androstenedione, and tetrahydrogestrinone)	Increase muscle mass and strength	Liver cysts; increased risk of cardiovascular disease, hypertension, and reproductive dysfunction; depression, sleep disturbances, mood swings (*roid rage*) *Illegal in the United States unless prescribed.*
Blood doping	Enhances aerobic capacity by increasing red blood cells	Blood thickening that strains the heart
Ephedrine (stimulant)	Increases muscle strength and power, promotes mental alertness and weight loss	Heart palpitations, anxiety, and death
Gamma hydroxybutyric acid (GHB)	Steroid alternative for bodybuilding	Vomiting, dizziness, tremors, seizures, and death
Growth hormone	Increases muscle mass and fat metabolism	Uncontrolled growth of the heart and other internal organs; death

Athletes should be skeptical of any substance until its ergogenic effect is scientifically validated. The U.S. Food and Drug Administration (FDA) has a limited ability to regulate these dietary supplements and the manufacturing processes for dietary supplements are not as tightly regulated by the FDA as they are for prescription drugs.

Some supplements contain substances that will cause athletes to test positive for various banned substances. This was demonstrated in the 2008 Summer Olympics, when swimmer Jessica Hardy tested positive for a banned substance that she inadvertently consumed as part of a dietary supplement. Studies consistently show that many supplements do not contain the substance and/or the amount listed on the label. Not only must athletes determine whether there is evidence that a dietary supplement is safe

and effective, but they must also question if the dietary supplement contains what it is supposed to contain.

Even substances whose ergogenic effects have been supported by scientific evidence should be used with extreme caution, as the testing conditions may not match those of the intended use. Extreme caution should be exercised when it comes to using the appropriate dose of supplements or using multiple types of supplements concurrently.[12]

Rather than waiting for a magic bullet to enhance performance, athletes are advised to concentrate their efforts on improving their training routines and sport techniques, while adhering to a well-balanced dietary pattern embracing whole foods as described in this chapter.

Summary (Numbers refer to numbered sections in the chapter.)

10.1 A gradual increase in regular physical activity is recommended for all persons. Benefits include improvements in cardiovascular health, gastrointestinal function, blood glucose regulation, mental health, quality of life, and sleep; reduced risk of certain cancers; and enhanced muscle and bone strength.

10.2 The Physical Activity Guidelines for Americans advise adults to do at least 150 minutes of moderate-intensity or 75 minutes of vigorous-intensity aerobic physical activity per week. In addition, adults should perform muscle-strengthening activities and flexibility exercises at least twice per week. Workouts should allow time for

warm-up exercises to increase blood flow and warm the muscles and then end with cooldown exercises, including stretching.

10.3 Human metabolic pathways extract chemical energy from carbohydrate, fat, and protein to yield ATP. Phosphocreatine is high-energy compound that can be used to resupply ATP during short, intense activities. The mix of macronutrients used for fuel depends on the intensity and duration of activity: short-term, intense exercises primarily use carbohydrate for fuel, whereas low- or moderate-intensity endurance exercises use more fat for fuel. Protein makes a minor contribution as a fuel source.

10.4 To support physical activity, athletes require 5 to 8 kcal per minute of activity above energy needs for a sedentary person. Monitoring weight changes over time is a good way to assess the adequacy of energy intake. Athletes should obtain energy from a varied diet that includes sources of carbohydrates (6 to 10 grams of carbohydrate per kilogram of body weight; usually 60% of total energy), protein (1.2 to 2.0 grams of protein per kilogram, depending on the type of training), and fat (up to 35% of energy, focusing on vegetable oils instead of solid fats). The increased overall food intake of athletes typically furnishes adequate vitamins and minerals. Some micronutrients of concern are iron and calcium, especially for women. Athletes should drink fluid before, during (to minimize loss of body weight), and after exercise (2 to 3 cups per pound lost). Sports drinks may help replace fluid, electrolytes, and carbohydrates lost during continuous workouts that last beyond 60 minutes.

10.5 Endurance athletes can delay or prevent fatigue by consuming enough fluids, electrolytes, and carbohydrates before, during, and after events. In addition, protein in the post-exercise period will aid muscle recovery. In addition to these strategies to maintain hydration and muscle glycogen stores, athletes who train to develop strength or power should place special emphasis on protein during the recovery period.

10.6 Athletes can benefit from ergogenic properties of sufficient water, electrolytes, and carbohydrates, and a balanced and varied diet consistent with the Dietary Guidelines and MyPlate. Although some ergogenic aids may be useful for enhancing athletic performance, extreme caution should be practiced as many ergogenic aids are dangerous. Protein and amino acid supplements are not necessary because athletes almost always meet protein needs from whole foods.

Check Your Knowledge (Answers are available at the end of this question set.)

1. An energy-rich compound, phosphocreatine (PCr), is found in _____ tissue.
   a. adipose
   b. muscle
   c. liver
   d. kidney

2. A physical activity program should include
   a. aerobic exercises 5 days per week.
   b. strength-training exercises 2 to 3 days per week.
   c. stretching exercises 2 to 3 days per week.
   d. all of these.

3. During muscle-building regimens, athletes should consume _____ grams of protein per kilogram body weight.
   a. 0.5 to 0.7
   b. 0.8
   c. 1.5 to 2
   d. 2 to 2.5

4. Which of these foods is the best choice for carbohydrate loading before endurance events?
   a. Potato chips
   b. French fries
   c. All-Bran® (high-fiber) cereal
   d. Rice

5. As the body adapts to regular exercise, the "training effect" results in
   a. decreased blood flow to muscles.
   b. increased lactic-acid production.
   c. decreased muscle triglyceride content.
   d. decreased resting heart rate.

6. A physically active lifestyle leads to
   a. increased bone strength.
   b. decreased risk of colon cancer.
   c. reduced anxiety and depression.
   d. all of these.

7. How many cups of fluid are required to replace each pound of weight lost during an athletic event or workout?
   a. 0.5 to 0.75 cup
   b. 1 to 1.5 cups
   c. 2 to 3 cups
   d. 4 to 5 cups

8. The benefit of a sports drink is to provide
   a. water to hydrate.
   b. electrolytes to enhance water absorption in the intestine and maintain blood volume.
   c. carbohydrate for energy.
   d. all of these.

9. Compared to anaerobic glucose metabolism, aerobic glucose metabolism produces more
   a. lactic acid.
   b. ATP.
   c. phosphocreatine.
   d. fatty acids.

10. Caffeine is used as an ergogenic aid by some athletes because it is thought to
    a. decrease fatigue.
    b. decrease the buildup of lactic acid.
    c. serve as an energy source.
    d. increase muscle mass and strength.

Answer Key: 1. b (LO 10.3), 2. d (LO 10.2), 3. c (LO 10.6), 4. d (LO 10.8), 5. d (LO 10.5), 6. d (LO 10.1), 7. c (LO 10.7), 8. d (LO 10.7), 9. b (LO 10.7), 10. a (LO 10.9)

Study Questions (Numbers refer to Learning Outcomes)

1. How does greater physical fitness contribute to better overall health? Explain the process. **(LO 10.1)**

2. You have set a goal to increase muscle mass and decrease body fat. Plan a weekly fitness regimen using the FITT principle. **(LO 10.2)**

3. How are carbohydrates, fat, and protein used to supply energy during a 100-meter sprint? During a weight-lifting session? During a 3-mile walk? **(LO 10.3)**

4. What is the difference between anaerobic and aerobic exercise? Explain why aerobic metabolism is increased by a regular exercise routine. **(LO 10.4)**

5. Is fat from adipose tissue used as an energy source during exercise? If so, when? **(LO 10.5)**

6. What are some typical measures used to assess whether an athlete's calorie intake is adequate? **(LO 10.6)**

7. List five nutrients of specific concern for athletes and the appropriate food sources from which these nutrients can be obtained. **(LO 10.6)**

8. Your neighbor is planning to run a 5-kilometer race. Summarize for her what you have learned about fluid intake before, during, and after the event. **(LO 10.7)**

9. You plan to participate in a half-marathon. Plan your menu for the day of the event, being sure to include appropriate levels of macronutrients and fluids before, during, and after the athletic event. **(LO 10.8)**

10. Should competitive athletes take amino acid supplements? Why or why not? **(LO 10.9)**

What the Dietitian Chose

In this chapter, you have learned that it's important to replenish carbohydrates, fluids, and electrolytes for optimal performance during endurance events, like this half-marathon. General guidelines are to consume ½ to 1 ½ cups of fluid every 15 minutes and 30 to 60 grams of carbohydrate per hour. Choosing a sports nutrition product is something you should try during training. With a few weeks to go, you have time to experiment with a product that can help you avoid "hitting the wall."

The PowerBar ProteinPlus® energy bar provides 210 kcal, 6 grams of fat, 25 grams of carbohydrate, and 20 grams of protein. This might be a convenient meal replacement during your busy weeks of training. Alternatively, it could serve as a recovery meal to help replenish your muscle glycogen stores after the race. However, during the race, its high fat and protein content would slow digestion, possibly leading to abdominal cramps. Furthermore, this product would not contribute to fluid replenishment.

The Essential Amino Energy drink provides 2 grams of carbohydrate and 5 grams of essential amino acids in free form, including branched-chain amino acids (BCAA). The drink may help meet fluid needs, but the carbohydrate content is not sufficient to maintain blood glucose during the race. It is true that BCAAs are utilized for fuel during endurance activities and they may enhance muscle building during weight training, but there is no consistent evidence that supplying BCAAs during endurance exercise enhances performance.

A sports drink, such as Powerade,® is superior to water for continuous and strenuous events lasting more than 60 minutes. The carbohydrates help to supply energy to the brain and muscles. The added flavor encourages consumption. The electrolytes replace those lost in sweating, increase fluid absorption, and stimulate thirst. A 32-ounce bottle of Powerade (4 servings) contains a total of 213 kcal and 56 grams of carbohydrate in 4 cups of fluid. One bottle of Powerade per hour while you compete would meet your fluid and carbohydrate needs but may be inconvenient to tote while running.

The energy gel is small enough to take along during the race. The label shows 110 kcal, 1.5 grams of fat, 22 grams of carbohydrate, 12 grams of sugar, and 100 milligrams of caffeine. A Clif Shot® Turbo during the race could help replenish blood glucose and electrolytes, but it definitely won't meet your fluid requirements while racing. However, there should be water available at numerous stops along the course.

Some energy gels are caffeine free, but this one contains as much caffeine as a strong cup of coffee. Research shows that caffeine can decrease feelings of fatigue and increase mental alertness among people who are not habitual caffeine consumers. On the other hand, negative effects of excessive caffeine can include dehydration, heart palpitations, and gastrointestinal discomfort, so moderation is necessary.

In summary, both the Powerade and the Clif Shot Turbo would replenish carbohydrates and electrolytes. The Powerade would also fulfill your fluid needs, whereas you'd need to grab water along the course if you choose the energy gel. The energy gel has the advantage of being light and portable, plus the caffeine may have an ergogenic effect. Give both the Powerade and the Clif Shot Turbo energy gel a trial run during your training sessions and see which one helps you most.

Further Readings

1. Garber CE and others: American College of Sports Medicine Position Stand: Quantity and quality of exercise for developing and maintaining cardiorespiratory, musculoskeletal, and neuromotor fitness in apparently healthy adults: Guidance for prescribing exercise. *Med Sci Sports Exerc* 2011; 43:1334.

2. U.S. Department of Health and Human Services. *2008 Physical Activity Guidelines for Americans.* Washington, DC: U.S. Department of Health and Human Services, 2008. ODPHP Publication No. U0036. http://www.health.gov/paguidelines. (Accessed August 6, 2015).

3. Thomas DT and others: Position of the Academy of Nutrition and Dietetics, Dietitians of Canada, and the American College of Sports Medicine: Nutrition and athletic performance. *J Acad Nutr Diet* 2016; 116:501.

4. Rosenfeld V and Wattenberg C: Weight loss in wrestling: Current state of the science. National Collegiate Athletic Association. Updated 2014. Available at http://www.scandpg.org/nutrition-info/nutrition-for-collegiate-sports-and-athletics/articles/

5. Burke LM and others: BJSM reviews: A–Z of nutritional supplements: Dietary supplements, sports nutrition foods and ergogenic aids for health and performance—Part 4. *Br J Sports Med* 2009; 43:1088.

6. Phillips SM and Van Loon LJC: Dietary protein for athletes: From requirements to optimum adaptation. *J Sports Sci* 2011; 29:S29.

7. Goodman C and others: A to Z of nutritional supplements: Dietary supplements, sports nutrition foods and ergogenic aids for health and performance—Part 21. *Br J Sports Med* 2011; 45:677.

8. Ormsbee MJ and others: Pre-exercise nutrition: The role of macronutrients, modified starches and supplements on metabolism and endurance performance. *Nutrients* 2014; 6:1782.

9. Slater G and Phillips SM: Nutrition guidelines for strength sports: Sprinting, weightlifting, throwing events, and bodybuilding. *J Sports Sci* 2011; 29:S67.

10. Stellingwerff T and others: Nutrition for power sports: Middle-distance running, track cycling, rowing, canoeing/kayaking, and swimming. *J Sports Sci* 2011; 29:S79.

11. Holway FE and Spriet LL: Sport-specific nutrition: Practical strategies for team sports. *J Sports Sci* 2011; 29:S115.

12. U.S. Department of Agriculture, National Agricultural Library. Ergogenic Aids. https://www.nal.usda.gov/fnic/ergogenic-aids. (Accessed 2/13/2017).

connect To get the most out of your study, visit Connect where you will find NutritionCalc Plus, SmartBook®, and many other dynamic tools.

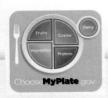

Rate Your Plate

Evaluating Protein Intake—A Case Study

Mark is a college student who has been lifting weights at the student recreation center. The trainer at the center recommended a protein drink to help Mark build muscle mass. Answer the following questions about Mark's current food intake and determine whether a protein drink is needed to supplement Mark's diet.

The following is a tally of yesterday's intake.

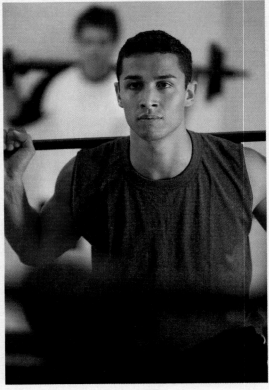

©Comstock Images/Jupiterimages RF

Breakfast	Frosted Mini-Wheats® cereal, 2 ounces 1% milk, 1 ½ cups Orange juice, 6 ounces Hard-boiled eggs, 2 Brewed coffee, 1 cup
Lunch	Double hamburger with condiments, 1 French fries, 30 pieces Cola, 12 ounces
Afternoon snack	Greek yogurt with honey, 1 cup Apple, 1 medium
Dinner	Frozen lasagna w/meat, 2 pieces 1% milk, 1 cup Loose-leaf lettuce, chopped, 1 cup Creamy Italian salad dressing, 2 tsp Tomato, 1/2 medium Carrot, 1 whole raw
Evening snack	Low-fat vanilla ice cream, 1 cup Hot fudge chocolate topping, 2 tsp

1. Evaluate Mark's diet using NutritionCalc Plus. Is he meeting the minimum recommendations of MyPlate's Daily Food Plan for his calorie needs?

    _____

2. Mark's weight has been stable at 70 kilograms (154 pounds). Determine his protein needs based on the RDA (0.8 gram per kilogram).
    a. Mark's estimated protein RDA: _____
    b. What are the maximum recommendations for protein intake for strength-training athletes?

    _____

    c. Calculate the maximum protein recommendation for Mark. _____

    _____

3. An analysis of the total calorie and protein content of Mark's current diet is 3400 kcal, 145 grams of protein (17% of total calories supplied by protein). This diet is representative of the food choices and amounts of food that Mark chooses on a regular basis.
    a. What is the difference between Mark's estimated protein needs as an athlete (from question 2) and the amount of protein that his current diet provides? _____
    b. Is his current protein intake inadequate, adequate, or excessive? _____

4. Mark takes his trainer's advice and goes to the supermarket to purchase a protein drink to add to his diet. Four products are available; they contain the following label information.

	Amino Fuel®	Joe Weider's® Sugar-Free 90% Plus Protein	Joe Weider's Dynamic Muscle Builder	Victory Super Mega Mass® 2000
Serving size	3 tbsp	3 tbsp	3 tbsp	¼ scoop
Kcal	104	110	103	104
Protein (grams)	15	24	10	5

The trainer recommends adding the supplement to Mark's diet two times a day. Mark chooses the Muscle Builder protein drink.

a. How much protein would be added to Mark's diet daily from two servings of the supplement alone (prior to mixing it with a beverage)?

b. Mark mixes the powder with the milk he already consumes at breakfast and dinner. How much protein total would Mark now consume in 1 day? (Add the protein amount from the nutrition analysis to the value from question 4a.)

c. What is the difference between Mark's estimated protein needs as an athlete and his total intake?

5. What is your conclusion—does Mark need the protein supplement?

Answers

1. Yes.
2. a. Mark's estimated protein RDA: 70 kilograms × 0.8 gram per kilogram = 56 grams.
   b. Maximum recommendation for protein intake for athletes = 2.0 grams per kilogram.
   c. Applied to Mark: 2.0 × 70 = 140 grams.
3. a. Difference between Mark's estimated maximum protein needs for muscle mass gain and the amount of protein provided by his current diet:
      145 − 140 = 5 grams.
   b. Mark's current protein intake exceeds maximum protein needs.
4. a. Two servings of protein supplement alone = 20 grams of protein.
   b. Mark's total protein consumption: 145 grams + 20 grams = 165 grams protein.
   c. Difference between Mark's estimated maximum protein needs for muscle mass gain and total protein consumption with protein supplement (from above): 165 grams − 140 grams = 25 grams protein.
5. No.

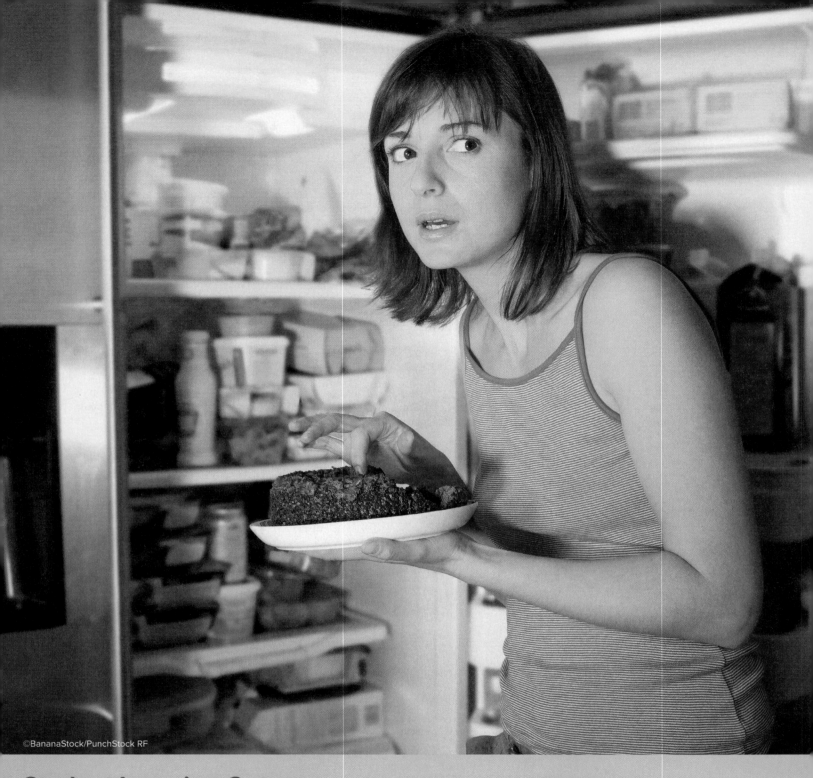

©BananaStock/PunchStock RF

Student Learning Outcomes

Chapter 11 is designed to allow you to:

11.1 Contrast healthy attitudes toward uses of food with behavior patterns that could lead to unhealthy uses of food.

11.2 Describe current hypotheses about the origins of eating disorders.

11.3 List physical and mental characteristics of anorexia nervosa, and outline current best practices for its treatment.

11.4 List physical and mental characteristics of bulimia nervosa, and outline current best practices for its treatment.

11.5 Enumerate physical and mental characteristics of binge eating disorder, and outline current best practices for its treatment.

Chapter 11
Eating Disorders

What Would You Choose?

Your college roommate has been acting strangely lately, and you are starting to suspect she has an eating disorder. Over the first few months at college, she gained the "freshman 15." She got kind of depressed about it when her jeans started to fit too snugly and declared she was going on a diet. Her weight has not really decreased much since then, but her eating behaviors certainly have changed. She stopped joining your group of friends for meals in the dining hall, opting instead to eat by herself in your dorm room. She has been spending at least 2 hours a day in the campus recreation center, sometimes going in the morning and evening. A few days ago, you thought you heard her throwing up in the restroom, but when she came out of the stall, she said she was fine. What would you choose to help your roommate?

- **a** Tell her she has bulimia and needs to get some treatment.
- **b** Give her some weight-management advice that you learned in Chapter 7.
- **c** Express your concern and ask her if you can go with her to the student health center to talk to someone about it.
- **d** Ignore her behavior; she is just trying to draw attention to herself, and this phase will pass in a few weeks.

Think about your choice as you read this chapter, then see What the Dietitian Chose at the end of the chapter.

Many of us occasionally eat until we're stuffed and uncomfortable, such as at Thanksgiving dinner. Faced with savory and tempting foods, we find that we cannot easily stop eating. Usually we forgive ourselves, vowing not to overeat the next time. Nevertheless, many of us have problems controlling our food intake and body weight. The combination of too many instances of simple overeating and too little physical activity eventually leads to progressive weight gain.

The obesity epidemic tends to upstage all other nutrition-related problems. However, the consequences of eating disorders are just as serious as obesity; indeed, if left untreated, eating disorders can be fatal. What is most alarming about these disorders—anorexia nervosa, bulimia nervosa, and binge eating disorder—is the increasing number of cases reported each year.

It is widely accepted that eating disorders arise as a result of interactions between brain biology and environmental influences. Successful treatment of eating disorders, therefore, is complex and must go beyond nutritional therapy. Keep in mind that eating disorders are not restricted to any socioeconomic class or ethnicity. They can also strike at any age in either females or males. Let us examine the causes, effects, and treatments of these conditions and consider strategies for prevention.

11.6 Describe other forms of eating disorders, including night eating syndrome and the female athlete triad.

11.7 Describe methods to reduce the development of eating disorders, including the use of warning signs to identify early cases.

449

11.1 From Ordered to Disordered Eating Habits

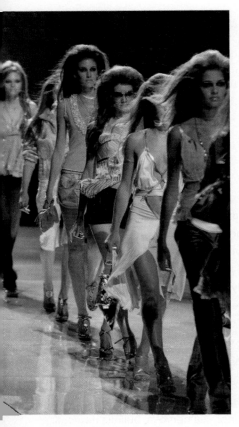

▲ Maintaining an ultraslim body type is an all-too-common goal in today's culture. The media and the fashion world bombard us with body images that are unrealistic for most people. ©Lars A. Niki RF

endorphins Natural body tranquilizers that may be involved in the feeding response and function in pain reduction.

disordered eating Mild and short-term changes in eating patterns that occur in relation to a stressful event, an illness, or a desire to modify one's diet for a variety of health and personal appearance reasons.

Eating—a completely instinctive behavior for animals—serves an extraordinary number of psychological, social, and cultural purposes for humans. Eating practices may take on religious meanings; signify bonds within families and ethnic groups; and provide a means to express hostility, affection, prestige, or class values. Within the family, supplying, preparing, and even withholding food may be a means of expressing love, hatred, or power.

We are bombarded daily with our society's portrayal of the "ideal" body. Dieting is promoted to achieve this ideal body—eternally young and admired. Television programs, billboard and Internet advertisements, video games, magazines, and movies suggest that an ultraslim body will bring happiness, love, admiration, and success. This fantasy notion is contradictory to the high rate of obesity in our society. In response to this social pressure, some individuals take an extreme approach: the pathological pursuit of weight control or weight loss.

Early in life, we develop images of "acceptable" and "unacceptable" body types. Of the attributes that constitute attractiveness, many people view body weight as the most important, partly because we can control our weight somewhat. Fatness is the most dreaded deviation from our cultural ideals of body image, the one most derided and shunned. In a study about weight bias conducted by researchers at Yale University, nearly half of survey respondents said they would rather give up 1 year of life than live with obesity.

It can be difficult to resist comparing your body to what the popular media portrays as "ideal." For some people, the disparity between their own body image and the perceived ideal may be enough to trigger an eating disorder.

FOOD: MORE THAN JUST A SOURCE OF NUTRIENTS

From birth, we link food with personal and emotional experiences. As infants, we associate milk with security and warmth, so the breast or bottle becomes a source of comfort. As noted in Section 1.1, even when older, most people continue to derive comfort and great pleasure from food. This is both a biological and a psychological phenomenon. Indeed, eating can stimulate the release of certain neurotransmitters (e.g., serotonin) and *natural opioids* (including **endorphins**), which produce a sense of calm and euphoria in the human body. Thus, in times of great stress, some people turn to food for its naturally calming, druglike effect.

Food is also used as a reward or a bribe. Perhaps some of the following comments sound familiar:

- You can have your dessert if you eat five more bites of your vegetables.
- You cannot play until you clean your plate.
- I will eat the broccoli if you let me watch TV.
- If you love me, you will eat your dinner.

On the surface, using food as a reward or bribe seems harmless. Eventually, however, this practice may encourage both caregivers and children to use food to achieve goals other than satisfying hunger and nutrient needs. Food may then become much more than a source of nutrients. Regularly using food as a bargaining chip can contribute to abnormal eating patterns. Carried to the extreme, these patterns can lead to **disordered eating.**

Disordered eating refers to short-term, mild changes in eating patterns that occur in response to a stressful event, an illness, or even a desire to modify the diet for a variety of health and personal appearance reasons. The problem may be no more than a bad habit, a style of eating adapted from friends or family members, or an aspect of preparing for athletic competition. While disordered eating can lead to weight fluctuations or nutrient deficiencies, it rarely requires in-depth professional attention. If, however, disordered eating becomes sustained or distressing, starts to interfere with everyday activities, or is linked to physiological changes, then it may require professional intervention.

ORIGINS OF EATING DISORDERS

Given the common practice of dieting in North America, it can sometimes be difficult to draw a definitive line between disordered eating and an **eating disorder.** Indeed, many eating disorders start with a simple diet. Eating disorders then go on to involve physiological changes associated with food restriction, binge eating, purging, and fluctuations in weight. They also involve a number of emotional and cognitive changes that affect the way a person perceives and experiences his or her body, such as feelings of distress or extreme concern about body shape or weight. Eating disorders are not due to a failure of will or behavior; rather, they are real, treatable medical illnesses in which certain maladaptive patterns of eating take on a life of their own.

People who suffer from eating disorders can experience a wide range of health complications, including heart conditions and kidney failure, which may even lead to death. Recognition of eating disorders as important and treatable diseases, therefore, is critical. The three main types of eating disorders are **anorexia nervosa, bulimia nervosa,** and **binge eating disorder.** Although it is convenient to label patients with a clear-cut diagnosis, the various types of eating disorders have more similarities than distinctions, particularly in their underlying biological and psychological processes.

Specific criteria from the *Diagnostic and Statistical Manual of Mental Disorders, 5th Edition (DSM-5)* are used by clinicians to diagnose eating disorders. As you read about the different eating disorders in this chapter, look for the relevant diagnostic criteria in Tables 11-1, 11-2, and 11-3. Keep in mind that individuals may exhibit a few symptoms of eating disorders but not enough to warrant a formal diagnosis. These people may be classified as having "subthreshold" eating disorders. Also, some people show characteristics of more than one eating disorder or may migrate from one disorder to another over time. Indeed, about half of women diagnosed as having anorexia nervosa eventually develop bulimic symptoms. Still, appreciating the differences between the disorders helps us to understand the various approaches to prevention and treatment.

Over the years, researchers have theorized that dysfunctional family interactions, especially between parents and adolescents, precipitate eating disorders. While unhealthy family relationships may lead to emotional distress, there is little scientific evidence that family functioning is a primary cause for eating disorders. In fact, insinuating that the family has caused a person's eating disorder leads to feelings of guilt and shame within the family that may actually hinder efforts at treatment.[1]

Scientists now recognize that genes bear much of the blame for eating disorders.[2] Twin studies have shown that when one of a set of identical twins (i.e., who have identical DNA) has an eating disorder, it is more likely that the other twin will also have an eating disorder—more likely than in sets of fraternal twins. Genetic factors account for an estimated 50% to 83% of the overall risk for developing an eating disorder.

A variety of genes could be involved in the development of eating disorders, including those responsible for the expression of hormones and neurotransmitters involved in weight regulation and eating behaviors (review Section 7.4). In about 80% of cases, eating disorders co-occur with other psychological disorders, such as anxiety disorders, major depression, and substance abuse disorders. It appears that genes influence the brain biology that determines how we perceive ourselves and respond to food stimuli or stress. In response to environmental triggers, some individuals may resort to self-destructive coping mechanisms, including disordered eating.

Because stressful life events may precipitate an eating disorder in genetically predisposed individuals, there is a strong association between eating disorders and a history of abuse. In fact, a history of physical and sexual abuse is about twice as common among people with eating disorders compared to the population as a whole.[3] Other stressful

eating disorder Severe alterations in eating patterns linked to physiological changes. The alterations are associated with food restriction, binge eating, inappropriate compensatory behaviors, and fluctuations in weight. They also involve a number of emotional and cognitive changes that affect the way a person perceives and experiences his or her body.

anorexia nervosa An eating disorder characterized by extreme restriction of energy intake relative to requirements leading to significantly low body weight.

bulimia nervosa An eating disorder characterized by recurrent episodes of binge eating followed by inappropriate compensatory behaviors to prevent weight gain.

binge eating disorder An eating disorder characterized by recurrent episodes of binge eating that are associated with marked distress and lack of control over behavior, but not followed by inappropriate compensatory behaviors to prevent weight gain.

Progression from Ordered to Disordered Eating

Attention to hunger and satiety signals; limitation of calorie intake to restore weight to a healthful level

↓

Some disordered eating habits begin as weight loss is attempted, such as very restricted eating.

↓

Clinically evident eating disorder recognized

epigenetics Heritable changes in gene function that are independent of DNA sequence. For example, malnutrition during pregnancy may modify gene expression in the fetus and affect long-term body weight regulation in the offspring.

life events, such as wartime military service, the death of a loved one, or constant social pressures to achieve thinness, are potential triggers for eating disorders.

In addition to genetics, researchers are studying **epigenetics** (heritable changes in gene expression that do not involve changes to the underlying DNA sequence), as it relates to the development of eating disorders.[4] Some studies suggest that maternal stress or hormone levels during pregnancy can predict the future development of an eating disorder in their children by affecting how the child's genes function.[5]

Overall, genes may set the stage for development of an eating disorder, but environmental factors also play a role. Identifying genes linked to eating disorders eventually could help in tailoring prevention and treatment efforts for at-risk individuals. However, the psychiatric counseling that is part of current therapy will still be of value.

THE CHANGING FACE OF EATING DISORDERS

If you were asked to paint a picture of a person with an eating disorder, who would you depict? The predominant stereotype is that eating disorders only affect young, white females of middle or upper socioeconomic status. However, the face of eating disorders is changing.

When it comes to anorexia and bulimia, women do outnumber men by about 9 to 1. Perhaps social pressures can account for part of this disparity: in the media, women are held to standards of unnatural thinness, whereas the image conveyed for men is big and muscular. However, men are affected by eating disorders as well. Among men, exercise status and sexual orientation are factors that particularly influence development of anorexia and bulimia. Male athletes are more prone than nonathletes to develop these eating disorders, especially those who participate in sports that require weight classes (e.g., boxers, wrestlers, and jockeys) or where judging is partly based on aesthetics (e.g., ice skating, diving, or dancing).[6] With reference to sexual orientation, the prevalence of eating disorders in gay men is two to three times that in heterosexual men.[7] Certain types of eating disorders are more common among men. While men make up less than 10% of cases of anorexia and bulimia, they account for about 40% of cases of binge eating disorder.

Eating disorders typically develop during adolescence or young adulthood. Adolescence is a period of turbulent sexual and social tensions. At this time of life, teenagers establish their own identities. While declaring independence, they seek acceptance and support from peers and parents and react strongly to how they think others perceive them. At the same time, their bodies are changing, and much of the change is beyond their control. This is a time when extreme dieting practices may take root. It is alarming that eating disorders are being diagnosed at earlier ages.[8] Note that calorie restriction is not always evidenced as weight loss; stunting (failure to grow in height) and delayed sexual maturation also could be signs of eating disorders among children and adolescents.

While much of the focus has been on youth, middle-aged and older adults are not immune to the devastating effects of eating disorders. In North America, aging baby boomers are the largest demographic group. Although eating disorders rarely make their first appearance late in adulthood, it may not be until later in adulthood that people who have suffered from eating disorders for years finally seek treatment. Furthermore, some recovered adults may relapse into former disordered eating practices.

Research reveals that disordered eating behaviors and dissatisfaction with body weight and shape are quite common among older women. In one study, binge eating was reported by 3.5% of a community-based sample of women over age 50; purging behaviors, such as excessive exercise, were employed by 7.8% of the women.[9] Negative body image can have a dramatic impact on self-esteem and overall quality of life at any age.

Until recently, most researchers have reported that eating disorders primarily affect middle- and upper-class Caucasian women. Now, studies show greater similarities in the rates of body dissatisfaction and disordered eating behaviors across ethnic and cultural groups. Perhaps minorities with eating disorders have been less likely to seek

▼ Individuals who participate in sports with weight classes, such as wrestling, may practice disordered eating behaviors in order to gain a competitive advantage over other athletes in a lower weight class. ©Rubberball/Getty Images RF

help in the past due to fear of shame or stigma, lack of resources, or language barriers. It seems more likely, however, that health care workers have been less likely to diagnose non-Caucasians as having eating disorders. Previously, it seemed that non-Caucasian cultures were more accepting of larger body shapes, but mainstream pressures for thinness now cut across cultural lines.

Do you know someone who is at risk for an eating disorder? If so, suggest that the person seek a professional evaluation because the sooner treatment begins, the better the chances for recovery. However, do not try to diagnose eating disorders in your friends or family members. Only a professional can exclude other possible diseases and correctly diagnose an eating disorder. Once an eating disorder is diagnosed, immediate treatment is advisable. As a friend, the best you can do is to encourage an affected person to seek professional help. Such help is commonly available at student health centers and student guidance/counseling facilities on college campuses.

> Our passion for thinness dates back to the Victorian era of the nineteenth century, which specialized in denying "unpleasant" physical realities, such as appetite and sexual desire. Flappers of the 1920s set the standard for the twentieth- and twenty-first-century trend for thinness. Since 1922, the BMI values of Miss America winners have steadily decreased; during the last three decades, most winners had a BMI in the "underweight" range (less than 18.5).

✓ CONCEPT CHECK 11.1

1. Differentiate between disordered eating and an eating disorder.
2. Describe how genetics and environment interact in the development of eating disorders.
3. Why are eating disorders more common among adolescents than other age groups?

11.2 Anorexia Nervosa

Anorexia nervosa is an eating disorder characterized by extreme weight loss, an irrational fear of weight gain, and a distorted body image. These three criteria are outlined in Table 11-1 and described in detail in this section. Anorexia nervosa affects an estimated 0.8% of American women.

First, people with anorexia nervosa severely restrict energy intake relative to requirements. The term *anorexia* implies a loss of appetite; however, a denial of one's appetite more accurately describes the behavior of people with anorexia nervosa. Low energy intake leads to a body weight that is significantly less than expected when compared to others of the same age, sex, stage of physical development, and activity level. While low body weight (i.e., less than 85% of expected body weight for a given age and sex or BMI of less than 17) may indicate anorexia nervosa, a variety of other medical conditions could also result in low body weight. The next two diagnostic criteria set anorexia nervosa apart from other problems related to poor food intake or low body weight.

The second key criterion for diagnosis of anorexia nervosa involves an intense fear of gaining weight or becoming obese. Some individuals with eating disorders may deny a fear of weight gain, so persistent behaviors that interfere with weight gain are also included in this criterion. To be diagnosed with anorexia nervosa, an individual must have experienced fear of weight gain or practiced behaviors to prevent weight gain at least 75% of the days in the last 3 months.

TABLE 11-1 ■ Diagnostic Criteria for Anorexia Nervosa

A. Extreme dietary restriction that leads to significantly low body weight
B. Overwhelming distress about weight gain (or avoidance of behaviors that may lead to weight gain) despite having a low body weight
C. Disturbed perception of one's own body weight or shape, overemphasis on body weight or shape in determining self-worth, or failure to recognize the dangers of extremely low body weight

Source: American Psychiatric Association, *Diagnostic and Statistical Manual for Mental Disorders, 5e*, 2013, American Psychiatric Association.

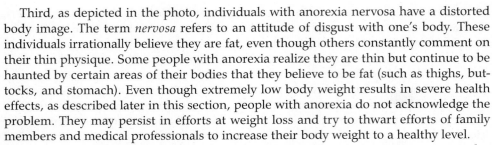

▲ For people with eating disorders, the difference between the real and desired body images may be too difficult to accept. See the website womenshealth.gov/body-image. ©Steve Niedorf Photography/Stone/Getty Images

Third, as depicted in the photo, individuals with anorexia nervosa have a distorted body image. The term *nervosa* refers to an attitude of disgust with one's body. These individuals irrationally believe they are fat, even though others constantly comment on their thin physique. Some people with anorexia realize they are thin but continue to be haunted by certain areas of their bodies that they believe to be fat (such as thighs, buttocks, and stomach). Even though extremely low body weight results in severe health effects, as described later in this section, people with anorexia do not acknowledge the problem. They may persist in efforts at weight loss and try to thwart efforts of family members and medical professionals to increase their body weight to a healthy level.

Note that there are two subtypes of anorexia nervosa: a restricting type and a binge eating/purging type. All individuals with anorexia nervosa severely restrict their calorie intake to achieve or maintain a low body weight. Men and women with the binge eating/purging type of anorexia nervosa also engage in episodes of binge eating followed by compensatory behaviors to rid the body of calories. One difference between bulimia nervosa and anorexia nervosa of the binge eating/purging subtype is that individuals with anorexia nervosa have low body weight (e.g., BMI < 17), while individuals with bulimia tend to have normal or high BMI.

COMMON BEHAVIORS OF ANOREXIA NERVOSA

Individuals who develop anorexia share some common traits. Take a young woman, for example, who is described by parents and teachers as responsible, meticulous, and obedient. She holds herself to high standards of performance and appearance. She is competitive and perfectionistic. At home, she may not allow clutter in her bedroom. Clinicians note that after a physical examination, she folds her examination gown very carefully and cleans up the examination room before leaving. As mentioned, both genetic and environmental factors contribute to both our self-perception and our responses to stress. These obsessive personality traits—rigidity and perfectionism—are related to the same brain biology that predicts development of eating disorders.

Anorexia nervosa may begin as a simple attempt to lose weight. A comment from a well-meaning friend, relative, or coach suggesting that the person seems to be gaining weight or is too fat may be all that is needed. The stress of having to maintain a certain weight to look attractive or perform better can also lead to disordered eating. Abusive experiences, a difficult breakup, or the stress of leaving home for college are examples of triggers for extreme dieting. Changing one's appearance might be viewed as a way to avoid future conflict or ensure success in a new situation.

Still, losing weight does not help people deal with anger, grief, anxiety, or depression. If these psychological issues are not addressed, individuals may intensify efforts to lose weight "to look even better," rather than work through unresolved psychological concerns. At first, dieting becomes the life focus. Such persons may derive a sense of achievement from their "success" at controlling body weight or perceive improvements in other areas of their life. What began as a diet leads to very abnormal self-perceptions and eating habits, such as cutting a pea in half before eating it.

Extreme dieting is the most important predictor of an eating disorder. (Adolescents expressing concern about their weight should be advised to focus on exercise, which does not appear to impart a risk for subsequent problems.) Once dieting begins, a person developing anorexia nervosa does not stop. As the disorder progresses, the range of foods eaten may narrow; the list of "safe foods" shortens, whereas the list of "unsafe foods" gets longer. Abnormal habits include hiding and storing food or spreading food around a plate to make it look as if much has been eaten. A person with anorexia nervosa may cook a large meal and watch others eat it while refusing to eat anything or may insist on having different meals from the rest of the family. Frequent weighing—multiple times per day—is common.[10]

As mentioned, among some people with anorexia nervosa, disordered eating behaviors may eventually include bingeing on large amounts of food in a short time and/or inappropriate behaviors to compensate for the large number of calories consumed. Covered further in Section 11.3, compensatory behaviors (sometimes called purging)

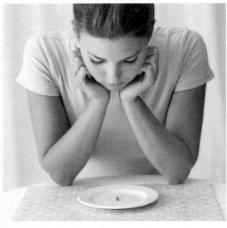

▲ Extreme dietary rules severely limit nutritional intake among people with anorexia nervosa. ©Stockbyte/PunchStock RF

include vomiting, using laxatives or diuretics, and excessive exercise. Thus, people with anorexia nervosa may exist in a state of continuous semistarvation or may alternate between periods of starvation and periods of bingeing and purging.

A state of semistarvation can cause depression, irritability, and hostility. People with anorexia may be excessively critical of themselves and usually withdraw from family and friends. Despite a strong drive for perfection, performance in school, sports, and work begins to deteriorate. (See Section 11.8 for a glimpse of the inner turmoil of a woman with anorexia nervosa.)

Ultimately, a person with anorexia nervosa eats very little food; 300 to 600 kcal daily is not unusual. In place of food, the person may consume up to 20 cans of diet soft drinks and chew many pieces of sugarless gum each day.

PHYSICAL EFFECTS OF ANOREXIA NERVOSA

The state of semistarvation disturbs many body systems as it forces the body to conserve energy stores as much as possible (Fig. 11-1). Many of the following complications

> A disturbing Internet trend is the attempt to promote eating disorders as a way of life. Some individuals with eating disorders have personified their illness into a role model named "Ana," who tells them what to eat and mocks them when they don't lose weight. Similarly, pro-"Mia" sites provide tips and encouragement for people with bulimia (e.g., how to induce vomiting and cover up evidence of compensatory behaviors). Pro-Ana and pro-Mia websites reject the serious health risks of eating disorders and instead dispense unsafe "thinspiration" to vulnerable individuals.[11]

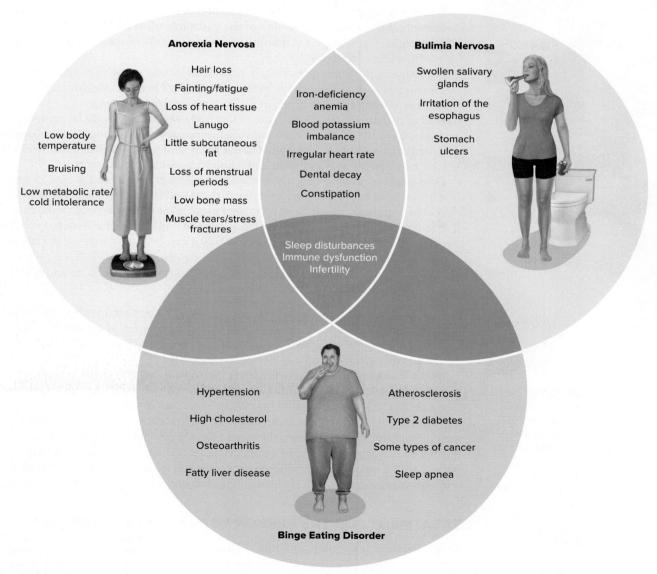

FIGURE 11-1 ▲ Physical effects of eating disorders. Although this figure contains many potential consequences, it is not an exhaustive list. Some of these physical effects can also serve as warning signs that a problem exists.

can be reversed by returning to a healthy weight, provided the duration of the semistarvation has not been too long.[12]

- Lowered body temperature and cold intolerance from loss of insulating fat layer
- Slowed metabolic rate from decreased synthesis of thyroid hormones
- Decreased heart rate as metabolism slows, leading to premature fatigue, fainting, and an overwhelming need for sleep (Other changes in heart function may occur as well, including loss of heart tissue, irregular heart rhythm, and low blood pressure.)
- Iron-deficiency anemia, which leads to further weakness
- Rough, dry, scaly, cracked, and/or cold skin, which may show multiple bruises because of the loss of the protective fat layer normally present under the skin
- Low white blood cell count, which increases the risk of infection—one cause of death in people with anorexia nervosa
- Abnormal feeling of fullness or bloating, which can last for several hours after eating
- Loss of hair from the head
- Appearance of **lanugo**—downy hairs on the body that trap air to partially counteract heat loss that occurs with loss of fat tissue
- Impaired swallowing ability due to loss of muscle tissue in the pharynx, which could lead to respiratory infections from aspiration of food and liquids into the lungs
- Constipation due to deterioration of the gastrointestinal tract and abuse of laxatives (In extreme cases, impaired motility can cause rupture of the GI tract, leading to infection and even death.)
- Low blood potassium, worsened by potassium losses during vomiting and use of some types of diuretics, which increases the risk of heart rhythm disturbances—another leading cause of death in people with anorexia nervosa
- Loss of menstrual periods because of low body weight, low body fat content, and the stress of the disease; accompanying hormonal changes contribute to bone loss
- Changes in brain size, blood flow to the brain, and neurotransmitter function, all of which contribute to depression and complicate treatment attempts
- Osteopenia or osteoporosis, which is evident in 85% of women and at least 25% of men with anorexia nervosa (Bone loss is due to decreased body weight and lean mass, several related hormonal changes, and prolonged use of some antidepressant medications.)
- Eventual loss of teeth caused by acid erosion of tooth enamel if frequent vomiting occurs (Tooth loss, along with low bone mass, can be lasting signs of the disease, even if other physical and mental problems are resolved.)
- Muscle tears and stress fractures in athletes because of decreased bone and muscle mass
- Sleep disturbances and depression

Many of the psychological and physical problems associated with anorexia nervosa arise from insufficient calorie intake, as well as deficiencies of nutrients such as thiamin, calcium, and iron. A person with this disorder is psychologically and physically ill and needs professional help.

About one-quarter of those with anorexia nervosa recover within 6 years, but many will struggle with the disease throughout life. Among all psychiatric diseases, anorexia nervosa has the highest mortality rate: 2% to 5% of people with anorexia nervosa eventually die from the disease—from heart ailments, infections, or suicide. The longer someone suffers from this eating disorder, the poorer the chances for complete recovery. A young patient with a brief episode and a supportive family has a better outlook than an older patient with a long history of disordered eating and no family support. Overall, prompt and vigorous treatment, and close long-term follow-up improve the chances for success.

TREATMENT FOR THE PERSON WITH ANOREXIA NERVOSA

People with anorexia often sink into shells of isolation and fear. They deny that a problem exists. Frequently, their friends and family members meet with them to confront the problem in a loving way. This is called an *intervention*. They present evidence of the problem and encourage immediate treatment.

lanugo Downlike hair that appears after a person has lost much body fat through semistarvation. The hair stands erect and traps air, acting as insulation for the body to compensate for the relative lack of body fat, which usually functions as insulation.

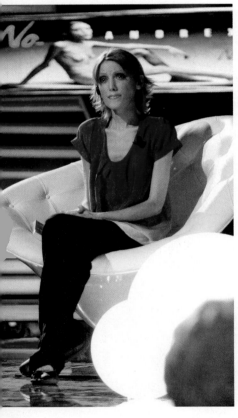

▲ In 2010, the death of French fashion model Isabelle Caro increased awareness of the serious nature of anorexia nervosa. In 2006, the 5-foot, 4-inch model was hospitalized when she slipped into a coma at her lowest weight of 55 pounds. After surviving the coma, she resolved to speak out against dieting in the fashion industry and posed for a controversial billboard ad under the words "No Anorexia." She also authored a book about her 15-year struggle with an eating disorder. Her weight had increased to at least 80 pounds by the filming of her interview for *National Geographic's Taboo: Beauty* documentary, but she died, at age 28, before it aired. ©Ernesto Ruscio/Getty Images

Treatment requires a multidisciplinary team of experienced physicians, registered dietitian nutritionists, psychologists, and other health professionals working together. An ideal setting is an eating disorders clinic in a medical center. Outpatient therapy generally begins first. This may be extended to 3 to 5 days per week. Day hospitalization (6 to 12 hours per day) is another option. Total hospitalization is necessary once a person falls below 75% of expected weight, experiences acute medical problems, and/or exhibits severe psychological problems or suicidal risk. Still, even in the most skilled hands at the finest facilities, efforts may fail. This tells us that the prevention of anorexia nervosa is of utmost importance.[13]

The health care team must gain the cooperation and trust of the person with anorexia and work together to restore body weight, correct medical complications, and treat mental illness. However, the individual who has been barely existing in a state of semistarvation cannot focus on much besides food. Dreams and even morbid thoughts about food will interfere with therapy until the person regains sufficient weight. Currently, the average time for recovery from anorexia nervosa is 7 years. Many insurance companies cover only a fraction of the estimated $150,000 cost of treatment.

Nutrition Therapy The ultimate goal of nutrition therapy is to restore body weight to a healthy range. The patient must increase oral food intake and gain enough weight to raise the metabolic rate to normal and reverse as many physical signs of the disease as possible. The refeeding plan is designed first to minimize or stop any further weight loss. Then, the focus shifts to restoring appropriate food habits. After this, the expectation can be switched to slowly gaining weight; 2 to 3 pounds per week is appropriate. Tube and/or intravenous (IV) feeding is used only if immediate renourishment is required, as this can frighten the person and cause him or her to distrust medical staff.

Persons with anorexia nervosa need considerable reassurance during the refeeding process because of uncomfortable and unfamiliar effects—such as bloating and increased body temperature. These symptoms occur because of starvation-related changes in GI tract function and will usually resolve over time, but they can be frightening for the person recovering from anorexia. Rapid changes in electrolytes and minerals in the blood associated with refeeding—especially potassium, phosphorus, and magnesium—can be dangerous. Therefore, monitoring blood levels of these minerals is of critical importance during the process of incorporating more food into the diet.

In addition to helping the person with anorexia nervosa reach and maintain adequate nutritional status, the registered dietitian nutritionist provides accurate nutrition information throughout the treatment, promotes a healthy attitude toward food, and helps the person learn to eat in response to natural hunger and satiety cues. The focus then turns to identifying healthy and adequate food choices that promote weight gain to achieve a BMI of 20 or more for adults or BMI-for-age between the 25th and 85th percentile for children (see Section 15.1). For children and adolescents, additional energy needs for growth must be considered.

As noted, nutrient deficiencies are commonly seen in patients with anorexia nervosa. As treatment progresses, the health care team will work with the patient to fully restore nutritional status. A multivitamin and mineral supplement will be added, as well as enough calcium to raise intake to about 1500 milligrams per day. Bone loss will not likely be completely restored, even if nutrition is adequate. Particularly in adolescent patients, a critical time for accrual of bone mass or gains in height may have been missed. However, supplementation with calcium and vitamin D is still necessary to prevent further bone loss.

Excessive physical activity prevents weight gain, so professionals must help people with anorexia nervosa to regulate their activity. At many treatment centers, moderate bed rest is used in the early stages of treatment to help promote weight gain.

Experienced professional help is the key for effectively treating anorexia nervosa.[14] Persons with anorexia may be on the verge of suicide and starvation, and may be very resistant to therapy. Surrendering control over eating can be scary and frustrating. They may try to hide weight loss by wearing many layers of clothes, putting coins in their pockets, and drinking numerous glasses of water before stepping on the scale.

Psychological Therapy Once the immediate physical problems of anorexia nervosa are addressed, the focus of treatment shifts to the underlying emotional problems that preceded the eating disorder. If therapists can discover the psychological conflicts that triggered the disorder, they can develop more effective treatment strategies. Education about the medical consequences of semistarvation is also helpful. A key aspect of psychological treatment is showing affected individuals how to regain control of other facets of their lives and cope with difficult situations. As eating evolves into a normal routine, they can turn to previously neglected activities.

Family-based therapy (usually 6 to 12 months) is the preferred method of psychological treatment for anorexia nervosa among *adolescents*.[14] Importantly, family-based therapy for anorexia nervosa absolves parents of blame for the eating disorder. Early treatment focuses on ways the family can help the person with anorexia achieve a healthy body weight. Eventually, responsibility for eating and weight control will be transferred back to the patient. Beyond eating behaviors, family-based therapy for anorexia nervosa also helps the patient to establish healthy relationships with parents and other family members.

At this time, there is not enough evidence to support one particular type of psychological therapy over another for *adults* with anorexia nervosa. Therapists may use **cognitive behavioral therapy,** which involves helping the person confront and change irrational beliefs about body image, eating, relationships, and weight. However, after subsisting in a starved state for months or years, the brain chemistry of a person with anorexia nervosa is so altered that attempts at cognitive restructuring are usually not effective in the early stages of illness. Underlying issues that may have triggered the

cognitive behavioral therapy
Psychological therapy in which the person's assumptions about dieting, body weight, and related issues are confronted. New ways of thinking are explored and then practiced by the person. In this way, an individual can learn new ways to control disordered eating behaviors and related life stress.

CASE STUDY Eating Disorders—Steps to Recovery

At age 16, Sarah suddenly became self-conscious about her body when her peers teased her about being overweight. She began exercising to an aerobics video for an hour each day and found that she had success in losing weight; this was the beginning of her obsession to be thin. Next, Sarah turned to eating less food to lose even more weight and began eliminating certain foods from her diet, such as candy and meat. She increased her water and vegetable intake and chewed sugarless gum to curb her appetite. Once she began dieting, it was impossible for her to stop. She enjoyed having a high degree of self-control over her body. Still, Sarah was literally obsessed with food, even staring at others while they were eating a meal. She occasionally cooked large meals and then refused to eat all but a few bites. By the time Sarah was 19 years old and 5 feet 6 inches tall, her weight had dropped from 150 to 105 pounds. Her family was concerned about her weight status, demanding that she go to a physician for an evaluation. Sarah was not happy about this idea because she worried the doctors would force her to eat and gain back unwanted weight, but she believed that her family would stop pestering her if she went. Sarah did not think she had a problem; she thought she was still grotesquely overweight. She did notice, however, that she always felt cold and was concerned that she had not menstruated in a year.

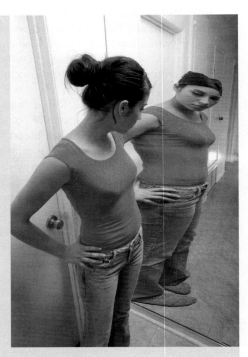
©Ted Foxx/Alamy

1. Sarah appears to have an eating disorder. Which eating disorder best describes her behavior?
2. List the behaviors that Sarah developed between ages 16 and 19 that are signs of the development of this eating disorder.
3. What physical symptoms of this disorder does Sarah have (review Fig. 11-1)?
4. Outline the therapies you think the physician will prescribe for Sarah. Where could she go for the therapy she needs? Which types of professionals would be involved?
5. Do you think Sarah has developed any vitamin or mineral deficiencies? Which ones would be most likely? How could these deficiencies be treated?
6. What is the likelihood that she will fully recover from her condition?

Complete the Case Study. Responses to these questions can be provided by your instructor.

eating disorder, such as sexual abuse, also must be identified and addressed by the therapist. Guided self-help groups for people with eating disorders, as well as their families and friends, represent additional nonthreatening first steps into treatment.

Pharmacological Therapy There are no medications approved by the U.S. Food and Drug Administration (FDA) specifically for the treatment of anorexia nervosa. Rather, food is the treatment of choice for people with this disorder. Generally, medications are not effective in managing the primary symptoms of anorexia nervosa. Fluoxetine (Prozac)® and related medications may stabilize recovery once 85% of expected body weight has been attained. These medications work by prolonging serotonin activity in the brain, which in turn regulates mood and feelings of satiety. A variety of other pharmacological agents, such as olanzapine (Zyprexa),® may have some role in treating mood changes, anxiety, or psychotic symptoms associated with anorexia nervosa, but they have limited value unless weight gain is also achieved.[14,15]

With professional help, many people with anorexia nervosa can lead normal lives. Although they may not be totally cured, recovering individuals no longer depend on unusual eating habits to cope with daily problems. They recover a sense of normalcy in their lives. Longer follow-up—sometimes several years—is associated with better outcomes. Recovery rates are around 20% to 30% for short-term therapy but increase to 70% to 80% with 8 years of follow-up. No universal approach exists because each case is unique. Establishing a strong relationship with either a therapist or another supportive person is especially important to recovery. Once people with anorexia nervosa feel understood and accepted by others, they can begin to build a sense of self and exercise some autonomy. As they learn alternative coping mechanisms, individuals with anorexia nervosa can relinquish dysfunctional relationships with food and instead develop healthy personal relationships.

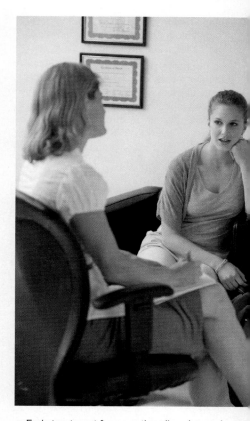

▲ Early treatment for an eating disorder, such as anorexia nervosa, improves chances of success.
©Tetra Images/Getty Images

✓ CONCEPT CHECK 11.2

1. Identify the three diagnostic criteria for anorexia nervosa.
2. List five physical effects of anorexia nervosa.
3. Describe elements of nutritional, psychological, and pharmacological therapy for anorexia nervosa.

11.3 Bulimia Nervosa

Literally translated, *bulimia* means ravenous (oxlike) hunger. This eating disorder is characterized by recurrent episodes of binge eating followed by some type of compensatory behavior to prevent weight gain (see Table 11-2). Also, as with anorexia nervosa, individuals with bulimia nervosa overvalue body weight and shape.

TABLE 11-2 ■ Diagnostic Criteria for Bulimia Nervosa

A. Repeated binge eating, characterized by:
   1. Eating a large amount of food in a short period of time (e.g., within 2 hours)
   2. Experiencing a loss of control over eating during binges

B. Repeated use of unsafe means of preventing weight gain (e.g., self-induced vomiting; inappropriate use of laxatives, diuretics, enemas, or other medications; fasting; or excessive exercise)
C. Binge-compensate cycles occur at least one time per week for 3 months
D. Undue influence of body weight or shape on self-evaluation
E. Behaviors are distinct from the binge eating/purging subtype of anorexia nervosa

Source: American Psychiatric Association, *Diagnostic and Statistical Manual for Mental Disorders*, 5e, 2013, American Psychiatric Association.

binge eating Consuming an abnormally large amount of food within a short time period (e.g., 2 hours).

compensatory behaviors Actions taken to rid the body of excess calories and/or to alleviate guilt or anxiety associated with a binge; examples include vomiting, misuse of laxatives, or excessive exercise.

Binge eating is defined as consuming an abnormally large amount of food within a short time period (e.g., 2 hours). These binges are characterized by a lack of control over the food consumed. **Compensatory behaviors** (also known as purging) used to rid the body of excess calories consumed during a binge may include vomiting; misuse of laxatives, diuretics, or enemas; or excessive exercise. For a diagnosis of bulimia nervosa, binge eating followed by inappropriate compensatory behaviors must take place at least four times per month over a period of 3 months or more.

It is likely that many people with bulimic behavior are never diagnosed. People with bulimia nervosa lead secret lives, hiding their abnormal eating habits. Moreover, it can be difficult to recognize the disorder based on appearance because people with bulimia nervosa are usually at or slightly above normal weight. By rough estimate, among North American women, approximately 2.6% will develop bulimia nervosa by the age of 20. An estimated 4% of college-age women have bulimia nervosa. About 10% of cases occur in men. However, most diagnoses of bulimia nervosa rely on self-reports, so the disorder may be much more widespread than commonly thought.

COMMON BEHAVIORS OF BULIMIA NERVOSA

Bingeing and purging (via vomiting) was evident in pre-Christian Roman times but was practiced in a group setting. The eating disorder bulimia nervosa is generally practiced in private. It was first described in the medical literature in 1979.

Bulimia nervosa involves episodes of binge eating followed by various means to rid the body of excess calories. Susceptible people often have genetic factors and lifestyle patterns that predispose them to becoming overweight, and many try frequent weight-reduction diets as teenagers. The person with bulimia nervosa may think of food constantly; however, unlike the person with anorexia nervosa, who turns away from food when faced with problems, the person with bulimia nervosa turns toward food in critical situations. Also, unlike those with anorexia nervosa, people with bulimia nervosa recognize their behavior as abnormal.

Individuals with bulimia nervosa tend to be impulsive, which may be expressed in behaviors such as stealing, increased sexual activity, drug and alcohol abuse (see the Newsworthy Nutrition in this section), self-mutilation, or attempted suicide. Some experts have suggested that part of the problem may actually arise from an inability to control responses to impulse and desire. Approximately half of the people with bulimia nervosa have major depression. Lingering effects of child abuse may be one reason for these feelings. Many people with bulimia nervosa report that they have been sexually abused. They appear competent to outsiders, while they actually feel out of control, ashamed, and frustrated.

For intake to qualify as a binge, an atypically large amount of food must be consumed in a short time and the person must exhibit a lack of control over the behavior. Among sufferers of bulimia nervosa, bingeing often alternates with attempts to rigidly restrict food intake. Elaborate food rules are common, such as avoiding all sweets. Thus, eating just one cookie or doughnut may cause individuals with this disorder to feel as though they have broken a rule. At that point, in the mind of a person with bulimia, the objectionable food must be eliminated. Usually this leads to further overeating, partly because it is easier to regurgitate a large amount of food than a small amount.

Binge-compensate cycles may be practiced daily, weekly, or across longer intervals. A specific time often is set aside. Most binge eating occurs at night, when other people are less likely to interrupt, and usually lasts from 30 minutes to 2 hours. A binge can be triggered by stress, boredom, loneliness, depression, or any combination thereof. It often follows a period of strict dieting and thus can be linked to intense hunger. The binge is not at all like normal eating; once begun, it seems to propel itself. The person not only loses control but generally does not even taste or enjoy food during a binge. This separates the practice from overeating.

Most commonly, individuals with bulimia consume cakes, cookies, ice cream, and other high-carbohydrate convenience foods during binges because these foods can be purged relatively easily and comfortably by vomiting. In a single binge, foods supplying 3000 kcal or more may be eaten. Compensatory behaviors follow in hopes that no weight will be gained; however, even when vomiting follows the binge, 33% to 75% of the calories taken in are still absorbed, inevitably causing some weight gain. When laxatives or enemas are

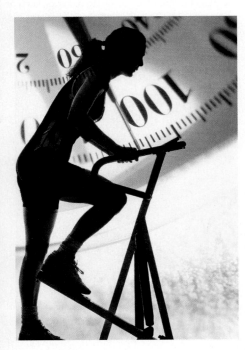

▲ Excessive exercise can be one component of bulimia if it is used as a way to offset the calorie intake from a binge. Exercise is considered excessive when it is done at inappropriate times or settings, or when a person does it despite injury or other medical complications.
©Comstock Images RF

used, about 90% of the calories are absorbed, as laxatives act in the large intestine, beyond the point of most nutrient absorption. The belief that purging soon after bingeing will prevent excessive calorie absorption and weight gain is a misconception.

At the onset of bulimia nervosa, sufferers often induce vomiting by placing their fingers deep into the mouth. They may bite down on these fingers inadvertently, resulting in bite marks and scars around the knuckles, a characteristic sign of this disorder. Once the disease is established, however, a person may be able to vomit simply by contracting the abdominal muscles. Vomiting may also occur spontaneously.

Another way a person with bulimia may attempt to compensate for a binge is by engaging in excessive exercise to expend a large amount of calories. In this practice, referred to as "debting," individuals try to estimate the amount of calories eaten during a binge and then exercise to counteract the excess.

People with bulimia nervosa are not proud of their behavior. After a binge, they usually feel guilty and depressed. Over time, they experience low self-esteem, feel hopeless about their situation, and are caught in a vicious cycle of obsession (Fig. 11-2). Compulsive lying, shoplifting to obtain food, and drug abuse can further intensify these feelings. A person discovered in the act of bingeing by a friend or family member may order the intruder to "get out" and "go away." Sufferers gradually distance themselves from others, spending more time preoccupied by and engaging in bingeing and compensating.

Because individuals with bulimia nervosa attempt to hide their behaviors, it may be difficult to identify them early in the disease process, when treatment is likely to be most effective. An early warning sign of bulimia is frequent trips to the bathroom during or after meals. To cover the sounds of vomiting, these individuals may run the bathroom fan or turn on the shower. Despite efforts to disguise the behavior with air fresheners, mouthwash, or breath mints, there may be a lingering odor of vomit. Be suspicious of packages or receipts for laxatives, diuretics, diet pills, or enemas. People who use exercise to compensate for binges are usually preoccupied with their workout schedule or might seem extremely stressed when they are unable to exercise. If you suspect someone is falling victim to bulimia nervosa, encourage the individual to get professional help. Early intervention can prevent some of the serious physical health effects described next.

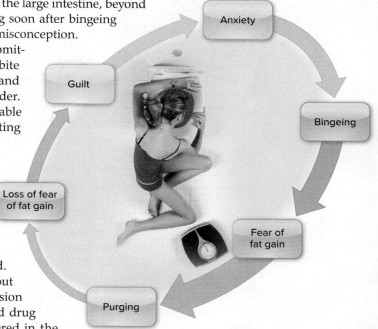

FIGURE 11-2 ▲ Bulimia nervosa's vicious cycle of obsession. ©Peter Dazeley/Getty Images

PHYSICAL EFFECTS OF BULIMIA NERVOSA

Repeated vomiting is a physically destructive method of purging. Indeed, the majority of health problems associated with bulimia nervosa, as noted here, arise from vomiting:[16]

- Repeated exposure of teeth to stomach acid causes demineralization (Fig. 11-3), making the teeth painful and sensitive to heat, cold, and acids. Eventually, the teeth may decay severely, erode away from fillings, and fall out. Dental professionals are sometimes the first health professionals to notice signs of bulimia nervosa.
- Blood potassium can drop significantly with regular vomiting or the use of certain diuretics. This can disturb the heart's rhythm and even produce sudden death.
- Salivary glands may swell as a result of infection and irritation from persistent vomiting.
- Ulcers, bleeding, and perforations may develop in the stomach or esophagus.
- Constipation may result as a complication of frequent laxative use.

The mortality rate for patients with bulimia nervosa is estimated around 0.4%. Patients with anorexia are about five times more likely to die from their disease than those with bulimia nervosa. Nonetheless, bulimia is a serious and potentially debilitating disorder that can lead to death, usually from suicide, cardiac arrest, or overwhelming infections.

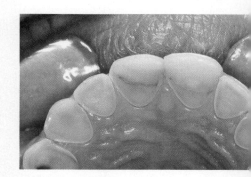

FIGURE 11-3 ▲ Dental erosion resulting from frequent episodes of self-induced vomiting by a patient with bulimia nervosa. Courtesy of Carl M. Allen, DDS, MSD

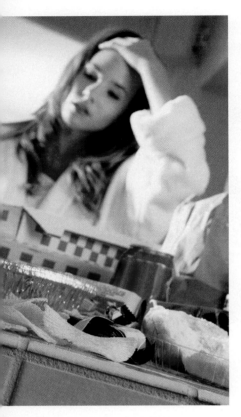

Developing regular eating habits helps a person with bulimia nervosa to stop the binge-purge cycle. ©Royalty-Free/CORBIS

TREATMENT FOR THE PERSON WITH BULIMIA NERVOSA

Therapy for bulimia nervosa, as for anorexia nervosa, requires a team of experienced clinicians.[15] Individuals with bulimia nervosa are less likely than those with anorexia nervosa to enter treatment in a state of semistarvation. However, if a person with bulimia nervosa has lost significant weight, this must be treated before psychological treatment begins. Although clinicians have yet to agree on the best therapy for bulimia nervosa, they generally agree that treatment should last at least 16 weeks. Hospitalization may be indicated in cases of extreme laxative abuse, regular vomiting, substance abuse, and depression, especially if physical harm is evident.

Nutritional Therapy Nutritional counseling by a registered dietitian nutritionist has two main goals: reestablishing regular eating habits and correcting misconceptions about food.

In general, the focus is not on stopping bingeing and purging per se, but on developing regular eating habits. Once this is achieved, the binge-purge cycle should start to break down. Initially, the registered dietitian nutritionist must help the person to decrease the amount of food in a binge. This will decrease the risk of esophageal tears from related purging by vomiting. A decrease in the frequency of this type of purging will also decrease damage to the teeth. Next, to develop a normal eating pattern, some specialists encourage their patients to develop daily meal plans and keep a food diary in which they record food intake, internal sensations of hunger, environmental factors that precipitate binges, and thoughts and feelings that accompany binge-compensate cycles.

Avoiding binge foods and not constantly stepping on a scale may be recommended early in treatment. Setting time limits for the completion of meals and snacks can also be important for people with eating disorders. Many individuals with bulimia eat quickly and have trouble interpreting satiety cues. Suggesting that they put their utensil down after each bite is a behavioral technique that a therapist might try

Newsworthy Nutrition

Substance use among adolescents with eating disorders

Previous research suggests a relationship between eating disorders and substance use. Between 2001 and 2012, researchers collected data from 290 adolescents (ages 12 to 18) with eating disorders who sought treatment at the University of Chicago Medical Center. Analyses showed that 24.6% of adolescents with anorexia nervosa and 48.7% of adolescents with bulimia nervosa had used substances. Alcohol was most commonly used, followed by cannabis, tobacco, and other illicit drugs. Binge drinking was reported by 27.5% of those who used alcohol. Substance use in this cohort was lower than use reported for the general population of adolescents, but this may be due to underreporting or the relatively young sample. It is notable that substance use was twice as common among adolescents with bulimia compared to anorexia. As hypothesized, the authors found that frequency of binge-purge cycles was directly related to substance use among adolescents with bulimia nervosa. The authors pointed out that the impulsive and risky nature of alcohol, tobacco, and other drug use is consistent with some behavioral traits of bulimia nervosa, which may be related to disruptions in neuroendocrine pathways. It is imperative to identify these behaviors early because the coexistence of eating disorders with substance use greatly increases health risks for adolescents.

Source: Mann AP, et al. "Factors associated with substance use in adolescents with eating disorders," *Journal of Adolescent Health* 55:182, 2014.

during recovery for bulimia. (In comparison, many people with anorexia eat in an excessively slow manner—for example, taking 1 hour to eat a muffin cut into tiny, bite-size pieces.)

Providing accurate information about bulimia nervosa and its consequences can help affected individuals to recognize the need to change the behavior. Over the long term, individuals are discouraged from following strict rules about dieting because this mimics the typical obsessive attitudes associated with bulimia nervosa. Rather, they must learn to honor internal hunger and satiety cues and to choose a variety of foods from each food group.

Psychological Therapy The primary aim of psychotherapy is to improve people's self-acceptance and to help them be less concerned about body weight. Cognitive behavioral therapy is generally used. Psychotherapy helps correct the all-or-none mentality that is typical of people with bulimia nervosa: "If I eat one cookie, I'm a failure and might as well binge." The premise of this psychotherapy is that if abnormal attitudes and beliefs can be altered, normal eating will follow. In addition, the therapist guides the person in establishing food habits that will minimize bingeing: to avoid fasting, to eat regular meals, and to use alternative methods—other than eating—to cope with stressful situations. Another goal of therapy is to help the person with bulimia to accept some depression and self-doubt as normal. Group therapy can be useful to foster strong social support.

> The binge-purge cycle can create an initial state of euphoria in the person. Giving up this euphoria has been equated to giving up an addiction.

Pharmacological Therapy Although pharmacological agents should not be used as the sole treatment for bulimia nervosa, studies indicate that some medications may be beneficial in conjunction with other therapies. Fluoxetine (Prozac)® is the only antidepressant that has been approved by the FDA for use in the treatment of bulimia nervosa (in combination with psychological therapy). It can help to increase feelings of satiety after eating and thereby reduce the frequency of binges. (Women of childbearing age should be cautious because fluoxetine has been linked to increased rates of miscarriages and other complications of pregnancy.) Physicians also may prescribe other similar forms of antidepressants, other classes of psychiatric medications, or certain antiseizure medications (e.g., topiramate [Topamax]).®

People with bulimia nervosa must recognize that they have a serious disorder that can have grave medical complications if not treated. Relapse is likely, so therapy should be long term. As seen with anorexia, earlier intervention and longer duration of treatment are associated with better outcomes. After just 1 year of therapy, about one-fourth of patients with bulimia nervosa experience recovery, but most will require many years of therapy. Those with bulimia nervosa need professional help because of their depression and high risk for suicide. About 50% of people with bulimia nervosa recover completely from the disorder. Others continue to struggle with it to varying degrees for a lifetime. Such a difficult course of treatment underscores the need for prevention.

✓ CONCEPT CHECK 11.3

1. Describe the eating behaviors of bulimia nervosa. What triggers them? What distinguishes them from simple overeating at a holiday meal?

2. What is a compensatory behavior? List at least three examples of inappropriate compensatory behaviors.

3. Describe at least three physical effects of bulimia nervosa.

4. Outline the basic components of nutritional therapy for people with bulimia nervosa. How do psychological and pharmacological therapies contribute to recovery?

Up to 25% of college-age women exhibit some degree of binge eating. Such behavior may have a negative impact on physical appearance, health, social life, and academics.

11.4 Binge Eating Disorder

First officially described in 1994, binge eating disorder is a growing, complex, and serious problem. Generally, binge eating disorder can be defined as binge eating episodes not accompanied by compensatory behaviors (as seen in bulimia nervosa) at least one time per week, on average, for at least 3 months. The diagnostic criteria for binge eating disorder are listed in Table 11-3.

While anorexia and bulimia disproportionately affect females, about 40% of people with binge eating disorder are males. For adults, the lifetime prevalence of binge eating disorder is estimated to be about 3.5% for women and about 2.0% for men. Among the general U.S. population, about 4 million have this disorder. However, many more people in the general population are likely to have less severe forms of the disorder that do not meet all the criteria described in Table 11-3. The number of cases of binge eating disorder is far greater than that of either anorexia nervosa or bulimia nervosa. This disorder is most common among the severely obese and those with a long history of frequent restrictive dieting, although obesity is not a criterion for having binge eating disorder. Compared to anorexia and bulimia, binge eating disorder tends to be diagnosed later in life, usually in the late 40s or early 50s.

Like anorexia and bulimia, binge eating disorder seems to arise when a person with a genetic predisposition for the disorder is stressed by an environmental trigger, such as emotional stress. Individuals with binge eating disorder may have disruptions in neurotransmitter function or altered activity in the part of the brain that responds to rewarding stimuli. There is a strong association between binge eating disorder and other psychological disorders, especially anxiety, depression, and addiction.[3,4]

COMMON BEHAVIORS OF BINGE EATING DISORDER

As described, a binge refers to the uncontrolled consumption of an unusually large amount of food within a discrete period of time. A binge can include any food, but most often consists of foods that carry the social stigma of "junk" or "bad" foods—ice cream, cookies, sweets, potato chips, and similar snack foods. During binges, food is eaten without regard to biological need and often in a recurrent, ritualized fashion. Unlike those with bulimia nervosa, people with binge eating disorder do not attempt to purge the excess calories.

Binge eating is usually triggered by negative emotions, such as stress, anxiety, loneliness, grief, or anger.[17] In fact, almost half of those with severe binge eating disorder

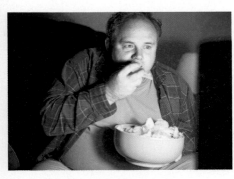

▲ Some experts describe binge eating disorder as an addiction to food, involving psychological dependence. The person becomes attached to the behavior and is driven to continue it, senses only limited control over it, and persists at it despite negative consequences. ©Ryan McVay/Getty Images RF

TABLE 11-3 ■ Diagnostic Criteria for Binge Eating Disorder

A. Recurrent binge eating, characterized by:
  1. Eating a large amount of food in a short period of time (e.g., within 2 hours)
  2. Experiencing a loss of control over eating during binges

B. Episodes of binge eating are associated with at least three of the following:
  1. Rapid rate of eating
  2. Continuing to eat beyond feelings of fullness
  3. Overeating in the absence of hunger
  4. Eating alone to avoid embarrassment
  5. Feelings of self-disgust, depression, or guilt after overeating

C. Extreme distress about binge eating

D. Binges occur at least one time per week for 3 months.

E. Behaviors are distinct from bulimia nervosa and anorexia nervosa.

Source: American Psychiatric Association, *Diagnostic and Statistical Manual for Mental Disorders*, 5e, 2013, American Psychiatric Association.

exhibit clinical depression. Often, people with binge eating disorder have not learned to express or appropriately deal with their feelings, so they turn to food to cope with stress or meet emotional needs. Those who regularly practice binge eating may grow up nurturing others instead of themselves, avoiding their own feelings and taking little time for themselves. Unfortunately, unresolved conflicts and unmet emotional needs will resurface. To make matters worse, binge eating itself brings added feelings of guilt, embarrassment, and shame.

Typically, binge eaters isolate themselves and eat large quantities of a favorite food. For example, a person might find comfort in consuming large quantities of food—such as a whole pizza in one sitting—when an emotional setback occurs. Other people with this disorder eat food continually over an extended period, called grazing. For instance, someone with a stressful or frustrating job might come home every night and graze until bedtime.

Many people with binge eating disorder have struggled to lose weight throughout their lives. As noted in Section 7.6, overly restrictive diets can lead to hunger and a sense of deprivation that triggers binge eating. People with binge eating disorder tend to perceive themselves as hungry more often than normal. During periods when little food is eaten, they get very hungry and obsessive about food. Restricting favorite foods, such as chocolate, leads to feelings of deprivation. When these individuals finally give themselves permission to eat a forbidden food or loosen up a rigid meal plan, they feel driven to eat in a compulsive, uncontrolled way. People with binge eating disorder usually began this cycle of strict dieting alternating with binge eating during adolescence or in their early twenties and have had little success with traditional weight-control programs.

PHYSICAL EFFECTS OF BINGE EATING DISORDER

Although obesity is not among the criteria for diagnosis of binge eating disorder, about 70% of those with the disorder are obese. The physical effects of the disorder reflect the comorbid conditions of obesity, which were extensively described in Table 7-2. The most deadly physical effects are listed here:

- Hypertension from excess body weight and high sodium intake
- Elevated cholesterol levels, which contribute to atherosclerosis (Binge eating may have a more severe effect on blood lipids than simply overeating by grazing throughout the day because large meals are linked to high insulin and high triglycerides.)
- Cardiovascular disease, which contributes to deaths from heart attacks and strokes
- Type 2 diabetes, which is strongly linked to obesity (An estimated one in five women with type 2 diabetes exhibits binge eating behaviors.)

TREATMENT FOR THE PERSON WITH BINGE EATING DISORDER

Approximately 30% of participants in organized weight-control programs have binge eating disorder. This means registered dietitian nutritionists and others who lead weight-management programs may be the first to identify binge eating disorder among their clients. As with anorexia and bulimia, binge eating disorder truly is a psychological problem with nutritional consequences. The success of traditional weight-loss therapies for people with binge eating disorder has been poor because these approaches fail to address the underlying psychological causes of the disorder. True, people with binge eating disorder will likely benefit from increased nutrition knowledge, but unless they find a way to manage or overcome negative emotions that underlie eating behaviors, the success of attempts to improve food choices and increase physical activity will be short lived. Thus, first addressing the psychological needs of individuals with binge eating disorder is essential to successful treatment.

The primary goal of treatment for people with binge eating disorder is to decrease and eventually eliminate episodes of binge eating. Losing excess body weight, alleviating

Mindfulness meditation is another strategy being studied to address the psychological issues that lead to bingeing. Mindful eating programs train a person to become aware of, accept, and acknowledge the daily experiences that can be triggers for binge eating but not to respond with emotional eating. Early studies show beneficial effects on body weight, stress, and symptoms of depression (review the discussion of mindful eating in Section 7.8).[19]

comorbid conditions of obesity, and improving psychological disturbances are secondary goals of therapy.[18]

Psychological Therapy Similar to treatments for bulimia nervosa, there is growing evidence that cognitive behavioral therapy techniques are useful for overcoming binge eating disorder. Many people with binge eating disorder may experience difficulty in identifying personal emotional needs and expressing emotions. This problem is a common predisposing factor in binge eating, so communication issues should be addressed during treatment. Binge eaters often must be helped to recognize their buried emotions in anxiety-producing situations and then encouraged to share them with their therapist or therapy group. Learning simple but appropriate phrases to say to oneself can help stop bingeing when the desire is strong. Even if negative situations cannot be changed, people must learn how to adapt to and bear with them effectively—not through self-destructive binge eating behaviors.

Cognitive behavioral therapy can be delivered in many forms. One-on-one sessions with a therapist and group therapy are the most common methods. Self-help groups such as Overeaters Anonymous® can also help. Their treatment philosophy, which parallels that of Alcoholics Anonymous,® is to create an environment of encouragement and accountability to overcome this eating disorder. Recently, even web-based adaptations of cognitive behavioral therapy have proved to be useful.

Although psychological therapy has been valuable for correcting binge eating behavior, it is not always successful at inducing weight loss among a population of overweight and obese individuals who may have one or more other health issues related to obesity. Thus, nutrition therapy is an important part of treatment for binge eating disorder.[18]

Nutrition Therapy Once effective coping mechanisms are learned, the registered dietitian nutritionist can educate the patient on developing normal eating patterns and making healthful food choices. First, those with binge eating disorder must learn to eat in response to hunger—a biological signal—rather than in response to emotional needs or external factors (such as the time of day, boredom, or the simple presence of food). Counselors often direct binge eaters to record their perceptions of physical hunger throughout the day and at the beginning and end of every meal. These people must learn to respond to a prescribed amount of fullness at each meal.

Individuals recovering from binge eating disorder should initially avoid weight-loss diets because feelings of food deprivation can trigger binge eating. Even if exposure to favorite binge foods is limited in the early stages of treatment, many experts feel that learning to eat all foods—but in moderation—is an effective long-term goal for people with binge eating disorder. This practice can prevent the feelings of desperation and deprivation that come from limiting particular foods.

Pharmacological Therapy Psychological and nutritional therapies are useful tools to treat binge eating disorder, but they are not 100% effective. Thus, there is growing interest in drug therapy.[18] As of 2015, the first drug to be approved for treatment of binge eating disorder is lisdexamfetamine dimesylate (Vyvanse),® a stimulant that has been used to treat attention-deficit hyperactivity disorder. Some antidepressants (e.g., fluoxetine [Prozac]® and duloxetine [Cymbalta])® and antiseizure medications (e.g., topamirate [Topamax])® have also demonstrated some success in reducing binge eating. Despite their usefulness for reducing binge eating, these medications still may not induce significant weight loss. Orlistat (Xenical)® and phentermine (Adipex-P),® discussed in Section 7.9, can assist with weight-loss efforts after binge eating is under control. The newest weight-loss medication, lorcaserin (Belviq),® has yet to be extensively tested for treatment of binge eating disorder.

Given the similarities between binge eating and other addictive behaviors, medications used to treat substance abuse (e.g., naltrexone) are being studied for use among patients with binge eating disorder. Another novel therapy that is currently being studied is Namenda,® which is used in patients with Alzheimer's disease.

ASK THE RDN   Intermittent Fasting

Dear RDN: I have had bad luck with traditional diets, but I've heard rave reviews of the "Fast Diet." Is an intermittent fasting program a good way to lose weight and keep it off?

There are three basic methods of intermittent fasting: whole-day fasting, alternate-day fasting, and time-restricted feeding. The definition of *fasting* can vary from one plan to the next; some plans allow only calorie-free beverages and sugar-free gum during fasts, whereas other plans recommend reducing energy intake to 20% to 25% of your usual intake (i.e., a modified fast) on fast days. Plans also differ in recommendations for food choices during feeding phases; some prescribe specific calorie and nutrient goals, while others allow unrestricted food intake during feeding phases. Proponents of intermittent fasting recommend that a person experiment to find the method that best fits his or her lifestyle.

With whole-day fasting, like the "Fast Diet," you would eat normally on most days of the week but undertake a complete or modified fast 1 or 2 days each week. With alternate-day fasting, days of normal eating alternate with complete or modified fasts. For time-restricted feeding protocols, you would delay the first meal of the day to achieve a fast of 14 to 20 hours (including overnight), but an unrestricted feeding period would be allowed for the remaining hours of the day.

Besides weight loss, purported benefits of intermittent fasting include improved insulin sensitivity, enhanced ability to use fat for energy, decreased triglyceride levels, and reduced inflammation—changes that may potentially decrease risks for chronic diseases and lead to a longer life. Much of the research to date, however, has been conducted in animals, with few controlled studies in humans.

Reviews of current (although sparse) studies of the effects of intermittent fasting suggest that it may be a reasonable alternative to the traditional weight-loss method of moderate daily calorie restriction for some people.[20,21] Weight loss and improvements in metabolic effects are similar with these two weight-loss methods. However, intermittent fasting is not a good fit for everyone. If you struggle with blood sugar control (e.g., hypoglycemia or diabetes) or are pregnant, you should not attempt intermittent fasting. Quite predictably, some side effects of any fasting regimen include hunger, headaches, fatigue, and irritability. Some critics of intermittent fasting point out that underfeeding in this way could lead to nutrient deficiencies. We, as registered dietitian nutritionists, can help you choose nutrient-dense foods during the feeding phases of any of these dietary patterns. Also, there is some concern that prolonged fasting may decrease your metabolic rate, which would make long-term weight maintenance very difficult. Because we have limited data on the long-term safety of intermittent fasting, it is not clear how much fasting is too much. Fasting too frequently may result in malnutrition, reduced immune function, organ damage, or eating disorders.

Wait—*eating disorders?*

Take a step back and look at the basic dietary patterns advocated here. Much like the dietary patterns of individuals with anorexia nervosa, intermittent fasting programs involve calorie counting and extended periods of hunger. For some plans, foods are classified as "safe" or "off limits," which promotes an unhealthy, dichotomous view of foods and ties eating into emotions such as guilt, shame, and fear. Intermittent fasting programs that advise fasting (deprivation) followed by several hours or days of unrestricted eating (indulgence) may foster binge eating. Participants may feel as if they've failed themselves and others when they have trouble adhering to a strict regimen. For a person who already exhibits anxiety, depression, or obsessive traits, intermittent fasting may be a gateway to pathological dieting and eating disorders.

Although intermittent fasting may be a reasonable alternative to daily moderate calorie restriction for some people, more research is needed to determine which protocol is best and if mental and physical health are affected over the long term. If you are determined to try intermittent fasting, continue to seek the advice of a registered dietitian nutritionist to ensure that your dietary pattern still meets your nutritional needs. Importantly, if you tend to obsess about food and body weight or you already have problems with depression or anxiety, steer clear of this dietary pattern. Recall what you learned in Section 11.1: eating disorders often begin with a simple diet. If efforts to control weight begin to interfere with daily activities and are linked to physiological and emotional changes, professional help will be needed to treat an eating disorder.

Fueling, not fasting,

Angela Collene, MS, RDN, LD, Author

Overall, people who have binge eating disorder are usually unsuccessful in controlling it on their own. Furthermore, unrecognized binge eating disorder will undermine the success of weight-loss therapies among many overweight and obese individuals who do seek professional help. By asking questions about eating patterns, feelings of loss of control over eating behaviors, and feelings of guilt after eating, health professionals can screen weight-loss clients for binge eating disorder and refer affected individuals to appropriate treatments.

> ✅ CONCEPT CHECK 11.4
>
> 1. What differentiates binge eating disorder from bulimia nervosa?
> 2. List at least three health effects that may result from binge eating disorder.
> 3. Why do people with binge eating disorder have little success in traditional weight-loss programs?

11.5 Other Eating Disorders

Besides those already covered, there are several lesser-known types of eating disorders. Some of these, such as **pica** (discussed next), rumination disorder, and avoidant/restrictive food intake disorder (discussed in Section 15.4), are distinct eating disorders with their own sets of diagnostic criteria. In *DSM-5*, the category of Other Specified Feeding or Eating Disorders encompasses several disorders that do not meet all of the criteria for diagnosis of anorexia, bulimia, or binge eating disorder. These include several categories of subthreshold eating disorders, **purging disorder,** and **night eating syndrome.**

PICA

Pica, which will be mentioned again in Section 14.5 as it relates to pregnancy, is a disorder in which a person persistently eats nonnutritive, nonfood substances over a period of at least 1 month. A few examples of nonfood substances ingested by people with pica are clay, dirt, ice, chalk, or wood. Pica could lead to some serious health consequences, including microbial infections, poisoning from toxins present in the nonfood material, gastrointestinal blockages, or nutrient deficiencies (in cases when nonfood substances displace nutritive foods in the diet). Pica tends to co-occur with other mental disorders, such as autism or obsessive-compulsive disorder.

OTHER SPECIFIED FEEDING OR EATING DISORDERS

Subthreshold Eating Disorders Individuals who meet some but not all of the criteria for diagnosis with anorexia nervosa, bulimia nervosa, or binge eating disorder may fall into one of five subthreshold classifications. For example, **atypical anorexia nervosa** describes a person who meets most of the criteria for diagnosis of anorexia nervosa but whose weight is still within a normal range. This could occur if an overweight person has just begun severely restricting calories. Despite significant weight loss, BMI may still fall within the healthy range of 18.5 to 24.9. Other diagnoses in this category include cases of bulimia nervosa or binge eating disorder in which episodes of binge eating occur less than once per week (**bulimia nervosa of low frequency** or **binge eating disorder of low frequency**) or have taken place for less than 3 months (**bulimia nervosa of limited duration** or **binge eating disorder of limited duration).**

Purging Disorder Purging disorder is the name given to the behavior of people who repeatedly purge (i.e., vomit) to promote weight loss even in the absence of binge eating.[22] This disorder is related to body dissatisfaction, anxiety, and depression. The physical effects of purging disorder are the same as those of bulimia nervosa and include dental problems, mouth sores, damage to the esophagus, constipation, dehydration, electrolyte imbalances, and overall malnutrition.

pica The practice of eating nonfood items, such as dirt, laundry starch, or clay.

purging disorder An eating disorder characterized by repeated purging (e.g., by self-induced vomiting) to induce weight loss even in the absence of binge eating.

night eating syndrome Eating a lot of food in the late evening and nocturnal awakenings with ingestion of food.

atypical anorexia nervosa A subthreshold eating disorder in which a person meets most of the criteria for diagnosis of anorexia nervosa, except weight is within a normal range.

bulimia nervosa of low frequency A form of other specified feeding or eating disorders in which a person meets all of the criteria for diagnosis of bulimia nervosa, except the frequency of binge-compensate cycles is less than once per week.

binge eating disorder of low frequency A form of other specified feeding or eating disorders in which a person meets all of the criteria for diagnosis of binge eating disorder—except the frequency of binges is less than once per week.

bulimia nervosa of limited duration A form of other specified feeding or eating disorders in which a person meets all of the criteria for diagnosis of bulimia nervosa—except the duration of the disordered eating behavior is less than 3 months.

binge eating disorder of limited duration A form of other specified feeding or eating disorders in which a person meets all of the criteria for diagnosis of binge eating disorder—except the duration of the disordered eating behavior is less than 3 months.

Night Eating Syndrome Night eating syndrome is characterized by recurrent episodes of night eating, manifested by eating after awakening from sleep or by excessive food consumption after the evening meal. With night eating syndrome, the person is fully aware of and able to recall the behavior, which results in marked distress. Although night eating syndrome was first observed among obese patients, it also occurs among nonobese people. It has been estimated to occur in 1.5% of the general population and in 8.9% of patients treated in obesity clinics; it tends to co-occur with other eating disorders. Some typical signs and symptoms of night eating syndrome include:

- Not feeling hungry in the morning and delaying the first meal until several hours after waking
- Overeating in the evening with more than 25% of daily food intake consumed after dinner
- Difficulty falling asleep and a need to eat something to help fall asleep faster
- Waking at least once during the night with a need to eat to be able to fall asleep again
- Eating behaviors produce feelings of guilt and shame
- Feeling depressed, especially at night

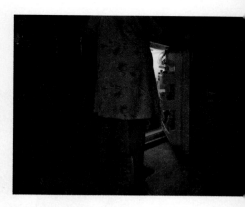

▲ Night eating syndrome is characterized by waking at least once during the night and needing to eat to be able to fall asleep again.
©Jim Corwin/ Alamy

Research shows that the circadian rhythm (your body's 24-hour clock) of food intake appears to be disturbed in night eating syndrome. Studies have also shown that night eating syndrome is prevalent among outpatients with sleep apnea, restless leg syndrome, or some psychiatric conditions. Behavioral changes, such as establishing and monitoring the sleep-wake schedule and performing regular exercise, can help. Symptoms are significantly improved with use of the antidepressant sertraline (Zoloft).®

✓ CONCEPT CHECK 11.5

1. List three ways pica could harm health.
2. Describe three different cases in which a person would be diagnosed with subthreshold eating disorders.
3. How is purging disorder similar to bulimia nervosa? How do these two disorders differ?
4. List three characteristics of night eating syndrome.

11.6 Additional Disordered Eating Patterns

There is a growing number of other patterns of disordered eating that have not yet been classified by *DSM-5* but are worthy of mention. Some of the patterns mentioned in this section, such as **female athlete triad,** have been the subject of much research. Others have been discussed mainly in popular media, yet health practitioners report encountering them regularly. Continued research is required to establish a set of diagnostic criteria, describe the course of the disorder, and establish evidence-based treatments.

female athlete triad A condition characterized by low energy availability, lack of menstrual periods (amenorrhea), and osteoporosis.

FEMALE ATHLETE TRIAD

Mentioned in Section 10.4, females participating in appearance-based and endurance sports are at heightened risk of developing eating disorders. One study of college-age female athletes found that 15% of swimmers, 62% of gymnasts, and 32% of varsity athletes exhibited disordered eating patterns.

Food restriction and stress can precipitate irregular menstruation among female athletes. When body fat is low, estrogen production decreases. Remember from Section 9.6, estrogen stimulates osteoblasts (bone-forming cells). In this way, low body fat impairs bone health. Some of these young women have bone mass measurements equivalent to those of 50- to 60-year-olds. This increases the risk for bone fractures during sports and general activities.

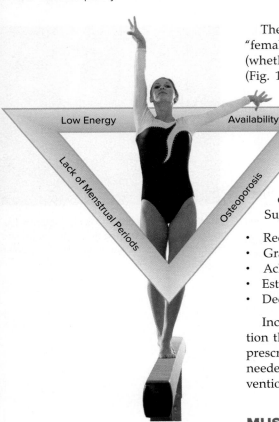

The American College of Sports Medicine (ACSM) has named this syndrome "female athlete triad" because it consists of three parts: low energy availability (whether intentional or unintentional), lack of menstrual periods, and osteoporosis (Fig. 11-4). Many coaches, trainers, and even some health professionals mistakenly believe that loss of menstrual periods is a normal consequence of a high level of physical activity. To combat misinformation, the ACSM has issued a plea to teachers, coaches, health professionals, and parents to educate female athletes about the triad and its health consequences.[23]

Those exhibiting symptoms of the female athlete triad should seek treatment from a multidisciplinary team of health professionals. Involving the coach or trainer in therapy is usually a key factor in the success of the treatment plan. Suggestions for treatment are as follows:

- Reduce preoccupation with food, weight, and body fat.
- Gradually increase meals and snacks to an appropriate amount.
- Achieve an appropriate weight for height.
- Establish regular menstrual periods.
- Decrease training time and/or intensity by 10% to 20%.

Increasing caloric intake will increase body weight and body fat. Estrogen production then increases and should stabilize bone mass. During therapy, a physician may prescribe a multivitamin and mineral supplement as well as calcium supplements as needed to maintain a daily calcium intake of 1200 to 1500 milligrams. Even with intervention, however, much of the bone loss that has already occurred is irreversible.

MUSCLE DYSMORPHIA

Muscle dysmorphia has gained attention as a psychological condition with many similarities to other eating disorders.[6,24] First identified among male bodybuilders in the 1990s, muscle dysmorphia was initially termed "reverse anorexia." Men (and some women) with this disorder perceive themselves as *too thin,* rather than too fat, and are preoccupied with strict weightlifting and diet regimens to achieve a high level of muscularity. Among high school and college-aged men, in particular, body dissatisfaction may lead to disordered eating and exercise practices.

In muscle dysmorphia, numerous hours are devoted to working out at the gym; planning and eating low-carbohydrate, high-protein meals; and keeping meticulous records of exercise, body measurements, and food intake. The dietary practices (e.g., high-volume eating, protein intakes of up to 5 grams per kilogram of body weight) and use of unproven ergogenic aids or anabolic steroids can result in physical impairment. Such exercise and eating routines also interfere with social, occupational, and recreational activities. People with muscle dysmorphia may avoid social contact, eating in restaurants, and being seen without clothes because of distress over appearing too thin. Considering its many similarities with anorexia nervosa and a tendency for people with muscle dysmorphia to cross over to other forms of eating disorders over time, some experts support recognition of muscle dysmorphia as an eating disorder.

DIABULIMIA

Adolescents with diabetes are at heightened risk of eating disorders.[22,25] As you learned in Chapter 4, when insulin is absent or when cells are insulin resistant, cells are unable to use glucose for energy. Weight loss occurs because carbohydrate calories essentially are wasted. After a person starts insulin or insulin-sensitizing therapy, cells are able to utilize glucose and store fat, so weight gain is a common side effect. About one in three teens with type 1 diabetes admits to intentionally skipping doses of insulin to induce weight loss. This practice, so-called "diabulimia," can lead to severe hyperglycemia and its myriad consequences, which include eye damage, kidney damage, diabetic coma, or

FIGURE 11-4 ▲ The female athlete triad occurs when the athlete has low energy availability (with or without an eating disorder), lack of menstrual periods, and osteoporosis. Stress fractures and chronic fatigue also occur. This triad often is seen in appearance-related sports, such as gymnastics. Long-term health is at risk; thus, prevention and early treatment are crucial. ©Juice Images Ltd/Shutterstock

The tragic case of Christy Henrich illustrates why anyone at risk for the female athlete triad should seek professional help. As a young teenager, Christy weighed 95 pounds and was 4 feet 11 inches tall. She showed promise as a gymnast but was told that she was too fat to excel in gymnastics. Christy continued her training but often starved herself, some days consuming just an apple and frequently purging by vomiting. Christy's eating disorder eventually rendered her too weak to compete. She was hospitalized after her weight had dropped to 47 pounds. She died, just after her twenty-second birthday, from the effects of long-term semistarvation.

death. On the other hand, about one in five teens with type 1 diabetes uses overdoses of insulin to compensate for episodes of binge eating, a practice that could lead to dangerously low levels of blood sugar. Among adolescents with type 2 diabetes, up to 25% show signs of binge eating disorder. For youth with diabetes, evidence of poor blood sugar control, frequently missed clinic visits, and the presence of depression can be warning signs of eating disorders.

ORTHOREXIA

As you have learned about nutrition in this course, you may have changed some of your own food choices. Obviously, a focus on healthy eating can help with weight management and prevention of disease, but when strict food rules begin to interfere with everyday life, they can be pathological. Some people worry excessively about the availability of food they permit themselves to eat, such as low-fat, sugar-free, or organic food choices. Although not currently classified as an eating disorder, orthorexia describes an emerging condition in which healthful eating becomes an obsession.[26,27] The term comes from Greek words meaning "straight or proper appetite." Unlike cases of anorexia or bulimia, orthorexia does not usually originate in the drive for thinness. Rather, a need for perfection or purity lies at the heart of orthorexia. Such extreme dietary perfectionism may be related to obsessive-compulsive disorder. Criteria to diagnose orthorexia have been proposed. These include interference of eating behaviors with normal activities of living and social activities, feelings of guilt or anxiety when eating "forbidden" foods, and physical signs of malnutrition.

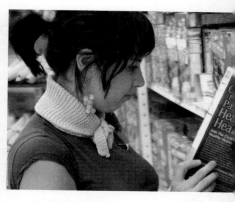

▲ Orthorexia describes a condition in which a person is unduly concerned with eating only healthful foods. ©McGraw-Hill Education/Andrew Resek, photographer

☑ CONCEPT CHECK 11.6

1. List the three components of the female athlete triad.
2. How is muscle dysmorphia similar to anorexia nervosa? How is it different?
3. What is diabulimia? List some of the harmful physical effects of such practices.
4. How would you distinguish between healthy eating and orthorexia?

11.7 Prevention of Eating Disorders

A key to developing and maintaining healthful eating behavior is to realize that some concern about diet, health, and weight is normal. It is also normal to experience variation in what we eat, how we feel, and even how much we weigh. For example, it is common to experience some minimal weight change (up to 2 to 3 pounds) throughout the day and even more over the course of a week. A large weight fluctuation or ongoing weight gain or weight loss is more likely to indicate a problem. If you notice a large change in your eating habits, how you feel, or your body weight, it is a good idea to consult your physician. Treating physical and emotional problems early helps lead you to peace of mind and good health.

With a view on society as a whole, many people begin to form opinions about food, nutrition, health, weight, and body image prior to or during puberty. Parents, friends, and professionals working with young adults should consider the following advice for preventing eating disorders:

- Discourage restrictive dieting and meal skipping. Fasting is also discouraged (except for religious occasions).
- Provide information about normal changes that occur during puberty.
- Correct misconceptions about nutrition, healthy body weight, and approaches to weight loss.
- Carefully phrase any weight-related recommendations and comments.

FARM to FORK   Apples

Grow
- Small apples (< 2 inches in diameter) are called crabapples. These are quite tart, but they are edible and actually contain more phytochemicals than larger apples.
- Apple trees can be grown from seeds, but the end product can be quite unpredictable. To ensure a desirable harvest, get a 2- or 3-year-old plant from a nursery. Advanced gardeners can try grafting a branch of an existing tree to the trunk of another apple tree.

Shop
- Many of the most common varieties of apples sold in the United States are quite low in phytochemicals. They have been bred to yield a large fruit with sweet flavor, but not necessarily for nutritional value!
- Common varieties with high phytochemical content include Cortland, Fuji, Granny Smith, and Honeycrisp. For the best phytochemical content, shop for varieties such as Haralson, Liberty, Northern Spy, and Ozark Gold at farmer's markets or specialty stores.
- Among the red apples, look for those with deep red color on all sides. This is an indication that the apples were exposed to lots of sunlight while growing. Sun exposure increases the phytochemical content of the fruit.
- When it comes to controlling calories, whole fruit is a better choice than fruit juice, but if you do shop for apple juice, choose a cloudy bottle! Filtering juice removes many healthy phytochemicals. If you hold the bottle up to the light, the juice should not be see-through and there should be some sediment at the bottom.

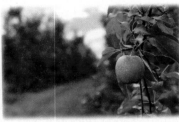
©Ingram Publishing

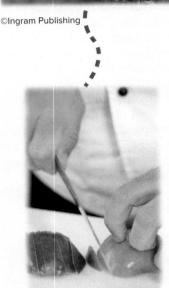
©Pixtal/AGE Fotostock

Store
- Store apples in the refrigerator, preferably in the crisper drawer, set to high humidity. These will last about 10 times longer than apples stored at room temperature.
- Apples harvested early in the season (July and August) can be stored for just 2 or 3 weeks before spoiling, but apples harvested late in the season (September, October, and November) store well for several months.

Prep
- Don't throw the skin in the compost bin! Many nutrients and phytochemicals are concentrated in the apple's skin. However, it is important to consider that apples are treated with pesticides. Scrubbing the fruit under running water is a good way to remove pesticide residues. If you can afford them, organic apples would be a great choice for reducing pesticide exposure.
- Apple skins can be pureed in a food processor and incorporated into recipes for baked treats and applesauce.
- To prevent sliced apples from browning, sprinkle with lemon juice. The citric acid inhibits the oxidase enzymes that cause browning.
- What can you do with crab apples? These small, tart fruits are excellent for use in making jams and jellies or sauces to cook with meats.

Source: Robinson J. "Apples: from potent medicine to mild-mannered clones," in *Eating on the Wild Side.* New York: Little, Brown and Company, 2013.

- Do not overemphasize numbers on a scale. Instead, teach the basics of proper nutrition and regular physical activity in school and at home.
- Encourage normal expression of disruptive emotions.
- Encourage children to eat only when they are hungry.
- Provide adolescents with an appropriate, but not unlimited, degree of independence, choice, responsibility, and self-accountability for their actions.
- Increase self-acceptance and appreciation of the power and pleasure emerging from one's body.
- Enhance tolerance for diversity in body weight and shape.
- Build respectful environments and supportive relationships.
- Encourage coaches to be sensitive to weight and body-image issues among athletes.
- Emphasize that thinness is not necessarily associated with better athletic performance.
- Support programs for eating disorder screening and prevention at high schools and colleges.

Our society as a whole can benefit from a fresh focus on nutritious food practices and a healthful outlook toward food and body weight (see Farm to Fork in this section). Not only is treatment of eating disorders far more difficult than prevention, but these disorders also have devastating effects on the entire family. For this reason, caregivers and health care professionals must emphasize the importance of an overall healthful dietary pattern that focuses on moderation, as opposed to restriction and perfection.

Overall, the challenge facing many North Americans is achieving a healthy body weight without excessive dieting. A growing number of health professionals support a nondiet approach to weight management. This means adopting and maintaining sensible eating habits, a physically active lifestyle, and realistic and positive attitudes and emotions while practicing creative ways to handle stress. Certain cultural ideals of beauty can trigger eating disorders; changing these values might reduce the pressures predisposing some people to various types of disordered eating behavior. The Health at Every Size® approach, discussed in Section 7.4, fights discrimination against overweight and obese people and asserts that each person should be free to find his or her natural weight. Women who combine careers and motherhood are saying that they have more important things to worry about. Some trendsetters in the fashion industry are tolerating more curves. We cannot change the genes that predispose people to eating disorders (at least not yet!), but we can make a difference in the environmental triggers that set these devastating disorders in motion.

These websites provide further information on eating disorders:
- Academy for Eating Disorders, www.aedweb.org
- The National Eating Disorders Association, www.nationaleatingdisorders.org
- National Institute of Mental Health's concise review of eating disorders, https://www.nimh.nih.gov/health/topics/eating-disorders/index.shtml

✓ CONCEPT CHECK 11.7

1. Why is prevention of eating disorders so important?
2. Imagine you are a coach for a high school girls' softball team. What could you do to foster an environment that prevents eating disorders among this group of adolescent girls?

Eating Disorder Reflections

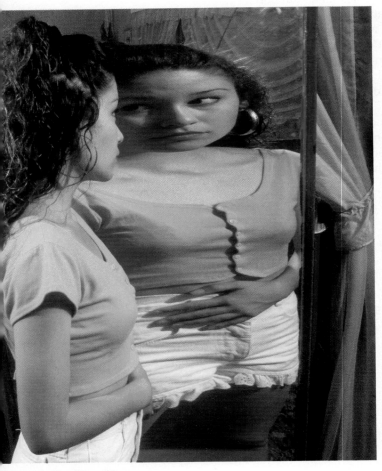

©Ted Foxx/Alamy RF

Reflections from a Woman with Anorexia Nervosa

It was the spring of my freshman year of high school, and I had just turned 15 years old. I was determined to land a leading role in the upcoming high school musical, *West Side Story*. I thought I should lose some weight to appear more attractive to the student director, Shawn, so I decided to give up "junk" food. The next day, my friend Sandra looked at my lunch, spread out neatly on a napkin before me, and squawked, "Dill pickles?! Who brings dill pickles for lunch in a Ziploc bag?" The other girls at the table fell into a fit of hysterics. "Casting for *West Side Story* is coming up," I said, "and I gave up 'junk' food to try to lose a few extra pounds." One of my friends thought it would be funny to give me one M&M—just to smell. Aren't they funny? So I put it in a little Tupperware container and kept it in my backpack as a reminder. Every once in a while, I did smell it.

For the next few weeks, there were times when I would find myself cracking open the refrigerator door and just staring at what I knew to be a deliciously crunchy, crisp, and cold Kit Kat bar in the dairy bin. I didn't eat it, though. At the mall with my friends, Bridgette and Nora wanted to stop and get a cinnamon bun. They chided me, but I didn't budge. The cinnamon bun smelled so good. But as I sat opposite them in the food court and watched them overdramatize its ooey-gooey goodness, I felt a sense of pride that I could make a decision and stick with it. I could see that they were jealous of my willpower.

When Easter came around, I took a look at the contents of the Easter basket my mom insisted on preparing and turned up my nose at it. I had proven to myself that I could resist temptation . . . why stop now?

After the musical, I started running with my friend Laura. She was getting in shape for the next season of field hockey. After school, we met in the locker room, changed out of our school clothes, and out we went. The running helped. Every morning, just after going to the bathroom and before getting any breakfast, I would pop onto the scale in my mom's bathroom. One hundred and fifteen pounds and still going. At 5 feet 7 inches, that wasn't too bad.

Cheese and butter had made it to the "no" list by the time I was 16 and down to 105 pounds. Fat-free was my mantra. For my sixteenth birthday, my friends threw a little surprise party for me. Nora, knowing I would put up a fight, made me a cake. "It's your birthday! You can have a piece of cake!" I politely said no, that I would cut it for everyone else, but I really didn't want any. They pestered me, and Nora started to feel offended, so finally I took a few bites, so she wouldn't burst into tears. It had been so long since I'd had so much sugar. I felt bloated and sick. I ate nothing for the rest of the day and only six saltines, an apple, and two stalks of celery the next day. Those foods were on the "yes" list. Salads also were okay but only with salt and vinegar. I told my parents that the dissections in biology class had given me a distaste for meat, but really, I just didn't want all those calories. For a while, I craved food day and night, but slowly, I was getting better and better at holding my ground.

By my senior year, I was skipping lunches altogether, opting instead to hang out in the library and read over my AP bio text. "Where were you at lunch today?" Bridgette would ask later. "Oh, I had some reading to do. The AP exam is going to be tough." At 100 pounds, I was getting closer to finding out what "tough" really meant.

Even though Laura moved out of state, I didn't give up on exercising. Now, my mom's stair stepper in the basement was my favorite. I'd take my biology notes, prop them up in front of me, and step-step-step until I had burned 400 kcal. I felt so efficient knowing that I could multitask. Sometimes I'd exercise twice a day. As senior year wore on, though, it got harder and harder to get up in the morning and put on my tennis shoes. And then one morning, in the shower, I just collapsed under the stream of hot water.

I ended up in this hospital bed with an IV in my arm. At 92 pounds, my body was starving. As it turns out, if you don't give your body enough fuel, you start to cannibalize yourself, in a sense. My body had been so hungry, my muscles had been wasting away, and the episode in the shower was due to a problem with my heart. It's a problem I have created . . . not my parents or my distant group of friends . . . only me. My mom was there, next to me, caressing the arm with the IV tube, putting her whole life on hold because of me. Isn't this what I'd wanted—to be in control of my own destiny?

Where do I go from here?

Thoughts of a Bulimic Woman

I am wide-awake and immediately out of bed. I think back to the night before when I made a new list of what I wanted to get done. My husband is not far behind me on his way into the bathroom to get ready for work. Maybe I can sneak onto the scale before he notices me. I am already in my private world. I am overjoyed when the scale says that I am the same weight as I was the night before, and I can feel that slightly hungry feeling. Maybe it will stop today, maybe today everything will change. What were the projects I wanted to do?

We eat the same breakfast, except that I take no butter on my toast, no cream in my coffee, and never take seconds (until he gets out the door). Today, I am going to be really good, which means eating certain predetermined portions of food and not taking one more bite than I think I am allowed. I am careful to see that I don't take more than he does. I can feel the tension building. I wish he'd hurry up and leave, so I can get going!

As soon as he shuts the door, I try to involve myself with one of the myriad of responsibilities on my list. But I hate them all! I just want to crawl into a hole. I don't want to do anything. I'd rather eat. I am alone, I am nervous, I am no good, I always do everything wrong anyway. I am not in control, I can't make it through the day—I know it. It has been the same for so long.

I remember the starchy cereal I ate for breakfast. I am back into the bathroom and onto the scale. It measures the same, but I don't want to stay the same! I want to be thinner! I look in the mirror. I think my thighs are ugly and deformed looking. I see a lumpy, clumsy, pear-shaped wimp. I feel frustrated, trapped in this body, and I don't know what to do about it.

I float to the refrigerator knowing exactly what is inside. I begin with last night's brownies. I always begin with the sweets. At first I try to make it look like nothing is missing, but my appetite is huge and I resolve to make another batch of brownies to replace the one I'm devouring. I know there is half of a bag of cookies in the trash, thrown out the night before, and I dig them out and polish them off. I drink some milk so my vomiting will be smoother. I like the full feeling I get after downing a big glass. I get out six pieces of bread and toast one side in the broiler, turn them over and cover them with butter and put them under the broiler again till they are

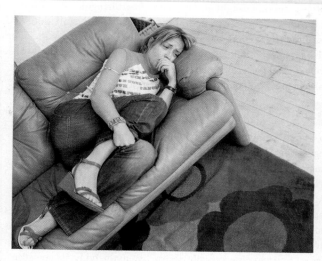

▲ Bulimic episodes add to the despair felt in this disorder. ©Royalty-Free/Corbis

bubbling. I take all six pieces on a plate to the television and go back for a bowl of cereal and a banana. Before the last toast is finished, I am already preparing the next batch of six more pieces. I might have another brownie or five from the new batch, and a couple large bowlfuls of ice cream, yogurt, or cottage cheese. My stomach is stretched into a huge ball below my rib cage. I know I'll have to go into the bathroom soon, but I want to postpone it. I am in never-never land. I am waiting, feeling the pressure, pacing the floor in and out of rooms. Time is passing. Time is passing. It is almost time.

I wander aimlessly through the living room and kitchen once more, tidying, making the whole house neat and put back together. Finally, I make the turn into the bathroom. I brace my feet, pull my hair back and stick my finger down my throat, stroking twice. I get up a huge gush of food. Three times, four, and another stream of partially digested food. I can see everything come back. I am glad to see those brownies, because they are SO fattening. The rhythm of the emptying is broken and my head is beginning to hurt. I stand up feeling dizzy, empty, and weak.

The whole episode has taken about an hour.

Source: Hall L. and Cohn L., *Bulimia—A Guide to Recovery*, Gurze Books: Carlsbad, CA. Pages xvii–xviii. Copyright ©2011 by Gurze Books. All rights reserved. Reprinted with permission.

Summary (Numbers refer to numbered sections in the chapter.)

11.1 Disordered eating encompasses mild and short-term changes in eating patterns that occur as a result of life stress, illness, or a desire to change body weight. When carried to the extreme, disordered eating may progress to an eating disorder in which severe changes in eating patterns have lasting and detrimental effects. Current research on the origins of eating disorders indicates that genetic factors dictate brain biology, which affects how certain individuals perceive their bodies and respond to life stresses. Thus, a person who is genetically predisposed to eating disorders may use disordered eating behaviors to cope with feelings of depression, anger, or guilt. The three main types of eating disorders are anorexia nervosa, bulimia nervosa, and binge eating disorder.

11.2 Anorexia nervosa is characterized by extreme weight loss (e.g., BMI of less than 17), a distorted body image, and an irrational fear of weight gain and obesity. Weight loss is achieved primarily by restricting food intake. Physical consequences include a profound decrease in body weight and body fat, heart irregularities, iron-deficiency anemia, impaired immunity, digestive dysfunction, and loss of menstrual periods. Treatment of anorexia nervosa includes increasing food intake to support gradual weight gain. Family-based psychological counseling can help anorexic individuals establish healthy eating behaviors and body image.

11.3 Similar to anorexia nervosa, bulimia is characterized by overvaluation of body weight and shape. However, the disordered eating patterns of bulimic individuals involve recurrent binge eating followed by compensatory behaviors. Binge eating is consuming an abnormally large amount of food within a short time period. A person with bulimia nervosa has lack of control over bingeing behaviors and feels extremely distressed after a binge. Inappropriate compensatory behaviors used to rid the body of excess calories include vomiting or misusing laxatives, diuretics, or enemas. Alternately, fasting and excessive exercise may be used. Vomiting as a means of purging is especially destructive to the body; it can cause severe tooth decay, stomach ulcers, irritation of the esophagus, low blood potassium, and other problems. Treatment of bulimia nervosa includes psychological and nutritional counseling. Prozac® is the only FDA-approved medication for treatment of bulimia nervosa, but other antidepressants and antiseizure medications are sometimes prescribed.

11.4 Binge eating disorder is the most widespread eating disorder. It tends to be diagnosed in middle age and affects men and women nearly equally. It is characterized by recurrent episodes of bingeing, which cause marked distress, but are not followed by compensatory behaviors. About 70% of people with binge eating disorder are obese. The health effects that stem from binge eating disorder are comorbid conditions of obesity, including hypertension, high blood cholesterol, cardiovascular disease, and type 2 diabetes. Treatment involves cognitive behavioral therapy and nutrition counseling. Vyvanse® is the only FDA-approved drug for treatment of binge eating disorder. Antidepressants and other medications may also be useful.

11.5 Pica is an eating disorder in which a person persistently ingests nonnutritive, nonfood items such as clay, dirt, or ice. Subthreshold eating disorders (e.g., atypical anorexia nervosa, bulimia nervosa of low frequency or limited duration, or binge eating disorder of low frequency or limited duration) capture those individuals who meet some but not all of the criteria for diagnosis of anorexia nervosa, bulimia nervosa, or binge eating disorder. People with purging disorder practice purging behaviors to achieve weight loss, but they do not exhibit the binge eating behaviors typical of bulimia nervosa. Individuals with night eating syndrome consume more than 25% of daily food intake after dinner, may have difficulty falling asleep without eating, and wake up at least once during the night to consume food.

11.6 Several additional disordered eating patterns that are not classified as eating disorders include the female athlete triad, muscle dysmorphia, diabulimia, and orthorexia. The female athlete triad consists of low energy availability, loss of menstrual periods, and osteoporosis. Muscle dysmorphia could be described as "reverse anorexia;" a person views him- or herself as less muscular than desired and resorts to patterns of disordered eating and obsessive exercise to achieve a muscular body shape. Diabulimia refers to the misuse of diabetes medication to regulate body weight. Some type 1 diabetic patients will skip doses of insulin to induce weight loss but then suffer the consequences of hyperglycemia. Alternatively, overdoses of insulin or glucose-lowering medications could be used to counter the effects of a binge. This practice could result in hypoglycemia. Orthorexia refers to an obsession with healthy eating such that overly restrictive food choices interfere with other aspects of life, such as social interactions.

11.7 Prevention of eating disorders is crucial because treatments are expensive, lengthy, and not 100% effective. Encouraging healthy attitudes about eating and exercise from a young age will aid in preventing the development of eating disorders. Those who work closely with children and young adults should encourage acceptance of diversity in body sizes and carefully phrase comments about body weight. Helping children to develop healthy ways to cope with emotions is also important.

11.8 Anorexia nervosa and bulimia nervosa are both biologically based disorders that are characterized by undue influence of body weight or shape on one's self-evaluation. The coping mechanisms (i.e., extreme dietary restriction versus binge-compensate cycles) used by people with these disorders can vary considerably.

Check Your Knowledge (Answers are available at the end of this question set.)

1. For 3 weeks leading up to her friend's wedding, Teresa skipped meals and restricted her food intake to 800 kcal per day so that she could fit into her bridesmaid dress. After the wedding, she resumed eating 2200 kcal per day. This is an example of
   a. disordered eating.
   b. an eating disorder.
   c. size acceptance.
   d. muscle dysmorphia.

2. Factors that could contribute to the development of eating disorders include
   a. genetics.
   b. social pressures to be thin.
   c. sexual abuse.
   d. all of these.

3. Anorexia nervosa can be defined as
   a. compulsive eating.
   b. hyperactivity.
   c. denial of appetite.
   d. purging.

4. The most likely long-term health consequence of anorexia nervosa is
   a. fractures resulting from bone loss.
   b. atherosclerotic heart disease.
   c. esophageal ulcers.
   d. cancer.

5. Bulimia is most frequently first recognized by a
   a. dietitian.
   b. physician.
   c. dentist.
   d. physical therapist.

6. The *most life-threatening* health risk from frequent vomiting due to bulimia nervosa is
   a. a drop in blood potassium.
   b. constipation.
   c. weight gain.
   d. swollen salivary glands.

7. Binge eating disorder can be characterized as
   a. bingeing accompanied by purging.
   b. secretive eating.
   c. eating to avoid feeling and dealing with emotional pain.
   d. the early phase of bulimia nervosa.

8. Night eating syndrome is characterized by
   a. eating dinner but no breakfast or lunch.
   b. the need to eat to fall asleep.
   c. waking at night to purge by vomiting.
   d. consuming all of the daily calories at night.

9. Female athlete triad consists of
   a. anorexia nervosa, lack of family support, and overtraining.
   b. disordered eating, overtraining, and lack of menstrual periods.
   c. osteoporosis, lack of menstrual periods, and low energy availability.
   d. osteoporosis, lack of sleep, and low energy availability.

10. If you were assigned to speak to a group of middle school 4-H students about healthy eating, which message would be best?
   a. Ask children to sort various snack ideas into "good" or "bad" groups.
   b. Illustrate how many minutes of exercise are needed to burn the calories in various snacks.
   c. Advise kids to restrict favorite treats (e.g., ice cream), except as a reward for reaching a goal, such as getting a good grade on a test.
   d. Emphasize that children should eat when they are hungry and stop eating when they are full.

Answer Key: 1. a (LO 11.1), 2. d (LO 11.2), 3. c (LO 11.3), 4. a (LO 11.3), 5. c (LO 11.4), 6. a (LO 11.4), 7. c (LO 11.5), 8. b (LO 11.6), 9. c (LO 11.6), 10. d (LO 11.7)

Study Questions (Numbers refer to Learning Outcomes)

1. What are the typical characteristics of a person with anorexia nervosa? What may influence a person to begin rigid, self-imposed dietary patterns? **(LO 11.3)**

2. List the detrimental physical effects of bulimia nervosa. Describe important goals of the psychological and nutrition therapy used to treat patients with bulimia nervosa. **(LO 11.4)**

3. What medications are currently used in the treatment of anorexia nervosa, bulimia nervosa, and binge eating disorder? **(LOs 11.3–11.5)**

4. Explain the role of excessive exercise in eating disorders. **(LO 11.1)**

5. How might parents or other role models contribute to the development of an eating disorder? Suggest an attitude that a parent or an adult friend of yours displayed that may not have been conducive to developing a healthy relationship with food. **(LO 11.7)**

6. Based on your knowledge of good nutrition and sound dietary habits, answer the following questions:
   a. How can repeated bingeing and purging lead to significant nutrient deficiencies?
   b. How can significant nutrient deficiencies contribute to major health problems in later life?
   c. A friend asks you if it is okay to "cleanse" the body by eating only grapefruit for a week. What is your response? **(LO 11.1)**

7. Provide an example of the way society contributes to development of eating disorders. **(LO 11.2)**

8. List the three components of the female athlete triad. What is the major health risk associated with loss of menstrual periods in the female athlete? **(LO 11.6)**

9. How does binge eating disorder differ from bulimia nervosa? Describe factors that contribute to the development of binge eating disorder. **(LO 11.5)**

10. Provide two recommendations to reduce the problem of eating disorders in our society. **(LO 11.7)**

What the Dietitian Chose

It can be uncomfortable to confront a friend about an unhealthy behavior. You may worry about compromising your friendship. The eating and excessive exercise behaviors you have witnessed may be short-term disordered eating and may pass in a few weeks. On the other hand, they might just be the tip of the iceberg. Ignoring her behavior will not make it go away. As you have learned in this chapter, eating disorders can have serious consequences, and the earlier they are treated, the better the outcome. If you feel unable to address your concerns one on one with your roommate, you can seek help from a resident assistant in your dorm, a school counselor, or a nurse

in the student health center. You will not be betraying your friendship; you will be showing how much you care about her by taking action.

Diagnosing an eating disorder is a complex task. People with eating disorders may deny the problem, hide their behaviors, and be irrational and uncooperative with those who try to help them. Do not try to diagnose your friend, but do try to keep the lines of communication open. Tell her what you have observed and ask her how you can help. She may open up to you and be glad she is not alone in her struggle. Then again, she may get angry and withdraw from you. Try to share what you know about eating

(continued)

disorders without lecturing or admonishing her. Also, be aware that your friend is going through a difficult emotional struggle that has probably been years in the making. Do not assume you know what she is going through.

Discussing healthy weight-management techniques with your roommate is not likely to help her if she has fallen prey to an eating disorder. She is already critical of her appearance and weight; your advice, although well intended and backed by the nutrition knowledge you have picked up in this course, may be construed as judgmental. Eating disorders are not about food. It is important to be supportive but not critical. Taking the focus off food and body weight is important. Do not try to force her to eat or slow down on her exercise. If you can help get your roommate to seek professional treatment, psychiatric counseling will help to address her unhealthy relationship with food; eventually, nutrition counseling will help her to establish better eating habits.

Get prepared before you confront your roommate. Find out what information and resources are available on campus so you can share them with her. Recognize that you are not going to cure her disorder—she needs professional help. You can be supportive and patient as she deals with her inner turmoil. Listen and offer to go with her to seek care. Someday, you may be a health professional who is able to diagnose and counsel victims of eating disorders. For now, leave it to a qualified professional.

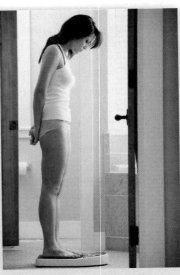
©Don Mason/Blend Images LLC RF

Further Readings

1. Le Grange D and others: Academy of Eating Disorders position paper: The role of the family in eating disorders. *Int J Eat Disord* 2010; 43:1.

2. Klump K and others: Academy for Eating Disorders position paper: Eating disorders are serious mental illnesses. *Int J Eat Disord* 2009; 42:97.

3. Mitchison D and Hay P: The epidemiology of eating disorders: Genetic, environmental, and societal factors. *J Clin Epidemiol* 2014; 6:89.

4. Campbell IC and others: Eating disorders, gene-environment interactions, and epigenetics. *Neurosci Biobehav Rev* 2011; 35:784.

5. Rivera HM and others: The role of maternal obesity in the risk of neuropsychiatric disorders. *Front Neurosci* 2015; 9.

6. Mitchison D and Mond J: Epidemiology of eating disorders, eating disordered behaviour, and body image disturbance in males: A narrative review. *J Eat Disord* 2015; 3:20.

7. Matthews-Ewald MR and others: Sexual orientation and disordered eating behaviors among self-identified male and female college students. *Eat Behav* 2014; 15:441.

8. Campbell K and Peebles R: Eating disorders in children and adolescents: State of the art review. *Pediatrics* 2014; 134:582.

9. Luca A and others: Eating disorders in late-life. *Aging Dis* 2015; 6:48.

10. Yeo M and Hughes E: Eating disorders: Early identification in general practice. *Aust Fam Physician* 2011; 40:108.

11. Borzekowski DLG and others: e-Ana and e-Mia: A content analysis of pro-eating disorder websites. *Am J Public Health* 2010; 100:1526.

12. Mehler PS and Brown C: Anorexia nervosa—medical complications. *J Eat Disord* 2015; 3:11.

13. Ozier AD and Henry BW: Position of the American Dietetic Association: Nutrition intervention in the treatment of eating disorders. *J Am Diet Assoc* 2011; 111:1236.

14. Zipfel S and others: Anorexia nervosa: Etiology, assessment, and treatment. *Lancet Psychiatry* 2015; 2:1099.

15. Waterhous T and others: Practice paper of the American Dietetic Association: Nutrition intervention in the treatment of eating disorders. *J Am Diet Assoc* 2011; 111:1261.

16. Mehler PS and Rylander M: Bulimia nervosa—medical complications. *J Eat Disord* 2015; 3:12.

17. Seher CL: Binge eating disorder—learning about this condition can help RDs counsel patients more effectively. *Today's Dietitian* 2012; 14:34.

18. Brownley KA and others: Pharmacological approaches to the management of binge eating disorder. *Drugs* 2015; 75:9.

19. Sojcher R and others: Evidence and potential mechanisms for mindfulness practices and energy psychology for obesity and binge eating disorder. *Explore* 2012; 8:271.

20. Orenstein BW: Intermittent fasting: The key to long-term weight loss? *Today's Dietitian* 2014; 26(12):40.

21. Patterson RE and others: Intermittent fasting and human metabolic health. *J Acad Nutr Diet* 2015; 115:1203.

22. Murray SB and Anderson LK: Deconstructing "atypical" eating disorders: An overview of emerging eating disorder phenotypes. *Curr Psychiatry Rep* 2015; 17:86.

23. Nattiv A and others: American College of Sports Medicine position stand: The female athlete triad. *Med Sci Sports Exerc* 2007; 39:1867.

24. Baghurst T: Muscle dysmorphia and male body image: signs and symptoms. *SCANS's Pulse* 2017; 36(1):5.

25. Colton PA and others: Eating disorders in girls and women with type 1 diabetes: A longitudinal study of prevalence, onset, remission, and recurrence. *Diabetes Care* 2015; 38:1212.

26. Dunn TM and Bratman S: On orthorexia nervosa: A review of the literature and proposed diagnostic criteria. *Eating Behaviors* 2016; 21:11–17.

27. Getz L: Understanding orthorexia—when healthful eating becomes an obsession. *Today's Dietitian* 2014; 16:18.

connect To get the most out of your study, visit Connect where you will find NutritionCalc Plus, SmartBook®, and many other dynamic tools.

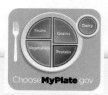

Rate Your Plate

Source: www.choosemyplate.gov

I. Assessing Risk of Developing an Eating Disorder

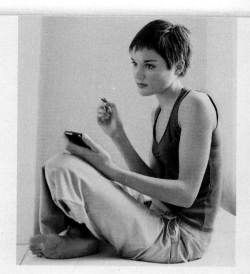

©Digital Vision/PunchStock RF

British investigators have developed a five-question screening tool called the SCOFF Questionnaire for recognizing eating disorders:*

1. Do you make yourself **Sick** because you feel full?

2. Do you lose **Control** over how much you eat?

3. Have you lost more than **One** stone (about 13 pounds) recently?

4. Do you believe yourself to be **Fat** when others say you are thin?

5. Does **Food** dominate your life?

Two or more positive responses suggest an eating disorder.

1. After completing this questionnaire, do you feel that you might have an eating disorder or the potential to develop one?

   _____

   _____

2. Do you think any of your friends might have an eating disorder?

   _____

   _____

3. What counseling and education resources exist in your area or on your campus to help with a potential eating disorder?

   _____

   _____

4. If a friend has an eating disorder, what do you think is the best way to assist him or her in getting help?

   _____

   _____

* Morgan JF and others: The SCOFF Questionnaire, *British Medical Journal*, 1999, 319:1467.

II. Helping Prevent Eating Disorders

You have been asked to speak to a junior high school class about eating disorders. What are four major points that you would make to help prevent disordered eating in this population?

1. _____

2. _____

3. _____

4. _____

Here are points you may consider:

1. Extreme thinness is oversold in the media. Extremely low weight (i.e., BMI of less than 17.5) is generally not healthy.

2. Self-induced vomiting is dangerous. Damage to the teeth, stomach, and esophagus often results.

3. Loss of menstrual periods is a sign of illness. It is important to see a physician about this. Bone deterioration is a common result.

4. The treatment of eating disorders in early phases aids success. These diseases are difficult to treat once firmly established.

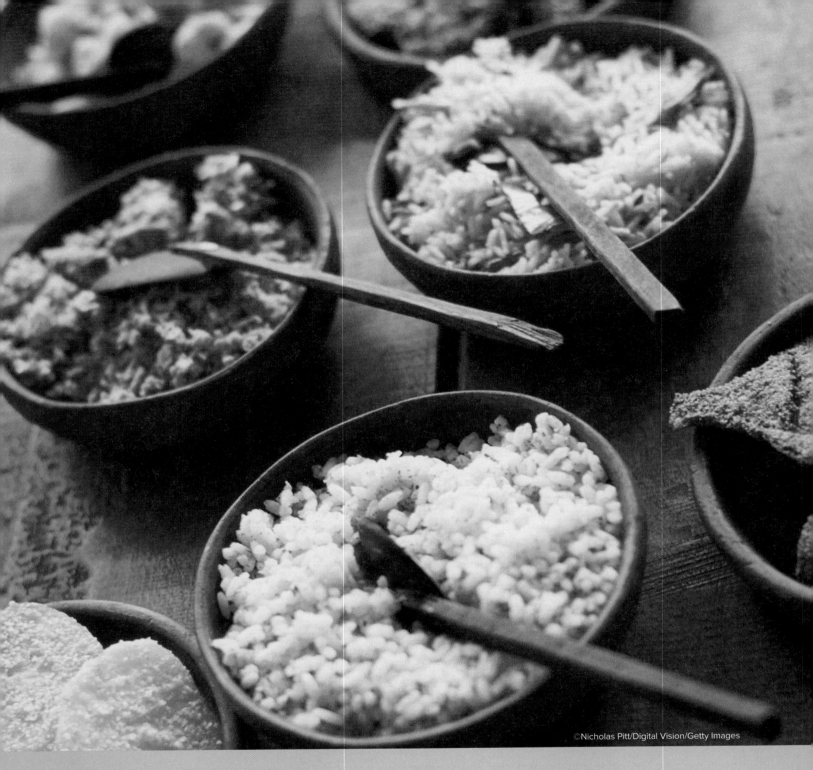

©Nicholas Pitt/Digital Vision/Getty Images

Student Learning Outcomes

Chapter 12 is designed to allow you to:

12.1 Define and characterize the terms *food insecure, nutrition security, hunger, malnutrition,* and *undernutrition.*

12.2 Examine undernutrition in the United States, and highlight several programs established to combat this problem.

12.3 Examine global nutrition, and evaluate the factors related to health impacts.

12.4 Outline some possible solutions to undernutrition in the developing world.

12.5 Evaluate the consequences of undernutrition during critical periods in a person's life.

Chapter 12
Global Nutrition

Global nutrition has never been more important than it is today. Currently, nearly one in nine people worldwide is chronically undernourished—too hungry to lead a productive, active life. The problems of poverty and undernutrition are widespread—even though there is enough food available to sufficiently feed all of us. Some progress has been made in decreasing the amount of poverty.

Within the developing world, over 795 million people are malnourished, with Asia having the largest number. This level of malnutrition is the main cause of lowered resistance to disease, infection, and death, with children under 5 years being the most susceptible.

This chapter examines global nutrition and focuses on the problem of undernutrition, contributing factors, and some solutions that are in progress. If we are to eradicate undernutrition, we all have to understand the problem. We must begin to assume responsibility today, not tomorrow, to work on solutions to hunger close to home and in faraway nations. It is important to recognize that many political, economic, and social factors worldwide, such as rising food prices, war, environmental catastrophes, and the global threat of AIDS, impact global nutrition. In 2015, the United Nations led the charge to adopt and promote a set of goals to alleviate global poverty, protect the planet, and ensure prosperity for all. These 17 goals, titled the *Sustainable Development Goals*, comprise the core of this new agenda. Each goal has measurable targets that will be analyzed over the next 15 years. To coordinate and achieve this initiative, stakeholders, governments, the private sector, society, and individuals (just like you) will be called on to support these sustainable goals, which are discussed in this chapter.

food insecure The state of being without reliable access to a sufficient quantity of affordable, nutritious food.

nutrition security Secure access to a nutritious diet coupled with a sanitary environment and adequate health services and care.

hunger The primarily physiological (internal) drive to find and eat food.

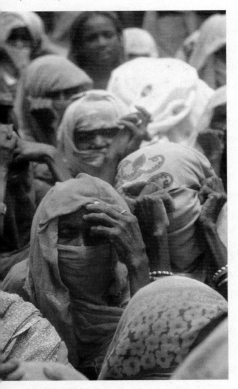

Malnutrition is associated with overpopulation in some developing countries. ©Getty Images

12.1 World Hunger: A Crisis of Nutrition Security

Uncertainty regarding the source of one's next meal remains a daily experience for close to 1 billion people around the world. This situation is troubling, considering that agriculture worldwide produces more than enough food to meet the energy requirements of each of the planet's 7 billion people. Even with this abundance, 795 million people—1 out of every 9 people on planet Earth—are still unable to access enough food to lead active, healthy lives. Hence, these individuals were **food insecure.** This statistic comes from the United Nations Food and Agriculture Organization (FAO), which measures undernutrition around the world. Availability, access, utilization, and stability are the four pillars of food security, which exists when people have physical, social, and economic access to sufficient, safe, and nutritious food to meet their dietary needs and food preferences for an active and healthy life (Fig. 12-1).[1]

Food security is actually a component of a larger concept called **nutrition security.** The FAO defines nutrition security as secure access to an appropriately nutritious diet (i.e., protein, carbohydrate, fat, vitamins, minerals, and water), coupled with a sanitary environment and adequate health services and care, in order to ensure a healthy and active life for all household members.[2] The combined term *food and nutrition security* is now preferred and can be used to emphasize both food and health requirements.[2]

The serious problems of food insecurity and malnutrition exist in virtually every nation in the world (Fig. 12-2). They are most common in regions of the developing world, with Asia and the Pacific having the largest number (520 million), along with sub-Saharan Africa (214 million), and Latin America and the Caribbean (37 million). Nearly all people suffering from food insecurity, hunger, or malnutrition are poor. There has been global interest in poverty and hunger for decades, and new development goals have been set forth by the United Nations (UN). In 2015, 17 Global Goals for Sustainable Development were implemented to improve people's lives by 2030. The goals are discussed in Section 12.4 of this chapter.

HUNGER

We will begin our look at the problem of world hunger and malnutrition by defining some key terms. The physiological state that results when not enough food is eaten to meet energy needs is **hunger.** This sensation is often is described as an uneasiness, discomfort, weakness, or pain caused by a lack of food. The medical and societal costs of the undernutrition that can result from hunger are high rates of preterm births, mental

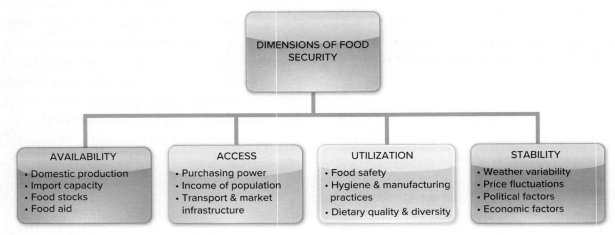

FIGURE 12-1 ▲ The four dimensions of food security.

Source: FAO, http://www.fao.org/docrep/013/al936e/al936e00.pdf

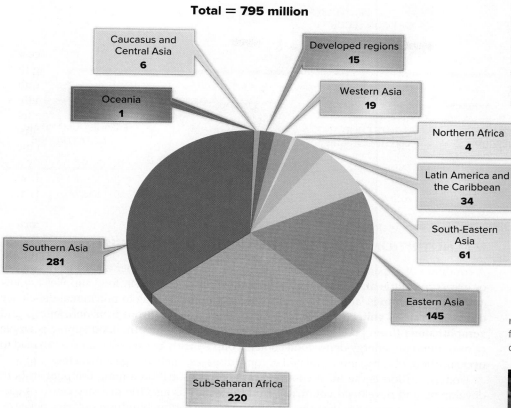

Total = 795 million

Caucasus and Central Asia
6

Developed regions
15

Oceania
1

Western Asia
19

Northern Africa
4

Latin America and the Caribbean
34

South-Eastern Asia
61

Southern Asia
281

Eastern Asia
145

Sub-Saharan Africa
220

FIGURE 12-2 ◀ Undernutrition by region (in millions). Regions have differed in their rates of progress toward reducing hunger. South-Eastern Asia, Eastern Asia, and Latin America and the Caribbean have seen the greatest decline, whereas the rates have increased in Southern Asia and sub-Saharan Africa.

Source: FAO

malnutrition Failing health that results from longstanding eating practices that do not coincide with nutritional needs.

disabilities, inadequate or stunted growth and development, poor academic performance, decreased work output, chronic disease, and many other preventable issues. Although **malnutrition** (both undernutrition and overnutrition) does occur in North America, it is typically not a result of extreme poverty over a large segment of the population. Instead, there are often specific causes, such as an eating disorder, alcoholism, unavailable or inadequate caregiving, or homelessness.[3] There is also some degree of moderate malnutrition in some of the poorer segments of North American society (i.e., those earning less than the current poverty level). Fortunately, there are *food safety nets*, such as food pantries and soup kitchens, though sometimes there are barriers to access for those in need. In addition, there is food insecurity, which is measured in the United States using the U.S. Department of Agriculture (USDA) Household Food Security Survey Module.[4] There are three levels of food insecurity: *food insecure, low food security*, and *very low food security*. In 2016, 12.3% of U.S. households (over 15.6 million households) reported experiencing food insecurity. However, the FAO cites five levels of food security (Fig. 12-3). The FAO's Integrated Food Security Phase Classifications are based on global mortality, malnutrition, food and water access and availability, dietary diversity, coping strategies, and livelihood assets.[1]

Poverty is a primary driver of malnutrition. In the United States, child poverty reached a record high level in 2014 and dropped in 2015, with 6.4 million children in families living below the federal poverty level. Poverty is defined as a family of four having an income less than of $24,600 per year in 2017. Research, however, estimates that families need an income of about twice that level to cover basic expenses. Living in poverty impairs a child's ability to learn and contributes to inadequate growth, behavioral problems, and poor health. The risks of poverty are greatest for young children. Fortunately, the United States does offer food assistance programs for low-income families. These programs do help shield children from hunger and will be discussed in Section 12.2.

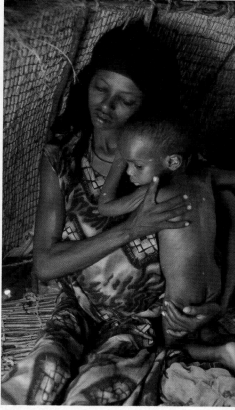

▲ Minimal intakes of protein and zinc limit the growth of children worldwide. About 25% of children in developing countries show evidence of inadequate growth and development. ©Mike Goldwater/Alamy

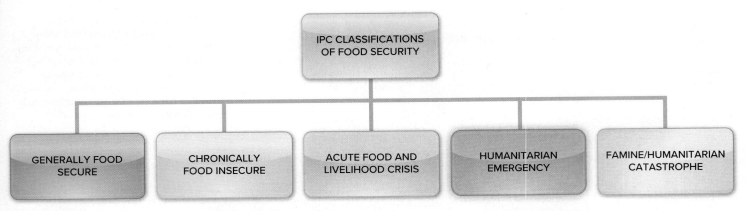

FIGURE 12-3 ▲ Integrated food security phase classifications.

Source: FAO, http://www.fao.org/docrep/013/al936e/al936e00.pdf

undernutrition Failing health that results from a longstanding dietary intake that is not enough to meet nutritional needs.

goiter An enlargement of the thyroid gland; this is often caused by insufficient iodine in the diet.

xerophthalmia Hardening of the cornea and drying of the surface of the eye, which can result in blindness.

The Irish potato famine of 1840 to 1850 caused an estimated 2 million deaths and resulted in nearly as many people emigrating to other countries. More than 3 million people may have perished in the great famine of 1943 in Bengal, India. China suffered a famine from 1959 to 1961 with mortality ranging from 20 to 43 million. In 1974, another 1.5 million starved in the country of Bangladesh.

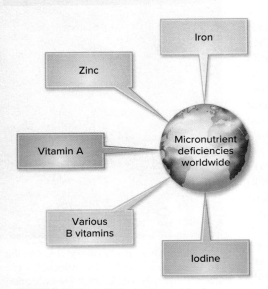

FIGURE 12-4 ▲ Critical micronutrient deficiencies worldwide.

MALNUTRITION AND MICRONUTRIENT DEFICIENCIES

A condition of impaired development or function caused by either a chronic deficiency or excess in calorie and/or nutrient intake is malnutrition. When food supplies are low and the population is large, **undernutrition** is common, leading to nutritional deficiency diseases, such as **goiter** (from iodine deficiency), anemia (from iron deficiency), and **xerophthalmia** (from poor vitamin A intake). However, when the food supply is ample or overabundant, energy-dense food choices coupled with an excessive intake can lead to overnutrition, obesity, and its related chronic diseases, such as type 2 diabetes.

Undernutrition is the most common form of malnutrition among the poor in both developing and developed countries. Undernutrition is also the primary cause of specific nutrient deficiencies that can result in muscle wasting, blindness, scurvy, pellagra, beriberi, anemia, rickets, goiter, and a host of other problems (Table 12-1).

The most critical micronutrients missing from diets worldwide (Fig. 12-4) are iron, vitamin A, iodine, zinc, and various B vitamins (e.g., folate), as well as selenium and vitamin C. About 1 billion people, mostly in the developing world, are affected by iron and zinc deficiencies. With poor iron status, cognitive development will likely be impaired, particularly if prolonged deficiency occurs during early infancy. An estimated 50 million people worldwide also suffer brain damage from preventable maternal iodine deficiency. It is estimated that in vitamin A–deficient areas, a large percentage of those who are deficient are pregnant women; and at least 250 million preschool children are vitamin A deficient. Although severe vitamin A deficiency, which causes blindness, is on the decline, up to 500,000 preschool-age children are still blinded by it each year, with half of them likely to die within 12 months of losing their sight. The United Nations Children's Fund (UNICEF) reports that the lives of one in three children could be saved annually in the developing world if vitamin A supplements were provided a few times each year. The annual cost per child is approximately 2 cents.

Of the 7.1 billion people in the world, about 2 billion may experience episodes of food shortages and be affected by some form of micronutrient malnutrition. Death and disease from infections, particularly those causing acute and prolonged diarrhea or respiratory disease, increase dramatically when the infections occur during a state of sustained undernutrition. Chronic undernutrition leaves many people in the developing world in a chronic state of depressed immunity, in turn greatly increasing the risk of death, especially during childhood.

Protein-calorie malnutrition (PCM) is a form of undernutrition caused by an extremely deficient intake of calories or protein and is generally accompanied by illness. The dramatic results of PCM—**kwashiorkor** and **marasmus**—were described in Chapter 6. This chapter focuses on the subtle effects of a chronic inadequate intake food.

TABLE 12-1 ■ **Nutrient-Deficiency Diseases That Commonly Accompany Undernutrition**

Disease and Key Nutrient Involved*	Typical Effects of Deficiency	Sources of Deficient Nutrient	Target Populations for Interventions
Xerophthalmia Vitamin A	Blindness from chronic eye infections, dryness, restricted growth, and keratinization of epithelial tissues	Fortified milk, sweet potatoes, spinach, greens, carrots, cantaloupe, and apricots	Asia and Africa
Rickets Vitamin D	Poorly calcified bones, bowed legs, and other bone deformities	Fortified milk, fish oils, and sun exposure	Asia, Africa, and parts of the world where religious dress prevents women and children from receiving adequate sun exposure; older adults in developed nations
Beriberi Thiamin	Nerve degeneration, altered muscle coordination, and cardiovascular problems	Sunflower seeds, pork, whole and enriched grains, and dried beans	Victims of famine in Africa and alcoholics worldwide
Ariboflavinosis Riboflavin	Inflammation of oral cavity; nervous system disorders	Milk, mushrooms, spinach, liver, and enriched grains	Victims of famine in Africa
Pellagra Niacin	Diarrhea, dermatitis, dementia, and death	Mushrooms, bran, tuna, chicken, beef, peanuts, and whole and enriched grains	Victims of famine in Africa and survivors of war-torn Eastern Europe
Megaloblastic anemia Folate	Enlarged red blood cells, fatigue, and weakness	Green leafy vegetables, legumes, oranges, and liver	Asia and Africa
Scurvy Vitamin C	Delayed wound healing, internal bleeding, and abnormal formation of bones and teeth	Citrus fruits, strawberries, broccoli, and tomatoes	Victims of famine in Africa
Iron-deficiency anemia Iron	Reduced work output, retarded growth, and increased health risk in pregnancy	Meats, seafood, broccoli, peas, bran, whole grains, and enriched products	Worldwide
Goiter Iodine	Enlarged thyroid gland in teenagers and adults, possible mental retardation, and congenital hypothyroidism	Iodized salt and saltwater fish	South America, Eastern Europe, and Africa

*Although the nutrients are listed separately to illustrate the important role of each one, often two or more nutrition-deficiency diseases are found in an undernourished person in the developing world.

FAMINE

Famine can lead to chronic hunger. Periods of famine are characterized by large-scale loss of life, climate change, social disruption, economic chaos, and political conflicts. As a result of these extreme events, the affected community may experience a downward spiral characterized by human distress; sales of land, livestock, and other farm assets; mass migration; division and impoverishment of the poorest families; crime; and humanitarian crises, as recently seen in Libya and Somalia with 90% of their population affected by violence and insecurity. In the midst of all this, undernutrition rates soar; infectious diseases, such as cholera, spread; and many people die.

Special efforts are needed to eradicate the fundamental causes of famine. These causes vary by region and decade, but the most common cause of famine is crop failure. The most obvious reasons are extreme weather conditions such as floods or drought, war, and civil strife. War deserves a special focus and will be specifically addressed in Section 12.3.

GENERAL EFFECTS OF SEMISTARVATION

In the initial stages, the results of undernutrition from semistarvation are often so mild that physical symptoms are absent and blood tests do not usually detect these slight

protein-calorie malnutrition (PCM) A condition resulting from regularly consuming insufficient amounts of calories and protein. The deficiency eventually results in body wasting, primarily of lean tissue, and an increased susceptibility to infections. Also known as *protein-energy malnutrition (PEM)*.

kwashiorkor A disease occurring primarily in young children who have an existing disease and consume a marginal amount of calories and insufficient protein in relation to needs. The child generally suffers from infections and exhibits edema, poor growth, weakness, and an increased susceptibility to further illness.

marasmus A disease resulting from consuming a grossly insufficient amount of protein and calories; one of the diseases classed as protein-calorie malnutrition. Victims have little or no fat stores, little muscle mass, and poor strength. Death from infections is common.

famine An extreme shortage of food, which leads to massive starvation in a population; often associated with crop failures, war, and political unrest.

Newsworthy Nutrition

Maternal iodine deficiency could lead to lower educational outcomes

The hypothesis of this study was that children born to mothers with mild iodine deficiency during pregnancy will have poorer educational outcomes in primary school than peers whose mothers did not have iodine deficiency during pregnancy. The study was a longitudinal design with follow-up when the children were 9 years old. The study participants were children born in Australia between 1999 and 2001. The mild iodine deficiency during pregnancy was followed with the children subsequently growing up in an iodine-adequate environment. Children whose mothers had mild iodine deficiency had reductions of 10.% in spelling, 7.6% in grammar, and 5.7% in English-literacy performance compared with children whose mothers were not iodine deficient. The authors conclude that even mild iodine deficiency during pregnancy can have long-term adverse impacts on fetal brain development that will affect cognition and are not improved by iodine sufficiency during childhood.

Source: Hynes KL, et al. "Mild iodine deficiency during pregnancy is associated with reduced educational outcomes in the offspring: 9-year follow-up of the gestational iodine cohort," *Journal of Clinical Endocrinology and Metabolism* 98(5):1954, 2013.

The effects of hunger are diverse, widespread, and devastating:

- Reduced energy and strength
- Diminished concentration
- Impaired learning
- Lowered productivity
- Progression of chronic disease
- Deterioration of mood
- Reduced immunity
- Decreased birth weights
- Stunted growth in infants and children

metabolic changes. Even in the absence of detectable symptoms, however, undernourishment may affect the ability to work, learn, reproduce, and recover from illnesses or injuries. Recall that as tissues continue to be depleted of nutrients, blood tests eventually detect biochemical changes, such as a drop in blood hemoglobin concentration. Physical symptoms, such as body weakness or fatigue, tend to follow with further depletion. Finally, the full-blown symptoms of the deficiency are recognizable, such as stunting or blindness (vitamin A deficiency).

When a few people in a population develop a severe deficiency, this may represent only the tip of the iceberg. Typically, a much greater number of individuals in that area may be suffering milder degrees of undernutrition. These deficiencies should not, therefore, be dismissed as trivial, especially in the developing world. In many low- and even middle-income countries, it is typical for a combination of micronutrient deficiencies to occur together. These are caused by any number of factors, including dietary patterns of poor nutritional quality related to seasonal variation in food availability, low bioavailability of nutrients from plant sources, cultural food practices, and poverty. It is becoming clear that combined deficiencies of specific vitamins and minerals (especially iron and zinc) can significantly reduce work performance, even in the absence of obvious physical symptoms. This resulting state of ill health, in turn, diminishes the ability of individuals, communities, and even whole countries to perform at peak levels of physical and mental capacity (Fig. 12-5). Because nutritional requirements are high during periods of rapid growth, pregnant women, infants, and children are especially vulnerable to the effects of undernutrition. Studies of pregnant women and children in developing countries have proven the negative impact of micronutrient deficiencies on birth size, length of gestation, growth, and intellectual development (Newsworthy Nutrition).

Added to their lack of nourishment, the inhabitants of poverty-stricken countries must also contend with recurrent infections, poor sanitation, extreme weather conditions, and regular exposure to infectious diseases. Deficiencies of micronutrients, especially iron and zinc, can lead to reduced immune function and thereby increase the risk of diseases, such as diarrhea and pneumonia.

Strategies to address the multiple nutrient deficiencies in developing countries have included supplementation and fortification of ready-to-use foods and beverages. Although supplementation has been the most widely practiced intervention, public health experts believe that fortification of a commonly consumed food could be a single, cost-effective intervention strategy that would target a larger population. Studies

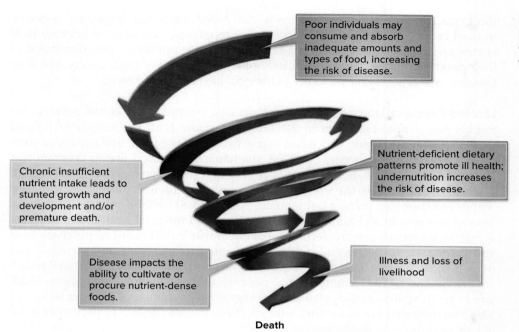

Poor individuals may consume and absorb inadequate amounts and types of food, increasing the risk of disease.

Chronic insufficient nutrient intake leads to stunted growth and development and/or premature death.

Nutrient-deficient dietary patterns promote ill health; undernutrition increases the risk of disease.

Disease impacts the ability to cultivate or procure nutrient-dense foods.

Illness and loss of livelihood

Death

FIGURE 12-5 ◄ The downward spiral of poverty and illness can ultimately end in death (Source: World Food Programme graphic).

of micronutrient supplementation during pregnancy have shown an increase in birth weight and a reduction in low birth weights but no impact on preterm births or perinatal mortality. In children, micronutrient supplementation with three or more nutrients has resulted in increases in height and weight.[5]

✓ CONCEPT CHECK 12.1

1. What are the characteristics of *hunger*?
2. What is the definition of *food insecure*?
3. Define the term *nutrition security*.
4. What are the health results of chronic hunger?
5. What is the primary cause of undernutrition?
6. At which stages of the life cycle is undernutrition especially damaging?
7. What are the effects of chronic undernutrition?

12.2 Undernutrition in the United States

In 2015, roughly 43.1 million (13.5%) people in the United States were living at or below the poverty level, estimated at about $24,300 annually for a family of four[6] between purchasing food and other essentials. According to the *Hunger in America 2016* report, 57% of households report choosing between purchasing food and housing costs, 69% between food and utilities, 66% between food and medicine, and 67% between food and access to transportation. While housing and utility costs, medical care, and transportation fares are nonnegotiable, a person can choose to eat less. Food is one of the few optional items in a household budget. The short-term consequences of eating less may be less dramatic than getting evicted, but the long-term cumulative effects are significant.

HELPING THE HUNGRY IN THE UNITED STATES

Until the twentieth century, individuals and a wide variety of charitable, often church-related organizations provided most of the help to poor, undernourished people in

Historical Research on Undernutrition

In the 1940s, a group of researchers led by Dr. Ansel Keys examined the general effects of undernutrition on adults. Previously healthy men were fed a diet averaging about 1800 kcal daily for 6 months. During this time, the men lost an average of 24% of their body weight. After about 3 months, the participants complained of fatigue, muscle soreness, irritability, intolerance to cold, and hunger pains. They exhibited a lack of ambition, self-discipline, and concentration, and were often moody, apathetic, and depressed. Their heart rate and muscle tone decreased, and they developed edema. When the men were permitted to eat normally again, feelings of recurrent hunger and fatigue persisted, even after 12 weeks of rehabilitation. Full recovery required about 8 months. This study helps us understand the general state of undernourished adults worldwide.

Source: Keys, A. "Will you starve that they be better fed?" *Brochure*, May 27, 1944

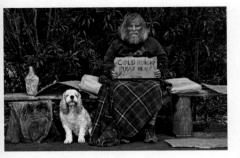

▲ This man is hoping to find work to fill his basic need of food. There are many federal food assistance programs for those in need. ©Jodi Cobb/Getty Images

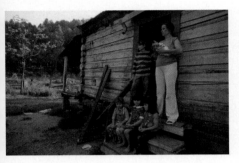

▲ Poverty aggravates the problem of hunger in the United States. ©DebbiSmirnoff/Getty Images

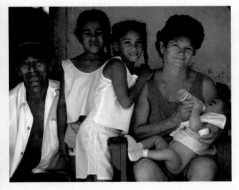

▲ Food insecurity is part of the North American landscape. A *safety net* of programs exists but fails to serve many households in need.

Source: USDA

the United States. Early programs rarely distributed direct cash payments to people in need because these were thought to reduce recipients' motivation to improve their circumstances or engage in negative behaviors, such as smoking, that contributed to their poverty. Beginning in the early 1900s, the involvement of local, county, and state governments in providing assistance to the poor has steadily increased.

Limited-Resource Households. After observing extensive hunger and poverty during his presidential campaign in the 1960s, President John F. Kennedy revitalized the Food Stamp Program, which had begun two decades earlier, and expanded commodity distribution programs. In 2008, the name of the Food Stamp Program was changed to the Supplemental Nutrition Assistance Program (SNAP) (Table 12-2). The new name reflects the program's focus on nutrition and putting healthy food within reach for low-income households. SNAP is a $74 billion program that helps low-income people and families buy food they need for good health. The program allows recipients to use an electronic benefit transfer (EBT) card to purchase food and garden seeds—but excludes tobacco, cleaning items, alcoholic beverages, and nonedible products—at stores authorized to accept them. The average SNAP recipient received about $127 a month ($4.23 per day). Over 43.2 million Americans—about one in seven adults—participated in this program in September 2015. Almost 70% of SNAP participants are in families with children; more than 25% of participants are elderly or those with disabilities.

A recent USDA report assessed the shopping cart of SNAP participants and found the top item purchased with SNAP dollars was soft drinks. The report compared SNAP households and non-SNAP households. While SNAP users purchased slightly more junk food and fewer vegetables, both groups purchased an abundant amount of sweetened drinks, candy, ice cream, and potato chips. SNAP households spent about 40 cents of each dollar on meat, fruits, vegetables, milk, eggs, and bread. Another 40 cents were spent on cereal, prepared foods, dairy products, rice, and beans. The final 20 cents was spent on highly processed and low nutrient-dense foods such as sweetened beverages, desserts, salty snacks, candy, and sugar.[7]

Other Food Assistance Programs. The U.S. Congress established the National School Lunch Program in the 1940s and the School Breakfast Program in the 1960s. School breakfast and lunch programs enable low-income students—14.6 million for breakfast and 30.3 million for lunch in 2016—to receive meals free or at reduced cost if certain income guidelines are met. The basis of eligibility for free and reduced-price meals can be determined by categorical, direct, community, or income-based eligibility.

The Older Americans Act (OAA) authorizes the elderly nutrition services program to reduce hunger and food insecurity, enhance socialization, promote health and well-being, and delay adverse health conditions for older individuals. Over 11 million (one in five) older adults are served annually by OAA programs such as congregate and home-delivered meals.

In 1972, the Special Supplemental Nutrition Program for Women, Infants, and Children (WIC) was authorized. This program provides food vouchers and nutrition education to low-income, nutritionally at-risk pregnant and lactating women and their young children. It serves 7.7 million women and children each month and remains the most successful federally-funded nutrition programs to date based upon health outcomes.

Food Assistance. Government food assistance programs are like a *safety net*: they are strong, yet porous. These programs were originally known as *welfare* and were designed to provide short-term relief for Americans suffering financial hardship. Now, many low- and middle-income U.S. households rely on food pantries and federal assistance chronically and for the majority of their nutritional needs. Feeding America® estimates that one in seven Americans—that is, 46 million people—rely on food pantries and emergency meal service programs to feed themselves and their households. Statistics show that most people requesting emergency food assistance are members of families. This

TABLE 12-2 ■ **Some Federally Subsidized Programs That Supply Food for People in the United States**

Program	Eligibility	Description
Supplemental Nutrition Assistance Program (formerly Food Stamp Program)	Low-income families	Electronic benefit transfer (debit) cards are given to purchase food at grocery stores; the amount is based on size of household and income.
The Emergency Food Assistance Program (TEFAP)	Low-income families	Provides nutrition assistance to needy Americans through distribution of USDA food commodities
Commodity Supplemental Food Program	Certain low-income populations, such as pregnant women, children up to the age of 6 years, and seniors	USDA surplus foods are distributed by county agencies; not found in all states; may be based on nutritional risk
Special Supplemental Nutrition Program for Women, Infants, and Children (WIC)	Low-income pregnant/lactating women, infants, and children less than 5 years at nutritional risk	Coupons are given to purchase milk, cheese, fruit juice, cereal, infant formula, and other specific food items at grocery stores; includes nutrition education component. Includes Farmers' Market Nutrition Program (FMNP)
National School Lunch Program	Low-income children of school age	Free or reduced-price lunch is distributed by the school; meal follows USDA pattern based on MyPlate; cost for the child depends on family income. For students who do not participate in the lunch program, special milk program may be available.
School Breakfast Program	Low-income children of school age	Free or reduced-price breakfast is distributed by the school; meal follows USDA pattern; and cost for the child depends on family income.
Child and Adult Care Food Program	Children enrolled in organized child-care programs and seniors in adult-care programs; income guidelines are the same as those for the National School Lunch Program	Reimbursement is given for meals supplied to children at the site; meals must follow USDA guidelines based on MyPlate.
Congregate Meals for the Elderly	Age 60 or over (no income guidelines)	Free noon meal is furnished at a site; meal follows specific pattern based on one-third of nutrient needs.
Home-Delivered Meals	Age 60 or over, homebound	Noon meal is delivered at no cost or for a donation at least 5 days a week. Sometimes additional meals for later consumption are delivered at the same time; often referred to as *Meals on Wheels*.
Summer Food Service Program	Residence in a low-income neighborhood or participation in a program	Free, nutritious meals and snacks are given to children in a low-income area at a central site, such as a school or a community center during long school vacations.
Food Distribution Program on Indian Reservations	Low-income American Indian and non-Indian households on reservations; members of federally recognized tribes	Alternative to Supplemental Nutrition Assistance Program, distributes monthly food packages; includes nutrition education component
Fresh Fruit and Vegetable Program	Low-income elementary schools	Provides free fresh fruits and vegetables to increase their consumption and combat childhood obesity

is not surprising considering that households with children report a higher rate of food insecurity than households without children, and the rate is even higher for households with children headed by single parents.

Undernutrition in North America is a much more subtle problem than in developing countries. To the untrained eye, undernourished children may just seem skinny, when, in fact, their growth is being stunted by insufficient nutrients. More likely, though, children from food-insecure households are prone to be overweight. This form of malnutrition may be the result of considerable reliance on highly processed convenience foods that provide excessive saturated fat and refined sugar. The availability of cooking facilities also affects nutrient intake among the poor. Without adequate cooking facilities, people may buy expensive convenience foods that require little to no preparation. These are typically highly processed foods that provide calories but are often lacking in nutrients.

SOCIOECOLOGICAL FACTORS RELATED TO UNDERNUTRITION

In the United States, poverty, psychosocial factors, and functional limitations all increase the risk of undernutrition. Extreme poverty used to be considered the root cause of hunger and undernutrition, but we now understand that hunger and undernutrition are also major causes of poverty. There appears to be a bidirectional relationship between these factors that is much more complex than once considered.

Poverty. Poverty is determined in the United States using poverty thresholds that are issued each year by the Census Bureau. Persons are designated as poor if they have income less than that deemed sufficient to purchase the basic needs of food, shelter, clothing, and other essentials. Poverty, however, is complex and does not mean the same thing to all people. Poverty can usually be characterized as *situational* or *generational.* Households can fall into situational poverty as the result of dire or unexpected circumstances, such as getting laid off from a job or a family member needing expensive medical treatment. Some have linked situational poverty to the *seven D's:* divorce, death, disease, downsizing, disablement, disasters, and debt. Situational poverty may be episodic or cyclical, may affect entire communities as a result of economic downturns, and may be alleviated by temporary social service programs. In contrast, generational poverty refers to a culture of persistent poverty passed from parents to children, with two or more generations living in poverty. Generational poverty is more complex because the cultures and traditions of previous generations are passed on to future generations and often include an undervaluation of the benefits of education and a lack of self-efficacy when it comes to changing one's economic circumstances.

A major driving force behind poverty is underemployment. This relationship increased significantly with the economic recession that caused unemployment to soar between December 2007 and September 2009, when 7.6 million jobs were lost across all major private-sector industries. The impact of unemployment was enhanced because many states cut their welfare assistance, resulting in more people living in poverty and in need of food assistance, at risk of homelessness, and without sufficient health care. Fortunately, the economy has more recently experienced some recovery.

Homelessness. The growing shortage of affordable rental housing and a simultaneous increase in poverty are the two trends largely responsible for the rise in homelessness over the past 25 years. In 2009, data from major cities indicated increases of homelessness by as much as 20% since the foreclosure crisis began in 2007. The homelessness created by the gap between the number of affordable housing units and the number of people needing them impacts the health and well-being of all individuals. Homeless children are most vulnerable and are twice as likely to experience hunger compared to children with a home.

Over 564,708 people experienced homelessness—meaning they were sleeping outside or in an emergency shelter or transitional housing program on any given night in 2015. Families most commonly become homeless as a result of an unexpected financial crisis that prevents them from retaining their housing. Events similar to those that cause situational poverty—a medical emergency, death in the family, loss of a job—can lead to homelessness. People in poverty must make difficult choices when limited resources cover only some necessities such as housing, food, child care, health care, and education. Because housing absorbs a high percentage of income, it is often sacrificed. Most situationally homeless families are able to quickly rebound from homelessness, requiring only short-term public assistance before returning to independence and stability.

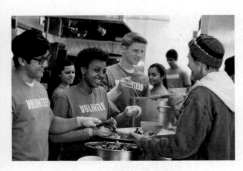

▲ Food pantries and soup kitchens are important sources of nutrients for a growing number of people in the United States. Consider volunteering some of your time to a local program. ©Ariel Skelley/ Getty Images

As the recession gripped America from 2007 to 2010, the number of people using shelters or transitional housing in suburban and rural areas increased 57% while the use of shelters in urban areas decreased. Regrettably, veterans make up over 8.6% of the homeless population, often due to war-related disabilities that affect their ability to work. In 2014, communities across America identified almost 50,000 homeless veterans during point-in-time counts.

Chronic homelessness is defined as involving either long-term and/or repeated occurrences of homelessness combined with physical and/or mental disability. Based on a single night in 2015, there were approximately 83,170 adults in America experiencing chronic homelessness. Chronically homeless individuals are more likely to be older, male, non-white, and experiencing long-term unemployment. Without access to health care, they may cycle through emergency departments and inpatient beds, detox programs, jails, prisons, and psychiatric institutions, all at high public expense. Fortunately, progress has been made in addressing chronic homelessness in the last decade, resulting in a 30% decline in this population.

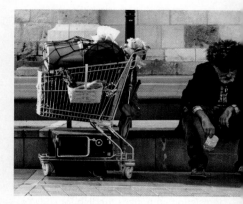

▲ Three-quarters, or about 75,000, of the chronically homeless are older men. ©Ruben Sanchez@lostintv/Getty Images RF

Access to Healthy Food. Access to affordable and nutritious foods from supermarkets, grocery stores, or other retailers is a challenge to many Americans, making it harder for them to eat a balanced, nutrient-dense dietary pattern. These impoverished areas with little access to healthy foods have been named **food deserts.** The USDA originally defined a food desert as a low-income area where a significant number of residents (33% or 500 people, whichever was less) lived far from a supermarket. "Far" was defined as more than a mile in an urban area or more than 10 miles in a rural area. USDA's online *Food Access Research Atlas,* presents a spatial overview of food access indicators for low-income and other census tracts. Measures include accessibility to sources of healthy food, as measured by distance to a store or by the number of stores in an area; individual-level resources that may affect accessibility, such as family income or vehicle availability; and neighborhood-level indicators of resources, such as the average income of the neighborhood and the availability of public transportation.[8]

food deserts Urban neighborhoods and rural towns without ready access to fresh, healthy, and affordable food.

The USDA's Fresh Fruit and Vegetable Program provides federal funding to elementary schools to serve fruits and vegetables as snacks to help children improve their dietary patterns.

The federal Healthy Food Financing Initiative (HFFI) provides government financing for developing and equipping grocery stores, small retailers, corner stores, and farmers markets selling healthy food in low-income communities. In addition, this initiative provides employment and business opportunities in underserved areas. Farmers markets are gaining attention as a simple and local approach in impacting hunger and health. Many farmers markets now participate in senior programs, WIC, SNAP, and the SNAP Double Dollar program, where shoppers using their SNAP EBT card will receive matching funds that can be redeemed for produce at that market.

POSSIBLE SOLUTIONS TO POVERTY AND HUNGER IN THE UNITED STATES

For many years, government-funded food assistance programs have helped to alleviate some problems of undernutrition in the United States.[9] An increasing number of people who are experiencing poverty are accessing the SNAP benefits

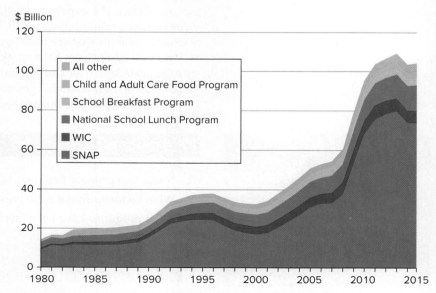

FIGURE 12-6 ▲ USDA expenditures for food and nutrition assistance, fiscal 1980–2015.

Source: USDA, Economic Research Service using data from USDA, Food and Nutrition Service. https://www.ers.usda.gov/data-products/ag-and-food-statistics-charting-the-essentials/food-security-and-nutrition-assistance/

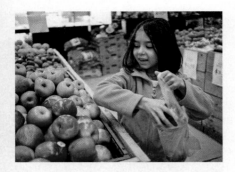

▲ Improving child nutrition is the goal of the Healthy, Hunger-Free Kids Act. This legislation authorizes funding for USDA's core child nutrition programs. ©Donald Iain Smith/Getty Images

and other federal assistance programs (Fig. 12-6). Obtaining adequate food to not only survive but thrive is a tremendous challenge, especially when homeless people are forced to live outside. Although many people assume that food pantries and soup kitchens are abundant and accessible for every needy person, there are many barriers to accessing these resources. The vast majority of food pantries are staffed by volunteers and dependent on food donations. They often have limited hours of operation, require appointments well in advance, often require proof of residence, and limit the amount of food patrons can take home per month. Homeless people often lack proper identification and proof of residence, do not have cooking facilities and equipment needed for food preparation, and do not have adequate storage to prevent foodborne illnesses and practice safe food-handling procedures. Food availability through soup kitchens is limited in most cities and absent in most rural areas.

An additional challenge is that a growing number of cities have taken strides to restrict or ban the act of food-sharing with the homeless. These laws are troubling, considering that most cities do not have adequate food resources to meet the needs of their poor and homeless. Advocates and food providers are eager to work with cities and other government agencies to help address the problems of hunger and homelessness by improving access to federal food benefits and other food resources. State governments have also begun moving to protect the right of individuals and groups to share excess food with others.

Through these recent efforts, lack of access to healthy food is now recognized as a solvable problem. The Healthy Food Financing Initiative (HFFI), a partnership between the U.S. Departments of Treasury, Agriculture and Health and Human Services, is a multiyear initiative that engages the private sector and aims to eliminate food deserts across the country. The HFFI attracts investment in underserved communities by providing financing tools such as low-cost loans, grants, tax credits, and technical assistance to healthy food retailers. The HFFI appears to be an effective and sustainable solution to the limited access to healthy foods. Its impact can be far reaching in terms of improving the nutritional status and overall health of families and children and reducing health disparities while creating jobs and stimulating the local economy in low-income areas.

Despite the highest motivation, the outlook is bleak for many people who attempt to gain independence from assistance programs. Teen pregnancy may have cut short the education or vocational training of one or both parents, thwarting efforts to earn adequate income. Often, the expense of reliable and reliable child care far exceeds the meager income from a minimum-wage job. Those that secure a part-time or entry-level position often lose benefits that are based upon income. Illness of either the parents or children may prevent adults from holding steady employment. Poor communication skills, inability to relocate, and a lack of economic reserves also complicate financial independence. Regardless of how wasteful government assistance appears to some people, welfare benefits will probably be maintained until there are widespread systematic changes.

✓ CONCEPT CHECK 12.2

1. Name two primary food assistance programs in the United States.
2. What factors influence the presence of poverty, hunger, and undernutrition?
3. What programs have been launched recently to provide long-term solutions to hunger?

12.3 Undernutrition in the Developing World

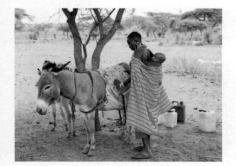

▲ This young Maasai woman, with her baby on her back, lives in Kenya, which is in a region with low contraceptive rates and the highest rates of maternal death. ©Britta Kasholm-Tengve/Getty Images

Undernutrition in the developing world is also tied to poverty, and any sustainable solution must address this issue. However, these countries have a multitude of problems so complex and interrelated that they cannot be treated separately. Programs that have proved helpful in the United States (and throughout the rest of North America) are only

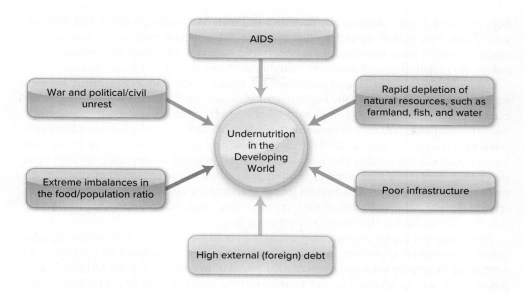

FIGURE 12-7 ◄ Many factors contribute to undernutrition in the developing world. Any solutions to the problem must take these multifaceted factors into consideration.

a starting point in this context. The major obstacles challenging those seeking a solution are illustrated in Figure 12-7 and require individual consideration.

FOOD/POPULATION RATIO

The world has over 7.4 billion inhabitants. Population growth exceeds economic growth in much of the developing world, and as a result, poverty is on the rise globally. This disrupts the balance in the food:population ratio, tipping it toward food shortages. If we want to ensure a decent life for a widening segment of humanity, many experts suggest that the growth in the earth's most vulnerable populations should slow.

According to 2015 statistics from the FAO, there are 795 million hungry people in the world and 98% reside in developing countries. More than 75% of all hungry people live in rural areas of Africa and Asia and remain totally dependent on local agriculture for all of their nutritional needs. Unfortunately, major food and health disparities continue to exist between developed and developing countries, among the rich and the poor, and even within the family unit (i.e., males may be fed before females).

Economists estimate that world food production will continue to increase more rapidly than the world population, allowing the food to population ratio to increase through the year 2020. This will come at a high cost in terms of the water, fertilizer, and chemicals (pesticides, fungicides, fertilizer) needed to allow for adequate food production. In the short term, the primary problem is not related to production but rather to the supply chain—both distribution and use. This reality is even more dire in poverty-stricken areas of developing nations. Unfortunately, many vulnerable people do not have the income to purchase their own farmland or the means to purchase food from nonlocal sources.

Most viable farmland in the world is already in use, and because of poor farming practices or competing land-use demands, the number of farmable acres is decreasing annually. For these reasons, *sustainable* world food output—an amount that does not deplete the earth's resources—is now running well behind food consumption. This discrepancy suggests that food production in less-developed countries will not keep up with population growth and will soon lag behind.

Responsible family planning can contribute to the reduction of poverty and hunger, and *decrease* the number of maternal and childhood deaths. On a daily basis, approximately 830 women die from preventable causes related to pregnancy and childbirth; 99% of these occur in developing countries. In addition, more than 225 million women in developing countries lack access to modern contraception. Global organizations are working to: (1) empower women and couples in developing countries to lead healthier

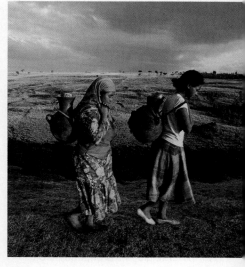

▲ Women in developing countries are forced to spend large parts of their day fetching water. ©68/Ocean/Corbis

global maternal mortality ratio The number of maternal deaths per 100,000 live births.

human immunodeficiency virus (HIV) The virus that leads to acquired immune deficiency syndrome (AIDS).

lives by increasing access to family planning and maternal health products and services; and (2) address policy, financing, delivery, and sociocultural barriers to women who desire access to such information, services, and supplies. Although strides have been made, the **global maternal mortality ratio** has declined by only 3.1% per year.

Promoting breastfeeding also contributes to infant health and birth control. Women who do not breastfeed generally begin to ovulate again within a month or so after childbirth. Although it is not a completely reliable method of contraception, exclusively breastfeeding an infant may delay ovulation after childbirth, thereby lowering the likelihood of fertilization. When childbirth is more widely spaced, not only do fewer total births occur, but the mother also has a longer period in which to physically recover from pregnancy, and the infant receives feeding priority for a longer period of time. When mothers are infected with the **human immunodeficiency virus (HIV),** the risk of transferring the virus through human milk is about 10%. Depending on the circumstances, this risk may outweigh the benefits of breastfeeding.

Increasing per capita income, improving the standard of living, and improving education, especially for women in developing nations, are considered to contribute to successful long-term solutions to excessive population growth. Global fertility is projected to decline to 2.5 children per woman birthed in 2010–2015 to 2.4 in 2025–2030. Yet even with these positive shifts, slower-than-projected fertility declines would still result in much higher population totals in subsequent time periods. The major concern remains whether there are enough resources worldwide to raise per capita income and provide enough education to slow total population growth.

WAR AND POLITICAL/CIVIL UNREST

Global military spending was $1.57 trillion in 2016. The five major contributors to military expenditures are the United States, China, Saudi Arabia, Russia, and the United Kingdom. In contrast, the 2015–2016 United Nations Peacekeeping operations budget is only $8.3 billion—less than half of 1% of all global military expenditures.

Aside from the economic impact of military spending, civil disruptions and wars continue to set back the progress of addressing poverty and contribute to massive undernutrition. Globally, 1 in every 113 humans is now either a refugee, internally displaced, or seeking political or religious asylum. In 2015, almost 12.4 million people became newly displaced—quadrupling from the previous year. The main reason for the acceleration has been the recent war in Syria, the world's largest driver of displacement.

In 2014, over 12.4 million people were uprooted by violence, mainly as war refugees in Syria, Afghanistan, and Somalia. These war-torn areas contribute to the 21.3 million refugees worldwide. Millions of deaths are anticipated and at least that many more displaced refugees. While war continues to rage, health, education, and public services continue to decline for affected populations. All the while, poverty and malnutrition increase.

War-related famine affects millions of people, mainly in South Asia, sub-Saharan Africa, and the Middle East. To assess hunger, the International Food Policy Research Institute annually calculates the *Global Hunger Index* (GHI), a tool designed to measure and track hunger worldwide. The GHI uses a multidimensional approach to assess hunger that includes population undernourishment, child wasting, child stunting, and child mortality. Eight countries, mainly in Africa, suffer from levels of hunger that are alarming. To date, GHI scores have not been calculated for Somalia due to data constraints, yet it is clearly considered one of the most vulnerable countries in the world.

Sadly, food has become a weapon in many wars. At the local level, fields are often mined and water wells intentionally contaminated. Even when food is readily available and accessible, political divisions may impede its distribution to the point that undernutrition will plague countries for years. Especially during emergencies, programs designed to aid the hungry have been undermined by unstable administrations, corruption, and political influence. During this chaos, relief agencies may be caught between warring factions and those attempting to alleviate suffering. The UN World

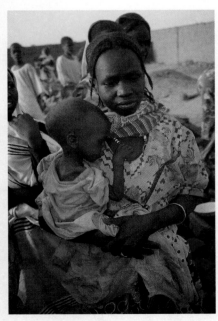

▲ This mother, holding her 27-month-old malnourished child at a camp for internally displaced persons in North Darfur, Sudan, is dependent on assistance from relief organizations that are often not welcome in the war-torn country. ©USAID

Food Programme recently reported that although 9 million people are in dire need of emergency food in Syria, it could reach only 4.5 million due to hostile ground conflicts and unsafe conditions.

During the 1960s and 1970s, the problem of undernutrition in developing countries was perceived as a technical one: how to produce enough food for the growing world population. The problem is now seen as largely political: how to achieve cooperation among and within nations, so that gains in food production and infrastructure are not weapons of war. The best answer may lie in a combination of approaches: finding technical solutions to address chronic hunger and poverty, and resolving political crises that push developing nations into a state of nutrition despair and chaos.

AGRICULTURE AND THE RAPID DEPLETION OF NATURAL RESOURCES

As we continue to deplete the Earth's resources, population control grows increasingly critical. Agriculture production is approaching its limits in many areas worldwide. Environmentally unsustainable farming methods have been undermining food production, especially in developing countries. In addition, climate change is increasingly linked to hunger and poverty. Climatic change patterns, characterized by drought, flooding, and severe storms, require significant alterations in farming practices.

The **green revolution** was a phenomenon that began in the 1960s when crop yields rose dramatically in some countries, such as the Philippines, India, and Mexico. The increased use of fertilizers and irrigation, and the development of superior crops through careful plant breeding made this boost in agricultural production possible. The green revolution was intended as a stopgap measure until world leaders could control population growth. Many of the technologies associated with the green revolution have now achieved their full potential. Additional gains in productivity and technology have been a challenge to accomplish because of the lack or loss of productive farmland.

The movement toward practices in **sustainable agriculture** and the development of new crops through food **biotechnology** have begun to improve crop yields on the shrinking amount of farmable land. Crops that are pest or chemical resistant or biofortified have been produced as a result of biotechnology. Controversy still surrounds the use of this technology, and more research is warranted on the effects of these crops on human health and the environment. Details of biotechnology are discussed in Section 12.4.

The world's fertile farmland is increasingly threatened by increased erosion, salinization, desertification, and deforestation. Other areas of the world remain uncultivated or ungrazed because they are too rocky, steep, infertile, dry, wet, or inaccessible to sustain farming. Agriculture is the largest user of freshwater resources. Nearly all global irrigation water is being used, and groundwater supplies are becoming depleted at rapid rates. The eventual water shortage is projected to increase war and civil unrest in arid areas of the world, such as Northern Africa and the Middle East. China, which has more than 20% of the world's irrigated land, is also plagued with a growing scarcity of fresh water. In the future, billions of people are expected to face ongoing water shortages.

In recent years, the amount of fish caught worldwide has leveled off as fish consumption has increased. Fish, once considered the poor person's protein, is quickly becoming depleted in our oceans. Fish farming simply cannot compensate for the degree of reduction in wild fish populations. Coastal fisheries in West Africa are overexploited, and in the past 30 years, stocks have declined by 50%. Yet 400 million people in Southeast Asia and Africa must depend on fish for their protein and nutritional needs.

We can only exploit the Earth's resources so far. If the world population continues to expand at its current rate, we face the potential threats of serious famine, disease, and death. A profound change is needed if we are to nourish an estimated 9.7 billion inhabitants of planet Earth by 2050. The FAO *State of Food Insecurity in the World* report calls for global sustainability support and practices. Agricultural systems should sustain the environment while providing adequate, healthy food. If food production is to keep

green revolution Refers to increases in crop yields that accompanied the introduction of new agricultural technologies in less-developed countries. The key technologies were high-yielding, disease-resistant strains of rice, wheat, and corn; greater use of fertilizer and water; and improved cultivation practices.

sustainable agriculture Agricultural system that provides a secure living for farm families; maintains the natural environment and resources; supports the rural community; and offers respect and fair treatment to all involved, from farm workers to consumers to the animals raised for food.

biotechnology A collection of processes that involves the use of biological systems for altering and, ideally, improving the characteristics of plants, animals, and other forms of life.

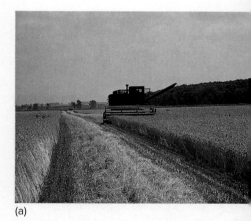

(a)

©Ohio State University Extension, outreach arm of the College of Food, Agricultural, and Environmental Sciences

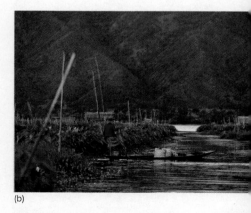

(b)

▲ Rich agricultural resources in North America, as seen in these wheat fields (a), contrast with gardens being tended by a farmer on a floating island in Myanmar (formerly Burma) (b). ©Getty Images

up with the expanding population, immediate action is needed to protect the Earth's already deteriorated environment from further destruction.[10]

INADEQUATE SHELTER AND SANITATION

When people die from undernutrition, other factors, such as inadequate shelter and sanitation, almost always contribute. No one can survive without clean water, nor can we stay healthy for any length of time without proper sanitation and shelter. Many more people suffer from the effects of poor sanitation and an unreliable water supply in developing countries than are affected by war and political/civil unrest. Without *w*ater, *s*anitation, and *h*ygiene (*WASH*), sustainable development remains impossible.

The tremendous movement of individuals to urban settings has caused a population redistribution that has challenged the capacity for shelter and sanitation. It is expected that in the next 30 years, most urban population growth will be in cities of developing countries, reaching almost 5.2 billion in 2050. Today, 54% of the world's population currently live in towns and cities, and by 2050, we can expect 70% of people to reside in urban areas. People go to the cities to find employment and resources the countryside can no longer provide. In developing countries, the poor make up most of the urban population, and their needs for housing and community services often exceed available governmental resources. Over 30% of current urban dwellers live in slums, totaling 1 billion people worldwide.

Most poverty-stricken urban residents live in overcrowded, self-made shelters, which lack a safe and adequate water supply and are only partially served by public utilities. The World Health Organization (WHO)/UNICEF Joint Monitoring Programme for Water Supply and Sanitation has estimated that as of 2015, 2.4 billion people lacked improved sanitation facilities, and 663 million people still use unsafe drinking water sources. The shantytowns and ghettos of the developing world are often worse than the rural areas the people left behind. The urban poor need resources to purchase food, so they often subsist on dietary patterns even more meager than the homegrown rural fare. Making matters worse, haphazard shelters often lack facilities to protect food from spoilage or damage by insects and rodents. This inability to protect food supplies in some developing countries leads to the loss of as much as 40% of all perishable foods.

The shift from rural to urban life takes its greatest toll on infants and children. WHO/UNICEF reports that inadequate access to safe water and sanitation services, combined with poor hygiene practices, kills and sickens thousands of children every day. For example, more than half of the 5.9 million deaths of children (under age 5 years) that occurred in developing countries could have been prevented by improving the standards of environmental hygiene. Contributing to this issue is the fact that infants are often weaned early from breast milk to infant formula, partly because the mother must find employment. Mothers may also be influenced by advertisements depicting images of sophisticated, formula-feeding women. Unfortunately, because infant formulas are expensive, food insecure parents may try to conserve the formula by either overdiluting the mixture or reducing the feeding volume to conserve formula. In addition, the water supply may not be safe, so the prepared formula is also likely to be contaminated with bacteria. Human milk, in contrast, is much more hygienic, readily available, and nutritious. It also provides infants with immunity to some ailments. In most situations, breastfeeding should be promoted as the safest and most nutritious choice for infant feeding.

Poor sanitation also creates a critical public health problem and, along with undernutrition, particularly raises the risk of infection. Inadequate sanitation is another example of the inferior infrastructure in the developing world. Human urine and feces are two of the most dangerous substances encountered in overcrowded urban areas. In addition, rotting garbage and associated insect and rodent infestations are potent sources of disease-causing organisms commonly seen in urban areas of the developing world. The inability to dispose of the massive numbers of deceased people (and animals) resulting from disease and wars causes additional sanitation problems. In some

Blood loss caused by intestinal and bloodborne parasite infections is a common cause of anemia among poor populations, especially when people do not wear shoes. Parasites, such as hookworms, can easily penetrate the soles of the feet and legs and enter the bloodstream. Although hookworm disease has been largely eradicated in the United States and other industrialized nations through improved sanitation, it continues to plague more than one-eighth of the world's population, mostly in tropical regions.

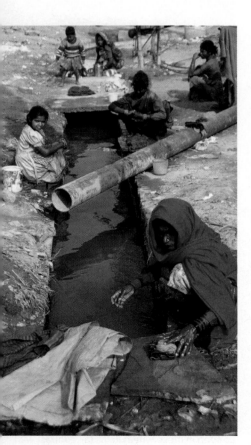

▲ Inadequate sanitation facilities and the consumption of contaminated water cause the majority of all diseases. ©Dr. Parvinder Sethi

developing countries, diarrheal diseases account for as many as one-third of all deaths in children younger than 5 years of age. Additional repercussions of poor sanitation are that children are denied access to education because their schools lack private and decent sanitation facilities.

Fortunately, organizations such as UNICEF are working in more than 100 countries across the globe to improve water supplies and sanitation facilities in schools and communities and to promote safe hygiene practices. The UNICEF WASH programs are designed to support the Sustainable Development Goal for clean water and sanitation, which aims to achieve universal and equitable access to safe and affordable drinking water for all by 2030. This goal can't come soon enough as 663 million people still lack access to safe water.

THE IMPACT OF AIDS WORLDWIDE

Nutrition security is impacted greatly in developing counties by the high prevalence of HIV infection and AIDS. HIV/AIDS impairs absorption of nutrients, increases nutrient requirements, and decreases the capacity to work. About 37 million people around the world were known to be infected with HIV or had gone on to develop AIDS from the infection in 2015. Cases in Sub-Saharan Africa account for almost 70% of the global total of new HIV infections.

An individual can be infected with HIV through contact with bodily fluids including blood, semen, vaginal secretions, and human milk. Thus, the virus can be transmitted through sexual contact, through blood-to-blood contact, and from a mother to an infant during pregnancy, delivery, or breastfeeding. The virus has a very limited ability to exist outside the body. Once infected with HIV, the individual is said to be HIV positive. If untreated, the viral disease progresses over the next few years, and the individual develops opportunistic infections with symptoms such as diarrhea, lung disease, weight loss, and a form of cancer. Once the individual has developed these symptoms, that person is said to have AIDS. Without treatment, an individual will likely die from AIDS within 4 to 5 years.

Ensuring healthy lives and promoting the well-being for all is one of the Sustainable Development Goals. This specific goal proposes to end the epidemics of AIDS, tuberculosis, malaria, and other tropical diseases and combat hepatitis, water-borne diseases, and other communicable diseases by 2030. Several countries have noted modest declines in the number of children newly infected with HIV, but the Middle East and North Africa have seen no reduction in the number of newly infected children (Fig. 12-8). Reductions in the number of adults who are newly infected with HIV, as well as the direct use of preventive antiretroviral medications, appear to be the reason for the reductions in the number of children acquiring HIV. Antiretroviral therapy (ART) is now credited for preventing more than 7.6 million deaths since 1995.

In the United States, it is estimated that more than 1.2 million people are infected with HIV, with one in eight (12.8%) unaware of their infections. Over 50,000 new cases of HIV infection are reported in the United States annually. HIV affects a large percentage of blacks in the United States, and gay and bisexual men are most seriously affected by HIV.

Toward Universal Treatment. Although no vaccine is available to prevent AIDS, the latest antiretroviral therapy (ART) can significantly slow the progression of the disease. Providing AIDS drugs to pregnant women is also an effective preventive measure. In pregnant women, a goal of therapy is prevention of perinatal HIV transmission and to maximize viral suppression to reduce the transmission of HIV to the fetus and newborn. Adverse effects have been noted during pregnancy so clinicians should follow the current perinatal ART guidelines.

Another barrier is economic: A typical drug regimen can cost over $10,000 per year, not including unforeseen hospital stays. Fortunately, drug companies and governments have worked successfully to lower the cost of AIDS drugs for developing nations. Most countries that aspire to expand access to treatment set a goal of providing ART to

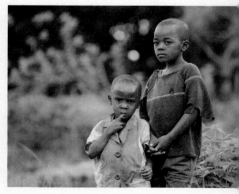

▲ A particularly sad consequence of AIDS in Africa is the number of AIDS orphans—children whose parents have both died of AIDS. These orphans then become responsible for the care of their siblings and other family members. ©RachelKolokoffHopper/Shutterstock

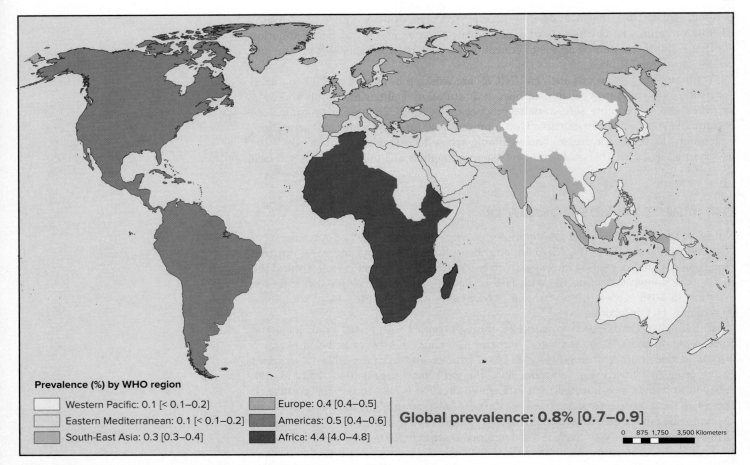

Prevalence (%) by WHO region

Western Pacific: 0.1 [< 0.1–0.2]	Europe: 0.4 [0.4–0.5]
Eastern Mediterranean: 0.1 [< 0.1–0.2]	Americas: 0.5 [0.4–0.6]
South-East Asia: 0.3 [0.3–0.4]	Africa: 4.4 [4.0–4.8]

Global prevalence: 0.8% [0.7–0.9]

0   875 1,750   3,500 Kilometers

FIGURE 12-8 ▲ Adult HIV prevalence (15–49 years) by WHO region, 2015.
Source: http://www.who.int/gho/hiv/en/. Reproduced with permission of the World Health Organization

around 80% of those in need. Although life-saving ART is reaching more individuals, global treatment is still reaching only 40% of those that need it, meaning there are still millions of people waiting to be treated. Progress to the goal of ensuring access to HIV treatment has been slower for children than for adults. Sadly, just 32% of HIV-infected children had access to antiretroviral therapy.

Nutrition and AIDS. Although adequate nutrition cannot prevent or cure HIV infection or AIDS, nutritional status can affect the progression of the disease. A focus on eliminating or reducing malnutrition can significantly slow disease progression and severity, and improve longevity. A dietary pattern adequate in energy, protein, and micronutrients can lessen the impact of infections associated with AIDS. Low levels of vitamins A and E can contribute to a more rapid onset of symptoms, including body wasting and fever. Maintenance of an optimal nutritional status should be an integral focus of the treatment for AIDS. Daily use of a balanced vitamin and mineral supplement has also been shown to slow health declines in people with HIV/AIDS. Nutritional counseling by a registered dietitian nutritionist (RDN) is paramount in assessing nutritional status, providing personalized education and recommendations, and monitoring outcomes. The main goals of nutritional treatment are to achieve and maintain a healthy body weight, body composition, and lab values; minimize nutrition-related side effects and complications; improve quality of life; and expand access to nutrition services.[11]

1. Why does undernutrition continue despite an adequate food supply in many areas?

2. What are some solutions to limiting population growth, especially in developing countries where birth rates are high?

3. How have war and declines in natural resources contributed to undernutrition in developing countries?

4. What effects have overpopulation and increased urbanization had on nutrition and disease risk?

5. How is HIV transmitted?

6. What role does nutrition play in combating AIDS?

12.4 Reducing Undernutrition in the Developing World

Reducing undernutrition in the developing world is quite complex and takes considerable time to accomplish. It has been a common practice for affluent nations to supply famine areas with direct food aid; however, this is not a long-term solution. Although it reduces the number of deaths from famine, it can also reduce incentives for local production by driving down food prices. In addition, the affected countries may have little or no means of transporting the food to those who need it most, and the donated foods may not be culturally acceptable or nutrient dense. In the short run or during a crisis, there is no choice: aid must be provided because people are starving.[3] Still, improving the infrastructure for poor people, especially rural people, needs to be the long-term focus.

With the adoption of the *Sustainable Development Goals* (Fig. 12-9) by all United Nations member states, world leaders committed to address the many dimensions of extreme poverty and create a better life for those in need by 2030. Pertinent hunger-related goals

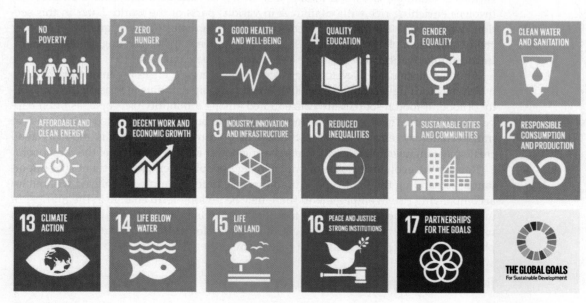

FIGURE 12-9 ▲ The United Nations Sustainable Development Goals: 17 goals to transform our world.

Source: United Nations/www.globalgoals.org

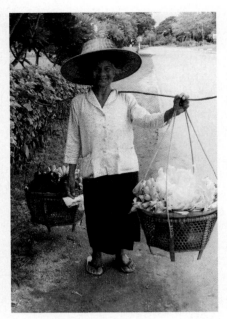

▲ Food security is fostered by communities raising and distributing locally grown food. ©Erin Koran

include reducing by half the proportion of men, women, and children of all ages living in poverty; eradicating extreme poverty for all, currently measured as people living on less than $1.25 a day; and ensuring that the poor and the vulnerable have equal rights to economic resources, as well as access to basic services, ownership and control over land and other forms of property, inheritance, natural resources, appropriate new technology, and financial services.

DEVELOPMENT TAILORED TO LOCAL CONDITIONS

Although world food supplies have grown faster than the population in recent years, an increase in malnutrition has resulted from inadequate of food distribution and access. In addition, millions of farmers are losing access to resources they need to be self-reliant. There is a growing realization that unless economic opportunities can be created as part of a plan for sustainable development, rural residents who do not own land will flock to the overcrowded cities.

For the most part, the sustainable solutions lie in helping people meet their own needs and directing them to resources and employment opportunities. Experience has shown that the provision of credit—along with education and training, food storage facilities, and marketing support—allows rural people to actively participate in their success, which benefits their families and communities. Understanding and appreciating the local conditions, including crop rotation, utilization of varieties of plants, and crop diversification, are essential to understanding barriers to success. Agroforestry initiatives and promotion of local and culturally sensitive foods are needed. Communities that have significant land and water limitations may require the intervention and assistance of local authorities.

One U.S. program, the *Peace Corps*, has helped to improve conditions in developing nations for over 50 years by providing education, distributing food and medical supplies, and building structures for local use. The aim of the Peace Corps is to help create independent, self-sustaining economies around the world. Becoming a Peace Corps volunteer is a meaningful way to make a difference around the world. Learn more about this program at www.peacecorps.gov.

Suitable technologies for processing, preserving, marketing, and distributing nutritious local staples also need to be encouraged, so that small farmers can flourish. Education on how to use whole foods to create healthful dietary patterns adds further benefit. Supplementing indigenous foods with nutrients that are in short supply, such as iron, various B vitamins, zinc, and iodine, also deserves consideration. One such program involves enriching rice with vitamin A in various parts of the world. Later in this section, we examine the role of biotechnology in improving nutrient quality and other characteristics of plants and animals, another positive step in lessening undernutrition. In addition, advances in water purification need to be employed.

Another Sustainable Development Goal aims to ensure environmental sustainability, which may include promoting extensive land ownership and thus increasing the availability of food. If food resources are concentrated among a minority of people, as often happens with unequal land ownership, food is unlikely to be equally distributed unless efficient transportation systems are in place. Small-scale industrial development is another way to create meaningful employment and purchasing power for vast numbers of the rural poor.

Raising the economic status of impoverished people by employing them is as important as expanding the food supply. If an increase in food supply is achieved without an accompanying rise in employment, there may be no long-term change in the number of undernourished people. Although food prices may fall with increased mechanization, use of fertilizers, and other modern farming technologies, these advances can also displace people from jobs, a result that may harm, rather than help, the population.

IMPROVING GENDER EQUALITY

Impoverished women are a special concern. In addition to working longer hours than men, they grow most of the food for family consumption and account for three-fourths

FARM to FORK　　Bananas

When you enjoy tropical fruits, you are eating globally. The most common tropical fruits are bananas, pineapples, mangos, and papayas—imported from Ecuador, Costa Rica, Mexico, and Hawaii. Bananas are the most consumed fruit in the United States—more than apples and oranges combined!

Grow

- Although bananas grow on "banana palms," bananas do not grow on trees. Banana palms are actually a perennial herb.
- Bananas do not grow from a seed but instead from a bulb or rhizome. After planting a banana palm in a subtropical environment, it can take up to 12 months to literally enjoy the fruits of your labor.
- Because bananas grow in tropical climates, they are not seasonal fruits but rather continue to grow all year long.

Shop

- There are two main categories of bananas. Plantains (or cooking bananas) are starchy, and Cavendish (or dessert bananas) are the sweet, yellow bananas most commonly sold at the supermarket.
- To increase your antioxidant content when eating bananas, look beyond Cavendish bananas. Red bananas and niños, or Lady Fingers, provide greater vitamin C, potassium, calcium, manganese, carotenoids, and zinc than the common Cavendish.

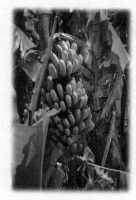

©Corey Hochachka/Design Pics

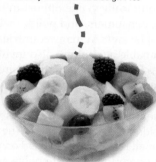

©Nataliia K/Shutterstock

Store

- Bananas continue to ripen after harvest and are often harvested when immature and green. These bananas will ripen in 5 to 7 days if left at room temperature.
- Store ripe bananas in the refrigerator. Although their skins will turn brown, the flesh will stay fresher for days.

Prep

- Plantains serve as the main carbohydrate source for 20 million individuals globally. Harvested when green, plantains are skinned, then steamed, baked, or fried.
- In the Caribbean, fried plantains are a staple. For a healthier recipe, try baked plantains. Use ripe plantains, spotted with brown or black spots, and slice after peeling. Coat a nonstick baking sheet with cooking spray and lay the plantains in rows. Cook at 450°F for 15 minutes, flipping them frequently.
- Celebrate bananas as the perfect on-the-go snack, lunch box treat, or sliced treat on top of cereal, yogurt, or whole wheat pancakes.

Source: Robinson J. "Tropical Fruits: Make the Most of Eating Globally," in *Eating on the Wild Side*. New York: Little, Brown and Company, 2013.

of the labor force in the informal sector of the economy and an increasing proportion in the formal sector. Of the 3 billion people in the world living on less than $2 a day, 70% are women. Clearly, economic opportunities for women and education regarding family planning must be augmented.

Empowerment of women is critical to improve the level of nutrition security, increase the production and distribution of food and other agricultural products, and enhance living conditions in general. Goal 5 of the Sustainable Development Goals aims to achieve gender equality and empower all women and girls. Increasing women's access to education, information and communication technologies, economic resources, and governance reduces poverty, promotes development, achieves gender equality, protects women's human rights, and eliminates violence against women. Although paid women workers outside of agriculture increased from 35% in 1990 to 41% in 2015, women continue to experience significant gaps in terms of poverty, labor market and wages, and participation in private and public decision making. There is still plenty of room for improvement.

SUSTAINABLE AGRICULTURE

Over the years, changes in agricultural practices have had many positive results on the availability of food around the world. Along with the positive effects on farming, however, there have been significant negative impacts. Most significant among these are the depletion of topsoil, contamination of groundwater, decline of family farms, neglect

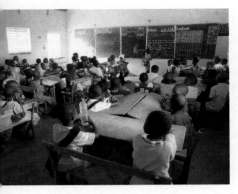

▲ This school teacher and her students are in a classroom in a village in Senegal, Africa. Eliminating gender disparity is a goal of the Sustainable Development Goals. ©Andia/UIG via Getty Images

sustainable development Economic growth that will simultaneously reduce poverty, protect the environment, and preserve natural capital.

genetic engineering Manipulation of the genetic makeup of any organism with recombinant DNA technology.

genetically modified organism (GMO) Any organism created by genetic engineering.

of living and working conditions for farm laborers, increasing costs of production, and lack of integration of economic and social conditions in rural communities.

As previously mentioned, the concept of **sustainable development** has been embraced as economic growth that will reduce poverty while, at the same time, protect the environment and preserve natural capital. The United Nations cites economic development, social development, and environmental protection as the *reinforcing pillars* of sustainable development. The role of the agriculture industry in promoting practices that contribute to environmental and social issues has been at the center of discussions of sustainable development. As a result, interest in alternative farming practices has grown and reinforced a movement toward sustainable agriculture. This type of agriculture describes farming systems that can indefinitely maintain their productivity and usefulness to society. Sustainable agriculture flows directly from the United Nation's Sustainable Development Goals to ensure sustainable consumption and production patterns globally. The targets depend on integration of several goals, including environmental health, economic profitability, and social and economic equity. Sustainable agriculture addresses many environmental and social concerns and offers innovative and economically viable opportunities for many in the food system, including growers, laborers, consumers, and policy makers. It is gaining support and acceptance from conventional farmers in many countries.

Sustainable agriculture also involves maintaining or enhancing the land and natural resources for use long into the future. It also requires consideration for human resources, including working and living conditions of laborers, the needs of rural communities, and consumer health and safety. The potential of sustainability is best understood when the consequences of farming practices on both human communities and the environment are considered. Farmers around the globe are transitioning to sustainable agriculture by taking small realistic steps based on their personal goals and family economics. Reaching the goal of worldwide sustainable agriculture requires participation by all stakeholders, including farmers, laborers, retailers, consumers, researchers, and policy makers.

BIOTECHNOLOGY

The ability of humans to modify natural resources has enabled us to improve the production and yield of many important foods. Traditional **biotechnology** is almost as old as agriculture itself. The first farmer to improve stocks by selectively breeding the best bull with the best cows was implementing biotechnology. The first baker to use yeast to make bread rise took advantage of biotechnology.

By the 1930s, biotechnology made possible the selective breeding of improved plant hybrids. As a result, corn production in the United States quickly doubled. Through similar methods, agricultural wheat was crossed with wild grasses to confer more desirable properties, such as greater yield, increased resistance to mildew and bacterial diseases, and tolerance to salt or adverse climatic conditions. Another type of biotechnology uses hormones rather than breeding. In the last decade, Canadian salmon have been treated with a hormone that allows them to mature three times faster than normal—without changing the fish in any other way. In general terms, biotechnology can be understood as the use of living things—plants, animals, bacteria—to manufacture novel products.

Biotechnology used in agriculture includes several methods that directly modify products. It differs from traditional methods because it directly changes some of the genetic material (DNA) of organisms to improve characteristics. Crossbreeding of plants or animals is no longer the only tool. Development of **genetic engineering** began in the 1970s. The field now features a wide range of cell and subcell techniques for the synthesis and placement of genetic material into organisms (Fig. 12-10). In comparison to modern biotechnology, conventional breeding is inefficient and has inconsistent results; biotechnology uses genetic material more precisely. Scientists select the traits they desire and genetically engineer or introduce the gene that produces that trait into plants or animals (called a **genetically modified organism [GMO]**). Genetic engineering has not replaced conventional breeding practices; both work together.

Biotechnology has been used to enhance crops in several categories. The primary category is the addition of a unique characteristic, called an *input trait,* to a crop. These enhanced input traits include herbicide (weed killer) tolerance, insect and virus protection, and tolerance to environmental stressors such as drought. Other categories are value-added *output traits,* such as plant oils with increased levels of omega-3 fatty acids, and crops that produce pharmaceuticals. Scientists have engineered plants that thrive with fewer pesticides, potatoes that can be stored longer, and apples that do not turn brown. In addition, biotechnology allows scientists to create fruits and grains with greater amounts of nutrients such as beta-carotene (e.g., *golden rice*) and vitamins E and C. Biotechnology is being used cautiously and conservatively, so the benefits are subtle. The ultimate benefits, however, could be significant in developing countries given the technology, training, and access.

Few consumers realize that over 92% of corn and 94% of soybeans produced in the United States have been genetically engineered to either resist certain insects, thereby reducing pesticide use, and/or survive when sprayed with herbicides that kill surrounding weeds. Papaya and sugar beet plants have been genetically engineered for viral resistance. Corn has been genetically altered by inserting a gene from the bacterium *Bacillus thuringiensis,* usually referred to as the *Bt gene,* into the corn DNA (Fig. 12-10). The gene allows the corn plant to make a protein lethal to predator caterpillars that destroy the crop. The Bt protein in the corn is present in low concentrations with no effect on humans; it is digested along with the other proteins in corn. In fact, for many years, organic farmers have used the Bt bacteria directly on plants to destroy pests without changing the DNA of the plant.

The FDA and the National Academy of Sciences are confident that approved varieties of genetically engineered foods are safe to consume. Food manufacturers, therefore, are not required to disclose the genetically modified ingredient content on food labels. However, surveys show that the majority of consumers request GMO labeling. Legislation will soon require future GMO food labeling, but it may not be printed on the package label. Instead, food manufacturers can make that information available through a QR code that can be scanned using a smartphone. Small food companies have the option of printing a website URL or a phone number that customers can call for more information. Consumers looking to avoid GMO food can buy certified organic food, since no GMO ingredients are permitted under the USDA's organic certification guidelines. The non-GMO verification seal (http://www.nongmoproject.org) is also an assurance that a product has been produced according to consensus-based best practices for GMO avoidance. The Ask the RDN in this section contains more information on GMOs.

Public response to use of biotechnology has been mixed. Even the scientific community has conflicting opinions about this technology, with supporters as convinced about the benefits as opponents are of the risks. The biggest debate in the United States surrounds the potential environmental hazards of introducing genes from one species to another. Some challengers even question the reduction in pesticide use that accompanies the cultivation of genetically modified crops. Although the use of genetically modified crops may reduce the need for environmentally harmful activities, such as spraying crops with pesticides, critics point out that seeds produced with additional insecticide, such as the Bt protein, may lead to rapid insect resistance because the insecticides are continuously emitted. Use of traditional pesticides involves prudent application, in part to avoid insect resistance. In addition, accidental release of genetically modified animals, such as fish, may go on to harm wild varieties.

Although the risks of biotechnology may appear to be momentarily negligible, they may be cumulative and therefore of concern in the long run. The FDA carefully examines all products developed using this technology and will enforce labeling of potential

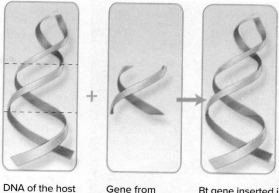

DNA of the host plant, corn

Gene from bacteria (Bt gene) that produces a protein toxic to the European corn borer

Bt gene inserted into DNA of corn plant. Now the corn plant is genetically modified. It makes the Bt toxin and so is resistant to the European corn borer.

FIGURE 12-10 ▲ Biotechnology involves various techniques for transferring foreign DNA into an organism. In this diagram, a sample of DNA is cleaved out of a larger DNA fragment and inserted into the DNA of a host cell. Thus, the host cell contains new genetic information, with the potential of providing the cell with new capabilities. For corn, this could mean resistance to the European corn borer, a plant predator that feeds on corn and attacks hundreds of crops. In another application, bacteria can be engineered to produce the human form of the hormone insulin.

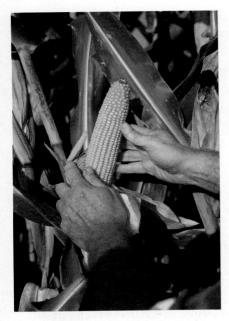

▲ Both traditional plant breeding and biotechnology have produced high-yielding and disease-resistant plant varieties, including new varieties of corn. ©Purestock/Getty Images

allergens that may be newly present in food altered by biotechnology. The public has long been opposed to processes perceived as harmful to the environment, such as producing unnatural products. Skepticism surrounds unnatural products, as exemplified by Western Europe's ban of hormones used in beef and milk production and of almost all genetically modified foods.

A global analysis of over 145 studies of biotechnology crops over the past 20 years confirmed the significant benefits of biotech crops. The study found that on average, GMO technology has reduced chemical pesticide use by 37%, increased crop yield by 22%, and increased farmer profits by 68%. This study estimated the value added to be over $133 billion for the years spanning 1996 to 2013.[12]

ROLE OF THE NEW BIOTECHNOLOGY IN THE DEVELOPING WORLD

Eighteen million farmers in 28 countries planted more than 181 million biotech crops in 2014. The top four GMOs include corn, soybean, alfalfa, and cotton. The United States maintained the largest growth of biotech crops with 180 million acres of corn, soybean, cotton, canola, sugar beet, alfalfa, papaya, and squash. Of the 18 million farmers that benefited from growing biotech crops in 2014, 16.5 million or 90% were small resource-poor farmers from developing countries.

Whether applications of genetic engineering will help to significantly reduce malnutrition in the developing world remains to be seen. Unless price cuts accompany the increased production, only landowners and suppliers of biotechnology will enjoy the benefits. Small farmers may benefit if they can afford to purchase the genetically modified seeds. This point deserves emphasis: the person who cannot afford to buy enough food today will still face that same predicament in the future. As with most innovations, the more successful farmers—often those with larger farms—will adopt new biotechnology first. Because of this, the present trend toward fewer and larger farms will continue in the developing world, a movement that undermines the solution to one of the most pressing undernutrition issues. Furthermore, biotechnology does not promise dramatic increases in the production of most grains and cassava, the primary food resources in developing parts of the world.

With the introduction of drought- and pest-resistant crops, as well as self-fertilizing crops, agricultural biotechnology may help to reduce world hunger. Perhaps the most promising potential of genetically modified foods today lies within the realm of plant breeding for micronutrients. Developing countries will have a tool to treat and prevent nutrient deficiencies among their populations if they have access to farming resources to increase the micronutrient composition of crops. In addition, greater yields for indigenous plants, such as tomatoes that tolerate high soil salinity, are another hopeful outcome. Biotechnology will likely be a useful tool against the complex scourge of world undernutrition. Improved crops produced by this technology, together with political and other efforts, can contribute to success in the battle against worldwide undernutrition.

CONCLUDING THOUGHTS

The economic loss from malnutrition is staggering, and the amount of human pain and suffering it causes is incalculable. With all the international relief efforts and assistance from governments and private organizations combined, the battle is far from over. Read more about the progress toward the Sustainable Development Goals and the ongoing challenges of hunger in several regions of the world, even as poverty has decreased at https://sustainabledevelopment.un.org/.[13]

Ultimately, the rapid depletion of world resources, massive debt incurred by poorer countries, threat of danger to more prosperous countries nearby, and toll of war and famine all affect the world economy and well-being. Planet Earth has enough food and the technical expertise to end hunger. With world leaders affirming the UN Sustainable Development Goals and working to achieve its targets by 2030, we have a promising

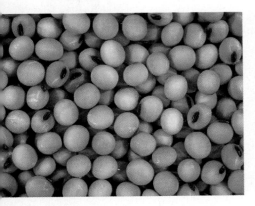

▲ Soybeans are a common GMO food in the marketplace. Over 94% of the soybeans grown in the United States are genetically modified. ©Ohio State University Extension, outreach arm of the College of Food, Agricultural, and Environmental Sciences

coordinated political effort that is making progress toward lasting reductions in hunger and optimal health for all.

ASK THE RDN Non-GMO Diet

Dear Author: Lately, my friends on social media have been discussing the hazards of genetically modified foods. Many of them promote a non-GMO lifestyle. Is this a nutritionally adequate eating pattern?

Great question! First, let me outline what science shows about their safety. Then you can make an informed decision.

Some benefits of genetic engineering in agriculture include increased crop yields, reduced food costs, diminished pesticide and chemical use, enhanced food safety and food security, and reductions in soil erosion and environmental stress. GMOs have created more tolerant crops that are able to grow where they might not otherwise flourish. Globally, the use of GMOs hold great promise for reducing the prevalence of nutrition-related deficiencies and disease. For example, vitamin A-enhanced rice, also known as *golden rice*, can correct vitamin A deficiencies and blindness for millions of people.

The FDA has approved GMOs for human consumption. Health experts cite hundreds of studies, spanning two decades, to support the safety of GMOs. Despite mounting evidence, the potential for unknown consequences remains. Some individuals believe that intentionally altering nature is intrinsically incorrect or immoral. Many groups are calling for clear labeling rules so consumers can make informed decisions when purchasing foods. Yet, in order to label products, there must be a clear definition and assessment of what constitutes a GMO.

Any alterations to an organism's natural state may affect metabolism, growth, and environmental outcomes. Potential health risks to humans include the possibility of exposure to new allergens or the advent of antibiotic-resistant organisms. Environmental concerns include the rise in *superweeds* requiring stronger pesticides or the possibility that genes may migrate to other species.

Yes, a non-GMO lifestyle can include a nutritionally adequate eating pattern, but it will require some inconvenience, extra costs, and close attention to food labels. Currently, up to 80% of conventionally processed food in the United States contains some genetically modified ingredients. The main tenets of a non-GMO dietary pattern align with the Dietary Guidelines, which emphasize a plant-based eating pattern—that is, rich in fiber and low in highly processed foods. Specific tips to reduce or avoid GMO exposure include:

- Focus on produce. Most fresh fruits and vegetables are non-GMO, yet some zucchini, squash, edamame, sweet corn, and papaya from Hawaii or China are considered high risk. Look for those products labeled "organic" because organic foods cannot contain GMOs.
- Look for the non-GMO-verified seal. Until GMO labeling is required, this seal can help you find GMO-free products.
- Embrace fiber. Most nuts, seeds, grains, and beans are GMO free.
- Avoid highly processed and packaged food. GMO food ingredients such as corn, canola oil, soy, and sugar beets are often used in food processing.
- Select wild-caught seafood. Some farm-raised seafood contains GMOs.

Balancing the pros and cons,

Colleen Spees, PhD, RDN, LD, FAND (author)

CRITICAL THINKING

Stan has read about various relief efforts to help undernourished people in developing countries, especially the emergency food aid programs for famine-ravaged areas. Yet many of these efforts appear temporary, and he wonders what long-range approaches might help alleviate the problem of undernutrition. What suggestions would you give Stan about possible long-term solutions for undernutrition in developing countries?

✅ CONCEPT CHECK 12.4

1. Why is development tailored to local conditions important in combating global hunger?
2. What is the definition of *sustainable agriculture*?
3. How is *biotechnology* used to enhance crops?

Undernutrition at Critical Life Stages

PREGNANCY

Undernutrition poses the greatest health risk during pregnancy. Every day, approximately 830 women die from preventable causes related to pregnancy and childbirth. A pregnant woman needs extra nutrients to meet both her own needs and those of her developing offspring. Nourishing the fetus may deplete maternal stores of nutrients. Maternal iron-deficiency anemia is one possible consequence of malnutrition during pregnancy.

Birth rates in Africa are the highest in the world. In Niger, for example, a woman gives birth to an average of nearly 8 children. Close behind are countries such as Chad, Somalia, Mali, and Nigeria, where an average of 6 to 7 children are born to each woman. Coupled with chronic malnutrition, a woman's risk of dying increases with every pregnancy and birth. This results in a strong connection between a high fertility rate and high maternal mortality rates. Although most of us consider pregnancy and childbirth as natural parts of life, for women living in developing countries and without access to health care, pregnancy and childbirth complications are among the leading causes of death. The cumulative effect of successive pregnancies does not allow the mother to recover key nutrients, such as iron and folate, lost during pregnancy and breastfeeding. Since 1990, the maternal mortality rate has been cut nearly in half. In South Asia, the maternal mortality rate has declined by 64% and in sub-Saharan Africa, it has fallen by 49%. The new Sustainable Development Goal is to reduce the global maternal mortality ratio to less than 70 per 100,000 live births by 2030.

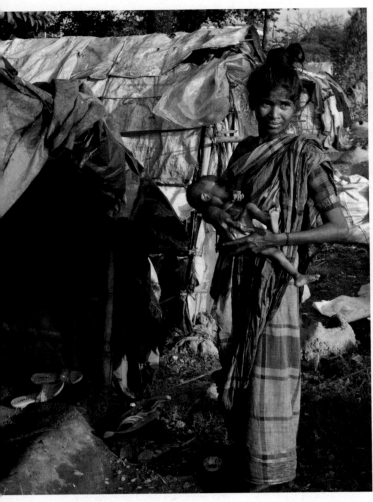

©Andrew Holbrooke/Corbis via Getty Images

Critical Life Stages When Undernutrition Is Particularly Devastating

Prolonged undernutrition is detrimental to many aspects of human health, resulting in increased maternal, infant, and child mortality; loss of parents (especially linked to AIDS); exploitation of women; reduced work capacity; reduced intellectual and social development; and overall human suffering, especially during a famine. It is particularly damaging during periods of growth and old age. A conceptual framework of malnutrition, developed by UNICEF, lists the immediate causes of malnutrition as inadequate dietary intake and unsatisfactory health. The underlying causes relate to families and include lack of access to food, inadequate care for women and children, and inadequate health services. Basic causes relate to human and economic resources and affect communities and nations. Effective strategies to combat malnutrition should embrace a life cycle approach. Public health programs should be complementary and comprehensive across vulnerable periods of the whole reproductive cycle.

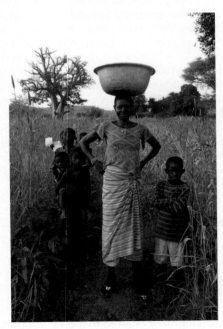

▲ This Lobi tribeswoman, standing with her six children in a grassy field in Burkina Faso, Africa, is an illustration of the typical birth rate in this region. Maternal nutrient levels become depleted with successive pregnancies followed by breastfeeding. ©Lissa Harrison

FETAL DEVELOPMENT AND INFANT STAGES

An unborn baby faces major health risks from undernutrition during gestation. To support growth and development of the brain and other body tissues, a growing fetus requires a rich supply of protein, vitamins, and minerals. When these nutrient needs are not met, the infant is often born before 37 weeks of gestation, well before the ideal 40 weeks. Preterm birth and low birth weight (5.5 pounds [2.5 kilograms] or less) contribute to 60% to 80% of all neonatal deaths. If the infant survives, abnormal growth and development can result. In extreme cases, low-birth-weight infants face 5 to 10 times the normal risk of dying before their first birthday, primarily due to complications of reduced lung development. When low birth weight is accompanied by other physical abnormalities, medical costs may exceed $200,000. Clearly, these costs can only be met in developed countries.

Worldwide, the incidence of infants born with low birth weight is 15%. Much higher rates, however, occur in developing countries, with the highest rates in Pakistan (32%), India (28%), Nanru China (27%), Niger (27%), and Haiti (25%). Undernutrition is a major contributor to these high rates of low birth weight in developing countries. About 8% of infants born in the United States and 6% in Canada have low birth weights. In the United States, low birth weight accounts for more than half of all infant deaths and 83% of deaths of infants younger than 1 month. Pregnancy during the teenage years, when a teen's body is still growing, contributes to low birth weight worldwide.

CHILDHOOD

Early childhood, when growth is rapid, is another period when malnutrition is extremely risky. The greatest impact of undernutrition occurs in the first 1000 days of life: from conception to a child's second birthday. Irreversible damage is the result if optimal nutrition is not available at critical times in development. The central nervous system—including the brain—is highly vulnerable because of rapid growth through early childhood. After the preschool years, brain growth and development slow dramatically. Nutritional deprivation, especially in early infancy, can lead to permanent brain impairment. Without an effective intervention, it is projected that ongoing undernutrition could leave more than 1 billion children with mental impairments by 2020.

In general, impoverished children are at the greatest risk for nutrient deficiencies and subsequent consequences. The WHO reports that nearly 165 million suffer from *stunted growth*. Iron-deficiency anemia is also more common among low-income children. This deficiency can lead to fatigue, reduced stamina, stunted growth, impaired motor development, and learning problems. Undernutrition in childhood can also weaken immune function and increase the risk of infection when nutrients such as protein, vitamin A, and zinc are low in a diet. Clearly, malnutrition and illness have a cyclical relationship. Not only does undernutrition lead to illness, but illness, particularly diarrheal and other infectious diseases, increases undernutrition. For this reason, millions of these children in developing countries are dying from the combination of malnutrition and infection. Conversely, when missing nutrients,

such as vitamin A and iron, are restored to a child's diet, improvements in health are evident.

Reducing stunting and wasting in children under 5 years of age and addressing the nutritional needs of adolescent girls are Sustainable Development Goals. Death rates have already been reduced from 90 to 43 per 1000 live births from 1990 to 2015. Despite this progress, 6 million children under 5 years of age died in 2015. Furthermore, the progress made in recent decades has been unequally distributed across regions and countries and within countries. India (21%) and Nigeria (13%) account for one-third of all under-5 deaths. These statistics indicate that undernutrition is one of the most important challenges to overcome because it is estimated to be an underlying cause in as many as 45% of the preventable deaths among children under age 5.

LATER YEARS

The WHO predicts a significant increase in the number of people age 65 years or older, from an estimate of 524 million in 2010 to almost 1.5 billion in 2050. Most of this increase in global aging will be in developing countries. Older adults, especially older women living alone in poverty, are at risk for undernutrition. All older adults require nutrient-dense foods in amounts dependent on their current health and degree of physical activity. Many older adults have fixed incomes and incur significant medical costs over time, so food often becomes a low-priority item. In addition, depression, social isolation, and declining physical and mental health can compound the problem of undernutrition in older adults.

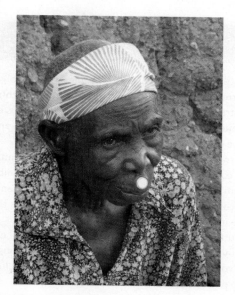

▲ This senior tribeswoman in Burkina Faso, Africa, with an ivory piercing in her upper lip, reminds us that the population of people aged 65 years or older will increase exponentially in developing countries. ©Lissa Harrison

CASE STUDY Undernutrition During Childhood

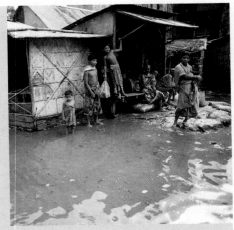

©Stockbyte/Getty Images RF

Jamal traveled to the Philippines with his church group last summer. During their stay, they helped build shelters in a village where, a few weeks before, a storm had destroyed several houses. Jamal noticed that many of the children were very short, much shorter than the children in his neighborhood in the United States. His group worked in a remote, low-elevation area where the storm and subsequent flooding had caused the most damage. On several occasions, he noticed young mothers crouched on curbs or in doorways, holding their children. These children rarely moved; they appeared pale and listless. In contrast to the children Jamal's group had met at a church in the capital city, most of the children in this village were not active and lively. One evening, a nurse from the local clinic came to speak to Jamal's group. She said that many children in this area do not get enough to eat and that undernutrition was rampant. She considered the recent storm a blessing in disguise, hoping it would spur the Philippine government to send supplies to the village, particularly food and medicines. Jamal was shocked by such a degree of suffering. He wonders why children in the Philippines can be starving to death while so many children in his hometown in the United States have more food than they need.

1. Which nutrients are likely to be deficient in the diets of these children?
2. Which nutrient deficiencies contribute to poor or *stunted* growth?
3. Which nutrient deficiencies may be reducing immune defenses?
4. Are these children likely to be consuming adequate calories? What effect does consumption of inadequate calories have on growth?
5. Why might the recent storm be a blessing for this small village?
6. List some reasons why the children in Jamal's neighborhood at home are more likely to be overweight than these children.

Complete the Case Study. Responses to these questions can be provided by your instructor.

Summary (Numbers refer to numbered sections in the chapter.)

12.1 Poverty is commonly linked to chronic or episodic undernutrition. Malnutrition includes both undernutrition and overnutrition and can occur when the food supply is either scarce or abundant. The resulting deficiency conditions and degenerative diseases contribute to poor health.

Undernutrition is the most common form of malnutrition in developing countries. It results from inadequate intake, absorption, or use of nutrients or food energy. Many nutrient deficiency conditions consequently appear, and infectious diseases thrive because the immune system is depressed.

Malnutrition diminishes both physical and mental capabilities. In poor countries, this is worsened by recurrent infections, unsanitary conditions, extreme weather, inadequate shelter, and exposure to pathogens and diseases.

12.2 In North America, famine is not seen, but food insecurity and undernutrition remain concerns, due in large part to poverty. Single mothers and their children are more likely to live in poverty. Soup kitchens, SNAP benefits the school lunch and breakfast programs, and WIC focus on improving the nutritional health of poor and at-risk people. When adequately funded, these programs have proved effective in reducing undernutrition.

12.3 Multiple factors contribute to the problem of undernutrition in the developing world. In densely populated countries, food resources, as well as the means for distributing food, may be inadequate. Environmentally unsustainable farming methods hamper future efforts to grow food. Limited water availability hinders food production. Natural disasters, urbanization, war, and disease all contribute to the major problem of undernutrition.

12.4 Proposed solutions to world undernutrition must consider multiple interacting factors, many thoroughly embedded in cultural traditions. Family planning efforts, for example, may not succeed until life expectancy increases. Through education and training, efforts should be made to upgrade farming methods, improve crops, limit pregnancies, encourage breastfeeding, and improve sanitation and hygiene.

Direct food aid is only a short-term solution. In what may appear to be a step backward, many experts recommend more subsistence-level sustainable farming. Small-scale industrial development is another way to create meaningful employment and purchasing power for vast numbers of the rural poor. Various biotechnology applications may also prove beneficial. The UN's 17 Sustainable Development Goals focus on global solutions.

12.5 The greatest risk of undernutrition occurs during critical periods of growth and development: gestation, infancy, and childhood. Low birth weight is a leading cause of infant deaths worldwide. Many developmental problems are caused by nutritional deprivation during critical periods of brain growth. People in their senior years are also at great risk.

Check Your Knowledge (Answers are available at the end of this question set.)

1. There are an estimated _____ chronically undernourished people in the world.
   a. 14 million
   b. 1 billion
   c. 3 billion
   d. 6 billion

2. The number one killer of children in developing countries is
   a. xerophthalmia.
   b. iron-deficiency anemia.
   c. iodine deficiency.
   d. diarrhea.

3. The human organism is particularly susceptible to the effects of undernutrition during
   a. pregnancy.
   b. infancy.
   c. childhood.
   d. all of these stages.

4. All of the following are barriers to solving undernutrition in the developing world *except*
   a. external debt.
   b. poor infrastructure.
   c. a lack of manpower.
   d. expanding population.

5. Many of the child deaths each year in developing countries could be prevented if
   a. technology were improved.
   b. doctors were more specialized.
   c. mothers would learn more about nutrition.
   d. sanitation and hygiene were improved.

6. The Supplemental Nutrition Assistance Program (SNAP) allows
   a. low-income families to buy surplus food at government stores with government-issued electronic benefit transfer cards.
   b. low-income people to purchase food, cleaning supplies, alcoholic beverages, and anything else sold in supermarkets with electronic benefit transfer cards.
   c. low-income people to turn in government-issued electronic benefit transfer cards for cash to buy food.
   d. low-income people to purchase food and seeds with government-issued electronic benefit transfer cards.

7. A long-term solution to world hunger is
   a. the green revolution.
   b. cash crops.
   c. jobs and self-sufficiency.
   d. government and private aid.

8. Bt corn has been genetically modified to make
   a. the bacterium *Bacillus thuringiensis*.
   b. a protein toxic to caterpillars that can destroy the corn plant.
   c. a sugar that makes the corn sweeter.
   d. a fat that makes corn oil healthier.

9. Genetically modified soybeans make up approximately _____% of the soybeans grown in the United States.
   a. 25
   b. 50
   c. 75
   d. 90

10. The FDA requires the statement "contains genetically modified ingredients" on the label of all foods containing genetically modified ingredients.
    a. True
    b. False

Answer Key: 1. b (LO 12.1), 2. d (LO 12.3), 3. d (LO 12.5), 4. c (LO 12.3), 5. d (LO 12.3), 6. d (LO 12.2), 7. c (LO 12.4), 8. b (LO 12.4), 9. d (LO 12.4), 10. b (LO 12.4).

Study Questions (Numbers refer to Learning Outcomes)

1. Describe the difference between malnutrition and undernutrition. (**LO 12.1**)

2. Describe, in a short paragraph, any evidence of undernutrition that you saw while you were growing up, in person or on television. What are or were the likely roots of these problems? (**LO 12.1**)

3. What do you believe are the major factors contributing to undernutrition in affluent nations, such as the United States? What are some possible solutions to this problem? (**LO 12.2**)

4. List three long-term consequences of undernutrition during fetal development or infancy. (**LO 12.5**)

5. What federal programs are available to address the problem of undernutrition in the United States? (**LO 12.2**)

6. Outline how war and civil unrest in developing countries have worsened problems of chronic hunger over the past few years. (**LO 12.3**)

7. How important is population control in addressing the problem of world hunger now and in the future? (**LO 12.3**)

8. Why is solving the problem of undernutrition a key factor in the ability of developing countries to reach their full potential? (**LO 12.3**)

9. Name three nutrients often lacking in the diets of undernourished people. What effects can be expected with each deficiency? (**LO 12.1**)

10. Describe how sustainable agriculture and biotechnology can improve food availability worldwide. (**LO 12.4**)

What the Dietitian Chose

The correct response for the question posed at the beginning of this chapter is *all of the above!* Do what comes naturally to you—whether it is donating your spare change or volunteering your spare time—to move thought into action against local and global hunger. Indeed, the need is great and opportunities to get involved abound.

As you learned in this chapter, there are basically two ways to address the problem of hunger: providing direct food aid and supporting organizations that provide education, training, and infrastructure support to those in need. Providing direct aid (e.g., donating money) is a short-term solution—one that necessarily fills an immediate gap between resources and requirements. In the long run, however, solving the problem of hunger will take bottom-up changes that enable struggling communities to provide and sustain their own food and clean water.

It may be easier and more comfortable to visualize the hunger problem in a faraway place, such as in a developing country. In reality, however, poverty and hunger lurk in your own community. You can help local efforts by donating nonperishable items to local food pantries, volunteering at summer feeding programs for school-age children, or simply by shopping for locally grown foods direct from farmers in your area.

In your quest to get involved, look for organizations whose focus is to help set up sustainable solutions in communities: empowering local citizens to grow their own food, maintaining their own clean water supplies, and building their own local economies:

- Action Against Hunger: www.actionagainsthunger.org
- The Alliance to End Hunger: www.alliancetoendhunger.org

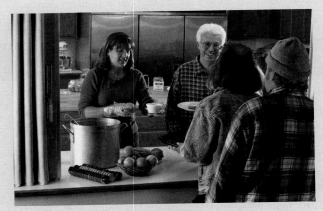

▲ Check out http://www.serve.gov/site-page/help-end-hunger to find a volunteer opportunity near you. ©Getty Images

- Blood: Water Mission: www.bloodwater.org
- Bread for the World: www.bread.org
- The Hunger Project: www.thp.org
- The International Food Policy Research Institute: www.ifpri.org
- MAZON: A Jewish Response to Hunger: http://mazon.org
- Stop Hunger Now: www.stophungernow.org

There are many creative ideas for raising funds and awareness to end world hunger. Check out the Rate Your Plate section at the end of this chapter for more ideas, and put your own talents and passions to work for a good cause!

Further Readings

1. Food and Agriculture Organization, International Fund for Agricultural Development, and WorldFood Programme: An introduction to the basic concepts of food security. http://www.fao.org/docrep/013/al936e/al936e00.pdf. (Accessed February 16, 2017).

2. Food and Agriculture Organization, International Fund for Agricultural Development, and World Food Programme: *The State of Food Insecurity in the World 2015.* Rome, Italy: FAO, 2015.

3. Academy of Nutrition and Dietetics: Position of the Academy of Nutrition and Dietetics: Nutrition security in developing nations: Sustainable food, water, and health. *J Acad Nutri Diet* 2013; 113:581.

4. Economic Research Service, U.S. Department of Agriculture: Food security in the U.S. survey tools. Updated October 4, 2016. https://www.ers.usda.gov/topics/food-nutrition-assistance/food-security-in-the-us/survey-tools/ (Accessed February 20, 2017).

5. Bhutta ZA and others: Meeting the challenges of micronutrient malnutrition in the developing world. *Br Med J* 2013; 106(1):7.

6. U.S. Census Bureau, Poverty in the U.S. Updated September 13, 2016. http://www.census.gov/topics/income-poverty/poverty.html (Accessed February 21, 2017).

7. U.S. Department of Agriculture: Foods typically purchased by Supplemental Nutrition Assistance Program (SNAP) households. Updated November 18, 2016. https://www.fns.usda.gov/snap/foods-typically-purchased-supplemental-nutrition-assistance-program-snap-households (Accessed February 21, 2017).

8. Economic Research Service, U.S. Department of Agriculture: Food access research atlas. March 11, 2015. http://www.ers.usda.gov/data-products/food-access-research-atlas.aspx (Accessed December 15, 2015).

9. American Dietetic Association: Position of the American Dietetic Association: Food insecurity in the United States. *J Am Diet Assoc* 2010; 110:1368.

10. Food and Agriculture Organization, International Fund for Agricultural Development, and World Food Programme: *The State of Food Insecurity in the World 2015.* Rome, Italy: FAO, 2015.

11. American Dietetic Association: Position of the Academy of Nutrition and Dietetics: Nutrition intervention and human immunodeficiency virus infection. *J Am Diet Assoc* 2010; 110:1105.

12. Klumper W and Qaim M: A meta-analysis of the impacts of genetically modified crops. *PLoS One* 2014; 160:9.

13. United Nations: Sustainable development goals: 17 goals to transform our world. 2016. http://www.un.org/sustainabledevelopment/ (Accessed February 21, 2017).

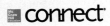 **To get the most out of your study, visit Connect where you will find NutritionCalc Plus, SmartBook®, and many other dynamic tools.**

I. Fighting World Undernutrition on a Personal Level

If you want to do something about world and domestic undernutrition, consider the following activities. It is a noble act to try to make a difference, even if you can take only one small step. As with any change in behavior, do not try to do too many things at once. Try one or two activities that represent your commitment to solving this problem.

1. Volunteer at a local soup kitchen, homeless shelter, or food pantry for a time (once a week for 1 month, for example). What insights did you gain?

2. Coordinate the efforts of a campus organization to donate money to an antihunger agency such as the following:

Antihunger Agencies	Web Address	Description
Bread for the World	www.bread.org	Bread for the World is a nationwide Christian citizens' movement seeking justice for the world's hungry people by lobbying our nation's decision makers.
CARE USA	www.care.org	CARE is one of the world's largest private international relief and development organizations, with the goal of saving lives, building opportunities, and bringing hope to people in need.
Catholic Relief Services	www.crs.org	This Catholic Charities organization started Food for All, a worldwide campaign to combat hunger.
EarthSave International	www.earthsave.org	This nonprofit agency seeks to improve the health of underserved populations, especially related to hunger and obesity.
Feeding America	www.feedingamerica.org	Feeding America, the largest domestic hunger-relief organization, shows you how to help online and has information about the latest updates.
UN Food and Agriculture Organization	www.fao.org	The Food and Agriculture Organization of the United Nations has worked to alleviate poverty and hunger by promoting agricultural development, improved nutrition, and the pursuit of food security. This website will keep you up-to-date on recent issues and provides an extensive list of publications related to food security.
Oxfam America	www.oxfamamerica.org	Oxfam works with people in more than 90 countries to create lasting solutions for hunger, poverty, and injustice.
Save the Children Foundation	www.savethechildren.org	Someone somewhere dies of hunger every 3.6 seconds. You can help stop the clock: go to and click on Donate Free Food to send a meal to someone in need. This site is affiliated with the UN World Food Programme, which tracks the number of clicks and then sends a bill to one of its corporate or nonprofit sponsors.
UN World Food Programme	www.wfp.org	The world's largest humanitarian agency fighting hunger worldwide.

3. Get on a hunger relief organization's mailing list, read its newsletters for information on upcoming fundraisers and other activities, and become involved.

4. Utilize your love of good food and healthy cooking to organize a local meal for the hungry or a benefit dinner to raise money for local food pantries. Resources to set up projects may be available from mission organizations. For example, with Blood: Water Mission's Lemon: Aid Project, students or families can use something as simple as the sale of a refreshing drink to fund potable drinking water in rural communities in Africa.

5. Participate in food drives organized by local community agencies by contributing food or services. Food-drive organizers may need volunteers to transport the donations to a food pantry. Pay attention to events around World Food Day, October 16.

6. Point, click, and fight hunger. Internet users can find information on hunger at several sites, including those listed throughout this chapter.

II. Joining the Battle Against Undernutrition

Imagine that you recently spent your summer vacation in a developing country and saw evidence of undernutrition and hunger. Then imagine that you are now asking a large corporation to support your efforts to ease hunger and suffering in this area. Develop a two-paragraph statement outlining why addressing hunger issues in this area is important. Include how the corporation could specifically assist and support you.

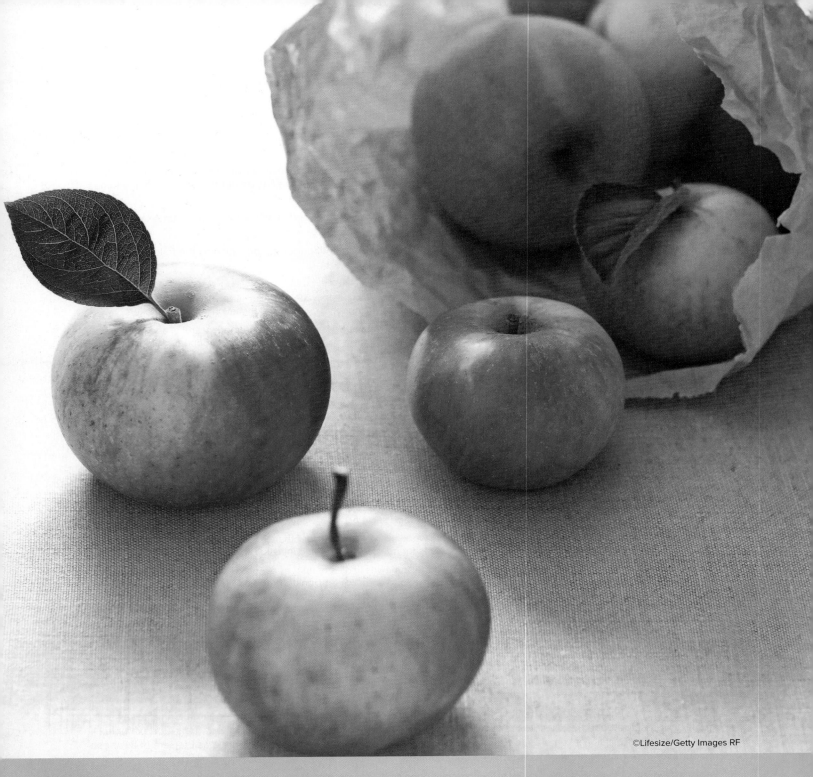

©Lifesize/Getty Images RF

Student Learning Outcomes

Chapter 13 is designed to allow you to:

13.1 List some types and common sources of viruses, bacteria, fungi, and parasites that can make their way into food.

13.2 Compare and contrast food preservation methods.

13.3 Understand the foodborne illnesses caused by bacteria, viruses, and parasites.

13.4 Describe the main reasons for using chemical additives in foods, the general classes of additives, and the functions of each class.

13.5 Identify sources of toxic environmental contaminants in food and the consequences of their ingestion.

Chapter 13
Protecting Our Food Supply

The first Food and Drug Act in the United States was passed over 110 years ago, in 1906, as a result of public pressure to improve food preparation standards. Today, warnings about the safety of food and water appear everywhere. While we are told to eat more fruits, vegetables, fish, and poultry and to drink more water, we are also warned that these may contain dangerous substances. Therefore, we still must ask, "How safe is our food and water?"

Scientists and health authorities agree that North Americans enjoy a relatively safe food supply, especially if foods are stored and prepared properly. Although tremendous progress has been made regarding food safety, microorganisms and certain chemicals in foods can still pose a health risk. As always, the nutritional and health benefits of food must be balanced against any food-related hazards. This chapter focuses on these hazards: how real they are and how you can minimize their effect on your life. You bear some responsibility for this; government agencies and industry can only do so much. The Dietary Guidelines encourage us to prepare and store foods safely. Which foods pose the greatest risk for foodborne illness? Is any food safe after being stored in the refrigerator for 6 months? Are food additives and pesticides an even greater day-to-day concern? Are there ways we can produce and eat food more sustainably? This chapter provides some answers.

13.6 Understand the reasons behind pesticide use, the possible long-term health complications, and the safety limits set for their use.

13.7 Understand the effects of conventional and sustainable agriculture on our food choices.

13.8 Describe the procedures that can be used to limit the risk of foodborne illness.

13.1 Food Safety: Setting the Stage

During the early stages of urbanization in North America, contaminated water and food, especially milk, were responsible for large outbreaks of devastating human diseases. These experiences led to the development of procedures for purifying water, treating sewage, and **pasteurizing** milk. Since that time, safe water and milk have become more universally available, yet not always accessible. The greatest health risk from food today is contamination of a variety of foods by **viruses** and **bacteria** and, to a lesser extent, by various forms of **fungi** and **parasites.** These microorganisms can all cause **foodborne illness.** The Centers for Disease Control and Prevention (CDC) estimates that foodborne illness affects about one in six Americans each year. We generally have a safe food supply, but there are occasional instances of foodborne illnesses.

Microbial contamination is still a concern today. Americans are also concerned about health risks from chemicals such as food additives, although they cause only about 4% of all cases of foodborne illness in North America. Microbial contamination of food is by far the more important issue for our short-term health, so it will be discussed first. This chapter will then cover chemical food-safety hazards, including the use and safety of food additives, and discuss the risks of pesticides in foods.

EFFECTS OF FOODBORNE ILLNESS

According to the CDC, foodborne illness causes 48 million illnesses, 128,000 hospitalizations, and 3000 deaths in the United States each year.[1,2] Some people are particularly susceptible to foodborne illness, including:

- Infants and children
- Older adults
- Those with liver disease, diabetes, HIV infection (and AIDS), or cancer
- Postsurgical patients
- Pregnant women
- People taking immunosuppressant agents (e.g., transplant patients)

Some bouts of foodborne illness, especially when coupled with ongoing health problems, are lengthy and lead to food allergies, seizures, blood poisoning (from **toxins** or microorganisms in the bloodstream), or other illnesses. Foodborne illnesses often result from the unsafe handling of food at home, so we each bear some responsibility for preventing them.[3,4] You cannot usually tell that a particular food contains harmful microorganisms by taste, smell, or sight; therefore, you might not even suspect that food has caused your distress. In fact, your last case of diarrhea may have been caused by foodborne illness.

In response to the significant public health burden of foodborne illness that is largely preventable, the FDA Food Safety Modernization Act of 2011 strengthened the food-safety system, enabling the U.S. Food and Drug Administration (FDA) to better protect public health.[5] It allows the FDA to focus on prevention of food-safety problems before they occur. The law provides new tools for inspection and compliance and for holding imported foods to the same standards as domestic foods.[5] The law directs the FDA to build a national food-safety system that is integrated and in partnership with state and local authorities. Several government agencies are at work on problems regarding food safety (Table 13-1). Of course, the work of these agencies does not substitute for individual safety efforts.

WHY IS FOODBORNE ILLNESS SO COMMON?

Foodborne illness is carried or transmitted to people by food. Most foodborne illnesses are transmitted through food in which microorganisms are able to grow rapidly. Unfortunately, this includes many of the foods we eat every day, such as meats, eggs, and dairy products.

pasteurizing The process of heating food products to kill pathogenic microorganisms and reduce the total number of bacteria.

virus The smallest known type of infectious agent, many of which cause disease in humans. A virus is essentially a piece of genetic material surrounded by a coat of protein. They do not metabolize, grow, or move by themselves. They reproduce only with the aid of a living cellular host.

bacteria Single-cell microorganisms; some produce poisonous substances, which cause illness in humans. Bacteria can be carried by water, animals, and people. They survive on skin, clothes, and hair, and thrive in foods at room temperature. Some can live without oxygen and survive by means of spore formation.

fungi Simple parasitic life forms, including molds, mildews, yeasts, and mushrooms. They live on dead or decaying organic matter. Fungi can grow as single cells, like yeast, or as a multicellular colony, as seen with molds.

parasite An organism that lives in or on another organism and derives nourishment from it.

foodborne illness Sickness caused by the ingestion of food containing harmful substances.

toxins Poisonous compounds produced by an organism that can cause disease.

TABLE 13-1 ■ **Agencies Responsible for Monitoring the U.S. Food Supply***

Agency	Responsibilities
U.S. Department of Agriculture (USDA) Food Safety and Inspection Service (FSIS) www.fsis.usda.gov	• The FSIS is the public health agency in the USDA responsible for ensuring that the nation's commercial supply of meat, poultry, and egg products is safe, wholesome, and correctly labeled and packaged.
Food and Drug Administration (FDA) www.fda.gov or call 1-800-FDA-4010 For the FDA Center for Food Safety and Applied Nutrition (CFSAN) information, call 1-888-SAFE-FOOD (1-888-723-3366)	• Protects consumers against impure, unsafe, and fraudulently labeled products • Sets standards for specific foods • The FDA Center for Food Safety and Applied Nutrition (CFSAN) regulates foods other than the meat, poultry, and egg products regulated by the FSIS.
Centers for Disease Control and Prevention (CDC) www.cdc.gov	• Leads federal efforts to gather data on foodborne illnesses, investigate foodborne illnesses and outbreaks, and monitor the effectiveness of prevention and control efforts in reducing foodborne illnesses • Plays a key role in building state and local health department capacity to support foodborne disease surveillance and outbreak response
Environmental Protection Agency (EPA) www.epa.gov	• Regulates pesticides • Establishes water quality standards
National Marine Fisheries Service or NOAA Fisheries www.nmfs.noaa.gov	• Domestic and international conservation and management of living marine resources • Voluntary seafood inspection program; can use official mark to show federal inspection
Bureau of Alcohol, Tobacco, Firearms and Explosives (ATF) www.atf.gov	• Enforces laws on alcoholic beverages
State and local governments www.FoodSafety.gov	• Regulate milk safety • Monitor food industry within their borders • Inspection of food-related establishments

*Government agencies responsible for monitoring food safety in Canada and the specific laws followed can be found at http://www.inspection.gc.ca/.

Microorganisms are able to grow rapidly in foods that are:

- generally moist.
- rich in protein.
- have a neutral or slightly acidic pH.

Our food industry tries whenever possible to prolong the shelf life of food products; however, a longer shelf life allows more time for bacteria in foods to multiply. Some bacteria even grow at refrigeration temperatures. Partially cooked—and some fully cooked—products pose a particular risk because refrigerated storage may only slow, not prevent, bacterial growth. Furthermore, we now know that besides serving as a good growth medium for microorganisms, food, especially seafood, is also a carrier of many microorganisms.

The following consumer and industry trends are increasing the risk of contracting foodborne illness:

1. Greater consumer interest in eating raw or undercooked animal products;
2. More foods prepared in kitchens outside the home;
3. Consumption of more imported ready-to-eat foods;
4. Centralization of food production;
5. Increased use of antibiotics in animal feeds;
6. More people taking medication that suppresses their ability to combat foodborne infectious agents; and
7. A continuing increase in the number of older adults in the population.

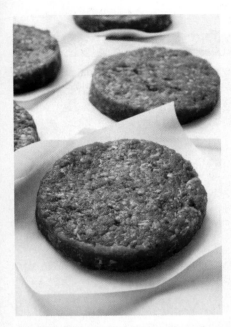

▲ Restaurants that choose to serve raw or undercooked foods of animal origin, such as eggs or meats, are required to have a consumer advisory on the menu warning customers of the health risks of ordering such foods. ©FoodCollection RF

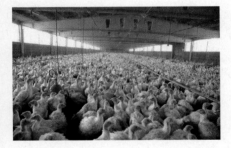

▲ Antibiotics may be given to animals, including turkeys, to prevent disease and increase feed efficiency. When antibiotics are used, a "withdrawal" period is required to ensure birds are free from any residues prior to slaughter. The USDA's Food Safety and Inspection Service randomly samples turkeys at slaughter to test for residues. If the bird is shown to contain antibiotic residues above established tolerance levels, it is deemed unfit for human consumption. ©Ingram Publishing/SuperStock

With the high number of two-income families, many people look for convenient and easy-to-prepare foods. Supermarkets have become an alternative to cooking at home by offering a variety of prepared foods from the meat departments, salad bars, and bakeries. Supermarkets offer entrées that can be served immediately or reheated. The foods are usually prepared in central kitchens or processing plants and shipped to individual stores. In 2015, an outbreak of *Escherichia coli (E. coli)* O157:H7 food poisoning was linked to rotisserie chicken salad made and sold in Costco Wholesale stores.

This centralization of food production by the food processing and restaurant industry enhances the risk of foodborne illness. If a food product is contaminated in a central processing plant, consumers over a wide area can suffer foodborne illness. For example, in 1994, a contaminated ice cream mix used in a Schwan® ice cream plant resulted in 224,000 suspected cases of *Salmonella* bacterial infections. The contamination was caused by an ice cream pre-mix that had been delivered to Schwan's in a truck that had not been properly washed after carrying raw, unpasteurized eggs. In 1992 and 1993, 4 children died and 732 became ill after eating undercooked hamburger contaminated with *E. coli* at one of 73 Jack in the Box® fast-food restaurants. Because restaurants are inspected by health departments only about every 6 months, we must rely on each restaurant to handle foods safely.

Greater consumption of ready-to-eat foods imported from foreign countries is another cause of increased foodborne illness in North America. In the past, food imports were mostly raw products processed here under strict sanitation standards. Now, however, we import more ready-to-eat processed foods—such as berries from Guatemala and shellfish from Asia—some of which are contaminated. U.S. authorities are reexamining inspection procedures for these imports. For example, a 2012 outbreak of *Listeria* was caused by contaminated ricotta cheese imported from Italy.

The use of antibiotics in animal feeds is also increasing the impact of outbreaks and the severity of cases of foodborne illness. The FDA reported that 17,000 tons of antibiotics approved for use in livestock were sold and distributed in the United States in 2015—a 1% increase from 2014. It is good to know that animals pass the antibiotics through their systems before they are slaughtered and animal products to be used for human consumption are tested for antibiotics. The real danger from such widespread use of antibiotics is that it encourages the development of antibiotic-resistant strains of bacteria. In other words, the animals may be a reservoir of pathogens that can grow even when exposed to typical antibiotic medicines. This issue of resistant bacteria in food-producing animals is receiving considerable attention by scientists. The CDC encourages the judicious use of antibiotics in humans and animals because both uses contribute to the emergence, persistence, and spread of resistant bacteria.

Every decade, the list of microorganisms suspected of causing foodborne illness lengthens. More cases of foodborne disease are reported now because health care providers are more likely to suspect foodborne contaminants as a cause of illness.

✓ CONCEPT CHECK 13.1

1. What are the annual rates of hospitalizations and deaths as a result of foodborne illnesses in the United States?
2. What lifestyle changes have made foodborne illness so common today?
3. What agencies are responsible for monitoring the safety of our food supply?

13.2 Food Preservation—Past, Present, and Future

For centuries, salt, sugar, smoke, fermentation, and drying have been used to preserve food. Ancient Romans used sulfites to disinfect wine containers and preserve wine. In the age of exploration, European adventurers traveling to the New World salted their meat to preserve it. Most preserving methods work on the principle of decreasing water content (Table 13-2). Bacteria need abundant stores of water to grow; yeasts and molds can grow with less water, but some is still necessary. Decreasing the water content of some high-moisture foods, however, would cause them to lose essential characteristics. Fermentation is an ancient preservation method using selected bacteria or yeast to ferment or pickle foods and producing pickles, sauerkraut, yogurt, and wine, from cucumbers, cabbage, milk and grape juice, respectively.

Today, we can add pasteurization, sterilization, refrigeration, freezing, canning, chemical preservation, and food **irradiation** to the list of food preservation techniques (Table 13-2). Two specific methods of food sterilization, **aseptic processing** and **ultra-high temperature (UHT) processing,** are especially useful for liquid foods, such as fruit juices. With aseptic packaging and UHT processing, boxes of sterile milk, smoothies, and juices can remain unrefrigerated on supermarket shelves, free of microbial growth, for many years.

irradiation A process in which radiation energy is applied to foods, creating compounds (free radicals) within the food that destroy cell membranes, break down DNA, link proteins together, limit enzyme activity, and alter a variety of other proteins and cell functions of microorganisms that can lead to food spoilage. This process does not make the food radioactive.

aseptic processing A method by which food and container are separately and simultaneously sterilized; it allows manufacturers to produce boxes of milk that can be stored at room temperature.

ultra-high temperature (UHT) processing Method of sterilizing food by heating it above 275°F (135°C) for 1 to 2 seconds. Also called *ultra-heat treatment.*

TABLE 13-2 ■ Food Preservation Techniques

Historic Methods	
Salt, sugar	Bind water; decease water available to microorganisms
Smoke	Heat kills microbes; chemicals in the smoke act as preservatives; water evaporates through drying.
Fermentation	Bacteria or yeast makes acids and alcohol; minimizes growth of other bacteria and yeast.
Drying	Evaporates water
Modern Methods	
Pasteurization	Moderately high (62°C to 100°C) temperatures are used for about 15 to 30 minutes to inactivate certain enzymes and kill microorganisms, especially in milk.
Refrigeration	Refrigeration slows down the deteriorative effects of microorganisms and enzymes. Household refrigerators are usually run at 40° to 45°F.
Freezing	Freezing stops the growth of microorganisms, which do not grow when the temperature of the food is below 15°F.
Canning	Food is heated in containers to a temperature that destroys microorganisms. Heating also causes air to be driven out of the container, forming a vacuum seal that prevents air and microorganisms from getting back into the product.
Chemical preservation	Many chemicals that kill microorganisms are permitted as food preservatives. Preservation is usually based on the combined or synergistic activity of several additives. Certain preservatives have been used for centuries and include salt, sugar, acids, alcohols, and components of smoke. Some other chemicals used include sulphur dioxide, benzoic acid, sorbic acid, and formic acid.
Irradiation	Radiation energy passes through food and controls growth of insects, bacteria, fungi, and parasites by breaking chemical bonds, destroying cell walls and cell membranes, breaking down DNA, and linking proteins together.
Sterilization: Aseptic processing	Food and package are sterilized separately before the food enters the package.
Sterilization: Ultra-high temperature processing	Food is sterilized by heating it above 275°F (135°C) for 1 to 2 seconds.

▲ The Radura® international label denotes prior irradiation of the food product. Source: USDA

radiation Literally, energy that is emitted from a center in all directions. Various forms of radiation energy include X rays and ultraviolet rays from the Sun.

foodborne infection Occurs when a person eats food containing harmful microorganisms, which then grow in the intestinal tract and cause illness.

toxin-mediated infection Occurs when a person eats food containing harmful bacteria. While in the intestinal tract, the bacteria produce toxins that cause illness.

foodborne intoxication Results when a person eats food containing toxins that cause illness.

Food irradiation is a preservation technique that could dramatically improve food safety because it takes minimal doses of radiation to control pathogens such as *E. coli* O157:H7 and *Salmonella*. In 1997, the FDA approved the use of irradiation for pathogen control in raw red meat to reduce risk of *E. coli* and other infectious microorganisms. Other additions to the approved list are eggs (still in the shell), seeds, other meats, spices, dry vegetable seasonings, and fresh fruits and vegetables. The **radiation** energy used does not make the food radioactive. The energy essentially passes through the food, as in microwave cooking, and no radioactive residues are left behind.

Irradiated food, except for dried seasonings, must be labeled with the international food irradiation symbol, the Radura, and a statement that the product has been treated by irradiation. Foods treated in this way are safe in the opinion of the FDA and many other health authorities, including the American Medical Association, World Health Association, and the International Atomic Energy Agency. Although the demand for irradiated foods is still low in the United States, other countries, including Canada, Japan, Italy, and Mexico, all use food irradiation technology widely. The safety of irradiated food has been evaluated and confirmed by the FDA for over 30 years. It has also been shown that irradiation does not compromise nutritional quality or noticeably change the taste, texture, or appearance of food. Harmful compounds are not found in irradiated food at any higher level than in foods that are not irradiated. Keep in mind that even when foods, especially meats, have been irradiated, it is still important to follow basic food-safety procedures, as later contamination during food preparation is possible.

✔ **CONCEPT CHECK 13.2**

1. What food preservation techniques have been used for centuries?
2. What is the UHT technique, and what types of foods are preserved with this process?
3. Why is irradiation considered a safe technique to preserve food?

13.3 Foodborne Illness Caused by Microorganisms

Most cases of foodborne illness are caused by specific viruses, bacteria, and other fungi. Prions—proteins involved in maintaining nerve cell function—can also turn infectious and lead to diseases such as bovine spongiform encephalopathy, better known as mad cow disease.

BACTERIA

Bacteria are single-cell organisms found in the food we eat, the water we drink, and the air we breathe. Many types of bacteria cause foodborne illness, including *Bacillus, Campylobacter, Clostridium, Escherichia, Listeria, Vibrio, Salmonella,* and *Staphylococcus* (Table 13-3). Bacteria are everywhere: each teaspoon of soil contains about 2 billion bacteria. Luckily, only a small number of all bacteria pose a threat.

Bacteria can cause foodborne illness in three ways:

1. **Foodborne infection.** Foodborne bacteria directly invade the intestinal wall.
2. **Toxin-mediated infection.** Foodborne bacteria produce a harmful toxin as they colonize the GI tract.
3. **Foodborne intoxication.** Bacteria secrete a toxin into food before it is eaten, which causes harm to humans after the food is ingested.

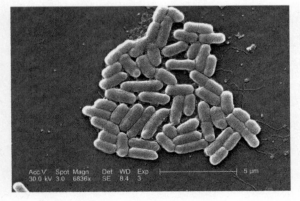

▲ An electron micrograph of *E. coli* bacteria, strain O157:H7, magnified 6836x. Although most strains of *E. coli* are harmless and live in the intestines of healthy humans and animals, this strain produces a toxin that causes severe illness. The first recognized outbreak of illness from *E. coli* O157:H7 occurred in 1982 from contaminated hamburgers and caused bloody diarrhea. Since then, most infections have been linked to eating undercooked ground beef. ©Janice Haney Carr/CDC

The main way to distinguish an infectious route from an intoxication is time: if symptoms appear in 4 hours or less, it is an intoxication. *Salmonella,* for example, causes an infection because the bacteria cause the illness. *Clostridium botulinum, Staphylococcus aureus,* and *Bacillus cereus* produce toxins and therefore cause illness from intoxication. In addition, whereas most strains of *E. coli* are harmless, *E. coli* O157:H7 and O104:H4 produce a toxin that can cause severe illness, including severe bloody diarrhea and the potentially fatal kidney complication known as **hemolytic uremic syndrome (HUS).**

hemolytic uremic syndrome (HUS) Disease characterized by anemia caused by destruction of red blood cells (hemolytic), acute kidney failure (uremic), and a low platelet count.

TABLE 13-3 ■ Bacterial Causes of Foodborne Illness

Bacteria	Illness and Food Sources	Outbreaks	Additional Information
Campylobacter jejuni 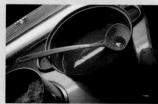 ©I. Rozenbaum/F. Cirou/Photo Alto RF	**Onset:** 2–5 days **Symptoms:** Muscle pain, abdominal cramping, diarrhea (sometimes bloody), and fever **Duration:** 2–7 days **Sources:** Raw and undercooked meat and poultry (more than half of raw poultry in the United States is contaminated), unpasteurized milk, and contaminated water	In March 2015, raw milk produced by Claravale Farm of San Benito County, California, tested positive for *Campylobacter* and was implicated in illnesses in six northern California residents diagnosed with campylobacteriosis.	Estimated 845,000 infections/year; produces a toxin that destroys intestinal mucosal surfaces; can cause Guillain-Barré syndrome, a rare neurological disorder that causes paralysis
Clostridium botulinum ©Kari Marttila/Alamy RF	**Onset:** 18–36 hours but can be 6 hours to 10 days **Symptoms:** Neurological symptoms—double and blurred vision, drooping eyelids, slurred speech, difficulty swallowing, muscle weakness, and paralysis of face, arms, respiratory muscles, trunk, and legs; can be fatal **Duration:** Days to weeks **Sources:** Improperly home-canned vegetables, meats, and fish; improperly canned commercial foods; herb-infused oils; bottled garlic; potatoes baked in foil and held at room temperature; honey	In April 2015, the largest botulism outbreak in the United States in nearly 40 years occurred among 77 persons who ate a church potluck meal in Fairfield County, Ohio. Consumption of homemade potato salad prepared with improperly home-canned potatoes was implicated as the vehicle for botulism. Of the 29 patients, 25 received botulinum antitoxin, and 11 required endotracheal intubation and mechanical ventilation; one patient died of respiratory failure shortly after arriving at the hospital emergency department.[6]	Estimated 100 cases/year; caused by a neurotoxin; *C. botulinum* grows only in the absence of air in non-acidic foods; incorrect home canning causes most botulism, but in 2007, commercially canned chili sauce caused an outbreak; honey can contain botulism spores and should not be given to infants younger than 1 year of age.
Clostridium perfringens ©Ingram Publishing/SuperStock RF	**Onset:** 8–24 hours **Symptoms:** Abdominal pain and diarrhea, usually mild; can be more serious in elderly or ill persons **Duration:** 1 day or less **Sources:** Beef, poultry, and gravy	In 2010, 42 residents and 12 staff members at a Louisiana state psychiatric hospital experienced vomiting, abdominal cramps, and diarrhea. Three patients died within 24 hours. Chicken that was cooked about 24 hours before serving and not cooled properly was associated with the illness. *C. perfringens* enterotoxin was detected in the chicken and stool specimens from ill residents and staff members.	Estimated 1 million cases/year; anaerobic bacteria widespread in soil and water; multiplies rapidly in prepared foods, such as meats, casseroles, and gravies, held for extended time at room temperature

(continued)

TABLE 13-3 ■ (*continued*)

Bacteria	Illness and Food Sources	Outbreaks	Additional Information
Escherichia coli (O157:H7, O104:H4, and other strains) 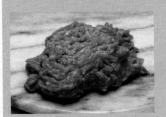 ©John A. Rizzo/Getty Images RF	**Onset:** 1–8 days **Symptoms:** Bloody diarrhea and abdominal cramps; in children under age 5 and the elderly, hemolytic uremic syndrome is a serious complication; red blood cells are destroyed and kidneys fail; can be fatal **Duration:** 5–10 days **Sources:** Undercooked ground beef; produce (e.g., lettuce, spinach, and sprouts); unpasteurized juice and milk	In 2015, rotisserie chicken salad made and sold in Costco Wholesale stores was the likely source of an outbreak of *E. coli* O157:H7 that affected 19 people in seven states; five people were hospitalized and two developed kidney failure. Also in 2015, a meal item or ingredient served at Chipotle Mexican Grill restaurants in nine states was the likely source of an outbreak of *E. coli* O157:H7. Of the 53 people infected, 20 were hospitalized. In 2009, prepackaged Nestle Toll House® refrigerated cookie dough was associated with an outbreak of *E. coli* O157:H7 in 30 states, with 72 persons infected from eating raw dough, 34 persons hospitalized, and 10 developing kidney failure. The deadliest outbreak of *E. coli* occurred from vegetable sprouts from a small, organic farm in Germany during the summer of 2011, with 3332 persons infected, more than 600 in intensive care, and a death toll of 36. The largest *E. coli* 0157:H7 outbreak in the United States affected 781 persons attending the Washington County Fair in upstate New York in 1999. The bacterium was found in infected well water, killed a 79-year-old man and a 4-year-old girl, and caused 10 other children to undergo kidney dialysis.	Leading cause of bloody diarrhea in the United States; estimated 100,000 illnesses/ year; lives in the intestine of healthy cattle; cattle and cattle manure are chief sources; illness caused by the powerful Shiga toxin made by the bacteria (so called because toxin is virtually identical to that produced by *Shigella dysenteria* toxin); petting zoos, lakes, and swimming pools can contain pathogenic *E. coli*.
Listeria monocytogenes 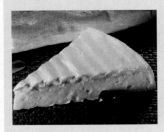 ©Digital Vision/Getty Images RF	**Onset:** 9–48 hours for early symptoms, 14–42 days for severe symptoms **Symptoms:** Fever, muscle aches, headache, vomiting; can spread to nervous system, resulting in stiff neck, confusion, loss of balance, or convulsion; can cause premature birth and stillbirth **Duration:** Days to weeks **Sources:** Unpasteurized milk and soft cheeses, raw meats, uncooked vegetables, ready-to-eat deli meats and hotdogs, and refrigerated smoked fish	In 2016, packaged salads produced at a Dole® facility in Ohio were linked to one death in Michigan and 12 people hospitalized in six states. In 2015, Blue Bell Creameries® products were implicated in an outbreak of listeriosis in 10 people from four states. All 10 victims were hospitalized. Five of the people contracted listeriosis while hospitalized for unrelated problems. While in the hospital, all had consumed milkshakes made with Blue Bell ice cream. Three of these people died as a result of their *Listeria* infection. In 2011, 147 persons in 28 states were infected with *Listeria* from cantaloupes. Most of those affected were older than 60 years; 143 were hospitalized and 33 died.	Estimated 1600 cases with 255 fatalities per year; widespread in soil and water and can be carried in healthy animals; grows at refrigeration temperatures; about one-third of cases occur during pregnancy; high-risk persons should avoid uncooked deli meats, soft cheeses (e.g., feta, Brie, and Camembert), blue-veined cheeses, Mexican-style cheeses (e.g., queso blanco made from unpasteurized milk), refrigerated meat spreads or pates, uncooked refrigerated smoked fish.

TABLE 13-3 ■ *(continued)*

Bacteria	Illness and Food Sources	Outbreaks	Additional Information
Salmonella species 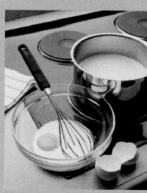 ©Photodisc/Getty Images	**Onset:** 12–72 hours **Symptoms:** Nausea, fever, headache, abdominal cramps, diarrhea, and vomiting; can be fatal in infants, the elderly, and those with impaired immune systems **Duration:** 4–7 days **Sources:** Raw and undercooked meats, poultry, eggs, and fish; produce, especially raw sprouts; peanut butter; unpasteurized milk	In 2016, eight people from three states were infected with an outbreak strain of *Salmonella*. Two people were hospitalized. Shell eggs distributed by Good Earth Egg Company in Missouri were the likely source of this outbreak. In 2015, 838 people from 38 states were infected with strains of *Salmonella Poona*. The outbreak was linked to cucumbers imported from Mexico and resulted in 165 hospitalizations and four deaths. In 2008–2009, one outbreak was traced to peppers imported from Mexico and led to 282 hospitalizations and two deaths, while another, traced to peanut butter from a processing plant in Georgia, may have caused at least eight deaths.	Estimated 1 million infections per year; bacteria live in the intestines of animals and humans; food is contaminated by infected water and feces; three strains of *Salmonella* account for almost 50% of cases; *S. enteritidis* infects the ovaries of healthy hens and contaminates eggs; almost 20% of cases are from eating undercooked eggs or egg-containing dishes; reptiles, such as turtles, also spread the disease.
Shigella species ©Comstock Images/PictureQuest RF	**Onset:** 1–3 days **Symptoms:** Abdominal cramps, fever, and diarrhea (often bloody) **Duration:** 5–7 days **Sources:** Fecal/oral transmission; water supplies, produce, and other foods contaminated by infected food handlers with poor hygiene	In October 2015, 190 people developed shigellosis after eating at Mariscos restaurant in San Jose, California. At least 11 of the *Shigella* victims were treated in hospital intensive care units. In 2001, a large multiple-restaurant outbreak of infection with *Shigella* was traced to tomatoes. A total of 886 restaurant patrons became ill. The illness was linked to bruised and overripe tomatoes that were purchased and served on a salad bar.	Estimated 448,000 cases/year in U.S.; humans and primates are the only sources; common in day care centers and custodial institutions from poor hygiene; traveler's diarrhea often caused by *S. dysenteriae*
Staphylococcus aureus ©Michael Lamotte/Cole Group/Getty Images RF	**Onset:** 1–6 hours **Symptoms:** Diarrhea, vomiting, nausea, and abdominal cramps **Duration:** 1–3 days **Sources:** Ham, poultry, egg salads, cream-filled pastries, custards, and whipped cream	In June 2015, 86 children were sickened and 30 were hospitalized as a result of *S. aureus* toxin found in several food products served at Sunnyside Child Care Centers in Montgomery, Alabama.	Estimated 241,148 cases per year; bacteria live on skin and within nasal passages of up to 25% of people; can be passed to foods; multiplies rapidly when contaminated foods are held for extended time at room temperature; illness caused by a heat-resistant toxin that cannot be destroyed by cooking

(continued)

TABLE 13-3 ■ *(continued)*

Bacteria	Illness and Food Sources	Outbreaks	Additional Information
Vibrio ©Rozenbaum/F. Cirou/Photo Alto RF	**Onset:** 1–2 days **Symptoms:** Vomiting, diarrhea, and abdominal pain; in more severe cases, bloodstream infection with fever, chills, decreased blood pressure, and blistering skin lesions **Duration:** 3 or more days **Sources:** *V. vulnificus:* raw and undercooked shellfish, especially oysters	In 2015, the number of *V. vulnificus* cases in Florida was 42, higher than any year since 2008. The death toll was 13, the highest since 2011. The majority of the illnesses were linked to eating raw oysters.	Estimated 95 cases/year; found in coastal waters; more infections in summer; those with impaired immune systems and liver disease at higher risk of infection; fatality rate of 50% with bloodstream infection
Yersinia enterocolitica ©Foodcollection RF	**Onset:** 4–7 days **Symptoms:** Fever, abdominal pain, and diarrhea (often bloody) **Duration:** Lasts 1–3 weeks or longer **Sources:** Raw or undercooked pork, particularly pork intestines (chitterlings); tofu; water; unpasteurized milk	In 2011, an outbreak of *Y. enterocolitica* was associated with drinking milk or eating ice cream made by the Brunton Dairy in Pennsylvania. Sixteen individuals were sickened. *Y. enterocolitica* was found in an unopened container of Brunton Dairy ice cream and was isolated from homemade yogurt made from the dairy's milk. In 2002, nine infants in Georgia developed gastroenteritis associated with *Y. enterocolitica.* Eight of the infants had been fed chitterlings, or chitlins. Most of the chitterlings had been purchased from the same grocery store chain.	Yersinosis most common in children under age 5 years; relatively rare; bacteria live mainly in pigs but can be found in other animals.

Bacterial foodborne illnesses typically cause gastrointestinal symptoms such as vomiting, diarrhea, and abdominal cramps. *Salmonella, Listeria, E. coli* O157:H7 and O104:H4, and *Campylobacter* are the bacterial foodborne illnesses of particular interest because they are the ones most often associated with death. *E. coli* O157:H7 and O104:H4 have caused deaths when HUS has developed. Listeriosis is of particular concern for pregnant women because they are about 20 times more likely to get this infection than other healthy adults, and listeriosis can cause spontaneous abortion or stillbirth because the *Listeria* bacteria can cross the placenta and infect the fetus.

Effects of Temperature: The Danger Zone To proliferate, bacteria require nutrients, water, and warmth. Most grow best in *danger zone* temperatures of 40 to 140°F (48 to 60°C). Pathogenic bacteria typically do not multiply when food is held at temperatures above 140°F (60°C) or stored at safe refrigeration temperatures, 32 to 40°F (0 to 4.4°C). One important exception is *Listeria* bacteria, which can multiply at refrigeration temperatures. Also note that high temperatures can kill toxin-producing bacteria, but any toxin produced in the food will not be inactivated by high temperatures. Most pathogenic bacteria also require oxygen for growth, but *Clostridium botulinum* and *Clostridium perfringens* grow only in **anaerobic** (oxygen-free) environments, such as those found in tightly sealed cans and jars. Food acidity can affect bacterial growth, too. Although most bacteria do not grow well in acidic environments, some, such as disease-causing *E. coli*, can grow in acidic foods, such as fruit juice.

anaerobic Requiring no oxygen.

aril Clear, ruby-colored fruit or seed pod that surrounds a tiny, crisp seed inside a pomegranate.

TABLE 13-4 ■ **Viral Causes of Foodborne Illness**

Viruses	Illness and Sources	Outbreaks	Additional Information
Norovirus (Norwalk and Norwalk-like viruses), human rotavirus ©lynx/iconotec.com/Glow Images	**Onset:** 1–2 days **Symptoms:** "Stomach flu"—severe diarrhea, nausea, vomiting, stomach cramping, low-grade fever, chills, and muscle aches **Duration:** 1–2 days or longer **Sources:** Foods prepared by infected food handlers; shellfish from contaminated waters; vegetables and fruits contaminated during growing, harvesting, and processing	In 2016, at least 120 Boston College students were sickened by Norovirus after eating at a Boston Chipotle® restaurant. Also in 2015, there were 12 outbreaks linked to Norovirus on international cruise ships reported to the Vessel Sanitation Program. These outbreaks occurred on six different cruise lines, affecting 1406 passengers and 130 crew members. The largest outbreak occurred on a Royal Caribbean® ship in January 2015, when 198 of 1948 passengers (10%) and 9 crew members became ill on the *Grandeur of the Seas.*	Estimated to cause over 20 million cases of gastroenteritis, 70,000 hospitalizations, and 800 deaths per year. Viruses found in stool and vomit of infected persons; food handlers can contaminate foods or work surfaces; Noroviruses are very infectious—as few as 10–100 particles can lead to infection; workers with Norovirus symptoms should not work until 2 or 3 days after they feel better.
Hepatitis A virus ©Foodcollection	**Onset:** 15–50 days **Symptoms:** Anorexia, diarrhea, fever, jaundice, dark urine, and fatigue; may cause liver damage and death **Duration:** Several weeks up to 6 months **Sources:** Foods prepared by infected food handlers, especially uncooked foods or those handled after cooking, such as sandwiches, pastries, and salads; shellfish from contaminated waters; vegetables and fruits contaminated during growing, harvesting, and processing	In 2013, 162 people were sickened, with 71 hospitalized, in 10 states by pomegranate **arils** in Townsend Farms® Organic Antioxidant Blend of frozen berries contaminated with hepatitis A and sold at Costco Warehouse® stores. In 2003, over 500 adults in the United States contracted hepatitis A after eating raw green onions in a Mexican restaurant. These were contaminated during growth in Mexico and not properly washed by food service workers.	Infected food handlers contaminate food and transmit the disease to dozens of persons; children and young adults are most susceptible; a vaccine is available, decreasing the number of infections dramatically; immunoglobulin given within 1 week to those exposed to hepatitis A virus can also decrease infection.

VIRUSES

Viruses, like bacteria, are widely dispersed in nature. Unlike bacteria, however, viruses can reproduce only after invading body cells, such as those that line the intestines. Experts speculate that about 70% of foodborne illness cases go undiagnosed because they result from viral causes, and there is no easy way to test for these pathogens. Table 13-4 describes the two most common viral causes of foodborne illness, Norovirus and Hepatitis A, along with typical food sources and symptoms and outbreaks of the illnesses they cause.

Norovirus is the number one pathogen contributing to cases of foodborne illnessses acquired in the United States. In 2014, there were 286 reported Norovirus outbreaks that caused 5553 illnesses, 65 hospitalizations, and 3 deaths. It causes an illness commonly misdiagnosed as the "stomach flu." Norovirus infection has a sudden onset and usually a short duration of only 1 to 2 days. Noroviruses cause almost all (over 90%) of the highly publicized diarrheal disease outbreaks on cruise ships. They are hardy and survive freezing, relatively high temperatures, and chlorination up to 10 parts per million. The most commonly reported Norovirus outbreaks from food contamination are at restaurants (Fig. 13-1).

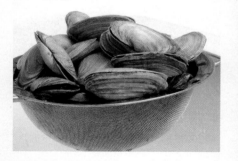

▲ Raw shellfish, especially bivalves (e.g., oysters and clams), present a particular risk related to foodborne viral disease. These animals filter feed, a process that concentrates viruses, bacteria, and toxins present in the water as it is filtered for food. Adequate cooking of shellfish will kill viruses and bacteria, but toxins may not be affected. It is important to buy shellfish from reliable sources that have harvested these foods from safe areas. ©Foodcollection

FIGURE 13-1 ▶ Settings of Norovirus outbreaks from food contamination in the United States in 2009–2012.

Source: CDC National Outbreak Reporting System, 2009–2012

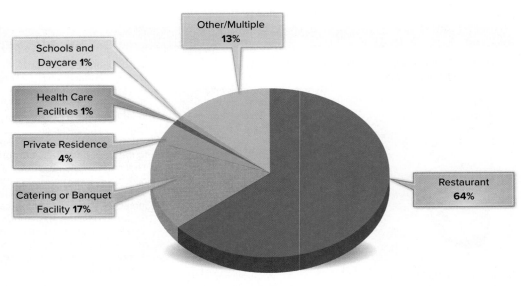

Other/Multiple **13%**

Schools and Daycare **1%**

Health Care Facilities **1%**

Private Residence **4%**

Catering or Banquet Facility **17%**

Restaurant **64%**

Norovirus Outbreaks

protozoa One-celled animals that are more complex than bacteria. Disease-causing protozoa can be spread through food and water.

helminth Parasitic worm that can contaminate food, water, feces, animals, and other substances.

PROTOZOAN AND HELMINTH PARASITES

Parasites live in or on another organism, known as the host, from which they absorb nutrients. Humans may serve as hosts to parasites. These tiny ravagers rob millions of people around the globe of their health and, in some cases, their lives. Those hardest hit live in tropical countries where poor sanitation fosters the growth of parasites.

The more than 80 foodborne parasites known to affect humans include mainly **protozoa** (one-celled animals), such as *Cryptosporidium* and *Cyclospora,* and **helminths,**

TABLE 13-5 ■ Parasitic Causes of Foodborne Illness

Parasite	Typical Food Sources	Illness	Additional Information
Trichinella spiralis ©Foodcollection RF	Pork, wild game	**Onset:** weeks to months **Symptoms:** GI symptoms followed by muscle weakness, fluid retention in the face, fever, and flu-like symptoms	The number of trichinosis infections has decreased greatly because pigs are now less likely to harbor this parasite; cooking pork to 160°F (72°C) will kill trichinella, as will freezing it for 3 days at −4°F (−20°C).
Anisakis ©Pixtal/Age Fotostock	Raw or undercooked fish	**Onset:** 12 hours or less **Symptoms:** Violent stomach pain, nausea, and vomiting	Caused by eating the larvae of roundworms; the infection is more common where raw fish is routinely consumed.

TABLE 13-5 ■ *(continued)*

Parasite	Typical Food Sources	Illness	Additional Information
Tapeworms ©Ingram Publishing	Raw beef, pork, and fish	**Symptoms:** Abdominal discomfort and diarrhea	Tapeworm larvae can get into the muscles of their hosts and cause infection when raw or undercooked meat from an infected animal is eaten.
Toxoplasma gondii ©Tetra Images/Alamy RF	Raw or undercooked meat, unwashed fruits and vegetables	**Onset:** 5–20 days **Symptoms:** Most people are asymptomatic; those with symptoms have fever, headache, sore muscles, and diarrhea; can be fatal to the fetus of pregnant women	Parasite is spread to humans from animals, including cats, the main reservoir of the disease; humans acquire the disease from ingesting contaminated meat or from fecal contamination from handling cat litter.
Cyclospora cayetanensis ©hadynyah/Getty Images	Water, contaminated food	**Onset:** 1 week **Symptoms:** Watery diarrhea, vomiting, muscle aches, fatigue, anorexia, and weight loss **Duration:** 10–12 weeks	Most common in tropical and subtropical areas, but since 1990, about a dozen outbreaks, affecting 3600 people, have occurred in the United States and Canada.
Cryptosporidium ©Ingram Publishing	Water, contaminated food	**Onset:** 2–10 days **Symptoms:** Watery diarrhea, abdominal pain, fever, nausea, vomiting, and weight loss; those with impaired immune systems become more ill **Duration:** 1–2 weeks in otherwise healthy people	Outbreaks occur worldwide; the largest U.S. outbreak was in 1993 in Milwaukee, with more than 443,000 persons affected; In August 2014, 11 persons in Idaho contracted cryptosporidiosis from drinking raw goat's milk. One patient was hospitalized. Also is causing an increasing number of outbreaks in U.S. water parks, community swimming pools, and spas.

such as tapeworms and the roundworm *Trichinella spiralis.* Table 13-5 describes common parasites and typical food sources and symptoms of the illnesses they cause. Parasitic infections spread via person-to-person contact and contaminated food, water, and soil.

✓ **CONCEPT CHECK 13.3**

1. What is the temperature "danger zone?"
2. What type of microorganisms pose the greatest risk for foodborne illness?
3. What is the setting for the most Norovirus outbreaks?

13.4 Food Additives

By the time you see a food item on the market shelf, it usually contains substances added to make it taste better, increase its nutrient content or shelf life, or make it easier to process. Other substances may have accidentally found their way into the foods you buy. All of these extraneous substances are known as **additives,** and, although some may be beneficial, others, such as sulfites, may be harmful for some people. All purposefully added substances must be evaluated by the FDA.

Food additives are classified into two types: **intentional food additives** (directly added to foods) and **incidental food additives** (indirectly added as contaminants). Both types of agents are regulated by the FDA in the United States. Currently, more than 2800 different substances are intentionally added to foods. As many as 10,000 other substances enter foods as contaminants. This includes substances that may reasonably be expected to enter food through contact with processing equipment or packaging materials.

WHY ARE FOOD ADDITIVES USED?

Most additives are used to limit food spoilage. Common food additives serve the general function of **preservatives,** which can extend the shelf life of some foods. For example, antioxidants (e.g., vitamin E and sulfites) prevent discoloration caused by exposure to oxygen and enzymes. Antimicrobial additives (e.g., potassium sorbate) retard the growth of microbes in food products. Table 13-6 describes common food additives in detail.

Additives are also used to reduce food spoilage caused by the activity of some enzymes that leads to undesirable changes in color and flavor in foods. This type of food spoilage occurs when enzymes in a food react to oxygen—for example, when apple and peach slices darken or turn rust color as they are exposed to air. Antioxidants are a type of preservative that slows the action of oxygen-requiring enzymes on food surfaces. These preservatives include vitamins E and C and a variety of sulfites.

additives Substances added to foods, either intentionally or incidentally.

intentional food additives Additives knowingly (directly) incorporated into food products by manufacturers.

incidental food additives Additives that appear in food products indirectly, from environmental contamination of food ingredients or during the manufacturing process.

preservatives Compounds that extend the shelf life of foods by inhibiting microbial growth or minimizing the destructive effect of oxygen and metals.

TABLE 13-6 ■ Types of Food Additives—Sources and Related Health Concerns

Food Additive Class	Attributes	Health Risks
Acidic or alkaline agents, such as citric acid, calcium lactate, and sodium hydroxide	Acids impart a tart taste to foods; inhibit mold growth; lessen discoloration and rancidity; and reduce the risk of botulism in naturally low-acid vegetables. Alkaline agents improve flavor by neutralizing acids produced during fermentation.	No known health risks when used properly
Alternative low-calorie sweeteners (see Table 4-2)	Sweeten foods without adding more than a few calories	Moderate use of these alternative sweeteners is considered safe (except for use of aspartame by people with the disease PKU).
Anticaking agents, such as calcium silicate	Absorb moisture to keep table salt and powdered food products free-flowing	No known health risks when used properly

©Karen Appleyard/Alamy

TABLE 13-6 ■ (*continued*)

Food Additive Class	Attributes	Health Risks
Antimicrobial agents, such as salt and sodium benzoate	Inhibit mold and fungal growth	Salt increases the risk of developing hypertension, especially in sodium-sensitive individuals; no known health risks from other agents when used properly
Antioxidants, such as BHA (butylated hydroxyanisole), BHT (butylated hydroxytoluene), vitamin E, vitamin C, and sulfites	Delay food discolorations from oxygen exposure; reduce rancidity from the breakdown of fats; maintain the color of deli meats; prevent the formation of cancer-causing nitrosamines	Sulfites can cause an allergic reaction in about 1 in every 100 people. Symptoms include difficulty breathing, wheezing, hives, diarrhea, abdominal pain, cramps, and dizziness. Salad bars, dried fruit, and wine are typical sources of sulfites.
Color additives, such as tartrazine ©Jules Frazier/Getty Images RF	Make foods more visually appealing	Tartrazine (FD&C yellow number 5) can cause allergic symptoms such as hives and nasal discharge, especially in people allergic to aspirin. FDA requires all forms of synthetic colors used in a food to be listed on its label.
Curing and pickling agents, such as salt, nitrates, and nitrites ©Renee Comet/National Cancer Institute (NCI)	Nitrates and nitrites act as preservatives, especially to prevent the growth of *Clostridium botulinum;* often used in conjunction with salt	Salt increases the risk of developing hypertension, especially in sodium-sensitive individuals. Nitrate and nitrite consumption has been associated with synthesis of nitrosamines. Some nitrosamines are cancer-causing agents. The American Institute for Cancer Research and World Health Organization recommend avoiding processed meats to lower colorectal cancer risk based on evidence that regular consumption of even small amounts of processed meats increase colorectal cancer risk.
Emulsifiers, such as monoglycerides and lecithins ©Karen Appleyard/Alamy	Suspend fat in water to improve uniformity, smoothness, and body of foods, such as baked goods, ice cream, and mayonnaise	No known health risks when used properly
Fat replacements, such as maltodextrins, emulsifiers, fiber, modified food starch, and engineered fats (see Section 5.3)	Limit calorie content of foods by reducing some of the fat content	Generally no known health risks when used properly; possible loss of fat-soluble vitamins and GI side effects if used in excess
Flavor and flavoring agents, such as natural and artificial flavors, sugar, and corn syrup	Impart more or improve flavor of foods	Sugar and corn syrup can increase risk for dental caries. Generally no known health risks for flavoring agents when used properly; possible weight gain and its comorbid conditions from excess calories

(*continued*)

TABLE 13-6 ■ (continued)

Food Additive Class	Attributes	Health Risks
Flavor enhancers, such as monosodium glutamate (MSG) and salt	Help bring out the natural flavor of foods, such as meats	Some people (especially infants) are sensitive to the glutamate in MSG and after exposure experience flushing, chest pain, facial pressure, dizziness, sweating, rapid heart rate, nausea, vomiting, increase in blood pressure, and headache. Affected individuals should look for the word *glutamate* on food labels, especially on labels for isolated protein, yeast extract, bouillon, and soup stock.
©Ingram Publishing/SuperStock		
Humectants, such as glycerol, propylene glycol, and sorbitol	Retain more moisture, texture, and fresh flavor in foods such as candies, shredded coconut, and marshmallows	No known health risk when used properly
Leavening agents, such as yeast, baking powder, and baking soda	Introduce carbon dioxide into food products	No known health risk when used properly
Maturing and bleaching agents, such as bromates, peroxides, and ammonium chloride	Shorten the time needed for maturation of flour to become usable for baking products	No known health risk when used properly
Nutrient supplements, such as vitamin A, vitamin D, and iodine	Enhance the nutrient content of foods such as margarine, milk, and ready-to-eat breakfast cereals	No known health risk if intake from such supplemental sources combined with other natural food sources of a nutrient does not exceed the Upper Level set for a particular nutrient
Sequestrants, such as EDTA and citric acid	Bind free ions to prevent them from causing rancidity in products containing fat	No known health risk when used properly
Stabilizers and thickeners, such as pectins, gums, gelatins, and agars	Impart a smooth texture and uniform color and flavor to candies, frozen desserts, chocolate milk, and beverages containing alternative sweeteners; prevent evaporation and deterioration of flavorings used in cakes, puddings, and gelatin mixes	No known health risk when used properly
©Lauri Patterson/Getty Images		

sequestrants Compounds that bind free metal ions. By so doing, they reduce the ability of ions to cause rancidity in foods containing fat.

generally recognized as safe (GRAS) A list of food additives that in 1958 were considered safe for consumption. Manufacturers were allowed to continue to use these additives, without special clearance, when needed for food products. The FDA bears responsibility for proving they are not safe and can remove unsafe products from the list.

Without the use of some food additives, it would be impossible to produce massive quantities of foods and safely distribute them nationwide or worldwide, as is now done. Despite consumer concerns about the safety of food additives, many have been extensively studied and proven safe when the FDA guidelines for their use are followed.

THE GRAS LIST

The Federal Food, Drug, and Cosmetic Act requires that any substance that is intentionally added to food is subject to review and approval by the FDA before it is used, unless the substance is generally recognized by qualified experts as having been adequately shown to be safe under the conditions of its intended use. In 1958, all food additives used in the United States and considered safe at that time were put on a **generally recognized as safe (GRAS)** list. The U.S. Congress established the GRAS list because it believed manufacturers did not need to prove the safety of substances that had been used for a long time and were already generally recognized as safe.

A substance can be removed from the GRAS list if the FDA can prove that it does *not* belong on the list. A few substances, such as cyclamates, failed the review process and were removed from the list. Red dye #3 was removed because it is linked to cancer. Many chemicals on the GRAS list have not yet been rigorously tested, primarily because of expense and because they have long histories of use without evidence of toxicity or their chemical characteristics do not suggest that they are potential health hazards. Substances may be added to the GRAS list if there are enough data to establish that the substance is safe under the conditions of its intended use.

The American Heart Association (AHA) and other experts have recently questioned the appropriateness of the GRAS listing for salt. They have suggested that sodium, one of the two components of salt, "has negative health consequences" and therefore does not meet the "safe" requirement of the GRAS. The AHA would like to see the FDA amend the GRAS listing for sodium chloride in an effort to reduce sodium content in processed foods.[7]

In a broader sense, the AHA and others are concerned that food manufacturers can make their own GRAS determinations, not needing to seek premarket approval from the FDA to use an additive in that way. The AHA would like to see improvements in the documentation of GRAS determinations and notification to the FDA. In 2010, the U.S. Government Accountability Office published the report "FDA Should Strengthen Its Oversight of Food Ingredients Determined to Be Generally Recognized as Safe (GRAS)" that supported the concerns of the AHA.[8]

ARE SYNTHETIC CHEMICALS ALWAYS HARMFUL?

Although human endeavors contribute some toxins to foods, such as synthetic pesticides and industrial chemicals, nature's poisons (see Section 13.5) are often even more potent and widespread. Nothing about a natural product makes it inherently safer than a synthetic product. Many synthetic products are laboratory copies of chemicals that also occur in nature. Some cancer researchers estimate that we ingest at least 10,000 times more (by weight) natural toxins produced by plants than we do synthetic pesticide residues. Plants produce these toxins to protect themselves from predators and disease-causing organisms. Some of these plant toxins are the beneficial phytochemicals we have already discussed (see Section 8.4). This comparison does not make synthetic chemicals any less toxic, but it does put them in perspective.

Lastly, toxicity is related to dosage. Consider vitamin E, often added to food to prevent rancidity of fats. This chemical is safe when used within certain limits. However, high doses have been associated with health problems, such as interfering with vitamin K activity in the body (review Section 8.5). Thus, even well-known, commonly used chemicals can be toxic in some circumstances and at some concentrations.

Sugar, salt, corn syrup, and citric acid constitute 98% of all additives (by weight) used in food processing.

TESTS OF FOOD ADDITIVES FOR SAFETY

Food additives are tested by the FDA for safety on at least two animal species, usually rats and mice. Scientists determine the highest dose of the additive that produces no *observable effects* in the animals. These doses are proportionately much higher than humans ever encounter. The maximum dosage that produced no observable effects is then divided by at least 100 to establish a margin of safety for human use. This 100-fold margin is used because it is assumed that we are at least 10 times more sensitive to food additives than laboratory animals and that any one person might be 10 times more sensitive than another. This broad margin essentially ensures that the food additive in question will cause no harmful health effects in humans.

One important exception applies to the procedure for testing intentional food additives: if an additive is shown to cause cancer, even though only in high doses, no margin of safety is allowed. The food additive cannot be used because it would violate

Delaney Clause A clause to the 1958 Food Additives Amendment of the Pure Food and Drug Act in the United States that prevents the intentional (direct) addition to foods of a compound shown to cause cancer in laboratory animals or humans.

Some important terms used by toxicologists:

toxicology	Scientific study of harmful substances
safety	Relative certainty that a substance will not cause injury
hazard	Chance that injury will result from use of a substance
toxicity	Capacity of a substance to produce injury or illness at some dosage

the **Delaney Clause** in the 1958 Food Additives Amendment. This clause prohibits intentionally adding to foods a compound introduced after 1958 that causes cancer at any level of exposure. Evidence for cancer could come from either laboratory animal or human studies. A few exceptions to this clause, including the curing and pickling agents nitrites and nitrates, are allowed.

Incidental food additives are another matter. The FDA cannot ban various industrial chemicals, pesticide residues, and mold toxins from foods, even though some of these contaminants can cause cancer. These products are not purposely added to foods. The FDA sets an acceptable level for these substances. An incidental substance found in a food cannot contribute to more than one cancer case during the lifetimes of 1 million people. If a higher risk exists, the amount of the compound in a food must be reduced until the guideline is met.

In general, if you consume a variety of foods in moderation, the chances of food additives jeopardizing your health are minimal. Pay attention to your body. If you suspect an intolerance or a sensitivity, consult your health care provider for further evaluation. Remember that in the short run, you are more likely to suffer from foodborne illness due to the microbial contamination of food than from consuming additives.

APPROVAL FOR A NEW FOOD ADDITIVE

Before a new food additive can be added to foods, the FDA must approve its use. Besides rigorously testing an additive to establish its safety margins, manufacturers must give the FDA information that (1) identifies the new additive; (2) gives its chemical composition; (3) states how it is manufactured; and (4) specifies laboratory methods used to measure its presence in the food supply at the amount of intended use.

Manufacturers must also offer proof that the additive will accomplish its intended purpose in a food, that it is safe, and that it is to be used in no higher amount than needed. Additives cannot be used to hide defective food ingredients, such as rancid oils; to deceive customers; or replace good manufacturing practices. A manufacturer must establish that the ingredient is necessary for producing a specific food product.

Worldwide Differences in Approval Despite these guidelines, many activists and public health watchdogs are not satisfied with the FDA procedures for regulating and monitoring the safety of food additives. These groups have urged the FDA and food manufacturers to stop the use of various chemicals until their safety can be more fully determined. A major incentive to these requests is the fact that many of the chemicals used in the United States are illegal to use as food additives in the countries of the European Union (EU) and others such as Brazil, Canada, India, and Japan.

Worldwide, there are differences in the approaches countries take to the approval of food additives. A key difference is that other countries do not rely on a GRAS list of compounds. An element that distinguishes the EU's approach from that of the United States is what the EU calls the precautionary principle. The EU believes that protective action or "precaution" should be taken when substantial, credible evidence of danger to human or environmental health is available, despite continuing scientific uncertainty. In contrast, the FDA's approach is that proof of harm must be demonstrated before regulatory action is taken. FDA approval is also unique in that when making determinations about additive safety, the FDA relies on studies performed by the companies seeking approval.

As an example, the artificial colors Red Dye No. 40 and Yellow Dyes No. 5 and No. 6 are allowed in the United States but have been taken off the market in the United Kingdom. In the rest of Europe, products that contain these dyes must carry labels warning of their potential adverse effect on children's attention and behavior. These differences stem from varying conclusions made by authorities in the United States and Europe after considering the results of a study published in 2007.[9] The study found that artificial colors or a sodium benzoate preservative (or both) in the diet resulted in increased hyperactivity in children. The study persuaded British authorities to ban use of these dyes as food additives, while the EU chose to require warning labels on products that contain them. In the United States, the colors remain in use because the FDA found the study inconclusive based on the fact that it examined effects of a mixture of additives rather than individual colorings.

Another example of differences is the status of "dough conditioners," additives to enhance flour's strength or elasticity. The International Agency for Research on Cancer considers one of these additives, potassium bromate, a possible carcinogen. This has led the EU, Canada, China, Brazil, and other countries to ban its use. Although the FDA limits the amount of dough conditioners that can be added to flour and has urged bakers to voluntarily discontinue their use, it has not banned them.

In the United States, several large companies and retailers have policies voluntarily barring some approved additives from their products. In 2014, the sandwich chain Subway announced that it would discontinue the use of the approved dough conditioner azodicarbonamide, whose breakdown product, urethane, has raised health concerns. Panera Bread went even further, announcing that food served in its cafes would be free of artificial additives by the end of 2016.

If you are bewildered or concerned about all the additives in your diet, you can easily avoid most of them by consuming unprocessed whole foods. However, no evidence shows that this will necessarily make you healthier, nor can you avoid all additives, because some, such as pesticides, are used even on whole foods. It amounts to a personal decision. Do you have confidence that the FDA and food manufacturers are adequately protecting your health and welfare, or do you want to take more personal control by minimizing your intake of compounds not naturally found in foods? Read about some "clean eating" strategies in the following Ask the RDN.

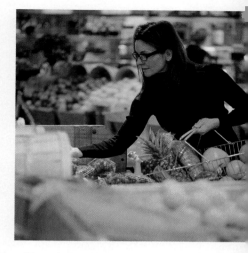

▲ Your choice to consume fresh rather than processed foods will lower your intake of food additives. Shop the perimeter of the grocery store for whole foods such as produce, meats, and dairy. ©Rob Melnychuk/Getty Images RF

ASK THE RDN   The *Eat-Clean® Diet*

Dear Author: *I have recently decided to "clean up my act" and avoid preservatives, artificial sweeteners, and other additives in my food. There is a* Clean Eating *magazine and an* Eat-Clean Diet. *Is the* Eat-Clean Diet *nutritionally sound or is it just another fad diet?*

Clean has become a popular term to describe some trendy lifestyle practices such as "clean eating" and "cleansing."[10] The *Eat-Clean Diet* by Tosca Reno has been around since 2007 and expanded into a lucrative business that sells many versions of her eating and fitness plan, as well as some pricey "raw food kits."

Reno describes her program as "a diet plan of unprocessed, whole foods like fruits, vegetables, whole grains, and lean meats, and void of artificial ingredients, preservatives, 'chemically charged foods,' sugars, saturated fat, and *trans* fat." She claims that the diet "allows you to eat more, weigh less, and become the healthiest you can be."

The specific principles include:

- Eat six small (i.e., 200 to 300 kcal) meals per day.
- Never miss a meal and eat breakfast within an hour of wakening.
- Eat lean protein (20 to 21 grams) and complex carbohydrates at every meal.
- Consume fresh fruits and vegetables.
- Control portions.
- Drink 2 to 3 liters of water (about 8 to 13 cups) every day.
- Consume 2 or 3 servings of healthy fats every day.

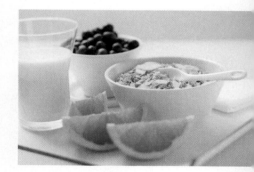

▲ One of the principles of the Eat-Clean Diet is to never miss a meal and to eat breakfast within an hour of wakening. ©FoodCollection

Do these recommendations sound familiar? They should because they are right in step with the eating patterns we have already recommended, including the *Dietary Guidelines for Americans*, the DASH Diet, and the Mediterranean diet. Thus, the key concepts embodied in the *Eat-Clean Diet* are not unique. Its tips for successful weight loss are basic to other credible plans: portion control; emphases on lean proteins, healthy fats, and minimally processed foods of plant origin; and plenty of water. Like any sound weight-loss program, the *Eat-Clean Diet* also encourages a routine of strength training and cardiovascular exercise.

Putting the "clean" in the *Eat-Clean Diet* comes down to stripping away:

1. Foods with chemical additives such as food dyes and sodium nitrite
2. Foods with preservatives
3. Artificial sweeteners
4. Sugary beverages, such as soda and juice
5. Highly processed foods, especially white flour and sugar
6. Artificial foods, such as processed cheese slices
7. Saturated fats and *trans* fats
8. Alcohol
9. "Anti-foods" (e.g., calorie-dense foods with no nutritional value)
10. Food that comes in a box or bag
11. Foods with more than one to three unpronounceable ingredients

Some of this advice is overly restrictive and may even contradict scientific evidence. For example, it is not necessary to totally eliminate saturated fats, and small amounts are typically unavoidable in a varied eating pattern. Also, there is evidence that small amounts of alcohol can provide cardiovascular benefits. In addition, Reno recommends several dietary supplements—advice that seems to counter the "clean" diet mantra to avoid all unnatural chemicals.

Clean eating can be achieved simply by being mindful of your food's origins. As nutrition experts, we encourage a "farm-to-fork" mindset. Simply stated, clean eating focuses on choosing foods as close to their original or natural form as possible. Think in terms of whole foods that have been minimally processed, if at all. This is why whole grains and fresh fruits and vegetables are on the top of the "clean" foods list. Remember that there is a large body of evidence that a plant-based diet—including whole grains, fruits, and vegetables—promotes good health and prevents disease.

Also, remember that "processing" is a broad term that might refer to something as minimal as adding salt or peeling a potato.[11] Cooking is another type of processing that alters the original form of a food. At the extreme is "ultra-processing," when ingredients are manipulated to produce a highly processed food, such as a diet soft drink. Minimally processed foods can certainly remain in your eating plan, but ultra- or highly processed foods should be avoided because they are likely to contain artificial ingredients and highly refined components. Unfortunately, many highly processed foods are deceptively marketed as being "healthy" or "nutritious" because they have been enriched or fortified with a selection of nutrients. Reading labels is the only method to ensure you are aware of the ingredients in a food or beverage.

Here is a simpler guide to "clean eating." When shopping or dining out, reach for:

Unprocessed foods:
- Fresh fruits and vegetables
- Dried beans
- Nuts and seeds
- Farm-fresh eggs

Minimally processed foods:
- Unrefined grains: whole wheat bread and pasta, popcorn, steel-cut oatmeal, quinoa, and brown rice
- Frozen fruits and vegetables without sauces or additives
- Unprocessed lean meats: wild or pastured
- Hormone-free dairy
- Plant oils
- For packaged foods, choose minimally processed foods with few ingredients (should be recognizable whole foods or spices).
- Focus on the perimeter of the grocery store for whole foods such as produce, meats, and dairy.
- A mix of raw and cooked foods. While cooking can lead to the loss of some nutrients, especially water-soluble vitamins, cooking enhances the absorption of fat-soluble vitamins and carotenoids, and makes many foods safer to eat. Choose quick cooking methods such as steaming or stir-frying to preserve nutrients and the natural state of the food.
- Control portion size to stay within your calorie needs.

Keeping it clean and simple,

Anne M. Smith, PhD, RDN, LD (author)

☑ **CONCEPT CHECK 13.4**

1. What are some of the functions of the additives used in food?
2. What is the difference between intentional and incidental additives?
3. How do scientists determine safe limits for the amount of additives that are allowed in foods?
4. What is the purpose of the Delaney Clause?

13.5 Natural Substances in Foods That Can Cause Illness

Foods contain a variety of naturally occurring substances that can cause illness. Table 13-7 shows some of the more important examples and the problems they can cause.

People have coexisted for centuries with these naturally occurring substances and have learned to avoid some of them and limit intake of others. They pose little health risk because we have developed cooking and food preparation methods to limit the potency of harmful substances, such as thiaminase. Spices are used in such small amounts that health risks do not result. Farmers know potatoes must be stored in the

TABLE 13-7 ■ Examples of Natural Substances in Foods That Can Cause Illness

Substance	Source	Effect
Safrole	Sassafras, mace, and nutmeg	Causes cancer when consumed in high doses
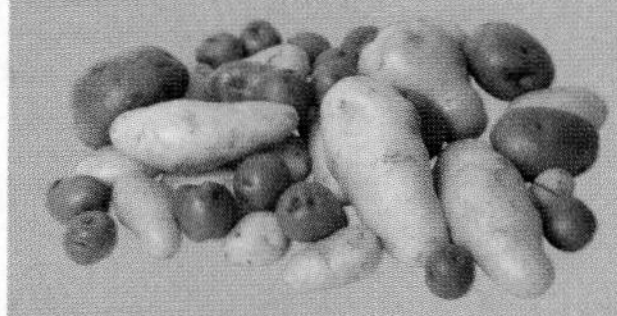 Solanine	Potato shoots and flesh when it has been stressed by exposure to light or pests and indicated by green spots on potato skins	Inhibits the action of neurotransmitters
©Ingram Publishing/Alamy		
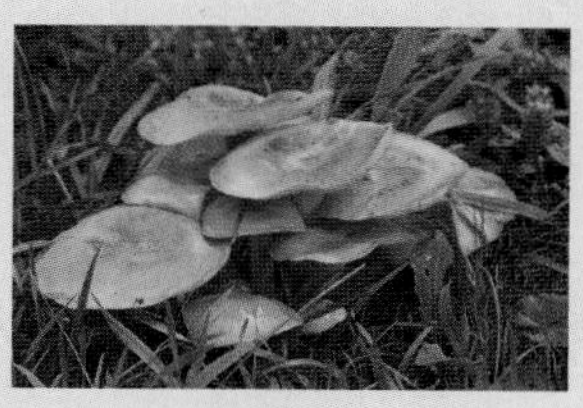 Mushroom toxins	Some species of mushrooms such as the jack-o'-lantern (shown here)	Stomach upset, dizziness, hallucinations, and other neurological symptoms. More lethal varieties can cause liver and kidney failure, coma, and even death. The FDA regulates commercially grown and harvested mushrooms. No systematic controls on individual gatherers harvesting wild species, except in Illinois and Michigan
©AwakenedEye/Getty Images		
Avidin	Raw egg whites (cooking destroys avidin)	Binds the vitamin biotin in a way that prevents its absorption, so a biotin deficiency may ultimately develop over the long term
Thiaminase	Raw fish, clams, and mussels	Destroys the vitamin thiamin
Tetrodotoxin	Puffer fish	Causes respiratory paralysis
Oxalic acid	Spinach, strawberries, sesame seeds	Binds calcium and iron in the foods and so limits absorption of these nutrients
Senna or comfrey	Herbal teas	Diarrhea and liver damage

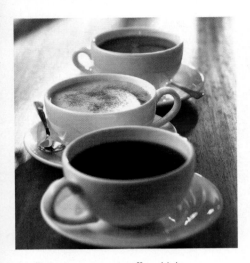

▲ Because gourmet coffee drinks are consumed several times a day, it is difficult to separate the effects of caffeine from the those of cream, sugar, chocolate, and other flavorings. ©Ingram Publishing/SuperStock

dark so that solanine will not synthesize. Nevertheless, it is important to understand that some potentially harmful chemicals in foods occur naturally.

IS CAFFEINE A CAUSE FOR CONCERN?

Why all the controversy over a cup of coffee? Researchers have spent a great deal of time on the study of caffeine, the substance of greatest concern in the favorite beverage of so many. Caffeine is a stimulant found as a natural or added ingredient in many beverages and chocolate. On average, we consume 75% of our caffeine intake as coffee, 15% as tea, 10% as soft drinks, and 2% as chocolate (Table 13-8). (For teenagers and young adults, this ratio is often relatively higher for soft drinks and lower for coffee.)

Caffeine is not often consumed by itself. With the popularity of trendy coffee shops that serve everything from mocha java to flavored lattes, it is difficult to separate the effects of caffeine intake from those of cream, sugar, alternative sweeteners, and flavorings. Although a 6-ounce cup of black coffee contains just 7 kcal, adding cream and sugar increases the kilocalorie count significantly. Adding half-and-half will give you an extra 46 kcal; liquid nondairy creamer adds 48 kcal; and 1 teaspoon of sugar adds about 23 kcal. So what is the health-conscious coffee drinker to think? Let us explore the myths and facts of caffeine intake.

Caffeine does not accumulate in the body and is normally excreted within several hours following consumption. Caffeine can cause anxiety, increased heart rate, insomnia, increased urination (possibly resulting in dehydration), diarrhea, and gastrointestinal upset in high doses. Those already suffering from ulcers or heartburn may experience irritation because caffeine relaxes sphincter muscles in the esophagus and increases acid production. Those who have anxiety or panic attacks may find that caffeine worsens their symptoms. Some people need little caffeine to feel such effects, and the threshold for children is likely even lower than that for adults.

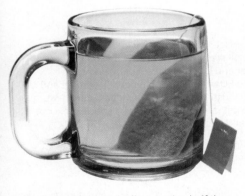

▲ A cup of tea typically contains half the amount of caffeine as coffee. ©John A. Rizzo/Getty Images RF

TABLE 13-8 ■ **Caffeine Content of Common Sources**

Item	Milligrams of Caffeine	
	Typical	Range*
Coffee (8 fl oz)		
Regular, brewed, drip method	85	65–120
Decaffeinated, brewed	3	2–4
Espresso (1 fl oz serving)	40	30–50
Teas (8 fl oz)		
Brewed, black tea	40	20–90
Brewed, green tea	20	8–30
Iced	25	9–50
Instant	28	24–31
Soft drinks (8 fl oz)	24	20–40
Coca-Cola®	23	
Mountain Dew®	36	
"Energy drinks" such as Red Bull® (8.3 fl oz)	80	0–80
Chocolate-flavored beverages (8 fl oz)		
Hot cocoa beverage	6	3–32
Chocolate milk beverage	5	2–7
Chocolate foods (1 oz)		
Milk chocolate	6	1–15
Dark chocolate, semisweet	20	5–35
Baker's® chocolate	26	26
Chocolate-flavored syrup	4	4

*For the coffee and tea products, the range varies due to brewing method, plant variety, brand of product, and so on.

For a more extensive list of caffeine content of food and drugs, visit www.cspinet.org/new/cafchart.htm.

Withdrawal symptoms are also real. Former coffee drinkers may experience head-ache, nausea, and depression for a short time after discontinuing use. These symptoms can be expected to peak at 20 to 48 hours following the last intake of caffeine. Symp-toms hold true even for those trying to quit as little as a cup of coffee per day. Slow tapering of use over a few days is recommended to avoid these problems.

Are there more serious consequences of consuming caffeine regularly? Although it has been hypothesized that caffeine consumption can lead to certain types of cancer, the association of caffeine with cancer has not been supported in recent literature. In fact, regular coffee consumption has been linked to a decreased risk of colon and liver cancer.[12]

Heavy coffee consumption does increase blood pressure for a short period of time, and coffee consumption has been linked to increased LDL-cholesterol and triglycerides in the blood. This association was found to be caused specifically by cafestol and kah-weol, two oils in ground coffee. However, filtered and instant coffees do not contain the harmful oils. It is prudent, though, to limit the amount of coffee in general, especially from French coffee presses and from espresso, as these beverages are not filtered.

Heavy caffeine use does mildly increase the amount of calcium excreted in urine. For this reason, it is important that heavy coffee drinkers check their diets for adequate cal-cium sources. Women are thought to be at higher risk for a variety of deleterious effects with caffeine consumption, including miscarriages, osteoporosis, and birth defects in their offspring. Some studies show a higher likelihood for miscarriages in women con-suming more than five 8-ounce cups of coffee per day (500 milligrams of caffeine). The position of the American College of Obstetricians and Gynecologists is that moderate caffeine intake, less than 200 milligrams a day, won't increase the risk of miscarriage, preterm birth, or birth defects (see Section 14.8).[13]

In contrast to these potential harmful effects of caffeine, coffee consumption has been linked to some beneficial effects, including reducing the risk of developing basal cell car-cinoma, depression, and cardiovascular disease. Swedish scientists recently found that women ages 40 to 83 who consumed more than a cup of coffee per day for 10 years had a 22% to 25% lower risk of stroke. Coffee consumption has also been shown to decrease a person's risk of type 2 diabetes and Parkinson's disease. Newer research findings sug-gest caffeine may reduce the risk of developing headaches, cirrhosis of the liver, some forms of kidney stones, gallstones, some nerve-related diseases, and type 2 diabetes.

Though the debate over caffeine will likely continue as long as North Americans drink coffee, research does not support many old misconceptions about caffeine. These studies are reinforcing the idea of moderation. A prudent dose of caffeine is 200 to 300 milligrams (about 2 to 3 cups of regular, brewed coffee) per day. Review Table 13-8 concerning the caffeine content of typical sources.

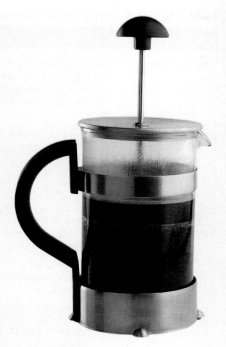

▲ The caffeine content of coffee varies with brewing method. Coffee made with a French press, shown here, is not filtered. ©lynx/iconotec.com/Glow Images

✔ CONCEPT CHECK 13.5

1. What are some examples of naturally occurring substances that can cause illness?
2. What is the typical caffeine content of 8-ounce cups of coffee and tea?
3. What are some of the negative effects of caffeine on the body?
4. Coffee consumption has been linked to a decreased risk of which disorders?

13.6 Environmental Contaminants in Food

A variety of environmental contaminants can be found in foods. Aside from pesticide residues, other potential contaminants that deserve attention are listed in Table 13-9. A general program to minimize exposure to environmental contaminants includes knowing which foods pose greater risks and consuming a wide variety of foods in moderation.

Lead Poisoning in Flint, Michigan

In December 2015, a state of emergency was declared in Flint, Michigan, when it was discovered that the proportion of infants and children with above-average levels of lead in their blood had nearly doubled since 2014, when the city switched from treated Lake Huron water (via Detroit) to using the Flint River as its water source. The Flint River water was deemed corrosive, causing lead to leach from aging pipes into the water supply. Lead contamination of the water supply was the suspected cause of extremely high blood lead levels and a variety of serious health problems in 6000 to 12,000 city residents. Flint officials have sought federal support to deal with the "irreversible" effects of lead exposure on the city's children. It is predicted that future needs will include an increase in special education and mental health services.

TABLE 13-9 ■ Potential Environmental Contaminants in Our Food Supply

Chemical Substance	Sources	Toxic Effects	Preventive Measures
Acrylamide	Fried foods rich in carbohydrate cooked at high temperatures for extended periods, such as French fries and potato chips	Known carcinogen for laboratory animals; relationship between acrylamide ingestion and development of cancer in humans has not been proven.	Limit intake of deep-fat fried foods rich in carbohydrate.
Bisphenol A (BPA)	Leaching of BPA from plastic food and beverage packages	Reproductive and developmental defects in animals	Use BPA-free bottles and cups. Consensus among regulatory agencies in the U.S. and Canada is that current levels of BPA exposure are not harmful, even for infants. To prevent exposure to BPA, do not microwave plastic containers, avoid plastic packaging with recycle codes 3 or 7, and reduce use of canned foods.
Cadmium	Plants grown in soil rich in cadmium Clams, shellfish, tobacco smoke Occupational exposure in some cases	Kidney disease Liver disease Prostate cancer (debatable) Bone deformities Lung disease (when inhaled)	Consume a wide variety of foods, including seafood sources.
Dioxin	Trash-burning incinerators Bottom-feeding fish from the Great Lakes Fat from animals exposed to dioxin via water or soil	Abnormal reproduction and fetal/infant development Immune suppression Cancer (only clearly shown in laboratory animals)	Pay attention to warnings of dioxin risks from local fish and limit intake as suggested. Consume a variety of fish from diverse water sources.
Lead	Contaminated water supply (see box, Lead Poisoning in Flint, Michigan) Lead-based paint chips and dust in older homes Occupational exposure (e.g., radiator repair) Lead caps on wine bottles Fruit juices and pickled vegetables stored in galvanized or tin containers or leaded glass Some solder used in joining copper pipes in older homes Mexican pottery dishes Some imported herbal remedies Leaded glass containers	Anemia Kidney disease Nervous system damage (tiredness and changes in behavior are symptoms) Reduced learning capacity in childhood (even from mild lead exposure)	Avoid paint chips and related dust in older homes; see information about programs to reduce lead-based paint hazards in homes at www.hud.gov/offices/lead. Meet iron and calcium needs to reduce lead absorption. Wipe the inside and outside neck of wine bottles before use if the bottle has a lead cap. Store fruit juices and pickled vegetables in glass, plastic, or waxed paper containers. Let water run 1 minute or so if off for more than 2 hours, and use only cold water for cooking; do not soften drinking water. Do not store alcoholic beverages in leaded glass containers.
Mercury	Swordfish, shark, king mackerel, and tilefish. Fresh and canned albacore tuna is also a possible source (light chunk tuna is very low in mercury).	Reduced fetal/child development; birth defects; toxic to nervous system	Consume affected food no more than once per week (no more than two times per week for albacore tuna). Pregnant and breastfeeding women as well as young children should avoid these species of fish, but some albacore tuna consumption is fine. Two to three fish meals per week is appropriate for pregnant (and nursing) women if different types of fish are eaten. Read more about mercury later in this section, in Environmental Contaminants in Fish.
Polychlorinated biphenyls (PCBs)	Fish from the Great Lakes and Hudson River Valley (e.g., coho salmon) Farmed salmon are a possible source.	Cancer has been shown in laboratory animals. Potential for liver, immune, and reproductive disorders	Pay attention to warnings of PCB contamination from local fish and limit intake as suggested on the fishing license or on state advisories. Choose a variety of fish from diverse water sources. Read more about PCBs later in this section, in Environmental Contaminants in Fish.
Urethane	Alcoholic beverages such as sherry, bourbon, sake, and fruit brandies	Cancer in laboratory animals	Avoid generous amounts of typical sources.

PESTICIDES IN FOOD

Pesticides used in food production produce both beneficial and unwanted effects. Most health authorities believe that the benefits outweigh the risks. Pesticides help ensure a safe and adequate food supply and help make foods available at reasonable cost. Nevertheless, consumers have come to assume that "synthetic" is dangerous and "organic" is safe. Some researchers believe that this sentiment is grounded in fear and fueled by unbalanced reports. Other scientists say concern about pesticides is valid and overdue.

Most concern about pesticide residues in food appropriately focuses on long-term rather than acute toxicity because the amounts of residue present, if any, are extremely small. These low concentrations found in foods are not known to produce adverse effects in the short term, although harm has been caused by the high amounts that occasionally result from accidents or misuse. For humans, pesticides pose a danger mainly in their cumulative effects, so their threats to health are difficult to determine. The contamination of underground water supplies and destruction of wildlife habitats indicate that the use of pesticides should be reduced. The U.S. federal government and many farmers are working toward that end. Section 12.4 discussed the latest use of biotechnology to reduce pesticide use.

WHAT IS A PESTICIDE?

Federal law defines a pesticide as any substance or mixture of substances intended to prevent, destroy, repel, or mitigate any pest. The built-in toxic properties of pesticides lead to the possibility that other, nontarget organisms, including humans, might also be harmed. The term *pesticide* tends to be used as a generic reference to many types of products, including insecticides (to kill insects), herbicides (to kill weeds), rodenticides (to kill rodents), and fungicides (to control fungi, mold, and mildew). A pesticide product may be chemical or bacterial, natural or synthetic.

For agriculture, the EPA allows about 10,000 pesticides to be used, containing some 300 active ingredients. The latest EPA report on pesticide use in the United States indicates that 762 million pounds of agricultural pesticide were used in 2012. Herbicides are the most widely used type of pesticide in the United States.

Once a pesticide is applied, it can turn up in a number of unintended and unwanted places. It may be carried in the air and dust by wind currents, remain in soil attached to soil particles, be taken up by organisms in the soil, decompose to other compounds, be taken up by plant roots, enter groundwater, or invade aquatic habitats. Each is a route to the food chain; some are more direct than others. A more recent concern is that pesticides are the probable cause of massive colony collapse disorder (CCD). CCD occurs when bees disappear from the colony and then die off en masse. It has been on the rise since 2006 and is a critical issue for our food supply because one-third of all food and beverages come from crops pollinated by honeybees.

WHY USE PESTICIDES?

The primary reason for using pesticides is economic: the use of agricultural chemicals increases production and lowers the cost of food, at least in the short run. Many farmers believe that it would be impossible to stay in business without pesticides. It is estimated that for every $1 that is spent on pesticides to increase crop yields, $4 are saved in crops. Farmers also rely more on pesticides to produce cosmetically attractive fruits and vegetables.

On the practical side, pesticides can protect against the rotting and decay of fresh fruits and vegetables. Also, food grown without pesticides can contain naturally occurring organisms that produce carcinogens at concentrations far above current standards for pesticide residues. For example, fungicides help prevent the carcinogen aflatoxin (synthesized by a fungus) from forming on some crops. Aflatoxin exposure in children is particularly harmful, leading to stunted growth, delayed development, liver damage,

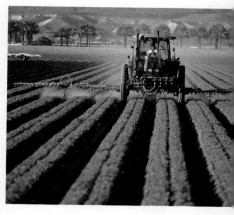
▲ There are risks and benefits associated with pesticide use. The greatest short-term risk is in rural communities, where exposure is more direct. These crops are being sprayed with pesticide.
Photo by Jeff Vanuga, USDA Natural Resources Conservation Service

One of the problems with pesticides is they create new pests when they destroy the predators (spiders, wasps, and beetles) that naturally keep most plant-feeding insect populations in check. In the United States, such major pests as spider mites and the cotton bollworm were merely nuisances until pesticides decimated their predators.

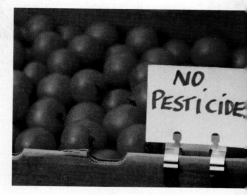
▲ Fruits and vegetables grown without use of synthetic pesticides are available and may bear an "organic" label (see Table 2-10 for rules regarding use of the term *organic* on food labels). These products generally are more expensive than conventional produce. Consumers need to decide if the potential benefits of the products are worth the extra cost.
©Nancy R. Cohen/Getty Images RF

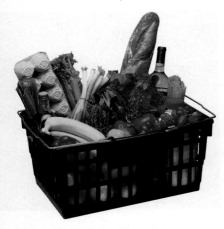

▲ The FDA's yearly evaluation of a **market basket** of typical foods shows that pesticide content is minimal in most foods. ©C Squared Studios/Getty Images RF

market basket Food the FDA buys, prepares, and analyzes as part of the ongoing Total Diet Study, which monitors levels of about 800 contaminants and nutrients in the average U.S. diet; the number varies slightly from year to year. About 280 kinds of foods and beverages from representative areas of the country are included four times a year.

and liver cancer. Thus, although some pesticides may do little more than improve the appearance of food products, others help keep foods fresher and safer to eat.

REGULATION OF PESTICIDES

The responsibility for ensuring that residues of pesticides in foods are below amounts that pose a danger to health is shared by the FDA, the EPA, and the Food Safety and Inspection Service of the USDA in the United States. Table 13-1 listed the roles of various food protection agencies. The FDA is responsible for enforcing pesticide tolerances in all foods except meat, poultry, and certain egg products, which are monitored by the USDA. A newly proposed pesticide must be tested extensively, perhaps over 10 years or more, before it is approved for use. The EPA must decide that the pesticide causes no unreasonable adverse effects on people and the environment and that benefits of use outweigh the risks of using it. The FDA tests thousands of raw products each year for pesticide residues. (A pesticide is considered illegal in this case if it is not approved for use on the crop in question or if the amount used exceeds the allowed tolerance.)

HOW SAFE ARE PESTICIDES?

Dangers from exposure to pesticides through food depend on how potent the chemical toxin is, how concentrated it is in the food, how much and how frequently it is eaten, and the consumer's resistance or susceptibility to the substance. As part of the FDA's Total Diet Study, typical foods are analyzed for elements, pesticides, and industrial chemicals four times per year. Specific foods are also analyzed for mercury. Accumulating information links pesticide use to increased cancer rates in farm communities. For rural counties in the United States, the incidence of lymph, genital, brain, and digestive tract cancers increases with higher-than-average pesticide use. Respiratory cancer cases increase with greater insecticide use. In tests using laboratory animals, scientists have found that some of the chemicals present in pesticide residues cause birth defects, sterility, tumors, organ damage, and injury to the central nervous system. Some pesticides persist in the environment for years.

Still, some researchers argue that the cancer risk from pesticide residues is hundreds of times less than the risk from eating such common foods as peanut butter, brown mustard, and basil. Plants manufacture toxic substances to defend themselves against insects, birds, and grazing animals (including humans). When plants are stressed or damaged, they produce even more of these toxins. Because of this, many foods contain naturally occurring chemicals considered toxic, and some are even carcinogenic.

The USDA Pesticide Data Program collects data on pesticide residues in food, particularly foods most likely consumed by infants and children. For samples collected in 2014, less than 1% of domestic and about 3% of imported samples had residues over tolerance. These findings are consistent with previous studies over the past 10 years. They indicate that, in general, pesticide residues in food are below EPA tolerances, confirming the safety of the food supply relative to pesticide residues. Visit the EPA website (https://www.epa.gov) for more information about pesticides and food.

PERSONAL ACTION

Every year, the Environmental Working Group (EWG) publishes a *Shopper's Guide to Pesticides in Produce.*™ The EWG is an environmental health research and advocacy organization whose mission is to serve as a watchdog to help Americans get factual information so they can make healthier choices and enjoy a cleaner environment. One of its goals is to help ensure that food products are free of harmful chemicals. Its *Shopper's Guide* includes a list of fruits and vegetables called "The Dirty Dozen" because they are most likely to contain the highest amounts of pesticide residue (Table 13-10). In 2016, strawberries topped the list, followed by apples, nectarines, peaches, celery, and grapes. Some key findings of the EWG testing found that in 2016, more than 98% of

TABLE 13-10 ■ The 2016 Dirty Dozen Fruits and Vegetables to Avoid (Unless Organically Grown) and the Clean 15 That Are Relatively Safe

Dirty Dozen	Clean 15
1. Strawberries	1. Avocados
2. Apples	2. Sweet corn
3. Nectarines	3. Pineapples
4. Peaches	4. Cabbage
5. Celery	5. Sweet peas (frozen)
6. Grapes	6. Onions
7. Cherries	7. Asparagus
8. Spinach	8. Mangos
9. Tomatoes	9. Papayas
10. Sweet bell peppers	10. Kiwi
11. Cherry tomatoes	11. Eggplant
12. Cucumbers	12. Honeydew melon
Dirty Dozen Plus	13. Grapefruit
Hot peppers	14. Cantaloupe
Kale/collard greens	15. Cauliflower

Source: Environmental Working Group, 2016 *Shopper's Guide to Pesticides.*

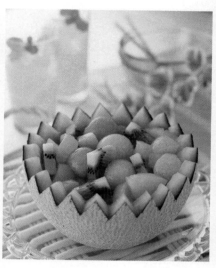

▲ This fruit salad is a healthy choice because cantaloupe, pineapple, and kiwi are some of the fruits found on the Clean 15 list. ©MIXA/Getty Images RF

strawberry, peach, nectarine, and apple samples tested positive for at least one pesticide residue. Single samples of strawberries showed 17 different pesticides, and single grape and sweet bell pepper samples each contained 15 pesticides. By weight, the potato had more pesticides than any other produce. The Dirty Dozen Plus category includes crops (hot peppers and kale/collard greens in 2016) that did not meet traditional Dirty Dozen criteria but were commonly contaminated with pesticides exceptionally toxic to the nervous system.

The *Shopper's Guide* also features a list of fruits and vegetables called "The Clean 15" because they are least likely to contain pesticide residues. To avoid pesticide exposure, consumers are encouraged to choose organic produce when buying anything on "The Dirty Dozen" list, whereas buying nonorganic produce from the "The Clean 15" group is relatively safe. Although sweet corn and papaya are found on the "The Clean 15" list, a small amount of these crops sold in the United States is produced from genetically engineered seeds. To avoid genetically engineered produce, buy organic varieties of these crops. Also keep in mind that produce on the "The Clean 15" list may also be susceptible to microbial contamination. Read about melons in the Farm to Fork feature and the potential for cantaloupes to harbor bacteria because of their "netted" surface. The EWG reminds consumers that "the health benefits of a diet rich in fruits and vegetables outweigh the risks of pesticide exposure."

The FDA and other scientific organizations believe that the hazards of pesticides are comparatively low and in the short run are less dangerous than the hazards of foodborne illness created in our kitchens. We can encourage farmers to use fewer pesticides to reduce exposure to our foods and water supplies, but we will have to settle for produce that is not perfect in appearance or that has been grown with the aid of biotechnology. (Read more about biotechnology used in agriculture in Chapter 12.) Additional advice for limiting exposure to pesticides is found in Table 13-11. Choosing organic

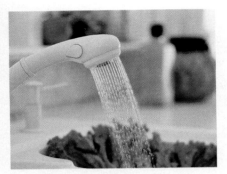

©Comstock Images/PictureQuest RF

TABLE 13-11 ■ What You Can Do to Reduce Exposure to Pesticides

WASH: Wash and scrub all fresh fruits and vegetables thoroughly under running water to remove bacteria and soil. Running water has an abrasive effect that soaking does not have. This will help remove bacteria and traces of chemicals from the surface of fruits and vegetables and dirt from crevices. Special antibacterial washing products are not necessary.

PEEL AND TRIM: Peel fruits and vegetables when possible to reduce dirt, bacteria, and pesticides. Discard outer leaves of leafy vegetables. Trim fat from meat and skin from poultry and fish because some pesticide residues collect in fat.

SELECT A VARIETY: Eat a variety of foods from a variety of sources to provide a better mix of nutrients and reduce your likelihood of exposure to a single pesticide.

CHOOSE ORGANIC: Choose organically grown and produced foods as a way to reduce exposure to synthetic pesticides. If cost is an issue, then choose organic for as many of the foods as you can from the Dirty Dozen.

USE INSECT REPELLENTS SAFELY: Read the label for pesticide safety information and apply insect repellents safely. See www.epa.gov/pesticides/factsheets/pest_ti.htm for more pesticide safety tips.

Source: U.S. Environmental Protection Agency

produce is one way to reduce your exposure to pesticide. A recent study found that people who report they "often or always" buy organic produce had significantly less insecticides in their urine samples, even though they reported eating 70% more servings of fruits and vegetables per day than adults reporting they "rarely or never" purchase organic produce.[14]

ENVIRONMENTAL CONTAMINANTS IN FISH

The presence of the environmental contaminants mercury and polychlorinated biphenyls (PCBs) in fish has caused some confusion regarding the risks and benefits of fish consumption. In our previous discussion of the benefits of omega-3 fatty acids (see Section 5.7), it was recommended that we include cold-water fatty fish, such as salmon or tuna, in our diet about twice a week. Conversely, you may have heard recommendations to eat less fish because they are a source of environmental contaminants. Balancing the benefits and risks of consuming fish is tricky, and not all experts agree.[15] For example, advice from the FDA and EPA indicates that salmon is safe to eat, even during pregnancy, because it is low in mercury. In contrast, the Environmental Defense Fund advocacy group recommends that all adults, not just pregnant women, limit consumption of wild salmon (except Alaskan) to only one serving per month and farmed salmon to no more than two servings a month (based on PCB contamination).

Mercury and PCBs are by-products of industrial processes and accumulate in fish tissue. PCBs were banned from use in 1979, but environmental levels have been decreasing very slowly and therefore still persist in our food supply, especially seafood. The contaminants become more concentrated in bigger fish as they eat smaller, contaminated fish. Fish are of primary concern because they are the only predators we eat regularly. The National Academy of Medicine, Food and Agriculture Organization, FDA, and EPA have issued similar guidelines for fish consumption. These groups advise pregnant women to eat up to 12 ounces of low-mercury fish per week and to avoid the four highest-mercury fish, which are swordfish, shark, tilefish, and king mackerel. For other adults, the basic recommendation is to "eat fish" but do not always eat the same type so you are not exposed to the same contaminants over and over.

Americans do not eat enough fish to cause concern about high intakes of environmental contaminants. On average, we consume only about 4 ounces of seafood per week. Around 80% of that is shrimp, canned tuna, salmon, and white fish, which are relatively low in environmental contaminants. Most Americans would benefit from eating more fish—a rich source of omega-3 fatty acids. Research shows that the risk of

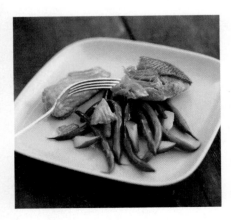

▲ This wild Alaskan salmon is a top choice among types of fish based on its high nutritional value and low mercury levels. ©Digital Vision/Getty Images RF

FARM to FORK   Melons

Americans eat, on average, 26 pounds of melons a year, making them one of our favorite fruits. They are about 95% water, so they are a great source of fluid but a diluted source of other nutrients. Most contain a reasonable amount of vitamin C and are a juicy, low-calorie treat. Honeydew and casaba melons are the sweetest melons, but are the least nutritious.

Grow
- Most melons available in the summer are grown in the United States. Most melons sold in spring, fall, and winter have been imported from Mexico.
- "Spitless" watermelons are the most popular, making up 50% of the world market.
- When buying melon seeds to plant in your garden, look for fruits with the deepest color.
- Watermelons can grow in your backyard garden when daytime temperatures are between 70 and 90°F and nighttime temperatures stay above 60°F.

Shop
- Fully ripe melons with deep colored flesh are the most nutritious and delicious. The darker the red flesh of watermelons, the greater the lycopene content, whereas deep orange cantaloupe flesh is high in overall carotenoid content.
- Melons presectioned into halves, quarters or wedges are typically fresh because they are cut up in the store and allow you to see the inside color before you buy them.

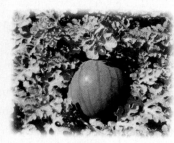

©Pixtal/Age Fotostock

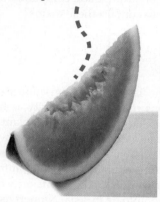

©lynx/iconotec/Glow Images

- Small watermelons are more nutritious that the large varieties.
- To find a ripe watermelon, look for one that has lost its gloss, has a yellow "ground spot," and has a deep sound when you thump it.
- A ripe cantaloupe will have a slight depression or "innie" at its stem end.

Store
- Storing watermelons at room temperature for a few days will increase its antioxidant value.
- Eat ripe cantaloupes as soon as possible. They will keep for up to five days in the drawer of the refrigerator.

Prep
- Scrub the outside of melons to remove any harmful soil bacteria they may have picked up while growing on the ground. Although cantaloupes are on the "Clean 15" list and are virtually free of pesticides, they can harbor more bacteria because of their "netted" surface and therefore need the most scrubbing.
- Once you have sliced open a melon, cover any uneaten portion and refrigerate it to inhibit the growth of bacteria. Eat within a day or two of slicing.

Source: Robinson J: Melons: Light in flavor and nutrition. In *Eating on the Wild Side*. Little Brown, New York, 2013.

dying from heart disease is about 50% greater among people who do not eat fish compared to those who eat one or two servings of fatty fish each week. Overall, it appears that the benefits of consuming fish twice per week outweigh the potential risks discussed in this section. Pregnant women should follow the FDA/EPA guidelines, and the rest of us should eat a variety of types of fish, focusing on the smaller, fatty fish at the bottom of the food chain. Read more recommendations about seafood consumption under Sustainable Seafood in Section 13.7.

AGROTERRORISM

A relatively recent addition to the list of food safety issues is agroterrorism. Agroterrorism is the deliberate introduction of harmful agents, biological and otherwise, into the agricultural and food processing system with the intent of causing actual or perceived damage. The potential target areas for agroterrorism are farm animals and livestock, plant crops, and the food processing, distribution, and retailing system. In response to acts of terrorism in 2001, the U.S. Congress passed the Public Health Security and Bioterrorism Preparedness and Response Act of 2002 (Bioterrorism Act). The Food Safety Modernization Act (FSMA) followed in 2011, giving the FDA increased power to monitor and control food in the United States. Although the United States has not been the victim of a agroterrorism attack, there are potential vulnerabilities within our agricultural and food processing systems. The goals of the Bioterrorism Act and FSMA include the establishment of a process for regulators, scientists, and public health officials to improve the defensive position of the agriculture industry and to reduce the threat of agroterrorism as much as possible.

> ### ✓ CONCEPT CHECK 13.6
>
> 1. What is a pesticide?
> 2. What are the benefits of pesticide use?
> 3. What agencies regulate the use of pesticides?
> 4. What foods are on the "Dirty Dozen" list?
> 5. What environmental contaminants can be found in fish, and which fish are most likely to contain these toxins?

13.7 Food Production Choices

During the last century, agriculture—the production of food and livestock—has seen tremendous rises in productivity as human labor has been replaced by machines and assisted by selective animal and plant breeding and synthetic fertilizers and pesticides. At one time, nearly everyone was involved in food production. Today, only about one in three people around the globe (less than 1% in the United States) is now involved in farming. Approximately 570 million farms, primarily run by individuals, produce about 80% of the world's food. The majority of large farms are in the Americas, whereas smaller farms predominate in Asia. Numerous advances in agricultural sciences are affecting our food supply; of particular note are organic food production, food biotechnology, and sustainable agriculture. Many of these new developments in agriculture are aimed at reducing the overall **carbon footprint** (carbon dioxide and methane emissions) generated on the road from the farm to the fork. At the same time, a growing area of concern relative to the economic and environmental impacts on our food supply is the issue of **food waste.**

carbon footprint The greenhouse gas emissions caused by an organization, event, product, or individual.

food waste Food that is edible or fit for consumption being discarded as plate waste by consumers and by retailers due to color or appearance.

ORGANIC FOODS

The term **organic food** refers to the way agricultural products are produced. Organic production relies on farming practices such as **biological pest management,** composting, manure applications, and crop rotation to maintain healthy soil, water, crops, and animals. Synthetic pesticides, fertilizers, and hormones; antibiotics; sewage sludge (used as fertilizer); genetic engineering; and irradiation are not permitted in the production of organic foods. However, many synthetic substances and natural pesticides may be used in organic crop production (see U.S. Organic Regulations at https://www.ams.usda.gov/grades-standards/organic-standards for more information). Additionally, organic meat, poultry, eggs, and dairy products must come from animals allowed to graze outdoors and consume only organic feed.

Interest in personal and environmental health has contributed to the increasing availability and sales of organic foods. Organic foods are increasingly available in supermarkets, specialty stores, farmers markets, and restaurants.[16] Consumers can select organic fruits, vegetables, grains, dairy products, meats, eggs, and many processed foods, including sauces and condiments, breakfast cereals, cookies, and snack chips. Direct marketing of farm products through farmers markets is a growing sales outlet for organic products nationwide. According to the Organic Trade Association, U.S. sales of organic foods exceeded $43 billion in 2016. This reflects an increase of 8.4% over the previous year. Canada's organic food and beverage market has also tripled since 2006, reaching $3 billion in 2012. Despite this rapid growth, only 4.2% of foods sold are organic. Organic foods, because they often cost more to grow and produce, are typically more expensive than comparable conventional foods.

organic food Food grown without use of pesticides, synthetic fertilizers, sewage sludge, genetically modified organisms, antibiotics, hormones, or ionizing radiation.

biological pest management Control of agricultural pests by using natural predators, parasites, or pathogens. For example, ladybugs can be used to control an aphid infestation.

The Organic Foods Production Act of 1990 established standards for the production of foods that bear the USDA Organic seal. Foods labeled and marketed as organic must be grown on farms that are certified by the USDA as following all of the rules established in the 1990 act. Products labeled "100% organic" may only contain organically produced ingredients and processing aids, excluding water and salt. No other ingredients or additives are permitted. Foods made from multiple ingredients (e.g., breakfast cereal) can be labeled as *organic* if at least 95% of their ingredients (by weight) meet organic standards. The term *made with organic ingredients* can be used if at least 70% of the ingredients are organic. Small organic producers and farmers with sales less than $5000 per year are exempt from the certification regulation. Some farmers use organic production methods but choose not to be USDA certified. Their foods cannot be labeled as organic, but many of these farmers market and sell to those seeking organic foods.

There has been an increase in USDA support and funding for research, cost-share assistance, and other organic food programs since 2002, when national organic standards were implemented. The organic food market grew exponentially in 2009, when the USDA offered $50 million in new funding to encourage greater production of organic food in the United States. With the additional financial support for farmers and ranchers, the number of certified organic operations in the United States increased to 21,781 in 2016, out of a global total of 31,160. Because most stores now offer organic products, consumers have the opportunity to compare products and prices. Increased availability and use of coupons, the proliferation of private label and store brands, and better-value products offered by major organic brands all have contributed to increased sales.

Organic Foods and Health Consumers may choose to eat organic foods to reduce their synthetic pesticide exposure, to protect the environment, and out of the belief that they will improve the overall nutritional quality of their diets. Organic produce typically carries fewer pesticide residues than conventional produce; however, the residues on both organic and nonorganic produce are tested annually by the USDA and remain below government safety thresholds. Cautious consumers may consider organic as a wise choice for vulnerable populations (e.g., young children, seniors) and opt for organic foods to encourage environmentally friendly **sustainable agriculture** practices.

In terms of nutritional quality, a large study examined 50 years' worth of scientific evidence about the nutrient content of organic and conventional foods. The researchers concluded that organic and conventional foods are not significantly different in their nutrient content or nutritional value.[17] At this point, it is not possible to recommend organic foods over conventional foods based on nutrient content: both can meet nutritional needs. A healthy dose of common sense also is important; an "organic" label does not change a less healthy food into a more healthy food. For example, organic potato chips have the same calorie and fat content as conventional potato chips.

One concern raised about organic foods is that food safety may be jeopardized because animal manures used for fertilizers may contaminate food with pathogens. Although reports of outbreaks of foodborne illness linked to organically grown foods have been increasing (see the Newsworthy Nutrition in this section), research does not show that certified organic food has higher contamination with bacterial pathogens. To avoid exposure to potential pathogens, consumers should wash or scrub all produce—organic and conventional—under running water. This safe food handling practice is critical for individuals with depressed immune systems.

Unlike the term *organic,* the term *natural* is not regulated by any federal agency. Products labeled as "natural" are generally those derived from natural ingredients, such as a plant source, which retain their native properties in the finished product. Meat or poultry labeled "natural" is expected to be minimally processed and contain no artificial flavoring, coloring, chemical preservative, or other artificial or synthetic ingredients. Also, many "natural" products, such as manure and arsenic, are detrimental to health and harmful if ingested. Unfortunately, few regulations are in place to ensure adherence to the policies, and there is debate over what constitutes "minimally processed." Although all organic products fit this definition of natural, not all natural products are necessarily organic.

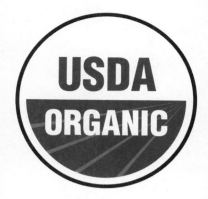

▲ The USDA organic seal identifies organic foods grown on USDA-certified organic farms. Source: USDA

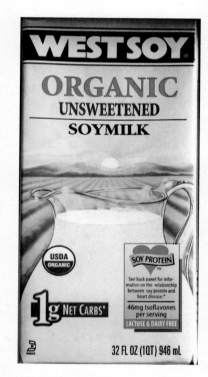

▲ USDA organic products have strict production and labeling requirements. Organic products must be (1) produced without excluded methods (e.g., genetic engineering, ionizing radiation, or sewage sludge); (2) produced using allowed substances; and (3) overseen by a USDA National Organic Program—authorized certifying agent, following all USDA organic regulations. ©McGraw-Hill Education/ Andrew Resek, photographer

sustainable agriculture Agricultural system that provides a secure living for farm families; maintains the natural environment and resources; supports the rural community; and offers respect and fair treatment to all involved, from farm workers to consumers to the animals raised for food.

Newsworthy Nutrition

Increase in foodborne illnesses associated with organic foods

Consumers often choose organic foods based on the perception that they are safer than conventionally produced foods. Organic standards, however, do not directly protect against microbial contamination. The aim of this study was to review outbreaks of foodborne illness reported to the CDC's Foodborne Disease Outbreak Surveillance System where the implicated food was reported to be organic. For each outbreak, information collected included the year, state, number of illnesses, pathogen, and implicated food. From 1992 to 2014, 18 outbreaks were identified that were caused by organic foods. These outbreaks resulted in 779 illnesses, 258 hospitalizations, and 3 deaths; 56% of outbreaks occurred more recently from 2010 to 2014.

Salmonella and *E. coli* O157:H7 were the most commonly occurring pathogens, resulting in 44% and 33% of the outbreaks, respectively. Produce items were implicated in eight of the outbreaks; unpasteurized dairy products in four; and eggs, nut and seed products, and multi-ingredient foods in two outbreaks each. Foods that were definitely or likely USDA-certified organic were linked to 15 (83%) outbreaks. These results indicate that an increase in foodborne outbreaks associated with organic foods has paralleled increases in organic food production and consumption in recent years. This study was unable to compare the risk of outbreaks due to organic foods with that of conventional foods because food production method is not systematically collected as part of foodborne outbreak surveillance. The authors conclude that consumers should focus attention on food safety regardless of whether foods are produced organically or conventionally and that consumers should be especially aware of the risk of milk and produce consumed raw, including organic.

Source: Harvey RR and others: Foodborne disease outbreaks associated with organic foods in the United States. *J Food Prot* 2016;79:1953.

FOOD BIOTECHNOLOGY

As discussed in Chapter 12, biotechnology differs from traditional methods of cross-breeding (or cross-hybridization) because it directly alters some of the genetic material of organisms to improve or enhance their characteristics. While conventional breeding has inconsistent results, biotechnology involves precision technologies. Scientists can select specific traits of interest and introduce the gene or genes that incorporate those characteristics into plants to produce a genetically modified organism (GMO). A major benefit of genetic engineering is the production of crops that resist predators, disease, and severe weather conditions—resulting in reductions in pesticide use and increases in crop yield and farmer profits. Skepticism over the use of biotechnology revolves around potential environmental hazards of introducing genes from one species to another, the opposition to production of unnatural products, and cumulative risks over a long period of time. Yet numerous scientific organizations have examined decades of research and found GMOs to be completely safe.

SUSTAINABLE AGRICULTURE

Conventional agriculture focuses on maximizing production through the use of large acreages, powerful machines, chemicals to control pests, and synthetic fertilizers to boost growth. A culture of sustainability has emerged, however, including a clear trend for sustainable food choices manufactured in an environmentally responsible way. Sustainable agriculture is an integrated system of plant and animal production that will, over the long term, have the following results:

- Satisfy human food needs
- Enhance environmental quality
- Efficiently use nonrenewable resources
- Sustain the economic viability of farm operations
- Enhance the quality of life for farmers and society as a whole

The United Nations Sustainable Development Goals (SDGs) include a goal aimed at promoting sustainable agriculture (see Section 12.4). In areas such as South America, successful sustainable practices have increased productivity. Sustainable farming practices include the following:

- Crop rotation, which protects the soil by reducing nutrient depletion of the soil
- Intercropping, or the growing of two or more crops in proximity, which encourages plants to thrive in varying soil characteristics
- Steppe farming, also known as terrace farming, which increases productivity by enabling planting on hillsides by terracing slopes to hold water for a long duration and retain the topsoil more effectively

Sustainable Living and Eating "Lifestyle of Health and Sustainability" describes a growing demographic group focused on sustainable living. An increasing number of today's college students are joining this market segment and developing behaviors associated with social responsibility. These consumers are driving changes in many areas, including the food industry. The food industry has responded with a move toward "green" initiatives that should be sustainable for the long term. Slow Food USA is an example of a nonprofit group dedicated to creating a framework for a deeper environmental connection to our food and aiming to inspire and empower Americans to build a food system that is sustainable, healthy, and delicious.

Eating sustainably is a major component of sustainable living and should be a significant part of our healthy eating pattern. Reducing the amount of food we waste is a big part of this equation and will go a long way in saving money and resources.[18] While the global population is growing and resources are becoming scarce, Americans are throwing away an enormous amount of food. It is estimated that we are discarding 30% to 40% of all food we grow, produce, package, and purchase.[19] Compared to the rest of the world, Americans are wasting the most food. Along with all that uneaten food goes wasted resources, including water, fertilizer, farmland, and energy.

Follow these strategies to reduce your food waste and eat more sustainably:

1. Do not shop for food while hungry. You will typically buy too many groceries or order too much food if you shop or dine out when very hungry. Buying less food will be easier on your budget and the environment.
2. Save and eat leftovers. Using food at home before buying more will save you money. This includes restaurant leftovers. Take them home and refrigerate within 2 hours of being served. Eat leftovers within 3 to 4 days or freeze.
3. Keep your refrigerator, freezer, and cupboards organized. Move older food products to the front and just-purchased items to the back. Use a permanent marker to write the date that you opened and first used the product. These hints will help you consume foods before they go bad.
4. Keep your eye on the garbage can and determine if you are frequently tossing the same foods. Use extra foods, especially produce, before they spoil. Add them to salads, soups, pasta, and casseroles; freeze them; or buy less of them.
5. Understand expiration dates. Most foods carry a "sell by, use by, best if used by" type of date stamp that is used by manufacturers to indicate peak quality. After this date, products may decline in flavor, texture, or color but are not necessarily unsafe to eat.
6. Donate excess food. Local food banks accept fresh produce, canned foods, dairy products, and juice within the expiration date.

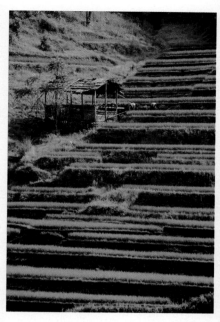

▲ Sustainable farming using terraced rice field in China. ©Bilderbuch/Design Pics

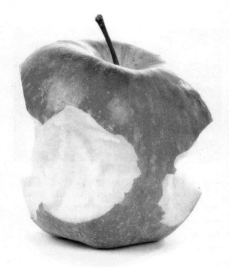

©Ingram Publishing/SuperStock

7. Compost excess food, scraps, and peels. Composting not only helps create nutrient-rich soil but also prevents food from rotting in landfills, which creates greenhouse gases.

8. Use an app such as the USDA Foodkeeper designed to help reduce food waste by helping you determine best storage practices, guidelines for using leftovers, and other tips for keeping food safe and around as long as possible.

Whether we reduce the amount of food we purchase, donate excess food to feed hungry people, compost scraps, or are more mindful of our shopping habits, reducing wasted food makes sense economically, environmentally, and socially.

Sustainable Seafood The challenge of increasing fish consumption, while also being wary of environmental contaminants in seafood, was discussed in Section 13.6. Seafood choices become even more complex when we consider the issue of overfishing and protecting endangered species of fish.[20] An "overfished" species is a population whose survival is jeopardized due to harvesting at a rate that exceeds the replenishing of stock. The good news is that fish production, whether farmed or wild caught, has a lower environmental cost compared to the production of meats. Fewer greenhouse gases are emitted, fewer chemicals and antibiotics are used, and fewer pounds of protein in feed are used than in beef, pork, or poultry production.

Fortunately, the United States has rigorous standards and closely monitors its fishing and aquaculture (fish farming) operations. The National Oceanic and Atmospheric Administration Fisheries establishes strict fishing catch levels in U.S. waters. As a result, when we buy U.S. wild-caught or farmed fish, we are making a sustainable choice. Look for the words "U.S. seafood product" on fish labels to ensure the fish or shellfish has been sustainably harvested.

The sustainable solution, however, is not that simple because the vast majority (90%) of the seafood we eat in the United States comes from international sources. About half of this seafood is from Southeast Asia, and a significant portion of it is caught by American fishermen, exported overseas for processing, and then imported back to the United States. Americans have a limited seafood palate, with only 10 species making up 90% of the seafood we eat. Fortunately, four of the most popular fish—shrimp, salmon, tilapia, and pangasius—are largely raised by certified and sustainable aquaculture operations. For example, salmon must be farmed to supply two-thirds of the 350 million tons of salmon that Americans consume annually. While many consumers perceive that wild-caught fish are the more environmentally friendly variety, many unregulated wild-caught fishing harvests have reached their peak capacity and are threatening future global seafood supplies. While sustainable seafood sourcing remains complex, both farmed and wild-caught fish can be healthy, sustainable, and economical choices.

LOCALLY GROWN FOODS

Consumers are demanding increased transparency in the food supply, and local food helps answer questions about where food comes from and how it was grown. Retailers are using the "locally grown" label to respond to consumer desires for fresh, safe products that also support small, local farmers and help the environment. Local products typically provide fresher options, do not have the added costs of long transportation and thus use less fossil fuel. Food service establishments are also placing greater emphasis on supporting local producers, encouraging a farm-to-fork approach.

Until recently, farmers markets were the typical way consumers had access to locally grown, farm-fresh produce. Farmers markets are also an integral part of the way that urban communities are linked to farms and continue to gain popularity. In 2016, there were 8669 farmers markets listed in USDA's National Farmers Market Directory.

The interest in "local" foods has become such a phenomenon that the term *locavore* was the 2007 Word of the Year in the *New Oxford American Dictionary*. A **locavore** is defined as someone who eats food grown or produced locally or within a certain radius from home, such as 50, 100, or 150 miles. The locavore movement has gained prominence due to food-safety concerns by consumers and the search for local, sustainable

Acceptable Fish

Groups such as the Natural Resources Defense Council (www.nrdc.org) and Seafood Watch (www.seafoodwatch.org) regularly update lists of acceptable fish.

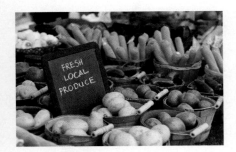

▲ The locavore movement is based on the assumption that local products are more nutritious and taste better and encourages consumers to buy from farmers markets or produce their own food. ©Arina P Habich/Shutterstock

locavore Someone who eats food grown or produced locally or within a certain radius such as 50, 100, or 150 miles.

foods. It also encourages consumers to buy from farmers markets or produce their own food, with the argument that fresh, local products are more nutritious and taste better.

There is no evidence, however, that locally grown products are safer. Although many small producers have proper food-safety practices, they often lack the expensive food-safety audits that are more common among big producers. Food-safety auditors evaluate evidence of insects on produce, sanitation practices, and similar food-safety criteria. Undetected foodborne illness outbreaks are more likely with "local" products delivered in small quantities and sold in a small area. Local products are not necessarily pesticide free and may not be cheaper, given that smaller growers lack the economic advantages of bigger growers.

Unlike organic products, there are no regulations specifying the meaning of "locally grown." Whole Foods Market, Inc., is the biggest retailer of natural and organic food and the most recognized for buying and selling locally grown produce. Whole Foods considers "local" to be anything produced within 7 hours of one of its stores, with most local producers located within 200 miles of a store. Walmart, the world's largest retailer, has also become a large buyer of locally grown fruits and vegetables and considers anything "local" if it is grown in the same state as it is sold. Searchable databases and mapping resources such as MarketMaker (https://foodmarketmaker.com) are available to connect growers with buyers, restaurants with distributors, and consumers with local farmers markets. These tools make it easier for people to find and sell locally grown foods. Positive attitudes toward organic, local, and sustainable food production practices are on the rise and appear to be increasing the conversations around dietary patterns and quality. For example, a study of college students in Minnesota showed that students who put a high importance on alternative food production methods had a higher-quality diet. They consumed more fruits and vegetables and dietary fiber, fewer added sugars and sugar-sweetened drinks, and less fat.

COMMUNITY SUPPORTED AGRICULTURE

Consumers are not only taking comfort in knowing where their food comes from but also becoming interested in community connections with local and regional farmers. Stemming from the interest in locally grown food, there is growing national support for local food collaboratives and community supported agriculture. **Community supported agriculture (CSA)** programs involve a partnership between local food producers and consumers. During each growing season, CSA farmers offer a share of foods to individuals, families, or companies that have pledged support to the CSA either financially and/or by working for the CSA.

Another example of a farm-community partnership is the National Farm to School Network, a nonprofit effort to connect farmers with nearby school (K–12) cafeterias. The objectives of this program are to serve healthy meals in school cafeterias; improve student nutrition; provide agriculture, health, and nutrition education opportunities; and support local and regional farmers. Between 1997 and 2014, this program grew from only 6 local programs to about 42,000 in all 50 states, incorporating the local bounty into their menus. Administrators of the program have found that if kids can meet the farmer who actually grew the food, they are much more likely to eat it.

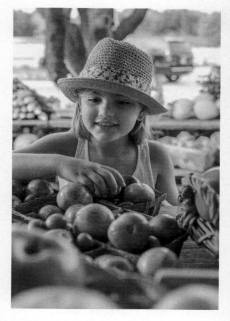

▲ Farmers participating in community supported agriculture and the National Farm to School Network offer other avenues for exposing customers to locally grown foods. ©Mark Edward Atkinson/Tracey Lee/Blend Images LLC

community supported agriculture (CSA) Partnership between local food producers and community members. Farmers offer a share of foods to individuals, families, or companies that have pledged support to the CSA either financially and/or by working for the CSA.

☑ CONCEPT CHECK 13.7

1. What are the basic requirements for foods to be labeled as organic?
2. What is the definition of *sustainable agriculture?*
3. What is the locavore movement, and what are its advantages?
4. What is a community supported agriculture program?

Visit www.localharvest.org to find farmers markets, family farms, and other sources of sustainably grown food in your area.

Look up www.farmtoschool.org to find a Farm to School Program near you.

13.8 Nutrition and Your Health
Preventing Foodborne Illness

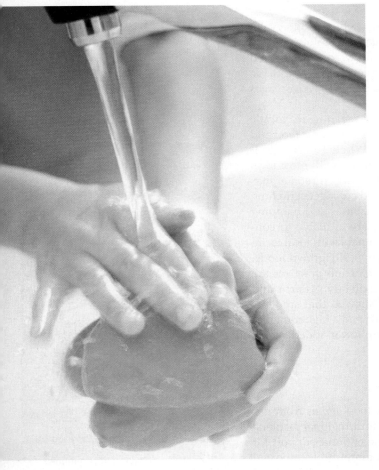

©White Rock/Getty Images RF

You can greatly reduce the risk of foodborne illness by following some important rules.[4,21] It is a long list because many risky habits need to be addressed.

Purchasing Food

- When shopping, select frozen foods and perishable foods such as meat, poultry, or fish last. Always have these products put in separate plastic bags, so that drippings do not contaminate other foods in the shopping cart. Do not let groceries sit in a warm car; this allows bacteria to grow. Get the perishable foods such as meat, eggs, and dairy products home and promptly refrigerate or freeze them.
- Do not buy or use food from damaged containers that leak, bulge, or are severely dented or from jars that are cracked or have loose or bulging lids. Do not taste or use food that has a foul odor or spurts liquid when the can is opened; the deadly *Clostridium botulinum* toxin may be present.
- Purchase only pasteurized milk and cheese (check the label). This is especially important for pregnant women because

highly toxic bacteria and viruses that can harm the fetus thrive in unpasteurized milk.
- Purchase only the amount of produce needed for a week's time. The longer you keep fruits and vegetables, the more time is available for bacteria to grow.
- When purchasing precut produce or bagged salad greens, avoid those that look slimy, brownish, or dry; these are signs of improper holding temperatures.
- Observe sell-by and expiration dates on food labels, and do not buy products that are near or past these dates.
- Follow food recalls because a Class I recall means that there is a "reasonable probability" that consuming the food will cause serious health consequences or death.

Preparing Food

- Thoroughly wash your hands for 20 to 30 seconds with hot, soapy water before and after handling food. This practice is especially important when handling raw meat, fish, poultry, and eggs; after using the bathroom; after playing with pets; or after changing diapers.
- Make sure counters, cutting boards, dishes, and other equipment are thoroughly sanitized and rinsed before use. Be especially careful to use hot, soapy water to wash surfaces and equipment that come in contact with raw meat, fish, poultry, and eggs as soon as possible to remove *Salmonella* bacteria that may be present. Otherwise, bacteria on the surfaces will infect the next foods that come in contact with the surface, a process called **cross-contamination.** In addition, replace sponges and wash kitchen towels frequently. (Microwaving sponges for 30 to 60 seconds helps rid them of live bacteria.)
- If possible, cut foods to be eaten raw on a clean cutting board reserved for that purpose. Then clean this cutting board using hot, soapy water. If the same board must be used for both meat and other foods, cut any potentially contaminated items, such as meat, last. After cutting the meat, wash the cutting board thoroughly. The FDA recommends cutting boards with unmarred surfaces made of easy-to-clean, nonporous materials such as plastic, marble, or glass. Wooden boards should be made of a nonabsorbent hardwood, such as oak, maple, or bamboo, and have no obvious seams or cracks. Recently, bamboo has become popular for cutting boards because its dense wood resists knife scarring and water penetration, leaving bacteria without a place to multiply. Keep a separate wooden cutting board for chopping produce and slicing bread to prevent cross-contamination. Furthermore, the FDA recommends that all cutting boards be replaced when they become streaked with hard-to-clean grooves or cuts, which may harbor bacteria. In addition, cutting boards should be sanitized once a week in a dilute bleach solution. Flood the board with the solution, let it sit for a few minutes, then rinse thoroughly.

cross-contamination Process by which bacteria or other microorganisms are unintentionally transferred from one substance or object to another, with harmful effect.

- Ignore the 5-second rule of eating food that has fallen on the floor because food picks up bacteria immediately upon contact.
- When thawing foods, do so in the refrigerator, under cold potable running water, or in a microwave oven. Also, cook foods immediately after thawing under cold water or in the microwave. Never let frozen foods thaw unrefrigerated all day or night. Also, marinate food in the refrigerator.
- Avoid coughing or sneezing over foods, even when you are healthy. Cover cuts on hands with a sterile bandage. This helps stop *Staphylococcus* bacteria from entering food.
- Carefully wash fresh fruit and vegetables under running water to remove dirt and bacteria clinging to the surface, using a vegetable brush if the skin is to be eaten. People have become ill from *Salmonella* introduced from melons used in making a fruit salad and from oranges used for fresh-squeezed orange juice. The bacteria were on the outside of the melons and oranges.

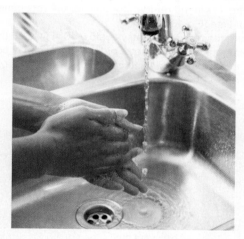

▲ Washing hands thoroughly (for at least 20 to 30 seconds) with hot water and soap should be the first step in food preparation. The four Fs of food contamination are fingers, foods, feces, and flies. Handwashing especially combats the finger and fecal routes. ©Dave & Les Jacobs/Getty Images

A tool used by the food service industry in the battle against foodborne illness is Hazard Analysis Critical Control Point (HACCP). By applying the principles of HACCP, food handlers critically analyze how they approach food preparation and what conditions may exist that might allow pathogenic microorganisms to enter and thrive in the food system. Once specific hazards and critical control points (potential problems) are identified, preventive measures can be used to reduce specific sources of contamination.

The USDA simplified the rules of foodborne illness prevention into four actions as part of its food-safety program (check out www.foodsafety.gov):

1. **Clean.** Wash hands and surfaces often.
2. **Separate.** Don't cross-contaminate.
3. **Cook.** Cook to proper temperatures.
4. **Chill.** Refrigerate promptly.

The Dietary Guidelines for Americans also stress the importance of these four actions.

The World Health Organization's Golden Rules for Safe Food Preparation:

1. Choose foods processed for safety.
2. Cook food thoroughly.
3. Eat cooked foods immediately.
4. Store cooked foods carefully.
5. Reheat cooked foods thoroughly.
6. Avoid contact between raw and cooked foods.
7. Wash hands repeatedly.
8. Keep all kitchen surfaces meticulously clean.
9. Protect foods from insects, rodents, and other animals.
10. Use pure water.

- Completely remove moldy portions of food, or do not eat the food. If a food is covered in mold, discard the food. Mold growth is prevented by properly storing food at cold temperatures and using the food promptly. Also discard soft foods with high moisture content such as bread, yogurt, soft cheeses, and deli meats if there are spots of mold on them. It is safe to trim off any moldy spots of dense foods such as hard cheeses or firm fruits and vegetables.
- Use refrigerated ground meat and patties in 1 to 2 days and frozen meat and patties within 3 to 4 months.

Cooking Food

- Cook food thoroughly and use a bimetallic thermometer to check for doneness, especially for fresh beef and fish (145°F [63°C]), pork (145°F [63°C]), and poultry (165°F [74°C]) (Fig. 13-2). Eggs should be cooked until the yolk and white are hard. The FDA does not recommend that eggs be prepared sunny-side up. Alfalfa sprouts and other types of sprouts should be cooked until they are steaming. Cooking is by far the most reliable way to destroy foodborne viruses and bacteria, such as Norovirus and toxic strains of *E. coli.* Freezing only temporarily halts viral and bacterial growth.

CLEAN   SEPARATE

COOK   CHILL

▲ Food safety logo of USDA. Source: USDA

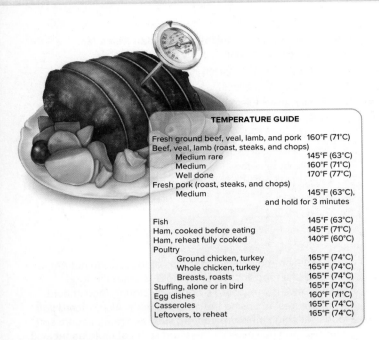

TEMPERATURE GUIDE

Fresh ground beef, veal, lamb, and pork	160°F (71°C)
Beef, veal, lamb (roast, steaks, and chops)	
Medium rare	145°F (63°C)
Medium	160°F (71°C)
Well done	170°F (77°C)
Fresh pork (roast, steaks, and chops)	
Medium	145°F (63°C), and hold for 3 minutes
Fish	145°F (63°C)
Ham, cooked before eating	145°F (71°C)
Ham, reheat fully cooked	140°F (60°C)
Poultry	
Ground chicken, turkey	165°F (74°C)
Whole chicken, turkey	165°F (74°C)
Breasts, roasts	165°F (74°C)
Stuffing, alone or in bird	165°F (74°C)
Egg dishes	160°F (71°C)
Casseroles	165°F (74°C)
Leftovers, to reheat	165°F (74°C)

FIGURE 13-2 ▲ Minimum internal temperatures when cooking or reheating foods. Source: USDA Food Safety and Inspection Service, Safe Minimum Internal Temperature Chart, www.fsis.usda.gov

Storing and Reheating Cooked Food

- Keep foods out of the "danger zone" (Fig. 13-3) by keeping hot foods hot and cold foods cold. Hold food below 40°F (4°C) or above 140°F (60°C). Foodborne microorganisms thrive in more moderate temperatures (60 to 110°F [16 to 43°C]). Some microorganisms can even grow in the refrigerator. Again, do not leave cooked or refrigerated foods, such as meats and salads, at room temperature for more than 2 hours (or 1 hour in hot weather) because that gives microorganisms an opportunity to grow. Store dry food at 60 to 70°F (16 to 21°C).
- Reheat leftovers to 165°F (74°C); reheat gravy to a rolling boil to kill *Clostridium perfringens* bacteria, which may be present. Merely reheating to a good eating temperature is not sufficient to kill harmful bacteria.
- Store peeled or cut-up produce, such as melon balls, in the refrigerator.
- Keep leftovers in the refrigerator only for the recommended length of time (Fig. 13-4).
- Make sure the refrigerator stays below 40°F (4°C). Either use a refrigerator thermometer or keep it as cold as possible without freezing milk and lettuce.

- A general precaution is to not eat raw animal products. As noted, many restaurants now include an advisory on menus stating that an increased risk of foodborne illness is associated with eating undercooked eggs. As long as restaurants provide this warning on their menus, however, they are allowed to cook eggs to any temperature requested by the consumer. The FDA warns us not to consume homemade ice cream, eggnog, and mayonnaise if made with unpasteurized, raw eggs because of the risk of *Salmonella* foodborne illness. The pasteurization of eggs or egg products kills *Salmonella* bacteria. Consuming raw seafood, especially oysters, also poses a risk of foodborne illness. Properly cooked seafood should flake easily and/or be opaque or dull and firm. If it is translucent or shiny, it is not done.
- Cook stuffing separately from poultry (or stuff immediately before cooking, and then transfer the stuffing to a clean bowl immediately after cooking). Make sure the stuffing reaches 165°F (74°C). *Salmonella* is the major concern with poultry.
- Once a food is cooked, consume it right away, or cool it to 40°F (4°C) within 2 hours. If it is not to be eaten immediately, in hot weather (80°F and above) make sure that this cooling is done within 1 hour. Do this by separating the food into as many shallow pans as needed to provide a large surface area for cooling. Be careful not to recontaminate cooked food by contact with raw meat or juices from hands, cutting boards, or other dirty utensils.
- Serve meat, poultry, and fish on a clean plate—never the same plate used to hold the raw product. For example, when grilling hamburgers, do not put cooked items on the same plate used to carry the raw product out to the grill.
- For outdoor cooking, cook food completely at the picnic site, with no partial cooking in advance.

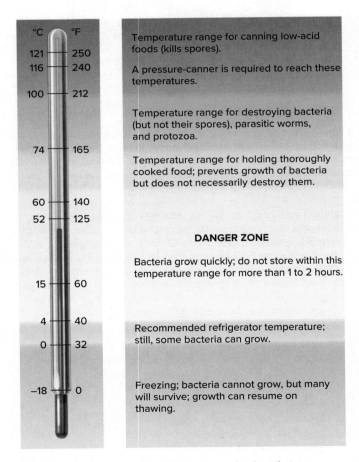

°C	°F	
121	250	Temperature range for canning low-acid foods (kills spores).
116	240	A pressure-canner is required to reach these temperatures.
100	212	
74	165	Temperature range for destroying bacteria (but not their spores), parasitic worms, and protozoa.
		Temperature range for holding thoroughly cooked food; prevents growth of bacteria but does not necessarily destroy them.
60	140	
52	125	
		DANGER ZONE
		Bacteria grow quickly; do not store within this temperature range for more than 1 to 2 hours.
15	60	
4	40	Recommended refrigerator temperature; still, some bacteria can grow.
0	32	
−18	0	Freezing; bacteria cannot grow, but many will survive; growth can resume on thawing.

FIGURE 13-3 ▲ Effects of temperature on microbes that cause foodborne illness. Source: USDA Food Safety and Inspection Service, Safe Minimum Internal Temperature Chart, www.fsis.usda.gov

When in doubt, throw it out!

Food	Refrigerator Storage Time (days)
Meats	
Cooked ground beef/turkey	3–4
Deli meat	2–3
Cooked pork	3–4
Cooked poultry	3–4
Cooked beef, bison, lamb	3–4
Seafood	
Raw (e.g. sushi/sashimi)	Must consume on day of purchase
Cooked	2
Other Entrees	
Pizza	1–2
Pasta/rice	1–2
Casserole	3–4
Soups and Chili	
Chili with meat	2–3
Chili without meat	3–4
Soup/stew	3–4
Side Dishes	
Fresh salad	1–2
Fresh vegetables	1–2
Pasta or potato salad	2–3
Deviled egg	2–3
Hard boiled egg	7
Potato (any style)	3–4
Cooked vegetables	3–4
Dessert	
Cream pie	2–3
Fruit pie	2–3
Pastries	7
Cake	7
Cheesecake	7

FIGURE 13-4 ▲ Length of time to keep leftovers in the refrigerator. Visit www.homefoodsafety.org for more tips on keeping your food safe.

- When the power goes out, keep the freezer and refrigerator doors closed as much as possible. Food can stay cold in an unopened refrigerator for about 4 hours; after 4 hours without power, discard perishable foods such as milk, meat, leftovers, and deli meats. Unopened freezers will keep food frozen for 2 days if full and 1 day if half full. Meat, poultry, and seafood can be refrozen if the freezer has not risen above 40°F.

Cross-contamination is not only a threat during food preparation; it can also become a problem during food storage. Make sure all foods, including leftovers, are contained and covered in the refrigerator to prevent drippings from uncooked and potentially hazardous foods from tainting other foods. It is a good idea to store foods likely to pose risk of foodborne illness on lower shelves of the refrigerator, beneath other foods to be eaten raw.

Raw fish dishes, such as sushi, can be safe for most people to eat if they are made with very fresh fish that has been commercially frozen and then thawed. The freezing is important to eliminate potential health risks from parasites. The FDA recommends that the fish be frozen to an internal temperature of −10°F for 7 days. If you choose to eat uncooked fish, purchase the fish from reputable establishments that have high standards for quality and sanitation. If you are at high risk for foodborne illness, it is wise to avoid raw fish products.

In summary, thoroughly cook all meat and poultry to reduce the risk of foodborne illness from *E. coli* and *Salmonella*. In addition, always separate raw meats and poultry products from cooked foods. To prevent foodborne intoxication from *Staphylococcus* organisms, cover cuts on hands and avoid sneezing on foods. To avoid intoxication from *Clostridium perfringens,* rapidly cool leftover foods and thoroughly reheat them. To avoid intoxication from *Clostridium botulinum,* carefully examine canned foods. Overall, do not allow cooked food to stand for more than 1 to 2 hours at room temperature. For other causes of foodborne illness, precautions already mentioned generally apply as well. In addition, thoroughly cook fish and other seafood; consume only pasteurized dairy products; wash all fruits and vegetables; and thoroughly wash your hands with soap and water before and after preparing food and after using the bathroom.

To reduce the risk of bacteria surviving during microwave cooking:

- Cover food with glass or ceramic when possible to decrease evaporation and heat the surface.
- Stir and rotate food at least once or twice for even cooking. Then, allow microwaved food to stand, covered, after heating is completed to help cook the exterior and equalize the temperature throughout.
- Use the oven temperature probe or a meat thermometer to check that food is done. Insert it at several spots.
- If thawing meat in the microwave, use the oven's defrost setting. Ice crystals in frozen foods are not heated well by the microwave oven and can create cold spots, which later cook more slowly.

CASE STUDY Preventing Foodbourne Illness at Gatherings

Nicole attended a gathering of her coworkers on a warm Saturday in July. The theme of the party was international dining. Nicole and her husband brought an Argentinian dish, potato and beef empanadas. They followed the recipe and cooking time carefully, removing the dish from the oven at 1 P.M. and keeping it warm by wrapping the pan in a towel. They traveled in their car to the party and set the dish out on the buffet table at 3 P.M. Dinner was to be served at 4 P.M. However, the guests were enjoying themselves so much lounging around the host's pool and drinking ginger beer (also on the menu) that no one began to eat until 6 P.M. Nicole made sure she sampled the empanadas that she and her husband made, but her husband did not. She also had some salad, garlic bread, and a sweet dessert made with coconut.

The couple returned home at 11 P.M. and went to bed. At about 2 A.M., Nicole knew something was wrong. She had severe abdominal pain and had to make a dash to the bathroom. She spent most of the next 3 hours in the bathroom with severe diarrhea. By dawn, the diarrhea subsided and she started to feel better. After a few cups of tea and a light breakfast, she was feeling like herself by noon. On Monday at work, she discovered that several of her coworkers also had diarrhea on Saturday night.

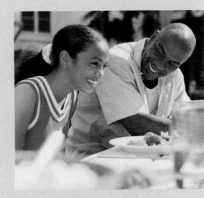
©Digital Vision RF

1. Based on her symptoms, what type of foodborne illness did Nicole contract?
2. Why is the beef the most likely vehicle for this type of foodborne illness?
3. Why is consuming food at large gatherings risky?
4. What precautions for avoiding foodborne illness were ignored by Nicole and the rest of the people at the party?
5. How could this scenario be rewritten to substantially reduce the risk of foodborne illness?

Complete the Case Study. Responses to these questions can be provided by your instructor.

Summary (Numbers refer to numbered sections in the chapter.)

13.1 Infants, children, older adults, postsurgical patients, immunosuppressed individuals, and pregnant women are most susceptible to foodborne illness. The risk of foodborne illness has increased as more of our foods are prepared outside of the home.

13.2 In the past, salt, sugar, smoke, fermentation, and drying were used to protect against foodborne illness. Today, careful cooking, pasteurization, irradiation, attention to food temperature, and thorough handwashing provide additional insurance.

13.3 Viruses, bacteria, and other microorganisms in food pose the greatest risk for foodborne illness. Major causes of foodborne illness are Norovirus and the bacteria *Campylobacter jejuni, Salmonella, Staphylococcus aureus,* and *Clostridium perfringens.* In addition, such bacteria as *Clostridium botulinum, Listeria monocytogenes,* and *Escherichia coli* have been found to cause illness.

13.4 Food additives are used primarily to extend shelf life by preventing microbial growth and the destruction of food components by oxygen, metals, and other substances. Food additives are classified as those intentionally added to foods and those that incidentally appear in foods. An intentional additive is limited to no more than one-one-hundredth of the greatest amount that causes no observed symptoms in animals. Under its jurisdiction in the United States, the Delaney Clause allows the FDA to ban the use of any intentional food additive that causes cancer.

13.5 Toxic substances occur naturally in a variety of foods, such as green potatoes, raw fish, mushrooms, and raw egg whites. Cooking foods limits their toxic effects in some cases; others are best to avoid altogether, such as toxic mushroom species and the green parts of potatoes.

13.6 A variety of environmental contaminants and pesticide residues can be found in foods. It is helpful to know which foods pose the greatest risks and act accordingly to reduce exposure, such as washing fruits and vegetables before use.

13.7 While conventional agriculture emphasizes large yields and low costs, the more recent trend toward sustainability considers the long-term environmental impact of agricultural practices. Consumers are driving up demand for organic and locally grown products.

13.8 Safe food handling can be summed up in four easy steps: (1) *clean* hands and surfaces often; (2) *separate* raw and ready-to-eat foods to prevent cross-contamination; (3) *cook* (and reheat) potentially hazardous foods thoroughly, measuring temperature with a food thermometer; and (4) *chill* foods by refrigerating promptly after eating. Two of these practices focus on food temperature; foods should not be held in the "danger zone" (40 to 140°F) for more than 2 hours.

Check Your Knowledge (Answers are available at the end of this question set.)

1. Nitrite prevents the growth of
   a. *Clostridium botulinum.*
   b. *Escherichia coli.*
   c. *Staphylococcus aureus.*
   d. yeasts.

2. Substances used to preserve foods by lowering the pH are
   a. smoke and irradiation.
   b. baking powder and soda.
   c. salt and sugar.
   d. vinegar and citric acid.

3. Food additives widely used for many years without apparent ill effects are on this list.
   a. FDA
   b. GRAS
   c. USDA
   d. Delaney

4. The four actions that are part of the USDA food-safety program are clean, _____, cook, and chill.
   a. sterilize
   b. separate
   c. pasteurize
   d. freeze

5. *Salmonella* bacteria are usually spread via
   a. raw meats, poultry, and eggs.
   b. pickled vegetables.
   c. home-canned vegetables.
   d. raw vegetables.

6. It is unwise to thaw meats or poultry
   a. in a microwave oven.
   b. in the refrigerator.
   c. under cool running water.
   d. at room temperature.

7. Milk that can remain on supermarket shelves, free of microbial growth, for many years has been processed by which of the following methods?
   a. Use of humectants
   b. Using antibiotics in animal feed
   c. Use of sequestrants
   d. Aseptic processing

8. Those at greatest risk for foodborne illness include
   a. pregnant women.
   b. infants and children.
   c. immunosuppressed individuals.
   d. all of these individuals.

9. Pasteurization involves the
   a. exposure of food to high temperatures for short periods to destroy harmful microorganisms.
   b. exposure of food to heat to inactivate enzymes that cause undesirable effects in foods during storage.
   c. fortification of foods with vitamins A and D.
   d. use of irradiation to destroy certain pathogens in foods.

10. Food can be kept for long periods by adding salt or sugar because these substances
    a. make the food too acidic for spoilage to occur.
    b. bind to water, thereby making it unavailable to the microorganisms.
    c. effectively kill microorganisms.
    d. dissolve the cell walls in plant foods.

Answer Key: 1. a (LO 13.4), 2. d (LO 13.2), 3. b (LO 13.4), 4. b (LO 13.8), 5. a (LO 13.1), 6. d (LO 13.8), 7. d (LO 13.2), 8. d (LO 13.3), 9. a (LO 13.2), 10. b (LO 13.4)

Study Questions (Numbers refer to Learning Outcomes)

1. What three trends in food purchasing and production have led to a greater number of cases of foodborne illness? **(LO 13.1)**

2. Which types of foods are most likely to be involved in foodborne illness? Why are they targets for contamination? **(LO 13.2)**

3. Identify three major classes of microorganisms responsible for foodborne illness. **(LO 13.3)**

4. Define the term *food additive,* and give examples of four intentional food additives. What are their specific functions in foods? What is their relationship to the GRAS list? **(LO 13.4)**

5. Describe the federal process that governs the use of food additives, including the Delaney Clause. **(LO 13.4)**

6. Put into perspective the benefits and risks of using additives in food. Point out an easy way to reduce the consumption of food additives. Do you think this is worth the effort in terms of maintaining health? Why or why not? **(LO 13.4)**

7. Name some substances that occur naturally in foods but may cause illness. **(LO 13.5)**

8. Describe four recommendations for reducing the risk of ill effects from environmental contaminants. **(LO 13.6)**

9. Describe some of the advances in agricultural science that are positively affecting our food supply. **(LO 13.7)**

10. List four techniques other than thorough cooking that are important in preventing foodborne illness. **(LO 13.8)**

What the Dietitian Chose

Exposure to environmental stressors may cause plants to produce more phytochemicals that have a positive impact on human health. However, current research is insufficient to recommend organic over conventional produce on the basis of nutrient content. The dietitian would choose canned and frozen fruits and vegetables, which have greater nutrient content compared to fresh or organic products that are harvested early and often purchased several days or weeks later. The ideal situation would be to grow our own produce or purchase it at a farmers market, allowing us to consume it very close to harvest. Recall from Section 8.1, maximal nutrient content coincides with the peak of ripeness. Thus, produce will have its highest vitamin and phytochemical content if it is harvested at peak ripeness.

Products labeled organic must comply with standards regarding use of fertilizers, pesticides, hormones, antibiotics, genetic engineering, and irradiation. Organic food producers may use natural preservatives. Buying fresh or frozen produce and preparing meals at home are the best ways to avoid excessive preservative intake.

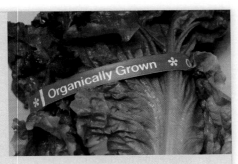

▲ Exposure to pesticides is lower from organic foods, although conventional foods remain well below the USDA pesticide residue limits. ©Ingram Publishing RF

Organic produce is no less likely to be contaminated with microorganisms than conventionally grown foods (recall the Newsworthy Nutrition in this chapter). Although manure is used as organic fertilizer, statistics show similar levels of foodborne illness organisms from either type of food. It is still important to follow food-safety advice, such as washing all fresh produce before eating it.

Further Readings

1. Scallan E and others: Foodborne illness acquired in the United States—Major pathogens. *Emerg Infect Dis* 2011;17:7.

2. Centers for Disease Control and Prevention: CDC estimates of foodborne illness in the United States. www.cdc.gov/foodborneburden. (Accessed February 16, 2017).

3. Glover L: How to avoid foodborne illness. *U.S. News & World Report*, August 2015. http://health.usnews.com/health-news/health-wellness/articles/2015/08/26/how-to-avoid-foodborne-illness

4. Kosa KM and others: Most Americans are not prepared to ensure food safety during power outages and other emergencies. *Food Protection Trends* 2011;31:428.

5. Academy of Nutrition and Dietetics: Position of the Academy of Nutrition and Dietetics: Food and water safety. *J Acad Nutr Diet* 2014;114:1819.

6. McCarty CL: Notes from the field: Large outbreak of botulism associated with a church potluck meal—Ohio, 2015. *CDC Morbidity and Mortality Weekly Report* 2015;64(29):802.

7. Institute of Medicine: *Strategies to reduce sodium intake in the United States.* Washington, DC: National Academies Press, April 20, 2010. www.iom.edu/Reports/2010/Strategies-to-Reduce-Sodium-Intake-in-the-United-states.aspx.

8. U.S. Government Accountability Office: FDA should strengthen its oversight of food ingredients determined to be generally recognized as safe (GRAS). GAO-10-246: February 3, 2010. Publicly released: March 5, 2010.

9. McCann D and others: Food additives and hyperactive behaviour in 3-year-old and 8-/9-year-old children in the community: A randomised, double-blinded, placebo-controlled trial. *Lancet* 2007;370(9598):1560.

10. Novella S: The clean eating delusion. *Science-Based Medicine,* January 20, 2016. https://www.sciencebasedmedicine.org/the-clean-eating-delusion/

11. Dennett C: Processed foods: Problem or panacea? *Today's Dietitian* 2015;17(8):40.

12. Setiawan VW: Association of coffee intake with reduced incidence of liver cancer and death from chronic liver disease in the US Multiethnic Cohort. *Gastroenterol* 2015;148(1):118.

13. Committee on Obstetric Practice: Moderate caffeine consumption during pregnancy. Committee Opinion No. 462. American College of Obstetricians and Gynecologists. *Obstet Gynecol* 2010;116:467.

14. Curl CL and others: Estimating pesticide exposure from dietary intake and organic food choices: The Multi-Ethnic Study of Atherosclerosis (MESA). *Environ Health Perspect* 2015;123:475.

15. Oken E and others: Which fish should I eat? Perspectives influencing fish consumption choices. *Environ Health Perspec* 2012;120:790.

16. Schardt D: Going organic: What's the payoff? *Nutr Action Healthletter* October 2012, p. 1.

17. Smith-Spangler C and others: Are organic foods safer or healthier than conventional alternatives?: A systematic review. *Ann Internal Med* 2012;157:348.

18. Vogliano C and Brown K: The state of America's wasted food and opportunities to make a difference. *J Acad Nutr Diet* 2016;116:1199.

19. Gunders D: Wasted: How America is losing up to 40 percent of its food from farm to fork to landfill. *Natural Resources Defense Council* 2012:1.

20. Geiger S: Eating seafood sustainably. *Today's Dietitian* 2012;14(6):38.

21. Schardt D: Safe at home: How to keep your kitchen from making you sick. *Nutr Action Healthletter,* November 2011 p. 3.

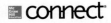 **To get the most out of your study, visit Connect where you will find NutritionCalc Plus, SmartBook®, and many other dynamic tools.**

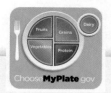

Rate Your Plate

Source: ChooseMyPlate.gov

I. Take a Closer Look at Food Additives

Evaluate a food label of a convenience food item (e.g., frozen entrée, ready-to-eat baked good) either in the supermarket or one you have available.

1. Write out the list of ingredients.

2. Identify the ingredients that you think may be food additives.

3. Based on the information available in this chapter, what are the functions of these food additives?

4. How might this food product differ without these ingredients?

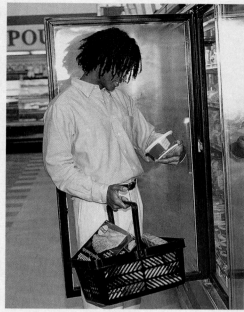

©Digital Vision/Getty Images RF

II. Take a Closer Look at Organic Foods

Visit one or more supermarkets to see what organic foods are available. Note your findings in the chart.

	Available	Not Available
Meat		
Poultry		
Milk		
Eggs		
Cheese		
Lettuce		
Apples		
Bananas		
Broccoli		
Other produce		
Breakfast cereal		
Snack chips		
Crackers		
Bread		
Pasta		

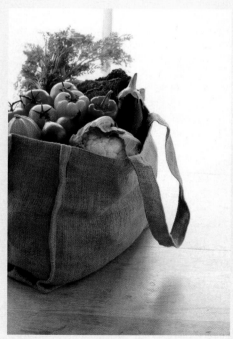

©David Buffington/Getty Images RF

Do you currently purchase organic foods? Why or why not?

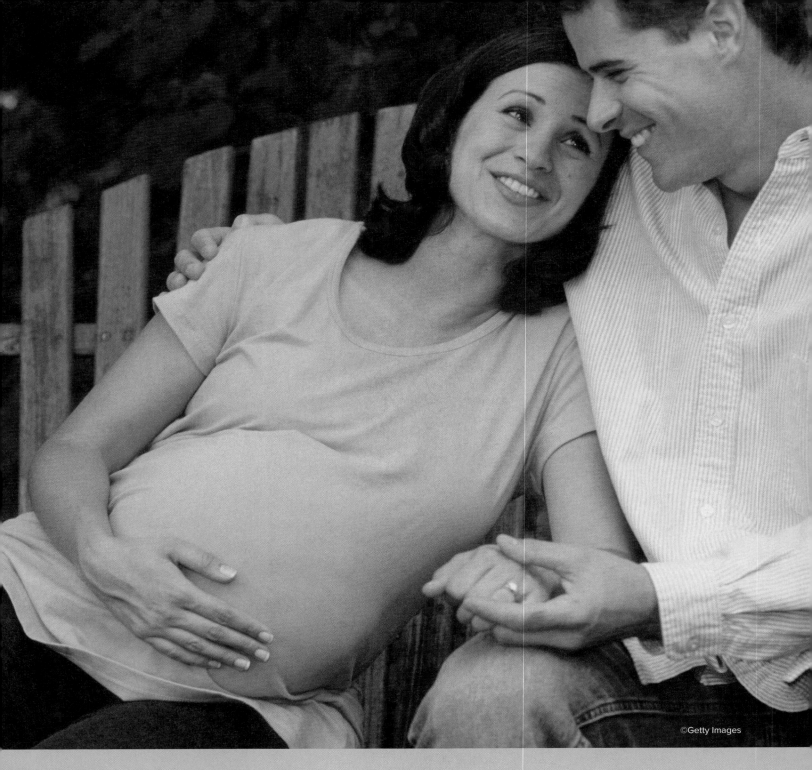

©Getty Images

Student Learning Outcomes

14.1 Describe how nutrition affects fertility.

14.2 Summarize the physiological changes of pregnancy and how they affect the nutrient requirements of a woman, and list nutrients that may need to be supplemented during pregnancy.

14.3 Define "success" in terms of positive health outcomes during pregnancy, and identify lifestyle factors that promote a successful pregnancy for both the mother and the infant.

14.4 Specify optimal ranges of weight gain during pregnancy for women with low, healthy, or high prepregnancy BMI.

14.5 Outline guidelines for exercise during pregnancy.

Chapter 14

Nutrition During Pregnancy and Breastfeeding

What Would You Choose?

As a pregnant vegetarian, which of the following meals would you choose as the best source of iron?

a Spinach salad with hard-boiled eggs and a whole wheat roll

b Lean hamburger with cheese, lettuce, and tomato, and roasted red potatoes

c Bean and cheese soft taco and stewed tomatoes

d Kellogg's® Smart Start® cereal, fat-free milk, and orange juice

Think about your choice as you read this chapter, then see What the Dietitian Chose at the end of the chapter.

The responsibility of nourishing and protecting a child is exhilarating and, at the same time, intimidating. Parents' desire to produce a healthy baby can arouse interest in nutrition and health information. They usually want to do everything possible to maximize their chances of having a healthy newborn.

Despite these intentions, the infant mortality rate in North America is higher than that seen in many other industrialized nations. In Canada, about 5 of every 1000 infants per year die before their first birthday, whereas in the United States, it is almost 6 infants. These are alarming statistics for two countries that have such a high per capita expenditure for health care compared to many other countries in the world. Comparatively, the rate of infant mortality in Sweden is less than 3 of every 1000 infants. In addition, in the United States, about 11% of pregnant women receive inadequate prenatal care.

Some aspects of fetal and newborn health are beyond our control. Still, conscious decisions about social, health, environmental, and nutritional factors during pregnancy significantly affect the baby's future. Choosing to breastfeed the infant adds further benefits. Let us examine how eating well during pregnancy and breastfeeding can help a baby to have a healthy start in life.

14.6 Describe the discomforts and complications of pregnancy that may be reduced by improving dietary patterns.

14.7 Summarize the physiological processes involved in breastfeeding and how breastfeeding affects the nutritional requirements of a woman.

14.8 Design an adequate, balanced meal plan for a pregnant or breastfeeding woman based on MyPlate.

14.9 List several advantages of breastfeeding for both the mother and the infant.

14.10 Relate the nutritional status of the parents to the risk of birth defects in the child.

14.1 Nutrition and Fertility

"Surprise, we're pregnant!" Considering the fact that only about half of all pregnancies are planned, a positive pregnancy test can be shocking news. Even when planned, women often do not suspect they are pregnant during the first few weeks after conception. They may not seek medical attention until 2 to 3 months after conception. Without fanfare, though, the **embryo** grows and develops daily. As you will learn in this chapter, the mother's nutritional status will affect the health of her baby before and long after birth. For that reason, the health and nutrition habits of a woman who is trying to become pregnant—or has the potential to become pregnant—are vitally important.

For up to 15% of couples who are planning for pregnancy, however, that pregnancy test shows a negative result month after month. **Infertility** refers to the inability of a couple to conceive after 1 year of unprotected intercourse. There are numerous possible causes for male and female infertility, many of which are outside the couple's control. In some cases, however, nutrition and lifestyle changes can improve a couple's chances of conceiving a child.

The nutritional status of both the mother- and the father-to-be can affect the likelihood of conception.[1] Some of the nutritional factors discussed in this chapter affect the hormone levels involved in reproduction. Others directly affect the viability of the egg or the sperm. Thus far, research clearly supports a link between body fat and fertility, and some evidence points to roles of certain dietary fats, carbohydrates, antioxidant nutrients, B vitamins, zinc, and iron.

ENERGY BALANCE

Recall from Section 7.1 that energy balance is the relationship between energy in and energy out. **Positive energy balance** describes a situation in which the amount of calories consumed exceeds the amount of calories required to support basic body processes and physical activity. Sustained over time, positive energy balance leads to gains in both lean mass and adipose tissue. **Negative energy balance** occurs when calorie intake falls short of calorie needs. Prolonged negative energy balance leads to loss of both lean and adipose tissue. At either extreme, prolonged energy imbalance can impair fertility.

It is important to note that adipose tissue serves as more than just a storage depot for energy; it also produces estrogen and other hormones and cellular signaling molecules with widespread effects. For example, leptin, a hormone produced primarily by adipose tissue, affects appetite, metabolic rate, immune function, growth, and reproduction.

Reproductive function is costly in terms of energy. Synthesis of reproductive hormones, maintenance of normal menstrual cycles, pregnancy, and breastfeeding require calories. With negative energy balance, little energy is available to maintain normal reproductive function. Consequently, many underweight women experience **amenorrhea,** a sign of impaired ovulation. Some causes of low energy availability are undernutrition that stems from poverty (see Section 12.5), an eating disorder (see Section 11.2), or high levels of athletic training (see Section 10.4). During World War II, for example, a famine in Holland drastically cut the calorie intake of women to about 1000 kcal per day. Many women became amenorrheic, and birth rates declined by about 50% during that time period. Studies in female athletes indicate that energy intake of at least 30 kcal per kilogram of lean mass is needed for normal reproductive function among women. For men, low body fat can decrease sex drive and sperm count.

On the opposite end of the spectrum, prolonged positive energy balance also decreases fertility. The extra adipose tissue affects the availability of reproductive hormones and induces insulin resistance. For women, these endocrine changes impair the success of ovulation and implantation. In fact, excess body fat is thought to cause about 25% of problems with ovulation that lead to infertility. Among men, excess body fat increases estrogen levels and decreases testosterone. Also, extra fat tissue increases the temperature of the testicular area. The changes in hormones and temperature result in

embryo In humans, the developing offspring in utero from about the beginning of the third week to the end of the eighth week after conception.

infertility Inability of a couple to conceive after 1 year of unprotected intercourse.

positive energy balance The state in which energy intake is greater than energy expended, generally resulting in weight gain.

negative energy balance The state in which energy intake is less than energy expended, resulting in weight loss.

amenorrhea Absence of menstrual periods in a woman of reproductive age.

lower sperm production. Excess body fat also increases oxidative stress, which damages DNA in both the egg and the sperm. For overweight or obese adults, studies show that losing just 5% to 10% of body weight can increase the chances of conception.

HORMONAL BALANCE

As we discuss the ways energy imbalances influence fertility, it is important to mention **polycystic ovary syndrome (PCOS).** Women with PCOS have hormonal imbalances that may lead to problems with ovulation, unusually high levels of androgen hormones (e.g., testosterone), and the presence of many tiny cysts that surround the ovaries like a strand of pearls. All women secrete some testosterone, but women with PCOS secrete more than normal. The high levels of male hormones lead to some of the signs and symptoms of PCOS: excess hair growth on the face, acne, and a tendency to deposit fat around the waist. Insulin resistance is another common feature of the syndrome. Thus, women with PCOS are at higher risk for diabetes (see Section 4.7), high blood pressure (see Section 9.17), and cardiovascular disease (see Section 5.8). Importantly for our discussion here, women with PCOS have irregular or absent periods, difficulty becoming pregnant, and higher-than-average rates of miscarriage. Indeed, PCOS is the leading cause of female infertility.[2]

Many dietary and lifestyle changes have been studied to see how they can alter the course of PCOS. To date, evidence most clearly indicates that weight loss is important to improve metabolic and fertility issues among overweight women with PCOS. If an overweight woman with PCOS loses just 5% of her body weight, regardless of diet composition, her chances of conception improve. Daily physical activity, known to improve insulin sensitivity, is a key component of any weight-management strategy (see Section 7.7).

In addition to managing body weight, the quality and quantity of carbohydrates may make a difference in controlling PCOS and improving fertility. Some experts recommend reducing carbohydrate intake to the lower end of the range recommended by the Food and Nutrition Board (about 45% of total kcal) and choosing low glycemic-index carbohydrates. For example, women with PCOS are urged to choose whole grains instead of refined grains and whole fruits and vegetables rather than juices, and to steer clear of sugar-sweetened beverages. There are claims that following a low-carbohydrate diet (less than 45% of total kcal) is useful for women with PCOS, but these claims are not well supported by research. Severely restricting carbohydrate choices could limit the intake of important nutrients, such as B vitamins.

KEY NUTRIENTS

Vitamins. Routine intake of a daily multivitamin and mineral supplement has been linked to improved fertility in many studies. There are a variety of micronutrients that may contribute, but folic acid tops the list for both men and women. As you learned in Section 8.12, folate is involved in DNA synthesis and the metabolism of homocysteine. For no other cells is proper DNA synthesis so important as for the egg and sperm, which transmit genetic information from one generation to the next! Foods such as leafy green vegetables, strawberries, and orange juice are sources of natural folate. The synthetic form, folic acid, can be found in dietary supplements and fortified foods, such as ready-to-eat breakfast cereals.

The chemical reactions of metabolism produce free radicals (molecules with unpaired electrons) that can damage cell membranes and DNA. The body has some antioxidant mechanisms that limit the activity of free radicals, but when the production of free radicals exceeds the antioxidant capacity of the body, oxidative damage to cells is likely. Free radicals can damage egg and (especially) sperm cells and can affect how well a fertilized egg implants and matures. Research studies show that dietary patterns rich in antioxidants—vitamin E, vitamin C, selenium, zinc, beta-carotene, and some other plant pigments—are linked to improved fertility for both men and women. Foods of plant

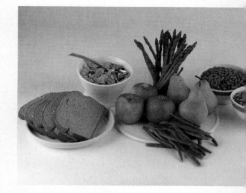

▲ Several studies show a link between a low glycemic-index eating pattern and improved fertility for women with PCOS.
©McGraw-Hill Education/Jill Braaten, photographer

polycystic ovary syndrome (PCOS)
A condition of hormonal imbalance (e.g., elevated testosterone and insulin) in a woman that can lead to infertility, weight gain in the abdominal region, excessive growth of body hair, and acne.

origin, including brightly colored fruits and vegetables, whole grains, and plant oils, are rich sources of antioxidant nutrients.

Minerals. Iron and zinc are two minerals that have been linked to fertility. Zinc appears to be especially important for male fertility. Not only is it involved as a cofactor in antioxidant reactions that could protect sperm from oxidative damage, but zinc is also required for normal sexual maturation and production of sperm and reproductive hormones. Men with poor zinc status may have poor sperm quality (e.g., low sperm production, impaired sperm motility, and/or damaged DNA). Studies have shown that zinc supplements can improve sperm quality in men who are deficient in zinc.

For women, iron and zinc are needed for normal ovulation. Data from a large observational study of nurses showed that use of iron supplements before conception was linked to improved ovulatory function and therefore better fertility. Interestingly, in this study, higher intakes of nonheme iron (from plant sources) were specifically related to improved fertility (see Ask the RDN in this section).

Dietary Fat. As recommended for the general population of healthy adults, men and women who are trying to conceive should try to limit sources of saturated and *trans* fats. For women, a diet rich in saturated and *trans* fat promotes insulin resistance and impairs ovulation. For men, high intakes of saturated and *trans* fat are linked to poor sperm quality. Instead of consuming the typical American fare of pizza and fast foods, men and women should emphasize plant oils and fish oils, which provide more unsaturated fats. Among men experiencing infertility, boosting intakes of omega-3 fatty acids, the type of polyunsaturated fatty acids found in fish oils and walnuts, can improve sperm quality.

ALCOHOL

While trying to conceive, it is safest to avoid alcohol. Most studies show that higher intakes of alcohol (i.e., more than one or two drinks per day) are related to lower rates of conception. Alcohol can decrease levels of estrogen and testosterone and can therefore disrupt the normal cycles of ovulation and sperm production. In Section 14.8, you will learn about the devastating effects of alcohol on the developing babies in utero. Given the fact that many women do not realize they are pregnant until several weeks after conception, it is best to avoid alcohol while trying to conceive.

When trying to conceive, should you switch to decaf? There has been some concern that caffeine could decrease fertility, but the evidence is mixed. In some studies, intake of more than 4 cups of coffee (about 500 mg caffeine) has been linked to decreased fertility, but most studies show no clear link between moderate caffeine intake and fertility.

ASK THE RDN The Fertility Diet

Dear RDN: My husband and I have been trying to conceive for 2 years. We have an appointment to see a fertility specialist, but I recently found The Fertility Diet. Is this a good resource for couples who are trying to get pregnant?

The Fertility Diet, written in 2007 by scientists from the Harvard School of Public Health, sums up findings from the Nurses' Health Study II regarding relationships between diet, lifestyle, and pregnancy success.[3] Based on extensive data collected from 18,555 women who were trying to conceive during the study, the authors boiled down their conclusions into 10 recommendations:

1. Avoid *trans* fats.
2. Use more unsaturated fats.
3. Eat more vegetable protein.
4. Choose "low and slow" carbohydrates (e.g., whole grains, foods with low glycemic index).
5. Temporarily trade in low-fat and fat-free dairy products for full-fat versions.
6. Use a daily multivitamin and mineral supplement that contains folic acid.
7. Ensure adequate iron intake from sources other than red meats.
8. Choose water for hydration; coffee, tea, and alcohol can be used in moderation, but sugar-sweetened beverages should be avoided.

9. Lose 5% to 10% of body weight (if overweight).
10. Incorporate moderate exercise.

With the exception of tip #5, all of these recommendations are in line with current dietary advice for Americans from major health authorities, including the *Dietary Guidelines*. For women who are trying to get pregnant, in particular, these recommendations are in agreement with the latest research on diet and fertility covered in this section.

What about #5? Grab an ice cream scoop? Public health messages have been telling us to choose low-fat and fat-free dairy foods for decades. Why might women seeking to become pregnant benefit from drinking whole milk and eating ice cream? The authors hypothesize that dairy fat, which does contain many hormones from lactating and sometimes pregnant cows, may influence the woman's hormone levels in a way that improves fertility. This is an intriguing hypothesis and one that certainly warrants further investigation. Notably, in their chapter on dairy choices, the authors also point out that dairy products may not be the best way for Americans to obtain calcium, in general. Instead, they advocate plant sources of calcium, dietary supplements, and a daily dose of sunshine to support bone health.

In addition to the tips offered in *The Fertility Diet,* I would also encourage you to find ways to include at least five servings per day of fruits and vegetables. These foods have much to offer in terms of the micronutrients that are needed to support a healthy pregnancy and can help with blood glucose control and weight management.

Research demonstrates that insulin resistance underlies many cases of infertility. Dietary changes that improve insulin sensitivity—losing excess body fat, choosing healthy fats, avoiding dramatic rises and falls in blood sugar throughout the day—can optimize a woman's chances of ovulating normally and becoming pregnant. Furthermore, adequate intake of several key micronutrients—iron and folic acid—are vital for growth and development of the fetus.

Keep in mind that the Nurses' Health Study (like most research on diet and fertility) is an observational study. Even though these dietary patterns are associated with improved fertility, they have not been tested as part of a controlled experiment. Also, the authors provide the rationale for these dietary and lifestyle strategies to counter ovulatory infertility only; dietary changes are less likely to help women with infertility due to structural abnormalities or other health conditions. In other words, neither *The Fertility Diet* nor any other diet or lifestyle change can guarantee a healthy pregnancy; however, this chapter does offer the best of what we know to enhance your chances of success.

In sum, *The Fertility Diet* provides excellent nutrition advice, backed by evidence from the Nurses' Health Study and many other research studies, that can be adopted by the whole family. The authors have a knack for explaining complex scientific concepts in terms nonscientists can understand. Furthermore, the book includes practical advice, meal plans, and recipes to help women translate science into food choices.

Wishing you pink or blue,

Angela Collene, MS, RDN, LD (author)

✓ CONCEPT CHECK 14.1

1. How is energy balance related to fertility?

2. What hormonal changes are characteristic of polycystic ovary syndrome? List two dietary or lifestyle modifications that may help a woman with PCOS.

3. List three nutrients that have been linked to fertility.

14.2 Prenatal Growth and Development

The length of a normal pregnancy is 38 to 42 weeks, measured from the first day of the woman's last menstrual period. For purposes of discussion, the duration of pregnancy is commonly divided into three periods, called **trimesters.** For 8 weeks after conception, a human embryo develops from a fertilized **ovum** into a **fetus.**

trimesters Three 13- to 14-week periods into which the normal pregnancy (on average, 40 weeks) is divided somewhat arbitrarily for purposes of discussion and analysis. Development of the offspring, however, is continuous throughout pregnancy, with no specific physiological markers demarcating the transition from one trimester to the next.

ovum The egg cell from which a fetus eventually develops if the egg is fertilized by a sperm cell.

fetus The developing organism from about the beginning of the ninth week after conception until birth.

FIGURE 14-1 ▶ The fetus in relationship to the placenta. The placenta is the organ through which nourishment flows to the fetus.

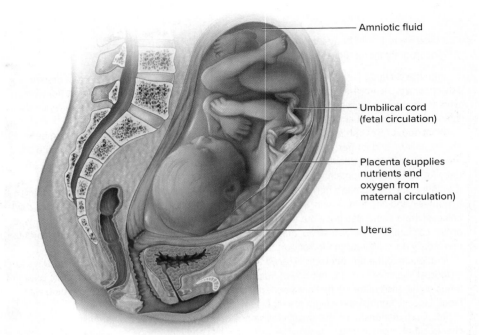

- Amniotic fluid
- Umbilical cord (fetal circulation)
- Placenta (supplies nutrients and oxygen from maternal circulation)
- Uterus

placenta An organ that forms in the uterus in pregnant women. Through this organ, oxygen and nutrients from the mother's blood are transferred to the fetus, and fetal wastes are removed. The placenta also releases hormones that maintain the state of pregnancy.

Until birth, the mother nourishes the fetus via a **placenta,** an organ that forms in her uterus to accommodate the growth and development of the fetus (Fig. 14-1). The role of the placenta is to exchange nutrients, oxygen, and other gases between the mother and fetus and to eliminate waste products. This occurs through a network of capillaries that bring the fetal blood close to the maternal blood supply, but the two blood supplies do not mix.

EARLY GROWTH—THE FIRST TRIMESTER IS A CRITICAL TIME

zygote The fertilized ovum; the cell resulting from the union of an egg cell (ovum) and sperm until it divides.

In the formation of the human organism, egg and sperm unite to produce the **zygote** (Fig. 14-2). From this point, the reproductive process occurs rapidly:

- Within 30 hours: the zygote divides in half to form two cells.
- Within 4 days: cell number climbs to 128 cells.
- At 14 days: the group of cells is called an embryo.
- Within 35 days: heart is beating, embryo is 1/30 of an inch (8 millimeters) long, eyes and limb buds are clearly visible.
- At 8 weeks: the embryo is known as a fetus.
- At 13 weeks (end of first trimester): most organs are formed, and the fetus can move.

Growth begins in the first trimester with a rapid increase in cell number. This type of growth dominates embryonic and early fetal development. The newly formed cells then begin to grow larger. Further growth is a mix of increases in cell number and cell size. By the end of 13 weeks—the first trimester—most organs are formed and the fetus can move (see Fig. 14-2).

spontaneous abortion Cessation of pregnancy and expulsion of the embryo or nonviable fetus prior to 20 weeks' gestation. This is the result of natural causes, such as a genetic defect or developmental problem; also called *miscarriage.*

As the embryo or fetus develops, nutritional deficiencies, toxicities, and other harmful environmental exposures have the potential to damage organ systems. For example, adverse reactions to medications, high intakes of vitamin A, exposure to radiation, or trauma can alter or arrest the current phase of fetal development, and the effects may last a lifetime (review Fig. 14-2). The most critical time for these potential problems is during the first trimester. Most **spontaneous abortions**—premature terminations of pregnancy that occur naturally—happen at this time. One-half or more pregnancies end in this way, often so early that a woman does not even realize she was pregnant. (An additional 15% to 20% are lost before normal delivery.) Early spontaneous abortions

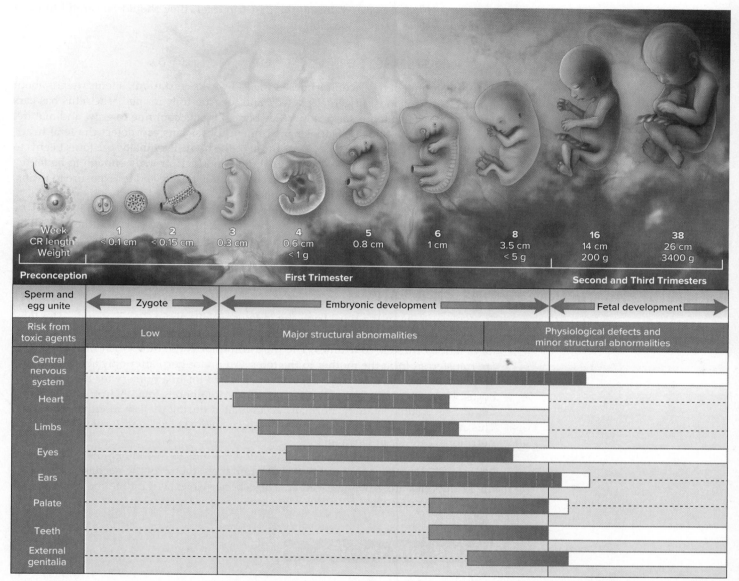

Week	1	2	3	4	5	6	8	16	38
CR length*	<0.1 cm	<0.15 cm	0.3 cm	0.6 cm	0.8 cm	1 cm	3.5 cm	14 cm	26 cm
Weight				<1 g			<5 g	200 g	3400 g

	Preconception	First Trimester		Second and Third Trimesters
Sperm and egg unite	←— Zygote —→	←———— Embryonic development ————→		←— Fetal development —→
Risk from toxic agents	Low	Major structural abnormalities		Physiological defects and minor structural abnormalities
Central nervous system				
Heart				
Limbs				
Eyes				
Ears				
Palate				
Teeth				
External genitalia				

FIGURE 14-2 ▲ Harmful effects of toxic agents during pregnancy. Vulnerable periods of fetal development are indicated with purple bars. The purple shading indicates the time of greatest risk to the organ. The most serious damage to the fetus from exposure to toxins is likely to occur during the first 8 weeks after conception, two-thirds of the way through the first trimester. As the white bars in the chart show, however, damage to vital parts of the body—including the eyes, brain, and genitals—can also occur during the later months of pregnancy.

*CR length = measurement from the crown (top of the head) to the rump (lowest part of the buttocks)

usually result from a genetic defect or fatal error in fetal development. Smoking (any form of nicotine or marijuana), alcohol abuse, use of aspirin and NSAIDs, and illicit drug use raise the risk for spontaneous abortion.

A woman should avoid substances that may harm the developing fetus, especially during the first trimester. This holds true, as well, for the time when a woman is trying to become pregnant. As previously mentioned, she is unlikely to be aware of her pregnancy for at least a few weeks. In addition, the fetus develops so rapidly during the first trimester that, if an essential nutrient is not available, the fetus may be affected even before evidence of the nutrient deficiency appears in the mother.

For this reason, the *quality*—rather than the *quantity*—of the woman's nutritional intake is most important during the first trimester. In other words, the mother should consume the same amount of calories as she did before she became pregnant, but she should focus on choosing more nutrient-dense foods. Although some women lose their appetite and feel nauseated during the first trimester, they should be careful to meet nutrient needs as much as possible.

SECOND TRIMESTER

gestation The period of intrauterine development of offspring, from conception to birth; in humans, normal gestation is 38 to 42 weeks.

By the beginning of the second trimester (i.e., 13 weeks' **gestation**), a fetus weighs about 1 ounce. Arms, hands, fingers, legs, feet, and toes are fully formed. The fetus has ears and begins to form tooth sockets in its jawbone. Organs continue to grow and mature, and, with a stethoscope or Doppler instrument, physicians can detect the fetal heartbeat. Most bones are distinctly evident through the body. Eventually, the fetus begins to look more like an infant. It may suck its thumb and kick strongly enough to be felt by the mother. As shown in Figure 14-2, the fetus can still be affected by exposure to toxins, but not to the degree seen in the first trimester.

During the second trimester, the mother's breast weight typically increases by approximately 30% due to the development of milk-producing cells and the deposition of 2 to 4 pounds of fat for **lactation.** This stored fat serves as a reservoir for the extra calories that will be needed to produce breast milk.

lactation The period of milk secretion following pregnancy; typically called *breastfeeding.*

THIRD TRIMESTER

By the beginning of the third trimester, a fetus weighs about 2 to 3 pounds. The third trimester is a crucial time for fetal growth. The fetus will double in length and increase its weight by three to four times. The third trimester is the time when many nutrients are transferred from the mother to the fetus. An infant born after only about 26 weeks of gestation has a good chance of surviving if cared for in a nursery for high-risk newborns. However, the infant will have low stores of minerals (mainly iron and calcium), fat, and fat-soluble vitamins normally accumulated during the last month of gestation. This and other medical problems, such as a poor ability to suck and swallow, complicate nutritional care for preterm infants.

By 40 weeks, the fetus usually weighs 7 to 9 pounds (3 to 4 kilograms) and is about 20 inches (50 centimeters) long. Soft spots (fontanels) on top of the head indicate where the skull bones are growing together. These bones close by the time the baby reaches 12 to 18 months of age.

✓ **CONCEPT CHECK 14.2**

1. What is the role of the placenta?
2. Describe how risks for fetal malformations vary throughout pregnancy.
3. During which trimester are most organs being formed?
4. During which trimester does fetal size increase the most?

14.3 Success in Pregnancy

The goal of pregnancy is to achieve optimal health for both the baby and the mother. For the mother, a successful pregnancy is one in which her physical and emotional health is protected so that she can return to her prepregnancy health status. For the infant, two widely accepted criteria are (1) a gestation period longer than 37 weeks; and (2) a birth weight greater than 5.5 pounds (2.5 kilograms). Sufficient lung development, likely to have occurred by 37 weeks of gestation, is critical to the survival of a newborn. The longer the gestation (up to 42 weeks), the greater the ultimate birth weight and maturation state, leading to fewer medical problems and better quality of life for the infant.

As you read this chapter, you will notice frequent references to lifelong effects of maternal nutrition, physical activity, and other lifestyle practices on the child. This

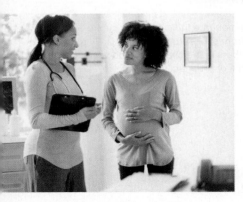

▲ To ensure optimal health and rapid treatment of medical conditions that develop during pregnancy, a pregnant woman should consult with her health care provider on a regular basis. Ideally, this consultation should begin before she becomes pregnant. ©JGI/Tom Grill/Blend Images/Corbis

is called the *developmental origins of health and disease hypothesis,* or more simply, the **fetal origins hypothesis.** Emerging evidence links prenatal influences, such as famines, fasting, exposure to alcohol, environmental pollution, and even stress to the child's risks for disease later in life (see Newsworthy Nutrition in Section 14.4). As we learn more about how environmental factors shape the ways our genes are expressed, it becomes increasingly evident that many aspects of our physical and mental health are programmed while we are yet in utero. What's more, these epigenetic changes may be passed down from generation to generation.

Overall, a successful pregnancy is the outcome of many complex gene-environment interactions. The decisions a mother and father make today can affect the health of their child for years to come. Although a mother's decisions, practices, and precautions during pregnancy contribute to the health of her fetus during all three trimesters, she cannot guarantee her fetus good health because some genetic and environmental factors are beyond her control. She and others involved in the pregnancy should not hold an unrealistic illusion of total control.

Low-birth-weight (LBW) infants are those weighing less than 5.5 pounds (2.5 kilograms) at birth. In the United States, 1 in 12 newborns is born LBW. Most commonly, LBW is associated with **preterm** birth. Medical costs during the first year of life for LBW infants are higher than those for normal-weight infants. In fact, hospital-related costs of caring for a preterm and/or LBW infant are more than $54,000 for the first year of life in the United States. For comparison, average medical costs during the first year of life for a healthy, full-term infant are around $4400. Overall, preterm births cost employers more than $12 billion in excess health care costs each year. (See the March of Dimes website at www.marchofdimes.org for additional information on preterm birth.)

Full-term and preterm infants who weigh less than the expected weight for their duration of gestation as a result of insufficient growth are described as **small for gestational age (SGA).** Thus, a full-term infant weighing less than 5.5 pounds at birth is SGA but not preterm, whereas a preterm infant born at 30 weeks' gestation is probably LBW without being SGA. Infants who are SGA are more likely than normal-weight infants to have medical complications, including problems with feeding, blood glucose control, temperature regulation, growth, and development in the weeks after birth.

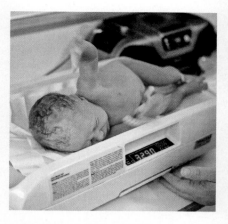

▲ A healthy newborn. At birth, a baby usually weighs about 7.5 pounds and is 20 inches long. ©Don Bayley/Getty Images

fetal origins hypothesis A theory that links nutritional and other environmental insults that occur during gestation to the future health of the offspring.

low birth weight (LBW) Referring to any infant weighing less than 2.5 kilograms (5.5 pounds) at birth; most commonly results from preterm birth.

preterm An infant born before 37 weeks of gestation; also referred to as *premature.*

small for gestational age (SGA) Referring to infants who weigh less than the expected weight for their length of gestation. This corresponds to less than 2.5 kilograms (5.5 pounds) in a full-term newborn.

PRENATAL CARE AND COUNSELING

Adequate prenatal care is a primary determinant of success in pregnancy. Ideally, women should receive examinations and counseling *before* becoming pregnant and continue regular prenatal care throughout pregnancy. If prenatal care is inadequate, delayed, or absent, untreated maternal nutritional deficiencies can deprive a developing fetus of needed nutrients. In addition, untreated health conditions, such as anemia, AIDS, hypertension, or diabetes, must be carefully addressed to minimize complications during pregnancy. Treating ongoing infections will also decrease risks of fetal damage. Without prenatal care, a woman is three times more likely to deliver a LBW baby—one who will be 40 times more likely to die during the first 4 weeks of life than a normal-birth-weight infant. Although the ideal time to start prenatal care is before conception, about 20% of women in the United States receive *no* prenatal care throughout the first trimester—a critical time to positively influence the outcome of pregnancy. One goal of *Healthy People 2020* is to increase by 10% the number of women who receive prenatal care beginning in the first trimester.

Food habits cannot be predicted from income, education, or lifestyle. Although some women already have good dietary habits, most can benefit from nutritional advice. All should be reminded of habits that may harm the growing fetus, such as severe dieting or fasting. By focusing on appropriate prenatal care, nutrient intake, and healthy habits, parents give their fetus—and later, their infant—the best chance of thriving. Overall, the chances of producing a healthy baby are maximized with education, an adequate diet, and early and consistent prenatal medical care.

A goal of *Healthy People 2020* is to reduce the number of live births that are LBW by 5% and preterm births by 10%. Currently, about 8% of live births are of low birth weight and about 10% are preterm.

EFFECTS OF MATERNAL AGE

The age of the mother is another factor that determines pregnancy outcome. The ideal age for pregnancy is between 20 and 35 years of age. Outside that age range—at either extreme—complications are more likely to arise. The rates of teen pregnancy have declined since 1990; still, approximately 250,000 babies are born to teen mothers in the United States each year—the highest of any industrialized country. Teen pregnancy increases risk for negative outcomes for both mother and child (Table 14-1) and costs taxpayers an estimated $9.4 billion each year.[4]

Pregnant teens frequently exhibit a variety of risk factors that can complicate pregnancy and pose risk to the fetus.[5] For instance, teenagers are more likely than adult women to be underweight at the start of pregnancy and to gain too little weight during pregnancy. In addition, their bodies may lack the physical maturity needed to carry a fetus safely. Even with prenatal care—and 7% of teenage mothers receive none at all—10% of children born to teenage mothers are of low birth weight and 14.5% are preterm.

Advanced maternal age also poses special risks for pregnancy. The likelihood of LBW and preterm delivery increases modestly, but progressively, with maternal age beyond 35 years. Given close monitoring, however, a woman older than 35 years has an excellent chance of producing a healthy infant.

CLOSELY SPACED AND MULTIPLE BIRTHS

The interval between the birth of one child and subsequent conception may affect the outcome of the latter pregnancy. Compared to those conceived at least 18 months following the birth of their older siblings, infants conceived less than 12 months after a previous birth have increased risks for preterm birth, LBW, SGA, birth defects, and developmental problems. These poor outcomes are probably related to insufficient time to rebuild nutrient stores depleted by the previous pregnancy. Similarly, multiple births (i.e., twins) increase the risk for preterm birth, LBW, and other medical complications for the mother and the offspring.

EXPOSURE TO TOXIC CHEMICALS

Figure 14-2 depicts how and when toxic agents can harm the developing fetus. In preparation for and during pregnancy, the mother should undoubtedly eliminate alcohol, tobacco, and illicit drugs (e.g., marijuana and cocaine). During organ development, exposure to these toxic chemicals can cause malformations. The adverse effects of fetal exposure to alcohol during gestation are discussed in Section 14.8. Smoking is linked to preterm birth and appears to increase the risk of birth defects, sudden infant death, childhood cancer, and disabilities.

Illicit drug use is particularly harmful during pregnancy. Many chemicals in recreational drugs cross the placenta and affect the fetus, whose detoxification systems are immature. Marijuana, the most common recreational drug used during the reproductive

Women with acquired immune deficiency syndrome (AIDS) may pass HIV to the fetus during pregnancy or delivery. About one in three infected newborns will develop AIDS symptoms and die within just a few years. Studies show that these odds of mother-to-child transmission can be cut significantly if the woman begins taking highly active antiretroviral therapy (HAART) and receiving routine obstetrical care. Before HAART was available, up to 45% of babies born to mothers with the AIDS virus were infected. Now, transmission is less than 2%. Thus, screening pregnant women for AIDS and providing HAART to those with AIDS are advocated by many experts. One target of the United Nations' recently released Sustainable Development Goals is to end the epidemic of AIDS by 2030.

TABLE 14-1 ■ **Effects of Teenage Pregnancy on Mother and Child**

For Mother	For Child
⬆ Depression and other mental health problems	⬇ Birth weight
⬆ Use of illicit drugs and alcohol	⬆ Premature birth
⬆ Poverty and reliance on public assistance	⬆ Infant mortality
⬇ Graduation rates from high school and college	⬆ Hospital admissions during childhood
⬆ Single parenthood	⬇ Academic performance
	⬇ Nutritional status
	⬆ Rates of imprisonment during adulthood

years, can result in reduced blood flow to the uterus and placenta, leading to poor fetal growth. Risks of low birth weight and preterm birth are increased for infants whose mothers used marijuana during pregnancy. Use of psychoactive drugs, such as cocaine and methamphetamines, restricts fetal growth and brain development, the effects of which may plague the child for a lifetime.

Even prescribed and common over-the-counter medications could have harmful effects on the developing fetus. Problem drugs include aspirin (especially when used chronically or heavily), hormone ointments, nose drops and related "cold" medications, rectal suppositories, weight-control pills, antidepressants, and medications prescribed for pre-existing illnesses. Some herbal therapies also have the potential to damage the fetus. Lower doses and/or safer alternatives should be substituted when a woman is planning to or has become pregnant.

In addition to these toxic chemicals, health hazards in the mother's environment, including job-related hazards and exposure to X rays, should be minimized.

FOOD SAFETY

Any foodborne illness during any stage of life is a concern. One type of foodborne illness that poses particular danger for pregnant women is caused by the bacterium *Listeria monocytogenes* (review Section 13.3). Infection with this microorganism typically causes mild flu-like symptoms, such as fever, headache, and vomiting, about 7 to 30 days after exposure. However, pregnant women and their offspring may suffer more severe symptoms, including fetal death. Unpasteurized milk, soft cheeses made from raw milk (e.g., brie, Camembert, feta, and blue cheeses), and some raw vegetables (e.g., cabbage and sprouts) can be sources of *Listeria* organisms, so it is especially important that pregnant women (and other people at high risk for infection) avoid these products. Experts advise consuming only pasteurized milk products and cooking meat, poultry, and seafood thoroughly to kill *Listeria* and other foodborne organisms. It is unsafe in pregnancy to eat any raw meats or other raw animal products, uncooked hot dogs, or undercooked poultry. These food safety recommendations are included in Appendix 14 of the *Dietary Guidelines for Americans*.

The U.S. Department of Agriculture (USDA) warns pregnant women to thoroughly cook (e.g., microwave) all ready-to-eat meats, including hot dogs and cold cuts, until they are steaming to reduce risk of *Listeria* infections.

PREPREGNANCY BMI

Women should aim to achieve a healthy body weight prior to becoming pregnant. Infants born to women who begin pregnancy substantially above or below a healthy weight are more likely to experience problems than those born to women who begin pregnancy at a normal weight. For instance, babies born to obese women are at increased risk of birth defects, death in the first few weeks after birth, and obesity in childhood. Many obese pregnant women experience high blood pressure, diabetes, and more difficult deliveries.

At the other extreme, women who begin pregnancy underweight (BMI under 18.5) are more likely to have infants who are low birth weight and preterm compared to women at a normal weight. These differences may be because underweight women tend to have lighter placentas and lower nutrient stores, especially iron, than heavier women, which could negatively affect fetal growth and development. An underweight woman can improve her nutrient stores and pregnancy outcome by gaining weight before pregnancy or gaining extra weight during pregnancy.

NUTRITIONAL STATUS

Is attention to good nutrition worth the effort? Yes! Extensive research suggests that an adequate vitamin and mineral intake at least 8 weeks before conception and throughout pregnancy can improve outcomes of pregnancy.[6] Extra nutrients and calories support fetal growth and development, of course, but also undergird the synthesis of maternal tissues. Her uterus and breasts grow, the placenta develops, her total blood volume

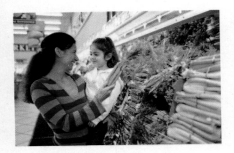

▲ In the United States, low-income pregnant women and their children benefit from the nutritional and medical attention provided by the WIC program. ©UpperCut Images/Getty Images

increases, the heart and kidneys work harder, and stores of body fat increase. In particular, meeting folate needs (400 micrograms of synthetic folic acid per day) helps to prevent birth defects such as neural tube defects (see Section 14.8) and decrease the risk of preterm delivery. Low intakes of calcium and iron or excessive intakes of vitamin A also are causes for concern during pregnancy.

Although it is difficult to predict the degree to which poor nutrition will affect each pregnancy, a daily diet containing only 1000 kcal has been shown to greatly restrict fetal growth and development. Increased maternal and infant death rates seen in famine-stricken areas of Africa provide further evidence.

Genetic background can explain little of the observed differences in birth weight between developed and developing countries. Both environmental factors and nutritional factors are important. The worse the nutritional status of the mother at the beginning of pregnancy, the more valuable a healthy prenatal diet and/or use of prenatal supplements are in improving the course and outcome of her pregnancy.

NUTRITION ASSISTANCE FOR LOW-INCOME FAMILIES

Poverty impacts pregnancy in many ways. Families of low socioeconomic status tend to receive inadequate health care. A lack of education, limited access to health care, or scant financial resources may contribute to poor health practices, such as dietary patterns that fail to meet the mother's increased nutrient requirements.

Several U.S. government programs provide high-quality health care and foods to reduce infant mortality. These government-subsidized programs are designed to alleviate the negative impact of poverty, insufficient education, and inadequate nutrient intake on pregnancy outcomes. An example of such a program is the Special Supplemental Nutrition Program for Women, Infants, and Children (WIC). This program offers health assessments and vouchers for foods that supply high-quality protein, calcium, iron, and vitamins A and C to pregnant women, infants, and children (up to 5 years of age) from low-income populations. The WIC program is available in all areas of the United States and has a staff trained to promote healthy behaviors during pregnancy. Participation in WIC has been shown to improve nutrient intakes of mothers, infants, and children.[7] More than 8 million women, infants, and young children are benefiting from this program, yet many eligible individuals are not participating.

✔ CONCEPT CHECK 14.3

1. In one or two sentences, how would you define success in pregnancy?
2. Define the terms *preterm, low birth weight,* and *small for gestational age.*
3. How is maternal age related to the outcome of pregnancy?
4. Is attention to good nutrition during pregnancy worth the effort? Why or why not?

14.4 Increased Nutrient Needs to Support Pregnancy

Pregnancy is a time of increased nutrient requirements. There are some general principles that are true for most women with regard to increased nutrient needs. However, recognize that each expectant mom will benefit from individualized counseling tailored to her unique nutritional and health needs.

CALORIE NEEDS

To support the growth and development of the fetus, pregnant women need to increase their calorie intake. Calorie needs during the first trimester are essentially the same as for nonpregnant women. However, during the second and third trimesters, it is necessary for a pregnant woman to consume approximately 350 to 450 kcal more per day than her prepregnancy needs (the upper end of the range is needed in the third trimester).

Rather than seeing this as an opportunity to fill up on sugary desserts or fat-filled snacks, pregnant women should consume these extra calories in the form of nutrient-dense foods. For example, throughout the day, about six whole wheat crackers, 1 ounce of cheese, and ½ cup of fat-free milk would supply the extra calories (and also some calcium). Although she "eats for two," the pregnant woman must not double her normal calorie intake. The "eating for two" concept refers more appropriately to increased needs for several vitamins and minerals. Micronutrient needs are increased by up to 50% during pregnancy, whereas calorie needs during the second and third trimesters represent only about a 20% increase.

If a woman is physically active during her pregnancy, she may need to increase her calorie intake by even more than the estimated 350 to 450 kcal per day. Her greater body weight requires more calories for activity. Many women find that they are not as active as usual during the later months, partly because of their increased size, so an extra 350 to 450 kcal in their daily diets is usually enough.

STAYING ACTIVE DURING PREGNANCY

Even though pregnancy is not the time to begin an intense fitness regimen, women can generally take part in most low- or moderate-intensity activities during pregnancy. In fact, the American College of Obstetrics and Gynecology recommends that pregnant women perform at least 30 minutes per day of moderate-intensity physical activity. Walking, cycling, swimming, or light aerobics for at least 150 minutes per week is generally advised. Such exercise may prevent pregnancy complications and promote an easier delivery.[8,9] Some research indicates that regular physical activity during pregnancy lowers a woman's risk of developing gestational diabetes by 50% and preeclampsia by 40%. These disorders of pregnancy are discussed further in Section 14.6. Figure 14-3 illustrates the broad range of benefits of exercise during pregnancy for both the mother and the baby.

Women who were highly active prior to pregnancy can maintain their activities as long as they remain healthy and review plans with their health care providers. Adequate

Why Exercise During Pregnancy?

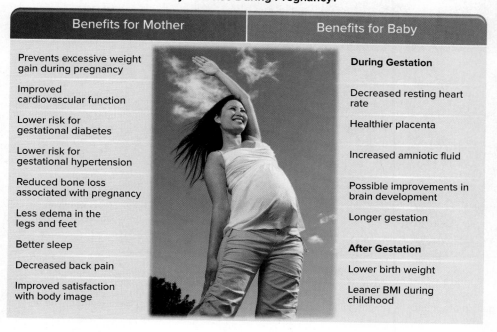

Benefits for Mother	Benefits for Baby
Prevents excessive weight gain during pregnancy	**During Gestation**
Improved cardiovascular function	Decreased resting heart rate
Lower risk for gestational diabetes	Healthier placenta
Lower risk for gestational hypertension	Increased amniotic fluid
Reduced bone loss associated with pregnancy	Possible improvements in brain development
Less edema in the legs and feet	Longer gestation
Better sleep	
Decreased back pain	**After Gestation**
Improved satisfaction with body image	Lower birth weight
	Leaner BMI during childhood

FIGURE 14-3 ◄ Benefits of exercise during pregnancy for the mother and baby. ©Tanya Constantine/Blend Images LLC

fluid intake before, during, and after physical activity is of heightened importance to regulate body temperature, because heat stress can be harmful to the developing fetus. Activities with inherent risk of falls or abdominal trauma—downhill skiing, horseback riding, and contact sports (e.g., soccer and basketball)—can potentially harm the fetus and should be avoided. In addition, pregnant women should avoid activities that require excess straining (e.g., heavy weightlifting) or exposure to extremes in air pressure (e.g., SCUBA diving).

Women with high-risk pregnancies, such as those experiencing premature labor contractions, may need to restrict physical activity. To ensure optimal health for both herself and her infant, a pregnant woman should first consult her primary care provider about physical activity and possible limitations.

OPTIMAL WEIGHT GAIN

Healthy prepregnancy weight and appropriate weight gain during pregnancy are excellent predictors of pregnancy outcome.[10,11] The mother's diet should allow for approximately 2 to 4 pounds (0.9 to 1.8 kilograms) of weight gain during the first trimester and then a subsequent weight gain of 0.8 to 1 pound (0.4 to 0.5 kilogram) weekly during the second and third trimesters (Fig. 14-4). A healthy goal for total weight gain for a woman of normal weight (based on prepregnancy BMI; Table 14-2) averages about 25 to 35 pounds (11.5 to 16 kilograms). Women of normal prepregnancy BMI carrying twins should aim to gain within the range of 37 to 54 pounds, whereas overweight or obese women pregnant with twins should gain less (31 to 50 pounds or 25 to 42 pounds, respectively).

For women who begin pregnancy with a low BMI, the goal for total weight gain increases to 28 to 40 pounds (12.5 to 18 kilograms). The goal decreases to 15 to 25 pounds (7 to 11.5 kilograms) for overweight women. Target weight gain for obese women is 11 to 20 pounds (5 to 9 kilograms). Figure 14-4 shows why the typical recommendation begins at 25 pounds.

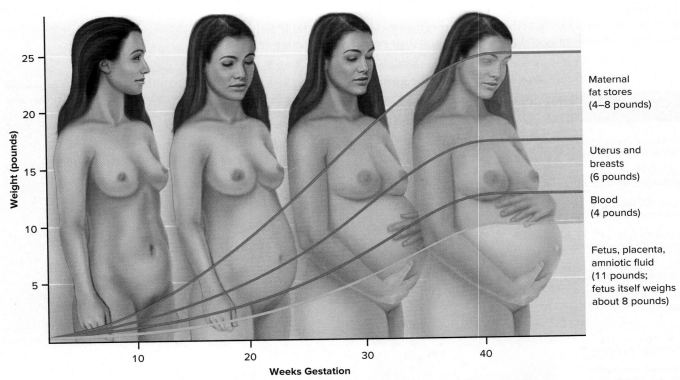

Maternal fat stores (4–8 pounds)

Uterus and breasts (6 pounds)

Blood (4 pounds)

Fetus, placenta, amniotic fluid (11 pounds; fetus itself weighs about 8 pounds)

FIGURE 14-4 ▲ The components of weight gain in pregnancy. A weight gain of 25 to 35 pounds is recommended for most women. The various components total about 25 pounds.

TABLE 14-2 ■ Recommended Weight Gain in Pregnancy Based on Prepregnancy Body Mass Index (BMI)

Prepregnancy BMI Category	Total Weight Gain*	
	(pounds)	(kilograms)
Low (BMI less than 18.5)	28 to 40	12.5 to 18
Normal (BMI 18.5 to 24.9)	25 to 35	11.5 to 16
High (BMI 25.0 to 29.9)	15 to 25	7 to 11.5
Obese (BMI greater than 30.0)	11 to 20	5 to 9

*The listed values are for pregnancies with one fetus. For women of normal BMI carrying twins, the range is 37 to 54 pounds (17 to 24.5 kilograms), or less for heavier women.

Source: Data from *Weight Gain During Pregnancy: Reexamining the Guidelines*, Copyright 2009 by the Institute of Medicine and National Research Council of the National Academies. National Academies Press, Washington, DC.

A weight gain of between 25 and 35 pounds for a woman starting pregnancy at normal weight has repeatedly been shown to yield optimal health for both mother and fetus if gestation lasts at least 38 weeks. The weight gain should yield a birth weight of 7.5 pounds (3.5 kilograms). Although some extra weight gain during pregnancy is usually not harmful (about 5 to 10 pounds), it can set the stage for a pattern of weight gain during the childbearing years if the mother does not return to her approximate prepregnancy weight after delivery.

Overweight and obesity do contribute to complications during pregnancy. Excess maternal body weight increases risk for diabetes, hypertension, blood clots, and spontaneous abortions during pregnancy. After childbirth, lasting effects of excess gestational weight gain for the mother include increased BMI, central body fat distribution, and elevated blood pressure. For the baby, there is a greater chance of birth defects and macrosomia, in which the fetus grows larger than average in utero. Larger infants contribute to a greater need for surgical delivery (i.e., Cesarean sections) among overweight and obese mothers. Over the long term, excessive maternal weight gain during pregnancy has been linked to increased risk for obesity and metabolic syndrome in the child.

Gestational weight gain is a key issue in prenatal care and a concern of many mothers-to-be. Even after the 2009 release of the weight gain guidelines summarized in Table 14-2, many women report receiving *no* guidance regarding weight gain from health care providers before or during pregnancy. Considering the extensive consequences of either inadequate or excessive weight gain during gestation, health professionals should take a more active role in educating pregnant mothers about what weight changes to expect, the consequences of too little or too much weight gain, and how to make corrections if the weight gain trajectory veers off course.[12,13] Weight gain during pregnancy should generally follow the pattern in Figure 14-4. Weekly monitoring of weight changes, especially on a chart that shows expected weight gains, can help a pregnant woman to assess how much to adjust her food intake and physical activity.

Realistic information about increased calorie requirements should be provided. Pregnant women need to understand that "eating for two" is more about increasing diet quality (i.e., choosing nutrient-dense foods) than diet quantity. Furthermore, as you learned in Section 7.8, successful weight management strategies involve a behavioral component; some women need to learn skills, such as self-monitoring of weight, dietary intake, and physical activity. Online tools (e.g., USDA's SuperTracker) and smartphone apps (e.g., Sprout Pregnancy) offer specialized tools to make self-monitoring tasks simple and social.

If a woman deviates from the desirable pattern, she should make appropriate adjustments, but weight loss during pregnancy is never advised. For example, if a woman begins to gain too much weight during her pregnancy, she should not lose weight to get back on track. Even if a woman gains 35 pounds in the first 7 months of pregnancy, she must still gain more during the last 2 months. She should, however, slow the increase in

Check out the pregnancy weight gain calculator at www.ChooseMyPlate.gov.

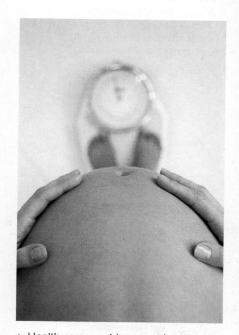

▲ Health care providers must be on the lookout for women who exhibit disordered eating behaviors during pregnancy. Although it is not yet recognized as a distinct diagnosis, *pregorexia* is gaining attention among practitioners who work with expectant moms. Some women are exceptionally concerned about weight gain and may restrict food intake, exercise excessively, or engage in other methods of purging excess calories to prevent weight gain. Inadequate weight gain during pregnancy puts the fetus at risk for growth restriction and birth defects.[14] ©John Slater/Getty Images

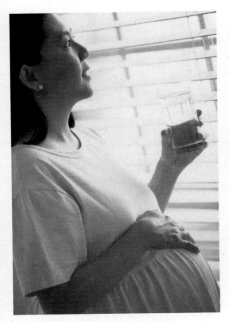

▲ During pregnancy, the Adequate Intake for total water increases 0.3 liter (1 ¼ cups) above prepregnancy needs to 3 liters (about 12 ½ cups) per day. For breastfeeding, consume 3.8 liters (16 cups) daily. ©Getty Images

Newsworthy Nutrition

Mothers' weight gain during pregnancy is linked to cognitive development of children

The Avon Longitudinal Study of Parents and Children includes 13,617 mother-offspring pairs in the United Kingdom who have been followed from pregnancy, through childbirth, and now into the offspring's young adulthood. In this analysis of gestational weight gain, children of mothers who gained less than recommended weight during pregnancy had lower School Entry Assessment scores at 4 years of age and lower performance on final examinations at 16 years of age. This study highlights the importance of adhering to the 2009 National Academy of Medicine recommendations for gestational weight gain. Appropriate weight gain during pregnancy improves multiple aspects of health for both the mother and the child.

Source: Gage SH, et al. "Associations of maternal weight gain in pregnancy with offspring cognition in childhood and adolescence: Findings from the Avon Longitudinal Study of Parents and Children." *American Journal of Epidemiology* 177:402, 2013.

weight to parallel the rise on the prenatal weight gain chart. In other words, the sources of the unnecessary calories should be found and minimized. On the other hand, if a woman has not gained the desired weight by a given point in pregnancy, she should not gain the needed weight rapidly. Instead, she should slowly gain a little more weight than the typical pattern to meet the goal by the end of the pregnancy. A registered dietitian nutritionist can help make any needed adjustments.

PROTEIN, CARBOHYDRATE, AND LIPID NEEDS

The RDA for protein increases by an additional 25 grams per day during pregnancy (Fig. 14-5). All women should check to make sure they are eating enough protein as well as enough calories (so that protein can be spared for synthesis of new tissue). However, many women already consume protein in excess of their needs and therefore do not need to focus specifically on increasing protein intake. Small changes are usually all that is necessary. For example, simply adding a cup of fat-free milk to the diet adds 90 nutrient-dense kilocalories and 8 grams of protein.

The RDA for carbohydrate increases to 175 grams daily, primarily to prevent ketosis. Ketone bodies, a by-product of metabolism of fat for energy, are poorly used by the fetal brain and may impair fetal brain development. Carbohydrate intakes of most women, pregnant or not, already exceed the RDA (see Fig. 14-5).

Fat intake should increase proportionally with calorie intake during pregnancy to maintain around 20% to 35% of total calories from fat. Pregnancy is not a time for a low-fat diet, as lipids are a source of extra calories and essential fatty acids needed during pregnancy. Recommendations for the types of lipids during pregnancy are generally the same as for nonpregnant adults: saturated fat should contribute no more than 10% of total calories and *trans* fat should be avoided.

During pregnancy, it is particularly important to make sure to consume adequate essential fatty acids—linoleic acid (omega-6) and alpha-linolenic acid (omega-3). As you learned in Section 5.2, essential fatty acids cannot be synthesized in the body and must be consumed in the diet. For the developing fetus, essential fatty acids are required for growth, brain development, and eye development. Children whose mothers consumed sources of omega-3 fatty acids during pregnancy tend to have better sleep patterns, better speech development, higher intelligence, and fewer behavioral problems as they grow and develop. For mothers, consuming omega-3 fatty acids during pregnancy may help to reduce postpartum depression.

Recommendations are slightly increased during pregnancy to 13 grams per day of linoleic acid and 1.4 grams per day of alpha-linolenic acid. These needs can be met by

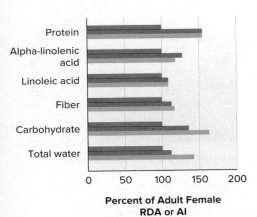

Percent of Adult Female RDA or AI

■ Adult female
■ Pregnancy
■ Breastfeeding

FIGURE 14-5 ▲ Relative macronutrient and water requirements for pregnancy and breastfeeding. Note that there is no RDA or AI for total fat; needs are based on 20% to 35% of overall energy intake.

consuming 2 to 4 tablespoons per day of plant oils. Consumption of two to three servings (8 to 12 ounces) per week of fish is recommended for meeting needs for essential fatty acids in the diet.[15] Women who choose not to eat fish can also obtain the same omega-3 fatty acids found in fish from specially raised eggs (it's in the chicken feed!) or fish oil supplements. For supplements, consumers should choose brands that have been distilled to remove environmental contaminants.[16] (See Section 14.8 for a discussion of mercury in fish.)

VITAMIN NEEDS

Vitamin needs increase from prepregnancy RDAs/AIs by up to 30% for most of the B vitamins, by 45% for vitamin B-6, and by 50% for folate (Fig. 14-6). Vitamin A needs only increase by 10%, so a specific focus on this vitamin is not needed. Recall from Section 8.2 that excess amounts of vitamin A are harmful to the developing fetus.

The extra amounts of vitamin B-6 and other B vitamins (except folate) needed in the diet are easily met via wise food choices, such as a serving of a typical ready-to-eat breakfast cereal and some lean animal protein sources. Folate needs, however, often merit specific diet planning and possible vitamin supplementation. The synthesis of DNA, and therefore cell division, requires folate, so this nutrient is especially crucial during pregnancy. Ultimately, both fetal and maternal growth depend on an ample supply of folate. Red blood cell formation, which requires folate, increases during pregnancy. Serious folate-related anemia therefore can result if folate intake is inadequate. The RDA for folate increases during pregnancy to 600 micrograms DFE per day (review Section 8.12 for calculation of DFE). This is a critical goal in the nutritional care of a pregnant woman. Increasing folate intakes to meet 600 micrograms DFE per day for a pregnant woman can be achieved through dietary sources (see the Farm to Fork in this section), a supplemental source of folic acid, or a combination of both. Choosing a diet rich in synthetic folic acid, such as from ready-to-eat breakfast cereals or meal replacement bars (look for approximately 50% to 100% of the Daily Value), is especially helpful in meeting folate needs. Recall from Section 8.12 that synthetic folic acid is much more easily absorbed than the various forms of folate found naturally in foods.[6]

Emerging evidence indicates that low maternal levels of vitamin D during pregnancy affect multiple health parameters in the offspring. About 54% of black women and 42% of white women have insufficient blood levels of the active form of vitamin D, even though many take a daily supplement containing 400 IU of vitamin D. Aside from its well-known roles in bone health and the incidence of rickets, poor vitamin D status is implicated in serious complications of pregnancy, including higher rates of blood sugar and blood pressure abnormalities during pregnancy and poor growth of the fetus.[17] Vitamin D's role in immune regulation is illustrated by higher rates of respiratory infections and mother-to-child transmission of HIV when its status is deficient. Because of the ability of vitamin D to modulate gene expression, vitamin D status is critically important during early fetal development through infancy. Diseases that develop later in childhood or adulthood, such as type 1 diabetes, multiple sclerosis, allergies, asthma, schizophrenia, and certain types of cancer, are associated with low vitamin D status during gestation. The RDA for pregnant women is 15 micrograms (600 IU) of vitamin D daily (the same as for nonpregnant women), but many experts advocate increasing this recommendation to 25 micrograms (1000 IU) or more.[18] Currently, there is no recommendation for universal vitamin D screening or supplementation, but the American College of Obstetricians and Gynecologists advises that for deficient individuals, 1000 to 2000 IU per day is a safe level of supplemental vitamin D during pregnancy.

MINERAL NEEDS

Mineral needs generally increase during pregnancy, especially the requirements for iodine, iron, and zinc (Fig. 14-7).[19] (Calcium needs do not increase but still may deserve special attention because many women find it difficult to meet their calcium needs in general.)

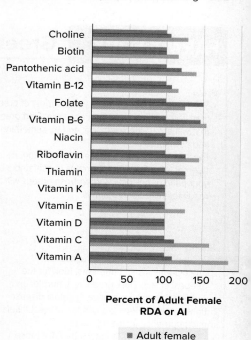

FIGURE 14-6 ▲ Relative vitamin requirements for pregnancy and breastfeeding.

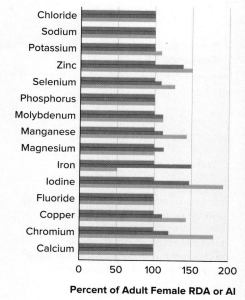

FIGURE 14-7 ▲ Relative mineral requirements for pregnancy and breastfeeding.

FARM to FORK   Greens

Grow
- Seed catalogs offer a much wider variety of greens than you can find in the grocery store. Find greens that will grow where you live, and try something new and nutritious!
- Even if you don't have space for gardening, it's easy to grow lettuce and other greens in containers on your patio or balcony. Garden-fresh greens will be ready to eat in 30 to 60 days.

Shop
- To identify greens that are highest in phytochemicals and nutrients, look for the deepest colors. Dark green, red, purple, and reddish-brown leaves have the most disease-fighting phytochemicals and the highest levels of micronutrients, including folate.
- Choose lettuces with leaves that are loose and open. These lettuce leaves produce more phytochemicals to protect themselves from the sun. Lettuces such as iceberg, with tightly wrapped leaves, provide only a fraction of the nutrients found in more colorful, loosely packed leaves.
- Fresh heads of lettuce or bunches of spinach tend to last longer than precut, prewashed greens sold in bags and plastic containers.

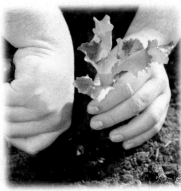

©Pixtal/Age Fotostock

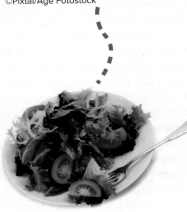

©D. Hurst/Alamy

Store
- Fresh greens need just the right amount of humidity and oxygen to stay fresh. After you bring home fresh greens, pull the lettuce apart, soak it in cold water for about 10 minutes, and spin it dry before storing. This increases the moisture content within the leaves but keeps the outside of the leaves dry, delaying spoilage.
- Use a pin to prick 10 to 20 holes in a gallon-size plastic bag. Store your greens in the perforated bag in the crisper drawer of your refrigerator to maintain optimal freshness. The bag helps the greens to retain their moisture. The tiny holes allow for some exchange of gases.

Prep
- Even though plants with the darkest colors have the most nutritional value, some people do not tolerate their somewhat bitter or peppery flavors. Harvesting the leaves early (i.e., baby lettuce greens) will yield a milder salad. Try mixing some bitter greens, such as arugula, with milder varieties, such as romaine or Bibb lettuce. Add sweet flavors, such as chopped fruit or a touch of honey in your salad dressing, to balance the stronger flavors.
- Don't skimp on the dressing! Many of the healthy compounds in these plants are fat-soluble. You will absorb more of the vitamin E and phytochemicals if you consume some fat as part of your meal. Olive oil is an excellent choice for homemade salad dressing.
- Boiling causes more than half of the nutrients to leach out of the vegetables and into the cooking water. If you cook your greens, sauté, steam, or microwave them.

Source: Robinson J. "From wild greens to iceberg lettuce: breeding out the medicine," in *Eating on the Wild Side*. New York: Little, Brown and Company, 2013.

congenital hypothyroidism The stunting of body growth and poor development in the offspring that result from inadequate maternal intake of iodine during pregnancy that impairs thyroid hormone synthesis (formerly called *cretinism*).

Pregnant women need extra iodine (RDA of 220 micrograms per day) to support thyroid hormone synthesis (for the mother and the developing fetus) and fetal brain development. If a mother is deficient in iodine during pregnancy, she may develop a goiter (see Section 9.12), and her child may suffer from a devastating birth defect called **congenital hypothyroidism** (formerly called *cretinism*). Section 14.8 provides further information on this and other nutrition-related birth defects. Typical iodine intakes are plentiful if the woman uses iodized salt.

The extra iron (RDA of 27 milligrams per day) is needed to synthesize a greater amount of hemoglobin during pregnancy and to provide iron stores for the fetus. About 2% of women begin pregnancy with clinically diagnosed iron-deficiency anemia, but an estimated one-third of pregnant women have poor iron stores, so heavy demands for iron during pregnancy cannot be met. The consequences of iron-deficiency anemia—especially during the first trimester—can be severe. Negative outcomes include preterm delivery, LBW infants, and increased risk for fetal death in the first weeks after birth.

Women often need a supplemental source of iron, especially if they do not consume iron-fortified foods, such as highly fortified breakfast cereals containing close to 100%

of the Daily Value for iron (18 milligrams). The American College of Obstetricians and Gynecologists recommends screening for iron deficiency for all pregnant women and provision of iron supplements for women who are deficient. In addition, most prenatal supplements contain iron. A potential pitfall is that iron supplements can decrease appetite and can cause nausea and constipation. To alleviate these problems, it may be helpful to take these supplements between meals or just before going to bed. Milk, coffee, or tea should not be consumed with an iron supplement because these beverages have compounds that interfere with iron absorption. Eating foods rich in vitamin C along with nonheme iron-containing foods and iron supplements helps increase iron absorption from those sources. Pregnant women who are not anemic may wait until the second trimester, when pregnancy-related nausea generally lessens, to start prenatal supplements if gastrointestinal side effects are a problem.

The RDA for zinc increases from 8 to 11 milligrams per day during pregnancy. Zinc is involved in many enzyme functions and protein synthesis. Zinc deficiency during pregnancy has been linked to preterm and LBW births. The zinc intakes of pregnant women in the United States are generally adequate, but low-income women and those who follow vegan or vegetarian diets are more susceptible to poor zinc status. Also, because iron and zinc compete for absorption, high levels of iron supplementation during pregnancy may impair zinc absorption. Incorporating lean animal proteins or a fortified ready-to-eat breakfast cereal in the diet is a good way to obtain enough extra zinc during pregnancy.

USE OF PRENATAL VITAMIN AND MINERAL SUPPLEMENTS

With the exceptions of folate, iron, and vitamin D, the vitamin and mineral intakes of pregnant women in developed countries are generally adequate.[20] Research evidence supports routine supplementation with folic acid and iron during pregnancy. Beyond these two nutrients, some studies indicate that use of a multivitamin and mineral supplement

Healthy People 2020 includes a goal of increasing by 10% the proportion of women of childbearing potential who consume at least 400 micrograms of folic acid per day. Currently, about 23% of women of childbearing age consume adequate folic acid from fortified foods or dietary supplements.

CASE STUDY Eating for Two

Lily and her husband have just found out that Lily is pregnant with their first child. She is 25 years old, weighs 135 pounds, and is 67 inches tall. Lily has been reading everything she can find on pregnancy because she knows that her health is important to the success of her pregnancy.

Lily knows she should avoid alcohol, especially because alcohol is potentially toxic to the growing fetus. Lily is not a smoker, does not take any medications, and limits her coffee intake to 4 cups a day and soft drink intake to 3 colas per day. Based on her reading, she has decided to breastfeed her infant and has already inquired about childbirth classes. She has modified her diet to include some extra protein, along with more fruits and vegetables. She has also started taking an over-the-counter vitamin and mineral supplement. Lily has always kept in good shape, and she is admittedly worried about gaining too much weight during pregnancy. Recently, she started a running program 5 days a week, and she plans to continue running throughout her pregnancy.

1. What recommendations do you have regarding Lily's use of dietary supplements?
2. What is Lily doing to prevent neural tube defects? What else could she do?
3. What recommendations would you make regarding Lily's caffeine consumption?
4. Should Lily include fish as a source of protein in her diet? Why or why not?
5. Constipation is a common complaint during pregnancy. What suggestions do you have to help Lily avoid this health concern?
6. What information would you share with Lily about appropriate weight gain during pregnancy?

Complete the Case Study. Responses to these questions can be provided by your instructor.

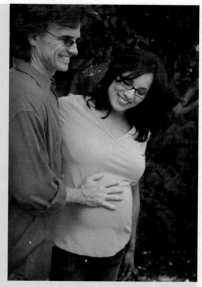

©Hill Street Studios/Blend Images LLC

is advantageous for reducing the number of LBW and SGA births. More research is needed to know if prenatal supplements are effective for reducing many other pregnancy complications.[21] To date, there is not enough evidence to recommend prenatal multivitamin and mineral supplements for all pregnant women, but they are prescribed routinely by most health care providers. Some supplements formulated for pregnancy are sold over the counter, while others are dispensed by prescription because of their high synthetic folic acid content (1000 micrograms), which could pose problems for others, such as older people. These supplements are high in iron (27 milligrams per pill). There is no evidence that use of such supplements causes significant health problems in pregnancy, with the possible exception of combined amounts of supplemental and dietary vitamin A (see Section 14.8).

Instances when prenatal supplements may especially contribute to a successful pregnancy are those involving women living in poverty, teenagers, women with an inadequate diet, women carrying multiple fetuses, women who smoke or use alcohol or illegal drugs, and vegans. In other cases, healthy diets can provide the needed nutrients. When choosing a multivitamin, rely on brands that display the USP symbol on their label, signifying that the supplement meets the content, quality, purity, and safety standards of the United States Pharmacopeial Convention (see Section 8.16). Of course, avoid megadoses of any nutrient. Skip supplements containing herbs, enzymes, and amino acids. Many of these ingredients have not been evaluated for safety during pregnancy or breastfeeding and may be toxic to the fetus. Furthermore, discard supplements that are past the expiration date, as some ingredients lose potency over time.

✔ CONCEPT CHECK 14.4

1. Patrice required 2200 kcal per day before she became pregnant. How many kilocalories will she need each day during her first, second, and third trimesters?

2. What is optimal weight gain during pregnancy for a woman who begins pregnancy at a healthy BMI? How does this differ for a woman who begins pregnancy underweight? Overweight? Obese?

3. List two nutrients that may need to be supplemented in the diet of a pregnant woman and the reason for each.

14.5 Eating Patterns for Pregnant Women

One dietary approach to support a successful pregnancy is based on MyPlate. For an active 24-year-old woman, about 2200 kcal is recommended during the first trimester (the same as recommended for such a woman when not pregnant). The plan should include 7 ounce equivalents from the grains group, 6 ounce equivalents from the protein foods group, 3 cups from the dairy group (or dairy alternatives), 3 cups of vegetables, and 2 cups of fruit. In addition, 6 teaspoons per day of vegetable oil, used in cooking or as salad dressing, will supply essential fatty acids. Figure 14-8 shows a balanced dietary pattern, based on MyPlate, for a pregnant woman in her first trimester. By selecting nutrient-dense foods from the food groups, the dietary pattern should be moderate in sodium (no more than 2300 milligrams per day), saturated fat (limit to 24 grams per day), and added sugars (limit to 55 grams per day).

In the second and third trimesters, about 2600 kcal is recommended for this woman. The plan should now include an additional 2 ounce equivalents from the grains group, an extra 1/2 ounce equivalent from the protein group, an additional 1/2 cup from the vegetables group, and 2 additional teaspoons of vegetable oil throughout the day. These additional servings are shown in lighter color in Figure 14-8.

Moms-to-be can personalize MyPlate for each trimester at www.choosemyplate.gov/moms-pregnancy-breastfeeding.

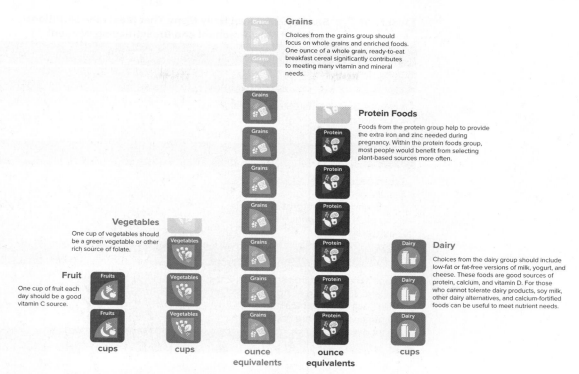

Grains
Choices from the grains group should focus on whole grains and enriched foods. One ounce of a whole grain, ready-to-eat breakfast cereal significantly contributes to meeting many vitamin and mineral needs.

Protein Foods
Foods from the protein group help to provide the extra iron and zinc needed during pregnancy. Within the protein foods group, most people would benefit from selecting plant-based sources more often.

Vegetables
One cup of vegetables should be a green vegetable or other rich source of folate.

Fruit
One cup of fruit each day should be a good vitamin C source.

Dairy
Choices from the dairy group should include low-fat or fat-free versions of milk, yogurt, and cheese. These foods are good sources of protein, calcium, and vitamin D. For those who cannot tolerate dairy products, soy milk, other dairy alternatives, and calcium-fortified foods can be useful to meet nutrient needs.

cups | cups | ounce equivalents | ounce equivalents | cups

FIGURE 14-8 ▲ Daily meal plan for a pregnant woman based on MyPlate. Servings per day for the first trimester (2200 kcal per day) are shown in dark colors. Additional servings per day for the second and third trimesters (2600 kcal per day) are shown in lighter colors.

Source: https://choosemyplate-prod.azureedge.net/sites/default/files/myplate/checklists/MyPlateDailyChecklist_2200cals_Age14plus.pdf

Table 14-3 illustrates one daily menu based on the 2600-kcal plan for pregnancy for women in the second or third trimesters. This menu meets the extra nutrient needs associated with pregnancy. Women who need to consume more than this—and some do for various reasons—should incorporate additional fruits, vegetables, and whole grain breads and cereals, not poor nutrient sources such as desserts and sugared soft drinks.

It is a common myth that women instinctively know what to eat during pregnancy. Cravings during the last two trimesters are often related to hormonal changes in the mother or family traditions. Some women crave nonfood items such as laundry starch, chalk, cigarette ashes, and soil (clay). This practice, known as **pica,** can be extremely harmful to the mother and the fetus. Following the nutrition advice of respected health professionals, such as registered dietitian nutritionists, is much more reliable than trusting cravings to meet nutrient needs.

PREGNANT VEGETARIANS

Women who are either **lactoovovegetarians** or **lactovegetarians** generally do not face special difficulties in meeting their nutritional needs during pregnancy. Like nonvegetarian women, they should be concerned primarily with meeting vitamin B-6, iron, folate, and zinc needs.

On the other hand, for a vegan, careful diet planning during preconception and pregnancy is crucial to ensure sufficient protein, vitamin D (particularly in the absence of sufficient sun exposure), vitamin B-6, iron, calcium, zinc, and especially a supplemental source of vitamin B-12. The basic vegan diet described in Section 6.8 should be modified to include more whole grains, beans, nuts, and seeds to supply the necessary extra amounts of some of these nutrients. As mentioned, use of a prenatal multivitamin and mineral supplement also is generally advocated to help fill micronutrient gaps.

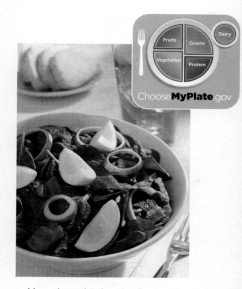

▲ How does this lunch of spinach and fruit salad and whole wheat toast compare to MyPlate? Is iced tea a good beverage choice? Why or why not? ©TheCrimsonMonkey/Getty Images

Source: www.choosemyplate.gov

pica The practice of eating nonfood items, such as dirt, laundry starch, or clay.

lactoovovegetarian A person who consumes plant products, dairy products, and eggs.

lactovegetarian A person who consumes plant products and dairy products.

TABLE 14-3 ■ Sample 2600-kcal Daily Menu That Meets the Nutritional Needs of Most Pregnant and Breastfeeding Women*

	Vitamin B-6	Folate	Iron	Zinc	Calcium
Breakfast					
1 cup Kellogg's® Smart Start® cereal	✓	✓	✓	✓	✓
1 cup orange juice		✓			
1 cup fat-free milk	✓				✓
Snack					
2 tbsp peanut butter	✓	✓	✓	✓	
2 stalks of celery		✓			
1 slice whole wheat toast		✓	✓	✓	
1 cup plain low-fat yogurt	✓				✓
½ cup strawberries		✓			
Lunch					
2 cups spinach and fruit salad with 2 tbsp oil and vinegar dressing		✓			✓
2 slices whole wheat toast		✓	✓	✓	
1 ½ ounces provolone cheese	✓				✓
Snack					
5 whole wheat crackers		✓	✓	✓	
1 cup grape juice					
Dinner					
2 bean burritos	✓	✓	✓	✓	✓
1 cup cooked broccoli		✓			✓
1 tsp soft margarine					
Unsweetened iced tea					
Snack					
Granola bar (2 ounces)	✓	✓	✓	✓	
½ banana					

*This diet meets nutrient needs for pregnancy and breastfeeding. Lack of a check (√) indicates a poor source of the nutrient. The vitamin- and mineral-fortified breakfast cereal used in this example makes an important contribution to meeting nutrient needs. Fluids can be added as desired. Total intake of fluids, such as water, should be 10 cups per day for pregnant women or about 13 cups per day for breastfeeding women.

However, although these are high in iron, this is not true for calcium (200 milligrams per pill). If iron and calcium supplements are used, they should not be taken together to avoid possible competition for absorption.

☑ CONCEPT CHECK 14.5

1. List three nutrients of special concern for a pregnant woman who practices a vegan lifestyle.
2. Modify the sample 2600-kcal daily menu in Table 14-3 so that it would be suitable for a pregnant vegan woman.
3. Michaela tells you about her pregnancy craving for ice cream. She says she has been eating one or two ice cream bars after lunch every day and usually stops for a milkshake at a fast-food restaurant on her way home from work. What nutrition information would you share with her?

14.6 Physiological Changes of Concern During Pregnancy

During pregnancy, fetal needs for oxygen and nutrients as well as excretion of waste products increase the burden on the mother's lungs, heart, and kidneys. Although a mother's organ systems work efficiently, some discomfort accompanies the changes her body undergoes to accommodate the fetus.

HEARTBURN, CONSTIPATION, AND HEMORRHOIDS

Hormones (such as progesterone) produced by the placenta relax smooth muscles in the uterus and the gastrointestinal tract. This often causes heartburn as stomach acid refluxes into the esophagus (review Section 3.12). When this occurs, the woman should avoid lying down after eating, eat less fat so that foods pass more quickly from the stomach into the small intestine, and avoid spicy foods, which can worsen symptoms. She should also consume most liquids between (rather than with) meals to limit the volume of stomach contents and thus relieve some of the pressure that encourages reflux. Women with more severe cases may temporarily need antacids or related medications.

The hormone-induced relaxation of muscles in the GI tract may also lead to constipation. This is especially likely to develop late in pregnancy, when the fetus competes with the GI tract for space in the abdominal cavity. To alleviate constipation, a woman should focus on consuming adequate fluid and fiber and should perform regular exercise. The AI for fiber in pregnancy is 28 grams, slightly more than for the nonpregnant woman. Fluid needs are 10 cups per day. The extra iron in prenatal supplements may also contribute to constipation. If this is the case, a clinician can reevaluate the woman's needs for supplemental iron. Alleviating constipation can also help to prevent hemorrhoids, which affect about one-third of pregnant women.

EDEMA

Placental hormones cause various body tissues to retain fluid during pregnancy. Blood volume also greatly expands during pregnancy. The extra fluid normally causes some swelling (edema). There is no reason to restrict salt severely or use diuretics to limit mild edema. However, the edema may limit physical activity late in pregnancy and occasionally requires a woman to elevate her feet or wear compression stockings to control the symptoms. Overall, edema is only a mild nuisance unless it is accompanied by hypertension and the appearance of extra protein in the urine (see Hypertensive Disorders of Pregnancy later in this section).

NAUSEA AND VOMITING OF PREGNANCY

About 70% to 85% of pregnant women experience nausea during the early stages of pregnancy. Nausea and vomiting of pregnancy are probably related to changes in GI motility induced by pregnancy-related hormones. Although commonly called "morning sickness," pregnancy-related nausea may occur at any time and persist all day. It is often the first signal to a woman that she is pregnant.

To help control mild nausea, pregnant women can try the following: avoiding nauseating foods, such as fried or greasy foods; cooking with good ventilation to dissipate nauseating smells; eating saltine crackers or dry cereal before getting out of bed; avoiding large fluid intakes early in the morning; and eating smaller, more frequent meals. The iron in prenatal supplements triggers nausea in some women, so changing the type of supplement used or postponing use until the second trimester may provide relief in some cases. If a woman thinks her morning sickness is related to her prenatal supplement, she should talk with her primary care provider about switching to another supplement.

CRITICAL THINKING

Sandy, 5 months pregnant, has been having heartburn and difficult bowel movements. As a student of nutrition, you understand the digestive system and the role of nutrition in health. What diet and lifestyle strategies might you suggest to Sandy to relieve her problems?

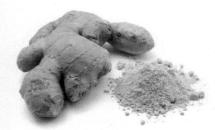

▲ Foods or dietary supplements made with ginger may alleviate nausea and vomiting of pregnancy for some women. ©Toltek/iStock/Getty Images

There is evidence that the following practices may also be useful for the prevention and treatment of nausea and vomiting of pregnancy; however, a pregnant woman should consult her primary care provider before trying any of these remedies:

- History of use of a balanced multivitamin and mineral supplement at the time of conception
- Use of megadoses of vitamin B-6 (10 to 25 milligrams taken three to four times a day), especially coupled with the antihistamine doxylamine (10 milligrams) with each dose
- Ginger may also be helpful (350 milligrams taken three times per day)

Usually, nausea is mild and stops after the first trimester. However, in up to 3% of pregnancies, nausea and vomiting are prolonged and severe enough to cause weight loss, dehydration, and dangerous electrolyte imbalances. In these cases, the preceding practices offer little relief; medical attention is needed to protect the health of the mother and her growing baby.

ANEMIA

physiological anemia The normal decrease in red blood cell levels in the blood due to increased blood volume during pregnancy; also called *hemodilution*.

To supply fetal needs, the mother's blood volume expands to approximately 150% of normal. The number of red blood cells, however, increases by only 20% to 30%, and this occurs more gradually. As a result, a pregnant woman has a lower ratio of red blood cells to total blood volume in her system. This hemodilution is known as **physiological anemia.** It is a normal response to pregnancy, rather than the result of inadequate nutrient intake.

However, if iron stores and/or dietary iron intake are not sufficient to meet her increased needs, the pregnant woman may develop iron-deficiency anemia. The *Dietary Guidelines for Americans* identify iron as a nutrient of public health concern because several population groups, including pregnant women, are likely to have low intakes of this nutrient. Iron-deficiency anemia requires medical attention at any stage of the life cycle, but consequences for the fetus are especially severe (see Section 14.4). Lean meats, beans, and fortified grains are nutrient-dense sources of iron that should be emphasized to prevent anemia during pregnancy (review Section 9.9). Importantly, once anemia has developed, dietary supplements will be needed to replete iron status; dietary changes alone are not sufficient to correct iron deficiency.

GESTATIONAL DIABETES

gestational diabetes A high blood glucose concentration that develops during pregnancy and returns to normal after birth; one cause is the placental production of hormones that antagonize the regulation of blood glucose by insulin.

Hormones synthesized by the placenta decrease the efficiency of insulin. This leads to a mild increase in blood glucose, which helps supply calories to the fetus. If the rise in blood glucose becomes excessive, this leads to **gestational diabetes,** often beginning between weeks 20 and 28, particularly in women who have a family history of diabetes or who are obese. Other risk factors include maternal age over 35 and gestational diabetes in a prior pregnancy.

In North America, gestational diabetes develops in as many as 10% of pregnancies (estimates vary based on the diagnostic criteria used). Today, pregnant women with risk factors for type 2 diabetes (e.g., obesity, family history) should be screened for undiagnosed type 2 diabetes at the first prenatal visit. Pregnant women without type 2 diabetes should be screened for gestational diabetes between 24 and 28 weeks using an oral glucose tolerance test (i.e., checking for elevated blood glucose concentration 1 to 2 hours after consuming a dose of glucose.[22] If gestational diabetes is detected, a special diet that distributes carbohydrates throughout the day needs to be implemented. Carbohydrate choices should be mostly whole, unprocessed grains, vegetables, fruits, and beans, which have a lower impact on blood glucose than refined grains or foods with lots of added sugars. Sometimes insulin injections or oral medications are also needed. Regular physical activity also helps to control blood glucose.[23]

The primary risk of uncontrolled diabetes during pregnancy is that the fetus can grow quite large. This is a result of the oversupply of glucose from maternal circulation coupled with an increased production of insulin by the fetus, which allows fetal tissues to take up an increased amount of building materials for growth. The mother may require a Cesarean section if the fetus is too large for a vaginal delivery. Another threat is that the infant may have low blood glucose at birth because of the tendency to produce extra insulin that began during gestation. Other concerns are the potential for early delivery, low iron stores, and increased risk of birth trauma and malformations.

Although gestational diabetes often disappears after the infant's birth, it increases the mother's risk of developing diabetes later in life, especially if she fails to maintain a healthy body weight. Uncontrolled blood sugar during gestation may have some long-term repercussions for the child, as well. Studies show that infants of mothers with gestational diabetes may also have higher risks of developing obesity, metabolic syndrome, and type 2 diabetes as they grow to adulthood. For all these reasons, proper control of blood glucose during pregancy is extremely important. Researchers are working to understand how breastfeeding may be helpful for women who had gestational diabetes. Some studies indicate that breastfeeding may lower the risk of developing type 2 diabetes later in life.[24]

HYPERTENSIVE DISORDERS OF PREGNANCY

Hypertension (blood pressure of 140/90 mmHg or higher) occurs in about 6% to 8% of pregnancies in the United States. Sometimes, women enter pregnancy with chronic hypertension. However, when hypertension first appears after 20 weeks of gestation, it is termed **gestational hypertension** (formerly called *pregnancy-induced hypertension*).

About half of women with gestational hypertension eventually develop **preeclampsia** (mild form) or **eclampsia** (severe form). Early symptoms include a rise in blood pressure, excess protein in the urine, edema, changes in blood clotting, headache, and visual disturbances. Very severe effects, including convulsions, can occur in the second and third trimesters. If not controlled, eclampsia eventually damages the liver and kidneys, and the mother and fetus may die.

The causes for hypertensive disorders of pregnancy are not well understood but likely involve interactions among genetics, certain environmental or lifestyle influences, and abnormal function of the placenta. The populations most at risk for these disorders are women under age 17 or over age 35, overweight or obese women, and those who have had multiple-birth pregnancies. A family history of gestational hypertension in the mother's or father's side of the family, diabetes, African-American race, and a woman's first pregnancy also raise risk.

Gestational hypertension resolves once the pregnancy ends, making delivery the most reliable treatment for the mother. However, if eclampsia develops before the fetus is ready to be born, medical intervention is necessary. Bed rest and administration of magnesium sulfate are the most effective treatment methods. Magnesium likely acts to relax blood vessels and so leads to a reduction in blood pressure. There is good evidence that adequate intakes of calcium and vitamin D are involved in reducing incidence of gestational hypertension. There is interest in the use of antioxidants to prevent or treat gestational hypertension, but current evidence does not support the use of antioxidant supplements for preventing these disorders. Several other treatments, such as various antiseizure and antihypertensive medications, fish oils, and selenium, are under study.[25]

✓ CONCEPT CHECK 14.6

1. What diet and lifestyle strategies would you suggest to a pregnant woman who complains of morning sickness?

2. Define *gestational diabetes*. What are the potential consequences of this disorder for the mother and baby?

3. Differentiate between chronic hypertension and gestational hypertension. Which two micronutrients may help to reduce risk for preeclampsia?

gestational hypertension Blood pressure of 140/90 mmHg or higher that is first diagnosed after 20 weeks of gestation. This may evolve into preeclampsia or eclampsia.

preeclampsia A form of gestational hypertension characterized by protein in the urine.

eclampsia A severe form of gestational hypertension characterized by protein in the urine and seizures (formerly called *toxemia*).

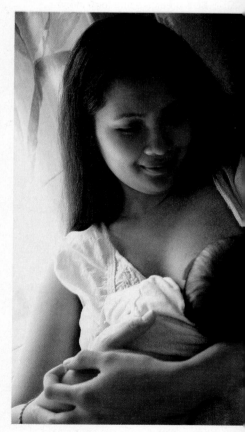

▲ Breastfeeding is the preferred way to feed a young infant. ©Diane Mcdonald/Getty Images

14.7 Breastfeeding

Breastfeeding the new infant complements the attention given to diet during pregnancy. The Academy of Nutrition and Dietetics (AND) and the American Academy of Pediatrics (AAP) recommend breastfeeding exclusively for the first 6 months, with the continued combination of breastfeeding and infant foods until 1 year.[26,27] The World Health Organization goes beyond that to recommend breastfeeding (with appropriate solid food introduction; see Section 15.3) for at least 2 years. Still, surveys show that only about 70% of North American mothers breastfeed their infants in the hospital, and at 4 and 6 months, only 33% and 20%, respectively, are still breastfeeding their infants. The number falls to 18% at 1 year of age. These statistics refer to Caucasian women; minority women are even less likely to be breastfeeding at these time intervals.

Women who choose to breastfeed usually find it an enjoyable, special time in their lives that strengthens the bond with their new infant. Although bottle feeding with an infant formula is also safe for infants, as discussed in Section 15.2, it cannot replicate all of the benefits derived from breastfeeding. If a woman does not breastfeed her child, milk production ceases within a few days after birth.

PLANNING TO BREASTFEED

Almost all women are physically capable of breastfeeding their children (see the later section "Medical Conditions Precluding Breastfeeding" for exceptions). In most cases, problems encountered in breastfeeding are due to a lack of knowledge or support. Anatomical problems in breasts, such as inverted nipples, can be corrected during pregnancy. Breast size generally increases during pregnancy and is no indication of success in breastfeeding. Most women notice a dramatic increase in the size and weight of their breasts by the third or fourth day of breastfeeding. If these changes do not occur, a woman needs to seek advice from her clinician or a lactation consultant.

Breastfed infants must be followed closely by caregivers over the first few days of life to ensure that feeding and weight gain are proceeding normally. Monitoring is especially important with a mother's first child because the mother will be inexperienced with the technique of breastfeeding. The infant is at risk of dehydration and blood clots if feeding does not proceed smoothly.

Although it is the most natural way to feed a newborn child, the *technique* does not always come naturally. Gathering information on breastfeeding, what obstacles to anticipate, and how to respond to such obstacles will help new mothers and their babies to succeed with breastfeeding. It also helps to have an experienced friend, family member, or a professional lactation consultant to call for advice when questions arise.

HUMAN MILK PRODUCTION

During pregnancy, breast weight increases by 1 to 2 pounds due to the action of placental hormones that stimulate the formation of milk-producing cells. Milk will be produced in the **lobules** (Fig. 14-9). A cluster of lobules forms a lobe. Ducts lead from each lobe to the nipple, where milk is ejected from the breast.

Most of the protein found in human milk is synthesized by breast tissue. Some proteins also enter the milk directly from the mother's bloodstream. These proteins include immune factors (e.g., antibodies) and enzymes. Some of the fats in human milk come from the mother's diet; other fats are synthesized by breast tissue. The sugar galactose is synthesized in the breast, whereas glucose enters from the mother's bloodstream. Together, these sugars form lactose, the main carbohydrate in human milk.

Lactation is regulated by two hormones: prolactin and oxytocin. **Prolactin** is the hormone that stimulates milk production in the lobules of the breast. As milk is produced between feedings, it is stored in the lobules. An important brain-breast connection—commonly called the **let-down reflex**—is necessary to release the milk stored in the lobules. This reflex occurs in response to the infant suckling at the breast. Stimulation of

Healthy People 2020 goals for breastfeeding:
- 82% of women breastfeeding their infants at time of hospital discharge
- 60% breastfeeding for 6 months
- 34% still breastfeeding at 1 year

lobules Saclike structures in the breast that store milk; also called *alveoli*.

prolactin A hormone secreted by the pituitary gland that stimulates the synthesis of milk in the breast.

let-down reflex A reflex stimulated by infant suckling that causes the release (ejection) of milk from milk ducts in the mother's breasts; also called *milk ejection reflex*.

oxytocin A hormone secreted by the pituitary gland. It causes contraction of the musclelike cells surrounding the ducts of the breasts and the smooth muscle of the uterus.

the nerves in the nipple area signals the pituitary gland to release **oxytocin,** which allows the lobules to contract and let down (release) stored milk (Fig. 14-10). The milk then travels via ducts to the nipple. The mother may feel a tingling sensation shortly before milk flow begins. Throughout the feeding, the suckling of the infant further stimulates prolactin release from the pituitary gland, so milk synthesis within the lobules continues. The more the infant suckles, the more milk is produced. Because of this, even twins (and triplets) can be breastfed adequately.

If the let-down reflex does not operate, little milk is available to the infant. The infant gets frustrated, which then frustrates the mother. The let-down reflex is easily inhibited by nervous tension, a lack of confidence, and fatigue. Mothers should be especially aware of the link between tension and a weak let-down reflex. They need to find a relaxed environment where they can breastfeed.

After a few weeks, the mother's let-down reflex becomes automatic. Milk ejection can be triggered just by thinking about her infant or seeing or hearing another one cry. At first, however, the process can be a bit bewildering. A mother cannot measure the amount of milk the infant takes in, so she may fear that she is not adequately nourishing the infant.

As a general rule, a well-nourished breastfed infant should (1) have 3 to 5 wet diapers per day by 3 to 5 days of age and four to six wet diapers per day thereafter; (2) show a normal pattern of weight gain; and (3) pass at least one or two stools per day that look like lumpy mustard. In addition, softening of the breast during the feeding indicates that enough milk is being consumed. Parents who sense their infant is not consuming enough milk should consult their primary care provider immediately because dehydration can develop rapidly. Losing more than 7% of birth weight indicates a feeding problem that requires intervention.

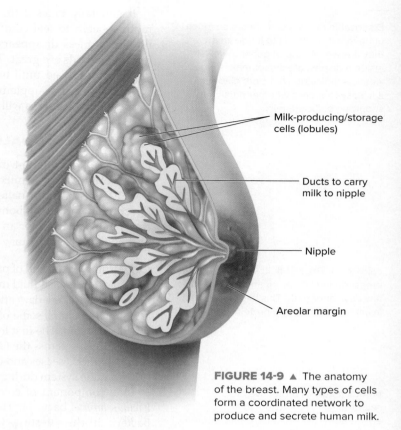

FIGURE 14-9 ▲ The anatomy of the breast. Many types of cells form a coordinated network to produce and secrete human milk.

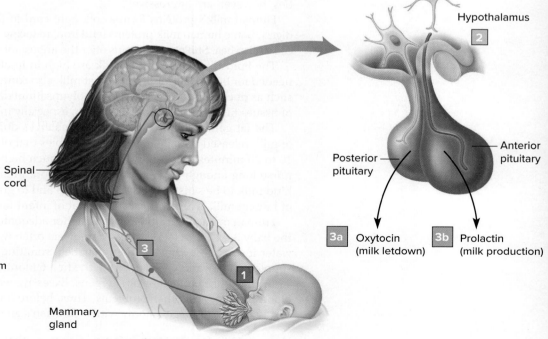

1. Suckling stimulates nerves in the nipple and areola that transmit impulses to the hypothalamus.

2. In response, the hypothalamus stimulates the posterior pituitary to release oxytocin and the anterior pituitary to release prolactin.

3. Oxytocin stimulates lobules in the breast to let down (release) milk from storage. Prolactin stimulates additional milk production.

FIGURE 14-10 ▲ Let-down reflex. Suckling sets into motion the sequence of events that lead to milk letdown, the flow of milk into ducts of the breast.

Disposable diapers can absorb so much urine that it is difficult to judge when they are wet. A strip of paper towel laid inside a disposable diaper makes a good wetness indicator. With cloth diapers, it is easy to assess whether nursing is supplying sufficient milk.

colostrum The first fluid secreted by the breast during late pregnancy and the first few days after birth. This thick fluid is rich in immune factors and protein.

bifidus factor A protective factor secreted in the colostrum that encourages growth of beneficial bacteria in the newborn's intestines.

It generally takes 2 to 3 weeks to fully establish the feeding routine: Infant and mother begin to feel comfortable, the milk supply meets infant demand, and initial nipple soreness disappears. Establishing the breastfeeding routine requires patience, but the rewards are great. The adjustments are easier if supplemental formula feedings are not introduced until breastfeeding is well established, after at least 3 to 4 weeks. Then it is fine if a supplemental bottle or two of infant formula per day is needed, but supplemental feedings will decrease milk production.

NUTRITIONAL QUALITIES OF HUMAN MILK

Human milk is different in composition from cow's milk. Unless altered (i.e., to make infant formula), cow's milk should never be used in infant feeding until the infant is at least 12 months old. Unaltered cow's milk is too high in minerals and protein and does not contain enough carbohydrate to meet infant needs. In addition, the major protein in cow's milk is harder for an infant to digest than the major proteins in human milk. The proteins in cow's milk may also spur allergies in some infants.

Colostrum. At the end of pregnancy, the first fluid made by the human breast is **colostrum.** This thick, yellowish fluid may leak from the breast during late pregnancy and is produced in earnest for a few days after birth. Colostrum contains antibodies, immune system cells, and growth factors, some of which pass intact through the infant's immature GI tract into the bloodstream. The first few months of life are the only time when we can readily absorb whole proteins across the GI tract. These immune factors and cells protect the infant from some GI tract diseases and other infectious disorders, compensating for the infant's immature immune system during the first few months of life.

One component of colostrum, the **bifidus factor,** encourages the growth of *Lactobacillus bifidus* bacteria. These beneficial bacteria limit the growth of potentially toxic bacteria in the intestine. Overall, breastfeeding promotes the intestinal health of the breastfed infant in this way.

Mature Milk. Human milk composition gradually changes until it achieves the normal composition of mature milk several days after delivery. Human milk looks very different from cow's milk. (Table 15-3 provides a direct comparison.) Human milk is thin and almost watery in appearance and often has a slightly bluish tinge. Its nutritional qualities, however, are impressive!

Human milk's proteins form a soft, light curd in the infant's stomach and are easy to digest. Some human milk proteins bind iron, reducing the growth of some bacteria that can cause diarrhea. Still other proteins offer the important immune protection already noted.

The lipids in human breast milk are high in linoleic acid and cholesterol, which are needed for brain development. Breast milk also contains long-chain omega-3 fatty acids, such as docosahexaenoic acid. This polyunsaturated fatty acid is used for the synthesis of tissues in the central nervous system, especially in the brain and the retina of the eye.

The fat composition of human milk changes during each feeding. The consistency of milk released initially (*fore milk*) resembles that of skim milk. The milk released after 10 to 20 minutes of feeding (*hind milk*) is much higher in fat-like cream. Babies need to nurse long enough (e.g., a total of 20 or more minutes) to get the calories in the rich hind milk to be satisfied between feedings and to grow well. The overall calorie content of human milk is about the same as that of infant formulas (67 kcal per 100 milliliters).

Human milk composition also allows for adequate fluid status of the infant, provided the baby is exclusively breastfed. Caregivers often wonder if the infant needs additional water if stressed by hot weather, diarrhea, vomiting, or fever. The AAP advises against supplemental water or juice during the first 6 months of life. The practice may unnecessarily introduce pathogens or allergens. Excessive water can lead to brain disorders, low blood sodium, and other problems. Thus, before 6 months of age, supplemental water and juice should be given only with a clinician's guidance.

Human Milk for Preterm Infants. Can a mother breastfeed her preterm infant? In some cases, human milk is the most desirable form of nourishment, depending on infant weight and length of gestation. Feeding of human milk to preterm infants has been linked to lower infant mortality, decreased risk of infections, reduced stays in the neonatal intensive care unit, fewer hospital readmissions, better growth, and improved brain development.[27]

Breastfeeding a preterm infant, however, demands great maternal dedication. Preterm infants sometimes have a weak or uncoordinated suck and swallow reflex, so it may be necessary to express milk from the breast and feed the infant through a tube until the infant's feeding ability develops. Fortification of the milk with calcium, phosphorus, sodium, and protein is often necessary to meet the needs of a rapidly growing preterm infant. In some cases, special feeding problems may prevent the use of human milk or necessitate supplementing it with specialized formula. Sometimes total parenteral nutrition (intravenous feeding) is the only option. Working as a team, the pediatrician, neonatal nurses, and registered dietitian nutritionist must guide the parents in this decision.

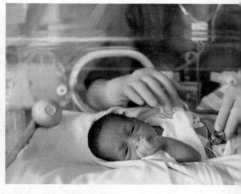

▲ If human milk is used to feed the preterm infant, fortification of the milk with certain nutrients is often needed. ©ERproductions Ltd/Blend Images LLC

EATING PATTERN FOR WOMEN WHO BREASTFEED

Nutrient needs for a breastfeeding mother change to some extent from those of the pregnant woman in the second and third trimester (see the DRI summary tables in Appendix G). Needs for folate and iron decrease while needs for calories, vitamins A, E, and C, riboflavin, copper, chromium, iodide, manganese, selenium, and zinc increase. Still, these increased needs of the breastfeeding mother will be met by the general diet plan proposed for a woman in the latter stages of pregnancy:

- 3 cups of calcium-rich foods such as from the dairy group or use of calcium-fortified foods to make up for any gap between calcium intake and need
- 6 ½ ounce equivalents from the protein group
- 3 ½ cups from the vegetables group
- 2 cups from the fruits group
- 9 ounce equivalents from the grains group
- 8 teaspoons of vegetable oil

Table 14-3 provided a menu for such a plan. As in pregnancy, a serving of a highly fortified ready-to-eat breakfast cereal (or use of a balanced multivitamin and mineral supplement) is helpful to meet extra nutrient needs. And, as mentioned for pregnant women, breastfeeding mothers should consume 8 to 12 ounces of low-mercury fish per week (or 1 gram per day of omega-3 fatty acids from a fish oil supplement) because the omega-3 fatty acids present in fish are secreted into breast milk and are likely to be important for development of the infant's nervous system.[15]

Milk production requires approximately 800 kcal every day. The estimated energy requirement during lactation includes an extra 400 to 500 kcal daily above prepregnancy recommendations. The difference between that needed for milk production and the recommended intake—about 300 kcal—should allow for a gradual loss of the extra body fat accumulated during pregnancy, especially if breastfeeding is continued for 6 months or more and the woman performs some physical activity. This shows just one of the natural benefits of following pregnancy with at least several months of breastfeeding.

After giving birth, women are often eager to shed the excess "baby fat." Breastfeeding, however, is no time for crash diets. A gradual weight loss of 1 to 4 pounds per month by the nursing mother is appropriate. At significantly greater rates of weight loss—when calories are restricted to less than about 1500 kcal per day—milk output decreases. A reasonable approach for a breastfeeding mother is to eat a balanced diet that supplies at least 1800 kcal per day; has moderate fat content; and includes a variety of dairy products, fruits, vegetables, and whole grains.

To promote the best possible feeding experience for the infant, there are several other dietary factors to consider. Hydration is especially important during breastfeeding; the woman should drink fluids every time her infant nurses. Drinking about 13 cups of fluids per day encourages ample milk production. Poor health habits, such as smoking cigarettes or drinking more than two alcoholic beverages a day, can decrease milk output. (Even less alcohol can have a deleterious effect on milk output in some women.) To avoid

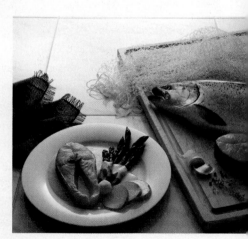

▲ Eating 8 to 12 ounces (2 to 3 servings) of fish per week will help breastfeeding women ensure that their infants receive ample omega-3 fatty acids. It is important, however, to avoid those fish likely to be contaminated with mercury (swordfish, shark, king mackerel, and tile fish). For more information about mercury in seafood, see Further Reading 15. ©Royalty-Free/Corbis

exposure to harmful levels of mercury, precautions concerning fish likely to contain mercury should extend past pregnancy for the breastfeeding mother. There is no evidence that maternal diet restrictions (e.g., peanuts, eggs, and fish) during pregnancy or breastfeeding prevent food allergies in infants. The American Academy of Allergy, Asthma, and Immunology recommends exclusive breastfeeding with the introduction of age-appropriate solid foods between 4 and 6 months of age for preventing **atopic diseases.**[29]

BREASTFEEDING TODAY

The vast majority of women are capable of breastfeeding and their infants would benefit from it (see Table 14-4).[27] Nonetheless, some circumstances may make breastfeeding impractical or undesirable for a woman. Mothers who do not want to breastfeed their infants should not feel pressured to do so. Breastfeeding provides advantages, but none so great that a woman who decides to bottle feed should feel she is compromising her infant's well-being.

Advantages of Breastfeeding. Human milk is tailored to meet infant nutrient needs for the first 4 to 6 months of life. In some cases, however, infant dietary supplements, used under a pediatrician's guidance, are recommended.

- The AAP recommends *all* infants, including exclusively breastfed infants, be given 400 IU of vitamin D per day, beginning shortly after birth and continuing until the infant consumes that much from food (e.g., at least 2 cups [0.5 liter] of infant formula per day). Some sun exposure also helps in meeting vitamin D needs.
- Full-term infants are usually born with adequate iron stores to last for the first 4 to 6 months of life. However, to prevent anemia, the AAP recommends iron supplements for exclusively breastfed infants starting at 4 months of age. More aggressive iron supplementation may be needed for infants born preterm, LBW, or to mothers with iron deficiency.[30]
- The AAP does not advise fluoride supplements before 6 months of age. After 6 months, the pediatrician or dentist may recommend supplemental fluoride if the

atopic disease A condition involving an inappropriate immune response to environmental allergens; examples include asthma, eczema, and seasonal allergies.

In the United States, although 70% of women initiate breastfeeding after birth, only about 20% of mothers are still breastfeeding their infants at 6 months of age. What if more women chose to breastfeed their infants? A recent analysis estimated the potential public health impact of near universal breastfeeding. By reducing the risk of problems such as gastrointestinal and respiratory infections, researchers projected that 823,000 infants deaths and 20,000 cases of breast cancer could be prevented per year.[28]

TABLE 14-4 ■ Advantages of Breastfeeding

For Infant
• Bacteriologically safe
• Always fresh and ready to go
• Provides antibodies and substances that contribute to maturation of the immune system
• Contributes to maturation of gastrointestinal tract via bifidus factor
• Decreases risk of infections, such as diarrhea, respiratory disease, and ear infections
• Reduces risk of food allergies and intolerances, as well as some other allergies
• Reduces risk of celiac disease and inflammatory bowel diseases
• Establishes habit of eating in moderation, linked to 15% to 30% lower risk of obesity and 40% lower risk of type 2 diabetes later in life
• Contributes to proper development of jaws and teeth for better speech development
• May enhance nervous system development and eventual learning ability
• Decreases risk of childhood leukemia and lymphoma

For Mother
• Contributes to earlier recovery from pregnancy due to the action of hormones that promote a quicker return of the uterus to its prepregnancy state
• Decreases risk of several chronic diseases later in life, including hypertension, cardiovascular disease, and diabetes
• Decreases the risk of ovarian and premenopausal breast cancer
• Potential for quicker return to prepregnancy weight
• Potential for delayed ovulation, thus reducing chances of pregnancy in the short term

infant's exposure to fluoride from drinking water, foods, and oral hygiene products is insufficient.

- Vitamin B-12 supplements are recommended for the breastfed infant whose mother is a complete vegetarian (vegan).

Fewer Infections. Due in part to the antibodies in human milk, breastfeeding reduces the infant's overall risk of developing infections. Breastfed infants also have fewer ear infections (otitis media) because they do not sleep with a bottle in their mouth. Experts strongly discourage allowing an infant to sleep with a bottle in the mouth; milk can pool in the mouth, throat, and inner ear, creating a growth medium for bacteria, which can lead to ear infections and dental caries. By reducing these common ailments, parents can decrease discomfort for the infant, avoid related trips to the doctor, and prevent possible hearing loss.

Lower Risk of Diseases. Research now links breastfeeding with reduced risks for many diseases. Breastfed infants may learn to self-regulate food intake and avoid overeating, which may explain the connection to lowered risk for obesity and type 2 diabetes among adults who were breastfed as infants. The immunologic benefits of breastfeeding seem to be involved in lowered rates of type 1 diabetes, celiac disease, and inflammatory bowel diseases. Reductions in risks of childhood leukemia and lymphoma have also been observed.

Fewer Allergies and Intolerances. Breastfeeding also reduces the chances of some allergies, especially in allergy-prone infants (see Section 15.7). The key time to attain this benefit from breastfeeding is during the first 4 to 6 months of an infant's life. A longer commitment is best, but breastfeeding for even a few weeks is beneficial. Infants are also better able to tolerate human milk than formulas. Formulas sometimes must be switched several times until caregivers find the best one for the infant.

Convenience and Cost. Breastfeeding frees the mother from the time and expense involved in buying and preparing formula and washing bottles. Human milk is ready to go and sterile. This allows the mother to spend more time with her baby.

Possible Barriers to Breastfeeding. Widespread misinformation, the mother's need to return to a job, and social reticence serve as barriers to breastfeeding.

Misinformation. The major barriers to breastfeeding stem from misinformation, such as the idea that one's breasts are too small, and the lack of role models. One positive note has been the widespread increase in the availability of lactation consultants over the past several years. First-time mothers who are interested in breastfeeding can find invaluable support from lactation consultants or by talking to women who have experienced it successfully. In almost every community, a group called La Leche League offers classes in breastfeeding and advises women who have problems with it (800-LALECHE or www.lalecheleague.org).

Return to an Outside Job. Working outside the home can complicate plans to breastfeed. One possibility after a month or two of breastfeeding is for the mother to express and save her own milk. She can use a breast pump or manually express milk into a sterile plastic bottle or nursing bag (used in a disposable bottle system). Federal legislation passed in 2010 requires employers to provide reasonable breaks and a private space (other than a bathroom) for breastfeeding mothers to pump milk.

Storing expressed human milk requires careful sanitation and rapid chilling. It can be stored in the refrigerator for 3 to 5 days or be frozen for 3 to 6 months. Thawed milk should be used within 24 hours.

There is a knack to learning how to express milk, but the freedom can be worth it, because it allows others to feed the infant the mother's milk. A schedule of expressing milk and using supplemental formula feedings is most successful if begun after 1 to 2 months of exclusive breastfeeding. After 1 month or so, the baby is well adapted to breastfeeding and probably feels enough emotional security and other benefits from nursing to feed both ways.

Some women can juggle both a job and breastfeeding, but others find it too cumbersome and decide to formula-feed. A compromise—balancing some breastfeedings,

Some researchers propose that the passage of flavors from the mother's diet into her milk affords an opportunity for the infant to learn about the flavor of the foods of its family long before solids are introduced. These researchers suspect that bottle-fed infants are missing significant sensory experiences that, until recent times in human history, were common to all infants.

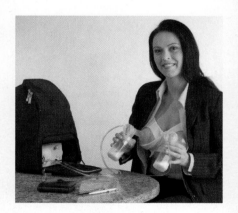

▲ Breast milk can be expressed by the mother using a manual, battery-operated, or electric (shown) breast pump. In 2010, President Barack Obama signed an amendment to the Fair Labor Standards Act that requires most U.S. employers to allow break time and a private setting for breastfeeding mothers to express milk. ©2008 Medela AG

perhaps early morning and night, with infant formula feedings during the day—is possible. However, too many supplemental infant formula feedings decrease milk production.

Social Concerns. Another barrier for some women is embarrassment about nursing a child in public. Historically, our society has stressed modesty and has discouraged public displays of breasts—even for as good a cause as nourishing babies. In the United States, no state or territory has a law prohibiting breastfeeding. However, indecent exposure (including the exposure of women's breasts) has long been a common law or statutory offense. Now, 49 states, the District of Columbia, and the Virgin Islands have specific laws that protect a woman's right to breastfeed in any location. Women who feel reluctant should be reassured that they do have social support and that breastfeeding can be done discreetly.

Medical Conditions Precluding Breastfeeding. Breastfeeding may be ruled out by certain medical conditions in either the infant or the mother. For example, breastfeeding is contraindicated for infants with galactosemia, an inherited disorder in which the body cannot break down galactose. Recall from Section 4.2 that lactose, the main carbohydrate in human breast milk, is made of glucose and galactose. When galactose is not properly broken down, its by-products can damage body organs.

Certain medications, which pass into the milk and adversely affect the nursing infant, are best avoided while breastfeeding. In addition, a woman in North America or other developed region of the world who has a serious chronic disease (such as tuberculosis, AIDS, or HIV-positive status) or who is being treated with chemotherapy medications should not breastfeed.

Cosmetic Alterations to the Breast. Nipple piercings should have no impact on a woman's ability to breastfeed, but the jewelry should be removed before each feeding. Repeated removal and reinsertion of the jewelry may be inconvenient and irritating, so it may be best to leave the jewelry out for the entire period of breastfeeding. Breast tattoos will not impair breastfeeding, either. However, getting a new nipple piercing or breast tattoo while breastfeeding is not advised due to the pain of healing and possibility of infection. Past breast augmentation or reduction surgeries may impair a woman's ability to breastfeed if milk-producing tissue was damaged during the surgery.

Environmental Contaminants in Human Milk. There is some legitimate concern over the levels of various environmental contaminants in human milk. However, the benefits of human milk are well established, and the risks from environmental contaminants are still largely theoretical. A few measures a woman could take to counteract some known contaminants are to (1) consume a variety of foods within each food group; (2) avoid freshwater fish from polluted waters; (3) carefully wash and peel fruits and vegetables (or choose organically raised produce, which has lower levels of pesticides than conventional produce); and (4) remove the fatty edges of meat, as pesticides concentrate in fat. In addition, a woman should not try to lose weight rapidly while nursing (more than 0.75 to 1 pound per week) because contaminants stored in her fat tissue might then enter her bloodstream and affect her milk. If a woman questions whether her milk is safe, especially if she has lived in an area known to have a high concentration of toxic wastes or environmental pollutants, she should consult her local health department.

> Phenylketonuria (PKU), a disorder of phenylalanine metabolism described in Section 6.1, was once thought to be a contraindication for breastfeeding. However, infants with PKU can enjoy the benefits of part-time breastfeeding in combination with specialized phenylalanine-free infant formulas.

✓ **CONCEPT CHECK 14.7**

1. What do AND and AAP recommend for duration of breastfeeding?
2. Describe the physiological processes of milk production and let down. Be sure to mention the hormones involved in these processes.
3. List three advantages of breastfeeding for the mother and three advantages for the infant.
4. Identify three micronutrients that may need to be supplemented in the diets of breastfed infants, and give the rationale for each.
5. Describe three potential barriers to breastfeeding, and suggest ways to overcome them.

Reducing the Risk of Birth Defects

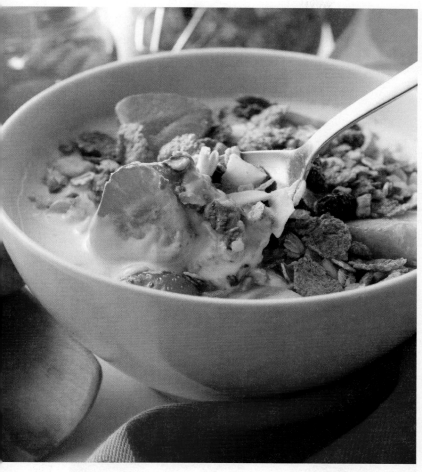

©Floortje/Getty Images

Eating well for a healthy pregnancy not only supplies materials for fetal growth and development, but also helps to direct the amazing process of building a new life. Considering the complexity of the human body and its more than 20,000 genes, it is not surprising that abnormalities of structure, function, or metabolism are sometimes present at birth. Birth defects impact 1 in every 33 babies born in the United States. In some cases, they are so severe that a baby cannot survive or thrive. Defects in embryonic or fetal development are the presumed cause of many spontaneous abortions and are at the root of about 20% of infant deaths before 1 year of age. However, many babies with birth defects can go on to live healthy and productive lives.

A wide range of physical or mental disabilities result from birth defects. Heart defects are present in approximately 1 in every 100 to 200 newborn babies, accounting for a large proportion of infant deaths. Cleft lip and/or cleft palate are malformations of the lip or roof of the mouth and occur in approximately 1 in 700 to 1000 births. Neural tube defects are malformations of the brain or spinal cord that occur during embryonic development. Examples include spina bifida, in which all or part of the spinal cord is exposed, and anencephaly, in which some or all of the brain is missing (Fig. 14-11).

Babies born with spina bifida can survive to adulthood but in many cases have disabilities, such as paralysis, incontinence, and cognitive disorders. Babies born with anencephaly die soon after birth. Neural tube defects occur in 1 in 1000 births. Down syndrome, a condition in which an extra chromosome leads to intellectual disability and other physical alterations, occurs in about 1 in 800 births. Other common birth defects include musculoskeletal defects, gastrointestinal defects, and metabolic disorders.

What causes a birth defect? About 15% to 25% of birth defects are known to be genetic (i.e., inherited or spontaneous mutations of the genetic code). Another 10% are due to environmental influences (e.g., exposure to **teratogens**). The specific cause of the remaining 65% to 75% of birth defects is unknown. Although the etiology of birth defects is multifactorial and many elements are beyond human control, good nutrition practices can positively influence the outcome of pregnancy.

Folic Acid

During the 1980s, researchers in the United Kingdom noticed a relationship between poor dietary habits and a high rate of neural tube defects among children of impoverished women. Subsequent intervention studies demonstrated that administration of a multivitamin supplement during the periconceptional period—the months before conception and during early pregnancy—reduced the recurrence of these birth defects. The specific link between dietary folic acid and neural tube defects was tested and confirmed in several follow-up studies. As you learned in Section 8.12, folate plays a leading role in the synthesis of DNA and the metabolism of amino acids. The rapid cell growth of pregnancy increases needs for folate during pregnancy to 600 micrograms DFE per day. Some women, for genetic reasons, may have an even higher requirement. Adequate folic acid in the periconceptional period decreases the risk of neural tube defects by about 70% and has also been associated with decreased risk of cleft lip/palate, heart defects, and Down syndrome.

In 1998, the U.S. Food and Drug Administration (FDA) mandated fortification of grain products to provide 140 micrograms of folic acid per 100 grams of grain consumed. In Canada, the level of fortification is 150 micrograms of folate per 100 grams of grain consumed. In general, this increases the average consumption of dietary folic acid by 100 micrograms per day.

Adequate folate status is crucial for all women of childbearing age because the neural tube closes within the first 28 days

In North America, maternal death as a result of childbirth is uncommon—only about 14 deaths in every 100,000 live births. The infant mortality rate, however, is much higher: for each 100,000 live births, about 600 infants die within the first year. The infant death rate among African-Americans is more than double the rates among whites and Hispanics in the United States.

teratogen A compound (natural or synthetic) that may cause or increase the risk of a birth defect. Exposure to a teratogen does not always lead to a birth defect; its effects on the fetus depend on the dose, timing, and duration of exposure.

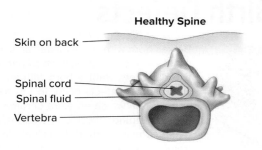
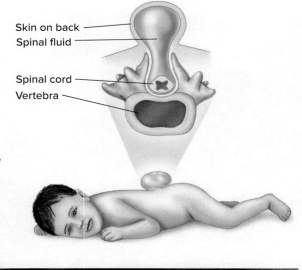

FIGURE 14-11 ▶ Spina bifida is one type of neural tube defect. Very early in fetal development, a ridge of neural-like tissue forms along the back of the embryo. As the fetus develops, this ridge develops into both the spinal cord and nerves at the lower end and the brain at the upper end. At the same time, the bones that make up the back gradually surround the spinal cord on all sides. In spina bifida, the backbones do not form a complete ring to protect the spinal cord. Deficient folate status in the mother during the beginning of pregnancy, especially in combination with a genetic abnormality in folate metabolism, greatly increases the risk of neural tube defects.

of pregnancy, a time when many women are unaware they are pregnant. A well-planned diet can meet the RDA for folic acid, but the U.S. Public Health Service, March of Dimes, and *Dietary Guidelines for Americans* recommend that all women of childbearing age take a daily multivitamin and mineral supplement that contains 400 micrograms of folic acid. Women who have already had a child with a neural tube defect are advised to consume megadoses of folic acid—4000 micrograms per day. They are to begin supplementation at least 1 month before any future pregnancy. This must be done under strict physician supervision.

Iodine

Low iodine status during the first trimester of pregnancy—a critical period of brain development—may lead to congenital hypothyroidism (formerly called *cretinism*).[31] If left untreated, consequences (which may vary in severity) include intellectual disability, stunting of growth, impaired hearing and speech, and infertility. Some other physical features are evident in Figure 14-12. When the defect is identified early (by newborn screening tests), these harmful effects can be prevented by treatment with thyroid hormones. With use of iodized salt, however, congenital hypothyroidism due to iodine deficiencies is rare.

Antioxidants

A case can be made for antioxidants in the prevention of birth defects as well. Free radicals are constantly generated within the body as a result of normal metabolic processes. An abundance of free radicals results in damage of cells and their DNA, which can lead to gene mutations or tissue malformations. Some research points to free radicals as a source of damage during embryo development and organogenesis. Antioxidant systems within the body act to minimize the damage caused by free radicals, and researchers hypothesize that dietary sources of antioxidants may aid in the prevention of birth defects. At this time, there is insufficient evidence to support supplementation of individual nutrients that participate in antioxidant systems—vitamin E, vitamin C, selenium, zinc, and copper—for the prevention of birth defects. However, use of a balanced multivitamin and mineral supplement while consuming a diet rich in whole grains,

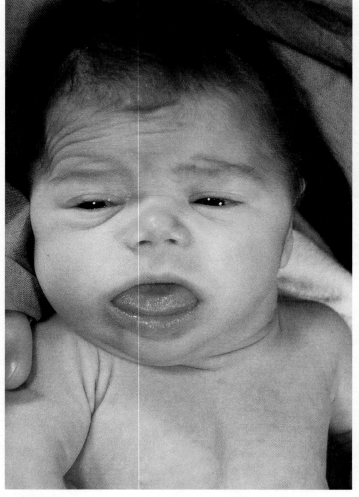

FIGURE 14-12 ▲ Child with congenital hypothyroidism due to maternal iodine deficiency. This birth defect leads to intellectual disability, stunting of growth, and other physical defects, such as large tongue, enlarged head, and puffy eyes. ©Mediscan/Alamy

legumes, and a variety of fruits and vegetables will provide enough of these nutrients to meet current recommendations.

Vitamin A

While the needs for most vitamins and minerals increase by about 30% during pregnancy, the requirement for vitamin A increases by only 10%. Studies have shown the teratogenic potential of vitamin A in doses as low as approximately 3000 micrograms RAE per day. This is just over three times the RDA of 770 micrograms RAE per day for pregnant adult women.

Fetal abnormalities resulting from vitamin A toxicity primarily include facial and cardiac defects, but a wide range of defects have been reported. It is rare that food sources of vitamin A would lead to toxicity. Recall from Section 8.2 that preformed vitamin A is found in liver, fish, fish oils, fortified milk and yogurt, and eggs. Carotenoids, found in fruits and vegetables, are precursors of vitamin A that are converted into vitamin A in the small intestine, liver, and kidneys. However, the efficiency of absorption of carotenoids decreases as intake increases. Vitamin A excesses typically arise from high-dose dietary supplements rather than food sources.

Typical North American diets supply adequate vitamin A from foods, so supplemental use is not generally necessary. During pregnancy, supplemental preformed vitamin A should not exceed 3000 micrograms RAE per day (15,000 IU per day). Most multivitamins and prenatal vitamins supply less than 1500 micrograms RAE per day. A balanced diet and prudent use of dietary supplements are actions that can sidestep potential problems with vitamin A toxicity.

Caffeine

Caffeine has been scrutinized for its safety during pregnancy, especially for any link with rate of birth defects. Caffeine decreases the mother's absorption of iron and may reduce blood flow through the placenta. In addition, the fetus is unable to detoxify caffeine. Research shows that as caffeine intake increases, so does the risk of miscarriage or delivering a LBW infant. Heavy caffeine use during pregnancy may also lead to caffeine withdrawal symptoms in the newborn. These risks are reported with caffeine intakes in excess of 500 milligrams, or the equivalent of about 5 cups of coffee per day. Moderate use of caffeine (up to 200 milligrams of caffeine, or the equivalent of 12 fluid ounces of regular coffee per day), however, is not associated with risk for birth defects.[6] Accounting for caffeine intake from tea, over-the-counter medicines containing caffeine, and chocolate is also important.

Aspartame

Phenylalanine, a component of the artificial sweetener aspartame (NutraSweet® and Equal),® is a cause for concern for some pregnant women. High amounts of phenylalanine in maternal blood disrupt fetal brain development if the mother has a disease known as *phenylketonuria* (see Obesity and Chronic Health Conditions in this section). If the mother does not have this condition, however, it is unlikely that the baby will be affected by moderate aspartame use.

For most adults, diet soft drinks are the primary source of artificial sweeteners. Of greater concern than the safety of sweeteners during pregnancy is the quality of foods and beverages consumed. A high intake of diet soft drinks may crowd out healthier beverages, such as water and low-fat milk.

Obesity and Chronic Health Conditions

Even before becoming pregnant, women of childbearing age should have regular medical checkups to keep an eye on any health conditions that already exist or to identify any developing health problems. In some cases, the condition itself increases risk for birth defects. Obesity, high blood pressure, and uncontrolled diabetes are common health problems known to increase the risk for birth defects, including neural tube defects. In other cases, medications used to control illnesses may pose a risk to the developing fetus. Other health issues, such as seizure disorders and metabolic disorders, could also affect fetal development. A preconception visit with a health professional can help to sort out and make plans to minimize such risks. Once a woman has become pregnant, early and regular prenatal care can aid in the success of a pregnancy.

Women with diabetes are two to three times more likely to give birth to a baby with birth defects compared to women with normal glucose metabolism. Examples of birth defects common in this group include malformations of the spine, legs, and blood vessels of the heart. Some experts speculate that the mechanism by which diabetes increases birth defects is via excessive free radicals, which lead to oxidative damage of DNA during early gestation. Careful control of blood glucose drastically lowers risk for women with diabetes. Optimal blood glucose control can be achieved through a combination of dietary modifications and medications. Given that diabetes is on the rise among women of childbearing age, this elevated rate of birth defects has become an area of heightened concern.

Another health condition for which maternal nutritional control is of utmost importance is PKU. Recall from Section 6.1 that PKU is an error of metabolism in which the liver lacks the ability to process phenylalanine, leading to an accumulation of this amino acid and its metabolites in body tissues. Babies born to women who have phenylketonuria that is not controlled by diet are at heightened risk for brain defects, such as microcephaly and intellectual disability.[32]

Alcohol

Conclusive evidence shows that repeated consumption of four or more alcoholic drinks at one sitting harms the fetus.[33] Such binge drinking is especially perilous during the first 12 weeks of pregnancy, as this is when critical early developmental events take place in utero. Experts have not determined a safe level of alcohol intake during pregnancy. Until a safe level can be established, women are advised not to drink any alcohol—from beverages, foods, or medications (check the label)—during pregnancy or when there is a chance of conception. The embryo (and, at later stages, the fetus) has no means of detoxifying alcohol.

Women with chronic alcoholism produce children with a variety of physical and intellectual problems collectively called **fetal alcohol spectrum disorders (FASDs)**. The most severe of these disorders is **fetal alcohol syndrome (FAS)**. A diagnosis of FAS is

fetal alcohol spectrum disorders (FASDs) A group of irreversible physical and mental abnormalities in the infant that result from the mother's consumption of alcohol during pregnancy.

fetal alcohol syndrome (FAS) Severe form of FASD that involves abnormal facial features and problems with development of the nervous system and overall growth as a result of maternal alcohol consumption during pregnancy.

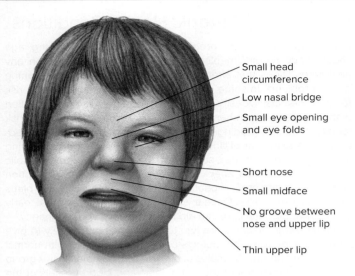

Small head circumference

Low nasal bridge

Small eye opening and eye folds

Short nose

Small midface

No groove between nose and upper lip

Thin upper lip

FIGURE 14-13 ▲ Fetal alcohol syndrome. The facial features shown are typical of affected children. Additional abnormalities in the brain and other internal organs accompany fetal alcohol syndrome but are not immediately apparent from simply looking at the child. Milder forms of alcohol-induced changes from a lower alcohol exposure to the fetus are known as alcohol-related neurodevelopmental disorders (ARNDs) and alcohol-related birth defects (ARBDs).

based mainly on poor fetal and infant growth, physical deformities (especially of facial features), and intellectual disability (Fig. 14-13). Irritability, hyperactivity, short attention span, and limited hand-eye coordination are other symptoms of FAS. Defects in vision, hearing, and mental processing may also develop over time. Other FASDs consist of some but not all of the defects of FAS. **Alcohol-related neurodevelopmental disorders (ARNDs)** include behavior and learning problems resulting from exposure to alcohol in utero. **Alcohol-related birth defects (ARBDs)** typically include malformations of the heart, kidneys, bones, and/or ears.

Exactly how alcohol causes these defects is not known. One line of research suggests that alcohol, or products of the metabolism of alcohol (e.g., acetaldehyde), cause faulty movement of cells in the brain during early stages of nerve cell development or block the action of certain brain neurotransmitters. In addition, inadequate nutrient intake, reduced nutrient and oxygen transfer across the placenta, cigarette smoking commonly associated with alcohol intake, drug use, and possibly other factors contribute to the overall result.

All major health authorities recommend that alcoholic beverages not be consumed by pregnant women. For more information about fetal alcohol syndrome, visit the website www.cdc.gov/ncbddd/fasd/.

alcohol-related neurodevelopmental disorders (ARNDs) One or more abnormalities of the central nervous system (e.g., small head size, impaired motor skills, hearing loss, or poor hand-eye coordination) related to confirmed alcohol exposure during gestation.
alcohol-related birth defects (ARBDs) One or more birth defects (e.g., malformations of the heart, bones, kidneys, eyes, or ears) related to confirmed alcohol exposure during gestation.

Environmental Contaminants

There is little evidence to link birth defects with the amounts of pesticides, herbicides, or other contaminants in foods or public water supplies in North America. However, evaluating such a link can be difficult, and many would argue that regulations concerning contaminants in the food and water supply are too permissive. Thus, it seems prudent to take measures to decrease intake of pesticides and other contaminants wherever possible. For fruits and vegetables, peeling, removing outer leaves, and/or thoroughly rinsing and scrubbing with a brush under running water will remove the majority of contaminants. In animal products, toxins are most likely to accumulate in fatty tissues. Therefore, removing skin, discarding drippings, and trimming visible fat will decrease exposure from meat, poultry, and fish.

For fish, mercury is of particular concern because it can harm the nervous system of the fetus. Thus, the FDA warns pregnant women to avoid swordfish, shark, king mackerel, and tilefish because of possible high mercury contamination. Largemouth bass are also implicated. In general, intake of other fish and shellfish should not exceed 12 ounces per week. Canned albacore tuna is a potential mercury source, so it should not be consumed in amounts exceeding 6 ounces per week.[15] Most experts agree that the benefits of consuming fish far outweigh the potential risks of environmental contaminants. As a rule of thumb, consuming a *variety* of foods minimizes risk of exposure to any one contaminant from the food supply.

In Summary

Although many risk factors for birth defects are beyond our control, a woman of childbearing potential can make some wise nutrition choices to improve her chances of having a healthy baby without birth defects. A varied and balanced diet, such as the food plan for pregnant women described in this chapter, along with a daily multivitamin and mineral supplement with 400 micrograms of folic acid will ensure adequate nutrient status. It is estimated that daily use of a multivitamin and mineral supplement containing folic acid will decrease the rate of all birth defects by 50%. Discuss use of any other dietary supplements with a primary care provider or registered dietitian nutritionist to be sure that the fetus will not be exposed to toxic levels of vitamin A or other dangerous food components. Early and consistent prenatal care can help control obesity and any chronic health conditions that may complicate a pregnancy. Also, avoiding alcohol during pregnancy will eliminate any risk for fetal alcohol spectrum disorders.

Although it seems that advice for a healthy pregnancy is always directed at the mother, fathers-to-be are not off the hook! Health is a family affair, so encouraging healthy eating habits and avoiding smoking and alcohol are important for fathers, too. As you read in the beginning of this chapter, the genetics of the baby are certainly an outcome of both parents. Indeed, inadequate supplies of zinc, folate, antioxidants, and omega-3 fatty acids affect the quality of sperm. Overall, the periconceptional period is a time for good nutrition and careful lifestyle practices for mothers- and fathers-to-be.

A goal of *Healthy People 2020* is 98.3% abstinence from alcohol, cigarettes, and illicit drugs by pregnant women, a 10% improvement over current statistics.

Summary

14.1 Energy imbalances can adversely affect fertility by altering hormone levels and promoting oxidative damage. Polycystic ovary syndrome, which tends to co-occur with upper-body obesity, is an condition of hormonal imbalance that causes infertility. Other than managing body weight, nutritional factors that may improve male and/or female fertility include low glycemic index carbohydrates, unsaturated fats, antioxidants, folate, iron, and zinc.

14.2 Pregnancy is arbitrarily divided into three trimesters of 13 to 14 weeks each. The first trimester is characterized by a rapid increase in cell number as the zygote grows to be an embryo, then a fetus. During the first trimester, the growing organism is most susceptible to damage from exposure to toxic agents or nutrient deficiencies. By the start of the second trimester, the organs and limbs have formed and will continue to grow and develop. The third trimester is marked by rapid fetal growth and storage of nutrients in preparation for life outside the womb.

14.3 A successful pregnancy results in optimal health for both the infant and the mother. Pregnancy success is defined as (1) gestation longer than 37 weeks; and (2) birth weight greater than 5.5 pounds (2.5 kilograms). Factors that predict pregnancy success include early and regular prenatal care, maternal age within the range of 20 to 35 years, and adequate nutrition. Factors that contribute to poor pregnancy outcome include inadequate prenatal care, obesity, underweight, teenage pregnancy, smoking, alcohol consumption, use of certain prescription medications and all illicit drugs, inadequate nutrition, heavy caffeine use, and various infections, such as listeriosis.

14.4 For women with a healthy prepregnancy BMI (18.5 to 24.9), total weight gain should be within the range of 25 to 35 pounds. Underweight women and those carrying multiple fetuses should gain more; overweight and obese women should gain less. During the first trimester, although she need not increase diet quantity, the woman should focus on diet quality to meet increased requirements for protein, carbohydrate, essential fatty acids, fiber, water, and many vitamins and minerals. A woman typically needs an additional 350 to 450 kcal per day during the second and third trimesters.

14.5 Following a plan based on the *Dietary Guidelines for Americans* as exemplified by MyPlate is recommended for pregnant and breastfeeding women. The mother-to-be should especially emphasize good sources of vitamin B-6, folate, vitamin D, iron, zinc, and calcium. Vegetarian diets are safe during pregnancy, but vegan mothers should specifically seek out good sources of vitamin B-12 and vitamin D. Prenatal multivitamin and mineral supplements are useful for meeting increased nutrient requirements during pregnancy.

14.6 Gestational hypertension, gestational diabetes, heartburn, constipation, nausea, vomiting, edema, and anemia are all possible discomforts and complications of pregnancy. Nutrition therapy can help minimize some of these problems.

14.7 Almost all women are physically able to breastfeed their infants. The nutritional composition of human milk is different from that of unaltered cow's milk; human milk is much more desirable for the infant.

For the infant, the advantages of breastfeeding over formula feeding are numerous, including fewer infections, reduced risk of allergies and food intolerances, and lower rates of obesity and type 2 diabetes throughout life. Benefits for the mother include reduced risk of certain cancers, earlier recovery from pregnancy, and faster return to prepregnancy weight. For mothers who choose not to breastfeed or have medical conditions that contraindicate breastfeeding (e.g., galactosemia), infants can be adequately nourished with formula.

14.8 There are several steps pregnant women can take to reduce the risk of birth defects. Achieve a healthy body weight before pregnancy and strive to gain weight within the ranges recommended by the National Academy of Medicine. Adequate intakes of folic acid, iodine, and antioxidant nutrients are essential for prevention of many types of birth defects. Excesses of vitamin A and caffeine should be avoided. There is no safe level of alcohol intake known during pregnancy. Dietary control of diseases (e.g., diabetes and PKU) will also protect the fetus.

Check Your Knowledge (Answers are available at the end of this question set.)

1. Which of the following nutrition interventions is most likely to improve fertility?
   a. Taking a vitamin E supplement
   b. Losing excess body fat
   c. Consuming a low-carbohydrate diet
   d. Taking an iron supplement

2. Increased carbohydrate needs during pregnancy are set to
   a. prevent ketosis.
   b. alleviate nausea.
   c. prevent gestational hypertension.
   d. supply adequate folate.

3. An infant born at 38 weeks' gestation weighing 5 pounds can be described as
   a. preterm.
   b. LBW.
   c. SGA.
   d. LBW and SGA.

4. If a woman is 5 feet 2 inches tall and weighs 150 pounds before becoming pregnant, how much weight should she gain during pregnancy?
   a. 28 to 40 pounds (12.5 to 18 kilograms)
   b. 25 to 35 pounds (11.5 to 16 kilograms)
   c. 15 to 25 pounds (7 to 11.5 kilograms)
   d. As little as possible

5. Benefits of exercise during pregnancy include
   a. preventing excessive gestational weight gain.
   b. improved sleep.
   c. lower risk for gestational diabetes.
   d. all of these.

6. Which of the following may help to alleviate nausea during pregnancy?
   a. Postponing meals until the afternoon
   b. Drinking large amounts of water
   c. Postponing use of iron supplements until the second trimester
   d. All of these

7. Physiologically, milk production requires _____ kcal per day.
   a. 300   c. 800
   b. 500   d. 1000

8. An eating pattern for a woman in the third trimester of pregnancy differs from her prepregnancy diet in that
   a. fluid needs are higher.
   b. additional oils are allowed.
   c. there are more servings from the grains group.
   d. all of these apply.

9. Advantages of breastfeeding include
   a. decreased ear infections in the infant.
   b. decreased diarrheal diseases in the infant.
   c. decreased risk of breast cancer for the mother.
   d. all of these.

10. Consuming a single cup of coffee per day is associated with
    a. spontaneous abortion.   c. birth defects.
    b. LBW.   d. none of these.

Answer Key: 1. b (LO 14.1), 2. a (LO 14.2), 3. d (LO 14.3), 4. c (LO 14.4), 5. d (LO 14.5), 6. c (LO 14.6), 7. c (LO 14.7), 8. d (LO 14.8), 9. d (LO 14.9), 10. d (LO 14.10)

Study Questions (Numbers refer to Learning Outcomes)

1. Provide three key pieces of nutrition advice for parents seeking to maximize their chances of conceiving. Why did you identify those specific factors? **(LO 14.1)**

2. Identify four key nutrients for which intake should be significantly increased during pregnancy. **(LO 14.2)**

3. Describe some nutritional concerns related to teenage pregnancy. At what age do you think pregnancy is ideal? Why? **(LO 14.3)**

4. Outline current weight-gain recommendations for pregnancy. What is the basis for these recommendations? **(LO 14.4)**

5. Suggest several safe exercises for a pregnant woman. **(LO 14.5)**

6. What nutrition advice would you give to a friend who suffers from morning sickness? **(LO 14.6)**

7. Describe the physiological mechanisms that stimulate human milk production and release. How can knowing about these help mothers breastfeed successfully? **(LO 14.7)**

8. A pregnant woman typically needs 350 to 450 kcal more than her usual needs. Suggest a combination of nutrient-dense foods that would supply these extra calories. **(LO 14.8)**

9. Give three reasons a woman should give serious consideration to breastfeeding her infant. **(LO 14.9)**

10. Describe the importance of folic acid for conception and fetal development. **(LO 14.10)**

What the Dietitian Chose

The spinach salad meal with hard-boiled egg and whole wheat roll provides only about 2 grams of iron. It is a healthy, nutrient-dense choice that provides some protein but does not make a significant contribution to meeting iron needs.

A hamburger is a source of iron—this meal would provide about 4.5 milligrams of iron—but it would not be a choice for a person who follows a vegetarian diet.

The bean and cheese taco option provides just as much iron (4.5 milligrams) as the hamburger meal and would be appropriate for a vegetarian. Even though the nonheme iron in beans is not as well absorbed as the heme iron in beef, the 20 milligrams of vitamin C in the stewed tomatoes will enhance iron absorption.

All of these meals, however, pale in comparison to the iron contribution of the fortified, ready-to-eat breakfast cereal. One cup of Kellogg's Smart Start cereal provides 18 milligrams of iron and the 72 milligrams of vitamin C in 1 cup of orange juice will enhance iron absorption. In one easy meal, any pregnant woman could obtain more than half of the 27-milligram RDA for iron during pregnancy.

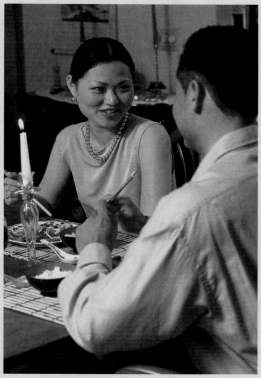
©Digital Vision/PunchStock

Further Readings

1. Swinney B: Eating to fuel fertility. *Today's Dietitian* 2013; 15:38.

2. Office on Women's Health: Polycystic ovary syndrome. May 27, 2016. https://www.womenshealth.gov/files/assets/docs/fact-sheets/polycystic-ovary-syndrome.pdf. (Accessed March 1, 2017).

3. Chavarro JE, and others: *The Fertility Diet: Groundbreaking Research Reveals Natural Ways to Boost Ovulation and Improve Your Chances of Getting Pregnant.* New York: The McGraw-Hill Companies, 2009.

4. Centers for Disease Control and Prevention: About teen pregnancy, April 2016. https://www.cdc.gov/teenpregnancy/about/. (Accessed March 1, 2017).

5. U.S. Department of Health and Human Services, Office of Adolescent Health: Teen pregnancy and childbearing, January 2017. https://www.hhs.gov/ash/oah/adolescent-health-topics/reproductive-health/teen-pregnancy/index.html. (Accessed March 1, 2017).

6. Academy of Nutrition and Dietetics: Position of the Academy of Nutrition and Dietetics: Nutrition and lifestyle for a healthy pregnancy outcome. *J Acad Nurti Diet* 2014; 114:1099.

7. Schultz DJ and others: The impact of the 2009 Special Supplemental Nutrition Program for Women, Infants, and Children food package revisions on participants: A systematic review. *J Acad Nutri Diet* 2015; 115:1832.

8. Committee on Obstetric Practice: Committee Opinion #650: Physical activity and exercise during pregnancy and the postpartum period. *Obstet Gynecol* 2015; 126:e135.

9. Van Pelt J: Exercise during pregnancy. *Today's Dietitian* 2014; 16:52.

10. Ferraro ZM and others: Gestational weight gain and medical outcomes of pregnancy. *Obstetric Medicine* 2015; 8(3): 133.

11. Institute of Medicine and National Research Council: *Weight gain during pregnancy: Reexamining the guidelines.* Washington, DC: National Academies Press, 2009.

12. Academy of Nutrition and Dietetics: Position of the Academy of Nutrition and Dietetics: Obesity, reproduction, and pregnancy outcomes. *J Acad Nutri Diet* 2016; 116:677.

13. Berenson AB and others: Obesity risk knowledge, weight misperception, and diet and health-related attitudes among women intending to become pregnant. *J Acad Nutri Diet* 2016; 116:69.

14. Getz L: Starving for two. *Today's Dietitian* 17:14, 2015.

15. U.S. Environmental Protection Agency and U.S. Food and Drug Administration: Advice about eating fish: What pregnant women and parents should know. January 2017. https://www.fda.gov/downloads/Food/FoodborneIllnessContaminants/Metals/UCM536321.pdf. (Accessed March 1, 2017).

16. Tone C: Omega-3 fats and pregnancy: Health benefits for both mom and baby. *Today's Dietitian* 18:14, 2016.

17. Wei S and others: Maternal vitamin D status and adverse pregnancy outcomes: A systematic review and meta-analysis. *J Matern Fetal Neonatal Med* 2013; 26:889.

18. De-Regil LM and others: Vitamin D supplementation for women during pregnancy. *Cochrane Database of Systematic Reviews* 2016; 2016:1.

19. Grieger JA, Clifton VL: A review of the impact of dietary intakes in human pregnancy on infant birthweight. *Nutrients* 2014; 7:153.

20. Blumfield ML and others: Micronutrient intakes during pregnancy in developed countries: Systematic review and meta-analysis. *Nutr Res* 2013; 71:118.

21. Lowensohn RI and others: Current concepts of maternal nutrition. *Obstet Gynecol Surv* 2016; 71:413.

22. Toiba R: Gestational diabetes. *Today's Dietitian* 2013; 15:48.

23. American Diabetes Association: Standards of medical are in diabetes—2017. *Diabetes Care* 2017; 40:S1.

24. Curry A: Special delivery: How diabetes affects the health of mother and child—and what you can do about it. *Diabetes Forecast* 2016; Sept/Oct 2016:51.

25. Xu H and others: Role of nutrition in the risk of preeclampsia. *Nut Res* 2009; 67:639.

26. Academy of Nutrition and Dietetics: Position of the Academy of Nutrition and Dietetics: Promoting and supporting breastfeeding. *J Acad Nutri Diet* 2015; 115:444.

27. Section on Breastfeeding: Policy Statement: Breastfeeding and the use of human milk. *Pediatrics* 2012; 129:e827.

28. Victora CG and others: Breastfeeding in the 21st century: Epidemiology, mechanisms, and lifelong effect. *The Lancet* 2016; 387:475.

29. Fleischer DM and others: Primary prevention of allergic disease through nutritional interventions. *J Allergy Clin Immunol: In Practice* 2013; 1:29.

30. Baker RD and others: Clinical report—diagnosis and prevention of iron deficiency and iron-deficiency anemia in infants and young children (0–3 years of age). *Pediatrics* 2010; 126:1040.

31. Zimmermann MB: The effects of iodine deficiency in pregnancy and infancy. *Pediatric Perinatal Epidemiology* 2012; 26 Suppl. 1:108.

32. Committee on Genetics: Policy Statement: Maternal phenylketonuria. *Pediatrics* 2008; 122:445. Reaffirmed January 2013.

33. Viteri OA and others: Fetal anomalies and long-term effects associated with substance abuse in pregnancy: A literature review. *Am J Perinatol* 2015; 32:405.

connect **To get the most out of your study, visit Connect where you will find NutritionCalc Plus, SmartBook®, and many other dynamic tools.**

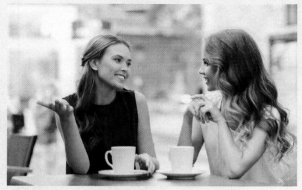

Rate Your Plate

Putting Your Knowledge About Nutrition and Pregnancy to Work

A college friend, Gayle, tells you that she is pregnant. The following is an example of her typical daily food choices:

Breakfast

Granola bar
Coffee

Lunch

Sweetened yogurt, 1 cup
Small bagel with cream cheese
Apple
Regular caffeinated soda, 12 ounces

Snack

Chocolate candy bar

©Syda Productions/Shutterstock

Dinner

2 slices of pizza
Regular caffeinated soda, 12 ounces

Snacks

Pretzels 1 ounce
Regular caffeinated soda, 12 ounces

1. Using the NutritionCalc Plus software, evaluate Gayle's usual menu. How do her intakes of protein, carbohydrates, folate, vitamin B-6, iron, calcium, and vitamin D compare with the recommended amounts for pregnancy?

   _____

   _____

   _____

2. Now redesign her diet, making sure that her intake meets pregnancy needs for protein, carbohydrate, folate, vitamin B-6, iron, calcium, and vitamin D. (Hint: Use of fortified foods, such as breakfast cereal, and a prenatal supplement will be useful.)

   _____

   _____

   _____

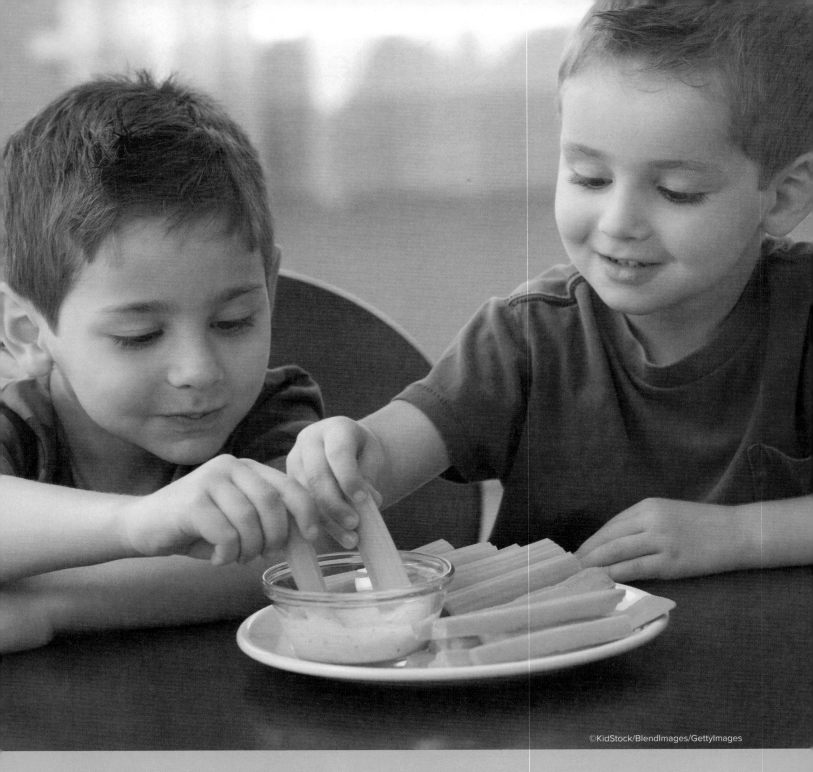

©KidStock/BlendImages/GettyImages

Student Learning Outcomes

Chapter 15 is designed to allow you to:

15.1 Describe the extent to which nutrition affects growth and physiological development from infancy through adolescence.

15.2 List specific nutrients often found to be lacking in the dietary patterns of infants, toddlers, preschoolers, and teenagers, and make recommendations to remedy the problems.

15.3 Identify dietary strategies to meet the basic nutritional needs for normal growth and development for an infant, and discuss some do's and don'ts associated with infant feeding.

15.4 Outline several challenges parents might face in dealing with eating habits during childhood and adolescence.

15.5 Describe the long-term effects of childhood obesity, and suggest ways to prevent or treat the problem.

15.6 Identify common food allergens, and suggest several practices that may reduce the risk of developing a food allergy.

Chapter 15
Nutrition from Infancy Through Adolescence

What Would You Choose?

Your brother and his wife have asked you to care for your 18-month-old niece, Lila, while they enjoy a weekend get-away at the lake to celebrate their anniversary. Before they drop her off, you make a trip to the grocery store to pick up some kid-friendly foods. Lila does not have any food allergies, but your brother warned you that she has developed some picky eating behaviors. Which of the following snack foods would you choose for your little houseguest?

a Reduced-fat popcorn

b Raw baby carrots with ranch dressing

c Fat-free light yogurt

d Whole grain crackers with sliced cheddar cheese

Think about your choice as you read this chapter, then see What the Dietitian Chose at the end of the chapter.

Children born in North America have access to some of the best health care in the world. Even so, the numbers of children and teenagers with obesity and type 2 diabetes are on the rise. Kids spend more time in their computer chairs and less time in active play. Soft drinks and energy drinks have replaced much of the milk that children and teenagers previously consumed daily. Consumption of fruits, vegetables, and whole grains—although these are abundantly available—consistently falls short of recommendations. Evidently, there is room for improvement in the dietary patterns of most American children. How can we influence healthy eating behaviors?

Education designed to change nutrition habits should start early and involve the family. During infancy and early childhood, the family controls food intake, informs food preferences, and models eating behaviors. Family mealtimes help children to establish healthy eating habits and aid in the prevention of childhood obesity. As children grow older, family meals are a time to teach children communication skills and improve self-esteem. Dietary habits and social skills learned early in life will equip children as they reach school age, when peer and media influences take on heightened importance. This chapter examines the dynamic nutritional needs of the growing years—from infancy through adolescence.

15.1 Assessing Growth

During infancy, future eating patterns and attitudes toward foods begin to take shape. If parents and other caregivers model good nutrition and are flexible, they can lead a child into lifelong healthful food habits. A family environment that encourages healthy eating will provide the nutrients needed to optimize physical growth and development. However, these advantages do not guarantee that a child will thrive.

Children also need specific attention focused on them; they need to grow in a stimulating environment, and they need a sense of security. For example, children hospitalized for growth failure gain weight more quickly when tactile stimulation, such as being held and rocked, accompanies needed nutrients.

THE GROWING INFANT

All babies seem to do is eat and sleep. There is a good reason for this! An infant's birth weight doubles in the first 4 to 6 months and triples within the first year. Never again is growth so rapid. Such rapid growth requires a lot of nourishment and sleep. After the first year, growth is slower; it takes 5 more years to double the weight seen at 1 year. An infant also increases in length in the first year by 50% and then continues to gain height through the teen years. These gains are not necessarily continuous; spurts of rapid growth alternate with periods of relatively little change. Height is typically maximized by age 19, although continued growth may occur in the early twenties, especially for boys. Head size in proportion to total height shrinks from one-fourth to one-eighth during the climb from infancy to adulthood.

The human body needs a lot more food to support growth and development than it does to merely maintain its size once growth ceases. When nutrients are missing at critical phases of this process, growth and development may slow or even stop. Adequate amounts of calories, protein, calcium, iron, and zinc are particularly important during these years. In developing nations, about one-third of the children under 5 years of age are short and underweight for their ages. Poor nutrition—called **undernutrition**—is at the heart of the problem. Undernourished children are smaller versions of nutritionally fit children. In poorer countries, when breastfeeding ceases, children are often fed a high-carbohydrate, low-protein diet (see Section 12.5). This diet supports some growth but does not allow children to attain their full genetic and developmental potential. Undernutrition occurs in North America, as well, but **overnutrition** is much more prevalent.

undernutrition Failing health that results from a long-standing dietary intake that is not enough to meet nutritional needs.

overnutrition A state in which nutritional intake greatly exceeds the body's needs.

EFFECT OF UNDERNUTRITION ON GROWTH

As with the fetus in utero, the long-term effects of nutritional problems in infancy and childhood depend on the severity, timing, and duration of the nutritional insult to cellular processes.

The single best indicator of a child's nutritional status is growth: gains in weight are a good reflection of growth in the short term, whereas gains in height are an indicator of growth over the long term. An inadequate dietary pattern during a critical stage of infancy or childhood hampers the cell division that should occur at that stage. Mild zinc deficiencies among North American children, for example, have been linked to diminished growth. Improving dietary patterns after a period of nutrient deficiency will not compensate for losses in physical or mental development, however, because the hormonal and other conditions needed for growth will not likely be present. In addition, gains in height are no longer possible after the skeleton reaches maturation. This happens as growth plates at the ends of the bones fuse, which begins around 14 years of age in girls and 15 years of age in boys. This process is complete by at about age 19 in girls and age 20 in boys. Furthermore, muscles can increase in diameter later in life, but their linear growth is limited by the length of the bone.

For these reasons, a 15-year-old Central American girl who is 4 feet 8 inches tall cannot attain the adult height of a typical North American girl simply by eating better. Girls experience their peak rate of growth right before the onset of menstrual periods. Once the time for growth ceases (in women, this is about 5 years after they start menstruating), a sufficient nutrient intake helps maintain health and weight but cannot make up for lost growth in height.

USING GROWTH CHARTS

Health professionals assess a child's pattern of growth by plotting measurements of height and weight on growth charts (Fig. 15-1). The charts contain **percentile** divisions, which represent the typical measurements for most children. A percentile represents the rank of the person among 100 peers matched for age and gender. If a young boy, for example, is at the 90th percentile of height-for-age, he is shorter than 10% and taller than 89% of children his age. A child at the 50th percentile is considered average. Fifty of 100 children will be taller than this child; 49 will be shorter.

A variety of growth charts for boys and girls are available from the Centers for Disease Control and Prevention (CDC) website (see Fig. 15-1). For children from birth to age 2, use the growth charts developed by the World Health Organization (WHO) in 2006 to assess length-for-age, weight-for-age, weight-for-length, and head-circumference-for-age

percentile Classification of a measurement of a unit into divisions of 100 units.

Children under 2 to 3 years of age are measured lying on their backs with legs fully extended, so the term *length* is used rather than *height* or *stature*.

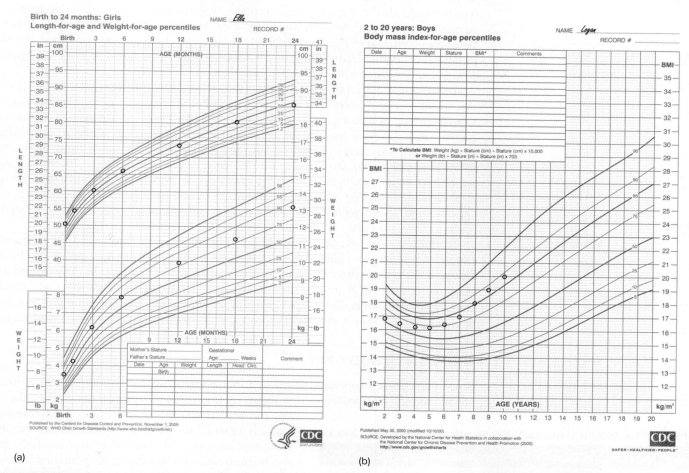

(a)

(b)

FIGURE 15-1 ▲ Growth charts for assessment of children in the growing years. The growth of a young girl and a boy is plotted to show how the charts are used in health care settings. For children from birth to age 2, CDC recommends using growth charts developed by WHO in 2006. For ages 2 to 20, use the CDC growth charts, developed by the National Center for Health Statistics and CDC in 2000. (a) Length-for-age and weight-for-age plotted for a young girl (Ella). A certain length (height) and weight correspond to a percentile value (i.e., a ranking of the individual among 100 peers). Ella has been tracking around the 50th percentile for length throughout the first 2 years of her life; her weight, which started out near the 50th percentile, is now between the 75th and 90th percentiles. (b) BMI-for-age plotted for a young boy (Logan) up to age 10. While Logan's BMI-for-age was around the 50th percentile when he was a preschooler, by age 10, he is above the 85th percentile. He would be classified as overweight according to his BMI-for-age. Source: (a) Centers for Disease Control and Prevention, based on WHO Child Growth Standards (2009); (b) Centers for Disease Control and Prevention (2000).

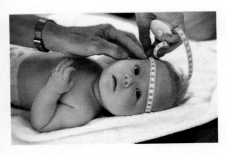

▲ Brain growth is faster in infancy than in any other stage of life. An infant's head needs to be large (about one-quarter of body length) to allow for such growth. By the time she reaches adulthood, this girl's head will only be about one-eighth of her height. ©Pixtal/Age Fotostock

measurements. WHO growth charts are based on data collected from children from various regions of the world who were raised *under conditions for optimal growth and development.* This means that they were breastfed as infants; had caregivers who followed recommended infant and child feeding practices set forth by WHO; had adequate health care; had mothers who did not use alcohol during pregnancy; and were not exposed to tobacco before or after birth. In contrast, older growth charts for young children were based on data from primarily white children who were mostly formula-fed during infancy. The WHO growth standards emphasize that breastfeeding is the biological norm for infant nutrition.

For children from ages 2 to 20, growth charts developed by the National Center for Health Statistics are available to assess weight-for-age and stature-for-age. However, the preferred way to assess weight status for children and adolescents is body mass index (BMI)-for-age. For adults, BMI has fixed cutoff points (e.g., a BMI of 25 for an adult is considered overweight). Please note, as Figure 15-1 shows, this is not true for children; BMI reference ranges are both gender- and age-specific.

In addition to taking measurements of weight and length, a health professional measures the infant's head circumference. Tracking head circumference-for-age on a growth chart (also available from CDC) is a means of assessing brain growth. The brain grows faster during the first year than at any other time of life. Unusual head circumference measurements can alert the health care team to a genetic disorder. A small head circumference could also be a result of malnutrition, infection, impaired mental development, or maternal substance abuse during pregnancy. An abnormally large measurement may be a sign of a tumor or fluid on the brain. Variations in head circumference may be due to harmless familial traits, but extreme deviations from the norm or rapid changes in percentiles over time warrant further investigation.

Infants and children should have their growth assessed during regular health checkups. It takes 1 to 3 years for the genetic potential (in terms of percentile ranking on growth charts) of infant growth to be established. By 3 years of age, a child's measurements, such as length (height) for age, should track consistently along an established percentile. If the child's growth measurements move up or down from his or her established percentile, the primary care provider needs to investigate whether a medical or nutritional problem is affecting growth. Likewise, when a child's BMI-for-age approaches the highest percentiles, caregivers should be concerned. A child between the 85th and 95th percentiles for BMI-for-age is considered overweight. At or above the 95th percentile, a child is considered obese (Table 15-1).

The growth charts available from the CDC are intended for healthy children; they may not be appropriate for children born at very low birth weight or who have special health care needs. Preterm infants tend to be smaller than full-term infants in the early months but typically catch up in growth within 2 or 3 years. Catch-up growth requires that the child move up in percentiles. Specialized growth charts have been developed for children with special health care needs that affect growth and development, such as Down syndrome.

GROWTH IN BODY FAT

Since 1970, researchers have speculated that overfeeding during infancy may increase the number of adipose tissue cells. Today, we know that the number of adipose cells can also increase as adulthood obesity develops. If energy intake is limited during infancy to minimize the number of adipose cells, the growth of other organ systems may also be severely restricted, especially brain and nervous system development. Furthermore, most overweight infants become normal-weight preschoolers without dietary restrictions. For these reasons, it is unwise for an infant's dietary pattern to be restrictive—especially fat intake. A healthy range of fat intake is 30% to 40% of total calories for ages 1 to 3 years and 25% to 35% of total calories for older children and teenagers.

TABLE 15-1 ■ **Weight Status Classifications for Children, Ages 2 to 20**

Weight Status Classification	BMI-for-Age Percentile
Underweight	<5th percentile
Healthy weight	5th up to 85th percentile
Overweight	85th up to 95th percentile
Obese	≥95th percentile

Source: Centers for Disease Control and Prevention.

FAILURE TO THRIVE

About 5% to 10% of infants or children do not grow as expected. An infant may fail to reach important milestones, such as doubling birth weight by 6 months of age. On growth charts, weight-for-age may track below the fifth percentile. This condition of inadequate growth is termed **failure to thrive.**[1]

In some cases, failure to thrive has a specific medical cause. Physical problems that may limit energy intake include improper development of the mouth or digestive tract or problems with breastfeeding (e.g., poor latch-on skills). Even if a child consumes enough food and beverages, growth may still falter if there are physical problems, such as celiac disease, which limit nutrient absorption. Lastly, some medical conditions, such as heart or lung disorders, lead to greatly increased kilocalorie requirements.

However, about 80% of infants or children who fail to thrive have no apparent disease; environmental or social problems are at the root of their undernutrition. Poverty is the biggest environmental risk factor for undernutrition leading to failure to thrive. Needing to stretch food dollars, caregivers may overdilute formula—a detrimental practice that fills the child up without providing adequate calories. Sometimes the cause is unhealthy infant-parent interaction, including situations of abuse or neglect. Either too little or too much concern over child feedings can lead to nutrition problems. Most poor interactions, however, arise from the parents' inexperience with infant feeding rather than from intentional negligence.

Whatever the cause, the consequences of failure to thrive are serious and far-reaching. Possible outcomes include poor physical growth, impaired mental development, and behavioral problems. When health professionals encounter an infant failing to thrive, the true causes need to be identified and then treated. If a lack of financial resources is at the root of the problem, appropriate referrals to social services should be made. Counseling about proper nutrition and the importance of healthy parent-child interactions can help to get a child's growth back on track.

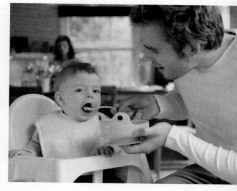

▲ Children older than 2 years are less likely to experience failure to thrive because they can often get food for themselves. Younger children, for the most part, are limited to what caregivers provide. ©ONOKY-Photononstop/Alamy

failure to thrive Condition of inadequate growth during infancy or early childhood caused by poor nutritional intake, inefficient nutrient absorption, or excessive energy expenditure; commonly defined as weight-for-age below the fifth percentile on multiple occasions or weight declining two or more major percentile lines on a standardized growth chart.

✓ CONCEPT CHECK 15.1

1. How do health care providers assess the growth of infants and children?
2. Define childhood overweight and obesity in terms of BMI-for-age.
3. If a female adolescent is short for her age due to a brief period of undernutrition between ages 10 to 12, can she catch up in growth after proper nutrition is restored? Why or why not?
4. What is failure to thrive? List some possible causes.

15.2 Infant Nutritional Needs

Infants' nutritional needs vary as they grow. For the first 4 to 6 months of life, human milk or infant formula supplies needed nutrients. Age-appropriate solid foods should be added to the infant's diet around 4 to 6 months of age. Even after solid foods are added, the basis of an infant's diet for the first year is still human milk or infant formula. Because of the critical importance of adequate nutrition in infancy and the difficulties encountered in feeding some infants, there is more discussion in this chapter on this developmental period than on the later periods of childhood.

ENERGY

Due to rapid growth and a high metabolic rate, the energy requirements per pound of body weight for an infant are the highest of any life stage (Table 15-2). For example, a 6-month-old infant requires two to four times more kilocalories per pound of body weight than an adult.

Healthy 6-month-old infant

$$\frac{700 \text{ kcal}}{15 \text{ pounds}} = \frac{47 \text{ kcal}}{\text{pound}}$$

Healthy 20-year-old woman

$$\frac{2200 \text{ kcal}}{135 \text{ pounds}} = \frac{16 \text{ kcal}}{\text{pound}}$$

Infants need a concentrated source of calories to meet these high demands. Exclusive feeding of either human milk or infant formula is ideal for the first 6 months of life; both are high in fat and supply about 640 kcal/quart (670 kcal/liter; Table 15-3). Beginning around 4 to 6 months of age, developmentally appropriate solid foods provide additional calories, nutrients, and variety for the developing infant.

CARBOHYDRATE

Carbohydrate needs in infancy are 60 grams per day at 0 to 6 months and 95 grams per day at 7 to 12 months. These needs are based on the typical intakes of human milk by breastfed infants and their eventual intake of solid foods. These carbohydrate goals are easily satisfied by the usual eating patterns of infants who are consuming a developmentally appropriate diet.

Do infants need fiber? There are no set AIs for fiber for infants and children younger than 2 years of age. For about the first 6 months of life, breast milk or formula, which contains no fiber, is adequate nutrition. As solid foods are introduced, include some fruits, vegetables, and whole grains. Some experts recommend working up to about 5 grams of fiber

TABLE 15-2 ■ Estimated Energy Requirements of Infants and Toddlers

Age	EER Equation
0 to 3 months	(89 kcal × weight in kilograms) + 75
4 to 6 months	(89 kcal × weight in kilograms) − 44
7 to 12 months	(89 kcal × weight in kilograms) − 78
13 to 35 months	(89 kcal × weight in kilograms) − 80

TABLE 15-3 ■ Composition of Human and Cow's Milk and Infant Formulas (per Liter)[a]

	Energy (kcal)	Protein (grams)	Fat (grams)	Carbohydrate (grams)	Minerals[b] (grams)
Milk					
Human milk	670[c]	11	45	70	2
Cow's milk, whole[d]	670	36	36	49	7
Cow's milk, fat-free[d]	360	36	1	51	7
Casein/Whey-Based Formulas					
Similac®	680	14	36	71	3
Enfamil®	670	15	37	69	3
Good Start®	670	16	34	73	3
Soybean Protein-Based Formulas					
ProSobee®	670	20	35	67	4
Isomil®	680	16	36	68	4
Transition Formulas/Beverages[e]					
Similac Go and Grow®	630	17	34	68	3
EnfaGrow® Next Step®	480	32	10	64	6

[a]At 3 months of age, infants typically consume 0.75 to 1 liter of human milk or formula per day.

[b]Calcium, phosphorus, and other minerals.

[c]Rough estimate; ranges from 650 to 700 kcal per liter.

[d]Not appropriate for infant feeding, based primarily on high protein and mineral content.

[e]For use after 6 months of age or later (see label).

per day by 1 year of age. Keep in mind that too much fiber can limit nutrient absorption because it binds to some minerals and speeds the passage of food through the GI tract. Let the child's bowel habits be your guide. If the child is constipated, try increasing fiber and fluid intakes. On the other hand, if the child is uncomfortably gassy or is having many soft bowel movements per day, decrease the amount of fiber in the diet.

PROTEIN

Daily protein needs in infancy are about 9 grams per day for younger infants and about 11 grams per day for older infants. These recommendations are based on the typical consumption of human milk by breastfed infants for 0 to 6 months and then on the increased protein needs for growth for older infants. About half of total protein intake should come from essential amino acids. As with carbohydrate, protein needs are easily satisfied by either human milk or infant formula. However, as you learned in Section 6.3, protein metabolism generates waste products that must be excreted by the kidneys. Dietary patterns that are excessive in protein may stress the infant's immature kidneys, so protein intake should not greatly exceed these recommendations.

In North America, infant protein deficiency is unlikely, except in cases of inappropriate formula preparation, such as when an infant's formula is excessively diluted with water. Protein deficiency may also be induced by elimination diets used to detect food **allergies.** As foods are eliminated from the diet, infants may not be offered enough protein to compensate for that supplied by the suspected food allergen (see Section 15.7).

allergy A hypersensitive immune response that occurs when the immune system identifies a harmless protein (e.g., a food protein) as a harmful pathogen (i.e., antigen) and attempts to destroy it.

FAT

Infants need about 30 grams of fat per day. Essential fatty acids should make up about 15% of total fat intake (about 5 grams per day). Both recommendations are again based on the typical consumption of human milk by breastfed infants and the eventual intake of solid foods. Fats are an important part of the infant's dietary pattern because they are vital to the development of the nervous system. Also, fats are a concentrated source of energy (9 kcal per gram). The stomach capacity of an infant is limited, so a concentrated source of calories is necessary to meet overall energy requirements. Thus, restriction of fat intake is not advised for infants or children under age 2 (Fig. 15-2).

Arachidonic acid (ARA) and docosahexaenoic acid (DHA) are two long-chain fatty acids that have important roles in infant development. These fatty acids can be made in the body from the essential fatty acids or they can be consumed as part of the diet. The nervous system, especially the brain and eyes, depends on these fatty acids for proper development. During the last trimester, DHA and ARA provided by the mother accumulate in the brain and retinas of the eyes in the fetus. Breastfed infants continue to acquire these fatty acids from human milk, especially if their mothers are regularly eating fish. Since 2002, infant formula manufacturers have been adding ARA and DHA to their products to match the average fatty acid composition of human milk. Such infant formulas are particularly useful for feeding preterm infants.

VITAMINS OF SPECIAL INTEREST

All of the essential vitamins play important roles in infant growth and development, but three vitamins—K, D, and B-12—are of special interest for infants because levels tend to be low and the consequences of deficiency are dire.

In Section 8.5, you learned about the role of vitamin K in blood clotting. Newborn infants have low levels of vitamin K because (1) limited amounts of this vitamin are transferred from the mother to the fetus during gestation; (2) breast milk is not particularly high in vitamin K; and (3) newborn infants lack the intestinal bacteria that synthesize vitamin K. Infant vitamin K deficiency can lead to a rare but potentially fatal bleeding problem. To prevent hemorrhage, vitamin K is routinely given by injection to all infants at birth.

For bone health, immune function, and chronic disease prevention, the American Academy of Pediatrics recommends that all infants and children consume 400 IU

FIGURE 15-2 ▶ The labels on infant foods, like those on adult foods, contain a Nutrition Facts panel; however, the information provided on infant food labels differs from that on adult food labels, (see Fig. 2-12 for a comparison). There are separate Daily Values set for infants through 12 months of age and children 1–3 years of age.

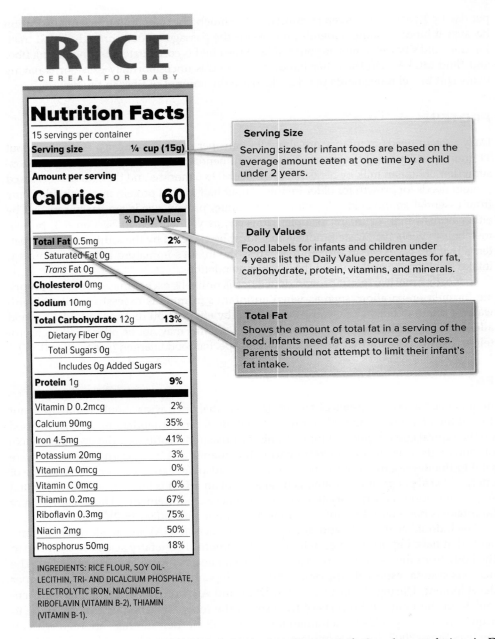

Serving Size
Serving sizes for infant foods are based on the average amount eaten at one time by a child under 2 years.

Daily Values
Food labels for infants and children under 4 years list the Daily Value percentages for fat, carbohydrate, protein, vitamins, and minerals.

Total Fat
Shows the amount of total fat in a serving of the food. Infants need fat as a source of calories. Parents should not attempt to limit their infant's fat intake.

vitamin D per day starting soon after birth (review Section 8.3). Supplemental vitamin D is necessary for all breastfed infants, as well as for formula-fed infants who consume less than 1 quart (approximately 1 liter) of formula per day.[2] However, no further benefits are seen beyond 400 IU per day, and toxicity is possible if intake exceeds 1000 IU per day. Any use of supplemental vitamin D can be discontinued when dietary sources provide at least 400 IU of vitamin D per day.

For breastfed infants whose mothers are total vegetarians (vegans), a supplemental source of vitamin B-12 is vitally important to prevent anemia, failure to thrive, and irreversible damage to the nervous system. Recall from Section 8.13 that vitamin B-12 is only found in foods of animal origin. Infant formula does contain vitamin B-12, but the breast milk of a mother who avoids all animal products will be deficient in vitamin B-12.

MINERALS OF SPECIAL INTEREST

Two minerals of special interest in the diets of infants are iron and fluoride. Infants also need adequate amounts of zinc (see Section 9.10) and iodine (see Section 9.12) to support growth. However, when human milk and infant formula are provided in quantities to meet kilocalorie needs, zinc and iodine requirements are generally met.

Infants are born with some internal stores of iron. However, if food sources of iron are not part of the infant's dietary pattern, body iron stores will be depleted by about 6 months of age. If the mother was iron deficient during the pregnancy, these iron stores will be exhausted even sooner. As you will recall from Section 9.9, iron-deficiency anemia can lead to poor mental development in infants. Several studies indicate that iron-deficiency anemia during infancy, even if corrected, has a lasting impact in terms of cognition, motor development, and behavior later in life.

To maintain a desirable iron status, the American Academy of Pediatrics recommends that formula-fed infants should be given an iron-fortified formula from birth. Years ago, low-iron formulas were prescribed for infants with gastrointestinal distress; however, current evidence shows that they do not improve GI symptoms but rather place an infant at risk for iron deficiency. Low-iron infant formulas are still available, but their use is strongly discouraged.

Breast milk is lower in iron than fortified infant formulas, but the form of iron in breast milk is much more bioavailable than the form in infant formula. Even so, by about 6 months of age, breastfed infants need solid foods to supply extra iron. This need for iron is a major consideration in the decision to introduce solid foods. To prevent iron deficiency, the American Academy of Pediatrics recommends that exclusively breastfed infants should receive iron supplements starting at 4 months of age and continuing until dietary sources of iron are introduced. Preterm and low-birth-weight infants, those with blood disorders, or infants born to anemic mothers may also need supplemental iron.[3]

Breast milk is a poor source of fluoride, and formula manufacturers use fluoride-free water in formula preparation, so intake of this mineral during the first 6 months of life is low. However, fluoride supplementation is not advised before 6 months of age. After 6 months, the pediatrician or dentist may recommend fluoride supplements to aid in tooth development if fluoride supplied by tap water, foods, and toothpaste is inadequate.

WATER

An infant needs about 3 cups (700 to 800 milliliters) of water per day to regulate body temperature and transport oxygen, nutrients, and wastes throughout the body. For the vast majority of infants, human milk or formula supply enough water to keep the infant well hydrated.

In infants, dehydration can occur rapidly and have devastating consequences. In the first few days after birth, improper feeding techniques can leave an infant deprived of water and nutrients. In addition, protracted episodes of vomiting or diarrhea can quickly deplete an infant of fluid and electrolytes.

To identify dehydration, look for these signs:

- More than 6 hours without a wet diaper
- Dark-yellow or strong-smelling urine
- Unusually tired and fussy
- Dry mouth and lips
- Absence of tears when crying
- Eyes and soft spot on the head appear sunken
- Cold and splotchy hands and feet

Severe dehydration can result in rapid loss of kidney function and warrants medical intervention. In some cases, hospitalization and intravenous rehydration may be necessary. Most of the time, dehydration can be corrected with special fluid-replacement formulas containing electrolytes, such as sodium and potassium. These oral rehydration solutions (e.g., Pedialyte)® are available in supermarkets and pharmacies to treat mild to moderate dehydration. A health care provider should guide any use of these products.

Caregivers often wonder if breast milk or formula is sufficient to keep an infant hydrated, especially in hot weather. They may be tempted to give an infant supplemental

The American Dental Association does not recommend fluoridated bottled water for use by infants because it heightens risk for enamel **fluorosis** during early tooth development.

fluorosis Discoloration of tooth enamel sometimes accompanied with pitting due to consuming a large amount of fluoride for an excessive period.

hyponatremia Dangerously low blood sodium level.

water or fruit juice. In some stores, bottled water products marketed specifically for infants may be placed alongside infant formulas and electrolyte-replacement solutions, giving the mistaken impression that bottled water products are an appropriate feeding supplement or substitute for fluid replacement for infants. Even in hot weather, the American Academy of Pediatrics does not recommend supplemental water or juice during the first 6 months. Excess water can cause **hyponatremia** in infants. It is important to remember that excessive fluid can be harmful, especially to the brain.

Overall, it is best to rely exclusively on breast milk or infant formula to meet infant fluid needs up to 6 months of age, unless a health care provider suggests otherwise. In sum, extremes in fluid intake—either too little or too much—can lead to health problems.

> ✅ **CONCEPT CHECK 15.2**
>
> 1. Using the EER equations listed in Table 15-2, calculate the kilocalorie needs of a healthy 4-month-old infant who weighs 15 pounds (6.8 kilograms).
> 2. Review Table 15-3. Why is unaltered cow's milk NOT recommended for infant feeding?
> 3. Do infants require any supplemental vitamins or minerals? If so, which ones? What is the rationale for their use?
> 4. You are planning a family trip to the zoo on a hot summer day. How can you keep your 3-month-old baby from becoming dehydrated?

15.3 Guidelines for Infant Feeding

Oral nutrition for infants comes in two forms: human breast milk or infant formula. As you learned in Section 14.7, breastfeeding is the preferred method of infant feeding (review Table 14-4). Besides its benefits for immune development, improved mother-infant bonding, and lower long-term risk for chronic diseases, breast milk offers optimal nutrition that is uniquely suited for human infants. For mothers who do not breastfeed, whether due to necessity or preference, infant formula is a workable substitute. In fact, formula manufacturers model their products on human milk. In areas of the world with safe water supplies, formula feeding is a safe and nutritionally adequate alternative to breastfeeding.

BREAST MILK IS THE BEST MILK

Human milk is uniquely suited to meet the nutritional needs of human infants. Table 15-3 gives the composition of human milk, but recognize that these numbers are just estimates. Maternal diet and nutritional status may impact the composition of breast milk, particularly for fatty acids and some micronutrients. In addition, the true composition of human milk changes over time as the infant matures and even within a feeding.

Breast milk provides up to 55% of total calories as fat. Fat is a dense source of calories, so it helps to meet the high energy needs of the growing infant even though the infant cannot consume a large volume of milk at one time. Interestingly, the fat content of breast milk changes within each feeding. When the baby first latches on and begins suckling, the consistency of breast milk is thin and watery; the infant takes in necessary carbohydrates, protein, vitamins, and minerals. As the feeding goes on, the fat content of the milk increases to fulfill energy needs and satisfy the infant's hunger for a few hours. The specific types of fat in human milk are ideal for infants, too. The short- and medium-chain fatty acids in breast milk are easily digested. Some of the fatty acids—ARA and DHA—are essential for proper brain and eye development. If the mother's dietary pattern is rich in these fats, her milk will be a better source of them for her infant as well.

Carbohydrates provide about 35% to 40% of the calories in human milk. The main carbohydrate in human milk is lactose, a disaccharide that tastes sweet and is easily

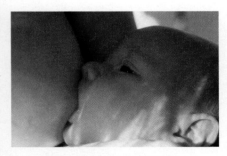

▲ Breastfeeding takes some skill and patience on the part of the mother, especially in the first few weeks, but the physical and emotional benefits are worth the effort. ©Getty Images

digested in the human infant's digestive tract. Although lactase production tends to decline later in life, lactose intolerance is quite rare among infants (review Section 4.4). Human milk also contains some oligosaccharides that have a **prebiotic** effect on the community of beneficial microorganisms in the infant's gut. A healthy microbial population in the GI tract influences development of the infant's immune system.

Protein supplies less than 10% of the total calories in human milk. The kidneys of the newborn infant are still immature, so they can be stressed by high protein intakes. The proteins that are present in human milk are easily digested and unlikely to trigger food allergies. These proteins do more than supply calories and building blocks for tissue synthesis. They also promote the proper development of the immune system and enhance nutrient absorption.

For the most part, the micronutrient needs of the infant can be met by human milk. A notable exception, described in Section 15.2, is vitamin D. Recall that the American Academy of Pediatrics recommends 400 IU per day of supplemental vitamin D for all infants (breastfed and formula-fed) until their dietary intake supplies this amount. For breastfed infants of mothers who follow a vegan diet, have had bariatric surgery, or have pernicious anemia, vitamin B-12 supplements are recommended. Last, if an infant has depleted iron stores (e.g., preterm birth or mother was deficient in iron during pregnancy), iron supplementation may be needed.

Breastfeeding during infancy impacts future feeding behaviors as well. Interesting research shows that the flavors of the mother's diet are transferred into her milk. This can positively affect the infant's acceptance of a variety of solid foods later in life. Breastfeeding also reinforces the natural ability of the infant or child to self-regulate food intake. The infant has to do some work to get milk from the mother's breast, so it is unlikely that the infant will override satiety cues and overeat from the breast. A growing body of research supports the hypothesis that breastfed infants learn to eat based on internal cues of hunger and satiety, leading to better body weight management and lower risk for cardiovascular diseases and type 2 diabetes throughout life.

FORMULA FEEDING FOR INFANTS

Young infants cannot tolerate unaltered cow's milk because of its high protein and mineral content. Cow's milk is perfect for the growth needs of calves but not for human infants! Thus, cow's milk must be altered by formula manufacturers to be safe for infant feeding. Altered forms of cow's milk, known as infant formulas, must conform to strict federal guidelines for nutrient composition and quality.

Formulas generally contain lactose and/or sucrose for carbohydrate, heat-treated proteins from cow's milk, and vegetable oils for fat (review Table 15-3). Soy protein–based formulas are available for vegan infants or those who cannot tolerate lactose or the types of proteins found in cow's milk. Infants with milk protein allergies are often sensitive to soy as well, so the best choice for infants with allergies is a **hydrolyzed protein formula**. In this type of formula, the proteins have been broken down into small polypeptides and amino acids. A variety of other specialized formulas are also available for specific medical conditions. In any case, it is important to use an iron-fortified formula unless a pediatrician recommends otherwise.

Some transition formulas/beverages have been introduced for older infants and toddlers (review Table 15-3). A few of these products are intended for use after 6 months of age if the infant is consuming solid foods, but most are intended for use only by toddlers (i.e., age 12 months and older). These transition products are lower in fat than human milk or standard infant formulas; their iron content is higher than that of cow's milk; and their overall mineral content is generally more like that of human milk than cow's milk. According to the manufacturers, the advantages of these transition formulas/beverages over standard formulas for older infants and toddlers include reduced cost and better flavor. Parents should consult their primary care provider with regard to the use of these products.

Infant formula comes in several different forms. Some infant formulas come in ready-to-feed, liquid form. These can be simply poured into a clean bottle and fed to the infant

prebiotic Selectively fermented ingredient that results in specific changes in the composition and/or activity of the gastrointestinal microbiota, thus conferring benefits upon the host.

hydrolyzed protein formula Infant formula in which the proteins have been broken down into smaller peptides and amino acids to improve digestibility and reduce exposure to potential food allergens; sometimes called *predigested* or *hypoallergenic infant formula*.

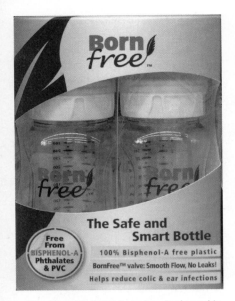

▲ Bisphenol A (BPA) is a chemical used in the production of many plastics. Human exposure to BPA, mainly through leaching of the chemical from packaging into foods and beverages, is widespread. Concern about exposure stems from animal studies that link high doses of BPA with reproductive and developmental defects and cancer. The consensus among regulatory agencies in the United States and Canada is that current levels of BPA exposure are not harmful, even for infants. Nevertheless, in response to public concern, the U.S. Food and Drug Administration (FDA) has banned the use of BPA in the manufacture of baby bottles, sippy cups, and packaging for infant formulas. ©McGraw-Hill Education/Mark Dierker, photographer

without further preparation. Powdered and concentrated fluid formula preparations are also commonly used. Powdered or concentrated formulas should be combined with clean, cold water, precisely following the directions on the formula label. The formula is then warmed, if desired, and fed immediately to the infant.

The following are some tips for safe preparation and storage of infant formula:

- All containers and utensils used to prepare formula should be washed with hot, soapy water and thoroughly rinsed with clean water before use. Household dishwashers are a good way to clean bottles and utensils, too. It is not necessary to boil the containers and utensils prior to use.
- Use cold water to prepare infant formula. Hot water that sits in a hot water heater or runs through pipes made with lead is more likely to accumulate contaminants than cold water (see Section 13.6). For homes with older plumbing systems, it is prudent to let cold tap water run for 1 to 2 minutes before filling a bottle or cup.
- If well water will be used to make infant formula, it should be tested regularly for contaminants, such as naturally occurring nitrates, which can lead to a severe form of anemia (especially among babies younger than 1 year).
- If microbial contamination of well water or municipal tap water is a concern, water should be brought to a rolling boil (for 1 minute) and then cooled to room temperature (for up to 30 minutes) before use in formula preparation. Caregivers should pay close attention to local water advisories. Some pediatricians recommend boiling (then cooling) the water to be used in formula preparation for infants up to 6 months of age, regardless of reports about water safety.
- The American Dental Association does not recommend that formula be mixed with bottled "nursery water," which can be found alongside infant formula in most supermarkets, to limit risk of tooth discoloration from high fluoride levels.
- To warm a bottle of formula, run hot water over it or place it briefly in a pan of simmering water. Infant formulas should not be heated in a microwave oven because hot spots may develop, which can burn the infant's mouth and esophagus.
- Refrigerating prepared formula for 1 day is safe. However, formula left over from a feeding should be discarded because it will be contaminated by bacteria and enzymes from the infant's saliva.

FEEDING TECHNIQUE

Infants swallow a lot of air as they ingest either formula or human milk. To alleviate discomfort, it is important to burp an infant during feeding (every 1 to 2 ounces) and again at the end of the feeding. Spitting up a bit of milk is normal at this time.

Formula intake and feeding frequency may vary considerably from one infant to another and also from one day to the next. In general, a formula-fed infant should consume about 2 1/2 fluid ounces (75 milliliters) of formula per pound of body weight each day (see Table 15-4), up to about 32 fluid ounces (960 milliliters) in one day. In most cases, however, the infant's appetite is a better guide than any standardized recommendations. When the infant begins acting full, bottle feeding should be stopped, even if some milk is left in the bottle. Common signals that an infant has had enough include turning the head

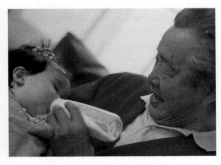

▲ Falling asleep while feeding is a sign that the infant has had enough to eat. ©Steve Mason/Getty Images

TABLE 15-4 ■ Typical Formula Intake of Infants

Age	Amount per Feeding	Frequency
<1 month	2 to 3 fluid ounces (60 to 90 ml)	Every 3 to 4 hours
1 to 6 months	4 to 6 fluid ounces (120 to 180 ml)	Every 4 to 6 hours
6 to 12 months	6 to 8 fluid ounces (180 to 240 ml)*	Every 4 to 6 hours

Source: Data from American Academy of Pediatrics: *Caring for your baby and young child: Birth to age 5*. 6th ed. New York: Bantam Books, 2014.

*With introduction of age-appropriate solid foods

away, being inattentive, falling asleep, or becoming playful. Breastfeeding infants usually have had enough to eat after about 20 minutes. Although it is difficult to tell how much milk breastfed infants are getting, they also give recognizable signs when they are full.

By carefully observing and responding appropriately to the cues of the bottle-feeding or breastfeeding infant, caregivers can (1) be assured that the infant's calorie needs are being met; (2) foster a climate of trust and responsiveness; and (3) help a child develop a habit of respecting internal cues of hunger and satiety.

EXPANDING THE INFANT'S MEALTIME CHOICES

By about 4 to 6 months of age, the infant is ready to start eating solid foods. Initially, solid foods add to—rather than replace—human milk or formula. In the first attempts to introduce solid foods, just getting the food into the infant's mouth may be a challenge. By the end of the first year, though, the infant should be eating a variety of protein sources, vegetables, fruits, and grains so that the diet begins to reflect a balanced pattern (Table 15-5). Throughout the process of expanding the infant's mealtime choices, the caregiver must proceed slowly and respond to the infant's cues that he or she is hungry or has had enough to eat. Feeding habits developed through early exposures to food will set the stage for healthy eating to last a lifetime.

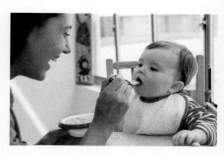

▲ Iron-fortified rice cereal is recommended as the first solid food to be fed to infants.
©E. Dygas/Getty Images

Recognizing the Infant's Readiness for Solid Foods. Parents may believe that the early addition of solid foods will help an infant sleep through the night. Actually, this achievement is a developmental milestone, and the type of food consumed by the infant is of little relevance to a good night's sleep. Before 4 months of age, infants are not physically mature enough to consume much solid food. Only occasionally does a rapidly growing infant need solid foods to meet calorie and nutrient needs before 6 months of age.

TABLE 15-5 ■ Sample Daily Menu for a 1-Year-Old Child*

Breakfast	Snack
1 to 2 tbsp unsweetened applesauce	½ ounce cheddar cheese
¼ cup Cheerios®	4 whole wheat crackers
½ cup whole milk	½ cup whole milk
Snack	**Dinner**
½ hard-cooked egg	1 ounce roasted turkey (finely diced)
½ slice whole wheat toast with ½ tsp butter	1 to 2 tbsp mashed potatoes with ½ tsp butter
½ cup mandarin orange segments	1 to 2 tbsp cooked carrots (cut in strips, not coins)
½ cup water	½ cup whole milk
Lunch	**Snack**
1 ounce roasted chicken, minced	½ banana
1 to 2 tbsp rice with ½ tsp butter	2 oatmeal cookies (no raisins)
1 to 2 tbsp cooked peas	½ cup whole milk
½ cup whole milk	

Nutritional Analysis	
Total energy (kcal)	1100
% energy from	
Carbohydrate	40%
Protein	19%
Fat	41%

*This diet is just a start. A 1 year old may need more or less food. In those cases, serving sizes should be adjusted. The milk can be fed by cup; some can be put into a bottle if the child has not been fully weaned from the bottle.

How does the caregiver know it is time to introduce solid foods? Infant size can serve as a rough indicator of readiness: reaching a weight of at least 13 pounds (6 kilograms) is a preliminary sign of readiness for solid foods. Another physiological cue is frequency of feeding, such as consuming more than 32 ounces (1 liter) of formula daily or breast-feeding more than 8 to 10 times within 24 hours. Underlying these noticeable signals are several important developmental factors:

1. *Nutritional need.* Before the infant is 6 months old, nutritional needs can generally be met with human milk and/or formula. After 6 months of age, however, many infants need additional calories. In terms of individual nutrients, iron stores are exhausted by about 6 months of age. Developmentally appropriate, nutrient-dense foods will help to meet the infant's calorie and iron needs.
2. *Physiological capabilities.* Before about 3 months of age, an infant's digestive tract cannot readily digest starch. Also, kidney function is limited until about 4 to 6 weeks of age. Until then, waste products from excessive amounts of dietary protein or minerals are difficult to excrete. As the infant ages, the ability to digest and metabolize a wider range of food components improves.
3. *Physical ability.* Three physical markers indicate that a child is ready for solid foods: (1) the disappearance of the extrusion reflex (thrusting the tongue forward and pushing food out of the mouth); (2) head and neck control; and (3) the ability to sit up with support. These usually occur around 4 to 6 months of age, but they vary with each infant.
4. *Allergy prevention.* Because a newborn's digestive system is still immature, whole proteins can readily be absorbed from birth until 4 to 5 months of age. If the infant is exposed too early to some types of proteins, the infant may be predisposed to future allergies and autoimmune conditions (e.g., type 1 diabetes). However, there is no benefit to delaying introduction of solid foods beyond 6 months of age.

With these considerations in mind—nutritional need, physiological and physical readiness, and allergy prevention—solid foods should be introduced between 4 and 6 months of age.

Foods to Match Needs and Developmental Abilities During the First Year. If solid foods are introduced before 6 months of age, the primary goal of the food should be to meet iron needs. Therefore, the first solid foods should be iron-fortified cereals. Some pediatricians may recommend lean ground (strained) meats for more absorbable forms of iron. Rice is the best cereal to begin with because it is least likely to trigger allergies.

When starting solid foods, begin with a teaspoon serving size of a single-ingredient food item, such as rice cereal, and increase the serving size gradually over the next few days. Once the new food has been fed for about a week without adverse effects, another food can be added to the infant's diet. At first, this can be another type of cereal or perhaps a cooked and strained (or mashed) vegetable, meat, fruit, or egg yolk.

Waiting about 7 days between the introduction of each new food is important because it can take that long for evidence of an allergy or intolerance to materialize. Also, it is best to avoid introducing mixed foods until each component of the combination dish has been given separately without an adverse reaction. Signs of food allergies include diarrhea, vomiting, a rash, or wheezing. If one or more of these signs appears, the suspected problem food should be avoided for several weeks and then reintroduced in a small quantity. If the problem continues, a pediatrician should be consulted. Fortunately, many babies outgrow food allergies later in childhood.

Until 2008, parents and caregivers were advised to avoid feeding children a wide range of potentially allergenic foods, including egg whites, chocolate, peanuts, tree nuts, fish, and other seafood. Now, the American Academy of Pediatrics acknowledges that there is no evidence that delaying introduction of solid foods—including these common food allergens—beyond 6 months of age is of any benefit for prevention of food allergies and other **atopic diseases.** Indeed, the most recent guidelines from the National Institute of Allergy and Infectious Diseases recommend early introduction of peanut protein—between 4 and 6 months of age—to infants at risk of food allergies.[4,5]

---

atopic disease A condition involving an inappropriate immune response to environmental allergens; examples include asthma, eczema, and seasonal allergies.

Example of Typical Solid Food Progression, Starting at 6 Months of Age*

Week 1	Rice cereal
Week 2	Add strained carrots
Week 3	Add applesauce
Week 4	Add oat cereal
Week 5	Add cooked egg yolk
Week 6	Add strained chicken
Week 7	Add strained peas
Week 8	Add plums

*Extending the rice cereal step for a month or so is advised if solid food introduction begins at 4 months of age. Also, if at any point signs of allergy or intolerance develop, substitute another similar food item.

Many strained foods for infant feeding are available at the supermarket. Single-food items are more desirable than mixed dinners and desserts, which are less nutrient dense. Most brands have no added salt, but some fruit desserts contain added sugar, which is not recommended for infant feeding.[6] Read food labels carefully to find the most nutrient-dense foods for infants.

As an alternative to store-bought baby foods, plain, unseasoned cooked foods—vegetables, fruits, and meats—can be ground up in an inexpensive baby food grinder at home. Another option is to puree a larger amount of food in a blender, freeze it in ice-cube portions, store in plastic bags, and defrost and warm as needed. Careful attention to food safety is necessary. Seasonings that may please the rest of the family should not be added to infant foods made at home. The infant does not notice the difference if salt, sugar, or spices are omitted. It is best to introduce infants to a variety of foods, so that by the end of the first year, the infant is consuming many foods—human milk or formula, meats, fruits, vegetables, and grains.

To ease early attempts at feeding solid foods, consider the following tips:

- Use a baby-sized spoon; a small spoon with a long handle is best.
- Hold the infant comfortably on the lap, as for breastfeeding or bottle feeding, but a little more upright to ease swallowing. When in this position, the infant expects food.
- Put a small dab of food on the spoon tip and gently place it on the infant's tongue.
- Convey a calm and casual approach to the infant, who needs time to get used to food.
- Expect the infant to take only two or three bites of the first meals.
- Present a new food on several consecutive days to aid an infant's acceptance of that food.

Self-feeding skills require coordination and can develop only if the infant is allowed to practice and experiment. By 6 to 7 months of age, the infant has learned to handle finger foods and transfer objects from one hand to the other with some dexterity. At about this time, teeth also begin to appear. By age 7 to 8 months, infants can push food around on a plate, play with a drinking cup, hold a bottle, and self-feed a cracker or a piece of toast. Through mastery of these manipulations, infants develop confidence and self-esteem. It is important that parents be patient and support these early self-feeding attempts, even though they appear inefficient.

At 9 to 10 months of age, the infant's desire to explore, experience, and play with foods may hinder feeding. Food is used as a means to explore the environment, and therefore, feeding time is often very messy—a bowl of macaroni may end up in the child's hair! Caregivers need to relax and take this phase of infant development in stride. By the end of the first year, finger-feeding becomes more efficient, and chewing is easier as more teeth erupt. Still, experimentation and unpredictability are to be expected.

WEANING FROM THE BREAST OR BOTTLE

Around the age of 6 months, expressed breast milk, formula, or water can be offered in a sippy cup with a wide, flat bottom. Drinking from a cup rather than from a bottle helps to prevent **early childhood caries** (Fig. 15-3). If an infant drinks continuously from a bottle, the carbohydrate-rich fluid bathes the teeth, providing an ideal growth medium for bacteria adhering to the teeth. These bacteria then make acids, which dissolve tooth enamel. To avoid dental caries, infants should not be put to bed with a bottle or placed in an infant seat with a bottle propped up.

By about 10 months of age, infants are learning to self-feed and likewise to drink independently from a cup. As children drink from a cup more frequently, fewer bottle feedings and/or breastfeedings are necessary. Infants should begin drinking from a cup by 1 year of age and should be completely weaned from a bottle by 18 months of age. The added mobility of crawling and walking should naturally lead to gradual weaning from the bottle or breast. Even so, getting a baby out of the bedtime-bottle habit can be difficult. Determined caregivers can either endure a few nights of their baby's crying or slowly wean the baby away from the bottle with either a pacifier or water (for a week or so).

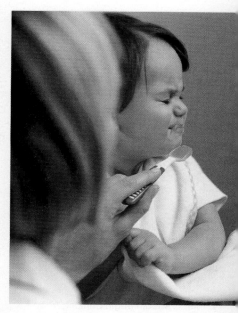

▲ Repeated exposure fosters acceptance of new tastes and textures. ©Corbis/ PictureQuest

early childhood caries Tooth decay that results from formula or juice (and even human milk) bathing the teeth as the child sleeps with a bottle in the mouth. The upper teeth are mostly affected as the lower teeth are protected by the tongue; formerly called *nursing bottle syndrome* and *baby bottle tooth decay*.

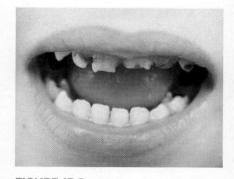

FIGURE 15-3 ▲ Early childhood caries. This type of tooth decay may have resulted from frequently putting the child to bed with a bottle. Some of the upper teeth have decayed almost all the way to the gum line. ©Zoonar/Ruslan Nassyrov/Alamy

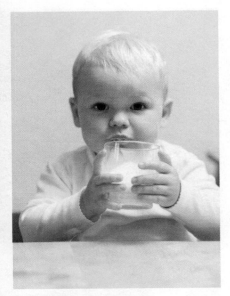

▲ Infants should begin drinking from a cup by 1 year of age. Cups with lids help to prevent spills, but caregivers should allow a toddler to practice without a lid as dexterity and coordination improve. ©StockFood/Getty Images

WHAT TO FEED AN INFANT

It can be difficult for new parents to make sense of nutrition goals for infants in the face of changing dietary recommendations from health authorities, cultural preferences, and outdated advice from friends and family. In response to various controversies surrounding infant feeding, the American Academy of Pediatrics has issued a number of statements concerning infant diets.[7] The following guidelines are based on these statements:

- *Build to a variety of foods.* For the first 6 months of life, human milk (or infant formula) is usually all an infant needs. (Vitamin D supplementation is an exception.) When the infant is ready, start adding new foods, one at a time. During the first year, the goal is to teach an infant to enjoy a variety of nutritious foods. A lifetime of healthy eating habits begins during infancy!
- *Pay attention to your infant's appetite to avoid overfeeding or underfeeding.* Feed infants when they are hungry. Never force an infant to finish an unwanted serving of food. Watch for signs that indicate hunger or fullness. This will reinforce the infant's natural ability to self-regulate food intake.
- *Infants need fat.* Although fat contributes to many adult health problems when it is consumed in excessive amounts, it is an essential source of calories for growing infants. Fat also helps the nervous system to develop.
- *Choose fruits, vegetables, and grains, but do not overdo high-fiber foods.* During the second half of the first year, infants should be fed a variety of fruits and vegetables. However, studies show that by 1 year of age, vegetable choices are dominated by white potatoes. Continuing to offer choices of colorful vegetables during late infancy and the toddler years will enhance intake of important vitamins, minerals, and phytochemicals. In terms of fiber, although many adults benefit from high-fiber diets, they are not ideal for infants. They are bulky, low in calories, and may limit absorption of minerals. The natural amounts of fiber and nutrients in fruits, vegetables, and grains are appropriate as part of a healthy infant diet.
- *Use sugars in moderation.* Sugars are a source of calories for active, rapidly growing infants. Foods such as human milk, fruits, and small portions of 100% juices are natural sources of sugars and other nutrients as well. On the other hand, an excessive intake of added sugars, particularly from sugar-sweetened beverages, contributes to the epidemic of childhood obesity. Caregivers should choose infant foods that do not contain added sugars. Foods that contain artificial sweeteners should also be avoided; they do not provide the calories or nutrients growing infants need.
- *Skip heavily seasoned and processed foods.* Sodium is an essential mineral found naturally in almost all foods. As part of a healthy diet, infants need sodium for their bodies to work properly. However, average intakes of sodium among infants and toddlers are above the AI. Caregivers should delay introduction of cow's milk (a natural source of sodium) until 1 year of age and refrain from offering heavily seasoned and processed foods.
- *Choose foods containing iron, zinc, and calcium.* Infants need good sources of iron, zinc, and calcium for optimum growth throughout the first 2 years. These minerals are important for healthy blood, optimal growth, and strong bones. Many infant and toddler foods (e.g., cereal, crackers, and biter biscuits) are fortified with these minerals.

WHAT *NOT* TO FEED AN INFANT

The following are several foods and practices to avoid when feeding an infant:

- *Excessive infant formula or human milk.* After 6 months of age, solid foods should play an increasing role in satisfying an infant's growing appetite. Age-appropriate solid foods provide necessary calories and iron, plus they help the infant to develop motor skills. About 24 to 32 ounces (¾ to 1 liter) of human milk or formula daily is ideal after 6 months, with complementary foods supplying the rest of the infant's energy needs.
- *Foods that tend to cause choking.* Foods that are round or ovoid in shape, larger than a half inch in diameter, or of a soft or sticky texture can easily get lodged in a child's throat. These foods include hot dogs, hard or gummy candies, whole nuts, grapes, coarsely cut

meats, raw carrots, popcorn, and peanut butter. Caregivers should not allow younger children to gobble snack foods during playtime and should supervise all meals.

- *Potential food allergens before 4 months of age.* Cow's milk, egg whites, peanuts, tree nuts, soy, and wheat are responsible for 90% of food allergies in childhood. If any solid foods are introduced before 4 months of age, they should be iron-fortified rice or oat cereals, pureed meats, vegetables, or fruits.

- *Cow's milk, especially low-fat or fat-free cow's milk.* The American Academy of Pediatrics strongly urges parents not to give children under age 2 fat-reduced, 1%, or fat-free milk. Before age 2, the amount of this milk needed to meet energy needs would supply too many minerals, which could overwhelm the kidneys. The lower fat intake might also harm nervous system development. Beyond 2 years, children can drink fat-reduced, 1%, or fat-free milk because by this age, they are consuming enough solid foods to meet calorie and fat needs.

- *Goat's milk.* Although perceived by some to pose lower risk for food allergies, goat's milk is low in folate, iron, vitamin C, and vitamin D, and should not be used as a source of nourishment for infants.

- *Excessive Fruit juice.* The fructose and sorbitol contained in some fruit juices, especially apple and pear juices, can lead to diarrhea because they are slowly absorbed. Also, if fruit juice or related drink products are replacing formula or milk in the diet, the infant may not be receiving adequate calories, calcium, or other nutrients essential for proper growth. Studies have shown a link between excessive amounts of fruit juice and failure to thrive, GI tract complications, obesity, short stature, and poor dental health. Fruit juice is not recommended at all for infants. After 1 year of age, limit fruit juice to 4 to 8 fluid ounces per day. See Sections 15.4 and 15.5 for age-specific recommendations.

- *Food safety hazards.* The immune system is still maturing during infancy and early childhood, so it is important to avoid potential sources of foodborne illness (review Chapter 13). For example, raw (unpasteurized) milk or soft cheeses (e.g., queso fresco) may be contaminated with bacteria or viruses. Meat, poultry, eggs, and seafood should be cooked to proper temperatures. In addition, honey may contain spores of *Clostridium botulinum,* which can lead to the potentially fatal foodborne illness known as *botulism.* Safe food handling starts with proper handwashing.

- *Excessive nutrient supplementation.* Intake of supplemental vitamins or minerals above 100% of the RDA or AI for age can increase risk for nutrient toxicities.

A Summary of Infant Feeding Recommendations

Breastfed Infants

- Breastfeed for 6 months or longer, if possible. Then introduce infant formula if and when breastfeeding declines or ceases. (Breast milk can also be pumped and placed in a bottle for later use.)
- Provide a vitamin D supplement (400 IU per day).
- Investigate the need for vitamin B-12, fluoride, and iron supplementation to prevent deficiencies.

Formula-Fed Infants

- Use iron-fortified infant formula for the first year of life.
- Provide a vitamin D supplement if formula intake provides less than 400 IU per day.
- Investigate the need for a fluoride supplement if the water supply is not fluoridated.

All Infants

- Introduce a variety of basic, soft foods starting between 4 and 6 months of age, advancing to a varied diet.
- Early solid food choices should include a source of iron, such as iron-fortified infant cereal.

CASE STUDY Undernutrition During Infancy

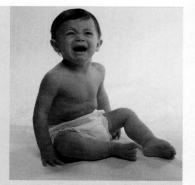

©Kwame Zikomo/PureStock/SuperStock

Damon is a 7-month-old boy who has been taken into a clinic for a routine checkup. On examination, he was found to be moderately underweight relative to his age and body length. His pediatrician scheduled a follow-up appointment in 3 months. At the 10-month visit, Damon appeared sluggish and was even more underweight for his age and length.

A registered dietitian nutritionist interviewed Damon's 16-year-old mother to collect information on Damon's dietary intake. His intake over the previous 24 hours consisted of two 8-ounce bottles of infant formula, three 8-ounce bottles of Kool-Aid,® and a hot dog. Damon may have been fed some additional items on the nights that his mother left him with a neighbor, so that she could go out with friends for a few hours. Thus, she was not aware of all that he ate.

1. Damon's mother did not specify what type of formula she gives to her child or how she prepares it. What questions would you ask about his formula?
2. What potential dangers await Damon if his growth continues to lag behind?
3. What foods should Damon's caregivers offer that are appropriate for his age and nutritional needs?
4. What problems might arise from consumption of sugary drinks from a bottle?
5. Does Damon need any vitamin or mineral supplements?

Complete the Case Study. Responses to these questions can be provided by your instructor.

✓ CONCEPT CHECK 15.3

1. List three similarities between human milk and infant formula. List three differences.
2. Describe four ways to assess an infant's readiness for solid foods.
3. Excessive intake of added sugars is common in late infancy. Describe several ways to limit intake of added sugars in an infant's diet.
4. List three foods to avoid feeding infants during the first year of life.

15.4 Toddlers and Preschool Children: Nutrition Concerns

Quick Guide to Child Nutrition Needs

Carbohydrates

- 130 grams per day to supply energy for the central nervous system and prevent ketosis

Protein

- 13 to 19 grams per day (ages 1 to 3)
- 34 to 52 grams per day (older children)

Fat

- 5 grams (minimum) per day of essential fatty acids
- 30% to 40% of total kcal (ages 1 to 3)
- 25% to 35% of total kcal (older children)

The rapid growth rate that characterizes infancy tapers off during the toddler and preschool years. The average annual weight gain is only 4.5 to 6.6 pounds (2 to 3 kilograms), and the average annual height gain is only 3 to 4 inches (7.5 to 10 centimeters) between the ages of 2 and 5. As the growth rate tapers off, energy needs decrease and eating behaviors change. For example, among toddlers, the decreased growth rate leads to a decreased appetite, often called "picky eating."

Energy needs (relative to body weight) gradually decline from approximately 100 kcal per kilogram during infancy to about 90 kcal per kilogram for the preschooler. As you can see in Table 15-6, as the child gets older, physical activity level is a consideration when determining energy requirements.

Except in cases of poverty or homelessness (review Section 12.2), the diets of toddlers and preschoolers in the United States and Canada are adequate in calories and most nutrients. A few nutrients of particular concern among this age group are iron, calcium, and sodium.[9]

Iron. Childhood iron-deficiency anemia is most likely to appear in children between the ages of 6 and 24 months—a time when iron stores from gestation have run out, but intake of iron from food sources may be inadequate. It can lead to decreases in both stamina and learning ability, as well as lowered resistance to disease. The targeted efforts of the Special Supplemental Nutrition Program for Women, Infants, and Children (WIC) have helped to decrease the occurrence of iron deficiency among children, but it still remains a problem for almost 16% of toddlers and about 5% of preschoolers.

The RDA for iron is 7 milligrams per day for children ages 1 to 3 and 10 milligrams per day for children ages 4 to 8. The best way to prevent iron-deficiency anemia in children is to provide foods that are adequate sources of iron. Even though some animal products are high in saturated fat and cholesterol, the high proportion of heme iron in many animal foods allows the iron to be more readily absorbed than is iron from plant foods.

TABLE 15-6 ■ **Approximate Energy Needs of Toddlers and Preschoolers**

Boys				Girls			
	Physical Activity				Physical Activity		
Age	Sedentary	Moderately Active	Active	Age	Sedentary	Moderately Active	Active
2	1000	1000	1000	2	1000	1000	1000
3	1000	1400	1400	3	1000	1200	1400
4	1200	1400	1600	4	1200	1400	1400
5	1200	1400	1600	5	1200	1400	1600

Source: Dietary Guidelines 2015–2020, *http://health.gov/dietaryguidelines/2015/guidelines/appendix-2/*

Focus on lean cuts of meat, such as ground sirloin. Fortified breakfast cereals also contribute to meeting iron (and other nutrient) needs. Consuming a source of vitamin C will aid absorption of the less readily absorbed iron in plants, fortified foods, and supplements. While dietary changes can be effective for preventing iron-deficiency anemia, supplementation will be required to correct existing anemia (review Section 9.9).

Calcium. Childhood is a period of rapid bone growth and mineralization. As you learned in Section 9.6, bone mass can only accrue until the early twenties; after age 30, bone mass starts to decline. It is vital, therefore, to maximize bone mass during childhood and adolescence. The RDA for calcium for ages 1 to 3 is 700 milligrams per day. Between the ages of 4 and 8, calcium needs increase to 1000 milligrams per day. However, national surveys of food intake show that the diets of children fall short of the RDA for this important nutrient.

Milk and other dairy products are the primary source of calcium in the diets of children, but unfortunately, milk consumption has declined as intake of sweetened beverages has increased. Two cups per day of milk will help toddlers and preschoolers meet their requirements for bone-building nutrients. Children up to 2 years of age should drink whole milk because they need the extra fat for energy, but after 2 years of age, reduced-fat or fat-free milk is preferred. For children who do not consume dairy products, whether due to choice or necessity, there are alternative sources of calcium and other bone-building nutrients. Fortified beverages, such as soy milk, almond milk, or orange juice, can supply as much calcium per serving as cow's milk. Some legumes and vegetables are sources of calcium, as well, but the mineral is not as bioavailable as it is from dairy foods.

Sodium. While iron and calcium intakes fall short of needs in preschool children, excessive sodium intake is a concern.[10] High intakes of fast foods and highly processed foods elevate sodium intakes to about 1000 milligrams per day *more* than preschoolers need. Caregivers can lower sodium intake by limiting salt added during cooking and at the table, by cutting back on use of highly processed foods (e.g., luncheon meats and hot dogs), by rinsing canned beans and vegetables before cooking, and by encouraging consumption of fruits, vegetables, and whole grains in place of prepackaged snacks.

Feeding skills are an important part of physical and cognitive development. Young children explore their environment through the tastes and textures of foods, develop dexterity using utensils and drinking from a cup, and begin to express their autonomy by refusing certain foods. At this time in life, children are also testing boundaries to find out what is acceptable in their little corner of the world. Messy mealtimes, food refusals, and **food jags** can be sources of tension in families. Creating a more harmonious family atmosphere at mealtime is an important way to keep these behaviors from becoming serious feeding problems (see "Understanding Picky Eating" later in this section). Caregivers must understand that these are normal phases of child development but should also be consistent about setting limits for behavior at the dinner table.

Because of the preschool child's reduced appetite, planning a dietary pattern that meets nutrient needs poses a special challenge to caregivers. Nutrient density is an important consideration for this age group. Overall, parents should focus on offering a variety of healthy choices, allowing the child to exert some autonomy over the specific type of food and the amount eaten.

MyPlate is a useful, easy-to-understand tool for children. The *proportions* apply to all ages, even though the *portions* will be smaller for children. Table 15-7 gives a general food plan that conforms to MyPlate proportions and is appropriate for preschool and school-age children. Until a child is about 5 years of age, a good starting point for portion sizes in the vegetables group,

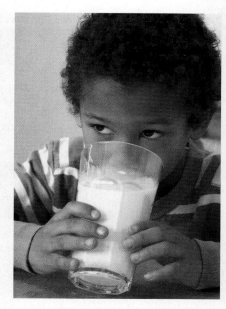

▲ Cow's milk is a source of bioavailable calcium and vitamin D for toddlers and preschoolers, but overreliance on milk can crowd out other nutrient-dense foods. Children who drink more than 3 cups of milk per day are likely to consume inadequate amounts of iron and fiber. ©Andrew Olney/age fotostock

food jag   A period of time (usually a few days or weeks) during which a person will eat only a limited variety of foods.

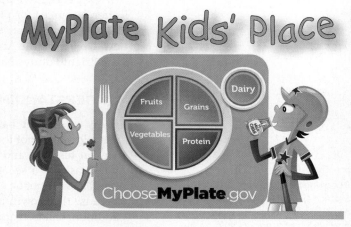

▲ MyPlate Kids' Place features educational games, music, and other activities. See http://www.choosemyplate.gov/kids.
Source: USDA

TABLE 15-7 ■ Food Plans for Children Based on MyPlate Daily Checklists

Food Group	Serving Size	Approximate Number of Servings[a]				
		Age 2[b]	Age 5[b]	Age 8[b]	Age 12[b,c]	Age 16[b,c]
Grains	ounce	3	5	5	6–7	6–10
Vegetables	cup	1	1.5	2	2.5–3	2.5–3.5
Fruits	cup	1	1.5	1.5	1.5–2	2–2.5
Dairy	cup	2	2.5	2.5	3	3
Protein	ounce	2	4	5	5–6	5.5–7
Food components to limit						
Sodium	milligrams	1500	1900	1900	2200	2300
Saturated fat	grams	11	16	18	20–24	22–31
Added sugar	grams	25	35	40	45–55	50–70

[a]Log on to www.chooseMyPlate.gov for other ages and other physical activity levels.

[b]Based on 30–60 minutes of physical activity per day.

[c]The lower amounts are appropriate for girls.

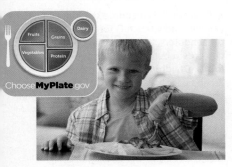

▲ How does this boy's dinner of broiled fish, broccoli, and carrots compare to MyPlate? Which groups are missing? ©Kidstock/Blend Images/Getty Images

Source: www.choosemyplate.gov

Renowned child nutrition expert Ellyn Satter, MS, RDN, explains, "Parents are responsible for the *what, when,* and *where* of feeding; children are responsible for the *how much* and *whether* of eating."

Source: www.ellynsatterinstitute.org

fruits group, and protein group is about 1 tablespoon per year of life. The serving sizes and the number of servings per day can be increased as needed to meet the recommendations outlined in Table 15-7. The same advice does not apply to the grains or dairy groups, but consuming too much milk can leave the diet short on iron.

Luckily, normal-weight children have a built-in feeding mechanism that adjusts hunger to regulate food intake at each stage of growth. If a child is developing and growing normally and the caregiver is providing a variety of healthful foods, all can be confident of the child's well-being.

It is important to promote a healthy attitude about eating. While caregivers will want to focus on nutrient-dense foods, there is no reason to be overly restrictive about child food choices. In fact, when parents are extremely controlling about the family's food intake, children may be at risk for body dissatisfaction and disordered eating. There is room for occasional indulgences, a skipped meal or two, or once in a while "less than ideal" choices. It is eating and lifestyle patterns over the course of a month (and lifetime) that matter. Children develop healthy eating habits when adults set a good example, provide opportunities to learn, give support for exploration, and limit inappropriate behavior.

Next, we will consider some typical complaints and concerns of parents, explore the causes, and make suggestions for achieving optimal nutrition during the toddler and preschool years. Beyond these pages, the U.S. Department of Agriculture's MyPlate (www.ChooseMyPlate.gov) and Team Nutrition (www.fns.usda.gov/tn/team-nutrition) offer resources for planning nutritious, age-appropriate meals and snacks. Additional nutrition guidance, starting with pregnancy and extending through adolescence, is available from the American Academy of Pediatrics' Bright Futures program. Download the Bright Futures Nutrition Pocket Guide from brightfutures.aap.org.

UNDERSTANDING PICKY EATING

Many parents are baffled by their toddler's erratic eating behaviors. Toddlers and preschoolers tend not to eat as much or as regularly as infants. One day, a young child may pick at his food and staunchly refuse to eat his green beans, but on the next day, he might ask for a second helping. Parents often need reminding that toddlers and preschoolers cannot be expected to eat as voraciously as infants or to eat adult-size portions. Because the growth rate slows after infancy, a toddler's drive to eat is not so intense. In addition, children are sometimes more interested in playing and exploring than eating!

Youngsters also tend to be wary of new foods. One reason is that they have more taste buds, and their taste buds are more sensitive than those of adults. A general distrust of unfamiliar things is common in this age group. Thus, familiarity plays an important role in food acceptance. Adults can encourage young children to broaden their food repertoire by repeating exposure to new food choices. It may take 10 or more exposures to a new food before a child finds it acceptable, but if adults can be patient and persevere, children will build good food habits.

Food preferences change rapidly in childhood and are influenced by food temperature, appearance, texture, and taste. The following are a few practical tips for improving acceptance of nutrient-dense foods.

- Build on what they know and accept. Pairing a new food item with a familiar one can help to foster acceptance of the new food.
- Enlist the child's aid in food selection and preparation. For example, let the child pick out the tomatoes and squash at the local farmers market.
- Serve meals on a sectioned plate. Sometimes children object to having foods mixed, as in stews and casseroles, even if they normally like the ingredients separately.
- Keep it crunchy. Certain food characteristics, such as crisp textures and mild flavors, are appealing to children. Kids who reject mushy, cooked carrots may enjoy them raw or lightly steamed. (After about age 4, children can safely eat raw vegetables without fear of choking.)
- Finger foods are fun. Preschoolers eventually develop skill with spoons and forks and can even use dull knives, but it is still a good idea to serve some finger foods, especially with healthy dips such as yogurt sauce or hummus.
- Save the best for last. If a child is prone to leave his or her chicken on the plate untouched, serve the chicken first. Hunger is the best means of getting a child to eat!

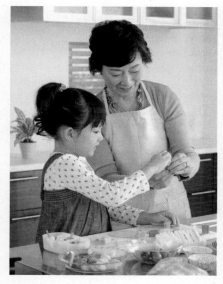

▲ Letting a child help select or prepare her food can increase the likelihood she will eat her food. ©Indeed/Aflo/Getty Images

The dinner table should not become a battleground. Caregivers should avoid nagging, forcing, and bribing children to encourage eating. Using dessert as leverage to get a child to eat vegetables tends to elevate the status of dessert, while making the vegetables seem less palatable. Indirectly, such tactics reinforce picky-eating behaviors due to the added attention given to them. In addition, pressuring children to clean their plates may teach them to override their internal cues for satiety. One reasonable policy is the one-bite rule: children should take at least one bite or taste of the foods presented to them. Also, caregivers should realize that what they *do* speaks louder than what they *say*; if caregivers eat a variety of nutrient-dense foods, children will imitate their behavior.

When a child refuses to eat, it is best not to overreact. Doing so may give the child the idea that not eating is a means of getting attention or manipulating a scene. Most children do not starve themselves to any point approaching physical harm. When children refuse to eat, have them sit at the table for a while; if they still are not interested in eating, remove the food and wait until the next scheduled meal or snack. Finally, instead of giving attention to negative behaviors, focus on positive behaviors when they occur. Praise a child for trying something new. Overall, mealtime should be a relaxed, pleasant opportunity to enjoy healthful foods and good company.[11]

Food jags, common among preschoolers, are typically no cause for alarm. A child may switch from one specific food focus to another with equal intensity (older infants may also act this way). If the caregiver continues to offer choices, the child will soon begin to eat a wider variety of foods again, and the specific food focus will disappear as suddenly as it appeared.

Although picky eating is usually just a manifestation of slower growth and a desire for autonomy, a child's sudden loss of appetite may be a sign of underlying illness, such as an infection or gastrointestinal problem. Be alert for signs of eating disorders, as well. Extreme, self-imposed dietary restrictions could be an early sign of anorexia nervosa (review Section 11.2). **Avoidant/restrictive food intake disorder (ARFID)** is an eating disorder primarily diagnosed among children. With this disorder, a child lacks interest in eating specific foods or all foods in general, which leads to weight loss or failure to grow as expected, as well as many nutrient deficiencies. The restricted food intake is much more severe than the picky eating or intermittent food refusal typical of childhood; children with this disorder become malnourished and may need tube feeding or intravenous feeding. It is most likely related to stress, anxiety, or depression. In some cases, the disorder may be a response to an adverse experience, such as choking or vomiting after eating a certain food.

avoidant/restrictive food intake disorder (ARFID) Eating disorder characterized by failure to meet energy or nutrient needs, resulting in significant weight loss, nutritional deficiencies, or dependence on tube or intravenous feeding; the eating disturbance is not better explained by lack of available food, a medical problem, or another eating disorder.

REDEFINE SNACKING

Parents may be concerned that frequent snacking will prevent children from eating well at mealtimes. However, children have small stomachs and need to eat every 3 to 4 hours. Sticking to three meals a day offers no special nutritional advantages; it is just a social custom.

Choking is a preventable hazard for young children. Some suggestions for caregivers include:

- Set a good example at the table by taking small bites and chewing foods thoroughly.
- Have children sit at the table, take their time, and focus on their food during meals and snacks.
- Avoid giving children any foods that are round, firm, sticky, or cut into large chunks, especially before molars emerge (around age 4). For toddlers and preschoolers, some examples of foods to avoid are nuts, grapes, raisins, popcorn, peanut butter, and hard pieces of raw fruits or vegetables.

Instead, offering five or six small meals can help children meet their nutritional requirements more successfully than limiting them to three meals each day.[12] If the stretch between lunch and dinner is 6 hours, an afternoon snack about 2 hours before dinner could provide some needed nutrients and may preempt a cranky attitude at the evening meal.

The location of snacking is important. Sitting calmly at the table instead of running around the house will decrease the risk for choking. Limiting distractions by turning off the television will help to prevent mindless eating. The caregiver could offer two or three nutrient-dense options and allow the child to choose one; responsibility for food choices by the child should start at an early age. Lastly, caregivers should promote hand-washing and good oral hygiene just as for a meal.

When we eat is not nearly as important as *what* we eat. Perhaps families simply need to redefine snacking altogether. A snack should not be synonymous with an indulgent dessert. Rather, a snack should be a small meal of nutrient-dense foods. Let hunger—not the clock—guide the timing of meals and snacks. It is important that these snack choices be planned ahead in order to have healthy foods available (Table 15-8). Fruits and vegetables (fresh, frozen, or canned) and whole grain breads and crackers are good snack choices (see the Farm to Fork in this chapter). Working parents should make sure their children are provided with nutritious snacks to tide them over until dinnertime.

CHOOSE DIETARY SUPPLEMENTS CAREFULLY

Major scientific groups, such as the Academy of Nutrition and Dietetics and the American Society for Nutrition, state that multivitamin and mineral supplements are generally unnecessary for healthy children; it is better to emphasize whole foods. In fact, consuming fortified foods and supplements may lead to intakes above the UL for some nutrients, such as vitamin A and zinc. Children's supplements that are made to look like candy may result in accidental overdose, particularly of iron. Fortified, low-sugar, ready-to-eat breakfast cereals with milk are especially helpful in closing any gap between current micronutrient intake and needs, such as for folate, vitamin D, vitamin E, iron, or zinc.

TABLE 15-8 ■ Twenty Healthy Snack Ideas for Children

	Iron	Zinc	Calcium	Vitamin C	Fiber
Almonds (1 oz)*			✓		✓
Unsweetened applesauce (1/2 cup)				✓	✓
Bean and cheese burrito (1)	✓	✓	✓		✓
Cheese (1 oz) and whole wheat crackers (6)	✓	✓	✓		✓
Reduced-sugar dried cranberries (1/4 cup)				✓	✓
Frozen fruit pieces (1 cup)				✓	✓
Fruit salad (1 cup)				✓	✓
Fruit smoothie with bananas and strawberries (1 cup)				✓	✓
Hard-boiled egg	✓	✓			
Hummus (2 tbsp) with bell pepper rings (1 cup)				✓	✓
Low-fat microwave popcorn (3 tbsp unpopped)*					✓
Mini-pizzas on whole grain English muffins (2)	✓	✓	✓	✓	✓
Peanut butter (2 tbsp) and apple slices (1 cup)*		✓			✓
Quick breads, such as banana bread, 1 slice	✓				✓
String cheese (1 stick)		✓	✓		
Trail mix (1/4 cup)*	✓	✓			✓
Tuna salad (1/2 cup) in whole wheat pita pocket	✓	✓			✓
Whole grain cereal (1 cup)	✓	✓		✓	✓
Whole wheat pasta salad with veggies (1 cup)	✓	✓			✓
Yogurt (6 oz) with granola (2 tbsp)			✓		✓

*Snack items that are best suited for children older than age 4 due to potential for choking.

FARM to FORK | Blueberries

From a health standpoint, it's tough to beat these AMAZING super fruits! The antioxidant and phytochemical activities of berries are four times greater than those of most other fruits, 10 times greater than those of most vegetables, and 40 times higher than those of most cereal grains. Berries may play a role in prevention of diabetes, cancer, high blood pressure, cardiovascular disease, and dementia!

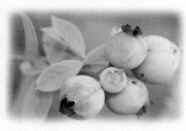

©U.S. Fish & Wildlife Service/Ryan Hagerty

Grow
- Many urban landscapes are adding attractive berry patches as part of an edible environment. Although most blueberries thrive in cooler climates, some varieties do fine in warmer climates.
- Children love to pick berries! If you don't have your own berry patch, consider finding a local U-pick farm for building great family memories.

Shop
- When shopping, examine the berries carefully and look for plump, firm, and colorful fruit.
- The most nutrient-dense frozen berries are flash-frozen to preserve phytochemicals and vitamin C. Flash-frozen wild berries are the best choice.
- If purchasing juice, read the ingredients to be sure it is 100% pure berry juice. Most berry

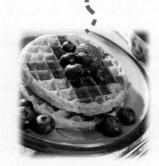

©Purestock/SuperStock

juices contain more juice from apples and white grapes than from berries.

Store
- If purchasing fresh, rinse berries just prior to eating and eat within several days to ensure the highest nutrient content.
- Before freezing your own berries, dust lightly with vitamin C powder or Fruit-Fresh® to retain nutrients.

Prep
- Berries may be enjoyed fresh, frozen, stewed, and dried. They can be used to sweeten any dish.
- Frozen berries thawed quickly in the microwave actually retain double the nutrient content as those thawed at room temperature or in the refrigerator.
- Cooked or canned berries actually increase the absorption of phytochemicals and key nutrients. Bottom line: eat more berries!

Source: Robinson J. "Blueberries and Blackberries: Extraordinarily nutritious," in *Eating on the Wild Side*. New York: Little, Brown and Company, 2013.

For a child who is ill, has a very erratic food preference pattern or appetite, or is on a weight-loss diet, the American Academy of Pediatrics states that the child may benefit from a children's multivitamin and mineral supplement not exceeding 100% of Daily Values for any nutrient. Still, as mentioned many times in this book, such a practice does not substitute for an otherwise healthy dietary pattern—children included. If current childhood feeding practices are to become more healthful, the focus should be on whole grain breads and cereals, fruits, vegetables, lean sources of protein, and low-fat milk and milk products.

REDUCE LEAD POISONING

Humans may be exposed to lead from drinking contaminated water, consuming or inhaling lead dust (e.g., from cracked and peeling lead paint), contaminated dietary supplements (e.g., calcium supplements derived from bone meal), or foods stored or prepared in lead-containing vessels. In the United States, nearly half a million children between the ages of 1 and 5 have unacceptably high blood lead levels. Young children are particularly vulnerable to lead poisoning because they are small, absorb lead quickly, spend a lot of time on the floor, and are apt to put objects in their mouths. In the short term, symptoms of lead poisoning include gastrointestinal distress, lack of appetite, irritability, fatigue, and anemia. Over the long term, devastating effects include intellectual and behavioral impairments and increased risk for several chronic diseases in adulthood.

Although it does not address the source of exposure, proper nutrition can reduce the risks of lead poisoning for children. Consuming regular meals with moderate fat intake and ensuring adequate iron and calcium status are dietary practices known to reduce lead absorption. Adequate zinc, thiamin, and vitamin E intakes also reduce the harmful

Between 2014 and 2015, the water supply in the city of Flint, Michigan, became contaminated with extremely high levels of lead. Read more about the far-reaching impact of this lead exposure in Section 13.6.

effects of absorbed lead. For lowest lead levels, only cold water should be used for drinking and preparation of formula or food. Letting cold water run from the tap for about 2 minutes after a long period of inactivity (e.g., overnight) will limit the amount of lead that has accumulated in tap water. If the public water supply contains a high concentration of lead, bottled water is a safer alternative, particularly for formula preparation. Overall, a balanced meal plan that offers a variety of whole grains, lean meats, and low-fat dairy products is especially useful for protecting children from lead poisoning.

ALLEVIATE CONSTIPATION WITH LIFESTYLE CHANGES

Constipation, a common problem among children, can be defined as hard, dry stools that are difficult to pass. Typically, a 4-year-old child has one bowel movement per day, but normal bowel habits vary widely. Therefore, the frequency of bowel movements is not as important as the consistency of stools. Pediatricians diagnose constipation after 2 or more weeks of delayed or difficult bowel movements. In rare situations, constipation can be a sign of a serious problem. If a child has a fever or vomiting along with constipation, if there is blood in the stool, or if the abdomen becomes swollen, caregivers should seek immediate medical attention.

What causes constipation? Although there could be a serious medical problem, most cases are related to lifestyle. Lack of physical activity contributes to constipation. Also, on average, children (and adults) in the United States barely obtain half of the AI for fiber. Altered bowel habits also may be a sign of a food allergy or intolerance to a food component such as cow's milk. The majority of the time, however, constipation results from the child withholding bowel movements. For children, a painful bowel movement can be so traumatic that they try to resist subsequent bowel movements. The longer they hold their stools, the harder and drier they get, leading to another painful movement. This cycle disrupts regular bowel habits, leading to distress and, if not treated, **fecal impaction.**

fecal impaction The presence of a mass of hard, dry feces that remains in the rectum as a result of chronic constipation.

When presented with a constipated child, a primary care provider first has to rule out a medical cause, such as an intestinal blockage. Treatment of fecal impaction may require evacuation of the bowels (e.g., with an enema). Once bowels have been evacuated, lifestyle changes are necessary to prevent future problems. Although various types of laxatives may be prescribed by the health care provider in the short term, diet and lifestyle are the safest strategies over the long term. First, regular bowel habits must be established. For example, parents should set aside time for the child to use the toilet, without rushing, after each meal. Rewards, such as stickers on a chart, may be used to reinforce good habits. Increasing physical activity while cutting back on sedentary activities (e.g., watching television or playing video games) can help to promote regular bowel movements. The primary dietary interventions to alleviate constipation include eating more fiber and drinking more fluids. In the initial stages of treatment, providing certain fruit juices (e.g., prune, grape, and apple) and substituting soy milk for cow's milk may relieve constipation.

Ultimately, whole fruits (e.g., plums, peaches, and apricots) are better choices than juices because whole fruits are less concentrated sources of calories. The American Academy of Pediatrics recommends limiting fruit juice to just 4 fluid ounces per day for toddlers (ages 1 to 3).[8] Other foods to emphasize for fiber include vegetables, whole grain breads and cereals, and beans. The daily fiber goals for children set by the Food and Nutrition Board vary by age (see accompanying note). Few children meet these goals. It is important to increase fluid consumption along with fiber to avoid another fecal impaction. Accompanying fluid recommendations are 4 cups (900 milliliters) per day for toddlers and about 5 cups (1200 milliliters) per day for older children.

PLAN VEGETARIAN DIETS APPROPRIATELY

Vegetarian diets can pose several risks for young children. These include the possibility of developing iron-deficiency anemia, a deficiency of vitamin B-12, and rickets from a vitamin D deficiency. During the first few years of life, children also may not consume enough calories when following a bulky vegetarian diet. These known pitfalls are easily avoided by informed diet planning (review Section 6.8). Dietary patterns for children who eat totally vegetarian fare should focus on the following:

Fiber Recommendations for Children

Young Children

1–3 years	19 grams/day
4–8 years	25 grams/day

Boys

9–13 years	31 grams/day
14–18 years	38 grams/day

Girls

9–13 years	26 grams/day
14–18 years	26 grams/day

Source: Food and Nutrition Board

- A variety of plant sources of protein to provide a full complement of essential amino acids (e.g., beans, nuts, and grains)
- A synthetic source of vitamin B-12 (e.g., dietary supplement or fortified breakfast cereal)
- Plenty of plant sources of iron (e.g., beans, dried fruits, and fortified grain products)
- Good sources of zinc (e.g., whole grains, beans, nuts, and seeds)
- Foods that are fortified with vitamin D (e.g., fortified orange juice), along with regular sun exposure
- Rich plant sources of calcium (e.g., fortified milk or juice), almonds, some forms of tofu, and green, leafy vegetables

PROMOTE GOOD ORAL HEALTH

A healthy dietary pattern goes a long way in reducing the risk for dental caries in young children. In addition to beginning oral hygiene when teeth start to appear and seeking early pediatric dental care, the following diet-related tips can help reduce dental problems in children:

- Drink fluoridated water (or any water) as opposed to carbohydrate-rich or acidic beverages (e.g., fruit juice, soft drinks, sports drinks, and energy drinks). If sugary or acidic beverages are consumed, it is better to drink them *with* meals rather than *between* meals. Sipping juice continuously between meals (e.g., from a sippy cup) exposes teeth to caries-promoting sugars and acids.
- Use small amounts of fluoridated toothpaste twice daily. In areas without fluoridated water, discuss fluoride needs with a dentist or pediatrician.
- Snack in moderation. Again, constant exposure of teeth to sugars and acids throughout the day (i.e., grazing) tends to promote caries.
- Make wise snack choices. We automatically think of sticky, sugary snacks as promoters of dental caries, but foods such as pretzels and popcorn provide a source of carbohydrates for oral bacteria, as well. In contrast, crunchy fruits and vegetables, such as apples or celery, can help to brush away sticky food particles. Snacking on dairy products, such as cheese, can actually buffer the acids that lead to tooth decay.
- If toddlers or preschoolers are chewing gum, sugarless gum is the best choice, as this has been shown to reduce the incidence of dental caries.

LINKS BETWEEN AUTISM AND NUTRITION

Autism spectrum disorder (ASD) is characterized by a range of problems with social interaction, verbal and nonverbal communication, and/or unusual, repetitive, or limited activities and interests. This disorder usually is diagnosed in early childhood and affects an estimated 1 in every 68 children, with higher prevalence in boys than girls. The causes for ASD are not well understood, but there is a definite genetic component.

ASD can both affect and be affected by nutritional status.[13] In addition to developmental and behavioral abnormalities, many children with ASD also experience GI disorders, such as constipation, diarrhea, or reflux disease. Such disorders may impair nutrient intake or absorption. Medications used to treat behavioral problems may alter appetite. Some children with ASD may have feeding problems related to developmental impairments. Also, selective eating behaviors may affect nutrient intake. Children with ASD can be very rigid with their food selections, rejecting foods or entire food groups based on sensory qualities such texture, color, and temperature. Thus, careful attention to nutrient-dense food choices is of prime importance.

There are many nutrient-based theories concerning the causes and treatment of ASD. Nutritional interventions, such as dietary restrictions or nutrient supplements, are commonly employed by families affected by ASD.[14] A widely used nutritional intervention is the gluten-free, casein-free (GFCF) diet, which eliminates all wheat, barley, rye, and milk products (see Ask the RDN in this section).[15] At this time, the American Academy of Pediatrics does not endorse any specific diet as a treatment for autism.

Other popular therapies for ASD include supplementation with probiotics, vitamins B-6 and B-12, folic acid, magnesium, and omega-3 fatty acids. Although sparse, research

ASK THE RDN | Autism Diet

Dear Author: *My 4-year-old son was just diagnosed with autism. He is a picky eater and often cries because his belly hurts, so I think he may have some food sensitivities. I read about an autism diet that is gluten free and casein free (GFCF). Could this diet help him feel better and treat his autism?*

A diagnosis of autism spectrum disorder can be bewildering, and the lack of treatment options may leave you feeling helpless. A dietary intervention may seem like a reasonable, low-risk option.

Proponents of the GFCF diet believe that some children have a "leaky gut," which allows food proteins to be absorbed intact from the GI tract into the bloodstream and possibly reach the brain. Certain proteins may cross the blood-brain barrier and exert drug-like effects, leading to the behaviors of autism spectrum disorder. They assert that by eliminating the offending food proteins, symptoms of autism may be reduced. This sounds scientifically plausible, yet there is little science to support this theory. The levels of these druglike proteins in body fluids are no higher among children with autism than normal-functioning children.

You mentioned that your son is known to be a picky eater. Many children on the autism spectrum display selective eating behaviors; they are more sensitive than other children to colors, tastes, temperatures, and textures. Also, children with autism prefer consistent routines and may refuse new foods. There is a strong possibility that the diet itself may prove disruptive and may affect your child's social and emotional functioning. Placing your son on a restrictive diet may further limit his food choices. Eliminating gluten will entail cutting out many types of breads, pastas, bakery products, crackers, and snack foods. Removing casein will require avoidance of milk, yogurt, cheese, butter, and many frozen desserts. By eliminating dietary sources of gluten and casein, your child is at risk for deficiencies of iron, calcium, vitamin D, and several B vitamins. Indeed, studies have shown that children with autism already have diets deficient in key nutrients. Children who follow a casein-free diet may have low bone mass or delayed bone development related to deficient intake of calcium and vitamin D. Children on a gluten-free diet have lower levels of folate and vitamin B-6, leading to elevated homocysteine. This can place them at risk for chronic disease as they age.

Clearly, the GFCF diet is not risk free. But would the risks be acceptable if the diet helps to improve symptoms? Unfortunately, there is very little evidence to support either the safety or the efficacy of the GFCF diet. The few studies that do show a positive outcome are of poor quality, meaning they were of short duration and had small numbers of subjects, poor study designs, and a high risk of bias.

Knowing that children with autism are at risk for dietary inadequacies, the best dietary strategy is to offer a variety of nutrient-dense foods at each meal. Consulting with a registered dietitian nutritionist would be helpful to assess your son's current dietary patterns and create a personalized plan to alleviate GI symptoms and ensure his nutritional needs are met. For a child with extremely limited dietary intake, multivitamin and mineral supplementation may be an option. Overall, a dietary restriction should only be used if there is evidence that your son has an allergy or intolerance to a food. If you are concerned that his GI distress may be due to a food allergy or intolerance, you should consult your primary care provider about allergy testing.

Despite the lack of evidence to support the GFCF diet for treatment of autism spectrum disorders, many parents will choose to try it anyway, hoping for positive results. There may, in fact, be a subset of children with autism who do respond to dietary treatments. If you are determined to try the GFCF diet, please seek the help of a registered dietitian nutritionist who can help you to plan meals and snacks that will still meet your son's nutrient needs while adhering to dietary restrictions.

Keeping it nutritious,

Angela Collene, MS, RDN, LD (author)

For children with ASD, exercise may improve more than just physical health. Some research shows that regular physical activity may improve attention, cognition, and behavior among children with ASD.[16]

on these therapies is encouraging. There is evidence of altered absorption or metabolism of nutrients among children with autism, so even with adequate nutrient intake, availability of some nutrients for metabolic processes may be low. Even though these supplements carry a low risk of adverse effects, caution is necessary to avoid overdose. Because of the rising incidence of ASD and the lack of curative treatments, nutritional interventions for ASD will continue to be an active area of research.

✓ **CONCEPT CHECK 15.4**

1. Why is picky eating common among preschoolers? Provide three or more suggestions to help a preschooler choose nutritious foods.

2. How often do preschoolers need to eat throughout the day? List three nutrient-dense snack ideas that would be appropriate for a 3-year-old child.

3. Should toddlers and preschoolers take a multivitamin and mineral supplement? Why or why not?

4. Explain the connections between nutrition and oral health. List three ways to reduce risk for dental caries with healthy eating habits.

5. What are some nutrition concerns of children with autism spectrum disorder?

15.5 School-Age Children: Nutrition Concerns

The dietary patterns of many school-age children can be improved, particularly with regard to fruit, vegetable, whole grain, and beverage choices. One survey of U.S. schoolchildren revealed that on the day of the survey, 40% of the children ate no vegetables, except for potatoes or tomato sauce, and 20% ate no fruits. Less than 20% of school-age girls consume adequate calcium. In general, the nutritional concerns and goals applicable to school-age children are the same as those discussed in relation to preschoolers. However, with the added pressures of peers, health messages from the media, and an increasing desire for independence, these goals may be harder to achieve as children grow older. MyPlate's daily food patterns, which are tailored to age, gender, height, weight, and activity level, continue to be a good basis for diet planning, with an emphasis on moderating fat and sugar intake and ensuring adequate iron, zinc, and calcium intake (Fig. 15-4). Now let us look at several nutritional issues of particular concern during the school-age years.

REVERSING TRENDS FOR OVERWEIGHT AND OBESITY

By far, the most troublesome nutritional problem facing children today is the rise in childhood obesity. Since the 1970s, the incidence of childhood overweight and obesity has more than tripled! In the past decade, the rate of childhood obesity has stabilized, but still, about one-third of U.S. school-age children are now classified as overweight or obese. The rates of childhood obesity are highest among children from low-income families and minority populations.

In the short run, the main consequences of childhood obesity are ridicule, embarrassment, possibly depression, and short stature linked to early puberty. In the long run, significant health problems associated with obesity, such as cardiovascular disease, type 2 diabetes, hypertension, cancer, and osteoarthritis may appear in adulthood or earlier. Childhood obesity is a serious health threat because about 40% of obese children (and about 80% of obese adolescents) become obese adults. To identify cases and reverse these trends, the United States Preventive Services Task Force recommends screening children for obesity starting at 6 years of age.[17]

Research points to many potential causes of childhood obesity. Recall the nature versus nurture discussion in Section 7.4. Some individuals are born with a genetic predisposition to obesity. They may experience lower metabolic rates, which means they use calories more efficiently and can store fat more easily. However, studies also suggest that genetic factors account for only one-third of individual differences in body weight.

Researchers believe that although diet is an important factor, inactivity is also a major contributor to the increase in childhood obesity. Studies show that as children age, physical activity steadily declines and screen time increases. Screen time includes time spent watching television, working at the computer, or using phones and other electronic devices. Only about one-half of children are getting the recommended 60 minutes of

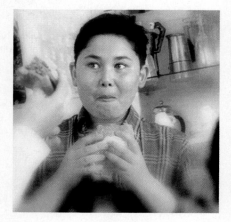

▲ Supersized portions of foods such as hamburgers and sugar-sweetened soft drinks are fueling a nation of supersized kids. ©image100/Corbis

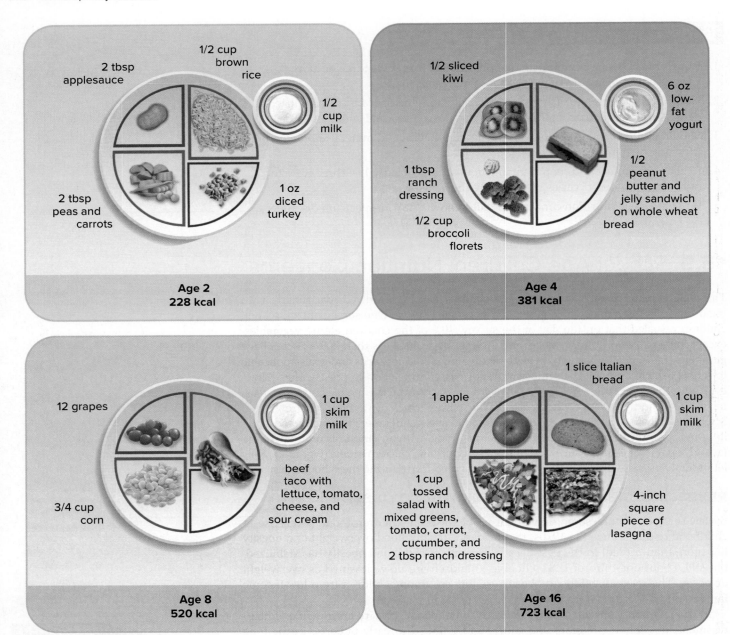

FIGURE 15-4 ▲ Using MyPlate to build a healthy meal for children. MyPlate is a useful tool for all Americans, ages 2 and older. MyPlate proportions apply to children as well as adults, but portion sizes and food choices vary by age.

exercise per day. It does not help that physical education classes are now elective in many high schools. Today's generation of children now engages in 7 hours per day of screen time, on average. The American Academy of Pediatrics recommends a limit of 1 hour per day of screen time for entertainment purposes for children 2 to 5 years of age. For school-age children, parents should set appropriate limits on screen time, making sure to encourage plenty of physical activity. In addition, excessive snacking, overreliance on fast-food restaurants, parental neglect, advertising and other messages in the media, lack of safe areas to play, and the abundant availability of high-calorie food choices contribute to childhood obesity. Soft drinks and other sugared beverages are especially implicated.

Recall from Section 12.4 that the United Nations Sustainable Development Goals call for efforts to control noncommunicable diseases, such as obesity. In 2016, WHO released its Report of the Commission on Ending Childhood Obesity (ECHO). The ECHO Report quantifies global rates of childhood obesity and recognizes the problems of an environment that promotes weight gain. To combat the global epidemic of childhood obesity, the commission recommends promoting healthy foods and physical activity beginning before conception (for the mother) and extending all the way through childhood. To access the full report, see http://www.who.int/end-childhood-obesity/final-report/en/.

The initial approach in treating an overweight or obese child is to assess physical activity. If a child spends too much time in sedentary activities (such as watching television or playing video games), more physical activities should be encouraged. The Physical Activity Guidelines for Americans recommend 60 minutes or more of moderate to vigorous physical activity per day for children and adolescents. Learning to engage in and enjoy regular physical activity will help children to maintain a healthy body weight throughout life. An increase in physical activity will not just happen; parents and other caregivers need to plan for it. Getting the family together for a brisk walk after dinner encourages healthy habits for all involved.[18] Age-appropriate activities for elementary school-age children include walking, dancing, jumping rope, and participation in organized sports that focus on fun rather than intense competition. For middle school–age children, more complex organized sports (e.g., soccer and basketball) are of interest, and some weight training with small weights can also be beneficial.

Moderation in calorie intake is important. High-calorie foods, such as sugar-sweetened soft drinks and whole milk, should be limited. The focus should be on more vitamin- and mineral-dense foods and healthy snacks. An emphasis on appropriate portion sizes may help youth learn to curb excessive food consumption. Making small changes, such as substituting low-fat for whole milk or fruit canned in its own juice instead of heavy syrup, can moderately cut calories without sacrificing taste or disrupting normal eating patterns. To specifically address the increased burden of overweight and obesity among minority populations, health professionals must become versed in varied cultural food preferences.

Resorting to a weight-loss diet is usually not necessary; it is best to change dietary and physical activity patterns to allow for weight maintenance. Children have an advantage over adults in dealing with obesity: their bodies can use stored energy for growth. An overweight child who maintains his or her body weight through a growth spurt will end up with a more favorable body composition. This is one reason it is desirable to address obesity in childhood. If weight loss is necessary in younger children, it should be gradual, about 0.5 to 1 pound per week. The child should be watched closely to ensure that the rate of growth continues to be normal; calorie intake should not be so low that gains in height diminish. In some cases, medications (e.g., orlistat [Xenical]) may be prescribed by a primary care provider. For the 1% to 2% of American children who are morbidly obese, bariatric surgery is an option for weight management.[19]

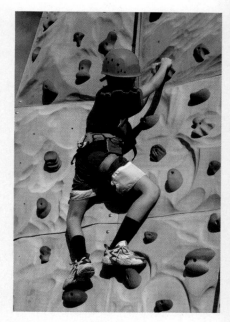

▲ To get kids involved in exercise, new physical education classes have been introduced into some schools. Lessons on rock climbing, in-line skating, and recreational jogging help to promote activity because they take the focus away from teams and competition, which often discourage and embarrass kids who lack athletic talent. ©Valerie Loiseleux/Getty Images RF

EARLY SIGNS OF CARDIOVASCULAR DISEASE

Parallel to the increase in childhood obesity, early signs of cardiovascular disease have become increasingly prevalent among children and adolescents. One in five American youths between the ages of 12 and 19 years has abnormal blood lipids. Therefore, lifestyle modifications to delay the progression of the disease are important throughout the life span. The American Academy of Pediatrics now recommends universal blood lipid screening for all children around the ages of 9 to 11. Even earlier screening is recommended for "at-risk" children who are overweight, have high blood pressure, smoke, or have diabetes; have a family history of cardiovascular disease; or whose family history is unknown. For children whose cholesterol is elevated, lifestyle approaches such as weight management through dietary modification and increased physical activity are the first line of therapy.[20] An eating pattern that is consistent with the Dietary Guidelines would be appropriate for prevention of cardiovascular disease. To complement modifications to fat and sodium intakes, the American Heart Association recently released guidelines for children to limit added sugar intake to 25 grams per day.[6] This is quite a reduction from the average 80 grams of added sugars consumed by children and adolescents per day!

TYPE 2 DIABETES AMONG YOUTH

Type 2 diabetes was once regarded as an adult condition. As reviewed in Section 4.7, it frequently occurs in overweight people over age 40. However, an alarming increase in the frequency of the disease among children (and teenagers) has been documented. This is primarily due to the rise in obesity in this age group. Up to 85% of children with the disease are overweight at diagnosis.

Starting at age 10, children who are overweight or obese and who have risk factors for type 2 diabetes should be screened for type 2 diabetes every 2 years. Besides obesity and a sedentary lifestyle, examples of risk factors include having a close relative with the disease or belonging to a nonwhite population. In 2013, the American Academy of Pediatrics released the first-ever guidelines for management of type 2 diabetes in children.[21] These guidelines provide recommendations for monitoring of blood glucose, use of medications, weight management, and physical activity. Dietary management strategies include a regular schedule of meals and snacks; education on appropriate portion sizes; limiting sugar-sweetened beverages, high-fat foods, snacks, and fast foods; and focusing on incorporating more fruits, vegetables, and low-fat or fat-free dairy products. For physical activity, experts advise children to engage in moderate- or vigorous-intensity physical activity for at least 60 minutes each day.

START THE DAY WITH BREAKFAST

You have heard it before: *Breakfast is the most important meal of the day.* Yet, as many as one-third of school-age children do not eat breakfast. The problem gets worse as children reach the teenage years. Children who skip breakfast are missing out on important nutrients that fuel the brain and the body. A fortified, low-sugar, ready-to-eat breakfast cereal is typically the greatest source of iron, vitamin A, and folic acid for children ages 2 to 18. Although there is disagreement over the true benefit of breakfast for cognitive ability, children who eat breakfast are more likely to meet their daily needs for vitamins and minerals compared to children not eating breakfast.[22] Also, a growing body of research shows that starting the day with breakfast reduces risk for obesity.

Fortified, low-sugar, ready-to-eat breakfast cereals offer lots of nutrition in a tasty and convenient package. Consumption of breakfast cereal is responsible for improved intakes of vitamin A and iron. Eating breakfast in general is linked to better intakes of vitamin A, vitamin C, calcium, iron, and fiber. Note that breakfast menus need not be limited to traditional fare. A little imagination can spark the interest of even the most reluctant eater. Instead of conventional breakfast foods, parents can offer leftovers from dinner, such as pizza, spaghetti, soups, yogurt topped with trail mix, chili with beans, or sandwiches. For lasting energy and satiety, combine traditional carbohydrate-rich breakfast foods with a source of protein, such as low-fat cheese, nuts, or eggs.

CHOOSE HEALTHY FATS

Dietary patterns of school-age children should include a variety of foods from each major group, not necessarily excluding any specific food because of its fat content. Overemphasis on fat-reduced diets during childhood has been linked to an increase in eating disorders and encourages an inappropriate "good food, bad food" attitude.

However, surveys of dietary intake among children show that they are consuming too much saturated fat, most of which comes from whole milk, other full-fat dairy products, and fatty meats. Furthermore, few children (or adults) meet recommendations to include two servings of fish per week to ensure adequate intake of omega-3 fats. Emphasizing low-fat dairy products (after age 2), offering broiled or baked fish, choosing leaner cuts of meat, trimming visible fat from meats, and removing the skin from poultry before serving foods will establish heart-healthy eating habits to last a lifetime. Snacks for children should include only moderate fat and sugar and emphasize fruit, vegetables, whole grain, and dairy choices. Ideas for healthy snacks are found in Table 15-8.

▲ For kids who complain about waking up early to make time for breakfast, consider preparing a portable breakfast (e.g., a sandwich bag full of dry cereal, nuts, and dried cranberries) the night before, for grab-and-go convenience the next morning. ©Ingram Publishing/SuperStock RF

SELECT APPROPRIATE BEVERAGES

Maintaining proper hydration is important for children. The fluid needs of school-age children range from approximately 1½ to 2½ liters per day, depending on age and gender. However, over the past 30 years, beverage choices have shifted from water and low-fat or fat-free milk to the empty calories provided by sugar-sweetened beverages. In fact, sugar-sweetened beverages (e.g, soft drinks, flavored fruit drinks, and sports drinks) and the sweeteners added to flavored milk account for about 200 empty kilocalories per day for school-age children.[23] The 135% increase in sugar-sweetened beverage consumption has paralleled the threefold rise in childhood obesity since the 1970s. Such high intakes of sugar-laden beverages are not only contributing excess calories, but are also linked to increased levels of inflammation and worsened blood lipid profiles among children.[24] Even 100% fruit juices, which are perceived by many to be an important source of vitamin C and potassium for children, have been linked to obesity, fatty liver, and metabolic syndrome.[25]

Replacing sugar-sweetened beverages with water and choosing unflavored, low-fat, or fat-free milk instead of flavored milk would reduce sugar intake by about 10½ teaspoons per day and shrink overall kilocalorie intake by about 10%. Furthermore, replacing 100% fruit juices with whole fruits would supply important nutrients in a lower-calorie package for children. Fruit juice should be limited to 6 fluid ounces per day for young children ages 4 to 6 or 8 fluid ounces per day for older children (ages 7 to 18).[8] Overall, children should be given water and low-fat or fat-free milk as primary beverage choices.

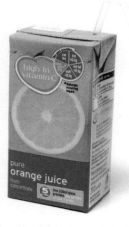

▲ The American Academy of Pediatrics recommends limiting fruit juice consumption.
— < 1 year: no fruit juice
— 1 to 3 years: no more than 4 fluid ounces per day
— 4 to 6 years: no more than 6 fluid ounces per day
— 7 to 18 years: no more than 8 fluid ounces per day

©Nikreates/Alamy

PROMOTE SOUND NUTRITION IN SCHOOLS

Children spend the majority of their waking hours in school, so it is a great place to learn about and practice healthy eating habits.[26] A strong emphasis on nutrition education in schools can help children understand why healthy dietary patterns will make them feel more energetic, look healthier, and work more efficiently. The USDA's Team Nutrition initiative supports child nutrition programs with education materials that promote healthy food choices and physical activity.

Most schools have included nutrition education in their health or science curricula, but until recently, these healthy nutrition messages were not consistently backed up by the food offerings in school cafeterias. In 2010, President Barack Obama signed into law the Healthy Hunger-Free Kids Act, which extended funding for the National School Lunch Program, School Breakfast Program, and several other federal nutrition programs. The law also authorized the USDA to make significant changes to the nutritional quality of foods provided in schools. Public school food service programs now have to meet nutrition standards that stipulate the inclusion of fruits, vegetables, and whole grains in meals. School cafeterias offer skim or 1% milk instead of whole milk. These standards also will gradually reduce the saturated fat, *trans* fat, and sodium content of meals over the coming years.

Breakfasts and lunches prepared by school cafeterias are not the only targets of school nutrition reforms. In 2014, new standards for the quality of competitive foods sold on school campuses (e.g., from snack bars and vending machines) went into effect. These guidelines set calorie limits on snacks and restrict the levels of saturated fat, sugar, and sodium in foods that can be sold to students.

These school nutrition regulations are based on research studies that show how changing the quality of foods offered to students at school can stem the rise in children's BMI. Students' food choices, however, depend a lot on how the food choices taste. School food service programs, although they receive some government reimbursement, often rely on cafeteria, snack bar, or vending machine sales to break even. It remains to be seen how these school nutrition reforms will influence children's eating behaviors. Some early research suggests that the new federal standards may increase vegetable consumption, but there is concern that requiring students to select a set amount of fruits and vegetables may contribute to food waste.[27]

> School breakfasts and lunches provided a nutritional safety net for more than 30 million students during the 2015–2016 school year. Of those meals, 72% were provided free or at reduced prices for children from low-income families.

If we are to reduce childhood obesity, improving nutritional awareness at school is only part of the solution. Positive nutrition influences must extend beyond the classroom and into the home. Caregivers and other adult role models need to create safe opportunities for children to be active and must practice what they preach when it comes to healthy habits at home.

✓ CONCEPT CHECK 15.5

1. Provide an example of a meal that resembles MyPlate and is appropriate for a 7-year-old child.
2. List three lifestyle changes to reduce childhood obesity. In what significant way do weight-management strategies for children differ from those for adults?
3. Describe appropriate beverage choices for school-age children. What are the implications of excessively consuming sugar-sweetened beverages?
4. Tim refuses to eat breakfast before school. He doesn't like cereal, toast, or any of the other usual breakfast foods. What can Tim's parents do to ensure that he eats nutritious foods before leaving for school?

15.6 Teenage Years: Nutrition Concerns

Teenagers are on the cusp of adulthood; parents and schools may still be providing healthful food choices for them, yet they are capable of acquiring and preparing food for themselves. They pursue their independence, experience identity crises, seek peer acceptance, and worry about physical appearance. Advertisers push a vast array of products—candy, fast foods, soft drinks, and energy drinks—at the teenage market. Frequently, these foods crowd out nutrient-dense foods, thus limiting intake of calcium, iron, zinc, fat-soluble vitamins, and folate.

Teens often do not think about the long-term benefits of good health. Developmentally, they have a hard time relating today's actions to tomorrow's health outcomes. Still, positive dietary patterns do not require giving up favorite foods. In moderation, small portions of fast foods and sweet treats can fit into a healthy dietary pattern based on abundant fruits and vegetables, lean sources of protein, fat-free and reduced-fat dairy products, and whole grain products.

One of the most salient nutritional changes among adolescents is an increase in kilocalorie intake. Most girls begin a rapid growth spurt between the ages of 10 and 13, and most boys experience rapid growth between the ages of 12 and 15. Early-maturing girls may begin their growth spurt as early as age 7 to 8, whereas early-maturing boys may begin growing by age 9 to 10. Nearly every organ and bone in the body grows during this adolescent growth spurt. Girls gain about 10 inches (25 centimeters) in height, and boys gain about 12 inches (30 centimeters). Girls tend to accumulate both lean and fat tissue, whereas boys tend to gain mostly lean tissue. This growth spurt provides about 50% of ultimate adult weight and about 15% of ultimate adult height (review Fig. 15-1).

As the growth spurt begins, teenagers begin to eat more. Physically active teenage boys, especially, seem driven to consume everything in sight! Teenage girls need 1800 to 2400 kcal per day, whereas teenage boys require 2200 to 3200 kcal per day. If teens choose nutrient-dense foods, they can take advantage of their ravenous appetites to easily satisfy their increased requirements for calcium, iron, and zinc. As discussed for younger age groups, MyPlate can serve as a guide (see Table 15-7 and Fig. 15-4). Unfortunately, teens very often meet (or exceed) their increased energy needs with empty calories rather than nutrient-dense food options. About one-third of their calories come from solid fats and added sugars.

Fruit and vegetable intake among teenagers is generally dismal; only about one-fourth of high school students regularly consume a minimum of five servings per day of fruits and vegetables. Sadly, potato chips and French fries make up more than one-third of the vegetable servings consumed by teens. Low consumption of fruits and vegetables

The physical changes of puberty cause body dissatisfaction for some adolescents. Late-blooming boys may be frustrated with slow gains in height and muscularity, whereas girls can be dissatisfied with gains in fat mass, which are a normal part of development. Be alert for signs of eating disorders (see Chapter 11).

correlates with inadequate intakes of vitamins A, C, and E, folate, magnesium, and fiber. Also, as teens (especially girls) trade their glasses of milk for bottles of soft drinks and other sugar-sweetened beverages, their intakes of calcium, phosphorus, and vitamin D fall short of recommendations. On the other hand, intakes of saturated fat, cholesterol, sodium, and sugars exceed the recommendations set by the American Heart Association, placing teens at risk for obesity and cardiovascular disease.

Childhood obesity, introduced in Section 15.5, continues to be a major nutritional problem into adolescence. Among children between the ages of 12 and 19, 17% are obese. There are gender and ethnic disparities for adolescent obesity: black females and Hispanic males are at highest risk. Overweight and obese teens are likely to become obese adults and to develop comorbid conditions, such as type 2 diabetes, hypertension, cardiovascular diseases, sleep apnea, and joint problems. If a teen is still growing, he or she has an advantage in terms of weight management; by holding body weight steady while height gains are achieved, body mass index will decrease over time. However, if a teen attains ultimate adult height and is still obese, a weight-loss regimen may be necessary. Weight loss should be gradual, perhaps 1 pound per week, and generally follow the advice in Chapter 7.

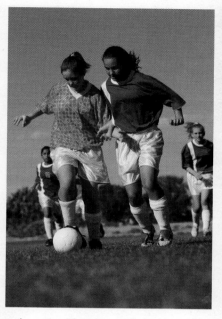

▲ An active lifestyle coupled with a healthy dietary pattern should be part of the teen years. Both habits contribute to bone development and strength. ©moodboard/Alamy

Calcium and Vitamin D. Over the last 20 years, soft drinks have been replacing milk as the preferred beverage among children. Intake of milk is especially poor among adolescent females, who may view dairy products as a source of unwanted calories. This trend in milk consumption begins early in childhood, but we discuss it here because the gap between needs and actual intake of bone-building nutrients is greatest during the adolescent growth spurt. Less than 10% of girls and less than 25% of boys meet recommendations for calcium intake. To make matters worse, one in five children is deficient in vitamin D. Meanwhile, the adolescent growth spurt marks a critical time for bone development. Calcium requirements for 14- to 18-year-old girls and boys are 1300 milligrams per day—higher than during any other time of life. As you learned in Section 9.6, failure to maximize bone mineralization during childhood sets the stage for development of osteoporosis later in life.

Three servings per day from the dairy group are recommended for all teenagers and young adults to meet calcium needs. If dairy products are not consumed, alternative calcium sources need to be included. Nondairy sources of calcium include almonds, legumes, some green vegetables, and fortified foods (e.g., fruit juices, cereal, and granola bars). However, it is important to note that these alternative sources of calcium may not provide other important nutrients supplied by dairy products, such as protein and vitamins A, D, and B-12.

Iron. About 10% of teenagers have low iron stores or iron-deficiency anemia. Iron-deficiency anemia is a highly undesirable condition for a teen. It can lead to fatigue and a decreased ability to concentrate and learn, such that academic and physical performance suffers. Iron-deficiency anemia sometimes appears in boys during their growth spurt, but adolescent females are at greatest risk of deficiency due to heavy menstrual flow and poor dietary intake. It is important that teenagers choose good food sources of iron, such as lean meats and fortified grain products. Teenage girls, in particular, need to eat good sources of iron (or regularly consume a balanced multivitamin and mineral supplement containing iron).

Many of the nutritional issues of adolescents—obesity, snacking, beverage choices, and skipping meals—have been adequately described with reference to younger children. Here, we present a few nutrition dilemmas that pertain especially to teenagers.

BREAK THE FAST-FOOD HABIT

It is convenient, casual, inexpensive, and all their friends work there. These are reasons why, on any given day, about 40% of the nation's youth eat food from a fast-food restaurant. Unfortunately, the average trip to a fast-food establishment yields about 300 extra kilocalories, 14 additional grams of fat, and 400 milligrams of sodium *in excess* of typical home-prepared meals for teenagers.[28,29]

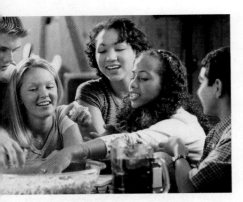

▲ The teenage years are noted for snacking. With reasonable food choices, teenagers can have healthful diets.
©SW Productions/Getty Images RF

With some small changes, teens can still enjoy dining out with friends without detriment to their health. When building a sandwich, opt for one layer of meat instead of double or triple patties, and select grilled instead of fried meat. For deli sandwiches, choose moderate portions of lean meats, such as roasted turkey or chicken, rather than fatty slices of bologna and salami. Skip the condiments or request them on the side; the mayonnaise on a typical fast-food sandwich supplies about 100 fat-laden kcal. Each slice of cheese supplies another 80 to 100 kcal. When it comes to choosing a side dish, a small baked potato or a garden salad with reduced-fat dressing will provide fewer calories and more nutrients than the typical 500-kcal large serving of fries. Calories from regular soft drinks—especially when free refills are available—can quickly add up. Teens should choose reduced-fat or fat-free milk as a nutrient-dense alternative or opt for water. Order a pizza with veggie toppings, low-fat cheese, and whole grain crust.

When burgers are measured in pounds instead of ounces, portion control is an issue. While already large, portion sizes at fast-food establishments continue to grow. Choosing items from the kids' menu can lessen the impact of dining out on adolescent wallets and waistlines. Supersized meals, while they may seem economical, should be avoided unless they are to be divided and shared among friends. All of us can benefit from the calorie information that many restaurants have already placed on their menus in anticipation of the mandatory posting that will soon be required (see Section 1.1).

CURB CAFFEINE INTAKE

The combined demands of school, work, extracurricular activities, social commitments, and late-night screen time leave many adolescents looking for a quick pick-me-up. Commonly, they are turning to caffeine, the most widely used stimulant on the planet. Soft drinks, a common choice among youth, provide about 25 milligrams of caffeine per serving. On average, 30% of adolescents report consuming energy beverages, which typically contain between 100 and 200 milligrams of caffeine per serving. Consumption of coffee and tea, which yield about 100 milligrams of caffeine per cup, is on the rise among teens. Various foods, including chocolate and some types of candies or sports nutrition products, contain caffeine as well. Average caffeine intake from all sources is just over 100 milligrams per day among teens. Many consumers are unaware of how much caffeine they are consuming; the exact amount of caffeine is not always listed on energy drink labels because (1) it is not currently required by food labeling laws; and (2) some manufacturers (especially of energy drinks) consider it to be part of a "proprietary blend."

For children, the American Academy of Pediatrics advises limiting caffeine intake to 100 milligrams per day, if it is used at all. Some of the negative effects of caffeine at any age are gastrointestinal distress, sleep disturbances, anxiety, increased blood pressure, and irregular heartbeat. For children, in particular, there is concern that excessive caffeine intake could affect normal neurological and cardiovascular development. Furthermore, disturbances in normal sleep patterns could affect growth and learning ability. Alarmingly, there have been thousands of reports of caffeine poisoning—and even some deaths—as a result of excessive intake of energy drinks. Clearly, excessive caffeine intake has no place in the diets of children.[30]

CHOOSING VEGETARIAN DIETS

Teenagers, who strive to forge an identity by adopting dietary patterns different from those of their families, may choose to follow vegetarian diets. As discussed in Section 6.8, vegetarians enjoy many health benefits, including lower body weight and better control of blood glucose and cholesterol. Indeed, an increased focus on plant foods is needed among adolescents, who often miss out on their recommended daily servings of fruits and vegetables. However, teens may not know enough about a vegetarian dietary pattern to keep from developing health problems, such as iron-deficiency anemia. The bulkiness of a plant-based diet is not as much of a concern for teens as it is for younger children with smaller stomach capacity, but a strictly vegetarian diet must be monitored for adequate energy, protein, iron, vitamin B-12, calcium, and vitamin D (the latter if sun exposure is not sufficient) at any age. These nutrients are particularly important in teenagers, as their diets are often already nutrient poor.

Teens often cite concern for the humane treatment of animals as their main reason for choosing vegetarian diets, but be observant of teens who choose vegetarianism as a method of weight loss. Vegetarianism is sometimes used as a socially acceptable way to restrict the diet and, for some, can be an early sign of disordered eating.

ALCOHOL ABUSE AMONG TEENS

In Section 15.5, we discussed how the beverage choices of school-age children are in need of improvement because they provide too much sugar and not enough micronutrients. The nutrient density of beverages continues to be a problem among teenagers, but a new problem arises: alcohol abuse. Developmentally, adolescents are prone to experimentation, rebellion, and risk taking, so use of this illegal and dangerous substance is common among teenagers. Results of the national Youth Risk Behavior Survey demonstrate that approximately 20% of teenagers have tried alcohol by the age of 13. At some point throughout the teenage years, about 70% of teens report drinking alcohol at least once, and 22% report binge drinking.

It is just harmless fun, right? Wrong! Alcohol use beginning in adolescence has severe consequences.[31] The adolescent's body and brain are still developing. Exposure to alcohol can decrease brain mass in the area of the brain involved in decision making, memory, and learning. This is evidenced by academic problems and poor decision making, which can lead to legal troubles, physical assault, and risky sexual behaviors. The most dangerous consequence of poor judgment is drinking and driving. About 1 in 10 teenagers admits to drinking and driving, a risky behavior that is implicated in about one-third of fatal motor vehicle accidents involving teens. Alcohol also contributes to other causes of accidental injuries and deaths, such as drowning, falls, and burns.

Adolescent alcohol abuse exacts a toll on long-term physical health, as well. Studies show that alcohol abuse beginning during adolescence is a strong predictor of alcohol abuse during adulthood. In Section 16.5, you will learn more about the effects of alcohol consumption on adults. Nutritional status can be affected because alcohol abuse is often accompanied by nutrient-poor diets. Also, weight gain from empty calories increases the risk for obesity-related diseases, such as hypertension and cardiovascular disease. These physical consequences may not surface until later in life, but it is certain that the effects of alcohol on the liver, brain, and cardiovascular system can start early.

Alcohol use by teenagers should not be viewed as a normal part of growing up. On the contrary, the physical, emotional, and intellectual consequences of underage drinking can be long-standing and devastating. Parents and other caregivers should talk to their children about the consequences of alcohol abuse, set clear rules, monitor their children's behavior, and be positive role models.

Newsworthy Nutrition

Glycemic index of food choices may influence acne

About 80% to 90% of teens experience acne to some degree. Although it is popularly believed that nuts, chocolate, and pizza contribute to acne, scientific studies have failed to show a strong role for any of these dietary factors. Based on the results of observational research, two dietary factors stand out as possible contributors to acne: foods with high **glycemic index (GI)** and high consumption of dairy products. Both of these dietary patterns are hypothesized to increase insulin levels, which through various mechanisms lead to increased sebum production and altered skin cell growth. To date, the highest-quality evidence supports the link between glycemic index of food choices and acne among males, but research on dairy products as well as on the fatty acid content of the diet is still underway. Whether or not it improves acne, changing the diet to include more whole grains, fruits, vegetables, and legumes would have multiple health benefits.

Source: Burris J, et al. "Acne: The role of medical nutrition therapy," *Journal of the Academy of Nutrition and Dietetics* 113:416, 2013.

glycemic index (GI) The blood glucose response of a given food, compared to a standard (typically, glucose or white bread). Glycemic index is influenced by starch structure, fiber content, food processing, physical structure, and macronutrients in the meal such as fat.

✓ CONCEPT CHECK 15.6

1. Which two minerals are most likely to be deficient in teen diets? Name two rich food sources of each of these minerals.

2. Design a meal for a teen that resembles MyPlate and can be purchased from a fast-food restaurant.

3. Are energy drinks safe for consumption by children of any age? Why or why not?

4. List three consequences of alcohol abuse that are specific to adolescents.

15.7 Nutrition and Your Health

Food Allergies and Intolerances

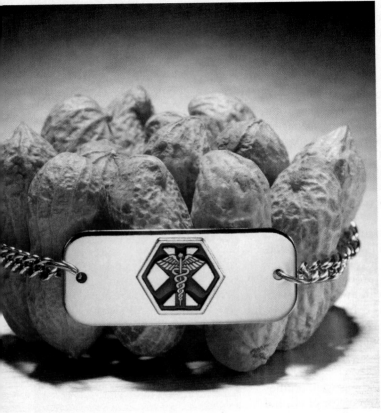

©FoodIngredients/Alamy RF

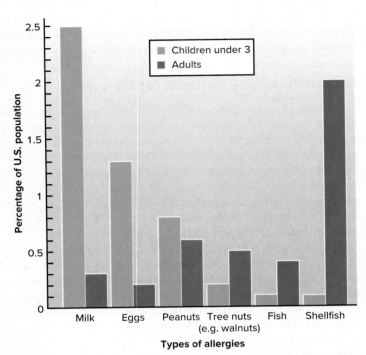

FIGURE 15-5 ▲ Types of allergies and percentage of U.S. population with those allergies. Source: *Journal of Allergy and Clinical Immunology* 2010; 125:S116. (study done by Mount Sinai School of Medicine).

Food allergies are on the rise. Between 1997 and 2011, food allergies among children increased by 50%. What used to be a rare medical incident is now the cause for 92,000 childhood emergency room visits and 84 child fatalities per year. Accounting for direct medical costs, special foods, and time lost from work, food allergies cost Americans $25 billion per year. Today, food allergies affect about 8% (5.9 million) of children in the United States, one-third of whom suffer from multiple food allergies.[32]

Adverse reactions to foods—indicated by sneezing, coughing, nausea, vomiting, diarrhea, hives, and other rashes—are broadly classed as **food allergies** (also called hypersensitivities) or **food intolerances.** The term *food sensitivity* is ill defined but generally refers to any symptom that is perceived to be food related. In our discussion, we group adverse food reactions into two categories. Those caused by an immune response are termed food allergies, and those not caused by an immune response are food intolerances.

Food Allergies: Symptoms and Mechanisms

Allergic reactions to foods are common (Fig. 15-5) and occur more frequently in females than males. Food allergies occur most often during infancy and young adulthood.

Symptoms of food allergies may affect the following:

- **Skin:** itching, tingling*, redness, hives, and swelling
- **GI tract:** nausea, vomiting, diarrhea, intestinal gas, bloating, pain, constipation, and indigestion
- **Respiratory tract:** runny nose, wheezing, congestion, and difficulty breathing*
- **Cardiovascular system:** low blood pressure* and rapid heart rate*

These symptoms usually set in shortly after consuming the offending food protein and may last for a few seconds or a few days. The symptoms marked with an asterisk (*) are signs of a rapid and potentially fatal type of allergic response called **anaphylaxis.** This severe allergic response results in low blood pressure and respiratory distress. A person who is extremely sensitive to a food may not be able to touch the food or even be in the same room where it is being cooked without reacting to it. Although any food can trigger anaphylaxis, the most common culprits are peanuts (a legume, not a nut), tree nuts (e.g., walnuts, pecans), shellfish, milk

food allergy An adverse reaction to food that involves an immune response; also called *food hypersensitivity.*

food intolerance An adverse reaction to food that does not involve an allergic reaction.

anaphylaxis A severe allergic response that results in lowered blood pressure and respiratory distress. This can be fatal.

(look for an ingredient called casein on the label), eggs (look for the ingredient albumin on the label), soybeans, wheat, and fish. Other foods frequently identified with adverse reactions include meat and meat products, fruits, and cheese. For a small number of people, avoiding foods such as peanuts or shellfish is a matter of life and death.

Basically, allergies are an inappropriate response of the immune system. When immune cells identify a harmful foreign protein **(antigen),** they destroy it and produce antibodies to it, so that the next response to the harmful substance will be swift and effective. Almost all food allergies are caused by proteins in foods that act as antigens (also called **allergens).** In these cases, the immune system mistakes the food protein for a harmful substance and mounts an immune response, leading to symptoms such as hives, runny nose, and GI disturbances.

No one is sure why the immune system sometimes overreacts to harmless proteins. The early introduction (e.g., before 4 months of age) of solid foods to infants may trigger food allergies. The reasoning is that the infant's GI tract is immature and "leaky," allowing some undigested proteins to be absorbed into the bloodstream. This is beneficial for the absorption of immune proteins from breast milk; however, if some food proteins are introduced before the GI tract has matured, these antigens may enter the bloodstream and stimulate an immune response.

The **hygiene hypothesis** offers another interesting explanation: in our "germophobic" society, with the protection of antibiotics, hand sanitizers, and antimicrobial soaps and cleaners, our immune systems are not vigorously challenged by antigens. As a result, the immune system may become sensitized to innocuous substances, such as food proteins. Current research supports the hygiene hypothesis. Children who grow up on farms or who have pets and are thereby exposed to many antigens have fewer allergies and asthma than children who grow up in more sterile environments.

Researchers are currently interested in the connection between a healthy gut microbiota and risk for food allergies. Also, researchers have proposed a link between low levels of vitamin D and food allergies. The relationship between vitamin D and food allergies may be mediated by the vitamin's role in immune function.

TESTING FOR A FOOD ALLERGY

The diagnosis of a food allergy can be a difficult task.[33] It requires the participation of a skilled clinician. To determine whether a food allergy is present, the health professional will record a detailed history of symptoms, including the time from ingestion to onset of symptoms, duration of symptoms, most recent reaction, food suspected of causing a reaction, and quantity and nature of food needed to produce a reaction. A family history of allergic diseases can also help, as allergies tend to run in families. A physical examination may reveal evidence of an allergy, such as skin diseases and asthma. Various diagnostic tests can rule out other conditions (Table 15-9).

If the patient history and physical exam suggest a food allergy, the health professional then faces the task of identifying the source of the food allergy. The first step in diagnosing a food allergy is to eliminate from the diet (for 1 to 2 weeks) all food components that appear to cause allergic symptoms. This is called an **elimination diet.** The person generally starts out eating foods to which almost no one reacts, such as rice, vegetables, noncitrus fruits, and fresh meats and poultry. If symptoms are still present, the person can more severely restrict the diet or even use special formula diets that are hypoallergenic.

Once a diet is found that causes no symptoms, foods can be added back one at a time. This type of food challenge is an option only when the culprit foods are known to pose no risk of anaphylaxis in the person. Doses of ½ to 1 teaspoon (2½ to 5 milliliters) are given at first. The amount is increased until the dose approximates usual intake. Any reintroduced food that causes significant symptoms to appear is identified as an allergen for the person.

Laboratory tests can also aid in diagnosis of food allergies. Skin testing involves pricking the skin with a small amount of purified food extract and observing any allergic response (e.g., a red eruption at the prick site). These types of tests are easy and safe, even for infants, but they may not clearly diagnose a food allergy. A positive skin-prick test merely indicates that a person has been sensitized to a food; it cannot definitively identify if that food is the cause

antigen Any substance that induces a state of sensitivity and/or resistance to microorganisms or toxic substances after a lag period; a foreign substance that stimulates a specific aspect of the immune system.

allergen A foreign protein, or antigen, that induces excess production of certain immune system antibodies; subsequent exposure to the same protein leads to allergic symptoms. Whereas all allergens are antigens, not all antigens are allergens.

hygiene hypothesis Assumption that reduced exposure to microorganisms in the environment (e.g., as a result of overuse of antibacterial soaps and antibiotics) impairs proper development of the immune system, making a person more susceptible to allergies and autoimmune diseases.

elimination diet A restrictive diet that systematically tests foods that may cause an allergic response by first eliminating them for 1 to 2 weeks and then adding them back, one at a time.

TABLE 15-9 ■ Diagnosing Food Allergies

History	Include description of symptoms, time between food ingestion and onset of symptoms, duration of symptoms, most recent allergic episode, quantity of food required to produce reaction, suspected foods, and allergic diseases in other family members.
Physical examination	Look for signs of an allergic reaction (rash, itching, intestinal bloating, etc.).
Elimination diet	Remove the suspected food allergen for 1 to 2 weeks or until symptoms clear.
Food challenge	Add back small amounts of excluded foods, one at a time, as long as anaphylaxis is not a possible consequence.
Blood test	Determine the presence of antibodies in blood that bind to food antigens tested.
Skin test	Place a sample of the suspected allergen under the skin and watch for an inflammatory reaction.

for the symptoms in question. Newer types of blood testing, however, have more diagnostic value. Blood tests estimate the blood concentration of antibodies that bind certain foodborne antigens.

LIVING WITH FOOD ALLERGIES

Once potential allergens are identified, dietary modifications must be made.[34] In some cases, small amounts of the offending food can be consumed without an observable reaction. Also, some food allergens are destroyed by heating, so cooking may eliminate the allergic response. This is effective primarily for allergies to fruits or vegetables, not for the more common allergies to milk, peanuts, or seafood. For most cases, though, complete avoidance of allergy-causing food ingredients is the safest course of action. This makes careful reading of food labels essential. The Food Allergen Labeling and Consumer Protection Act of 2006 requires manufacturers to clearly identify the presence of major food allergens (milk, eggs, fish, shellfish, peanuts, tree nuts, wheat, and soy) on food product labels. Some advocacy groups have petitioned to see sesame seeds added to the list of food allergens that must be listed on food labels.

A major challenge when treating a person with a food allergy is to make sure that what remains in the dietary pattern can still provide essential nutrients. The small food intake of children permits less leeway in removing offending foods that may contain numerous nutrients. A registered dietitian nutritionist can help guide the diet-planning process to ensure that the remaining food choices still meet nutrient needs or to guide supplement use, if that is necessary.[35]

Studies show that about 25% of young children with food allergies outgrow them. Parents should be made aware of this and not assume the allergy will be lifelong. Food allergies diagnosed after 3 years of age are often longer lived, but not always. It is common for children to outgrow allergies to milk, soy, or eggs, but allergies to peanuts, tree nuts, and shellfish are likely to endure. Periodic reintroduction of offending foods can be tried every 6 to 12 months

> People with a history of serious allergic reactions and those who have asthma should carry a self-administered form of epinephrine, such as EpiPen,® to subside an episode of anaphylaxis, should it occur.

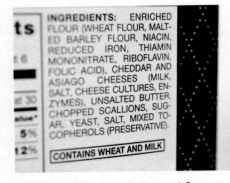

▲ In 2006, the Food Allergen Labeling and Consumer Protection Act mandated that food manufacturers make consumers aware of the presence of highly allergenic ingredients in their products. ©FoodIngredients/Alamy

Newsworthy Nutrition

Early introduction of peanut protein reduces peanut allergy

Based on a hypothesis that early introduction of food proteins in infants' diets increased risk for food allergies, pediatricians once advised parents to delay introduction of potential food allergens (e.g., 2 years for eggs and 3 years for peanuts, tree nuts, and fish). However, in the 1990s, evidence started to accumulate that delaying introduction of a variety of foods provided no benefit for preventing food allergies. For instance, Jewish children raised in the United Kingdom, where peanuts were not introduced until after 1 year of age, were 10 times more likely to develop peanut allergies than Jewish children raised in Israel, where peanut-based foods are introduced within the first year of life. The Learning Early About Peanut allergy (LEAP) trial aimed to see if early introduction of peanut protein could prevent peanut allergies among at-risk children. The randomized, controlled trial included 640 infants between 4 and 11 months of age who were at risk for food allergies (based on existing allergies, severe eczema, or both). Participants were divided into two groups based on previous sensitization to peanut protein (i.e., skin testing showed if the infants' immune systems had already reacted to peanut protein from dietary, skin, or respiratory exposure). Then, the infants were randomized to treatment or control groups. The treatment group received at least 6 grams of peanut protein per week in the form of a peanut-based snack food or smooth peanut butter, while the control group was advised to avoid dietary exposure to peanuts. At 5 years of age, the children were tested for peanut allergy using an oral food challenge. Among the children who were not sensitized to peanuts at baseline, peanut consumption reduced the risk of developing peanut allergy by 86.1% compared to controls. Among the children who were initially sensitized to peanut protein, treatment with peanut protein reduced the risk of developing peanut allergy by 70%. The researchers concluded that early (< 11 months), sustained peanut consumption reduced peanut allergy among children at risk of food allergies.

Source: Du Toit G, et al. "Randomized trial of peanut consumption in infants at risk for peanut allergy," *New England Journal of Medicine* 372:803, 2015.

or so, to see whether the allergic reaction has decreased. If no symptoms appear, tolerance to the food has developed.

Several strategies are under study to ease the dietary restrictions imposed by food allergies. One possibility includes treatment with antibodies that will increase the threshold at which an allergic response occurs. For a person with an allergy to peanuts, for

> Free information on food allergies is available by contacting Food Allergy Research and Education. The telephone number is (800) 929-4040; the website is www.foodallergy.org.

example, this would alleviate some anxiety about severe reactions to trace amounts of peanuts found in foods. Similarly, immunotherapy, which exposes allergic individuals to very small but progressively larger amounts of food allergens, may help some people build up a tolerance to certain food components. Vaccines are another area of research. Also, scientists are working on genetically engineered foods that do not contain common allergens.

PREVENTING FOOD ALLERGIES

With the rising number of cases of food allergies, many new parents wonder when and how to introduce new foods during infancy and early childhood. It is evident that introducing foods other than human milk or infant formula before 4 months of age is associated with higher risk of allergic diseases. Most experts, including the American Academy of Pediatrics and the American Academy of Allergy, Asthma, and Immunology, advise waiting to introduce solid foods until 4 to 6 months of age for lowest risk of food allergies. Delaying introduction of solid foods beyond 6 months of age is not advised.

Any food can contain a potential allergen, but certain foods have been found to have high allergenic potential. The eight leading food allergens in the United States are milk, eggs, peanuts, tree nuts, fish, shellfish, wheat, and soy. The American Academy of Pediatrics and the National Institute of Allergy and Infectious Diseases no longer advise delaying the introduction of highly allergenic foods beyond 6 months of age, even for infants with a family history of food allergies (see the Newsworthy Nutrition in this section).

Until recently, allergy-prone women were advised to avoid highly allergenic foods during pregnancy and breastfeeding. Allergens can cross the placenta during pregnancy and are secreted in breast milk. However, research does not demonstrate a benefit of maternal dietary restrictions in preventing food allergies in infants.

The best course of action is to breastfeed the infant exclusively for 6 months and continue to breastfeed through 12 months with appropriate introduction of solid foods to meet the infant's nutritional needs. Human milk contains factors that play a role in the maturation of the small intestine. Formula-fed infants, especially those on cow milk-based formulas, have a greater risk for developing food allergies. There is evidence that hydrolyzed infant formulas (in which the large proteins have been broken down into smaller peptides) may be useful in allergy prevention for infants at risk of developing food allergies. However, hydrolyzed formulas are about three times as costly as cow milk-based formulas.

FOOD INTOLERANCES

Food intolerances are adverse reactions to foods that do not involve immunologic mechanisms. Generally, larger amounts of an offending food are required to produce the symptoms of an intolerance than to trigger allergic symptoms. Common causes of food intolerances include:

- Constituents of certain foods (e.g., red wine, tomatoes, and pineapples) that have a drug-like activity, causing physiological effects such as changes in blood pressure
- Certain synthetic compounds added to foods, such as sulfites, food-coloring agents, and monosodium glutamate (MSG)
- Food contaminants, including antibiotics and other chemicals used in the production of livestock and crops, as well as insect parts not removed during processing
- Toxic contaminants, which may be ingested with improperly handled and prepared foods containing *Clostridium botulinum, Salmonella* bacteria, or other foodborne microorganisms (see Section 13.3)
- Deficiencies in digestive enzymes, such as lactase (review Section 4.4)

Almost everyone is sensitive to one or more of these causes of food intolerance, many of which produce GI tract symptoms. Sulfites, added to foods and beverages as antioxidants, cause flushing, spasms of the airway, and a loss of blood pressure in susceptible people. Wine, dehydrated potatoes, dried fruits, gravy, soup mixes, and restaurant salad greens commonly contain sulfites. A reaction to MSG may include an increase in blood pressure, numbness, sweating, vomiting, headache, and facial pressure. MSG is commonly found in restaurant food and many processed foods (e.g., soups). A reaction to tartrazine, a yellow food-coloring additive, includes spasm of the airway, itching, and reddening skin. Tyramine, a derivative of the amino acid tyrosine, is commonly found in "aged" foods such as cheeses and red wines. This natural food constituent can cause high blood pressure in people taking monoamine oxidase (MAO) inhibitor medications, which may be prescribed for clinical depression.

The basic treatment for food intolerances is to avoid specific offending components. However, total elimination often is not required because people generally are not as sensitive to compounds causing food intolerances as they are to allergens.

Summary (Numbers refer to numbered sections in the chapter.)

15.1 Growth is rapid during infancy; birth weight doubles by 6 months of age, and length increases by 50% in the first year. An adequate dietary pattern, especially in terms of calories, protein, iron, and calcium, is essential to support normal growth. Growth charts can be used to assess changes in body weight, height (or length), head circumference, and body mass index over time.

15.2 The energy needs of infants are highest per kilogram of body weight compared to any other life stage (about 100 kcal per kilogram). Fat should make up about 50% of total energy intake. DHA and ARA are important fatty acids for nervous system development. Carbohydrate needs range from 60 grams per day for younger infants to 95 grams per day for older infants. Protein needs are 9 grams per day for younger infants and 11 grams per day for older infants. Supplementation with vitamin D, iron, and fluoride may be appropriate for some infants. Adequate hydration can be maintained using only breast milk or formula; supplemental water is not recommended during the first 6 months of life.

15.3 Infant nutrient needs can usually be met by human milk or iron-fortified infant formula for the first 6 months of life. Introduction of solid foods should begin between 4 and 6 months of age, based on an infant's nutritional needs, physical abilities, and developmental readiness. Solid foods should be introduced one at a time, starting with iron-fortified infant cereals or ground meats (sources of iron). Some foods to avoid giving infants in the first year include honey, unaltered cow's milk (especially fat-reduced varieties), foods with added salt or sugar, and foods that may cause choking.

15.4 A slower growth rate results in decreased appetite among preschool children. Other common nutrition-related concerns include iron-deficiency anemia, constipation, and dental caries. With smaller portion sizes and picky eating behaviors, it is crucial to offer several small meals and snacks with a variety of nutrient-dense foods. Follow the example set forth by MyPlate, but use smaller portions (e.g., 1 tablespoon of food per year of life). For autism spectrum disorders, several nutritional interventions, including the gluten-free, casein-free diet, are under study, but none are endorsed by the AAP.

15.5 Among school-age children, excessive energy and fat intakes coupled with low levels of physical activity have led to an alarming increase in overweight, obesity, type 2 diabetes, and cardiovascular disease. Parents can provide healthful food choices and encourage at least 60 minutes of physical activity per day. When controlled early through dietary and exercise interventions, the problem of obesity may correct itself as the child continues to grow in height. Other important nutrition strategies for school-age children include starting the day with breakfast and selecting low-fat or fat-free milk or water instead of sugar-sweetened beverages. Recent changes in meal offerings through schools are aimed at curtailing the rise in childhood obesity.

15.6 During the adolescent growth spurt, both boys and girls have increased needs for iron, calcium, and overall calories. Inadequate calcium intake by teenage girls is a major concern because it can set the stage for the development of osteoporosis later in life. Adolescents need to limit their intakes of high-fat and high-sugar fast foods and snacks and use caffeine in moderation (if at all). Alcohol abuse during adolescence has many severe consequences, including impaired brain development and increased risk for liver and cardiovascular diseases in adulthood.

15.7 The most common food allergies are associated with peanuts, tree nuts, shellfish, milk, eggs, soybeans, wheat, and fish. Food allergies occur most often during infancy and young adulthood. Dietary treatment for food allergies involves complete avoidance of the food allergen.

Check Your Knowledge (Answers are available at the end of this question set.)

1. Inadequate intake of which of the following results in poor growth?
   a. Calories
   b. Iron
   c. Zinc
   d. All of these

2. Cow's milk is a nutrient-dense source of all of the following except
   a. protein.
   b. iron.
   c. calcium.
   d. zinc.

3. To ensure adequate vitamin and mineral intake for a picky eater,
   a. provide a fortified breakfast cereal.
   b. promise dessert as a reward for eating meats and vegetables.
   c. use a multivitamin and mineral supplement.
   d. avoid all of these.

4. An 11-month-old girl who weighs 19 pounds needs approximately ___ kcal per day.
   a. 690
   b. 810
   c. 845
   d. 930

5. Introduction of cow's milk should be delayed until 12 months of age because it
   a. contains too much fat.
   b. supplies too much lactose.
   c. contains too much protein.
   d. does all of these.

6. Your niece breaks out in hives and feels nauseous after eating a salad containing mango. She probably has a food
   a. sensitivity.
   b. allergy.
   c. intolerance.
   d. All of these are correct.

7. Which of the following are benefits of consuming a fortified, ready-to-eat breakfast cereal instead of skipping breakfast?
   a. Improved academic performance
   b. Meeting RDAs for iron and calcium
   c. Lower risk for childhood obesity
   d. All of these

8. A gluten-free, casein-free diet has been studied for treatment of
   a. rickets.
   b. anemia.
   c. lead poisoning.
   d. autism.

9. If moderate weight loss is needed, a school-age child should
   a. eat fewer meals.
   b. follow a low-carbohydrate eating plan.
   c. exercise for 60 minutes per day or more.
   d. avoid dairy products.

10. You are trying to introduce an apple and blueberry puree to a 7-month-old infant, but she rejects it. You should
    a. assume she doesn't like apples and blueberries.
    b. offer the food again on another day.
    c. force a spoonful into her mouth.
    d. do none of these.

Answer Key: 1. d (LO 15.1), 2. b (LO 15.2), 3. a (LO 15.2), 4. a (LO 15.3), 5. c (LO 15.3), 6. b (LO 15.6), 7. d (LO 15.4), 8. d (LO 15.4), 9. c (LO 15.5), 10. b (LO 15.3)

Study Questions (Numbers refer to Learning Outcomes)

1. List two factors that limit "catch-up" growth when a nutrient-deficient dietary pattern has been consumed throughout childhood. **(LO 15.1)**

2. A 3-month-old infant is taken to a clinic with failure to thrive. What are two possible explanations? **(LO 15.1)**

3. Which two nutrients are of particular concern in planning dietary patterns for teenagers? Why does each deserve to be singled out? **(LO 15.2)**

4. List three nutrients of concern for a child who chooses a vegetarian lifestyle. **(LO 15.2)**

5. Outline three key factors that help to determine when to introduce solid foods into an infant's dietary pattern. **(LO 15.3)**

6. Compare the guidelines for infant feeding summarized in this chapter with the *Dietary Guidelines for Americans* for children over age 2 and adults discussed in Chapter 2. Which guidelines are similar? Do any contradict each other? If so, why? **(LO 15.3)**

7. Describe the pros and cons of snacking. What is the basic advice for healthful snacking from childhood through the teenage years? **(LO 15.4)**

8. List three reasons why preschoolers are noted for picky eating. For each, describe an appropriate parent response. **(LO 15.4)**

9. What three factors are likely to contribute to obesity in a typical 10-year-old child? **(LO 15.5)**

10. List evidence-based strategies to reduce the risk of food allergies in infants. **(LO 15.6)**

What the Dietitian Chose

At 18 months of age, Lila's dietary pattern should include small portions of a variety of foods from each MyPlate food group. She should have several teeth by now, but her chewing ability is still limited. As a young child, Lila has high nutrient needs and yet has a small stomach capacity, so snacking makes an important contribution to meeting overall nutrient needs.

Reduced-fat popcorn is a healthy, low-fat snack for older children and adults. Feeding children bulky foods with low energy density, however, can lead to fullness without meeting nutritional needs. Furthermore, popcorn is a choking hazard.

Although baby carrots with ranch dressing would be a good source of beta-carotene and plant oils, toddlers are not expert chewers just yet, and large pieces of hard, crunchy foods present a choking hazard. Slicing the carrots into long, thin strips would be a better idea.

Fat-free, light yogurt is a good source of calcium and vitamin D for building healthy bones and certainly does not present a choking risk; however, infants and toddlers need the fat and sugar in dairy products to supply calories for their growing bodies. Whole-milk

yogurt such as YoBaby® would be a better choice.

Whole grain crackers with sliced cheddar cheese would be an excellent snacking option for Lila. This snack provides a healthy balance of carbohydrates, protein, and fat. Using whole grain crackers, rather than those made with refined flour, will boost the vitamin and mineral content (review Section 4.3).

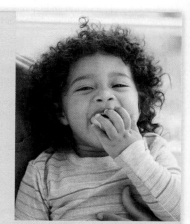
©Hero/Corbis/Glow Images

Toddlers are known for picky eating behaviors. Lila's slower pace of growth may reduce her appetite, and she may be more interested in exploring the world around her than sitting down for a meal. Make sure Lila sits down to eat and supervise her while she is eating. Finally, be a good role model. If she sees you eat the healthy snacks you have offered, she will be more likely to accept them.

Further Readings

1. Cole SZ and Lanham JS: Failure to thrive: An update. *Am Fam Physician* 2011; 83:829.

2. Wagner CL and others: Prevention of rickets and vitamin D deficiency in infants, children, and adolescents. *Pediatrics* 2008; 122(5):1142.

3. Baker RD and Greer FR: Clinical report—diagnosis and prevention of iron deficiency and iron-deficiency anemia in infants and young children (0–3 years of age). *Pediatrics* 2010; 126:1040.

4. Abrams EM: Introducing solid foods: Age of introduction and its effect on risk of food allergy and other atopic diseases. *Can Fam Physician* 2013; 59:721.

5. Togias A and others: Addendum guidelines for the prevention of peanut allergy in the United States: Report of the National Institute of Allergy and Infectious Disease–sponsored expert panel. *Ann Allergy Asthma Immunol* 2017; 118:166.

6. American Heart Association: Added sugars and cardiovascular disease risk in children: A scientific statement from the American Heart Association. *Circulation* 2016; 134:1.

7. American Academy of Pediatrics: *Bright futures nutrition: Pocket guide,* 3rd ed. 2011. https://brightfutures.aap.org/Bright%20Futures%20Documents/BFNutrition3rdEdPocketGuide.pdf (Accessed March 9, 2017).

8. Heyman MB and others: Fruit juice in infants, children, And adolescents: Current recommendations. *Pediatrics* 2017; 139(6):e20170967.

9. Moag-Stahlberg A: *The state of family nutrition and physical activity: Are we making progress? Report of the American Dietetic Association and American Dietetic Association Foundation,* 2011. http://eatrightfoundation.org/wp-content/uploads/2016/10/fnpa-report_2011.pdf (Accessed September 15, 2017).

10. Ford CN and others: Trends in dietary intake among US 2–6-year-old children, 1989–2008. *J Acad Nutr Diet* 2013; 113:35.

11. Academy of Nutrition and Dietetics: Position of the American Dietetic Association: Nutrition guidance for healthy children ages 2 to 11 years. *J Acad Nutr Diet* 2014; 114:1257.

12. Palmer S: Snacking in young children. *Today's Dietitian* 2016; 18:8.

13. Privett D: Autism spectrum disorder: Research suggests good nutrition may manage symptoms. *Today's Dietitian* 2013; 15:46.

14. Stewart PA and others: Dietary supplementation in children with autism spectrum disorders: Common, insufficient, and excessive. *J Acad Nutr Diet* 2015; 115:1237.

15. Mari-Bauset S and others: Evidence of the gluten-free and casein-free diet in autism spectrum disorders: A systematic review. *J Child Neurol* 2014; 29:1718.

16. Van Pelt J: Exercise as autism therapy. *Today's Dietitian* 2016; 18:48.

17. Grossman DC and others: Screening for obesity in children and adolescents: US Preventive Services Task Force recommendation statement. *JAMA* 2017; 317:2417.

18. Schaeffer J: Family-based weight loss. *Today's Dietitian* 2014; 16:26.

19. World Health Organization: *Report of the Commission on Ending Childhood Obesity.* Geneva: WHO Document Production Services, 2016.

20. Kavey RW and others: Expert panel on integrated guidelines for cardiovascular health and risk reduction in children and adolescents: Summary report. *Pediatrics* 2011; 128:S213.

21. Copeland KC and others: Management of newly diagnosed type 2 diabetes mellitus (T2DM) in children and adolescents. *Pediatrics* 2013; 131:364.

22. Williams PG: The benefits of breakfast cereal consumption: A systematic review of the evidence base. *Adv Nutr* 2014; 5:636S.

23. Briefel RR and others: Reducing calories and added sugars by improving children's beverage choices. *J Acad Nutr Diet* 2013; 113:269.

24. Kosova EC and others: The relationship between sugar-sweetened beverage intake and cardiometabolic markers in young children. *J Acad Nutr Diet* 2013; 113:219.

25. Wojcicki JM and Heyman MB: Reducing childhood obesity by eliminating 100% fruit juice. *Am J Public Health* 2012; 102:1630.

26. Briggs M and others: Position of the American Dietetic Association, School Nutrition Association, and Society for Nutrition Education: Comprehensive school nutrition services. *J Am Diet Assoc* 2010; 110:1738.

27. Cullen KW and Dave JM: The new federal school nutrition standards and meal patterns: Early evidence examining the influence on student dietary behavior and the school food environment. *J Acad Nutr Diet* 2017; 117:185.

28. Powell LM and Nguyen BT: Fast-food and full-service restaurant consumption among children and adolescents: Effect on energy, beverage, and nutrient intake. *JAMA Pediatrics* 2013; 167:14.

29. Quader ZS and others: Sodium intake among US school-aged children: National Health and Nutrition Examination Survey, 2011–2012. *J Acad Nutr Diet* 2017; 117:39.

30. Committee on Nutrition and the Council on Sports Medicine and Fitness: Sports drinks and energy drinks for children and adolescents: Are they appropriate? *Pediatrics* 2011; 127:1182.

31. Office of Juvenile Justice and Delinquency Prevention: Effects and consequences of underage drinking. *Juvenile Justice Bulletin* 2012. http://www.ojjdp.gov/pubs/237145.pdf. (Accessed September 15, 2017).

32. Gupta RS and others: Childhood food allergies: Current diagnosis, treatment, and management strategies. *Mayo Clin Proc* 2013; 88:512.

33. National Institute of Allergy and Infectious Diseases: Guidelines for the diagnosis and management of food allergy in the United States: Report of the NIAID-sponsored expert panel. *J Allergy Clin Immunol* 2010; 126:S1.

34. Orenstein BW: Pediatric food allergies. *Today's Dietitian* 2014; 16:12.

35. Academy of Nutrition and Dietetics: Practice paper of the Academy of Nutrition and Dietetics: Role of the registered dietitian nutritionist in the diagnosis and management of food allergies. *J Acad Nutr Diet* 2016; 116:1621.

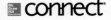 **To get the most out of your study, visit Connect where you will find NutritionCalc Plus, SmartBook®, and many other dynamic tools.**

Getting Young Bill to Eat

Bill is 3 years old, and his mother is worried about his eating habits. He refuses to eat vegetables, meat, and dinner in general. Some days he eats very little food. He wants to eat snacks most of the time. Mealtime is a battle because Bill says he is not hungry, and his mother wants him to sit down and eat all of his lunch and dinner to make sure he gets all the nutrients he needs. He drinks five or six glasses of whole milk per day because that is the one food he likes.

When his mother prepares dinner, she makes plenty of vegetables, boiling them until they are soft, hoping this will appeal to Bill. Bill's dad waits to eat his vegetables last, regularly telling the family that he eats them only because he has to. He also regularly complains about how dinner has been prepared. Bill saves his vegetables until last and usually gags when his mother orders him to eat them. Bill has been known to sit at the dinner table for an hour until the war of wills ends. Bill's mother serves casseroles and stews regularly because they are convenient. Bill likes to eat breakfast cereal, fruit, and cheese, and regularly requests these foods for snacks. However, his mother tries to deny his requests, so that he will have an appetite for dinner. Bill's mother comes to you and asks you what she should do to get Bill to eat.

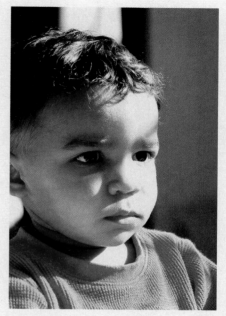

©McGraw-Hill Education/Jill Braaten, photographer

Analysis

1. List four mistakes Bill's parents are making that contribute to Bill's inadequate eating pattern.

   _____

   _____

   _____

2. List four strategies they might try to promote good eating habits in Bill.

   _____

   _____

   _____

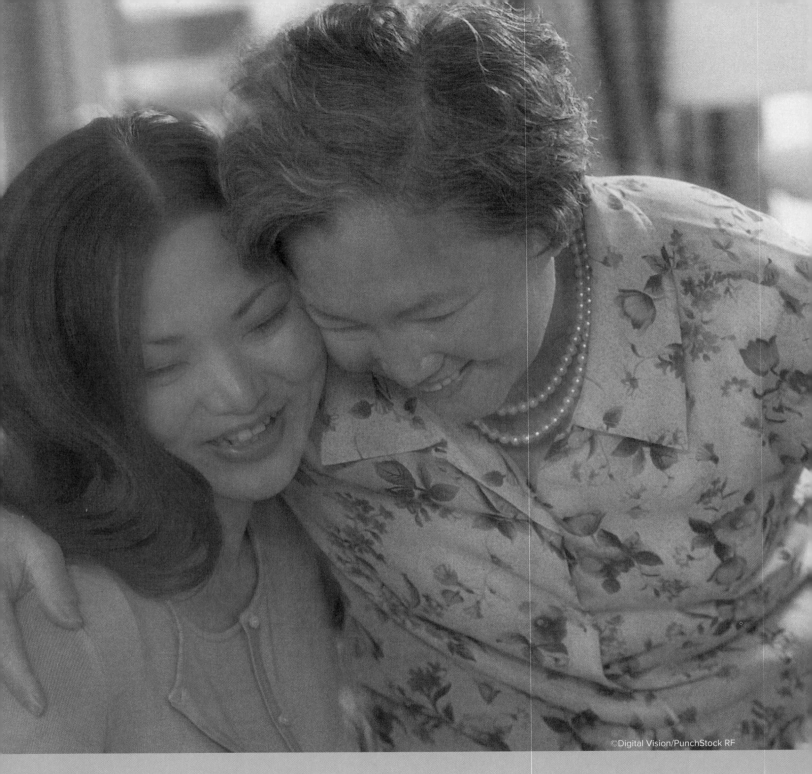

©Digital Vision/PunchStock RF

Student Learning Outcomes

Chapter 16 is designed to allow you to:

16.1 Discuss demographic trends among adults in North America and how they impact health care.

16.2 List several hypotheses about the causes of aging.

16.3 Describe how physiological changes of aging affect the nutritional status of adults.

16.4 Compare the dietary intake of adults with current recommendations.

16.5 Identify nutrition-related health conditions of the adult years, and describe the prevention and treatment options.

16.6 List several nutritional programs available to help meet the nutritional needs of older adults.

16.7 Compare benefits of moderate alcohol use to the risks of alcohol abuse.

Chapter 16
Nutrition During Adulthood

Eating is one of our great pleasures. Guided by common sense and moderation, eating well is also a means to good health. Most of us want a long, productive life, free of illness. Unfortunately, many people from adulthood onward suffer from obesity-related diseases such as cardiovascular disease, hypertension, stroke, type 2 diabetes, osteoporosis, and cancer. We can slow the development of—and in some cases, even prevent or slow the progression of—these diseases by following a dietary pattern such as that exemplified by MyPlate or the Mediterranean diet. The cumulative effect of such a dietary pattern is most profitable if we begin early and continue throughout adulthood. We serve ourselves best—as individuals and as a nation—by striving to maintain vitality even in the later decades of life. This concept was first explored in Chapter 1 and is discussed again in this chapter, in light of the nutritional needs of adults.

Keep in mind that today's behaviors can significantly influence your health years from now. Although genes do play a role, as discussed previously, many of the health problems that occur with age are not inevitable; they result from diet-related disease processes that influence physical and mental health. Much can be learned from healthy older people whose attention to healthy dietary and activity patterns—along with a little help from genetics—keeps them active and vibrant well beyond the average life span. Successful aging is the goal. Age quickly or slowly: it is primarily your choice.

16.1 The Graying of North America

Due to advances in health care and sanitation, the demographics of developed countries are shifting so that, as a population, we are getting older. In North America, the group constituting those aged 85+ years is the fastest growing segment. Between 1997 and 2050, the population aged 85+ years in the United States is expected to increase from 3.4 to 19 million (Fig. 16-1). Even more amazing, 1 million or more people in the United States could be over 100 years old in 2050.

This *graying* of North America poses some problems. Although people older than age 65 account for just 13.8% of the U.S. population, they account for more than 33% of all prescription medications used, 35% of acute hospital stays, and 30% of the federal health budget. Hip fractures alone cost the nation about $12 billion per year. Of older persons, 80% or more have chronic conditions, such as cardiovascular disease, type 2 diabetes, hypertension, and osteoporosis.

Preventing or postponing the onset of these chronic diseases for as long as possible will help control health care costs and improve quality of life. Health and independence contribute quality—not just quantity—to life and lessen the load on an already overburdened health care system. Keep in mind that aging alone is not a disease. Furthermore, diseases that commonly accompany old age—osteoporosis, cancer, and atherosclerosis, for example—are not an inevitable part of aging. Many can be prevented or managed.

THE CAUSES OF AGING

Adulthood, the longest stage of the normal life cycle, begins when an adolescent completes his or her physical growth. Unlike earlier stages of the life cycle, nutrients are used primarily to maintain the body rather than support physical growth. Pregnancy is the only time during adulthood when substantial amounts of nutrients are used for growth. As adults get older, nutrient needs change. For example, vitamin D needs increase for older adults.

Aging can be defined as the physical and physiological changes in body structure and function that occur throughout adulthood as humans mature and become older. One view of aging describes it as a process of slow cell death, beginning soon after fertilization.

aging Time-dependent physical and physiological changes in body structure and function that occur normally and progressively throughout adulthood as humans mature and become older.

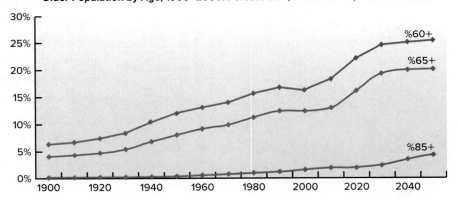

Older Population by Age, 1900–2050: Percent 60+, Percent 65+, and Percent 85+

FIGURE 16-1 ▲ **Growth of the U.S. Population of Older Adults.** This chart shows that the proportion of the total U.S. population composed of older adults has been steadily increasing over the past century and how these trends are expected to continue. The 85+ demographic group (green line), although still the smallest group in total numbers, is experiencing the most rapid rate of growth. Enhancements in health care and sanitation, as well as the baby boom that occurred after World War II, are contributing to the graying of North America. Conversely, most demographic groups under the age of 45 are shrinking as a percentage of overall population (not shown here). This means that fewer young people will be available to care for a growing population of older adults in years to come.

Source: U.S. Administration on Aging

When we are young, aging is not apparent because the major metabolic activities are geared toward growth and maturation. We produce plenty of active cells to meet physiological needs. During late adolescence and adulthood, the body's major task is to maintain cellular function. From the beginning of adulthood until age 30 or so, the body operates at peak performance: stature, stamina, strength, endurance, efficiency, and health. During this time, rates of cell synthesis and breakdown are balanced in most tissues.

Inevitably, though, cells age and die. After about age 30, the rate of cell breakdown slowly begins to exceed the rate of cell renewal, leading to a gradual decline in organ size and efficiency. Eventually, the body cannot adjust to meet all physiological demands, and body functioning begins to decrease (Fig. 16-2). Still, body systems and organs usually retain enough **reserve capacity** to handle normal, everyday demands throughout one's entire lifetime. Problems caused by diminished capacity typically do not arise unless severe demands are placed on the aging body. For example, alcohol intake can overtax an aging liver. The stress of shoveling a snow-covered sidewalk can exceed the capacity of the heart and lungs. Coping with an illness also can push an older body beyond its capacity.

The causes of aging remain a mystery. Most likely, the physiological changes of aging are the sum of automatic cellular changes, lifestyle practices, and environmental influences, as listed in Table 16-1. Even with the most supportive environment and healthy lifestyle, cell structure and function still decline over time. The eventual death of deteriorating cells can be beneficial in preventing diseases such as cancer. Unfortunately, there are negative consequences to this natural cell progression because, as more and more cells in an organ die, organ function declines. For example, **kidney nephrons** are continually lost as we age. In some people, this loss exhausts the kidneys' reserve capacity and ultimately leads to kidney dysfunction or failure.

The diseases and degenerative processes commonly observed in older people have long been assumed to be unavoidable consequences of aging. Certainly, some of the declines we blame on aging may be inevitable, such as gradual reductions in tissue and organ cell numbers, graying hair, and reduced lung capacity. However, many age-related changes can, in fact, be minimized, prevented, and/or reversed by healthy lifestyles (e.g., eating a nutritious diet, exercising regularly, and getting enough sleep) and avoiding adverse environmental factors (e.g., excessive exposure to sunlight and tobacco). These discoveries have led researchers to introduce the concepts of *usual aging* and *successful aging*.

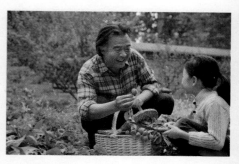

▲ The first baby boomers turned 70 in 2016, resulting in an increase in demand for attention to the health concerns of this aging population. ©XiXinXing/Getty Images

reserve capacity The extent to which an organ can preserve essentially normal function despite decreasing cell number or cell activity.

kidney nephrons The units of kidney cells that filter wastes from the bloodstream and deposit them into the urine.

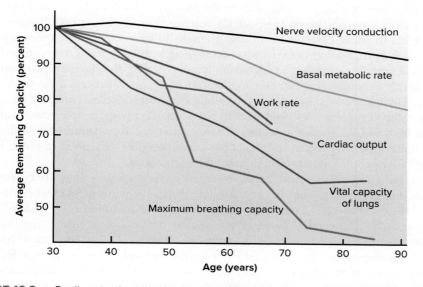

FIGURE 16-2 ▲ Declines in physiological function seen with aging. The decline in many body functions is especially evident in sedentary people.

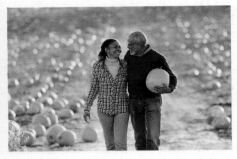

▲ Adopting eating patterns and lifestyle behaviors that minimize a decline in body function is an investment in your future health. Visit www.nia.nih.gov for many free resources on healthy aging. ©Image Source, all rights reserved

glycosylation The process by which glucose attaches to (glycates) other compounds, such as proteins.

TABLE 16-1 ■ Current Hypotheses About the Causes of Aging

Genetic mutations in DNA.
Copy errors in the cell cycle can lead to mutations that cause protein dysfunction, resulting in cell death.

Connective tissue stiffens.
Parallel protein strands, found mostly in connective tissue, cross-link to each other, resulting in reduced flexibility in key body components.

Oxidative free radicals damage cellular components.
Electron-seeking free radicals can break down cell membranes and proteins.

Hormonal changes.
Concentrations of many hormones, such as testosterone in men and estrogen in women, decline during the aging process.

Glycosylation of proteins.
Chronically elevated blood glucose attaches to various blood and body proteins, causing dysfunction and promoting an immune response.

Immune system inefficiency.
With advancing age, the immune system is less able to recognize and counteract foreign substances, such as viruses, that enter the body.

Autoimmune malfunctions.
Autoimmune reactions occur when the immune system malfunctions and begins to attack healthy cells, resulting in inflammation and cell damage or death.

Programmed cell death.
Each human cell can divide about 50 times before it automatically succumbs.

Excess calorie intake promotes more rapid aging.
Reduced caloric intake, by about 30%, in studied rodents results in significantly longer life spans than for their well-fed counterparts. Calorie restriction is currently the only known method to substantially slow the aging process.[1]

USUAL AND SUCCESSFUL AGING

Body cells eventually age, despite what health practices we follow. However, to a considerable extent, you can choose how quickly you age throughout your adult years. *Usual aging* refers to those changes commonly thought to be a typical or expected part of aging, such as increasing body fatness, decreasing lean body mass, rising blood pressure, declining bone mass, and increasingly poor health. Researchers point out that many of these changes represent an acceleration of the aging process induced by modifiable lifestyle choices, adverse environmental exposures, and/or chronic disease. For instance, blood pressure does not tend to rise with age among people who maintain a healthy body weight, engage in regular physical activity, and consume a primarily plant-based dietary pattern low in sodium. Lean body mass is maintained at much higher rates in older people who exercise than in those who do not.

Successful aging, on the other hand, describes physiological declines that occur only because one grows older, not because lifestyle choices, environmental exposures, and chronic disease have accelerated the aging process and assaulted body tissues. Those who are successful agers experience age-related declines at a slower rate and the onset of chronic disease symptoms at a later age than usual agers. Striving to have the greatest number of healthy years and the fewest years of illness is often referred to as **compression of morbidity.** In other words, a person tries to delay the onset of disabilities and discomforts caused by chronic disease and to compress significant sickness related to aging into the last few years—or months—of life.

compression of morbidity Delay of the onset of disabilities caused by chronic disease.

FACTORS AFFECTING THE RATE OF AGING

Life span refers to the maximum number of years a human can live. The longest human life documented to date is 122 years for a woman and 116 years for a man. **Life expectancy,** alternatively, is the time an average person born in a specific year can expect to live. Life expectancy in North America is about 76 years for men and about 81 years for women, with a span of *healthy years* of about 64. Furthermore, most people who survive to age 80 can expect to live an additional 7 to 10 years.

The rate at which one ages is individual; it is determined by genetics, lifestyle, and environment. With the exception of genetics, most of the factors that influence the rate of aging are directly linked to choices that are largely under our control.

Genetics Living to an old age tends to run in some families. If your parents and grandparents lived a long time, you are likely to have the potential to live to an old age, too. Studies of twins indicate that about 20% to 30% of longevity can be attributed to genetics.

One of the most obvious genetic characteristics influencing longevity is gender. In the case of humans, as well as most other species, females tend to live longer than males. Another genetic characteristic that may influence longevity is metabolic efficiency. Some researchers hypothesize that individuals with a **thrifty metabolism** require fewer calories for metabolic processes and are able to store body fat more easily than those with faster metabolic rates. Throughout history, it was the individuals with thrifty metabolism who tended to live the longest because they efficiently stored fat during times of plenty and thus had the energy stores needed to survive frequent periods of food scarcity. In today's environment of labor-saving devices and abundant, energy-dense foods, however, a thrifty metabolism may actually reduce longevity. Accumulation of excessive body fat increases the risk of developing health problems that reduce life expectancy (e.g., heart disease, hypertension, and many cancers).

Is DNA your destiny? Although genetics remain largely unchangeable, let us examine how you can exert greater control over your lifestyle and environment.

Lifestyle Lifestyle is one's pattern of living; it includes food choices, physical activity, and substance use (e.g., alcohol, drugs, and tobacco). Lifestyle choices can have a major impact on health and longevity, partly by regulating gene expression. If individuals have a family history of premature heart disease, they can adjust their dietary and activity patterns, and decrease tobacco use to slow the progression of the disease and possibly extend their lifetime. The converse is true, too. That is, lifestyle choices (e.g., high saturated-fat dietary pattern and sedentary lifestyle) can increase susceptibility to diseases that hasten the rate of aging, ultimately shortening life expectancy, even if a person is free from a genetic predisposition to disease.

In an effort to unlock the secrets to living a long and healthy life, researchers have been very interested in studying lifestyle patterns of communities in which life expectancy is higher than average. Several communities in which people quite often live to see their 90th and 100th birthdays include Okinawa, Japan; some parts of the Mediterranean region; and areas of California that are home to members of the Seventh-day Adventist religious denomination. Recall the 9 common lifestyle behavior traits of these *Blue Zone* communities were presented in Chapter 7.

Worldwide, the highest average life expectancy (86.8 years for women and 80.5 years for men) is in Okinawa, in southern Japan. The Okinawan dietary pattern is based on rice, fish, vegetable protein sources, fruits, vegetables, tea, herbs for seasonings, and small amounts of meat. Alcohol and salt intake is minimal. The low energy density translates into a generally low calorie intake, and the average BMI is 21. A desire to mimic their weight-management success, compression of morbidity, and extended longevity has given rise to several popular books and websites that promote Okinawan dietary practices.

Followers of the traditional Mediterranean diet enjoy some of the lowest recorded rates of chronic disease in the world. As previously mentioned, the Mediterranean diet features abundant daily intake of fruits, vegetables, whole grains, beans, nuts, and

life span The potential oldest age a person can reach.

life expectancy The average length of life for a given group of people born in a specific year.

thrifty metabolism A genetic tendency toward efficient use of energy that results in below-average energy requirements and increased storage of calories as fat.

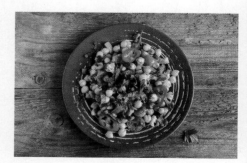

▲ A plant-based diet, exemplified by this dinner of couscous, chickpeas, and vegetables, is a common feature among populations who enjoy long, healthy lives. ©Mizina/iStock/Getty Images Plus

Besides having other long-lived family members, *centenarians*, or people who live to 100 years, generally:

- Do not use tobacco or drink heavily
- Maintain healthy weight
- Eat many fruits and vegetables
- Perform daily physical activity
- Challenge their minds
- Have a positive outlook
- Maintain close friendships and social networks
- Are or were married (especially for men)

seeds. Olive oil, a source of heart-healthy monounsaturated fat, is the main dietary fat. Beans and fish are emphasized as sources of protein, whereas dairy products, eggs, poultry, and meats are consumed less frequently. Daily exercise is a way of life. In addition, many Mediterraneans consume wine in moderation at mealtimes.

Loma Linda, California, is a town with a large population of Seventh-day Adventists, a Christian religious denomination that emphasizes stewardship of the mind and body as a way to honor God. Men in this group live about 7 years longer and women live about 4 years longer than average Americans. About 30% of Seventh-day Adventists follow a vegetarian dietary pattern, but even for those who occasionally consume animal products, the focus is on unprocessed plant foods. In particular, regular consumption of nuts and whole grains have emerged as dietary patterns that predict the lower rates of chronic diseases observed in this population. Unlike the Mediterraneans, most Seventh-day Adventists avoid alcohol. Other salient aspects of the Seventh-day Adventist lifestyle that are associated with longevity include daily physical activity, avoidance of tobacco, strong faith, and strong social support networks within a tight-knit community.

Note the similarities in lifestyle behaviors of these groups of healthy agers. All tend to focus on unprocessed, fiber-rich foods, healthy sources of fat (e.g., vegetable oils and fish), and plant-based or lean sources of protein. Besides dietary patterns, physical activity is a major component of their daily routines.

Environment Income, education level, health care, shelter, and socioecological factors exert a powerful influence on the rate of aging. For instance, being able to access and purchase nutritious foods, obtain optimal health care, and reside in safe housing decreases the rate of aging. Having the education to earn sufficient living wages, as well as the knowledge to make wise lifestyle choices, also can slow the aging process.

Newsworthy Nutrition

Low animal protein intake is associated with a major reduction in mortality

Caloric restriction (CR) without malnutrition has consistently shown to increase longevity in a variety of animal models. However, the effect of CR on the lifes pan of humans remains controversial. The aim of this study was to combine epidemiological data with both animal and cellular study results to understand the link between protein intake, aging, disease, and mortality. Over 6380 U.S. adults, aged 50 and older, from the National Health and Nutrition Examination Survey (NHANES), were included in the sample. Mortality data was available for NHANES III participants through 2006 and covered an 18-year span. After follow-up, respondents, aged 50 to 65, with a high protein intake (> 20% calories) had a 75% increase in overall mortality and a four-fold increase in cancer death. In respondents over 65, however, high protein intake was associated with reduced cancer and overall mortality. It is believed that these results are related to regulation of circulating insulin and inflammation. The authors speculate that vulnerable and often underweight seniors are more susceptible to protein malnourishment. It is also possible that other factors, such as inflammation or genetics, may contribute to the varying protein sensitivity in the elderly subjects. These results align with those of other studies showing that the amount of proteins derived from animal sources accounted for a significant proportion of the negative associations between overall protein intake and mortality. The authors are clear to point out that plant-based proteins are likely to maximize health benefits in all age groups and should be enjoyed. In summary, these results suggest that low animal protein intake (< 10% calories) during middle age followed by moderate to high protein consumption in old adults may optimize health span and longevity.

Source: Levine ME and others: Low protein intake is associated with a major reduction in IGF-1, cancer, and overall mortality in the 65 and younger but not older population. *Cell Metabolism* 19:407, 2014.

In addition, the ability and willingness to seek health care promptly when it is needed, the health literacy to understand a health care provider, and the ability to accept the responsibility for one's own health can slow the rate of aging. Likewise, safe shelter that protects individuals from physical danger, environmental toxins, climate extremes, and sun exposure helps slow the aging process. Allowing people to make at least some decisions for themselves and control their own activities (autonomy), and providing psychosocial support (informational and emotional resources) promote successful aging and psychological well-being. In contrast, aging is likely to accelerate if any or all of the converse are true—that is, insufficient income, low education level, lack of health care, inadequate shelter, and/or lack of autonomy and psychosocial support.

✓ CONCEPT CHECK 16.1

1. Describe three current hypotheses about the causes of aging.
2. What is the difference between *usual* and *successful* aging?
3. Discuss how genetics, lifestyle, and environment influence aging.

16.2 Nutrient Needs During Adulthood

The challenge of the adult years is to maintain the body, preserve optimal function, and avoid chronic disease; that is, to age successfully. A healthy dietary pattern can help achieve this goal. One blueprint for a healthy diet comes from the *Dietary Guidelines for Americans*. The advice from those guidelines included the following goals:

1. Follow a healthy eating pattern across the life span.
2. Focus on variety, nutrient density, and amount.
3. Limit calories from added sugars and saturated fats and reduce sodium intake.
4. Shift to healthier food and beverage choices.

Overall, good nutrition benefits adults in many ways. Meeting nutrient needs delays the onset of certain diseases; improves the management of some existing diseases; speeds recovery from many illnesses; increases mental, physical, and social well-being; and often decreases the need for and length of hospitalization.[2] As you know, American adults remain overweight. Common dietary excesses are calories, saturated fat, sodium, and, for some, alcohol. The dietary patterns of adult women tend to fall short of the recommended amounts of vitamins D and E, folate, magnesium, calcium, zinc, and fiber. The dietary patterns of adult men tend to be low in the same nutrients, except vitamin D, which becomes more problematic after age 50.[3] The iron intake of most women during their childbearing years (ages 19 to 50) is insufficient to meet their needs; however, due to a reduced iron need after **menopause,** older women do get enough iron.

People age 65 and up, particularly those in long-term care facilities and hospitals, are the single largest group at risk of malnutrition. They often are underweight and show signs of numerous micronutrient deficiencies (e.g., vitamins B-6, B-12, folate). To pinpoint those over age 65 at risk of nutrient deficiencies, the American College of Physicians, American Academy of Family Physicians, Academy of Nutrition and Dietetics, and National Council on Aging developed the *DETERMINE Nutrition Checklist* for Older Adults (Fig. 16-3). Older Americans, family members, and health care providers can use the DETERMINE checklist to identify those at nutritional risk before health deteriorates significantly. Registered dietitian nutritionists can offer professional and personalized advice to help adults achieve a healthful dietary pattern.

The DRIs for adults (Appendix G) are divided by gender and by age. The intervals encompassing ages 19 through 50 are often referred to as *young adulthood,* 51 to 70 as *middle adulthood,* and beyond 70 years of age as *older adulthood.* These changes in nutrient needs take into consideration aging-related physiological alterations in body composition, metabolism, and organ function.

menopause The cessation of the menstrual cycle in women, usually beginning at about 50 years of age.

FIGURE 16-3 ▶ DETERMINE: A nutrition checklist for older adults.

Source: From the Nutrition Screening Initiative, a project of the American Academy of Family Physicians, Academy of Nutrition and Dietetics and the National Council on Aging, Inc., and funded part by a grant from Abbott Nutrition

Nutrition Checklist for Older Adults: DETERMINE Mnemonic

Here's a nutrition check for anyone over age 65. Circle the number of points for each statement that applies. Then compute the total and check it against the nutritional score.

Possible Problem	Points	
Disease	2	1. The person has a chronic illness or current condition that has changed the kind or amount of food eaten.
Eating Poorly	3	2. The person eats fewer than two full meals per day.
	2	3. The person eats few fruits, vegetables, or milk products.
	2	4. The person drinks three or more servings of beer, liquor, or wine almost every day.
Tooth Loss/ Mouth Pain	2	5. The person has tooth or mouth problems that make eating difficult.
Economic Hardship	4	6. The person does not have enough money for food.
Reduced Social Contact	1	7. The person eats alone most of the time.
Multiple Medications	1	8. The person takes three or more different prescription or over-the-counter drugs each day.
Involuntary Weight Loss/Gain	2	9. The person has unintentionally lost or gained 10 pounds within the last 6 months.
Needs Assistance In Self Care	2	10. The person cannot always shop, cook, or feed himself or herself.
Total		

Nutritional score:

0–2: Good. Recheck in 6 months.

3–5: Marginal. A local agency on aging has information about nutrition programs for the elderly. The National Association of Area Agencies on Aging can assist in finding help; call (800) 677-1116. Recheck in 6 months.

6 or more: High risk. A doctor should review this test and suggest how to improve nutritional health.

CALORIES

After age 30 or so, total calorie needs of physically inactive adults fall steadily throughout adulthood. There are a variety of explanations for the lower calorie requirements of older adults. Basal metabolic rate declines by about 2% per decade after age 30, such that overall energy needs of a 70-year-old man are reduced by 100 to 150 kcal per day compared to those of a 30-year-old man. Losses of lean body mass and decreases in physical activity also tend to accompany aging. To a considerable extent, adults can exert control over this reduction in calorie need by exercising. Physical activity can halt, slow, and even reverse reductions in lean body mass and subsequent declines in energy needs. Being able to consume more calories makes it much easier to meet micronutrient needs without dietary supplements.

PROTEIN

The protein intake of younger adults in North America typically exceeds the current RDA (0.8 gram per kilogram of body weight) and falls within the recommended range of 10% to 35% of total calories. However, several studies indicate that consuming protein in amounts slightly higher than the RDA (in the range of 1.0 to 1.2 grams per kilogram of body weight) may help preserve muscle and bone mass among older adults.[4,5] As with calorie needs, protein requirements should be determined in relation to routine physical activity.

Furthermore, current research is focusing on the benefits of older adults consuming an adequate amount (25–30 grams) of high-quality protein at each meal, which, in combination with physical activity, may delay the onset of muscle loss, slow its progression, and reduce the magnitude of its functional consequences. Breakfast provides a great opportunity for increased high-quality protein intake because many individuals, including older adults, typically start their day with a meal that is low in protein and dominated by carbohydrate. It is hypothesized that an even distribution of protein throughout the day along with physical activity will promote anabolism in older adults.[6]

Inclusion of animal proteins may be important because they generally have a higher proportion of the amino acid leucine, which plays a key role in stimulating muscle protein growth. Yet plant-based proteins such as soy products (tofu, soy milk, and soy yogurt), lentils, beans, nuts, and seeds are excellent choices for vegetarians. Adults who have limited food budgets, have difficulty chewing meat, or are lactose intolerant may not get enough protein, especially animal protein. On the other end of the spectrum, recall that any protein consumed in excess of that needed for the maintenance of body tissue will be broken down and used as energy or stored as fat. The waste products of metabolism of protein must be removed by the kidneys; excessive protein intake may accelerate kidney function decline.

FAT

The fat intake of adults of all ages is often at or above the 20% to 35% of total calories recommended by the Food and Nutrition Board. It is a good idea for almost all adults to reduce their fat intake because of the strong link between high saturated fat and obesity, heart disease, and certain cancers. The *Dietary Guidelines* describe a healthy eating pattern as one that includes plant-based oils (27 grams or 5 teaspoons per day) and limits saturated fats and *trans* fats. A key recommendation is to consume less than 10% of calories per day from saturated fats.

CARBOHYDRATES

Although total carbohydrate intake of adults of all ages in North America is adequate, the intake of whole grains remains inadequate. Many adults need to shift the carbohydrate composition of their diets to emphasize complex carbohydrates and whole grains while minimizing intake of sugary, refined simple carbohydrates. Remember that the healthy eating pattern described in the *Dietary Guidelines* limits added sugars to 10% of calories per day but emphasizes the following carbohydrates:

- A variety of vegetables from all of the subgroups: dark green, red and orange, legumes (beans and peas), starchy, and other
- Fruits, especially whole fruits
- Grains, at least half of which are whole grains
- Low-fat dairy, including milk, yogurt, cheese, and/or fortified soy beverages

About 35% of Americans follow the advice to *make half your grains whole grains*. A diet rich in complex carbohydrates helps us meet our nutrient needs without excess calories. Replacing sweets and refined carbohydrates with foods rich in complex carbohydrates also improves blood glucose control. This is particularly helpful because inactivity and increasing body fatness are connected to insulin resistance. Carbohydrate metabolism dysfunction is so common that more than 25% of those age 65 years or older have diabetes. A diet rich in fiber helps adults reduce their risk of cancer and heart disease, lowers blood cholesterol levels, and minimizes constipation. The typical American adult gets slightly more than half the recommended amount of dietary fiber. Americans could benefit from incorporating more whole grains into their dietary patterns.

Home-Delivered Meal Kits

Approximately 8 million U.S. consumers have purchased meal kit delivery services accounting for $1.5 billion in sales in 2016. With over 100 companies occupying this growing space, these kits are attractive for busy consumers with little time or novice cooking skills. Benefits include convenience, minimal food waste, portion control, and meal variety—often at a lower cost than the same meal served at a restaurant.

Eight of the most popular services are:

HelloFresh

Blue Apron

Plated

Terra's Kitchen

Martha & Marley Spoon

PeachDish

Chef'd

Green Chef

ostomy Surgically created short circuit in intestinal flow where the end point usually opens from the abdominal cavity rather than the anus; for example, a colostomy.

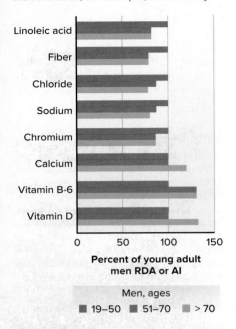

FIGURE 16-4 ▲ Relative nutrient requirements for aging adult men. Only nutrients that vary by age are shown.

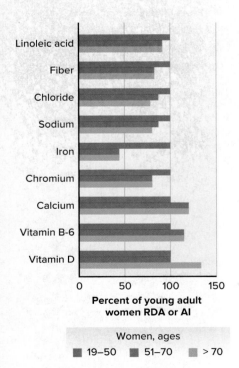

FIGURE 16-5 ▲ Relative nutrient requirements for aging adult women. Only nutrients that vary by age are shown.

WATER

Many adults, especially those in the later years, fail to consume adequate quantities of water. In fact, many are in a constant state of mild dehydration and at risk of electrolyte imbalances. Low fluid intakes in older adults may be caused by a fading sensitivity to thirst sensations, chronic diseases, and/or conscious reductions in fluid intake in order to reduce the frequency of urination. Some may have increased fluid output because they are taking certain medications (i.e., diuretics and laxatives), have an **ostomy,** and/or experience an age-related decline in the kidneys' ability to concentrate urine. Dehydration is very dangerous and, among other symptoms, can cause disorientation and mental confusion, constipation, fecal impaction, and death. Initiatives to improve fluid intake, especially in older adults, should include assessments of barriers to drinking, hydration education, close intake monitoring, frequent prompting, offering a choice of healthy drinks, and addressing continence issues.

MINERALS AND VITAMINS

Dietary requirements for many nutrients change throughout the adult years (Figs. 16-4 and 16-5). The micronutrients that need special attention because they tend to be present in less than optimal amounts in the diets of many adults are calcium, vitamin D, iron, zinc, magnesium, folate, and vitamins B-6, B-12, and E. Adults with impaired absorption or who are unable to consume a nutritious diet may benefit from mineral or vitamin supplements matched with their needs. In fact, many nutrition experts recommend a daily balanced multivitamin and mineral supplement for older adults, especially for those 70 years of age and older (see AARP's guide to supplements at http://www.aarp.org/health/drugs-supplements/info-09-2010/vitamins_from_a_to_z.html). Supplements or fortified foods can be especially helpful when it comes to meeting vitamin D and vitamin B-12 needs.

Calcium and Vitamin D These bone-building nutrients tend to be low in the dietary patterns of all adults. They become particularly problematic after age 50. Inadequate intake of these nutrients, combined with their reduced absorption, the reduced synthesis of vitamin D in the skin, and the kidneys' decreased ability to put vitamin D in its active form, greatly contributes to the development of osteoporosis. Getting enough of these nutrients is a challenge for many older adults because food sources of vitamin D are limited and the major sources—fatty fish and fortified milk—are not widely consumed by older adults. Plus, with increasing age, lactase production frequently decreases. As you know, one of the richest and most absorbable sources of these nutrients—milk—contains lactose. To get the vitamin D and calcium needed, many with lactose intolerance can consume small amounts of milk at mealtime with no ill effects. Calcium-fortified foods, cheese, yogurt, fish eaten with bones (e.g., canned sardines or salmon), and dark, green leafy vegetables can help those with lactose intolerance meet calcium needs—but these foods often do not provide vitamin D. Just 10 to 15 minutes per day of sunlight can make a large difference in vitamin D status.

Iron Iron deficiency is the most common type of malnutrition during the adult years. Recall that iron deficiency can impair red blood cell synthesis, which leads to weakness, fatigue, shortness of breath, and *brain fog*. Iron deficiency is found most frequently in women in their reproductive years because their dietary patterns do not provide enough iron to compensate for the iron lost monthly during menstruation. Other common causes of iron deficiency in adults of all ages include digestive tract injuries that cause bleeding (i.e., bleeding ulcers or hemorrhoids) and the use of medicines, such as aspirin, that cause blood loss. Impaired iron absorption due to age-related declines in stomach-acid production may contribute to iron deficiency in older adults. Remember that iron deficiency can be present before the actual signs of anemia. Dietary sources of iron include fortified grains; meat, fish and poultry; seafood; beans; dark-green leafy vegetables; and peas.

Zinc In addition to less than optimal dietary zinc intake during adulthood, zinc absorption declines as stomach-acid production diminishes with age. Poor zinc status may contribute to the taste sensation losses, mental lethargy, declines in immune function, and the delayed wound healing many elderly adults experience. Some dietary sources of zinc include oysters, beef, seafood, fortified grains, pork, yogurt, and chickpeas.

Magnesium This mineral tends to be low in the adult diet. Inadequate magnesium intakes may contribute to the bone loss, muscular weakness, and mental confusion seen in some elderly adults. It also can lead to sudden death from poor heart rhythm and is linked to cardiovascular disease, osteoporosis, and diabetes. The best source of magnesium is the food because supplements can cause diarrhea. Dietary sources of magnesium include nuts, spinach, soy milk, beans, and peanut butter.

Sodium Average sodium intakes of American adults are about 3400 milligrams per day—more than two times the AI. A heavy reliance on highly processed foods and restaurant meals are mostly to blame for the high sodium intakes of Americans.[7] Data from the What We Eat in America, National Health and Nutrition Examination Survey (NHANES) 2009–2010 indicate that sandwiches are major contributors of sodium in the dietary patterns of American adults.[7]

The declining sense of taste that typically accompanies aging could also contribute to a preference for highly salted foods. The Dietary Guidelines advise adults to consume less than 2300 milligrams of sodium per day. For adults over age 50; those with existing hypertension, prehypertension, diabetes, or kidney diseases; and all African-Americans, the upper limit is even lower: 1500 milligrams per day. These groups of people are especially sensitive to the effects of sodium on blood pressure. Less than 10% of adults, however, keep their sodium intakes below the UL. Recall that there are specific sodium AIs for young, middle-aged, and older adults (see margin box). The most widely recognized consequence of high sodium intake is hypertension, but high sodium intake has also been linked to osteoporosis secondary to increased calcium excretion in the urine and may overtax poorly functioning kidneys of older adults.

Even though excessive sodium receives most of the attention, low blood sodium (*hyponatremia*) is also a concern for older adults. Adults older than age 70, especially those who take diuretic medications or who have poor kidney function, are at increased risk for hyponatremia. The consequences of mild hyponatremia include lightheadedness, confusion, and unsteady gait, which can certainly increase the risk for falls among older adults. Other problems include fatigue, muscle cramps, and lack of appetite. There is no reason to severely restrict sodium among older adults who do not have kidney disease, but lowering sodium intakes closer to the AI would improve health for most adults.

Folate and Vitamins B-6 and B-12 Sufficient folate, because of its role in prevention of neural tube defects, is very important to women during the childbearing years. In later years, folate and vitamins B-6 and B-12 are especially important because they are required to clear homocysteine from the bloodstream. Elevated blood concentrations of homocysteine are associated with the increased risk of cardiovascular disease, stroke, bone fracture, and neurological decline seen in some elderly people. Vitamin B-12 is a particular problem for the older population because a deficiency may exist even when intake appears to be adequate. As people age, the stomach slows its production of acid and intrinsic factor, which leads to poor absorption of vitamin B-12. If vitamin B-12 is depleted, anemia and nerve damage could result. Adults age 51 years and older often must meet vitamin B-12 needs with supplements or fortified foods because synthetic vitamin B-12 is more readily absorbed than natural forms of B-12.

Vitamin E The dietary intake of most of the population falls short of recommendations for vitamin E. Low vitamin E intake means that the body has a reduced supply of antioxidants, which may increase the degree of cell damage caused by free radicals,

Sodium

AI

  9–50 years: 1500 milligrams

  51–70 years: 1300 milligrams

  > 70 years: 1200 milligrams

DV: 2400 milligrams

UL: 2300 milligrams

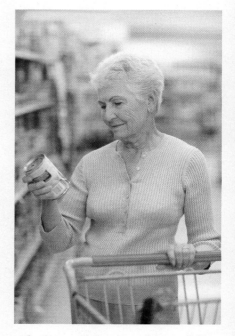

▲ Sodium needs for older adults are 1200 to 1300 milligrams per day. Older adults routinely consume at least this much sodium. Potassium needs are 4700 milligrams per day. Many older adults do not meet this goal.
©Blend Images/Getty Images Plus

FARM to FORK | Grapes and Raisins

Thompson seedless grapes are the nation's most popular variety of grapes, outselling others by 1000 to 1. Yet the red, purple, and black varieties have 50% to 75% more phytochemicals than the pale Thompson. Sun-dried raisins, from Thompson grapes, are the most popular dried fruit in the United States. Both are fantastic sources of nutrients and fiber for all ages.

Grow
- Grapevines are often ornamental and serve as excellent shade protection or living screens when properly trained to climb stable structures.
- A well-maintained grapevine can produce up to 20 pounds of grapes per year for over 50 years!

Shop
- As with many fruits, grapes are often harvested well before maximum ripeness to ensure stability during shipping.
- When shopping, look for vine-ripe organic grapes for maximum flavor and texture. Look for grapes that are firm and plump. Stems should be bright green and flexible, not dry and brittle. To check freshness, give the stem a gentle shake, and the grapes should remain on the vine.

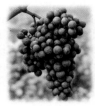

©Getty Images/Flickr RF

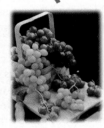

©Pixtal/Age Fotostock

Store
- Once harvested, cool grapes quickly in the coldest part of the refrigerator to extend shelf life and nutrient content.
- Store grapes in the plastic grape bag from the grocery.
- Rinse grapes just prior to eating to reduce decay.

Prep
- The beauty of grapes is that they are a no-prep healthy snack for any time of the day!
- To add variety, try frozen grapes, grapes or raisins in salads, or pair with low-fat cheeses.
- Home drying can be accomplished in a dehydrator or oven, or by baking in the sun.

Source: Robinson J. "Grapes and raisins: From muscadines to Thompson seedless," in *Eating on the Wild Side.* New York: Little, Brown and Company, 2013.

promote the progression of chronic diseases and cataracts, and accelerate the aging process. In addition, low vitamin E levels can lead to declines in physical abilities.

Carotenoids Dietary intakes of certain carotenoids have been shown to have a variety of important antiaging, anticancer, and other health protective effects. Specifically, lutein and zeaxanthin have been linked with the prevention of cataracts and age-related macular degeneration. Diets high in fruit and vegetables, the major sources of carotenoids and other beneficial phytochemicals, are consistently shown to be protective against a wide variety of age-related conditions.

ARE ADULTS FOLLOWING CURRENT DIETARY RECOMMENDATIONS?

In general, adults in North America are trying to follow many of the dietary recommendations described in this chapter. Since the mid-1950s, they have consumed less saturated fat as more people substitute fat-free and low-fat milk for cream and whole milk. However, they eat more cheese, usually a concentrated form of saturated fat. Since 1963, they have eaten less butter, fewer eggs, less animal fat, and more vegetable oils and fish. These changes generally comply with recommendations to reduce the intake of saturated and *trans* fat in favor of unsaturated fat choices. Animal breeders are raising much leaner animals than those produced in 1950, which also helps reduce saturated fat intake.

Other aspects of the average adult diet are still in need of improvement. The latest nutrition survey of eating habits in the United States shows that the major contributors of calories to the adult dietary pattern are white bread, beef, doughnuts, cakes and cookies, soft drinks, milk, poultry, cheese, alcoholic beverages, salad dressing, mayonnaise, potatoes, and sugars/syrups/jams. If Americans were truly lowering their intakes of sugar, saturated fat, and sodium while increasing their intakes of fiber, many of these foods would not appear at the top of the list.

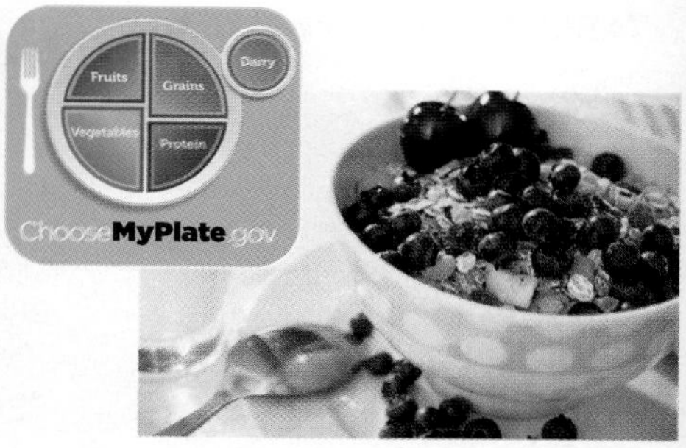

✅ **CONCEPT CHECK 16.2**

1. Is the current adult RDA for protein appropriate for older adults? Why or why not?
2. Which nutrients should be limited in the dietary patterns of most American adults? Suggest three specific dietary changes that would help to limit these food components.
3. Name three nutrients that are commonly lacking in the dietary patterns of adults. Suggest one rich food source of each of these nutrients.

▲ How does this breakfast of whole grain cereal, fruit, and milk compare to MyPlate? Source: www.choosemyplate.gov; ©Image Source/Getty Images

16.3 Factors Related to Nutritional Status of Adults

Dietary adequacy is influenced by physiological, psychosocial, and economic factors. Table 16-2 summarizes the nutritional implications of many of the physiological changes that occur during adulthood. Some of the changes listed (e.g., tooth loss and changes in perceptions of taste and smell) can directly influence dietary intake. Other changes (e.g., loss of lean body tissue) can alter nutrient and/or calorie needs. Some body changes (e.g., reduced stomach acidity, diminished kidney function) can affect nutrient utilization. Furthermore, chronic diseases and the medications used to manage them may influence food intake and nutrient needs. The following section details the influences of several of these factors on nutritional status during adulthood.

TABLE 16-2 ■ Physiological Changes of Aging

Physiological Changes	Recommendations
⤵ Appetite	Monitor changes in weight over time.
	Eat small, frequent meals throughout the day.
	Use supplemental nutritional drinks, such as Boost® and Ensure Plus.®
⤵ Sense of taste and smell	Vary the colors and textures of foods.
	Experiment with sodium-free herbs and spices.
⤵ Chewing or swallowing ability	Work with a dentist or therapist to maximize chewing and swallowing ability.
	Modify food consistency as necessary.
⤵ Sense of thirst	Monitor fluid intake.
	Stay alert for evidence of dehydration (e.g., dark-colored urine).
⤵ Stomach acidity	Include lean meats and iron-fortified foods in the dietary pattern.
	Ask health care team to monitor iron status.
	Consume a source of vitamin C to enhance absorption of nonheme iron from foods.
	Choose foods fortified with vitamin B-12 or use a supplemental source of vitamin B-12.

(continued)

TABLE 16-2 ■ (*continued*)

⬇ Bowel function	Emphasize fruits, vegetables, and whole grains in the diet. Meet fluid needs. Increase physical activity.
⬇ Lactase production	Reduce serving sizes of milk with meals. Substitute yogurt or cheese for milk. Use reduced-lactose or lactose-free products. Seek nondairy calcium sources.
⬇ Liver function	Consume alcohol in moderation, if at all. Avoid consuming dietary supplements that contain more than 100% of the Daily Value of nutrients, especially vitamin A.
⬇ Insulin function	Maintain healthy body weight. Choose whole grains and limit refined grains. Perform regular physical activity.
⬇ Kidney function	If necessary, work with primary care provider and registered dietitian nutritionist to modify protein and other nutrients in the dietary pattern.
⬇ Immune function	Meet nutrient needs, especially protein, vitamin E, vitamin B-6, and zinc. Perform regular physical activity.
⬇ Lung function	Avoid tobacco products. Perform regular physical activity.
⬇ Vision	Choose a dietary pattern rich in fruits, vegetables, and whole grains, which are natural sources of carotenoids, vitamin C, vitamin E, and zinc. Regularly consume fatty fish, a source of omega-3 fatty acids. Wear sunglasses in sunny conditions. Avoid tobacco products. Perform regular physical activity to improve insulin sensitivity.
⬇ Lean tissue	Meet nutrient needs, especially protein and vitamin D. Perform regular physical activity, including strength training.
⬇ Cardiovascular function	Achieve and maintain a healthy body weight. Choose a dietary pattern based on fruits, vegetables, whole grains, plant sources of protein, and fatty fish. Adhere to prescribed medications to keep blood lipids and blood pressure within desirable ranges. Stay physically active.
⬇ Bone mass	Meet nutrient needs, especially protein, calcium, and vitamin D (regular sun exposure). Perform regular physical activity, especially weight-bearing physical activity. Aim to maintain a healthy body weight (i.e., BMI between 18.5 and 24.9).
⬇ Mental function	Choose a dietary pattern rich in fruits, vegetables, whole grains, beans, and legumes, which are natural sources of antioxidant nutrients. Consume seafood, a source of omega-3 fatty acids, twice per week. Discuss the possible need for vitamin B-12 supplements with a primary care provider. Strive for lifelong learning. Perform regular physical activity. Obtain adequate sleep.
⬇ Fat stores	Avoid overeating. Perform regular physical activity.

BODY COMPOSITION

The primary changes in body composition that occur with aging are diminished lean body mass, increased fat stores, and decreased body water. A focus on physical activity, as detailed in a later section, can attenuate many of these unwanted changes.

The loss of lean body mass is termed **sarcopenia.** Some muscle cells shrink, others are lost as muscles age, and some muscles lose their elasticity as they accumulate fat and collagen. Loss of muscle mass leads to a decrease in basal metabolism, muscle strength, and energy needs. Less muscle mass also leads to lower fitness performance, which makes the prognosis for maintaining muscle even worse. Clearly, it is best to prevent this downward spiral.

As lean tissue declines with age, body fat often increases, a condition called **sarcopenic obesity.**[8] Much of this increase in body fat results from overeating and limited physical activity, although even physically fit men and women typically gain some additional body fatness after age 50. A small fat gain in adulthood may not compromise health, but large gains are problematic. Recall that obesity increases risks for hypertension, cardiovascular disease, type 2 diabetes, osteoarthritis, cancers, and many other serious chronic conditions. Ultimately, these changes in body composition may diminish a person's ability to perform daily tasks, such as getting up from a chair and climbing a flight of stairs.

On the other hand, decreases in body weight can also be a problem for adults age 70 and older. About 2% of older adults are underweight (BMI less than 18.5). Unintended weight loss increases the risk of malnutrition, which alters an individual's ability to cope with illnesses and injuries and could ultimately lead to death. Potential causes for unintended weight loss among older adults (many of which can be detected using the DETERMINE nutrition screening tool in Figure 16-3) include:

- Mental or physical illness
- Depression/social isolation
- Side effects of medications
- Changes in taste or smell
- Reduced chewing ability
- Limited financial resources
- Decreased dexterity or strength
- Transportation barriers

sarcopenia In general, loss of muscle tissue. Among older adults, this loss of lean mass greatly increases their risk of illness and death.

sarcopenic obesity Loss of muscle mass accompanied by gains in fat mass.

Researchers believe that maintaining lean muscle mass may be the most important strategy for successful aging because doing so:
- Maintains basal metabolic rate, which helps to decrease the risk of obesity
- Keeps body fat low, which helps in the management of blood lipids and blood glucose
- Maintains body water, which decreases the risk of dehydration and improves body temperature regulation

BONES AND JOINTS

Recall that some bone loss is an expected consequence of aging. In women, bone loss rapidly occurs after menopause. For men, bone loss is slow and steady from middle age throughout later life. Many older adults may suffer from undiagnosed **osteomalacia,** a condition mainly caused by insufficient vitamin D. Osteoporosis can limit the ability of older people to shop, prepare food, and engage in physical activity. Consuming adequate vitamin D, calcium, and protein; not smoking; drinking alcohol moderately or not at all; and engaging in weight-bearing exercises can help preserve bone mass. Medications also can help lessen bone loss.

There are over 100 forms of arthritis, a disease that causes the degeneration and roughening of the cartilage that covers and cushions the joints. Such changes in the joints cause them to ache and become inflamed and painful to move. Severe arthritis can cause permanent joint changes, and some types of arthritis affect the heart, eyes, lungs, kidneys, and skin in addition to the joints. Over 53 million U.S. adults suffer from some type of arthritis. **Osteoarthritis,** which affects about 30 million U.S. adults, is the leading cause of disability among older persons. **Rheumatoid arthritis,** which affects about 1.5 million U.S. adults, is more prevalent in younger adults. **Gout,** a very painful form of arthritis that comes on suddenly and can be related to changes in the diet, affects about 6 million men and 2 million women in the United States.

Although precise causes or cures are unknown, many unproven arthritis *remedies* have been publicized. Unproven diets, food restrictions, and nutrient supplementation are some of the more popular treatments. Maintaining a healthy weight, which reduces stress on painful arthritic joints, is the best evidence-based diet-related strategy

osteomalacia Adult form of rickets. The bones have low mineral density and subsequently are at risk for fracture.

osteoarthritis A degenerative joint condition caused by a breakdown of cartilage in joints. It often results from *wear and tear* due to repetitive motions or the pressure of excess body weight.

rheumatoid arthritis A degenerative joint condition resulting from an autoimmune disease that causes inflammation in the joints and other sites of the body.

gout A form of arthritis caused by the buildup of uric acid crystals in the joints.

to offer relief from arthritis. Although no special diet, food, or nutrient has been proven to reliably prevent, relieve, or cure arthritis in humans, some research shows that a dietary pattern (e.g., Mediterranean diet) that is rich in antioxidant nutrients, anti-inflammatory phytochemicals, and omega-3 fatty acids can help to reduce the inflammation that underlies these conditions.[9] As far as supplements go, glucosamine and chondroitin have been most extensively studied in relation to arthritis. Results remain controversial, but some studies demonstrate that these supplements can relieve pain, slow the progression of joint degeneration, or rebuild cartilage.

ASK THE RDN — Anti-Inflammatory Diet

Dear Author: *My mother has been battling osteoarthritis for several years and wonders if Dr. Weil's Anti-Inflammatory Diet can help her cope with her disease. How is Dr. Weil's plan different from the Mediterranean diet?*

When you are sick or injured, chronic inflammation wreaks havoc on the body and is now thought to be at the root of many chronic diseases, including heart disease, Alzheimer's disease, and arthritis.

There is good evidence that an anti-inflammatory eating pattern may reduce inflammation, the risk of chronic diseases, and some symptoms of arthritis. The basic principles of an anti-inflammatory eating plan include:

- Eating plenty of fruits, vegetables, and whole grains
- Limiting or avoiding saturated and *trans* fats
- Including good sources of omega-3 fatty acids
- Choosing lean sources of protein instead of red or processed meats
- Avoiding refined carbohydrates and highly processed foods
- Including herbs and spices with known anti-inflammatory effects

To ease arthritis, the #1 thing you can do is to keep your weight within a healthy range. Although Dr. Weil's plan is not aimed at weight loss, it is not surprising that when individuals consume a primarily plant-based diet and reduce their intakes of solid fats and highly processed foods, they often drop some pounds.

Carbohydrates make up 40% to 50% of daily calories on Dr. Weil's plan. Whole or cracked grains, beans, and abundant fruits and vegetables are recommended. When it comes to selecting produce, go for a wide variety of colorful fruits and vegetables. Many of the phytochemicals in colorful plant foods have anti-inflammatory effects.

Dr. Weil also emphasizes healthy fats, which should account for about 30% of your daily calories. He recommends seeking out sources of omega-3 fatty acids, which are found in foods such as avocados; nuts and nut butters; fortified eggs; flaxseeds; hemp seeds; and fish such as salmon, sardines, black cod, and herring. Extra-virgin olive oil is the preferred oil for cooking and flavoring foods.

Protein should make up 20% to 30% of your daily calories on Dr. Weil's plan, but he stresses the importance of plant sources of protein. In fact, he recommends limiting most animal proteins to two servings per week. Instead, choose beans and products made from soybeans along with fish as sources of protein.

If the Anti-Inflammatory Diet sounds a lot like the Mediterranean diet you read about earlier, that's because Dr. Weil based his plan on this healthy dietary pattern! He also adds specific advice about anti-inflammatory herbs and spices, such as garlic, ginger, and turmeric and touts the health benefits of tea and small amounts of dark chocolate.

As RDNs, we fully support this food-based strategy to fight chronic diseases. However, we would be cautious when it comes to purchasing dietary supplements, including fish oil, ginger, turmeric, and several antioxidant compounds. There is little evidence that these supplements will provide benefits beyond what whole foods supply.

Wholesome thoughts,

Colleen Spees, PhD, RDN, LD, FAND (author)

PHYSICAL ACTIVITY

Many physical changes of aging can be traced back to a sedentary lifestyle. As you might predict, an active lifestyle helps preserve muscle mass and decrease body fat. Physical activity increases muscle strength and mobility, improves balance and decreases the risk of falling, eases daily tasks that require strength, improves sleep, slows bone loss, and increases joint movement, thus reducing injuries. It also has a positive impact on a person's mental outlook. Ideally, an active lifestyle should be maintained throughout life and include activities to build endurance, strength, balance, and flexibility. The *Physical Activity Guidelines for Americans* provide the following guidelines specifically for older adults.

Aerobic Activity All adults should engage in moderate-intensity aerobic physical activity for at least 150 minutes per week, vigorous-intensity aerobic activity for 75 minutes per week, or an equivalent combination of the two. This amount of aerobic activity improves endurance and aids in prevention of chronic diseases. A longer duration of daily physical activity may be required for weight loss or weight maintenance. Weight-bearing exercises are particularly helpful for preservation of bone mass. For older adults who have not been physically active, it is important to increase the pace gradually. Even small bouts (e.g., 10 minutes) of physical activity are better than no exercise at all!

Strength Training To maintain lean tissue and basal metabolic rate, strength training should include 8 to 10 different exercises (each with two sets of 8 to 15 repetitions), performed two to three times per week. Exercises that involve the large muscle groups (e.g., arms, back, and legs) and exercises that enhance grip strength should be emphasized. Start slowly, concentrate on breathing, rest between sets, avoid locking joints in the arms and legs, and stop an exercise if it becomes painful.

Balance Exercises For those over age 65 who are at risk for falling, exercises that improve balance are recommended. Tai chi and yoga are a few types of exercise that can improve balance, but even standing on one foot or getting up from a chair without using hands can be a good start.

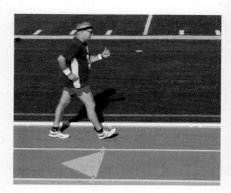

▲ Endurance, strength, balance, and flexibility are the four elements of the Go4Life campaign from the National Institute on Aging. Download a free copy of Exercise and Physical Activity: Getting Fit for Life at www.nia.nih.gov. ©Anne Smith

Flexibility Exercises Stretching each major muscle group should accompany aerobic or strength training at least 2 days per week. Improving flexibility can make it easier to perform many simple tasks, such as tying one's shoes.

All older adults should avoid inactivity. Having a comprehensive physical activity plan, developed with a health professional to accommodate individual health risks and needs, will enhance success for older adults. Men older than age 40; women older than age 50; those with heart conditions, diabetes, or joint problems; and anyone who has been sedentary should consult a primary care provider before beginning a physical activity program. The Go4Life campaign from the National Institute of Aging encourages older adults to become more active and provides many practical tips for exercising safely. Learn more at go4life.nia.nih.gov.

DIGESTIVE SYSTEM

As you recall from earlier chapters, digestion begins in the mouth. About 27% of older adults have no natural teeth, and many more are missing some teeth. The problem of tooth loss is worse among low-income populations. Even with properly fitting dentures, chewing ability may be limited. Older adults with poor dentition avoid meats or crunchy fruits and vegetables, thereby missing out on important nutrients such as protein, iron, and zinc (from meat) as well as potassium and fiber (from fruits and vegetables). Ground meats and cooked vegetables are easier options for older adults with chewing problems.[10]

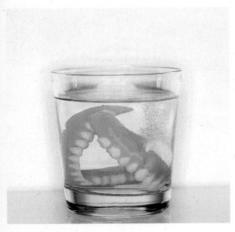

▲ Poor dentition contributes to decreased food intake and digestive problems. Serve softer, easier-to-chew foods and allow extra time for chewing and swallowing. ©Stockbyte/Getty Images

Further along the GI tract, the production of HCl, intrinsic factor, and some digestive enzymes (e.g., lactase) declines with advancing age.[11] In addition, some medications affect acid production. As a result of low acid production, absorption of some minerals, such as iron, is impaired. Low levels of acid and intrinsic factor reduce the digestion and absorption of vitamin B-12. Thus, even with adequate intakes of iron and vitamin B-12, older adults may become anemic. Symptoms of lactose intolerance can lead to avoidance of dairy products, which can limit the availability of bone-building nutrients. Fortified foods or supplements can help older adults overcome these problems with digestion and absorption of nutrients.

Constipation is the main intestinal problem for older people. To prevent constipation, older people should have a primarily plant-based dietary pattern to meet fiber needs, drink enough fluids, and engage in regular physical activity. Fiber supplements, may be useful when overall food consumption does not allow for adequate fiber intake. Because some medications can be habit forming, a primary care provider should be consulted to determine if a laxative or stool softener is needed.

In addition to changes in the GI tract, the functions of the accessory organs decline as we age. For instance, the liver functions less efficiently. A history of significant alcohol consumption or liver disease will intensify any existing problems with liver function. As liver efficiency declines, its ability to detoxify substances, including medications, alcohol, and vitamin and mineral supplements, drops. This increases the possibility for vitamin toxicity.

The gallbladder also functions less efficiently in later years. Gallstones can block the flow of bile out of the gallbladder into the small intestine, thereby interfering with fat digestion. Obesity is a major risk factor for gallbladder disease, especially in older women. A low-fat diet or surgery to remove the gallbladder may be necessary.

Although pancreatic function may decline with age, this organ has a large reserve capacity. One sign of a failing pancreas is high blood glucose, although this can occur as the result of several conditions. The pancreas may be secreting less insulin, or cells may be resisting insulin action (as is commonly seen in people with android obesity). Where appropriate, improved nutrient intake, regular physical activity, and loss of excess body weight can improve insulin action and blood glucose regulation.

NERVOUS SYSTEM

A gradual loss of nerve cells that transmit signals may decrease taste and smell perceptions and impair neuromuscular coordination, reasoning, and memory. Both hearing and vision decline with age. Hearing impairment is the greatest in those who have been exposed consistently to loud noises, such as urban traffic, lawnmowers, and loud music. Because they cannot hear well, older people may avoid social contacts, which increases their risk of inadequate dietary patterns.

Declining eyesight, frequently caused by retina degeneration and cataracts, can affect a person's abilities to grocery shop, locate desired foods, read labels for nutritional content, and prepare foods at home. Vision losses also may cause people to curtail social contacts, reduce physical activity, and not practice daily personal health and grooming routines. Age-related macular degeneration, a common cause of failing eyesight in old age, affects about 2 million U.S. adults. A major risk factor is cigarette smoking. Diets rich in carotenoids and omega-3 fatty acids help to reduce the risk of certain eye diseases among older adults.[12]

Neuromuscular coordination losses may make it difficult to shop for and prepare food. Physical tasks as simple as opening food packages can become so difficult that individuals restrict dietary intake to foods that require little preparation and depend on others to provide food that is ready to eat. Eating may become difficult, too. Loss of coordination makes it a challenge to grasp cup handles and manipulate eating utensils. As a result, older adults may avoid foods that can be easily spilled (e.g., soups and juices) or that need to be cut (e.g., meats, large vegetable pieces). Some may even withdraw from social interaction and eat alone, which often means eating less.

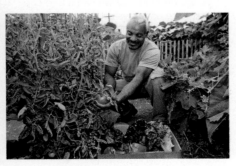

▲ Immune function declines with age, so food safety becomes increasingly important for older adults. ©Blend Images-Peathegee Inc/Getty Images

IMMUNE SYSTEM

With age, the immune system often operates less efficiently. Consuming adequate protein, vitamins (especially folate and vitamins A, D, and E), iron, and zinc helps maximize immune system function. Recurrent illnesses and delayed wound healing are warning signs that nutrient deficiencies (especially of protein and zinc) may be hindering immune function. On the other hand, overnutrition appears to be equally harmful to the immune system. For example, obesity and excessive fat, iron, and zinc intakes can suppress immune function.

ENDOCRINE SYSTEM

As adulthood progresses, the rate of hormone synthesis and release can slow. Declining thyroid hormone production, for example, can decrease basal metabolic rate, leading to unexpected weight gain. A decrease in insulin release or sensitivity to insulin, for instance, means that it takes longer for blood glucose levels to return to normal after a meal. Maintaining a healthy weight, exercising regularly, adhering to a dietary pattern that is low in saturated fat and high in fiber, and avoiding highly processed foods can enhance the body's ability to use insulin and restore elevated blood glucose levels to normal after a meal.

CHRONIC DISEASE

The prevalence of obesity, heart disease, osteoporosis, cancer, hypertension, and diabetes rises with age. More than half of older adults have one of these chronic and potentially debilitating diseases. Six out of 10 elderly people have at least two chronic conditions. One small change can trigger a chain of events or *domino effect* that results in poor health (Fig. 16-6). Chronic diseases may have a strong impact on dietary patterns. For instance, obesity, heart disease, and osteoporosis may impair physical mobility to the extent that victims are unable to shop for and prepare food. Chronic disease also can influence nutrient and calorie needs. Cancer, for example, boosts these needs. Hypertension may indicate a need to lower sodium intake. Nutrient utilization can be affected by chronic disease, too. For instance, diabetes alters the body's ability to utilize glucose. In addition, the effects of heart disease on the kidneys may impair their ability to reabsorb glucose, amino acids, and vitamin C.

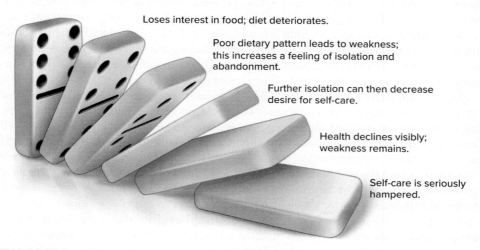

Social isolation; perhaps spouse has died.

Loses interest in food; diet deteriorates.

Poor dietary pattern leads to weakness; this increases a feeling of isolation and abandonment.

Further isolation can then decrease desire for self-care.

Health declines visibly; weakness remains.

Self-care is seriously hampered.

FIGURE 16-6 ▲ The decline of health often seen in older adults. A small change leads to a chain of events or *domino effect* that results in poor health. Early detection and intervention can prevent declines in physical health related to psychosocial factors.

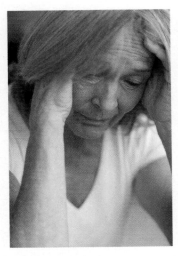

▲ The most commonly cited dietary triggers for migraine headaches are chocolate, cheese, citrus, alcohol, and coffee. ©Ian Hooton/Science Source

MIGRAINE HEADACHES

A migraine is a severe, intense, and recurring throbbing pain affecting one or both sides of the head in 38 million adults and children in the United States. Migraines interfere with quality of life in 90% of sufferers. Depression, anxiety, and sleep disturbances are common for those with chronic migraines. Other potentially debilitating neurological symptoms may include visual disturbances; nausea and vomiting; dizziness; sensitivity to sound, light, touch, and smell; and tingling or numbness in the extremities or face.

Both biologic and lifestyle factors contribute to migraines: family history, age, gender, hormonal changes, genetics, and lifestyle behaviors. Obese individuals are at increased risk of migraines, possibly related to higher levels of inflammation.

In susceptible individuals, potential dietary triggers for migraine headaches appear to be associated with foods that precipitate changes in blood flow and neurotransmitter release in the brain. Tyramine is a substance found naturally in foods such as aged cheese; aged, canned, cured, or processed meats; beans such as fava, garbanzo, pinto, and broad; pickles; and canned soups. Nitrates from processed meats and monosodium glutamate (MSG) from soy sauce, Asian dishes, and packaged foods have also been implicated as potential migraine triggers. Other food-related triggers include chocolate, nuts, olives, black tea, bananas, onions, raisins, apple skins, canned soups, red wine, and sulfites. Caffeine withdrawal, dehydration, meal skipping, supplements, and medications can also be overlooked culprits. Although there is some evidence that a low-fat, vegan dietary pattern reduces migraine frequency and severity,[13] a dietary pattern that complies with the Dietary Guidelines—that is, high in fruits, vegetables, whole grains, and legumes but low in sodium, solid fats, alcohol, and added sugars—has also been linked to fewer complaints of migraine headaches.

DEPRESSION

Major depressive disorders affect nearly 1 in 10 adults in the United States. Clinical depression is more than just a *case of the blues*. It is characterized by feelings of sadness, hopelessness, or despair that last for more than 2 weeks and interfere with daily living. Some symptoms of depression include loss of interest in activities that were once enjoyable (e.g., work, hobbies), changes in sleep habits (sleeping either too much or too little), and changes in appetite, which can lead to either weight loss or weight gain.

The causes of depression are varied. Stress, grief, illness, substance abuse, and some medications may certainly lead to depression, but biological changes in the brain are also implicated. For example, people who experience depression may have altered synthesis or activity of hormones (e.g., cortisol) or neurotransmitters (e.g., serotonin).

The B vitamins, folic acid, vitamin B-6, and vitamin B-12 are involved in the synthesis and activity of neurotransmitters and have been studied most extensively in relation to depression. Research also suggests that vitamin D and zinc may be particularly important in the prevention or treatment of depressive disorders.

Evidence supports a role of omega-3 fatty acids in the prevention or treatment of depression. The importance of omega-3 fatty acids to brain health is threefold. First, long-chain polyunsaturated fatty acids, particularly DHA, are incorporated into cell membranes throughout the brain. The fatty-acid composition of phospholipids affects the fluidity of cell membranes, which influences how well substances and signals are transported across the cell membrane. Membrane fluidity may affect how well chemical signals are transmitted by neurotransmitters from nerve cells to target cells. Second, omega-3 fatty acids improve vascular health by reducing the risk of blood clots and atherosclerosis. These changes ensure an adequate blood supply to the brain. Third, omega-3 fatty acids are involved in biochemical pathways that decrease inflammation and are associated with a reduction in depression.

When it comes to overall dietary patterns, several studies have shown that following a plant-based diet—one naturally rich in folate and vitamin B-6—may reduce depression and anxiety. Emphasizing healthy sources of fat, such as walnuts, canola oil, flaxseed, oil, and fatty fish, will boost levels of omega-3 fatty acids in the body. In some cases, supplementation with omega-3 fatty acids may be appropriate. Conversely, dietary patterns that are high in added sugars may be a risk factor for depression. Rapid rises and falls in blood sugar may deprive the brain of glucose and negatively affect mood. Carbohydrates also influence the production of serotonin, a neurotransmitter that is associated with pleasure.

NEURODEGENERATIVE DISEASES

Neurodegenerative disease is a term that encompasses a variety of conditions characterized by gradual, progressive deterioration of neurons. Alterations of these cells result in abnormal functioning, plaque formation, and eventual cell death. The most common neurodegenerative diseases in the United States include Alzheimer's disease, **Parkinson's disease, Creutzfeldt-Jakob disease,** and **multiple sclerosis.** In the past, research focused on genetics and aging as the primary risk factors for diseases of the brain. Now, researchers are turning their focus to lifestyle choices, with energy balance and optimal body fatness viewed very important for optimizing brain health. Research actually links both undernutrition and overnutrition to reduced cognitive function, via mechanisms that involve changes in hormone levels in the body.[14] Obese adults are three times more likely to suffer impaired cognitive function and dementia.

The most common neurodegenerative disease is Alzheimer's disease, diagnosed in about 5.1 million adults in the United States. It is an irreversible, progressive deterioration of the brain that causes victims to steadily lose the ability to remember, reason, and comprehend, often taking a terrible toll on the mental and eventual physical health of older people. Scientists have proposed various causes, including alterations in cell development or protein production in the brain, strokes, altered blood lipoprotein composition, poor blood glucose regulation (e.g., diabetes), high blood pressure, viral infections, and high free radical levels. The 10 warning signs of Alzheimer's disease are listed in the margin.

Early efforts at prevention of Alzheimer's disease should receive the most attention because the process of cognitive decline begins 10 to 20 years before warning signs appear. Preventive measures for Alzheimer's disease focus on eating a diet rich in fruits and vegetables, maintaining brain activity through lifelong learning, and taking ibuprofen. Fruits and vegetables provide antioxidant nutrients, such as vitamin C, vitamin E, and selenium, that help to protect the body from the damaging effects of free radicals. In addition, various phytochemicals with antioxidant and anti-inflammatory properties, including polyphenols and carotenoids (e.g., lutein and zeaxanthin), have been shown to protect the brain throughout life. Good food sources of lutein and zeaxanthin include green leafy vegetables, yellow-orange fruits and vegetables, and egg yolks. Polyphenols are found in foods such as berries, coffee, green or black tea, and chocolate.

Adequate intakes of folate, vitamin B-6, vitamin B-12, and choline are important to decrease blood homocysteine, which is a risk factor for neurodegenerative and cardiovascular disease (see Newsworthy Nutrition). Dietary fats, too, may play a role in keeping Alzheimer's disease at bay. Individuals with diets rich in omega-3 fatty acids and low in saturated and *trans* fatty acids have a reduced risk of Alzheimer's disease.[14] The role of nutrition in preventing or minimizing the risk of this disease continues to be studied.

The *MIND Diet* is a dietary intervention that shows promising results for protecting the brain against cognitive decline. MIND stands for *Mediterranean-DASH Intervention for Neurodegenerative Delay,* a hybrid of the nutrient-rich Mediterranean eating pattern with the low-calorie, low-sodium DASH Diet. The MIND diet's 10 *brain-healthy* foods include green leafy vegetables, other vegetables, nuts, berries, beans, whole grains, fish, poultry, olive oil, and wine. The five foods to limit include red meats, butter and stick margarine, cheese, pastries and sweets, and fried or fast food. Each day, followers of the MIND Diet should consume a minimum of three servings of whole grains, a salad plus

Parkinson's disease Disease that belongs to a group of conditions called *motor system disorders,* which are the result of the loss of dopamine-producing brain cells. The four primary symptoms of PD are tremor, or trembling in hands, arms, legs, jaw, and face; rigidity, or stiffness of the limbs and trunk; bradykinesia, or slowness of movement; and postural instability, or impaired balance and coordination.

Creutzfeldt-Jakob disease A rare, degenerative, invariably fatal brain disorder. Symptoms include problems with muscular coordination, personality changes including progressive and severe mental impairment, impaired vision that may lead to blindness, and involuntary muscle jerks.

multiple sclerosis An unpredictable disease of the central nervous system that can range from relatively benign to somewhat disabling to devastating, as communication between the brain and other parts of the body is disrupted.

Ten Warning Signs of Alzheimer's Disease

1. Recent memory loss that affects job performance
2. Difficulty performing familiar tasks
3. Problems with language
4. Faulty or decreased judgment
5. Problems with abstract thinking
6. Tendency to misplace things
7. Changes in mood or behavior
8. Changes in personality
9. Loss of initiative
10. Withdrawal from work or social activities

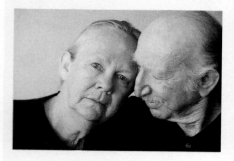

▲ Patients with advanced dementia may be easily distracted during meals, forget to eat, be unable to prepare food safely, and have trouble feeding themselves or swallowing. Caregivers and health care providers need to monitor the patient's weight to ensure maintenance of a healthy weight and nutritional state.
©Ingram Publishing

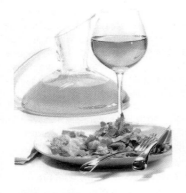

▲ The MIND Diet includes three servings of whole grains, a salad plus one other vegetable, and a glass of wine each day. ©Ingram Publishing

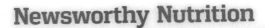

Newsworthy Nutrition

Folic acid and Vitamin B-12 may prevent cognitive decline

Folic acid and vitamin B-12 may be effective in the prevention of cognitive impairment and dementia based on their ability to lower homocysteine concentrations and reduce vascular risk factors. This randomized controlled trial was designed to assess the effects of folic acid and vitamin B-12 on depression. Nine hundred and nine older adults in Australia (aged 60 to 74 years) received either a placebo or a dietary supplement containing 400 micrograms folic acid and 100 micrograms vitamin B-12 for 24 months. A secondary analysis revealed that subjects who received folic acid and vitamin B-12 performed better on tests of short- and long-term recall, which was also related to smaller increases in plasma homocysteine levels over time. Supplementation with these B vitamins may help older adults maintain cognitive functioning as they age.

Source: Walker JG, et al. "Oral folic acid and vitamin B-12 supplementation to prevent cognitive decline in community dwelling older adults with depressive symptoms—the Beyond Ageing Project: A randomized controlled trial," *American Journal of Clinical Nutrition* 95:194, 2012.

one other vegetable, and one glass (5 oz.) of red wine. Nuts, beans, poultry, and berries are recommended regularly, but butter, cheese, and fast food are strictly limited.[15] Adults who adhered to the MIND Diet had 54% lower rates of Alzheimer's disease. Even more surprising, those that followed the MIND pattern, even periodically, also reduced their risk of the disease by 35%.

MEDICATIONS

Older adults are major consumers of medications (prescription and over-the-counter) and nutritional supplements. About 90% of older adults take at least one prescription medication daily, and half of all people over age 65 take several medicines each day. The rate of supplement use increases throughout adulthood such that by age 50, approximately half of all adults are using supplements daily. Physiological declines that occur during aging (e.g., reduced body water and reduced liver and kidney function) exaggerate and prolong the effects of medications and nutrient supplements in older adults.

Medications can eradicate infections and control chronic diseases, but some also adversely affect nutritional status, particularly of those who are older and/or take many different medications. For instance, some medications depress taste and smell acuity or cause anorexia or nausea that can blunt interest in eating and lead to reduced dietary intake. Some medications alter nutrient needs. Aspirin, for example, increases the likelihood of stomach bleeding, so long-term use may elevate the need for iron, as well as other nutrients. Antibiotics kill beneficial bacteria along with pathogens, so they can limit the amount of vitamin K that is synthesized by bacteria in the large intestine. Some medications may impair nutrient utilization; diuretics and laxatives may cause excessive excretion of water and minerals. Even vitamin and mineral supplements may have unanticipated effects on nutritional status. Iron supplements taken in large doses can interfere with the functioning of zinc and copper. Folate supplements can mask vitamin B-12 deficiencies.

People who must take medications should eat nutrient-dense foods and avoid any specific food or supplement that interferes with the function of their medications. For example, vitamin K can reduce the action of oral anticoagulants, aged cheese can interfere with certain drugs used to treat hypertension and depression, and grapefruit can interfere with medications such as tranquilizers and those that lower cholesterol levels. A registered dietitian nutritionist can help to plan a dietary pattern that meets nutritional needs while avoiding harmful food/medication interactions.

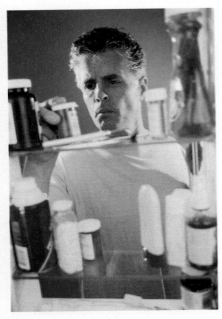

▲ About one-third of older adults take eight or more medications each day. In some cases, drugs can affect nutrient status. For example, certain diuretics may increase excretion of minerals in the urine. Other times, nutrients and other food components can impact the effectiveness of drugs. Vitamin K, for example, can affect the action of anticlotting medications. ©Ingram Publishing

COMPLEMENTARY AND ALTERNATIVE MEDICINE

At least half of adults report using some kind of dietary, botanical, or herbal supplement. Herbal dietary supplement sales in the United States increased by 7.5% in 2015. Recall that the safety, purity, and effectiveness of dietary supplements are not tightly monitored by the FDA. Table 16-3 reviews some popular herbal products used by older adults. Note from the table that these products can pose health risks in certain people. In addition, they may be expensive—in some cases, more than $100 per month—and are not covered by health insurance plans. In recent years, the use of many herbal products has declined because of expense and negative effects. Instead, consumers are opting to spend their money on products with more credible research results, such as multivitamins, vitamin D, omega-3 fatty acids, fiber, and probiotics.

When it comes to herbal products, proceed with caution. Significant health risks—including death—have been associated with the use of many herbal products. The FDA advises anyone who experiences adverse side effects from an herbal product to contact a primary care provider. Clinicians are then encouraged to report adverse events to the FDA, state and local health departments, and consumer protection agencies.

TABLE 16-3 ■ **A Closer Look at Popular Herbal Products**

Product	Purported Effects[a]	Side Effects	Vulnerable Population Groups
Black cohosh	• Mild reduction of postmenopausal symptoms in some studies	• Nausea • Liver damage	• Women who have had breast cancer • Pregnant women • Anyone taking estrogen, or hypertension or blood-thinning medications[b] • Anyone with abnormal liver function
Chondroitin sulfate	• Possible pain relief from osteoarthritis	• GI tract discomfort • Swelling • Hair loss • Irregular heartbeat	• People with asthma • Men with prostate cancer • Anyone taking blood-thinning medications
Cranberry	• Prevention or treatment of urinary tract infections (possibly effective) • Prevention of *Helicobacter pylori* infections of the stomach, with the aim of reducing the risk for ulcers (some evidence of efficacy)	• Gastrointestinal upset and diarrhea • Use of concentrated tablets may increase the risk of kidney stones	• People susceptible to kidney stones • Anyone taking antidepressants or prescription painkillers • Anyone taking blood thinners
Echinacea	• Prevention or treatment of colds or other infections (possibly effective)	• Nausea • Skin irritation • Allergic reactions • Minor GI tract upset • Increased urination	• Anyone with an autoimmune disease • Pre- or postsurgical patients • Anyone with allergies to daisies
Garlic	• Antifungal properties (possibly effective) • Reduction of blood cholesterol or blood pressure (possibly effective)	• GI tract upset (e.g., heartburn, flatulence) • Unpleasant odor • Allergic reactions	• Pre- or postsurgical patients • Perinatal women • Anyone taking blood-thinning medications or AIDS medications
Ginger	• Relief of nausea and vomiting (possibly effective)	• Heartburn • Diarrhea • Increased menstrual bleeding	• Pregnant women should proceed with caution due to possible risks for bleeding. • People with bleeding disorders or who take blood-thinning medications • Anyone with a heart condition • People taking blood glucose-lowering medications

(continued)

TABLE 16-3 ■ (continued)

Product	Purported Effects[a]	Side Effects	Vulnerable Population Groups
Ginkgo biloba	• Increased circulation (possibly effective) • Improvement of memory (especially for people with Alzheimer's disease; low evidence of efficacy)	• Mild headache • GI tract upset • Allergic reactions • Irritability • Reduced blood clotting • Seizures (if contaminated with toxic ginkgo seeds)	• People with bleeding disorders • Pre- or postsurgical patients • Anyone with allergies to the plant • Concurrent use of feverfew, garlic, ginseng, dong quai, or red clover • Anyone taking diabetes medications, blood-thinning medications, vitamin E supplements, antidepressants, or diuretics
Ginseng	• Lowering blood sugar (possibly effective) • Increased energy (possibly ineffective)	• Hypertension • Asthma attacks • Irregular heartbeat • Hypoglycemia • Insomnia • Headache • Nervousness • GI tract upset • Reduced blood clotting • Menstrual irregularities and breast tenderness	• Anyone who takes a prescription drug • Women who have had breast cancer • Anyone with chronic GI tract disease • Anyone with uncontrolled hypertension
Glucosamine sulfate	• Prevention and treatment of osteoarthritis (likely effective)	• GI tract upset	• People with asthma or shellfish allergies
St. John's wort	• Alleviation of mild to moderate depression (likely effective)	• Mild GI tract upset • Rash • Tiredness • Restlessness • Increased sensitivity to sunlight	• Anyone who takes a prescription drug • People with UV sensitivity, including that induced by medications or other treatments[c] • People with bipolar disorder, major depression, schizophrenia, and Alzheimer's disease • Anyone recovering from a graft or organ transplant
Turmeric	• Pain relief from osteoarthritis (possibly effective)	• GI tract upset • Dizziness	• People with gallbladder problems • People with GERD • Pre- or postsurgical patients
Valerian	• Alleviation of insomnia (possibly effective) • Reduction of anxiety (insufficient evidence to rate effectiveness)	• Impaired attention • Headache • Morning grogginess • Irregular heartbeat • GI tract upset • Disagreeable odor • Withdrawal delerium	• Anyone taking anesthetics or central nervous system depressants[d] • Anyone who drinks alcohol • People about to operate heavy machinery or drive

[a]Ratings of effectiveness from MedlinePlus and/or NCCAM; [b]Coumadin,® aspirin, Heparin,® Lovenox,® or Fragmin;® [c]Sulfa medications, anti-inflammatory medications, or acid-reflux medications; [d]Valium, halcion, seconal.

Pregnant or breastfeeding women, children under 2 years of age, anyone over the age of 65 years, and anyone with a chronic disease should never take supplements unless under the guidance of a primary care provider. A concern has been raised with regard to patients who abruptly end alternative medicines at the start of hospital treatments or deny that they are using alternative therapy. Interactions between alternative therapies and pharmaceutical drugs can be drastic and include complications such as delirium, clotting abnormalities, and rapid heartbeat, resulting in the need for intensive care. Full disclosure of all prescription and nonprescription treatments aids in prevention of such complications. Experts recommend that, if time permits, patients stop taking herbal products for about a week before a scheduled surgery or otherwise take all original supplement containers to the hospital, so that the anesthesiologist can evaluate what was taken.

If you decide to consume an herbal or botanical product, only ingest one product at a time, keep a diary of symptoms, and definitely check with your primary care provider before discontinuing any prescribed medication. In particular, avoid the following herbal ingredients:

Chaparral	Kava kava	Paraguay tea	Stephania
Comfrey	Kombucha tea	Penny-royal	Tung shueh
Germander	Lobelia	Pokeroot	Willow bark
Hai gen fen	Magnolia	Sassafras	Yohimbe
Jin bu huan	Mandrake	Senna	

> For additional information about herbal products, access the following websites:
>
> National Institutes of Health
> National Center for Complementary and Integrative Health
> https://nccih.nih.gov
>
> National Institutes of Health
> Office of Dietary Supplements
> www.ods.od.nih.gov
>
> Natural Medicines
> www.naturalmedicines.therapeuticresearch.com/

✔ CONCEPT CHECK 16.3

1. What is sarcopenia? What diet and lifestyle changes would you suggest to avoid this condition?

2. Describe three ways aging affects the processes of digestion, absorption, and utilization of nutrients.

3. How does depression influence nutritional status?

4. List two types of complementary and alternative medicine adults may use to improve health.

16.4 Ensuring a Healthful Dietary Pattern for the Adult Years

Recommended dietary practices for later years would be to increase the diet's nutrient density and to make sure fiber and fluid intakes are adequate. In addition, some protein should come from lean meats to help meet protein, vitamin B-6, vitamin B-12, iron, and zinc needs.

Singles of all ages face logistical barriers obtaining adequate nutrients: purchasing, preparing, storing, and using food with minimal waste can be challenging. Value-priced packages of meats and vegetables are normally too large to be useful for a single person. Many singles live in small dwellings, some without kitchens and freezers. Creating an adequate dietary pattern to accommodate a limited budget and a single appetite requires special considerations. The following are some practical suggestions for diet planning for singles. Table 16-4 provides additional ideas for eating healthfully in later years.

- If you have access to a freezer, cook large amounts, divide into single-serve portions, and freeze.
- Buy only what you will use; small containers may be expensive, but letting food spoil is also costly.
- Ask the grocer to divide family-sized packages of wrapped meat or fresh vegetables, separate, and wrap into smaller units.
- Buy smaller amounts of fruit—perhaps one ripe, one medium-ripe, and one unripe—so that the fruit can be eaten over a period of several days.
- Keep a box of dry milk handy to add nutrients to recipes for baked foods and other foods for which this addition is acceptable.

TABLE 16-4 ■ Guidelines for Healthful Eating in Later Years

- Eat regularly; small, frequent meals. Use plant-based nutrient-dense foods as a basis for menus.

- Use labor-saving cooking methods and healthier convenience foods, but try to incorporate fresh foods into daily menus.

- Try new foods, new seasonings, and new ways of preparing foods. Use low-sodium canned goods or frozen produce in cooking.

- Keep easy-to-prepare foods on hand for times when you feel tired.

- Have a treat occasionally, perhaps an expensive cut of fish or a favorite fresh fruit.

- Eat in a well-lit or sunny area; serve meals attractively; and experiment with different flavors, colors, shapes, textures, and smells.

- Arrange kitchen and eating area so that food preparation and cleanup are simple.

- Eat with friends, relatives, or at a community center when possible.

- Share cooking responsibilities with a neighbor or close friend.

- Use community resources for help with shopping and other daily care needs.

- Stay physically active and well hydrated.

- If possible, take a walk before eating to stimulate the appetite.

- When necessary, chop, grind, or blend hard-to-chew foods. Softer, protein-rich foods (e.g., beans, shredded meats, eggs) can be substituted for whole pieces of meat when poor dentition prevents normal food intake. Prepare soups, stews, cooked whole grains, and casseroles.

Nutritional deficiencies and protein-calorie malnutrition have been identified among some aging populations, particularly those in hospitals, nursing homes, or long-term care facilities. The DETERMINE Nutrition Checklist for Older Adults shown in Figure 16-3 can be used to identify older adults at nutritional risk. Malnutrition increases the risk for infections and bed sores (pressure ulcers) and compromises recovery from illness and surgery. Friends, relatives, and health care professionals should monitor nutrient intake in older people, including those who live in long-term care facilities. Family members can play a valuable role in making sure nutrient needs are met by looking for weight maintenance based on regular, healthful meal patterns. If problems arise in consuming a healthful dietary pattern, a registered dietitian nutritionist can assess nutrition concerns and offer professional and personalized advice.

Older adults benefit from good nutrition in many ways. Meeting nutrient needs delays the onset of some diseases; improves the management of some existing diseases; hastens recovery from many illnesses; increases mental, physical, and social well-being; and often decreases the need for and length of hospitalization. MyPlate is a useful guide for planning healthy meals, but older adults must be sure to emphasize certain nutrients: potassium, calcium, vitamin D, vitamin B-12, vitamin C and fiber. In 2016, Tufts University released an updated MyPlate for Older Adults that illustrates nutrient-dense food choices that are accessible and appealing for this population group (Fig. 16-7). The graphic also affirms the importance of adequate fluid intake and modified physical activity goals. In some cases, dietary supplementation may be appropriate to address the unique needs of older adults.

Obtaining enough food may be difficult for some older persons, especially if they have a low income, are unable to drive, or do not have social networks that can assist with cooking or shopping. For an older person, a request for help may be equated to a loss of independence. Pride or fear may stand in the way of much-needed aid.

The World Health Organization recommends eating 5 portions of fruit and vegetables every day, but a new meta-analysis[16] found that eating 10 portions of fruit and vegetables a day could significantly reduce the risk of:

- Cardiovascular disease by 28%
- Stroke by 33%
- Cancer by 13%
- Early death by 31%
- 7.5 million premature deaths globally

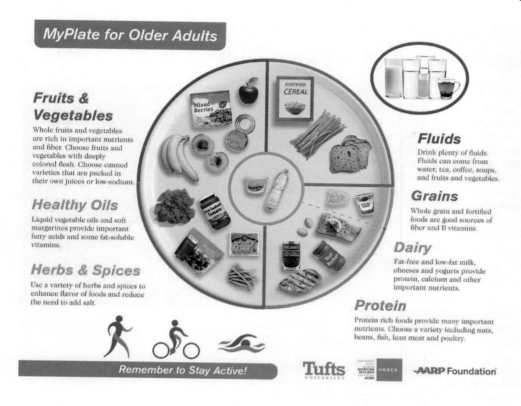

MyPlate for Older Adults

Fruits & Vegetables

Whole fruits and vegetables are rich in important nutrients and fiber. Choose fruits and vegetables with deeply colored flesh. Choose canned varieties that are packed in their own juices or low-sodium.

Healthy Oils

Liquid vegetable oils and soft margarines provide important fatty acids and some fat-soluble vitamins.

Herbs & Spices

Use a variety of herbs and spices to enhance flavor of foods and reduce the need to add salt.

Fluids

Drink plenty of fluids. Fluids can come from water, tea, coffee, soups, and fruits and vegetables.

Grains

Whole grain and fortified foods are good sources of fiber and B vitamins.

Dairy

Fat-free and low-fat milk, cheeses and yogurts provide protein, calcium and other important nutrients.

Protein

Protein rich foods provide many important nutrients. Choose a variety including nuts, beans, fish, lean meat and poultry.

Remember to Stay Active!

Tufts | AARP Foundation

In these cases, family and friends can be a big help. Special transportation arrangements may also be available through community agencies, local transit companies, or lift services. Indeed, many eligible older people are missing meals and are poorly nourished because they do not realize that programs are available to help them. Irregular meal patterns and weight loss are warning signs that malnutrition may be developing. An effort should be made to identify poorly nourished seniors and inform them of available community services.

COMMUNITY NUTRITION SERVICES FOR OLDER ADULTS

Health care advice and services for older people can come from clinics, private practitioners, hospitals, and health maintenance organizations. Home health care agencies, adult day care programs, adult overnight-care programs, and **hospice care** (for the terminally ill) also provide daily care for those who qualify.

One in five adults (about 11 million) are served by the Older Americans Act (OAA). Originally enacted in 1965, the OAA supports a range of home and community-based services, including Meals on Wheels and other nutrition programs. The OAA nutrition programs serve about 242 million meals each year to U.S. adults over the age of 60. Federal standards mandate that these meals supply at least one-third of adult energy and nutrient requirements.

Some meals, such as Meals on Wheels, are delivered directly to older adults in their homes. Although home-delivered meals can make a valuable contribution to the positive nutritional status of home-bound older adults, services are usually limited to one or two meals per day. If a recipient has a poor appetite, the food may end up stored for later or simply thrown away. If foods are not eaten on delivery and not stored properly, risk for foodborne illness could be a concern. Other meals are provided by congregate meal programs, which usually serve lunch at a central location. With congregate meals, the social aspect of eating tends to improve nutritional intake. However, programs generally provide just one meal per day on 5 days per week. Where can older adults with limited resources find additional nutrition assistance?

hospice care A program offering care that emphasizes comfort and dignity at the end of life.

To learn more about resources available for older adults in your area, check out the following websites:

Food Assistance Programs for Seniors:
www.nutrition.gov/
food-assistance-programs

Elder Care Locator:
www.eldercare.gov

National Institute on Aging:
www.nia.nih.gov

American Geriatrics Society:
www.americangeriatrics.org

Administration on Aging:
www.aoa.gov

CASE STUDY Dietary Assistance for an Older Adult

Frances is an 82-year-old woman who suffers from macular degeneration, osteoporosis, and arthritis. Since her husband died a year ago, she has moved from their family home to a small one-bedroom apartment. Her eyesight is progressively getting worse, making it difficult to go to the grocery store or even to cook (for fear of burning herself). She is often lonely; her only son lives an hour away and works two jobs, but he visits her as often as he can. Frances has lost her appetite and, as a result, often skips meals during the week. She has resorted to eating mostly cold foods. These are simple to prepare but seriously limit the variety and palatability of her diet. Also, she wears dentures and has trouble chewing tough meats and foods with crisp textures. She is slowly losing weight as a result of her eating patterns and loss of appetite.

Her typical diet usually consists of a breakfast that may include 1 slice of wheat toast with margarine, honey, and cinnamon, and 1 cup of hot tea. If she has lunch, she normally has a can of peaches, half of a turkey sandwich, and a glass of water. For dinner, she might have half of a tuna fish sandwich made with mayonnaise and 1 cup of iced tea. She usually includes one or two soft cookies at bedtime.

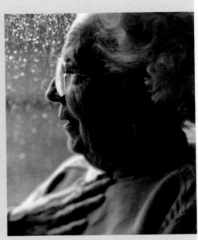
©Getty Images

1. What nutrients are likely to be inadequate in Frances's current diet?
2. What potential effects will Frances's limited dietary pattern have on her health status?
3. Which physiological changes of aging will add to the effects of her inadequate dietary intake (review Table 16-2)?
4. What other questions would you ask Frances to get a better sense of her nutrition status?
5. What services are available in the community that could help Frances improve her diet?
6. What other convenience foods could be included in her diet to make it more healthful and more varied?

Complete the Case Study. Responses to these questions can be provided by your instructor.

In addition to congregate and home-delivered meals, federal commodity distribution is available in some areas of the United States to low-income older people. Such individuals whose incomes are below the poverty level can benefit from the SNAP program (previously known as *food stamps*). The Senior Farmers Market Nutrition Program provides low-income seniors with coupons that can be exchanged for eligible foods (fruits, vegetables, honey, and fresh-cut herbs) at farmers markets, roadside stands, and community-supported agriculture programs. Food cooperatives and a variety of clubs and religious and social organizations provide additional aid.

✓ CONCEPT CHECK 16.4

1. Gerald is a 76-year-old man whose wife recently passed away. He now lives alone for the first time in his life and is not accustomed to preparing meals for himself. What three pieces of advice would you give Gerald about eating well?

2. List three possible nutrition resources for an older adult with limited financial means.

16.5 Nutrition and Your Health

Nutrition Implications of Alcohol Consumption

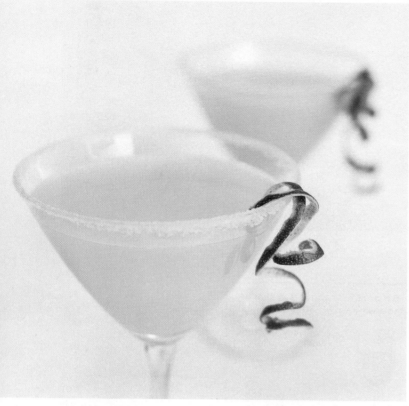
©Digital Vision/Getty Images

(BAC) rises above the legal limit of 0.08 gram per deciliter. This usually correlates to five or more drinks for men or four or more drinks for women. Although binge drinking is certainly linked to negative effects on physical and emotional health, it is not necessarily an alcohol use disorder, which will be discussed next.

Moderate consumption of alcohol by a person of legal drinking age is an acceptable practice and even has some health benefits.[17] However, only about half of alcohol consumed is done so in moderation. About one in four people over the age of 12 report binge drinking in the last 30 days. Problem drinking that becomes severe is given the medical diagnosis of **alcohol use disorder**. About 15 million people in the United States suffer from alcohol use disorders (often referred to as *alcoholism*). By far, alcohol is the most commonly abused drug.

How Alcoholic Beverages Are Produced

The basis of alcohol production is fermentation, a process by which microorganisms break down simple sugars (e.g., glucose or maltose) to alcohol, carbon dioxide, and water in the absence of oxygen. High-carbohydrate foods encourage the growth of yeast, the microorganism responsible for alcohol production. Wine is formed by the fermentation of grape or other fruit juices. Beer is made from malted cereal grain. Distilled spirits (e.g., vodka, gin, and whiskey) are made from any number of fruits, vegetables, and grains. Production temperatures, the composition of the food used for fermentation, and aging techniques determine the characteristics of the product.

Given the wide spectrum of alcohol use and abuse, knowledge of alcohol consumption and its relationship to overall health is essential to the study of nutrition. Alcoholic beverages contain the chemical form of alcohol known as **ethanol.** Although not a nutrient per se, alcohol is a source of calories (about 7 kcal per gram). Over half of American adults drink alcohol. On average, alcohol accounts for about 4.7% of total calories in the average North American diet (Table 16-5).

A *standard drink* contains about 14 grams alcohol. For beer or wine coolers, this equates to a 12-fluid-ounce serving. Most cans of beer are 12 fluid ounces, but some cans or bottles may contain as much as 40 fluid ounces. Malt liquor has a slightly higher alcohol content than beer, so the standard drink size is 8 to 9 fluid ounces. For wine, a 5-fluid-ounce glass is standard. A standard drink of hard liquor, such as whiskey or rum, is the size of a shot glass—1.5 fluid ounces. Standard drink sizes are depicted in Figure 16-8.

Moderate drinking is defined by single-day and weekly amounts. To be classified as a moderate drinker, an individual must meet both criteria. For men, moderate drinking is no more than 4 drinks in 1 day AND no more than 14 drinks per week. For women, moderate drinking is no more than 3 drinks in 1 day AND no more than 7 drinks per week. **Heavy drinking** encompasses all patterns of alcohol consumption in excess of moderate drinking. **Binge drinking** is characterized by drinking so much within a short period of time (usually within 2 hours) that blood alcohol concentration

> Alcohol proof represents twice the volume of alcohol in percentage terms. Thus, 80 proof vodka contains 40% alcohol.

ethanol Chemical term for the form of alcohol found in alcoholic beverages.

moderate drinking For men, consuming no more than 4 drinks in 1 day AND no more than 14 drinks per week; for women, consuming no more than 3 drinks in 1 day AND no more than 7 drinks per week.

heavy drinking Any pattern of alcohol consumption in excess of 4 drinks in 1 day or 14 drinks per week for men or 3 drinks in 1 day or 7 drinks per week for women.

binge drinking Drinking sufficient alcohol within a 2-hour period to increase blood alcohol content to 0.08 grams per deciliter or higher; for men, consuming 5 or more drinks in a row; for women, consuming 4 or more drinks in a row.

alcohol use disorder A psychiatric disorder characterized by a problematic pattern of alcohol use that leads to significant impairment or distress.

TABLE 16-5 ■ Approximate Alcohol, Carbohydrate, and Calorie Content of Alcoholic Beverages*

Beverage	Amount (fluid ounces)	Alcohol (grams)	Carbohydrates (grams)	Calories (kcal)
Beer				
Regular	12	13	13	146
Light	12	11	5	99
Distilled Spirits				
Gin, rum, vodka, bourbon, whiskey (80 proof)	1.5	15	—	105
Wine				
Red/white/rosé	5	15	4	125
Dessert and sweet	5	23	17	225
Other Alcohol Drinks				
Daiquiri	7	20	33	259
Martini	3	27	—	189
Hard lemonade	11.2	13	34	228
Cream liqueur (34 proof)	1.5	6.5	10	154

*There is little to no fat or protein contribution to calorie content.

Source: USDA

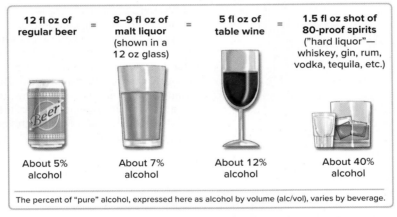

12 fl oz of regular beer	=	8–9 fl oz of malt liquor (shown in a 12 oz glass)	=	5 fl oz of table wine	=	1.5 fl oz shot of 80-proof spirits ("hard liquor"— whiskey, gin, rum, vodka, tequila, etc.)
About 5% alcohol		About 7% alcohol		About 12% alcohol		About 40% alcohol

The percent of "pure" alcohol, expressed here as alcohol by volume (alc/vol), varies by beverage.

FIGURE 16-8 ▲ The standard drink sizes shown provide about 14 grams of alcohol. Keep in mind that alcoholic beverages served in bars and restaurants can be 20% to 45% larger than a standard drink.

Source: NIAAA

Absorption and Metabolism of Alcohol

Alcohol requires no digestion. It is absorbed rapidly from the GI tract by diffusion, making it the most efficiently absorbed of all calorie sources. Once absorbed, alcohol is freely distributed into all the fluid compartments within the body. About 1% to 3% of alcohol is excreted via urine and about 1% to 5% evaporates via the breath, the basis for the breathalyzer test. Most alcohol (90% to 98%), however, is metabolized. The liver is the primary site for alcohol metabolism, and some may also be metabolized by the cells lining the stomach. The main pathway of alcohol metabolism involves the enzymes **alcohol dehydrogenase** and **acetaldehyde dehydrogenase.** Alcohol cannot be stored in the body, so it takes absolute priority over other energy sources for metabolism.

As a person's alcohol consumption exceeds the body's capacity to metabolize it, blood alcohol concentration rises, the brain is exposed to alcohol, and symptoms of intoxication appear (Table 16-6). Absorption and metabolism of alcohol depend on numerous factors: genetics, gender, body size, physical condition, meal composition, gastric emptying rate, the alcohol content of the beverage, use of certain drugs, chronic alcohol use, and even how much sleep one has had. Women absorb and metabolize alcohol less efficiently than men. The amount of alcohol metabolized by the cells lining the stomach is greater in men than in women. Women also have less body water in which to dilute the alcohol than do men. Overall, women develop chronic alcohol-related ailments, such as cirrhosis of the liver, more rapidly than men do with the same alcohol-consumption habits.

alcohol dehydrogenase An enzyme used in alcohol (ethanol) metabolism that converts alcohol into acetaldehyde.

acetaldehyde dehydrogenase An enzyme used in ethanol metabolism that eventually converts acetaldehyde into carbon dioxide and water.

TABLE 16-6 ■ Blood Alcohol Concentration and Symptoms

Concentration[a]	Sporadic Drinker	Chronic Drinker	Hours for Alcohol to Be Metabolized[b]
50 (0.05%)	Congenial euphoria, decreased tension, and noticeable impairment in driving and coordination	No observable effect	2–3
75 (0.075%)	Gregarious	Often no effect	3–4
80–100 (0.08%–0.1%)	Uncoordinated, 0.08% is legal driving limit in U.S. and Canada	Minimal signs	4–6
125–150 (0.125%–0.15%)	Unrestrained behavior, episodic uncontrolled behavior	Pleasurable euphoria or beginning of uncoordination	6–10
200–250 (0.2%–0.25%)	Alertness lost, lethargic	Effort is required to maintain emotional and motor control	10–24
300–350 (0.3%–0.35%)	Stupor to coma	Drowsy and slow	10–24
> 500 (> 0.5%)	Some will die.	Coma	> 24

[a]Milligrams of alcohol per 100 milliliters of blood.

[b]For a social drinker; alcohol metabolism is somewhat faster in chronic alcohol abusers.

Source: Modified from Goldman L, Schafer AI: *Goldman's Cecil Medicine,* 24th edition. Philadelphia: Elsevier Health Sciences, 2012.

Benefits of Moderate Alcohol Use

When used in moderation, alcohol is linked to several health benefits. Benefits of alcohol use are associated with specific intakes of no more than two drinks per day for men and no more than one drink per day for women. Socialization and relaxation are among the intangible benefits of moderate alcohol use by people of legal drinking age. In terms of physiological benefits, moderate drinkers experience lower risk of developing cardiovascular diseases and type 2 diabetes. However, recent reports suggest that just one drink per day can increase the risk for breast cancer. Previous consumers of alcohol no longer experience the benefits of alcohol when consumption ceases. See Table 16-7 for benefits of moderate alcohol consumption.

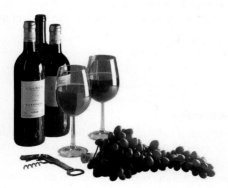

▲ Of all the alcohol sources, red wine in moderation is often singled out as the best choice because of the added bonus of the many studied phytochemicals present (e.g., resveratrol). These are leached out from the grape skins as the red wine is fermented. Dark beer is also a source of phytochemicals. ©Ingram Publishing/Alamy

Risks of Heavy Drinking

An alcohol use disorder is a formal psychiatric diagnosis defined in the latest edition of the *Diagnostic and Statistical Manual of Mental Disorders (DSM-5)* as a problematic pattern of alcohol use leading to significant impairment or distress. This new definition integrates both alcohol abuse and alcohol dependence into a single disorder with mild, moderate, and severe sub-classifications. According to *DSM-5,* diagnosis depends on meeting two or more of the following criteria within the past year:

- Use of alcohol in larger amounts or over a longer period than intended
- Persistent desire or unsuccessful efforts at cutting down or controlling alcohol use
- Spending a great deal of time obtaining, using, and recovering from the effects of alcohol
- Experiencing cravings for alcohol
- Repeated use of alcohol that results in failure to fulfill major obligations at school, work, or home
- Continued use of alcohol despite personal problems created by the effects of heavy drinking
- Avoiding social, occupational, or recreational activities due to use of alcohol
- Recurrent alcohol use in situations in which it is physically hazardous
- Continuing to use alcohol even after realizing one has a problem caused by heavy drinking
- Developing a **tolerance** to the effects of alcohol
- Experiencing symptoms of **withdrawal** in the absence of alcohol use

Alcohol use disorders affect about 17% of adult men and about 8% of adult women at some point in their lives. Studies suggest

tolerance Needing more of a substance to achieve the desired effect (e.g., intoxication) or experiencing diminished effects of a given amount of a substance after repeated use.

withdrawal Physical symptoms related to cessation of substance use, such as sweating, rapid pulse, shakiness, insomnia, nausea and vomiting, anxiety, and even seizures.

cirrhosis A loss of functioning liver cells, which are replaced by nonfunctioning connective tissue. Any substance that poisons liver cells can lead to cirrhosis. The most common cause is a chronic, excessive alcohol intake. Exposure to certain industrial chemicals also can lead to cirrhosis.

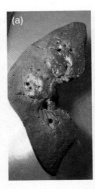 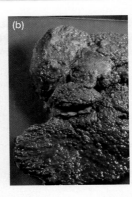

FIGURE 16-9 ▲ Effects of alcohol on the liver. Alcohol is particularly damaging to this organ. Pictured are (a) a healthy liver, and (b) a liver with cirrhosis. There is no cure for this disease except a liver transplant. ©Arthur Glauberman/Science Source

that about 40% of a person's risk for developing these disorders is genetic. Therefore, people with a family history of heavy drinking, particularly children of alcoholics, should be especially aware of their alcohol consumption.

Early diagnosis of alcohol use disorders can prevent multiple health problems and save millions in health care costs. Asking a person about the quantity and frequency of alcohol consumption is an important means of detecting problematic behaviors (see CAGE Questionnaire below). Observable warning signs of an alcohol use disorder may include an alcohol odor on the breath, flushed face and reddened skin, nervous system disorders (such as tremors), unexplained work absences, frequent accidents, and falls or injuries of vague origin. Laboratory evidence (e.g., impaired liver function, enlarged red blood cells, and elevated triglycerides) is also helpful for diagnosis of alcohol use disorders.

Despite the few benefits of regular, moderate use, the risks of heavy drinking are more numerous and harmful. Although it is one of the most preventable health problems, excessive consumption of alcohol contributes significantly to 5 of the 10 leading causes of death in North America: heart failure, certain forms of cancer, **cirrhosis** of the liver, motor vehicle and other accidents, and suicides (Table 16-7 lists additional health risks). In the United States, about $249 billion is spent annually in terms of lost productivity, medical care, and property damage associated with alcohol use disorders. Overall, alcohol use disorders typically reduce a person's life expectancy by up to 30 years.

Alcohol is most damaging to the liver. Cirrhosis develops in up to 20% of cases of alcohol use disorders and is the second leading reason for liver transplants, affecting about 2 million people in the United States. This chronic and usually relentlessly progressive disease is characterized by fatty infiltration of the liver. Fatty liver occurs in response to increased synthesis of fat and decreased use of it for energy by the liver. Eventually, the enlarged fat deposits choke off the blood supply, depriving the liver cells of oxygen and nutrients. Liver cells can accumulate so much fat that they burst, die, and are replaced by connective (scar) tissue. At this stage, the liver is deemed cirrhotic (Fig. 16-9). Early stages of alcoholic liver injury are reversible, but advanced stages are not. Once a person has cirrhosis, there is a 50% chance of death within 4 years, a far worse prognosis than many forms of cancer. While no specific level of alcohol consumption guarantees cirrhosis, some evidence suggests that damage is caused by a dose as low as 40 grams per day for men (3 beers) and 20 grams per day for women (1.5 beers).

Alcoholic beverages have little nutritional value, and thus, nutrient deficiencies are a common result of alcohol use disorders. The protein and vitamin content is extremely low, except in beer, where it is marginal at best. Iron content varies widely between drinks, with red wine ranking especially high in iron. Deficiencies arise mainly from poor nutrient intakes, but increased urinary losses and fat malabsorption (linked to poor pancreatic function) also contribute. Vitamins most susceptible to depletion from heavy drinking include vitamins A, D, E, and K; thiamin; niacin; folate; vitamins B-6 and B-12; and vitamin C. Mineral deficiencies of calcium, phosphorus, potassium, magnesium, zinc, and iron are also possible. Conversely, vitamin and mineral toxicity is also of concern with heavy drinking. Damage to the GI tract and liver, as well as high levels of some minerals in alcoholic beverages, may lead to toxicity of vitamin A, iron, lead, or cobalt. In nutritional treatment of alcohol use disorders, the immediate aim is eliminating alcohol intake, followed by restoration of nutrient stores.

CRITICAL THINKING

For many people, drinking and smoking go hand in hand. What health problems arise from the combination of these behaviors?

Cage Questionnaire

The CAGE Questionnaire is used to identify alcohol use disorders. More than one positive response suggests an alcohol problem.

C: Have you ever felt you ought to *cut* down on drinking?

A: Have people *annoyed* you by criticizing your drinking?

G: Have you ever felt bad or *guilty* about your drinking?

E: Have you ever had a drink first thing in the morning to steady your nerves or get rid of a hangover (an *eye-opener*)?

TABLE 16-7 ■ Effects of Moderate Versus Heavy Drinking

	Moderate Drinking	Heavy Drinking
Coronary heart disease	Decreased risk of death in those at high risk for coronary heart disease–related death, primarily by increasing HDL-cholesterol, decreasing blood clotting, and relaxing blood vessels	Heart rhythm disturbances, heart muscle damage, increased blood triglycerides and blood clotting
Hypertension and stroke	Mild decrease in blood pressure, lower rates of ischemic stroke in people with normal blood pressure	Increased blood pressure (hypertension), more ischemic and hemorrhagic stroke
Peripheral vascular disease	Decreased risk due to reduced blood clotting	No benefit
Blood glucose regulation and type 2 diabetes	Decreased risk of developing type 2 diabetes, decreased risk of death from cardiovascular disease among those diagnosed with diabetes	Hypoglycemia, reduced insulin sensitivity, and damage to pancreas
Bone and joint health	Some increase in bone mineral content in women, linked to estrogen output	Loss of active bone-forming cells and eventual osteoporosis, increased risk of gout
Brain health	Enhanced brain function and decreased risk of dementia by increasing brain blood circulation	Brain tissue damage and decreased memory
Skeletal muscle health	No benefit	Skeletal muscle damage
Cancer	Decreased risk of colon, basal cell, ovarian, and prostate cancers; increased risk of breast cancer	Increased risk of at least 11 cancers
Liver function	No benefit	Fatty infiltration and eventual liver cirrhosis (especially if a person is also infected with hepatitis C), iron toxicity
GI tract health	Decreased risk of certain bacterial infections in the stomach	Inflammation of the stomach and pancreas, absorptive cell damage leading to malabsorption of nutrients
Immune system function	No benefit	Reduced function and increased infections
Nervous system function	No benefit	Loss of nerve sensation and nervous system control of muscles
Sleep disturbances	Some relaxation	Fragmented sleep patterns; worsens sleep apnea
Impotence and decreased libido	No benefit	Contributes to the problem in both men and women
Obesity	No benefit	Increased abdominal fat deposition; contributes to weight gain
Dietary intake	May supply some B vitamins, phytochemicals, and iron	Leads to numerous nutrient deficiencies: protein, vitamins, and minerals
Fetal health	No benefit	Variety of toxic effects on the fetus when alcohol is consumed by pregnant women
Socialization and relaxation	Provides some benefit to socialization and leads to relaxation by increasing brain neurotransmitter activity	Contributes to violent behavior and agitation

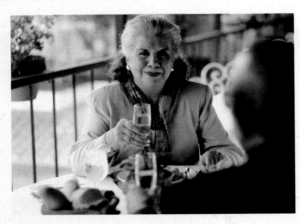

▲ The limit for alcohol intake for older adults is one drink per day.
©Steve Mason/Getty Images

Older adults are uniquely vulnerable to alcohol use disorders, perhaps due to an abundance of free time, social events involving drinking, interactions with medications, loneliness, or depression. Common symptoms of alcohol use disorders—trembling hands, slurred speech, sleep problems, memory loss, and unsteady gait—can be easily overlooked as signs of aging. Slower alcohol metabolism and decreased body water allow older adults to become intoxicated from a smaller amount of alcohol than their younger counterparts. Even moderate alcohol consumption can exacerbate some chronic health conditions, such as diabetes and osteoporosis. As well, even small amounts of alcohol can react negatively with various medications used by older persons. The adverse health effects of drinking may be amplified in older adults, so people over the age of 65 should limit alcohol consumption to no more than one drink per day.

Once a diagnosis of an alcohol use disorder is established, a primary care provider can arrange appropriate treatment and counseling for the person and his or her family. Treatment often

Ethnicity plays an important role in both the probability of becoming a heavy drinker and the negative health risks associated with heavy drinking. Native Americans suffer the highest rates of unintentional injuries, suicide, homicide, and domestic abuse related to alcohol use. African-Americans with alcohol use disorders are at greater risk than other racial groups for tuberculosis, hepatitis C, HIV/AIDS, and other infectious diseases. Hispanic Americans are at particular risk for cirrhosis-related death.

includes the use of targeted medications, counseling, and social support. Total abstinence must be the ultimate objective. *Alcoholics Anonymous* or other reputable therapy programs can support those struggling with alcohol use disorders and their families as they recover from this devastating disease.

Guidance Regarding Alcohol Use

No government agencies recommend drinking alcohol. The *Dietary Guidelines for Americans* provide the following advice regarding use of alcoholic beverages:

- If alcohol is consumed, it should be in moderation—no more than one drink per day for women and no more than two drinks per day for men—and only by adults of legal drinking age.
- For those who choose to drink, moderate alcohol consumption can be incorporated within the calorie limits of most healthy eating patterns.
- The *Dietary Guidelines* do not recommend that individuals who do not drink alcohol start drinking for any reason.
- Many individuals should not consume alcohol, including individuals who are taking certain over-the-counter or prescription medications or who have certain medical conditions, those who are recovering from alcoholism or are unable to control the amount they drink, and anyone younger than 21 years.
- Individuals should not drink if they are driving, planning to drive, or are participating in other activities requiring skill, coordination, and alertness. The National Transportation Safety Board is calling for states to lower BAC limits from 0.08 to 0.05 gram per deciliter.
- Women who are or who may be pregnant should not drink. Drinking during pregnancy, especially in the first few months of pregnancy, may result in negative behavioral or neurological consequences in the offspring. Women who are breastfeeding should consult with their health care provider regarding alcohol consumption.

As the understanding of the relationship between drinking alcohol and health grows, registered dietitian nutritionists and other health professionals can promote healthy lifestyle—not by encouraging indiscriminate drinking, but by reassuring adults that moderate alcohol consumption may have beneficial health outcomes.

To learn more about alcohol use disorders, visit these websites:

- National Institute on Alcohol Abuse and Alcoholism: www.niaaa.nih.gov
- American Society of Addiction Medicine: www.asam.org
- Centers for Disease Control and Prevention: www.cdc.gov/alcohol

Summary (Numbers refer to numbered sections in the chapter.)

16.1 Although maximum life span has not changed, life expectancy has increased dramatically over the past century. For many societies, this means that an increasing proportion of the population is over 65 years of age. As health care costs rise, the goal of delaying adequate treatment of chronic disease becomes critically important.

The physiologic changes of aging are the sum of cellular changes, lifestyle practices, and environmental influences. Many of these changes can be minimized, prevented, and/or reversed by healthy lifestyles. Usual aging refers to the age-related physical and physiological changes that are commonly thought to be typical of aging. Successful aging describes the declines in physical and physiological function that occur because one grows older. Striving to have the greatest number of healthy years and the fewest of illness is referred to as compression of morbidity.

16.2 A dietary pattern based on MyPlate and the *Dietary Guidelines for Americans* can help one to preserve body function, avoid chronic disease, and age successfully. American adults are fairly well nourished, although common dietary excesses are calories, saturated fat, sodium, and, for some, alcohol. Common dietary inadequacies include vitamins D and E, folate, magnesium, calcium, zinc, and fiber. People ages 65 and older, particularly those in long-term care facilities and hospitals, are at risk for malnutrition. The DETERMINE Nutrition Checklist for Older Adults can help to identify older adults at risk of nutrient deficiencies. The DRIs for adults are divided by gender and age to reflect how nutrient needs change as adults grow older. These changes in nutrient needs take into consideration the aging-related physiological alterations in body composition, metabolism, and organ function.

16.3 Chronic diseases, changes in body composition, and declining function of body systems can influence nutritional status. Of particular concern is sarcopenia, or loss of muscle mass that frequently accompanies aging. The use of high-quality protein intakes, prescription medications, and multivitamin and mineral supplements can improve health and quality of life, but some also adversely affect nutritional status. Herbal products should be used with extreme caution.

16.4 Dietary patterns for adults should be based on nutrient-dense foods and need to be individualized for existing health problems, physical abilities, the presence of drug-nutrient interactions, possible depression, and economic constraints. Community nutrition assistance programs, including congregate or home-delivered meal systems, SNAP, and commodity distribution make wholesome, nutritious foods accessible for low-income and older adults.

16.5 Alcohol requires no digestion and is metabolized primarily in the liver. The benefits of alcohol use are associated with low to moderate alcohol consumption. These benefits include the pleasurable and social aspects of alcohol use, a reduction in various forms of cardiovascular disease, increase in insulin sensitivity, and protection against some harmful stomach bacteria. Heavy drinking, however, contributes significantly to 5 of the 10 leading causes of death in North America. If alcohol is consumed, it should be consumed in moderation with meals. Women (and older adults, in general) are advised to drink no more than 3 drinks in 1 day and no more than 7 drinks per week; men should drink no more than 4 drinks in 1 day and no more than 14 drinks per week.

Check Your Knowledge (Answers are available at the end of this question set.)

1. The reason the incidence of obesity increases with age is that
   a. the basal metabolic rate decreases with age.
   b. physical activity often decreases with age.
   c. energy intake exceeds energy expenditure.
   d. any of these can occur.

2. Congregate meal programs provide
   a. 100% of nutrient needs.
   b. a social atmosphere for eating.
   c. food stamps.
   d. all of these.

3. Among the older population of the United States, the age of the fastest growing segment is _____ years.
   a. 65
   b. 74
   c. 79
   d. 85+

4. Which of the following accurately portrays a theory about the causes of aging?
   a. Increases in testosterone and estrogen affect cell processes.
   b. Blood sugar decreases, failing to supply adequate energy to brain cells.

   c. Inadequate calorie intake speeds body breakdown.
   d. Excess free radicals damage cell components.

5. The immune system becomes less efficient with age, so it is especially important to consume adequate _____ and _____, nutrients that contribute to immune function.
   a. vitamin A, potassium
   b. protein, zinc
   c. zinc, iodide
   d. vitamin A, vitamin K

6. Which of the following is a useful strategy to prevent or delay the onset of Alzheimer's disease?
   a. Avoid stressing the brain with challenging mental tasks.
   b. Limit intake of dairy products.
   c. Consume adequate B vitamins, such as folate, B-6, and B-12.
   d. Increase the ratio of omega-6 to omega-3 fatty acids in the diet.

7. To maintain optimal nutritional status and healthy weight, the diet of an older person should have a _____ nutrient density and be _____ in energy content.
   a. low, high
   b. low, low
   c. high, moderate
   d. high, high

8. Donald has been diagnosed with cirrhosis. To cope with his impaired liver function, he will need to
   a. take high doses of vitamin and mineral supplements.
   b. minimize alcohol intake.
   c. limit his intake of dietary fiber.
   d. do all of these.

9. Alcohol is digested in the
   a. stomach.
   b. small intestine.
   c. liver.
   d. None of these is correct, because alcohol requires no digestion.

10. Alcohol is most damaging to the
    a. brain cells, because alcohol can be used as an energy source even before glucose.
    b. kidney cells, because this is where alcohol is excreted.
    c. cells of the gastrointestinal tract, because they are in direct contact with ingested alcohol.
    d. liver cells, because this is where alcohol is metabolized.

Answer Key: 1. d (LO 16.5), 2. b (LO 16.6), 3. d (LO 16.1), 4. d (LO 16.2), 5. b (LO 16.3), 6. c (LO 16.3), 7. c (LO 16.4), 8. b (LO 16.5), 9. d (LO 16.7), 10. d (LO 16.7)

Study Questions (Numbers refer to Learning Outcomes)

1. What is the difference between life span and life expectancy? **(LO 16.1)**

2. Describe two hypotheses proposed to explain the causes of aging, and note evidence for each in your daily life experiences. **(LO 16.2)**

3. List four organ systems that can decline in function in later years, along with an eating pattern lifestyle response to help cope with the decline. **(LO 16.3)**

4. Defend the recommendation for regular physical activity during older adulthood, including some resistance activity (weight training). **(LO 16.5)**

5. List four warning signs of undernutrition in older people that are part of the acronym DETERMINE. Briefly justify the inclusion of each. **(LO 16.2)**

6. List three important points made by the *Dietary Guidelines for Americans* for the general population, and give an example of why each one may be difficult for older adults to implement. What are some suggestions for overcoming these barriers? **(LO 16.4)**

7. How might the nutritional needs of older people differ from those of younger people? How are their needs similar? Be specific. **(LO 16.4)**

8. List three common herbal remedies. What are the possible benefits and risks of each one? If your grandmother were considering using any of these herbal remedies, what advice would you give her? **(LO 16.6)**

9. What three resources in a community are widely available to aid older adults in maintaining nutritional health? **(LO 16.6)**

10. List two benefits of moderate alcohol intake. List two risks of heavy drinking. Should a nondrinker take up drinking for the health benefits? **(LO 16.7)**

What the Dietitian Chose

As far as nutrient deficiencies go, vitamin B-12 deficiency is relatively common. About 6% of older adults are deficient in vitamin B-12, and many more likely have marginal B-12 status. Older adults are at particular risk of vitamin B-12 deficiency because stomach production of acid and intrinsic factor, which are required for vitamin B-12 absorption, tends to decline with age. In addition, certain medications can reduce acid production and thereby affect B-12 absorption.

As you learned earlier, foods of animal origin are the only natural sources of vitamin B-12. Although the leafy green vegetables would be an excellent source of folate—another B vitamin that is required for red blood cell health—they are not a good food source of vitamin B-12.

A 3-ounce serving of pot roast provides about 100% of the 2.4 micrograms of vitamin B-12 needed per day. However, recall that stomach acid is needed to cleave vitamin B-12 from protein in food sources. Even though beef is a rich source of vitamin B-12, with reduced stomach-acid secretion, not much

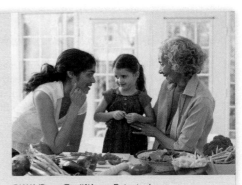

©LWA/Dann Tardif/Aage Fotostock

of the vitamin B-12 will be absorbed.

Synthetic vitamin B-12—the form found in dietary supplements and fortified foods—is actually better absorbed than the natural form of the vitamin. This is because synthetic vitamin B-12 does not have to be cleaved from food proteins before it can bind with intrinsic factor and be absorbed in the ileum of the small intestine. A fortified breakfast cereal, provides about 80% of the RDA for vitamin B-12, and because this vitamin B-12 is not protein bound, it is efficiently absorbed. Thus, the fortified cereal would be a good way to boost vitamin B-12 status.

A dietary supplement formulated for older adults, such as Centrum® Silver® Adults 50+, provides 25 micrograms of efficiently absorbed, synthetic vitamin B-12. That's 10 times the RDA! Is it a problem to consume this megadose of vitamin B-12? Actually, no Upper Level has been set for vitamin B-12, and no toxicity has ever been reported. To correct your existing vitamin B-12 deficiency, the high dose of vitamin B-12 in this supplement would be most effective. After your nutrition status is back to normal, you could switch to a fortified food, such as breakfast cereal, to keep your red blood cells healthy with adequate B-12 and other micronutrients.

Further Readings

1. Fontana L and others: Promoting health and longevity through diet: From model organisms to humans. *Cell* 2015; 161:1.

2. Bernstein M and others: Position of the Academy of Nutrition and Dietetics: Food and nutrition for older adults: Promoting health and wellness. *J Acad Nutri Diet* 2012; 112:1255.

3. Thalheimer JC: Nutrition and healthy aging for men. *Today's Dietitian* 2015; 17(6):44.

4. Berner LA and others: Characterization of dietary protein among older adults in the United States: Amount, animal sources, and meal patterns. *J Acad Nutri Diet* 2013; 113:809.

5. Genaro P and others: Dietary protein intake in elderly women: Association with muscle and bone mass. *Nutr Clin Pract* 2015; 30:283.

6. Paddon-Jones D and others: Protein and healthy aging. *Am J Clin Nutr* 2015; 101:s1339.

7. Sebastian RS and others: Sandwiches are major contributors of sodium in the diets of American adults: Results from What We Eat in America, National Health and Nutrition Examination Survey 2009–2010. *J Acad Nutri Diet* 2015; 115:272.

8. Buch A and others: Muscle function and fat content in relation to sarcopenia, obesity and frailty of old age—an overview. *Exp Geront* 2016; 16(10).

9. Oliviero F and others: How the Mediterranean diet and some of its components modulate inflammatory pathways in arthritis. *Swiss Medical Weekly* 2015; 145:w14190.

10. Touger-Decker R and Mobley C: Position of the American Academy of Nutrition and Dietetics: Oral health and nutrition. *J Acad Nutri Diet* 2013; 113:693.

11. Scarlata K: Digestive wellness: The link between aging and digestive disorders. *Today's Dietitian* 2015; 17(7):12.

12. Broadhead GK and others: Dietary modification and supplementation for the treatment of age-related macular degeneration. *Nutr Res* 2015; 73:448.

13. Bunner AE and others: Nutrition intervention for migraine: A randomized crossover trial. *Journal of Headache and Pain* 2014; 15:69.

14. Dauncey MJ: Nutrition, the brain and cognitive decline: Insights from epigenetics. *Eur J Clin Nutri* 2014; 68:1179.

15. Marcason W: What are the components to the MIND diet? *J Acad Nutri Diet* 2015; 115:1744.

16. Aune D and others: Fruit and vegetable intake and the risk of cardiovascular disease, total cancer and all-cause mortality—a systematic review and dose-response meta-analysis of prospective studies. *Int J Epidemiol,* 2016.

17. National Institute on Alcohol Abuse and Alcoholism: Rethinking drinking: Alcohol and your health. December 2015. http://pubs.niaaa.nih.gov/publications/RethinkingDrinking/Rethinking_Drinking.pdf. (Accessed February 4, 2016).

connect To get the most out of your study, visit Connect where you will find NutritionCalc Plus, SmartBook®, and many other dynamic tools.

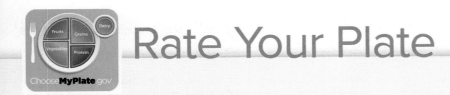
I. Am I Aging Healthfully?

Take Control of Your Aging by Dr. William B. Malarkey (Wooster Book Co., Wooster, OH, 1999) includes a plan that incorporates various diet and lifestyle factors associated with successful aging. Indicate the degree to which you are following such a plan (or alternatively, fill this out with a parent or another older relative in mind).

Physical: Do you eat a well-balanced diet, exercise on a regular basis, remain free of illness, abstain from smoking, refrain from drinking alcohol excessively, and experience refreshing sleep?

_____

_____

Intellectual: Are you analytical, do you read regularly, do you learn new things each day, do you engage your mental ability, and do you often reflect on your life?

_____

_____

_____

Emotional: Are you at peace, do you like who you are, are you optimistic, and do you laugh and relax regularly?

_____

_____

_____

Relational: Are you a good listener, do you feel supported by friends, do you attend social functions, do you talk with family members often, and do you feel close to others?

_____

_____

_____

Spiritual: Do you appreciate nature, give to or serve others, meditate or seek religious worship, and feel life has meaning?

_____

_____

_____

The more of these factors that you include in your life, the more well rounded your plan is for maintaining overall health. Any one of the five areas in which you are not achieving success should show you characteristics to work on in the future.

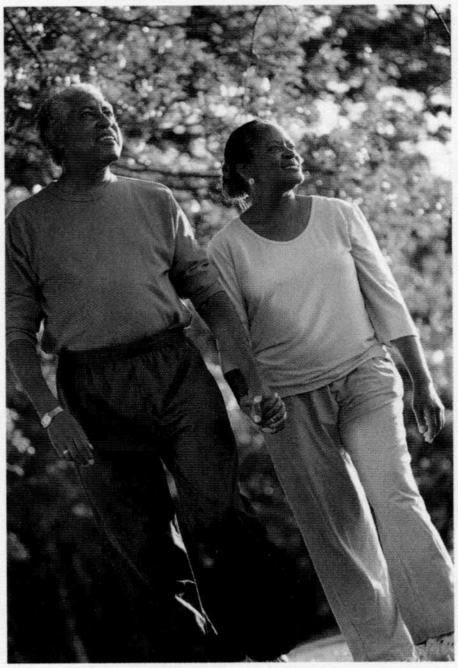

©Royalty-Free/CORBIS

II. Helping Older Adults Eat Better

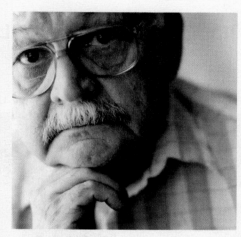

©Mel Curtis/Getty Images

During their lifetimes, most people usually eat meals with families or loved ones. As people reach older adulthood, many of them are faced with living and eating alone. In a study of the diets of 4400 older adults in the United States, one man in every five living alone and over age 55 ate poorly. One of four women between the ages of 55 and 64 years followed a low-quality diet. These poor dietary patterns can contribute to deteriorating mental and physical health. Consider the following example of the living situation of an older adult.

Neal, a 70-year-old man, lives alone in his home in a local suburb. His wife died 1 year ago. He does not have many friends; his wife was his primary confidante. His neighbors across the street and next door are friendly, and Neal used to help them with yard projects in his spare time. Neal's health has been good, but he has had trouble with his teeth recently. His diet has been inadequate, and in the past 3 months, his physical and mental vigor has deteriorated. He has been slowly lapsing into a depression, so he keeps the shades drawn and rarely leaves his house. Neal keeps very little food in the house because his wife did most of the cooking and shopping, and he just is not that interested in food.

If you were one of Neal's relatives and learned of Neal's situation, what six things could you do or suggest to help improve his nutritional status and mental outlook? Look back into this chapter to get some ideas.

1. _____
2. _____
3. _____
4. _____
5. _____
6. _____

Appendix A

Daily Values Used on Food Labels

TABLE A-1 ■ Daily Values Used on Food Labels in the United States, with a Comparison to the Latest RDAs and Other Nutrient Standards*

Dietary Constituent	Unit of Measure	Current Daily Values for People Over 4 Years of Age	RDA or Other Current Dietary Standard	
			Males 19–30 Years Old	Females 19–30 Years Old
Total fat[†]	g	78	—	—
Saturated fatty acids[†]	g	< 20	—	—
Protein[†]	g	50	56	46
Cholesterol[§]	mg	< 300	—	—
Carbohydrate[†]	g	275	130	130
Added Sugars	g	50	—	—
Dietary fiber	g	28	38	25
Vitamin A	mcg Retinol Activity Equivalents (RAE)	900	900	700
Vitamin D	mcg	20	15	15
Vitamin E	mg alpha tocopherol	15	15	15
Vitamin K	mcg	120	120	90
Vitamin C	mg	90	90	75
Folate	mcg Dietary Folate Equivalents (DFE)	400	400	400
Thiamin	mg	1.5	1.2	1.1
Riboflavin	mg	1.7	1.3	1.1
Niacin	mg	20	16	14
Vitamin B-6	mg	2	1.3	1.3
Vitamin B-12	mcg	6	2.4	2.4
Biotin	mcg	300	30	30
Pantothenic acid	mg	10	5	5
Calcium	mg	1300	1000	1000
Phosphorus	mg	1250	700	700
Iodine	mcg	150	150	150
Iron	mg	18	8	18
Magnesium	mg	420	400	310
Copper	mg	2	0.9	0.9
Zinc	mg	15	11	8
Sodium[‡]	mg	< 2300	1500	1500
Potassium[‡]	mg	4700	4700	4700
Chloride[‡]	mg	3400	2300	2300
Manganese	mg	2.3	2.3	1.8
Selenium	mcg	70	55	55
Chromium	mcg	120	35	25
Molybdenum	mcg	75	45	45

* Daily Values are generally set at the highest nutrient recommendation in a specific age and gender category. Some changes were made recently to the Daily Values and their units as part of the new Nutrition Facts Label. Most changes occurred because of the dietary related diseases that are common in the United States and to more closely match the RDA or AI values for the nutrient.

† These Daily Values are based on a 2000-kcal diet, instead of RDAs, with a caloric distribution of 30% from fat (and one-third of this total from saturated fat), 60% from carbohydrate, and 10% from protein.

§ Based on recommendations of U.S. federal agencies.

‡ The considerably higher Daily Values for sodium and chloride are there to allow for more diet flexibility, but the extra amounts are not needed to maintain health.

Appendix B

Diabetes Menu-Planning Tools

Lists, Choices, and Exchanges: Making Sense of Meal Planning for Diabetes

Registered dietitian nutritionists and other diabetes educators work closely with their patients to help them understand how the foods they eat directly impact their day-to-day quality of life. **Food lists** (also known as *exchange lists*) are one way diabetes educators can help people to plan their dietary patterns to better manage their blood sugar. The first exchange lists for people with diabetes were developed by the American Dietetic Association (now the Academy of Nutrition and Dietetics), American Diabetes Association, and U.S. Public Health Service over 50 years ago. Since then, they have been revised to reflect advances in nutrition recommendations and the ever-expanding variety of foods in the marketplace. The most recent version, *Choose Your Foods: Food Lists for Diabetes,* was published in 2014.

Food lists organize the many details of the nutrient composition of foods into a manageable framework based on calorie and macronutrient content. In the *Food Lists for Diabetes,* individual foods are placed into three broad groups: carbohydrates, proteins, and fats. Within these groups are lists that contain foods of similar macronutrient composition: various types of milk and milk substitutes, fruits, vegetables, starches, other carbohydrates, proteins, and fats. There are even lists that show how to account for alcohol, combination foods (e.g., casseroles), and a wide variety of fast foods. These lists are designed so that when the given serving size is observed, each food on a list provides roughly the same amount of carbohydrate, protein, fat, and kilocalories. The patient and a registered dietitian nutritionist first tailor a healthy eating pattern to meet the client's energy and specific macronutrient needs. Then, the client can select **choices** (i.e., *exchanges*) from each of the various lists that fit into the plan without having to look up or memorize the nutrient values of numerous foods.

Table B-1 summarizes the basic nutrient composition of foods in each food list. The serving sizes of individual foods in a list may vary, but general estimates are given. The protein and milk and milk substitutes lists are divided into subclasses, which vary in fat content and, thus, in the amount of kilocalories they provide. You can see that each food list is unique in the kilocalories and macronutrients it supplies. A healthy meal plan should include foods from each of the lists to ensure nutrient adequacy. Study Table B-1 to become familiar with the food groupings, the approximate size of choices on each food list, and the amounts of carbohydrate, protein, fat, and kilocalories per choice.

Because the *Food Lists for Diabetes* offer a quick way to estimate the calorie, carbohydrate, protein, and fat content in any food or meal, they are a valuable menu-planning tool for individuals without diabetes, as well. In fact, the Academy of Nutrition and Dietetics and the American Diabetes Association have published a related guide, *Choose Your Foods: Food Lists for Weight Management.*

Recognize that the *Food Lists for Diabetes* group foods somewhat differently than MyPlate. For the *Food Lists,* we care more about nutrient composition and the food's eventual physiological effect on blood sugar than its plant or animal origin. For example, the starch list includes not only bread, dry cereal, cooked cereal, rice, and pasta but also baked beans, corn on the cob, and potatoes. Although potatoes and corn are vegetables, their macronutrient composition resembles that of bread more than that of broccoli. In addition, many foods that would traditionally be categorized as dairy products do not appear with the milk and milk substitutes list. Instead, cheeses are grouped as proteins, whereas cream and cream cheese show up on the fats lists.

food lists A system for classifying foods into numerous lists based on the foods' macronutrient composition, and establishing serving sizes, so that one serving of each food on a list contains the same amount of carbohydrate, protein, fat, and calorie content; also called *exchange lists.*

choice The serving size of a food on a specific exchange list; formerly called *exchange.*

TABLE B-1 ■ Approximate Nutrient Composition of Food Choices from *Choose Your Foods: Food Lists for Diabetes, 2014*

Groups/Lists	Household Measures*	Carbohydrate (g)	Protein (g)	Fat (g)	Energy (kcal)
Carbohydrates					
Starch (e.g., bread, cereal, pasta, rice, crackers, and beans)	1 slice, ¾ cup raw, or ½ cup cooked	15	3	1 or less†	80
Fruits	1 small/medium piece	15	—	—	60
Milk and milk substitutes	1 cup				
Fat-free, low-fat		12	8	0–3†	100
Reduced-fat		12	8	5	120
Whole		12	8	8	160
Nonstarchy vegetables	1 cup raw or ½ cup cooked	5	2	—	25
Sweets, desserts, and other carbohydrates	Varies	15	Varies	Varies	Varies
Proteins	1 ounce				
Lean		—	7	2	45
Medium fat		—	7	5	75
High fat		—	7	8	100
Plant-based		Varies	7	Varies	Varies
Fats	1 teaspoon	—	—	5	45
Alcohol	Varies	Varies	—	—	100

*An estimate; see food lists for actual amounts.

†Calculated as 1 gram for purposes of calorie contribution.

Source: *Choose Your Foods: Food Lists for Diabetes*, 2014 which is the basis of a meal planning system designed by a committee of the American Diabetes Association and the Academy of Nutrition and Dietetics.

In some instances, a food counts for more than one choice at a time. In the category of sweets, desserts, and other carbohydrates, you will find a variety of snack items and condiments that count as carbohydrates and fats. The food lists also provide the user with some guidance on accounting for a wide variety of combination foods, such as pizza, casseroles, and soups. A list of free foods includes choices such as reduced-fat or fat-free foods, condiments, seasonings, and sugar-free drinks that, when consumed in moderation, have little or no impact on energy intake and blood sugar.

USING THE *FOOD LISTS* TO DEVELOP DAILY MENUS

Now let us use the *Food Lists* to plan a 1-day menu. Our kilocalorie target will be 2000 kcal, with 55% derived from carbohydrates (1100 kcal), 15% from protein (300 kcal), and 30% from fat (600 kcal). This can be achieved with 2 reduced-fat milk choices, 3 non-starchy vegetable choices, 5 fruit choices, 11 starch choices, 4 lean protein choices, and 6 fat choices (Table B-2). This is just one of many possible combinations; the *Food Lists* offer great flexibility. For example, more protein choices could be included if less milk were used.

Table B-3 arbitrarily distributes these choices into breakfast, lunch, dinner, and a snack. Breakfast includes 1 reduced-fat milk choice, 2 fruit choices, 2 starch choices, and 1 fat choice. Drawing from the food lists, this plan could be achieved with ¾ cup of a ready-to-eat breakfast cereal, 1 cup of reduced-fat milk, 1 slice of bread with 1 teaspoon margarine, and 1 cup of orange juice.

TABLE B-2 ■ Possible Food Choice Patterns That Yield 55% of Calories as Carbohydrate, 30% as Fat, and 15% as Protein

Food List	1200*	1600*	2000	2400	2800	3200	3600
Milk (reduced-fat)	2	2	2	2	2	2	2
Nonstarchy vegetable	3	3	3	4	4	4	4
Fruit	3	4	5	6	8	9	9
Starch	5	8	11	13	15	18	21
Protein (lean)	4	4	4	5	6	7	8
Fat	2	4	6	8	10	11	13

*Calorie intakes of 1200 and 1600 kcal contain 20% of calories as protein and 50% of calories as carbohydrate to allow for greater flexibility in diet planning.

TABLE B-3 ■ **Sample 1-Day 2000-kcal Menu Based on the Food Lists for Diabetes Plan***

Breakfast
1 reduced-fat milk choice	1 cup reduced-fat milk (some on cereal)
2 fruit choices	1 cup orange juice
2 starch choices	¾ cup ready-to-eat breakfast cereal and 1 piece whole wheat toast
1 fat choice	1 teaspoon soft margarine on toast

Lunch
4 starch choices	2 slices whole wheat bread and 6 graham crackers (2½ inches by 2½ inches)
2 fat choices	1 slice bacon, 1 teaspoon mayonnaise
1 nonstarchy vegetable choice	1 sliced tomato
2 fruit choices	1 banana (9 inches)
1 reduced-fat milk choice	1 cup reduced-fat milk

Snack
1 starch choice	¾ ounce pretzels

Dinner
4 lean protein choices	4 ounces lean steak (well trimmed)
2 starch choices	1 medium baked potato
1 fat choice	1 teaspoon soft margarine
2 nonstarchy vegetable choices	1 cup cooked broccoli
1 fruit choice	1 kiwi fruit
	Coffee (if desired)

Snack
2 starch choices	½ large bagel
2 fat choices	2 tablespoons regular cream cheese

*The target plan was a 2000-kcal intake, with 55% of calories from carbohydrate, 15% from protein, and 30% from fat. Computer analysis indicates that this menu yielded 2040 kcal, with 53% of calories from carbohydrate, 16% from protein, and 31% from fat—in close agreement with the targeted goals.

This 1-day menu is only one of endless possibilities with the *Food Lists for Diabetes*. Apple juice could replace the orange juice; two apples could be exchanged for the banana. For simplicity, we have used a variety of individual foods to achieve the total number of choices for this healthy eating plan. However, the *Food Lists* also include some commonly used combination foods. For instance, a 1-cup serving of lasagna typically provides 2 medium-fat meat choices plus 2 carbohydrate choices. With practice, you will be able to estimate the choices from complex foods on your own (Fig. B-1). For now, using individual foods makes learning the *Food Lists* much easier. Finally, you might want to prove to yourself that the food choices listed in Table B-3 really fulfill the plan set forth in Table B-2.

Food List	Total Food Choices to Be Consumed Daily	Food Choices Consumed at Each Meal			
		Breakfast	Lunch	Dinner	Snacks
Milk and milk substitutes					
Nonstarchy vegetables					
Fruits					
Starch					
Proteins					
Fats					

FIGURE B-1 ◄ Record the *Food Lists for Diabetes* pattern you have chosen in the left-hand column. Then distribute the food choices throughout the day, noting the food to be used and the serving size.

Examples of Food Choices from
Food Lists for Diabetes

In this section, you will find just a few examples of the many food choices that are included in the most recent edition of *Choose Your Foods: Food Lists for Diabetes* from the American Diabetes Association. For complete information, you can order your own copy of the booklet at http://www.shopdiabetes.org.

Starches

Starches provide 15 grams of carbohydrate, 0 to 3 grams of protein, 0 to 1 gram of fat, and about 80 kcal per serving. Keep in mind that the serving sizes for starch choices on these food lists are usually smaller than those recommended by MyPlate. Also, some foods with high fat content may be counted as 1 starch plus 1 or 2 fats. Beans, peas, and lentils count as 1 starch plus 1 lean protein choice.

BREAD

Serving Size	Food
¼	Bagel, large (about 4 oz)
1 slice	Bread
½	English muffin
1	Pancake (4-inch diameter)
1	Tortilla, flour (6-inch diameter)
⅓	Tortilla, flour (10-inch diameter)
3¼-inch square	Naan
½	Hamburger bun

CEREALS

Serving Size	Food
½ cup	Cooked cereal (e.g., oatmeal)
¼ cup	Granola cereal
1½ cups	Puffed cereal (e.g., puffed rice)
½ cup	Sweetened cereal (e.g., Frosted Flakes)®
¾ cup	Unsweetened ready-to-eat cereal (e.g., Cheerios)®

GRAINS

Serving Size	Food
⅓ cup	Rice, cooked (e.g., white and brown)
⅓ cup	Pasta, cooked
½ cup	Wild rice, cooked
⅓ cup	Quinoa, cooked

STARCHY VEGETABLES

Serving Size	Food
½ cup	Corn
1 cup	Mixed vegetables (e.g., corn, peas, and carrots)
½ cup	Spaghetti sauce
¼ large	Potato, baked
½ cup	Potatoes, mashed
1 cup	Winter squash (e.g., acorn and butternut)
½ cup	Sweet potato

CRACKERS AND SNACKS

Serving Size	Food
8	Animal crackers
3 2½-inch squares	Graham crackers
6	Saltines
6	Butter crackers (e.g., Ritz®; count as 1 starch + 1 fat)
3 cups	Popcorn (no fat added)
¾ ounce	Pretzels
8	Baked snack chips
13	Tortilla or potato chips (count as 1 starch + 2 fats)

BEANS, PEAS, AND LENTILS
(count as 1 starch and 1 lean protein)

Serving Size	Food
⅓ cup	Baked beans
½ cup	Beans, cooked or canned (e.g., black, garbanzo, and kidney)
½ cup	Lentils, cooked
½ cup	Peas, cooked (e.g., black-eyed and split)

Fruits

One choice from the Fruits list provides 15 grams of carbohydrate, 0 grams of protein, 0 grams of fat, and 60 kcal. Typically, 1 fruit choice is equal to ½ cup of canned or frozen fruit, 1 small fresh fruit, ½ cup of unsweetened fruit juice, or 2 tablespoons of dried fruit. Recognize that the fruit you buy at the grocery store may amount to more than one fruit choice; a large banana, for example, counts for 2 fruit choices. The serving sizes of fruit juices and dried fruit are small because these are more concentrated sources of carbohydrates and energy.

FRUITS

Serving Size	Food	Serving Size	Food
1 small	Apple (about 4 oz)	½ cup	Kiwi, sliced
½ cup	Applesauce, unsweetened	1 medium	Orange
1 extra small	Banana (about 4 inches)	½ cup	Pineapple, canned
1 cup	Blackberries	3	Prunes
¾ cup	Blueberries	½ cup	Pomegranate seeds (arils)
12	Cherries	1 ¼ cup	Strawberries, whole
17	Grapes	1 ¼ cup	Watermelon, diced
1 cup	Honeydew melon, diced		

FRUIT JUICE

Serving Size	Food
½ cup	Apple juice or apple cider
⅓ cup	Grape juice
½ cup	Orange juice
⅓ cup	Prune juice

Milk and Milk Substitutes

Milk and milk substitutes are divided into subcategories based on their fat content. All milk and yogurt products provide 12 grams of carbohydrate and 8 grams of protein but may vary in fat content from 0 to 8 grams per choice. The subcategory of other milk foods and milk substitutes includes some products that may be used in place of milk in the diet (e.g., soy milk), but have a slightly different nutrient profile than traditional milk and yogurt products. Those foods, as indicated below, are counted as a combination of carbohydrate (15 grams of carbohydrate, 70 kcal) and fat (5 grams of fat, 45 kcal) choices. Please note that other products used as dairy alternatives (e.g., almond milk) are listed with fat choices.

FAT-FREE (SKIM) AND LOW-FAT MILK AND YOGURT
(12 grams of carbohydrate, 8 grams of protein, 0–3 grams of fat, and 100 kcal)

Serving Size	Food
1 cup	Fat-free (skim) milk, 1% milk, or buttermilk
½ cup	Canned, evaporated, fat-free milk
⅔ cup	Yogurt (fat-free plain or fat-free Greek, unsweetened or artificially sweetened)

REDUCED-FAT (2%) MILK AND YOGURT
(12 grams of carbohydrate, 8 grams of protein, 5 grams of fat, and 120 kcal)

Serving Size	Food
1 cup	2% milk, acidophilus milk, or kefir
⅔ cup	Yogurt (reduced-fat, plain)

WHOLE MILK AND YOGURT
(12 grams of carbohydrate, 8 grams of protein, 8 grams of fat, and 160 kcal)

Serving Size	Food
1 cup	Whole milk, buttermilk, or goat's milk
½ cup	Evaporated whole milk
1 cup	Yogurt (whole milk, plain)

OTHER MILK FOODS AND MILK SUBSTITUTES

Serving Size	Food	Choices
⅓ cup	Eggnog (made from whole milk)	1 carbohydrate + 1 fat
1 cup	Rice drink, plain, fat-free	1 carbohydrate
1 cup	Rice drink, flavored, low-fat	2 carbohydrates
1 cup	Soy milk, plain, low-fat	½ carbohydrate + ½ fat
1 cup	Soy milk, regular, plain	½ carbohydrate + 1 fat
⅔ cup	Yogurt with fruit, low-fat	1 fat-free milk + 1 carbohydrate

Nonstarchy Vegetables

Nonstarchy vegetables still provide carbohydrates, but not as much as their starchy counterparts. One nonstarchy vegetable provides 5 grams of carbohydrate, 2 grams of protein, 0 grams of fat, and 25 kcal. Typically, a choice is equal to ½ cup of cooked vegetables or 1 cup of raw vegetables. Large servings of nonstarchy vegetables (i.e., three choices) should be counted as one carbohydrate choice (15 grams of carbohydrate, 70 kcal) rather than multiple nonstarchy vegetables. Because of their low carbohydrate content, salad greens (e.g., iceberg, romaine, and endive) actually count as free foods. To comply with advice from the Dietary Guidelines for Americans, it is important to select a variety of starchy and nonstarchy vegetables each day because each has a distinct micronutrient and phytochemical profile. Take extra care to select vegetables with deep colors, such as spinach, carrots, and beets.

Serving Size	Food
½ cup	Asparagus, cooked
1 cup	Sliced carrots, raw
½ cup	Beets, cooked
½ cup	Broccoli, cooked
½ cup	Collard greens, cooked
1 cup	Cucumber, raw slices
½ cup	Green beans, cooked
½ cup	Summer squash, cooked
½ cup	Tomatoes, stewed

Sweets, Desserts, and Other Carbohydrates

Foods on this list may not match the nutrient profiles of other starches, but they are commonly consumed and must be accounted for in diet planning. Sweetened beverages, desserts, and sweeteners and condiments that we add to foods can be counted as a combination of carbohydrate (15 grams of carbohydrates, 70 kcal) and fat (5 grams of fat, 45 kcal) choices.

BEVERAGES, SODA, AND SPORTS DRINKS

Serving Size	Food	Choices
½ cup	Cranberry juice cocktail	1 carbohydrate
1 cup	Fruit drink or lemonade	2 carbohydrates
1 can (12 oz)	Soft drink, regular	2 ½ carbohydrates
1 cup	Sports drink (e.g., Gatorade)®	1 carbohydrate

BROWNIES, CAKE, COOKIES, GELATIN, PIE, AND PUDDING

Serving Size	Food	Choices
1 ¼-inch square	Brownie, unfrosted	1 carbohydrate + 1 fat
¹⁄₁₂ cake	Angel food cake, unfrosted	2 carbohydrates
2-inch square	Cake, frosted	2 carbohydrates + 1 fat
2	Chocolate chip cookies	1 carbohydrate + 2 fats
5	Vanilla wafers	1 carbohydrate + 1 fat
½ cup	Gelatin, regular	1 carbohydrate
⅛ pie	Pumpkin pie	1 ½ carbohydrates + 1 ½ fats
½ cup	Pudding, regular, made with 2% milk	2 carbohydrates

CANDY, SPREADS, SWEETS, SWEETENERS, SYRUPS, AND TOPPINGS

Serving Size	Food	Choices
5	Chocolate kisses	1 carbohydrate + 1 fat
2 tbsp	Liquid nondairy coffee creamer	1 carbohydrate
1 tbsp	Honey	1 carbohydrate
1 tbsp	Jam or jelly, regular	1 carbohydrate
1 tbsp	Pancake syrup, regular	1 carbohydrate

CONDIMENTS AND SAUCES

Serving Size	Food	Choices
3 tbsp	Barbecue sauce	1 carbohydrate
½ cup	Gravy	½ carbohydrate + ½ fat
3 tbsp	Salad dressing, fat-free, cream-based	1 carbohydrate

DOUGHNUTS, MUFFINS, PASTRIES, AND SWEET BREADS

Serving Size	Food	Choices
1	Glazed doughnut	2 carbohydrates + 2 fats
1 (4 oz)	Muffin, regular	4 carbohydrates + 2 ½ fats
1 (2 ½ oz)	Danish	2 ½ carbohydrates + 2 fats

FROZEN BARS, FROZEN DESSERTS, FROZEN YOGURT, AND ICE CREAM

Serving Size	Food	Choices
1 (3 oz)	Frozen 100% fruit juice bar	1 carbohydrate
½ cup	Ice cream, no sugar added	1 carbohydrate + 1 fat
½ cup	Ice cream, regular	1 carbohydrate + 2 fats
½ cup	Sherbet	2 carbohydrates
½ cup	Greek frozen yogurt, low-fat	1 ½ carbohydrates

Protein

Similar to the choices on the Milk and Milk Substitutes list, protein choices vary in fat and kilocalorie content. Lean protein choices, such as egg whites and skinless poultry, provide 0 grams of carbohydrate, 7 grams of protein, 2 grams of fat, and 45 kcal. Medium-fat protein choices, such as whole eggs and poultry with skin, provide 0 grams of carbohydrate, 7 grams of protein, 5 grams of fat, and 75 kcal. High-fat protein choices, including many types of sausage and bacon, provide 0 grams of carbohydrate, 7 grams of protein, 8 grams of fat, and 100 kcal. Plant-based protein choices usually contain some carbohydrates, so they count as a combination of carbohydrate or starch and protein choices. Note that choices are very small; a typical hamburger would count as 3 or 4 protein choices.

LEAN PROTEIN (0 grams of carbohydrate, 7 grams of protein, 2 grams of fat, and 45 kcal)

Serving Size	Food
1 oz	Beef with 10% or lower fat (e.g., round and sirloin)
1 oz	Cheese with 3 grams of fat or less (e.g., fat-free mozzarella)
1 oz	Fish, not fried (e.g., catfish, cod, and tuna canned in water)
2	Egg whites
1 oz	Wild game (e.g., buffalo and venison)
1 oz	Lean pork (e.g., ham and tenderloin)
1 oz	Poultry, without skin
1 oz	Deli meats with 3 grams of fat or less per serving (e.g., turkey and ham)
1 oz	Shellfish (e.g., shrimp and crab)

MEDIUM-FAT PROTEIN (0 grams of carbohydrate, 7 grams of protein, 5 grams of fat, and 75 kcal)

Serving Size	Food
1 oz	Beef with 15% or lower fat (e.g., rib roast and ground beef)
1 oz	Cheese with 4 to 7 grams of fat per ounce (e.g., feta and mozzarella)
1	Egg
1 oz	Fish, fried
1 oz	Pork (e.g., cutlet and shoulder roast)
1 oz	Poultry, with skin

HIGH-FAT PROTEIN (0 grams of carbohydrate, 7 grams of protein, 8 grams of fat, and 100 kcal)

Serving Size	Food
2 slices	Bacon, pork
1 oz	Cheese (e.g., American, Cheddar, Parmesan, and Swiss)
1	Hot dog
1 oz	Deli meats with 8 grams of fat or more per serving (e.g., bologna and salami)
1 oz	Sausage (e.g., bratwurst and summer sausage)

PLANT-BASED PROTEIN

Serving Size	Food	Choices
⅓ cup	Baked beans	1 starch + 1 lean protein
½ cup	Beans, cooked or canned (e.g., black, kidney, and pinto)	1 starch + 1 lean protein
½ cup	Edamame, shelled	½ carbohydrate + 1 lean protein
⅓ cup	Hummus	1 carbohydrate + 1 medium-fat protein
3 oz	Meatless burger, soy-based	½ carbohydrate + 2 lean proteins
½ cup	Tofu	1 medium-fat protein

Fats

One fat choice is 5 grams of fat and 45 kcal. Fats are subdivided into unsaturated fats, which come mainly from plant sources, and saturated fats, which come mainly from animal sources. In line with recommendations from other major health authorities, the *Food Lists for Diabetes* advises people to choose unsaturated fats in place of saturated fats and to avoid *trans* fats.

UNSATURATED FATS—MONOUNSATURATED FATS (5 grams of fat and 45 kcal)

Serving Size	Food
1 cup	Almond milk, unsweetened
2 tbsp	Avocado
1½ tsp	Nut butter (e.g., almond and peanut)
6	Almonds
10	Peanuts
16	Pistachios
1 tsp	Oil (e.g., canola and olive)

UNSATURATED FATS—POLYUNSATURATED FATS (5 grams of fat and 45 kcal)

Serving Size	Food	Serving Size	Food
1 tbsp	Low-fat vegetable oil spread	1 tsp	Oil (e.g., corn, safflower, and sunflower)
1 tsp	Margarine	2 tbsp	Salad dressing, reduced-fat (may contain carbohydrate)
1 tbsp	Low-fat mayonnaise	1 tbsp	Salad dressing, regular
1 tsp	Mayonnaise	1 tbsp	Flaxseed, ground

SATURATED FATS (5 grams of fat and 45 kcal)

Serving Size	Food
1 slice	Bacon
1 tbsp	Butter, reduced-fat

Serving Size	Food
1 tsp	Butter, regular
2 tbsp	Coconut, shredded

Free Foods

A *free food* is any food or drink that contains less than 20 kcal or less than 5 grams of carbohydrate per serving. When eaten in small amounts throughout the day, these foods have little impact on blood sugar. Foods with a serving size listed should be limited to 3 servings per day. Foods listed without a serving size (indicated with a)* can be eaten as often as you like. However, many free foods are high in sodium, so moderation is important.

LOW-CARBOHYDRATE FOODS

Serving Size	Food
1 piece	Candy, hard or sugar-free
2 tsp	Jam or jelly, light or no-sugar-added type
*	Gelatin, sugar-free
*	Salad greens (no dressing)

Serving Size	Food
*	Sugar substitutes
½ cup	Raw nonstarchy vegetables (e.g., broccoli, carrots, cucumber, and tomato)
¼ cup	Cooked nonstarchy vegetables (e.g., carrots, cauliflower, and green beans)

REDUCED-FAT OR FAT-FREE FOODS

Serving Size	Food
1 tbsp	Cream cheese, fat-free
4 tsp	Coffee creamer, liquid, sugar-free, flavored
1 tsp	Margarine spread, reduced-fat

Serving Size	Food
1 tbsp	Mayonnaise, fat-free
1 tbsp	Salad dressing, fat-free
2 tbsp	Whipped topping, light or fat-free

CONDIMENTS

Serving Size	Food
2 tsp	Barbecue sauce
1 tbsp	Ketchup
*	Hot pepper sauce
*	Mustard (e.g., brown, Dijon, or yellow)

Serving Size	Food
1 tbsp	Parmesan cheese, grated
1 ½	Dill pickles (medium)
1 tbsp	Soy sauce

DRINKS/MIXES

Serving Size	Food
*	Bouillon or broth
*	Club soda
*	Diet soft drinks, sugar-free

Serving Size	Food
*	Coffee, unsweetened or artificially sweetened
*	Water
*	Water, flavored, sugar-free

SEASONINGS

Serving Size	Food
*	Garlic, fresh or powder
*	Herbs, fresh or dried
*	Spices

Combination Foods

These foods contain a mixture of ingredients and cannot be grouped into one food list. Many of these foods are high in sodium.

ENTREES

Serving Size	Food	Choices
1 cup (8 oz)	Casserole-type entrees (e.g., tuna noodle, lasagna, and spaghetti with meatballs)	2 carbohydrates + 2 medium-fat proteins
1 cup (8 oz)	Stews (meat and vegetables)	1 carbohydrate + 1 medium-fat protein + 0 to 3 fats

FROZEN MEALS/ENTREES

Serving Size	Food	Choices
1 (5 oz)	Burrito (beef and bean)	3 carbohydrates + 1 lean protein + 2 fats
9–12 oz	Dinner-type healthy meal (fewer than 400 kcal)	2 to 3 carbohydrates + 1 to 2 lean proteins + 1 fat
¼ of a 12-inch	Pizza with thin crust and meat toppings	2 carbohydrates + 2 medium-fat proteins + 1½ fats
1 (4½ oz)	Pocket sandwich	3 carbohydrates + 1 lean protein + 1 to 2 fats

SALADS (DELI-STYLE)

Serving Size	Food	Choices
½ cup	Coleslaw	1 carbohydrate + 1½ fats
½ cup	Macaroni salad	2 carbohydrates + 3 fats
½ cup (3½ oz)	Tuna salad or chicken salad	½ carbohydrate + 2 lean proteins + 1 fat

SOUPS

Serving Size	Food	Choices
1 cup (8 oz)	Bean, lentil, or split pea soup	1½ carbohydrates + 1 lean protein
1 cup (8 oz)	Chowder (made with milk)	1 carbohydrate + 1 lean protein + 1½ fats
1 cup (8 oz)	Ramen noodle soup	2 carbohydrates + 2 fats
1 cup (8 oz)	Tomato soup (made with water)	1 carbohydrate
1 cup (8 oz)	Broth-based soups with vegetables and meat	1 carbohydrate + 1 lean protein

Fast Foods

Fast foods are high in sodium and fat. These should be consumed in moderation, if at all. It is much easier to control carbohydrate, fat, sodium, and kilocalorie intake when you prepare your own foods at home rather than relying on restaurants.

MAIN DISHES/ENTREES

Serving Size	Food	Choices
1 (7 oz)	Chicken breast, breaded and fried	1 carbohydrate + 6 medium-fat proteins
6	Chicken nuggets or tenders	1 carbohydrate + 2 medium-fat proteins + 1 fat
1 (2 oz)	Chicken wing, breaded and fried	½ carbohydrate + 2 medium-fat proteins
⅛ of 14-inch	Pizza, thick crust with or without meat toppings	2½ carbohydrates + 1 high-fat protein + 1 fat

ASIAN

Serving Size	Food	Choices
1 cup (6 oz)	Meat with vegetables in sauce	1 carbohydrate + 2 lean proteins + 1 fat
1 (3 oz)	Egg roll with meat filling	1½ carbohydrates + 1 lean protein + 1½ fats
1 cup	Fried rice, meatless	2½ carbohydrates + 2 fats
1 cup	Lo mein or chow mein	2 carbohydrates + 2 fats

MEXICAN

Serving Size	Food	Choices
1 (6 oz)	Burrito with beans and cheese	3½ carbohydrates + 1 medium-fat protein + 1 fat
8	Nachos with cheese	2½ carbohydrates + 1 high-fat protein + 2 fats
1 (3 oz)	Crisp taco with meat and cheese	1 carbohydrate + 1 medium-fat protein + ½ fat
1 lb	Taco salad with chicken and tortilla bowl	3½ carbohydrates + 4 medium-fat proteins + 3 fats

SANDWICHES

Serving Size	Food	Choices
1 (4 oz)	Breakfast burrito with sausage, egg, and cheese	1½ carbohydrates + 2 high-fat proteins
1 (7 oz)	Grilled chicken sandwich	3 carbohydrates + 4 lean proteins
1 (5 oz)	Fried fish fillet sandwich with cheese and tartar sauce	2½ carbohydrates + 2 medium-fat proteins + 1½ fats
1 (8 oz)	Cheeseburger (4 oz) with condiments	3 carbohydrates + 4 medium-fat proteins + 2½ fats
1 6-inch	Submarine sandwich (no cheese or sauce)	3 carbohydrates + 2 lean proteins + 1 fat

SIDES/APPETIZERS

Serving Size	Food	Choices
1 medium (5 oz)	French fries	3½ carbohydrates + 3 fats
8 (5 oz)	Onion rings	3½ carbohydrates + 4 fats
1 small	Side salad (no cheese, croutons, or dressing)	1 nonstarchy vegetable

BEVERAGES AND DESSERTS

Serving Size	Food	Choices
12 fl oz	Coffee, latte, with fat-free milk	1 fat-free milk
16 fl oz	Milk shake	7 carbohydrates + 4 fats
1 small	Ice cream cone	2 carbohydrates + ½ fat

Alcohol

For people with diabetes, up to 1 or 2 drinks per day for women and men, respectively, can safely fit into a healthy eating plan. Alcohol itself does not raise blood glucose, but alcoholic drinks often contain carbohydrates that must be counted. One alcohol equivalent provides 100 kcal. One carbohydrate choice provides 15 grams of carbohydrate and 70 kcal. Alcohol should be consumed with a meal to lower the risk of hypoglycemia.

Serving Size	Drink	Choices
12 fl oz	Beer, regular	1 alcohol equivalent + 1 carbohydrate
1½ fl oz	Distilled spirits (e.g., rum and vodka)	1 alcohol equivalent
5 fl oz	Champagne	1 alcohol equivalent
3½ fl oz	Dessert wine	1 alcohol equivalent + 1 carbohydrate

Appendix C
Dietary Assessment

Although it may seem overwhelming at first, it is easy to track the foods you eat. One tip is to record all foods and beverages as soon as possible after consumption.

I. **Fill in the food record form that follows.** Appendix C contains a blank copy, Table C-2 (see the completed example in Table C-1). Your instructor may ask you to record 1 day or several days. To get a good estimate of your usual nutrient intake, it is best to record several days (e.g., 2 weekdays and 1 weekend day). As you record your intake for use on the nutrient analysis form that follows, consider the following tips:
- Measure and record the amounts of foods eaten in portion sizes of cups, teaspoons, tablespoons, ounces, slices, or inches (or convert metric units to these units).
- Record brand names of all food products, such as "Quick Quaker Oats."®
- Measure and record all those little extras, such as gravies, salad dressings, taco sauces, pickles, jelly, sugar, ketchup, and butter.
- For beverages:
  - List the type of milk, such as whole, fat-free, 1%, evaporated, chocolate, or reconstituted dry.
  - Indicate whether fruit juice is fresh, frozen, or canned.
  - Indicate type for other beverages, such as fruit drink, fruit-flavored drink, Kool-Aid,® and hot chocolate made with water or milk.
- For fruits:
  - Indicate whether fresh, frozen, dried, or canned.
  - If whole, record number eaten and size with approximate measurements (such as 1 apple—3 inches in diameter).
  - Indicate whether processed in water, light syrup, or heavy syrup.
- For vegetables:
  - Indicate whether fresh, frozen, dried, or canned.
  - Record as portion of cup, teaspoon, or tablespoon, or as pieces (such as carrot sticks—4 inches long, ½ inch thick).
  - Record preparation method.
- For cereals:
  - Record cooked cereals in portions of tablespoon or cup (a level measurement after cooking).
  - Record dry cereal in level portions of tablespoon or cup.
  - If butter, milk, sugar, fruit, or something else is added, measure and record amount and type.
- For breads:
  - Indicate whether whole wheat, rye, white, and so on.
  - Measure and record number and size of portion (biscuit—2 inches across, 1-inch thick; slice of homemade rye bread—3 inches by 4 inches, ¼-inch thick).
  - Sandwiches: list all ingredients (lettuce, mayonnaise, tomato, and so on).
- For meat, fish, poultry, and cheese:
  - Give size (length, width, and thickness) in inches or weight in ounces after cooking for meat, fish, and poultry (such as cooked hamburger patty— 3 inches across, ½-inch thick).
  - Record measurements only for the cooked, edible part—without bone or fat left on the plate.
  - Describe how meat, poultry, or fish was prepared.
  - Give size (length, width, and thickness) in inches or weight in ounces for cheese.

- For eggs:
  - Record as soft or hard-cooked, fried, scrambled, poached, or omelet.
  - If milk, butter, or drippings are used, specify types and amount.
- For desserts:
  - List commercial brand or "homemade" or "bakery" under brand.
  - Purchased candies, cookies, and cakes: specify kind and size.
  - Measure and record portion size of cakes, pies, and cookies by specifying thickness, diameter, and width or length, depending on the item.

TABLE C-1 ■ Example of a 1-Day Food Record

Time	Minutes Spent Eating	M or S*	H† (0–3)	Activity While Eating	Place of Eating	Food and Quantity	Others Present	Reason for Choice
7:10 A.M.	15	M	2	Standing, fixing lunch	Kitchen	Orange juice, 1 cup	—	Health
						Crispix cereal, 1 cup		Habit
						Nonfat milk, ½ cup		Health
						Sugar, 2 tsp		Taste
						Black coffee, 1 cup		Habit
10:00 A.M.	4	S	1	Sitting, taking notes	Classroom	Diet cola, 12 oz	Class	Weight control
12:15 P.M.	40	M	2	Sitting, talking	Student union	Chicken sandwich with lettuce and mayonnaise (3 oz chicken, 2 slices of whole wheat bread, and 2 tsp mayonnaise)	Friends	Taste
						Pear, 1 medium		Health
						Nonfat milk, 1 cup		Health
2:30 P.M.	10	S	1	Sitting, studying	Library	Regular cola, 12 oz	Friend	Hunger
6:30 P.M.	35	M	3	Sitting, talking	Kitchen	Pork chop, broiled, 1	Boyfriend	Convenience
						Baked potato, 1		Health
						Butter, 2 tbsp		Taste
						Lettuce and tomato salad, 1 cup		Health
						Ranch dressing, 2 tbsp		Taste
						Peas, steamed, ½ cup		Health
						Whole milk, 1 cup		Habit
						Cherry pie, 1 piece		Taste
						Iced tea, 12 oz		Health
9:10 P.M.	10	S	2	Sitting, studying	Living room	Apple, 1 medium	—	Weight control
						Water, 1 cup		Weight control

*M or S: Meal or snack.

†H: Degree of hunger (0 none; 3 maximum).

TABLE C-2 ■ 1-Day Food Record

Time	Minutes Spent Eating	M or S*	H† (0–3)	Activity While Eating	Place of Eating	Food and Quantity	Others Present	Reason for Choice

*M or S: Meal or snack.

†H: Degree of hunger (0 none; 3 maximum).

II. **Enter all the foods and beverages you consumed into NutritionCalc Plus** (see Fig. C-1). As you get started, you will find many useful tutorial videos on the NutritionCalc Plus site. If you have not already done so, you will need to create a profile in NutritionCalc Plus. For each food or drink, select the meal or snack and the appropriate serving size. If you have data for more than 1 day, be sure to enter your foods and beverages on separate days. If the NutritionCalc Plus database does not contain the exact food or drink you consumed, you may need to enter a reasonably close substitute. For example, the chicken sandwich from the student union in the food record example in Table C-1 was entered as a Subway® 6" chicken sandwich on white bread.

FIGURE C-1 ▶ Entering food and beverage intake data using NutritionCalc Plus.

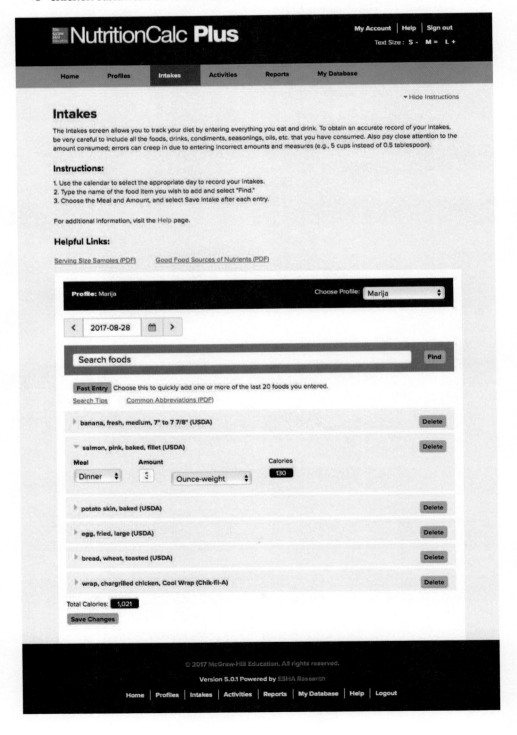

III. **Use NutritionCalc Plus to generate a report of your nutrient intake** (see Fig. C-2). After you have finished entering all the foods and beverages you consumed, save your intake data and click on the **Reports** tab. Select **Bar Graph** to see a report of your nutrient intake for a particular day or several days compared to your nutrient needs. Be sure to enter your student ID information (name, instructor, and course), choose the correct profile for comparison, then select the day(s) and meals(s) you would like to analyze. Then you may save your report as a PDF or Excel spreadsheet or e-mail it as an attachment to yourself or your instructor.

FIGURE C-2 ◄ Sample Bar Graph Report from NutritionCalc Plus.

Bar Graph Report

The Bar Graph Report displays graphically the amount of the nutrient consumed and compares that to the dietary intake recommendations.

Profile Info

Personal: Marija   Female   34 yrs   6 ft   170 lb

Day(s): 2017 Jun 29, Aug 28 (All)

Activity Level: Low Active   (Strive for an Active activity level.)

BMI: 23.1   Normal is 18.5 to 25.

Weight Change: Lose 2 lb per week   Best not to exceed 2 lbs per week.

Nutrient	Value	DRI Goal	Percent	0 50 100 150
Basic Components				
Calories	798.92	1,414.74	56 %	
Calories from Fat	228.45	396.13	58 %	
Calories from SatFat	69.52	127.33	55 %	
Protein (g)	53.86	61.69*	87 %	
Protein (% Calories)	26.97	17.44*	155 %	
Carbohydrates (g)	94.30	194.53	48 %	
Carbohydrates (% Calories)	47.22	55.00	86 %	
Total Sugars (g)	13.78 ^			
Dietary Fiber (g)	13.59	19.81	69 %	
Soluble Fiber (g)	0.42			
InSoluble Fiber (g)	1.83			
Fat (g)	25.38	44.01	58 %	
Fat (% Calories)	28.60	28.00	102 %	
Saturated Fat (g)	7.72	14.15	55 %	
Trans Fat (g)	0.43			
Mono Fat (g)	6.90	15.72	44 %	
Poly Fat (g)	4.27	14.15	30 %	
Cholesterol (mg)	409.86	300.00~	137 %	
Water (g)	851.72	2,700.00	32 %	
Vitamins				
Vitamin A - RAE (mcg)	374.88	700.00	54 %	
Vitamin B1 - Thiamin (mg)	0.50	1.10	46 %	
Vitamin B2 - Riboflavin (mg)	0.94	1.10	86 %	
Vitamin B3 - Niacin (mg)	10.32	14.00	74 %	
Vitamin B6 (mg)	1.18	1.30	91 %	
Vitamin B12 (mcg)	3.05	2.40	127 %	
Vitamin C (mg)	76.08	75.00	101 %	
Vitamin D - mcg (mcg)	8.02	15.00	53 %	
Vitamin E - a-Toco (mg)	2.04	15.00	14 %	
Folate (mcg)	234.45	400.00	59 %	
Minerals				
Calcium (mg)	406.46	1,000.00	41 %	
Iron (mg)	9.24	18.00	51 %	
Magnesium (mg)	125.29	320.00	39 %	
Phosphorus (mg)	610.36	700.00	87 %	
Potassium (mg)	1,359.51	4,700.00	29 %	
Sodium (mg)	977.30	2,300.00~	42 %	
Zinc (mg)	3.33	8.00	42 %	

IV. **Use NutritionCalc Plus to compare your dietary pattern to the dietary pattern recommended by the Dietary Guidelines for Americans** (see Fig. C-3). On the **Reports** tab, choose **MyPlate.** Enter your student information, choose the correct profile for comparison, and select the day(s) and meal(s) you would like to analyze. You may save your report, print it, or e-mail it as an attachment to yourself or your instructor.

FIGURE C-3 ▶ Sample MyPlate Report from NutritionCalc Plus.

MyPlate

The MyPlate report graphically compares the food list to the latest USDA Dietary Guidelines (see ChooseMyPlate.gov for more info).

Profile Info

Personal: Marija   Female   34 yrs   6 ft   170 lb

Day(s): 2017 Jun 29, Aug 28 (All)

Activity Level: Low Active   (Strive for an Active activity level.)

BMI: 23.1   Normal is 18.5 to 25.

Weight Change: Lose 2 lb per week   Best not to exceed 2 lbs per week.

Intake vs. Recommendation
1400 Calorie Pattern

Group	Percent Comparison	Amount *
Grains Intake	61 %	3.0 oz equivalent
Grains Recommendation		5.0 oz equivalent
Vegetables Intake	72 %	1.1 cup equivalent
Vegetables Recommendation		1.5 cup equivalent
Fruits Intake	26 %	0.4 cup equivalent
Fruits Recommendation		1.5 cup equivalent
Dairy Intake	36 %	0.7 cup equivalent
Dairy Recommendation		2.0 cup equivalent
Protein Foods Intake	146 %	5.8 oz equivalent
Protein Foods Recommendation		4.0 oz equivalent

Make Half Your Grains Whole

Aim for at least 2.5 oz equivalents whole grains a day

Oils & Empty Calories

Aim for 4.0 teaspoons of oils a day

Limit your extra fats & sugars to 171 Calories a day

Vary Your Vegetables

Dark Green Vegetables	1.5	cups weekly
Orange Vegetables	1.0	cups weekly
Dry Beans & Peas	1.0	cups weekly
Starchy Vegetables	2.5	cups weekly
Other Vegetables	4.5	cups weekly

* oz equivalent is a 1 ounce estimate, rounded to consumer friendly units. For example, an oz equivalent of Grains is a 1 slice of bread, or 1/2 cup of rice. An oz equivalent of Protein Foods 1 oz of meat, 1 egg, or 1/4 cup cooked beans.

V. **Evaluate your dietary pattern.** Answer the following questions about the results of your own dietary assessment and suggest ways that you could improve your dietary pattern.

1. How did your kilocalorie intake compare to the goal recommended by Nutrition-Calc Plus? If it was much higher or lower than your goal, what specific changes could you make to adjust your energy intake?

2. Do your meals usually resemble MyPlate? If not, what specific changes could you make to improve your meal planning?

3. Use the worksheet below to calculate your fat intake as a percentage of total kilocalories. How does this compare to the Acceptable Macronutrient Distribution

Range (AMDR) of 20% to 35% of total kilocalories from fat (review Chapter 5, Section 5.7)? If your fat intake does not fall within the AMDR, what specific changes could you make?

> Calculating Percent of Kilocalories from Fat:
>
> _____ grams of fat × 9 kcal per gram = _____ kcal from fat
>
> _____ kcal from fat / _____ total kcal = _____% of kcal from fat

4. Use the worksheet below to calculate your saturated fat intake as a percentage of total kilocalories. How does this compare to the Dietary Guidelines' recommendation to limit saturated fat to 10% of total kilocalories? If your intake of saturated fat was higher than 10% of total kcal, what specific dietary changes could you make to lower your intake of saturated fat?

> Calculating Percent of Kilocalories from Saturated Fat:
>
> _____ grams of saturated fat × 9 kcal per gram = _____ kcal from saturated fat
>
> _____ kcal from saturated fat / _____ total kcal = _____% of kcal from saturated fat

5. The Dietary Guidelines advise Americans to limit their consumption of added sugars. What were some sources of added sugars in your diet on the days you recorded? List several nutrient-dense food choices you could use to replace sources of added sugars in your dietary pattern.

6. What was your average fiber intake for the 3 days? How close did you come to meeting the AI for fiber? If your intake of fiber was lower than the AI, what specific dietary changes could you make to improve your intake of fiber?

7. How did your average intake of sodium compare to your AI and UL for sodium? If your sodium intake was higher than the UL, what specific dietary changes could you make to lower your intake of sodium?

8. Are your intakes of any vitamins or minerals less than 75% of the RDA or AI? Choose one of these nutrients and discuss how you could change your *dietary* habits to increase your intake of this nutrient.

9. Besides sodium, do your intakes of any vitamins or minerals exceed the UL? (Also consider any micronutrients consumed in supplement form.) If so, what negative consequences could this have for your health?

10. If you consume alcohol, are your drinking habits consistent with the Dietary Guidelines' recommendations to limit alcohol to 1 drink per day (women) or 2 drinks per day (men)? List one potential benefit of moderate alcohol consumption. List one negative consequence of excessive alcohol consumption.

Appendix D

Chemical Structures Important in Nutrition

Amino Acids

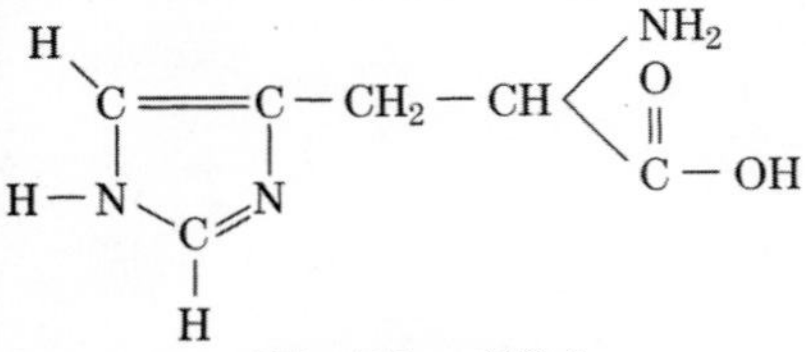

Histidine (His)
(essential)

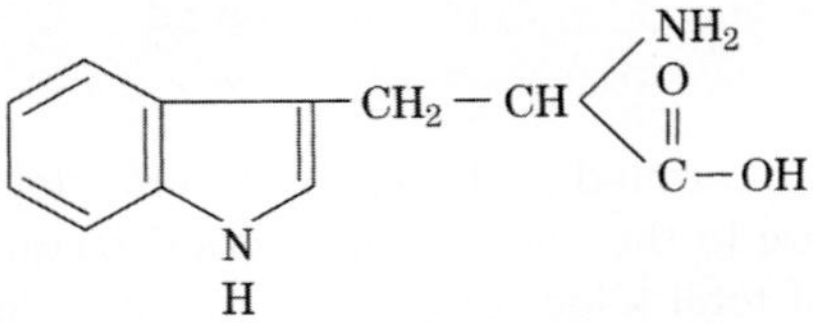

Tryptophan (Trp)
(essential)

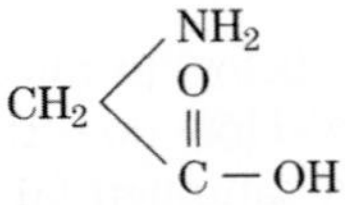

Glycine (Gly)

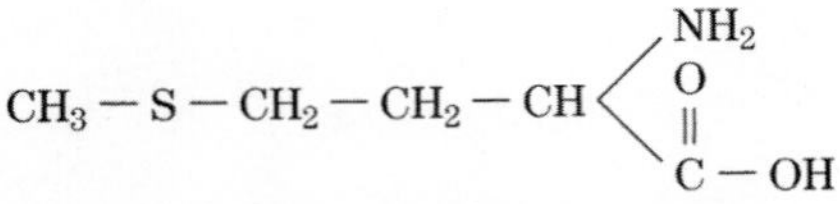

Methionine (Met)
(essential)

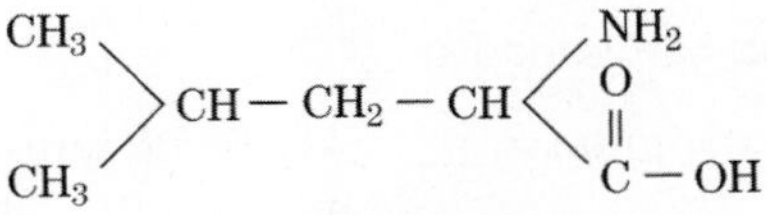

Leucine (Leu)
(essential)

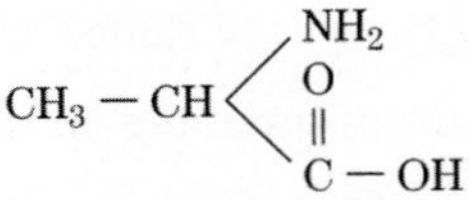

Alanine (Ala)

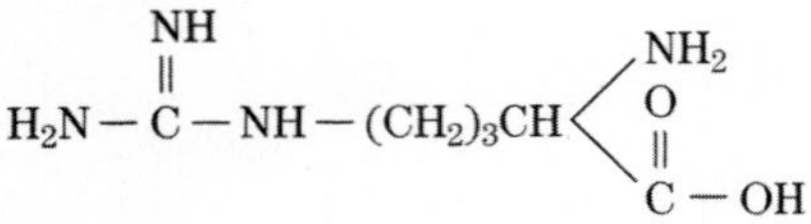

Arginine (Arg)
(essential in infancy)

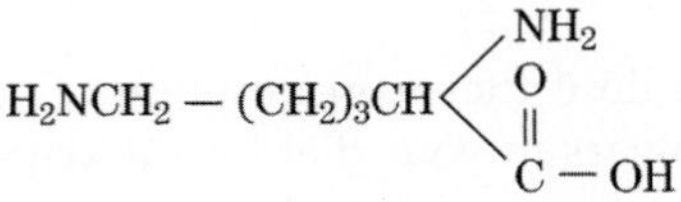

Lysine (Lys)
(essential)

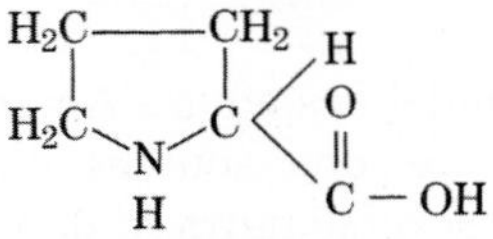

Proline (Pro)

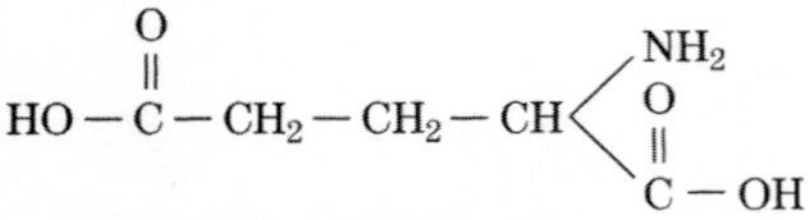

Glutamic Acid (Glu)

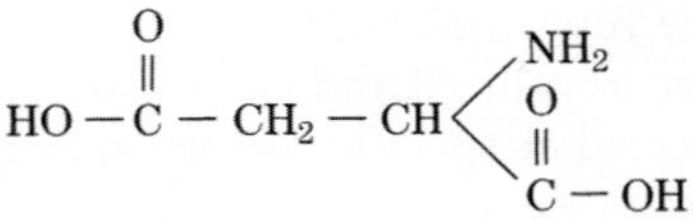

Aspartic Acid (Asp)

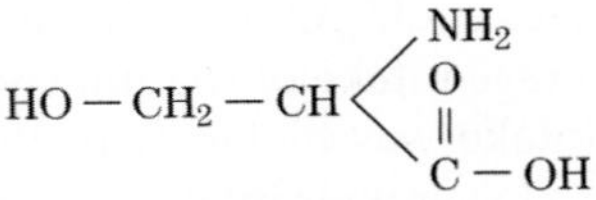

Serine (Ser)

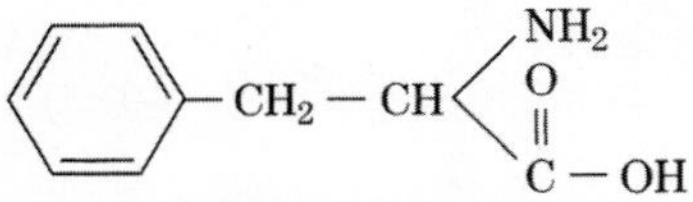

Phenylalanine (Phe)
(essential)

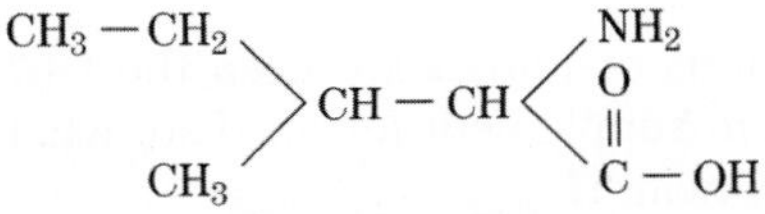

Isoleucine (Ile)
(essential)

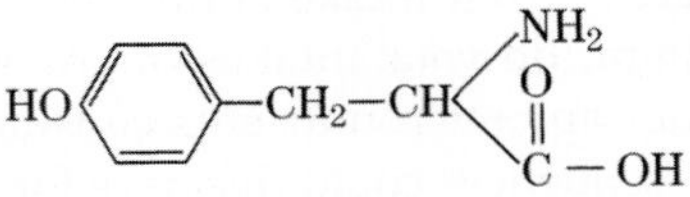

Tyrosine (Tyr)

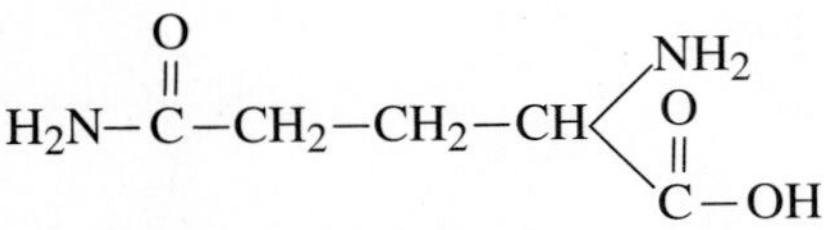

Glutamine (Gln)

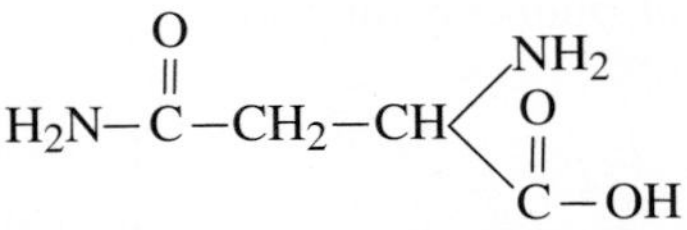

Asparagine (Asn)

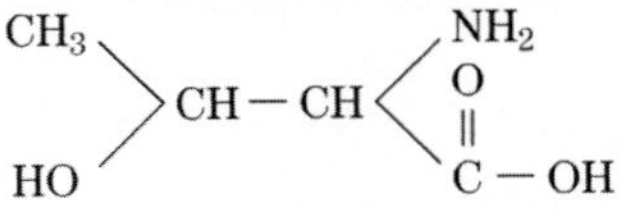

Threonine (Thr)
(essential)

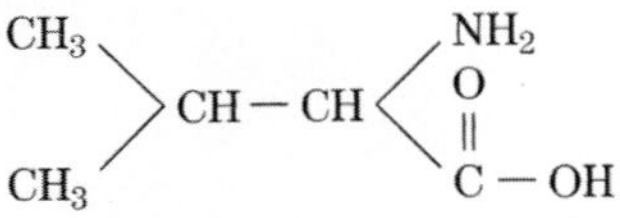

Valine (Val)
(essential)

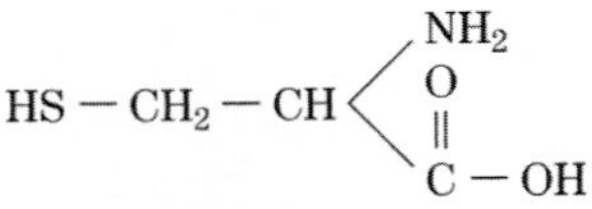

Cysteine (Cys)

Vitamins

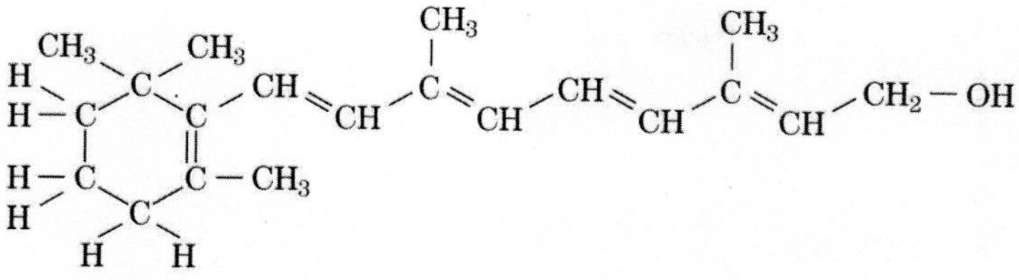

Vitamin A: retinol

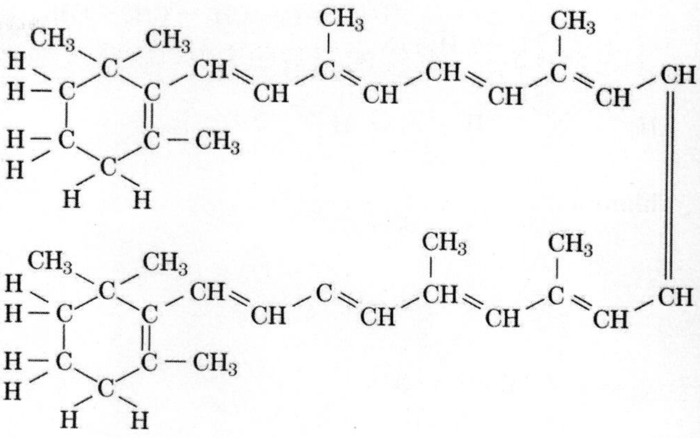

Beta-carotene

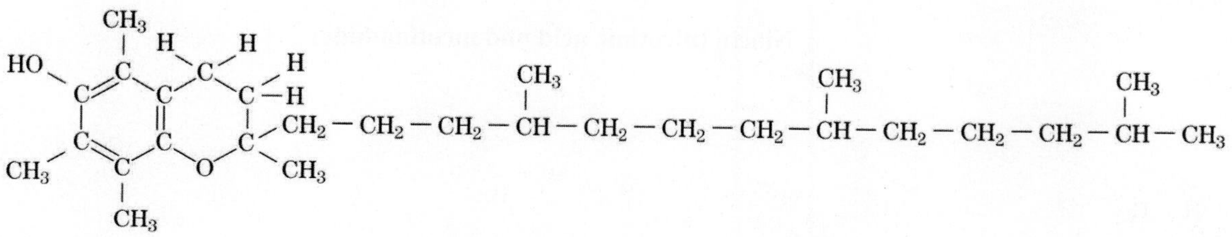

Vitamin E

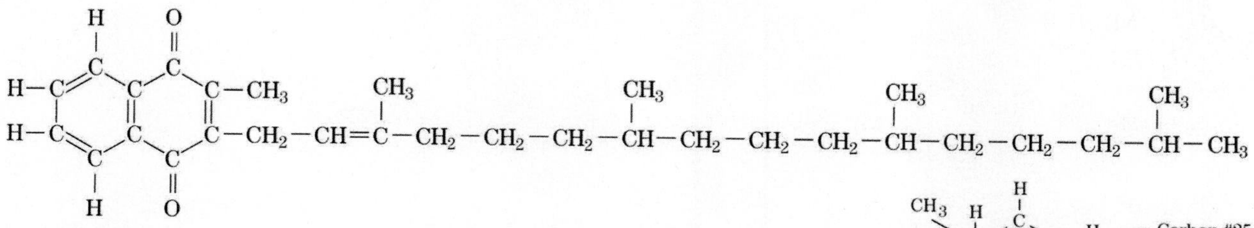

Vitamin K

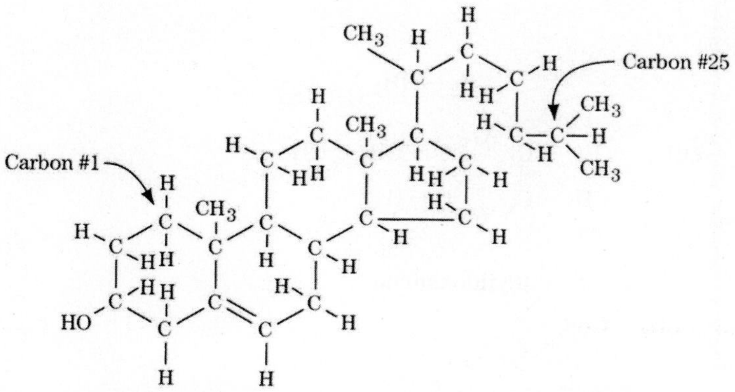

7-Dehydrocholesterol

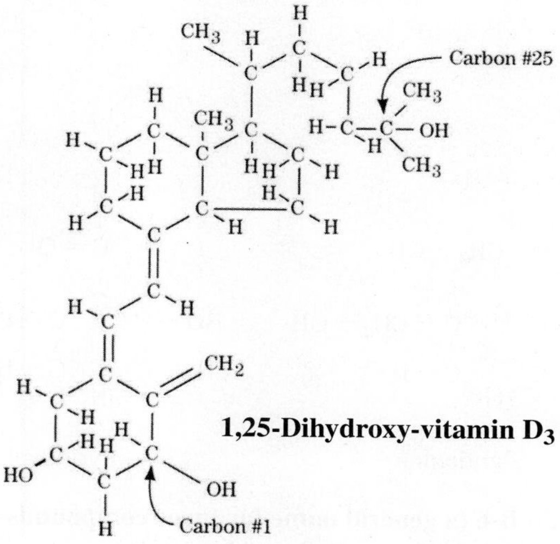

1,25-Dihydroxy-vitamin D$_3$ (calcitriol)

Active vitamin D (calcitriol) and its precursor 7-dehydrocholesterol

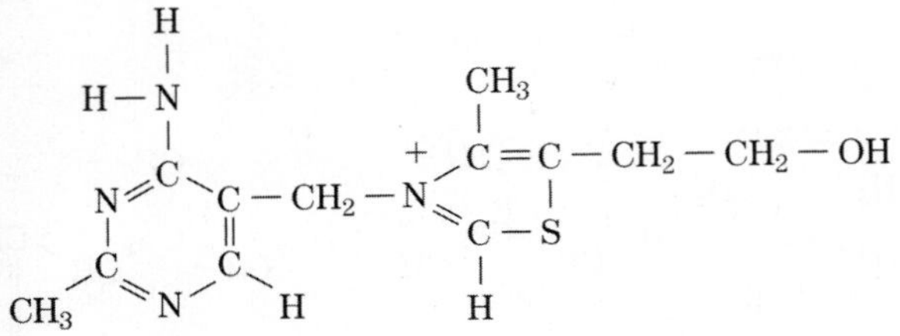

Thiamin

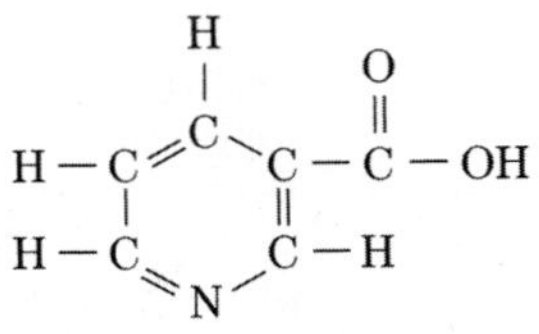

Niacin (nicotinic acid and nicotinamide)

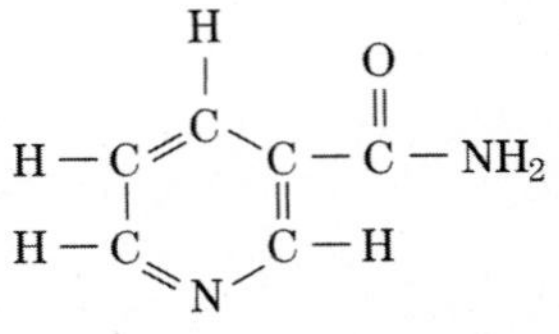

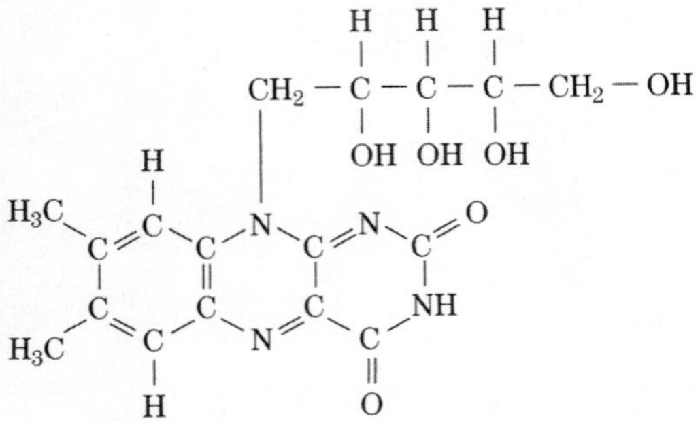

Nicotinic acid

Nicotinamide

Riboflavin

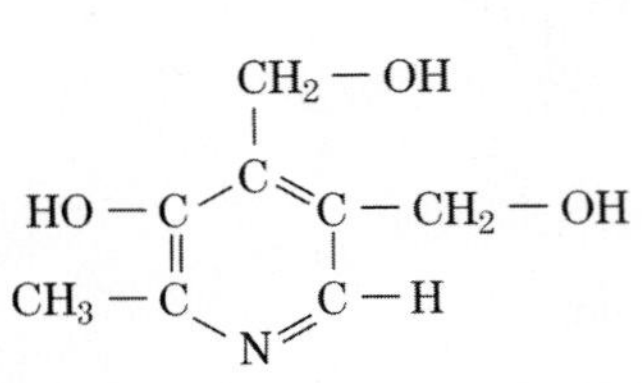

Pyridoxine

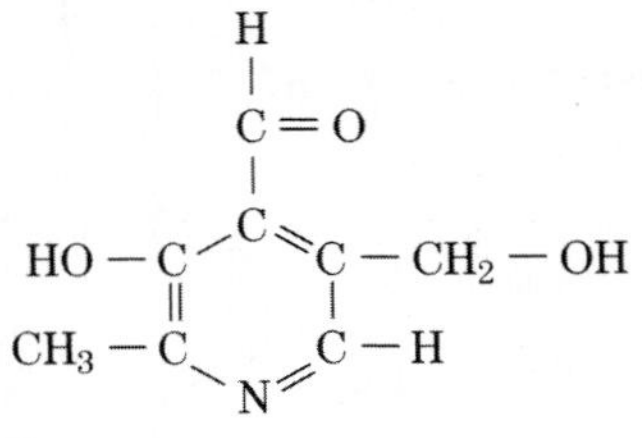

Pyridoxal

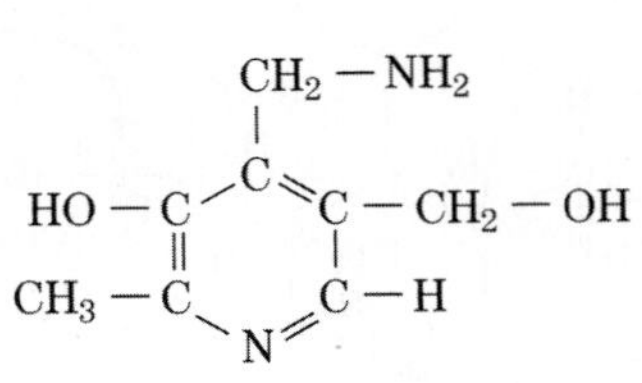

Pyridoxamine

**Vitamin B-6 (a general name for three compounds—
pyridoxine, pyridoxal, and pyridoxamine)**

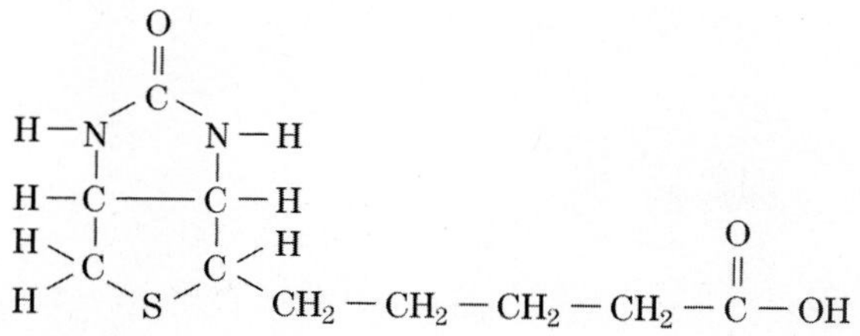

Biotin

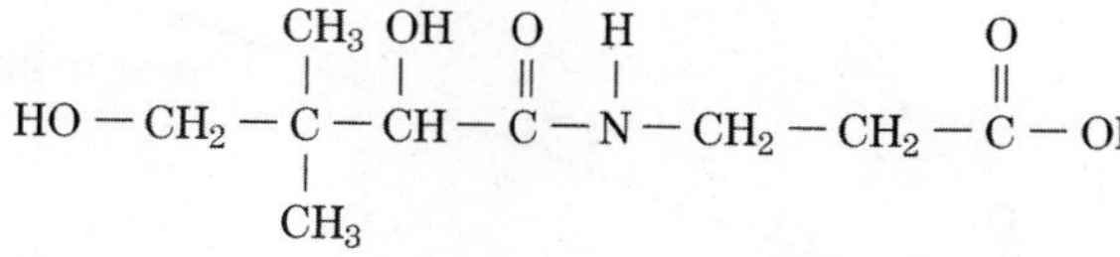

Pantothenic acid

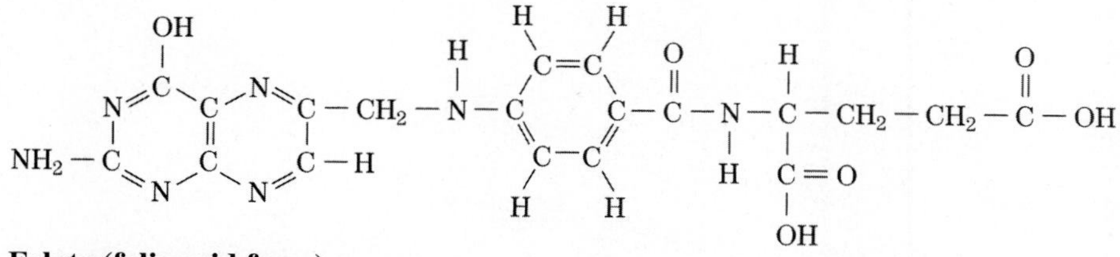

Folate (folic acid form)

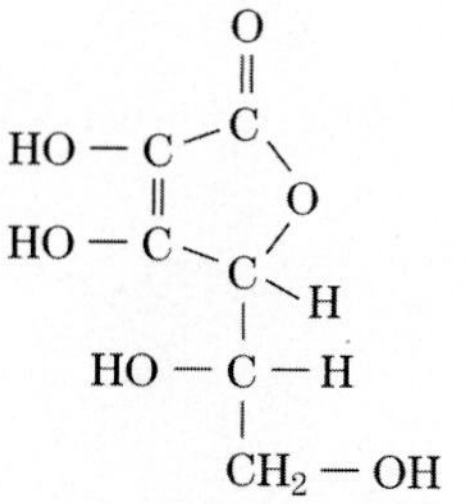

Vitamin C (ascorbic acid)

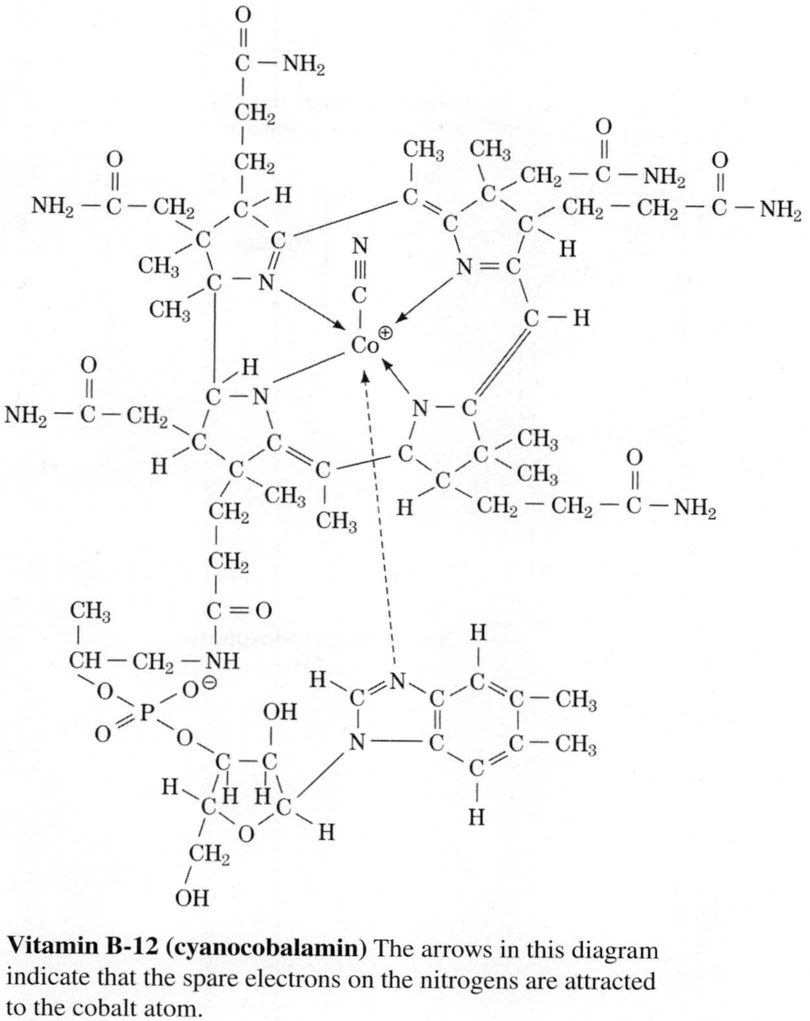

Vitamin B-12 (cyanocobalamin) The arrows in this diagram indicate that the spare electrons on the nitrogens are attracted to the cobalt atom.

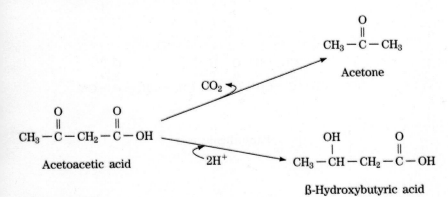

Ketone bodies

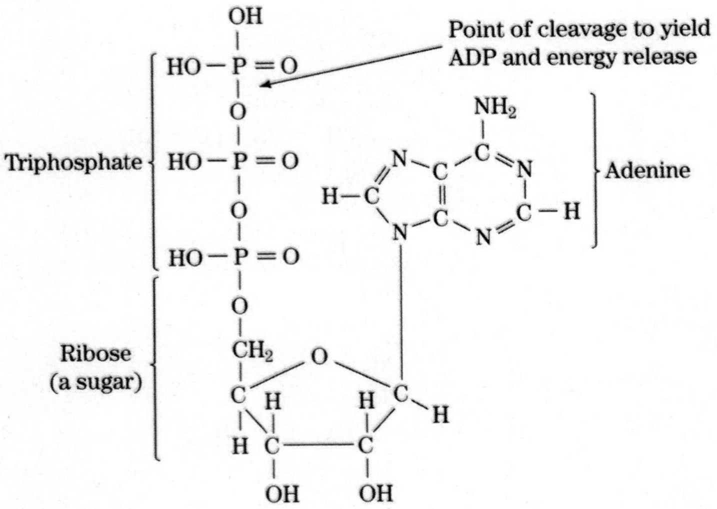

Acetone

CH_3-C-CH_3

Acetoacetic acid

CH_3-C-CH_2-C-OH

CO_2

$2H^+$

β-Hydroxybutyric acid

$CH_3-CH-CH_2-C-OH$

Point of cleavage to yield
ADP and energy release

Triphosphate

$HO-P=O$
$HO-P=O$
$HO-P=O$

Adenine

Ribose
(a sugar)

OH OH

**Adenosine triphosphate
(ATP)**

Appendix E

Sources of Nutrition Information

Consider the following reliable sources of food and nutrition information:

Journals That Regularly Cover Nutrition Topics

*American Family Physician**
American Journal of Clinical Nutrition
American Journal of Epidemiology
American Journal of Medicine
American Journal of Obstetrics and Gynecology
American Journal of Public Health
American Scientist
Annals of Internal Medicine
Annual Review of Medicine
Annual Review of Nutrition
Appetite
Archives of Disease in Childhood
British Journal of Nutrition
BMJ (British Medical Journal)
Canadian Journal of Dietetic Practice and Research
Cancer Research
Clinical Nutrition
Critical Reviews in Food Science and Nutrition
Current Opinion in Clinical Nutrition and Metabolic Care
Current Opinion in Endocrinology, Diabetes and Obesity

Diabetes
Diabetes Care
Food and Chemical Toxicology
Gastroenterology
International Journal of Behavioral Nutrition and Physical Activity
International Journal of Obesity
*Journal of the Academy of Nutrition and Dietetics**
*Journal of the American College of Nutrition**
Journal of the American Geriatrics Society
JAMA (Journal of the American Medical Association)
Journal of Clinical Investigation
Journal of Food Science
Journal of Functional Foods
Journal of Human Nutrition and Dietetics
JNCI (Journal of the National Cancer Institute)
Journal of Nutrition
*Journal of Nutrition Education and Behavior**
Journal of Nutrition in Gerontology and Geriatrics

Journal of Pediatrics
The Lancet
Maternal and Child Health
Medicine & Science in Sports & Exercise
Nature
The New England Journal of Medicine
Nutrition
Nutrition & Dietetics
*Nutrition in Clinical Practice**
Nutrition Journal
Nutrition, Metabolism and Cardiovascular Diseases
Nutrition Research Reviews
Nutrition Reviews
*Nutrition Today**
Obesity
Pediatric Obesity
Pediatrics
Proceedings of the Nutrition Society
Public Health Nutrition
Science
*Science News**
Scientific American
*Today's Dietitian**

The majority of these journals are available in college and university libraries or in a specialty library on campus, such as one designated for health sciences. Most of them are now available online. As indicated, a few journals will be filed under their abbreviations, rather than the first word in their full name. A reference librarian can help you locate any of these sources. The journals with an asterisk (*) are ones you may find especially interesting and useful because of the number of nutrition articles presented each month or the less technical nature of the presentation.

Textbooks and Other Sources for Advanced Study of Nutrition Topics

Erdman JW and others: *Present knowledge in nutrition.* 10th ed. Washington, DC: International Life Sciences and Wiley-Blackwell, 2012.

Gropper SS and others: *Advanced nutrition and human metabolism.* 7th ed. Boston, MA: Cengage Learning, 2013.

Mahan LK and Raymond JL: *Krause's food and the nutrition care process,* 14th ed. St. Louis: Elsevier Saunders, 2017.

Rodwell VW and others: *Harper's illustrated biochemistry.* 30th ed. New York: McGraw-Hill Education, 2015.

Ross AC and others: *Modern nutrition in health and disease.* 11th ed. Philadelphia: Lippincott, Williams & Wilkins, 2012.

Stipanuk MH and Caudill MA: *Biochemical, physiological, and molecular aspects of human nutrition.* 3rd ed. St. Louis: Philadelphia: Elsevier Saunders, 2012.

Newsletters That Cover Nutrition Issues on a Regular Basis

Berkeley Wellness
University of California at Berkeley
www.berkeleywellness.com
Consumer Health Digest
www.consumerhealthdigest.com
ENC Blog
Egg Nutrition Center
www.eggnutritioncenter.org/blog

Environmental Nutrition
www.environmentalnutrition.com

Harvard Health Letter (and others)
Harvard Medical School
www.health.harvard.edu/newsletters

Health & Nutrition Letter
Tufts University
www.nutritionletter.tufts.edu

Mayo Clinic Health Letter
Mayo Clinic
www.healthletter.mayoclinic.com

Nutrition Action Healthletter
Center for Science in the Public Interest
www.cspinet.org

Soy Connection
United Soybean Board
www.soyconnection.com

Women's Nutrition Connection Newsletter
Weill Cornell Medical College
www.womensnutritionconnection.com

Professional Organizations

Academy of Nutrition and Dietetics
www.eatright.org

American Academy of Pediatrics
www.aap.org

American Cancer Society
www.cancer.org

American College of Sports Medicine
www.acsm.org

American Dental Association
www.ada.org

American Diabetes Association
www.diabetes.org

American Geriatrics Society
www.americangeriatrics.org

American Heart Association
www.heart.org

American Institute for Cancer Research
www.aicr.org

American Medical Association
www.ama-assn.org

American Public Health Association
www.apha.org

American Society for Nutrition
www.nutrition.org

Canadian Nutrition Society
www.cns-scn.ca

Diabetes Canada
www.diabetes.ca

Dietitians of Canada
www.dietitians.ca

Environmental Working Group
www.ewg.org

Institute of Food Technologists
www.ift.org

National Academy of Medicine
https://nam.edu

National Council on Aging
www.ncoa.org

National Osteoporosis Foundation
www.nof.org

Society for Nutrition Education and
  Behavior
www.sneb.org

**Professional Organizations with a
Commitment to Nutrition Issues**

Bread for the World Institute
www.bread.org

Food Research & Action Center
frac.org

Institute for Food and
  Development Policy
foodfirst.org

La Leche League International
www.llli.org

March of Dimes
www.marchofdimes.org

National Council Against
  Health Fraud
www.ncahf.org

National WIC Association
www.nwica.org

Overeaters Anonymous
www.oa.org

Oxfam America
www.oxfamamerica.org

**Local Resources for Advice on
Nutrition Issues**

Cooperative extension agents in county
  extension offices
Nutrition faculty affiliated with
  departments of food and nutrition,
  and dietetics
Registered dietitian nutritionists
  (RDNs) in health care, city, county,
  or state agencies, as well as in
  private practice

**Government Agencies Concerned
with Nutrition Issues or That Distribute
Nutrition Information**

United States
Agricultural Research Service
United States Department of Agriculture
www.ars.usda.gov

Federal Citizen Information Center
publications.usa.gov

Food and Drug Administration
www.fda.gov

Food Safety and Inspection Service
United States Department
  of Agriculture
www.fsis.usda.gov

MyPlate
www.choosemyplate.gov

National Agricultural Library
www.nal.usda.gov

National Cancer Institute
www.cancer.gov

National Center for Health Statistics
www.cdc.gov/nchs

National Heart, Lung, and Blood Institute
www.nhlbi.nih.gov

National Institute on Aging
www.nia.nih.gov

U.S. Government Publishing Office
www.gpo.gov

Canada
Canadian Food Inspection Agency
www.inspection.gc.ca

Health Canada
www.hc-sc.gc.ca

United Nations
Food and Agriculture Organization
www.fao.org

World Health Organization
www.who.int

**Trade Organizations and Companies
That Distribute Nutrition Information**

Abbott Nutrition
abbottnutrition.com

American Institute of Baking
www.aibonline.org

Beech-Nut Nutrition
www.beechnut.com

Campbell Soup Company
www.campbells.com/campbell-soup

Dannon Company
www.dannon.com

Del Monte Foods
www.delmonte.com

General Mills/Pillsbury
www.generalmills.com

Gerber
www.gerber.com

Idaho Potato Commission
www.idahopotato.com

Kellogg Company
www.kelloggs.com

Kraft Foods Group, Inc.
www.kraftrecipes.com

Kraft Heinz
www.heinzbaby.com/en-ca/

Mead Johnson Nutrition
www.meadjohnson.com

National Dairy Council
www.nationaldairycouncil.org

North American Meat Institute
www.meatinstitute.org

Sunkist Growers
www.sunkist.com

Appendix F

English-Metric Conversions and Metric Units

Metric-English Conversions

LENGTH

English (USA) | **Metric**
inch (in) | = 2.54 cm, 25.4 mm
foot (ft) | = 0.30 m, 30.48 cm
yard (yd) | = 0.91 m, 91.4 cm
mile (statute) (5280 ft) | = 1.61 km, 1609 m
mile (nautical) (6077 ft, 1.15 statute mi) | = 1.85 km, 1850 m

Metric | **English (USA)**
millimeter (mm) | = 0.039 in (thickness of a dime)
centimeter (cm) | = 0.39 in
meter (m) | = 3.28 ft, 39.37 in
kilometer (km) | = 0.62 mi, 1091 yd, 3273 ft

WEIGHT

English (USA) | **Metric**
grain | = 64.80 mg
ounce (oz) | = 28.35 g
pound (lb) | = 453.60 g, 0.45 kg
ton (short—2000 lb) | = 0.91 metric ton (907 kg)

Metric | **English (USA)**
milligram (mg) | = 0.002 grain (0.000035 oz)
gram (g) | = 0.04 oz (1/28 of an oz)
kilogram (kg) | = 35.27 oz, 2.20 lb
metric ton (1000 kg) | = 1.10 tons

VOLUME

English (USA) | **Metric**
cubic inch | = 16.39 cc
cubic foot | = 0.03 m^3
cubic yard | = 0.765 m^3
teaspoon (tsp) | = 5 ml
tablespoon (tbsp) | = 15 ml
fluid ounce | = 0.03 liter (30 ml)*
cup (c) | = 237 ml
pint (pt) | = 0.47 liter
quart (qt) | = 0.95 liter
gallon (gal) | = 3.79 liters

Metric | **English (USA)**
milliliter (ml) | = 0.03 oz
liter (L) | = 2.12 pt
liter | = 1.06 qt
liter | = 0.27 gal

1 liter ÷ 1000 = 1 milliliter or 1 cubic centimeter (10^{-3} liter)
1 liter ÷ 1,000,000 = 1 microliter (10^{-6} liter)

* Note: 1 ml = 1 cc.

Metric and Other Common Units

Unit/Abbreviation	Other Equivalent Measure
milligram/mg	1/1000 of a gram
microgram/µg	1/1,000,000 of a gram
deciliter/dl	1/10 of a liter (about ½ cup)
milliliter/ml	1/1000 of a liter (5 ml is about 1 tsp)
International Unit/IU	Crude measure of vitamin activity generally based on growth rate seen in animals

Fahrenheit-Celsius Conversion Scale

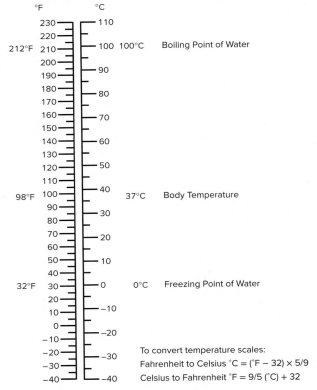

To convert temperature scales:
Fahrenheit to Celsius °C = (°F − 32) × 5/9
Celsius to Fahrenheit °F = 9/5 (°C) + 32

Household Units

3 teaspoons	= 1 tablespoon	= 15 grams
4 tablespoons	= ¼ cup	= 60 grams
5 ⅓ tablespoons	= ⅓ cup	= 80 grams
8 tablespoons	= ½ cup	= 120 grams
10 ⅔ tablespoons	= ⅔ cup	= 160 grams
16 tablespoons	= 1 cup	= 240 grams
1 tablespoon	= ½ fluid ounce	= 15 milliliters
1 cup	= 8 fluid ounces	= 15 milliliters
1 cup	= ½ pint	= 240 grams
2 cups	= 1 pint	= 480 grams
4 cups	= 1 quart	= 960 grams = 1 liter
2 pints	= 1 quart	= 960 grams = 1 liter
4 quarts	= 1 gallon	= 3840 grams = 4 liters

DIETARY REFERENCE INTAKES (DRIs): RECOMMENDED INTAKES FOR INDIVIDUALS, VITAMINS

Food and Nutrition Board, Institute of Medicine, National Academies

Life Stage Group	Vitamin A (µg/d)[a]	Vitamin C (mg/d)	Vitamin D (µg/d)[b,c]	Vitamin E (mg/d)[d]	Vitamin K (µg/d)	Thiamin (mg/d)	Riboflavin (mg/d)	Niacin (mg/d)[e]	Vitamin B-6 (mg/d)	Folate (µg/d)[f]	Vitamin B-12 (µg/d)	Pantothenic Acid (mg/d)	Biotin (µg/d)	Choline (mg/d)[g]
Infants														
0–6 mo	400*	40*	10	4*	2.0*	0.2*	0.3*	2*	0.1*	65*	0.4*	1.7*	5*	125*
7–12 mo	500*	50*	10	5*	2.5*	0.3*	0.4*	4*	0.3*	80*	0.5*	1.8*	6*	150*
Children														
1–3 y	300	15	15	6	30*	0.5	0.5	6	0.5	150	0.9	2*	8*	200*
4–8 y	400	25	15	7	55*	0.6	0.6	8	0.6	200	1.2	3*	12*	250*
Males														
9–13 y	600	45	15	11	60*	0.9	0.9	12	1.0	300	1.8	4*	20*	375*
14–18 y	900	75	15	15	75*	1.2	1.3	16	1.3	400	2.4	5*	25*	550*
19–30 y	900	90	15	15	120*	1.2	1.3	16	1.3	400	2.4	5*	30*	550*
31–50 y	900	90	15	15	120*	1.2	1.3	16	1.3	400	2.4	5*	30*	550*
51–70 y	900	90	15	15	120*	1.2	1.3	16	1.7	400	2.4[h]	5*	30*	550*
>70 y	900	90	20	15	120*	1.2	1.3	16	1.7	400	2.4[h]	5*	30*	550*
Females														
9–13 y	600	45	15	11	60*	0.9	0.9	12	1.0	300	1.8	4*	20*	375*
14–18 y	700	65	15	15	75*	1.0	1.0	14	1.2	400[i]	2.4	5*	25*	400*
19–30 y	700	75	15	15	90*	1.1	1.1	14	1.3	400[i]	2.4	5*	30*	425*
31–50 y	700	75	15	15	90*	1.1	1.1	14	1.3	400[i]	2.4	5*	30*	425*
51–70 y	700	75	15	15	90*	1.1	1.1	14	1.5	400	2.4[h]	5*	30*	425*
>70 y	700	75	20	15	90*	1.1	1.1	14	1.5	400	2.4[h]	5*	30*	425*
Pregnancy														
≤18 y	750	80	15	15	75*	1.4	1.4	18	1.9	600[j]	2.6	6*	30*	450*
19–30 y	770	85	15	15	90*	1.4	1.4	18	1.9	600[j]	2.6	6*	30*	450*
31–50 y	770	85	15	15	90*	1.4	1.4	18	1.9	600[j]	2.6	6*	30*	450*
Lactation														
≤18 y	1200	115	15	19	75*	1.4	1.6	17	2.0	500	2.8	7*	35*	550*
19–30 y	1300	120	15	19	90*	1.4	1.6	17	2.0	500	2.8	7*	35*	550*
31–50 y	1300	120	15	19	90*	1.4	1.6	17	2.0	500	2.8	7*	35*	550*

mg = milligram, µg = microgram

NOTE: This table (taken from the DRI reports; see www.nap.edu) presents Recommended Dietary Allowances (RDAs) in **bold type** and Adequate Intakes (AIs) in ordinary type followed by an asterisk (*). RDAs and AIs may both be used as goals for individual intake. RDAs are set to meet the needs of almost all (97 to 98%) individuals in a group. For healthy breastfed infants, the AI is the mean intake. The AI for other life stage and gender groups is believed to cover needs of all individuals in the group, but lack of data or uncertainty in the data prevents being able to specify with confidence the percentage of individuals covered by this intake.

aAs retinol activity equivalents (RAEs). 1 RAE = 1 µg retinol, 12 µg β-carotene, 24 µg α-carotene, or 24 µg β-cryptoxanthin. To calculate RAEs from REs of provitamin A carotenoids in foods, divide the REs by 2. For preformed vitamin A in foods or supplements and for provitamin A carotenoids in supplements, 1 RE = 1 RAE.

bcholecalciferol. 1 µg cholecalciferol = 40 IU vitamin D.

cIn the absence of adequate exposure to sunlight.

dAs α-tocopherol. α-Tocopherol includes RRR-α-tocopherol, the only form of α-tocopherol that occurs naturally in foods, and the 2R-stereoisomeric forms of α-tocopherol (RRR-, RSR-, RRS-, and RSS-α-tocopherol) that occur in fortified foods and supplements. It does not include the 2S-stereoisomeric forms of α-tocopherol (SRR-, SSR-, SRS-, and SSS-α-tocopherol), also found in fortified foods and supplements.

eAs niacin equivalents (NE). 1 mg of niacin = 60 mg of tryptophan; 0–6 months = preformed niacin (not NE).

fAs dietary folate equivalents (DFE). 1 DFE = 1 µg food folate = 0.6 µg of folic acid from fortified food or as a supplement consumed with food = 0.5 µg of a supplement taken on an empty stomach.

gAlthough AIs have been set for choline, there are few data to assess whether a dietary supply of choline is needed at all stages of the life cycle, and it may be that the choline requirement can be met by endogenous synthesis at some of these stages.

hBecause 10 to 30% of older people may malabsorb food-bound B-12, it is advisable for those older than 50 years to meet their RDA mainly by consuming foods fortified with B-12 or a supplement containing B-12.

iIn view of evidence linking folate intake with neural tube defects in the fetus, it is recommended that all women capable of becoming pregnant consume 400 µg from supplements or fortified foods in addition to intake of food folate from a varied diet.

jIt is assumed that women will continue consuming 400 µg from supplements or fortified food until their pregnancy is confirmed and they enter prenatal care, which ordinarily occurs after the end of the periconceptional period—the critical time for formation of the neural tube.

Adapted from the Dietary Reference Intakes series, National Academies Press. Copyright 1997, 1998, 2000, 2001, 2011, by the National Academy of Sciences. The full reports are available from the National Academies Press at www.nap.edu.

DIETARY REFERENCE INTAKES (DRIs): RECOMMENDED INTAKES FOR INDIVIDUALS, ELEMENTS
Food and Nutrition Board, Institute of Medicine, National Academies

Life Stage Group	Calcium (mg/d)	Chromium (µg/d)	Copper (µg/d)	Fluoride (mg/d)	Iodine (µg/d)	Iron (mg/d)	Magnesium (mg/d)	Manganese (mg/d)	Molybdenum (µg/d)	Phosphorus (mg/d)	Selenium (µg/d)	Zinc (mg/d)
Infants												
0–6 mo	200*	0.2*	200*	0.01*	110*	0.27*	30*	0.003*	2*	100*	15*	2*
7–12 mo	260*	5.5*	220*	0.5*	130*	11	75*	0.6*	3*	275*	20*	3
Children												
1–3 y	700	11*	340	0.7*	90	7	80	1.2*	17	460	20	3
4–8 y	1000	15*	440	1*	90	10	130	1.5*	22	500	30	5
Males												
9–13 y	1300	25*	700	2*	120	8	240	1.9*	34	1250	40	8
14–18 y	1300	35*	890	3*	150	11	410	2.2*	43	1250	55	11
19–30 y	1000	35*	900	4*	150	8	400	2.3*	45	700	55	11
31–50 y	1000	35*	900	4*	150	8	420	2.3*	45	700	55	11
51–70 y	1000	30*	900	4*	150	8	420	2.3*	45	700	55	11
> 70 y	1200	30*	900	4*	150	8	420	2.3*	45	700	55	11
Females												
9–13 y	1300	21*	700	2*	120	8	240	1.6*	34	1250	40	8
14–18 y	1300	24*	890	3*	150	15	360	1.6*	43	1250	55	9
19–30 y	1000	25*	900	3*	150	18	310	1.8*	45	700	55	8
31–50 y	1000	25*	900	3*	150	18	320	1.8*	45	700	55	8
51–70 y	1200	20*	900	3*	150	8	320	1.8*	45	700	55	8
> 70 y	1200	20*	900	3*	150	8	320	1.8*	45	700	55	8
Pregnancy												
≤18 y	1300	29*	1000	3*	220	27	400	2.0*	50	1250	60	12
19–30 y	1000	30*	1000	3*	220	27	350	2.0*	50	700	60	11
31–50 y	1000	30*	1000	3*	220	27	360	2.0*	50	700	60	11
Lactation												
≤18 y	1300	44*	1300	3*	290	10	360	2.6*	50	1250	70	13
19–30 y	1000	45*	1300	3*	290	9	310	2.6*	50	700	70	12
31–50 y	1000	45*	1300	3*	290	9	320	2.6*	50	700	70	12

NOTE: This table presents Recommended Dietary Allowances (RDAs) in **bold type** and Adequate Intakes (AIs) in ordinary type followed by an asterisk (*). RDAs and AIs may both be used as goals for individual intake. RDAs are set to meet the needs of almost all (97 to 98%) individuals in a group. For healthy breastfed infants, the AI is the mean intake. The AI for other life stage and gender groups is believed to cover needs of all individuals in the group, but lack of data or uncertainty in the data prevents being able to specify with confidence the percentage of individuals covered by this intake.

Sources: *Dietary Reference Intakes for Calcium, Phosphorus, Magnesium, Vitamin D, and Fluoride* (1997); *Dietary Reference Intakes for Thiamin, Riboflavin, Niacin, Vitamin B-6, Folate, Vitamin B-12, Pantothenic Acid, Biotin, and Choline* (1998); *Dietary Reference Intakes for Vitamin C, Vitamin E, Selenium, and Carotenoids* (2000); *Dietary Reference Intakes for Vitamin A, Vitamin K, Arsenic, Boron, Chromium, Copper, Iodine, Iron, Manganese, Molybdenum, Nickel, Silicon, Vanadium, and Zinc* (2001); and *Dietary Reference Intakes for Calcium and Vitamin D* (2011). These reports may be accessed via www.nap.edu.

Adapted from the Dietary Reference Intake series, National Academies Press. Copyright 1997, 1998, 2000, 2001, and 2011 by the National Academy of Sciences. The full reports are available from the National Academies Press at www.nap.edu.

DIETARY REFERENCE INTAKES (DRIs): RECOMMENDED INTAKES FOR INDIVIDUALS, MACRONUTRIENTS
Food and Nutrition Board, Institute of Medicine, National Academies

Life Stage Group	Carbohydrate (g/d)	Total Fiber (g/d)	Fat (g/d)	Linoleic Acid (g/d)	α-Linolenic Acid (g/d)	Protein[a] (g/d)
Infants						
0–6 mo	60*	ND	31*	4.4*	0.5*	9.1*
7–12 mo	95*	ND	30*	4.6*	0.5*	**11.0**
Children						
1–3 y	130	19*	ND[b]	7*	0.7*	**13**
4–8 y	130	25*	ND	10*	0.9*	**19**
Males						
9–13 y	130	31*	ND	12*	1.2*	**34**
14–18 y	130	38*	ND	16*	1.6*	**52**
19–30 y	130	38*	ND	17*	1.6*	**56**
31–50 y	130	38*	ND	17*	1.6*	**56**
51–70 y	130	30*	ND	14*	1.6*	**56**
>70 y	130	30*	ND	14*	1.6*	**56**
Females						
9–13 y	130	26*	ND	10*	1.0*	**34**
14–18 y	130	26*	ND	11*	1.1*	**46**
19–30 y	130	25*	ND	12*	1.1*	**46**
31–50 y	130	25*	ND	12*	1.1*	**46**
51–70 y	130	21*	ND	11*	1.1*	**46**
>70 y	130	21*	ND	11*	1.1*	**46**
Pregnancy						
14–18 y	175	28*	ND	13*	1.4*	**71**
19–30 y	175	28*	ND	13*	1.4*	**71**
31–50 y	175	28*	ND	13*	1.4*	**71**
Lactation						
14–18 y	210	29*	ND	13*	1.3*	**71**
19–30 y	210	29*	ND	13*	1.3*	**71**
31–50 y	210	29*	ND	13*	1.3*	**71**

NOTE: This table presents Recommended Dietary Allowances (RDAs) in **bold type** and Adequate Intakes (AIs) in ordinary type followed by an asterisk (*). RDAs and AIs may both be used as goals for individual intake. RDAs are set to meet the needs of almost all (97 to 98%) individuals in a group. For healthy breastfed infants, the AI is the mean intake. The AI for other life stage and gender groups is believed to cover needs of all individuals in the group, but lack of data or uncertainty in the data prevents being able to specify with confidence the percentage of individuals covered by this intake.

[a]Based on 0.8 g protein/kg body weight for reference body weight.

[b]ND = not determinable at this time.

Sources: *Dietary Reference Intakes for Energy, Carbohydrate, Fiber, Fat, Fatty Acids, Cholesterol, Protein, and Amino Acids* (2002). This report may be accessed via www.nap.edu.

Adapted from the *Dietary Reference Intake series*, National Academies Press. Copyright 1997, 1998, 2000, 2001, by the National Academy of Sciences. The full reports are available from the National Academies Press at www.nap.edu.

DIETARY REFERENCE INTAKES (DRIs): RECOMMENDED INTAKES FOR INDIVIDUALS, ELECTROLYTES AND WATER
Food and Nutrition Board, Institute of Medicine, National Academies

Life Stage Group	Sodium (mg/d)	Potassium (mg/d)	Chloride (mg/d)	Water (L/d)
Infants				
0–6 mo	120*	400*	180*	0.7*
7–12 mo	370*	700*	570*	0.8*
Children				
1–3 y	1000*	3000*	1500*	1.3*
4–8 y	1200*	3800*	1900*	1.7*
Males				
9–13 y	1500*	4500*	2300*	2.4*
14–18 y	1500*	4700*	2300*	3.3*
19–30 y	1500*	4700*	2300*	3.7*
31–50 y	1500*	4700*	2300*	3.7*
51–70 y	1300*	4700*	2000*	3.7*
> 70 y	1200*	4700*	1800*	3.7*
Females				
9–13 y	1500*	4500*	2300*	2.1*
14–18 y	1500*	4700*	2300*	2.3*
19–30 y	1500*	4700*	2300*	2.7*
31–50 y	1500*	4700*	2300*	2.7*
51–70 y	1300*	4700*	2000*	2.7*
> 70 y	1200*	4700*	1800*	2.7*
Pregnancy				
14–18 y	1500*	4700*	2300*	3.0*
19–50 y	1500*	4700*	2300*	3.0*
Lactation				
14–18 y	1500*	5100*	2300*	3.8*
19–50 y	1500*	5100*	2300*	3.8*

NOTE: The table is adapted from the *DRI reports*. See www.nap.edu. Adequate Intakes (AIs) are followed by an asterisk (*). These may be used as a goal for individual intake. For healthy breastfed infants, the AI is the average intake. The AI for other life stage and gender groups is believed to cover the needs of all individuals in the group, but lack of data prevent being able to specify with confidence the percentage of individuals covered by this intake; therefore, no Recommended Dietary Allowance (RDA) was set.

Source: *Dietary Reference Intakes for Water, Potassium, Sodium, Chloride, and Sulfate* (2005). This report may be accessed via www.nap.edu.

ACCEPTABLE MACRONUTRIENT DISTRIBUTION RANGES

	Range (percent of energy)		
Macronutrient	Children, 1–3 y	Children, 4–18 y	Adults
Fat	30–40	25–35	20–35
omega-6 polyunsaturated fats (linoleic acid)	5–10	5–10	5–10
omega-3 polyunsaturated fats[a] (α-linolenic acid)	0.6–1.2	0.6–1.2	0.6–1.2
Carbohydrate	45–65	45–65	45–65
Protein	5–20	10–30	10–35

[a]Approximately 10% of the total can come from longer-chain n-3 fatty acids.

SOURCE: *Dietary Reference Intakes for Energy, Carbohydrate, Fiber, Fat, Fatty Acids, Cholesterol, Protein, and Amino Acids* (2002). The report may be accessed via www.nap.edu.

Adapted from the *Dietary Reference Intakes series,* National Academies Press. Copyright 1997, 1998, 2000, 2001, 2011, by the National Academy of Sciences. The full reports are available from the National Academies Press at www.nap.edu.

DIETARY REFERENCE INTAKES (DRIs): TOLERABLE UPPER INTAKE LEVELS (UL[a]), VITAMINS
Food and Nutrition Board, Institute of Medicine, National Academies

Life Stage Group	Vitamin A (µg/d)[b]	Vitamin C (mg/d)	Vitamin D (µg/d)	Vitamin E (mg/d)[c,d]	Vitamin K	Thiamin	Riboflavin	Niacin (mg/d)[d]	Vitamin B-6 (mg/d)	Folate (µg/d)[d]	Vitamin B-12	Pantothenic Acid	Biotin	Choline (g/d)	Carotenoids[e]
Infants															
0–6 mo	600	ND[f]	25	ND	ND	ND	ND	ND	ND	ND	ND	ND	ND	ND	ND
7–12 mo	600	ND	38	ND	ND	ND	ND	ND	ND	ND	ND	ND	ND	ND	ND
Children															
1–3 y	600	400	63	200	ND	ND	ND	10	30	300	ND	ND	ND	1.0	ND
4–8 y	900	650	75	300	ND	ND	ND	15	40	400	ND	ND	ND	1.0	ND
Males, Females															
9–13 y	1700	1200	100	600	ND	ND	ND	20	60	600	ND	ND	ND	2.0	ND
14–18 y	2800	1800	100	800	ND	ND	ND	30	80	800	ND	ND	ND	3.0	ND
19–70 y	3000	2000	100	1000	ND	ND	ND	35	100	1000	ND	ND	ND	3.5	ND
>70 y	3000	2000	100	1000	ND	ND	ND	35	100	1000	ND	ND	ND	3.5	ND
Pregnancy															
≤18 y	2800	1800	100	800	ND	ND	ND	30	80	800	ND	ND	ND	3.0	ND
19–50 y	3000	2000	100	1000	ND	ND	ND	35	100	1000	ND	ND	ND	3.5	ND
Lactation															
≤18 y	2800	1800	100	800	ND	ND	ND	30	80	800	ND	ND	ND	3.0	ND
19–50 y	3000	2000	100	1000	ND	ND	ND	35	100	1000	ND	ND	ND	3.5	ND

[a]UL = The maximum level of daily nutrient intake likely to pose no risk of adverse effects. Unless otherwise specified, the UL represents total intake from food, water, and supplements. Due to lack of suitable data, ULs could not be established for vitamin K, thiamin, riboflavin, vitamin B-12, pantothenic acid, biotin, or carotenoids. In the absence of ULs, extra caution may be warranted in consuming levels above recommended intakes.

[b]As preformed vitamin A only.

[c]As α-tocopherol; applies to any form of supplemental α-tocopherol.

[d]The ULs for vitamin E, niacin, and folate apply to synthetic forms obtained from supplements, fortified foods, or a combination of the two.

[e]β-Carotene supplements are advised only to serve as a provitamin A source for individuals at risk of vitamin A deficiency.

[f]ND = Not determinable due to lack of data of adverse effects in this age group and concern with regard to lack of ability to handle excess amounts. Source of intake should be from food only to prevent high levels of intake.

SOURCES: Dietary Reference Intakes for Calcium and Vitamin D (2011); Dietary Reference Intakes for Calcium, Phosphorus, Magnesium, Vitamin D, and Fluoride (1997); Dietary Reference Intakes for Thiamin, Riboflavin, Niacin, Vitamin B-6, Folate, Vitamin B-12, Pantothenic Acid, Biotin, and Choline (1998); Dietary Reference Intakes for Vitamin C, Vitamin E, Selenium, and Carotenoids (2000); and Dietary Reference Intakes for Vitamin A, Vitamin K, Arsenic, Boron, Chromium, Copper, Iodine, Iron, Manganese, Molybdenum, Nickel, Silicon, Vanadium, and Zinc (2001). These reports may be accessed via www.nap.edu.

Adapted from the Dietary Reference Intakes series, National Academies Press. Copyright 1997, 1998, 2000, 2001, 2011, by the National Academy of Sciences. The full reports are available from the National Academies Press at www.nap.edu.

DIETARY REFERENCE INTAKES (DRIs): TOLERABLE UPPER INTAKE LEVELS (UL[a]), ELEMENTS AND ELECTROLYTES[b,c]
Food and Nutrition Board, Institute of Medicine, National Academies

Life Stage Group	Arsenic[b]	Boron (mg/d)	Calcium (g/d)	Copper (µg/d)	Fluoride (mg/d)	Iodine (µg/d)	Iron (mg/d)	Magnesium (mg/d)[d]	Manganese (mg/d)	Molybdenum (µg/d)	Nickel (mg/d)	Phosphorus (g/d)	Selenium (µg/d)	Vanadium (mg/d)[e]	Zinc (mg/d)	Sodium (mg/d)	Chloride (mg/d)
Infants																	
0–6 mo	ND[f]	ND	1	ND	0.7	ND	40	ND	ND	ND	ND	ND	45	ND	4	ND	ND
7–12 mo	ND	ND	1.5	ND	0.9	ND	40	ND	ND	ND	ND	ND	60	ND	5	ND	ND
Children																	
1–3 y	ND	3	2.5	1000	1.3	200	40	65	2	300	0.2	3	90	ND	7	1500	2300
4–8 y	ND	6	2.5	3000	2.2	300	40	110	3	600	0.3	3	150	ND	12	1900	2900
Males, Females																	
9–13 y	ND	11	3	5000	10	600	40	350	6	1100	0.6	4	280	ND	23	2200	3400
14–18 y	ND	17	3	8000	10	900	45	350	9	1700	1.0	4	400	ND	34	2300	3600
19–70 y	ND	20	2.5[g]	10000	10	1100	45	350	11	2000	1.0	4	400	1.8	40	2300	3600
>70 y	ND	20	2	10000	10	1100	45	350	11	2000	1.0	3	400	1.8	40	2300	3600
Pregnancy																	
≤18 y	ND	17	3	8000	10	900	45	350	9	1700	1.0	3.5	400	ND	34	2300	3600
19–50 y	ND	20	2.5	10000	10	1100	45	350	11	2000	1.0	3.5	400	ND	40	2300	3600
Lactation																	
≤18 y	ND	17	3	8000	10	900	45	350	9	1700	1.0	4	400	ND	34	2300	3600
19–50 y	ND	20	2.5	10000	10	1100	45	350	11	2000	1.0	4	400	ND	40	2300	3600

[a]UL = The maximum level of daily nutrient intake that is likely to pose no risk of adverse effects. Unless otherwise specified, the UL represents total intake from food, water, and supplements. Due to lack of suitable data, ULs could not be established for arsenic, chromium, and silicon. In the absence of ULs, extra caution may be warranted in consuming levels above recommended intakes.

[b]Although a UL was not determined for arsenic, there is no justification for adding arsenic to food or supplements.

[c]Although silicon has not been shown to cause adverse effects in humans, there is no justification for adding silicon to supplements.

[d]The ULs for magnesium represent intake from a pharmacological agent only and do not include intake from food and water.

[e]Although vanadium in food has not been shown to cause adverse effects in humans, there is no justification for adding vanadium to food and vanadium supplements should be used with caution. The UL is based on adverse effects in laboratory animals and this data could be used to set a UL for adults but not children and adolescents.

[f]ND = Not determinable due to lack of data of adverse effects in this age group and concern with regard to lack of ability to handle excess amounts. Source of intake should be from food only to prevent high levels of intake.

[g]Upper Limit declines to 2 after age 50.

SOURCES: Dietary Reference Intakes for Calcium and Vitamin D (2011); Dietary Reference Intakes for Calcium, Phosphorus, Magnesium, Vitamin D, and Fluoride (1997); Dietary Reference Intakes for Thiamin, Riboflavin, Niacin, Vitamin B-6, Folate, Vitamin B-12, Pantothenic Acid, Biotin, and Choline (1998); Dietary Reference Intakes for Vitamin C, Vitamin E, Selenium, and Carotenoids (2000); Dietary Reference Intakes for Vitamin A, Vitamin K, Arsenic, Boron, Chromium, Copper, Iodine, Iron, Manganese, Molybdenum, Nickel, Silicon, Vanadium, and Zinc (2001); and Dietary Reference Intakes for Water, Potassium, Sodium, Chloride, and Sulfate (2004). These reports may be accessed via www.nap.edu. The full reports are available from the National Academies Press. Copyright 1997, 1998, 2000, 2001, 2011, by the National Academy of Sciences.

Adapted from the Dietary Reference Intakes series, National Academies Press. Copyright 1997, 1998, 2000, 2001, 2011, by the National Academy of Sciences. The full reports are available from the National Academies Press at www.nap.edu.

Glossary

1,25-dihydroxyvitamin D$_3$ (calcitriol) Biologically active form of vitamin D.

25-hydroxyvitamin D$_3$ (calcidiol or calcifediol) Form found in blood. Sometimes shortened to 25(OH)D$_3$.

7-dehydrocholesterol Precursor of vitamin D found in the skin.

absorption The process by which substances are taken up from the GI tract and enter the bloodstream or the lymph.

absorptive cells Also known as *enterocytes*; the intestinal cells that line the villi and participate in nutrient absorption.

Acceptable Daily Intake (ADI) Estimate of the amount of a sweetener that an individual can safely consume daily over a lifetime. ADIs are given as milligrams per kilogram of body weight per day.

acesulfame-K Alternative sweetener that yields no energy to the body; 200 times sweeter than sucrose.

acetaldehyde dehydrogenase An enzyme used in ethanol metabolism that eventually converts acetaldehyde into carbon dioxide and water.

acid group In chemistry, a functional group that consists of a carbon atom that shares bonds with two oxygen atoms. This is the site where fatty acids are linked to glycerol to form triglycerides.

action potential Change in the electrical charge of the nerve cell membrane resulting in an electrical signal that can be transmitted from one nerve cell to the next.

active absorption Movement of a substance across a semipermeable membrane from an area of lower solute concentration to an area of higher solute concentration. This type of transport requires energy and a carrier.

adaptive thermogenesis This term refers to the ability of humans to regulate body temperature within narrow limits (thermoregulation). Two visible examples of thermogenesis are fidgeting and shivering when cold.

additives Substances added to foods, either intentionally or incidentally.

adenosine diphosphate (ADP) A breakdown product of ATP. ADP is synthesized into ATP using energy from foodstuffs and a phosphate group (abbreviated P$_i$).

adenosine triphosphate (ATP) The main energy currency for cells. ATP energy is used to promote ion pumping, enzyme activity, and muscular contraction.

Adequate Intake (AI) Nutrient intake amount set for any nutrient for which insufficient research is available to establish an RDA. AIs are based on estimates of intakes that appear to maintain a defined nutritional state in a specific life stage.

adipose tissue Connective tissue made up of cells that store fat and also cushions and insulates the body.

aerobic Requiring oxygen.

aging Time-dependent physical and physiological changes in body structure and function that occur normally and progressively throughout adulthood as humans mature and become older.

air displacement A method for estimating body composition that makes use of the volume of space taken up by a body inside a small chamber (Bod Pod®). This tool is also known as air displacement plethysmography.

alcohol Ethyl alcohol or ethanol (CH$_3$CH$_2$OH) is the compound in alcoholic beverages.

alcohol dehydrogenase An enzyme used in alcohol (ethanol) metabolism that converts alcohol into acetaldehyde.

alcohol use disorder A psychiatric disorder characterized by a problematic pattern of alcohol use that leads to significant impairment or distress.

alcohol-related birth defects (ARBDs) One or more birth defects (e.g., malformations of the heart, bones, kidneys, eyes, or ears) related to confirmed alcohol exposure during gestation.

alcohol-related neurodevelopmental disorders (ARNDs) One or more abnormalities of the central nervous system (e.g., small head size, impaired motor skills, hearing loss, or poor hand-eye coordination) related to confirmed alcohol exposure during gestation.

aldosterone A hormone produced by the adrenal glands when blood volume is low. It acts on the kidneys to conserve sodium (and therefore water) to increase blood volume.

allergen A foreign protein, or antigen, that induces excess production of certain immune system antibodies; subsequent exposure to the same protein leads to allergic symptoms. Whereas all allergens are antigens, not all antigens are allergens.

allergy A hypersensitive immune response that occurs when the immune system identifies a harmless protein (e.g., a food protein) as a harmful pathogen (i.e., antigen) and attempts to destroy it.

alpha-linolenic acid An essential omega-3 fatty acid with 18 carbons and three double bonds.

amenorrhea Absence of menstrual periods in a woman of reproductive age.

amino acid The building block for proteins containing a central carbon atom with nitrogen and other atoms attached.

amylase Starch-digesting enzyme produced by the salivary glands and the pancreas.

amylopectin A digestible branched-chain type of starch composed of glucose units.

amylose A digestible straight-chain type of starch composed of glucose units.

anaerobic Requiring no oxygen.

anal sphincters A group of two sphincters (inner and outer) that help control expulsion of feces from the body.

anaphylaxis A severe allergic response that results in lowered blood pressure and respiratory distress. This can be fatal.

anemia A decreased oxygen-carrying capacity of the blood. This can be caused by many factors, such as iron deficiency or blood loss.

anencephaly Birth defect characterized by the absence of some or all of the brain and skull.

angiotensin A hormone produced by the liver and activated by enzymes from the kidneys. It signals the adrenal glands to produce aldosterone also and directs the kidneys to conserve sodium (and therefore water). Both of these actions have the effect of increasing blood volume.

animal model Use of animals to study disease to understand more about human disease.

anorexia nervosa An eating disorder characterized by extreme restriction of energy intake relative to requirements leading to significantly low body weight.

anthocyanins Flavonoid plant pigments that appear red, purple, or blue and are found in berries, grapes, and red cabbage.

anthropometric assessment Measurement of body weight and the lengths, circumferences, and thicknesses of parts of the body.

antibody Blood protein that binds foreign proteins found in the body.

antibody-mediated immunity A process in which one type of lymphocyte produces antibodies that bind to specific antigens, thus marking foreign proteins or pathogens for destruction by other white blood cells.

antidiuretic hormone (ADH) A hormone that is secreted by the pituitary gland when blood concentration of solutes is high. It causes the kidneys to decrease water excretion, which increases blood volume.

antigen Any substance that induces a state of sensitivity and/or resistance to microorganisms or toxic substances after a lag period; a foreign substance that stimulates a specific aspect of the immune system.

antioxidant A substance that has the ability to prevent or repair the damage caused by oxidation.

anus Last portion of the GI tract; serves as an outlet for the digestive system.

appetite The primarily psychological (external) influences that encourage us to find and eat food, often in the absence of obvious hunger.

arachidonic acid (AA) An omega-6 fatty acid made from linoleic acid with 20 carbon atoms and four carbon-carbon double bonds.

ariboflavinosis Riboflavin-deficiency disease resulting in irritation of the skin, mouth, and throat; usually accompanied by low overall intakes of calories and protein.

aril Clear, ruby-colored fruit or seed pod that surrounds a tiny, crisp seed inside a pomegranate.

artery A blood vessel that carries blood away from the heart.

ascending colon Segment of the large intestine that carries feces from the cecum, up the right side of the abdomen, to the transverse colon.

aseptic processing A method by which food and container are separately and simultaneously sterilized; it allows manufacturers to produce boxes of milk that can be stored at room temperature.

aspartame Alternative sweetener made of two amino acids and methanol; about 200 times sweeter than sucrose.

atherosclerosis A buildup of fatty material (plaque) in the arteries, including those surrounding the heart.

atom Smallest combining unit of an element, such as iron or calcium. Atoms consist of protons, neutrons, and electrons.

atopic disease A condition involving an inappropriate immune response to environmental allergens; examples include asthma, eczema, and seasonal allergies.

atypical anorexia nervosa A subthreshold eating disorder in which a person meets most of the criteria for diagnosis of anorexia nervosa, except weight is within a normal range.

avoidant/restrictive food intake disorder (ARFID) Eating disorder characterized by failure to meet energy or nutrient needs, resulting in significant weight loss, nutritional deficiencies, or dependence on tube or intravenous feeding; the eating disturbance is not better explained by lack of available food, a medical problem, or another eating disorder.

bacteria Single-cell microorganisms; some produce poisonous substances, which cause illness in humans. Bacteria can be carried by water, animals, and people. They survive on skin, clothes, and hair, and thrive in foods at room temperature. Some can live without oxygen and survive by means of spore formation.

bariatrics The medical specialty focusing on the treatment of obesity.

basal metabolism The minimal amount of calories the body uses to support itself in a fasting state when resting and awake in a warm, quiet environment. It amounts to roughly 1 kcal per kilogram per hour for men and 0.9 kcal per kilogram per hour for women; these values are often referred to as *basal metabolic rate (BMR)*.

basophil The white blood cell that controls inflammation; level increases with poisoning.

benign Noncancerous; tumors that do not spread.

beriberi The thiamin-deficiency disorder characterized by muscle weakness, loss of appetite, nerve degeneration, and sometimes edema.

beta-carotene The orange-yellow pigment in carrots; beta-carotene is the only carotenoid that can be sufficiently absorbed and converted into retinol in the body.

BHA, BHT Butylated hydroxyanisole and butylated hydroxytoluene: two common synthetic antioxidants added to foods.

bifidus factor A protective factor secreted in the colostrum that encourages growth of beneficial bacteria in the newborn's intestines.

bile A liver secretion stored in the gallbladder and released through the common bile duct into the first segment of the small intestine. It is essential for the digestion and absorption of fat.

bile acid A compound produced by the liver. Bile acids are the main component of bile, which aids in emulsification of fat during digestion in the small intestine.

binge drinking Drinking sufficient alcohol within a 2-hour period to increase blood alcohol content to 0.08 grams per deciliter or higher; for men, consuming 5 or more drinks in a row; for women, consuming 4 or more drinks in a row.

binge eating Consuming an abnormally large amount of food within a short time period (e.g., 2 hours).

binge eating disorder An eating disorder characterized by recurrent episodes of binge eating that are associated with marked distress and lack of control over behavior, but not followed by inappropriate compensatory behaviors to prevent weight gain.

binge eating disorder of limited duration A form of other specified feeding or eating disorders in which a person meets all of the criteria for diagnosis of binge eating disorder, except the duration of the disordered eating behavior is less than 3 months.

binge eating disorder of low frequency A form of other specified feeding or eating disorders in which a person meets all of the criteria for diagnosis of binge eating disorder, except the frequency of binges is less than once per week.

bioavailability The degree to which an ingested nutrient is absorbed and available to be utilized by the body.

biochemical assessment Measurement of biochemical functions (e.g., concentrations of nutrient by-products or enzyme activities in the blood or urine) related to a nutrient's function.

bioelectrical impedance (BIA) The method to estimate total body fat that uses a low-energy electrical current. The more fat storage a person has, the more impedance (resistance) to electrical flow will be exhibited.

biological pest management Control of agricultural pests by using natural predators, parasites, or pathogens. For example, ladybugs can be used to control an aphid infestation.

biotechnology A collection of processes that involves the use of biological systems for altering and, ideally, improving the characteristics of plants, animals, and other forms of life.

bisphosphonates Drugs that bind minerals and prevent osteoclast breakdown of bone. Examples are alendronate (Fosamax) and risedronate (Actonel).

body mass index (BMI) Weight (in kilograms) divided by height (in meters) squared; a value of 25 and above indicates overweight and a value of 30 and above indicates obesity.

bolus A moistened mass of food swallowed from the oral cavity into the pharynx.

bomb calorimeter An instrument used to determine the calorie content of a food.

bond A linkage between two atoms formed by the sharing of electrons, or attractions.

bone marrow The spongy tissue in flat bones and trabecular bone that contains stem cells.

bone mineral density Total mineral content of bone at a specific bone site divided by the width of the bone at that site, generally expressed as grams per cubic centimeter.

bone remodeling The chemical process by which bone is broken down and replaced by new bone.

branched-chain amino acids Amino acids with a branching carbon backbone; these are leucine, isoleucine, and valine. All are essential amino acids.

brown adipose tissue A specialized form of adipose (fat) tissue that produces large amounts of heat by metabolizing energy-yielding nutrients without synthesizing much useful energy for the body. The unused energy is released as heat.

buffer Compounds that cause a solution to resist changes in acid–base conditions.

bulimia nervosa An eating disorder characterized by recurrent episodes of binge eating followed by inappropriate compensatory behaviors to prevent weight gain.

bulimia nervosa of limited duration A form of other specified feeding or eating disorders in which a person meets all of the criteria for diagnosis of bulimia nervosa, except the duration of the disordered eating behavior is less than 3 months.

bulimia nervosa of low frequency A form of other specified feeding or eating disorders in which a person meets all of the criteria for diagnosis of bulimia nervosa, except the frequency of binge-compensate cycles is less than once per week.

cancer A condition characterized by uncontrolled growth of abnormal cells.

capillary A microscopic blood vessel that connects the smallest arteries and veins; site of nutrient, oxygen, and waste exchange between body cells and the blood.

capillary bed Network of one-cell-thick vessels that create a junction between arterial and venous circulation. It is here that gas and nutrient exchange occurs between body cells and the blood.

carbohydrate A compound containing carbon, hydrogen, and oxygen atoms. Most are known as *sugars, starches,* and *fibers.*

carbohydrate loading A process in which a high-carbohydrate diet is consumed for 6 days before an athletic event while tapering exercise duration in an attempt to increase muscle glycogen stores.

carbon footprint The greenhouse gas emissions caused by an organization, event, product, or individual.

carbon skeleton Amino acid structure that remains after the amino group ($-NH_2$) has been removed.

cardiovascular disease A general term that refers to any disease of the heart and circulatory system. This disease is generally characterized by the deposition of fatty material in the blood vessels (hardening of the arteries), which in turn can lead to organ damage and death. Also termed coronary heart disease (CHD), as the vessels of the heart are the primary sites of the disease.

cardiovascular system The body system consisting of the heart, blood vessels, and blood. This system transports nutrients, waste products, gases, and hormones throughout the body and plays an important role in immune responses and regulation of body temperature.

carotenoids Precursors of vitamin A found in plant foods.

case-control study A study in which individuals who have a disease or condition, such as lung cancer, are compared with individuals who do not have the condition.

catalase Enzyme that catalyzes the decomposition of hydrogen peroxide into water and oxygen.

cecum A pouch at the first part of the large intestine that houses many bacteria.

celiac disease Chronic, immune-mediated disease precipitated by exposure to dietary gluten in genetically predisposed people.

cell The structural basis of plant and animal organization. In animals it is bounded by a cell membrane. Cells have the ability to take up compounds from and excrete compounds into their surroundings.

cell nucleus Membrane-bound organelle that contains genetic information (DNA) for protein synthesis and cell replication.

cell-mediated immunity A process in which certain white blood cells come in contact with the invading cells to destroy them.

cellular differentiation The process of a less-specialized cell becoming a more specialized type such as stem cells in the bone marrow becoming red and white blood cells.

cellulose An undigestible, nonfermentable, straight-chain polysaccharide made of glucose molecules.

cerebrovascular accident (CVA) Death of part of the brain tissue due typically to a blood clot. Also termed a *stroke.*

ceruloplasmin Copper-containing protein in the blood; functions in the transport of iron.

chain-breaking Breaking the link between two or more behaviors that encourage overeating, such as snacking while watching television.

cheilosis Inflammation of the skin at one or both corners of the mouth; may be a nonspecific symptom of a nutrient deficiency or just opportunistic infection; also called *angular cheilitis.*

chemical reaction An interaction between two chemicals that changes both chemicals.

chlorosis In traditional medical terminology, a form of iron-deficiency anemia characterized by pale or greenish skin, weakness, fatigue, and shortness of breath. In modern medical literature, chlorosis is termed *hypochromic anemia.*

choice The serving size of a food on a specific exchange list; formerly called *exchange.*

cholesterol A waxy lipid found in all body cells. It has a structure containing multiple chemical rings that is found only in foods of animal origin.

chromosome A single, large DNA molecule and its associated proteins; contains many genes to store and transmit genetic information.

chronic Long-standing, developing over time. When referring to disease, this term indicates that the disease process, once developed, is slow and lasting. A good example is cardiovascular disease.

chylomicron Lipoprotein made of dietary fats surrounded by a shell of cholesterol, phospholipids, and protein. Chylomicrons are formed in the absorptive cells of the small intestine after fat absorption and travel through the lymphatic system to the bloodstream.

chylomicron remnant Lipoprotein that remains after triglycerides have been removed from a chylomicron; composed of protein, phospholipids, and cholesterol.

chyme A mixture of stomach secretions and partially digested food.

cirrhosis A loss of functioning liver cells, which are replaced by nonfunctioning connective tissue. Any substance that poisons liver cells can lead to cirrhosis. The most common cause is a chronic, excessive alcohol intake. Exposure to certain industrial chemicals also can lead to cirrhosis.

***cis* fatty acid** A form of an unsaturated fatty acid that has the hydrogens lying on the same side of the carbon-carbon double bond.

clinical assessment Examination of general appearance of skin, eyes, and tongue; sense of touch; ability to cough and walk; and evidence of rapid hair loss.

coagulation Formation of a blood clot.

coenzyme An organic compound that combines with an inactive enzyme to form a catalytically active form. In this manner, coenzymes aid in enzyme function.

cofactor An inorganic compound (e.g., mineral) that combines with an inactive enzyme to form a catalytically active form.

cognitive behavioral therapy Psychological therapy in which the person's assumptions about dieting, body weight, and related issues are confronted. New ways of thinking are explored and then practiced by the person. In this way, an individual can learn new ways to control disordered eating behaviors and related life stress.

cognitive restructuring Changing one's frame of mind regarding eating; for example, instead of using a difficult day as an excuse to overeat, a person would substitute other pleasures for rewards, such as a relaxing walk with a friend.

collagen Hard, insoluble and fibrous protein found in connective tissue, bone, teeth, tendons, and blood vessels.

colostrum The first fluid secreted by the breast during late pregnancy and the first few days after birth. This thick fluid is rich in immune factors and protein.

community supported agriculture (CSA) Partnership between local food producers and community members. Farmers offer a share of foods to individuals, families, or companies that have pledged support to the CSA either financially and/or by working for the CSA.

compensatory behaviors Actions taken to rid the body of excess calories and/or to alleviate guilt or anxiety associated with a binge; examples include vomiting, misuse of laxatives, or excessive exercise.

complementary proteins Two food protein sources that make up for each other's inadequate supply of specific essential amino acids; together, they yield a sufficient amount of all nine and so provide high-quality (complete) protein for the diet.

complex carbohydrate Carbohydrate composed of many monosaccharide molecules. Examples include glycogen, starch, and fiber.

compression of morbidity Delay of the onset of disabilities caused by chronic disease.

conditionally essential amino acids Amino acids that must be made from essential amino acids if insufficient amounts are eaten.

congenital hypothyroidism The stunting of body growth and poor development in the offspring that result from inadequate maternal intake of iodine during pregnancy that impairs thyroid hormone synthesis (formerly called *cretinism*).

congenital lactase deficiency Birth defect resulting in the inability to produce lactase, such that a lactose-free diet is required from birth.

connective tissue Protein tissue that holds different structures in the body together. Some body structures are made up of connective tissue—notably, tendons and cartilage. Connective tissue also forms part of bone and the nonmuscular structures of arteries and veins.

constipation A condition characterized by infrequent bowel movements (i.e., fewer than three bowel movements per week).

contingency management Forming a plan of action to respond to a situation in which overeating is likely, such as when snacks are within arm's reach at a party.

control group Participants in an experiment who are not given the treatment being tested.

cortical bone The compact or dense bone found on the outer surfaces of bone.

creatine An organic (i.e., carbon-containing) molecule in muscle cells that serves as part of a high-energy compound (termed creatine phosphate or phosphocreatine) capable of synthesizing ATP from ADP.

Creutzfeldt-Jakob disease A rare, degenerative, invariably fatal brain disorder. Symptoms include problems with muscular coordination, personality changes including progressive and severe mental impairment, impaired vision that may lead to blindness, and involuntary muscle jerks.

cross-contamination Process by which bacteria or other microorganisms are unintentionally transferred from one substance or object to another, with harmful effect.

cytokines Chemical messengers that regulate immune responses.

cytoplasm The fluid and organelles (except the nucleus) in a cell; also called cytosol.

dehydration Inadequate intake of water to replace losses.

Delaney Clause A clause to the 1958 Food Additives Amendment of the Pure Food and Drug Act in the United States that prevents the intentional (direct) addition to foods of a compound shown to cause cancer in laboratory animals or humans.

dementia A general loss or decrease in mental function.

denaturation Alteration of a protein's three-dimensional structure, usually because of treatment by heat, enzymes, acid or alkaline solutions, or agitation.

dental caries Erosions in the surface of a tooth caused by acids made by bacteria as they metabolize sugars.

deoxyribonucleic acid (DNA) The site of hereditary information in cells; DNA directs the synthesis of cell proteins.

depolarization During nerve impulse transmission, the process in which the resting state of the nerve cell membrane (slightly negative inside the cell membrane) is temporarily disrupted.

descending colon Segment of the large intestine that carries feces from the transverse colon, down the left side of the abdomen, to the sigmoid colon.

diabetes A group of diseases characterized by high blood glucose. Type 1 diabetes involves insufficient or no release of the hormone insulin by the pancreas and therefore requires daily insulin therapy. Type 2 diabetes results from either insufficient release of insulin or general inability of insulin to act on certain body cells, such as muscle cells. Persons with type 2 diabetes may or may not require insulin therapy.

diarrhea Increased fluidity, frequency, or amount of bowel movements (i.e., three or more loose stools per day).

diastolic blood pressure The pressure in the arterial blood vessels when the heart is between beats.

dietary assessment Estimation of typical food choices relying mostly on the recounting of one's usual intake or a record of one's previous days' intake.

dietary fiber Fiber found in food.

Dietary Reference Intakes (DRIs) Term used to encompass nutrient recommendations made by the Food and Nutrition Board of the Institute of Medicine. These include RDAs, AIs, EERs, and ULs.

digestion Process by which large ingested molecules are mechanically and chemically broken down to produce basic nutrients that can be absorbed across the wall of the GI tract.

digestive system System consisting of the gastrointestinal tract and accessory structures (liver, gallbladder, and pancreas). This system performs the mechanical and chemical processes of digestion, absorption of nutrients, and elimination of wastes.

diglyceride A breakdown product of a triglyceride consisting of two fatty acids bonded to a glycerol backbone.

direct calorimetry A method of determining a body's energy use by measuring heat released from the body. An insulated chamber is typically used.

disaccharide Class of sugars formed by the chemical bonding of two monosaccharides.

disordered eating Mild and short-term changes in eating patterns that occur in relation to a stressful event, an illness, or a desire to modify one's diet for a variety of health and personal appearance reasons.

diuretic A substance that increases the volume of urine.

diverticula Pouches that protrude through the exterior wall of the large intestine.

diverticulitis Inflammation of the diverticula caused by acids produced by bacterial metabolism inside the diverticula.

diverticulosis The condition of having many diverticula in the large intestine.

docosahexaenoic acid (DHA) An omega-3 fatty acid with 22 carbons and six carbon-carbon double bonds. It is present in large amounts in fatty fish and is slowly synthesized in the body from alpha-linolenic acid. DHA is especially present in the retina and brain.

double-blind study An experimental design in which neither the participants nor the researchers are aware of each participant's assignment (test or placebo) or the outcome of the study until it is completed. An independent third party holds the code and the data until the study has been completed.

dual energy x-ray absorptiometry (DEXA) A scientific tool used to measure bone mineral density and body composition.

duodenum First segment of the small intestine that receives chyme from the stomach and digestive juices from the pancreas and gallbladder. This is the site of most chemical digestion of nutrients; approximately 10 inches in length.

early childhood caries Tooth decay that results from formula or juice (and even human milk) bathing the teeth as the child sleeps with a bottle in the mouth. The upper teeth are mostly affected as the lower teeth are protected by the tongue; formerly called *nursing bottle syndrome* and *baby bottle tooth decay*.

eating disorder Severe alterations in eating patterns linked to physiological changes. The alterations are associated with food restriction, binge eating, inappropriate compensatory behaviors, and fluctuations in weight. They also involve a number of emotional and cognitive changes that affect the way a person perceives and experiences his or her body.

eclampsia A severe form of gestational hypertension characterized by protein in the urine and seizures (formerly called *toxemia*).

edema The buildup of excess fluid in extracellular spaces.

eicosanoids A class of hormone compounds, including the prostaglandins, derived from the essential polyunsaturated fatty acids. These signaling compounds are involved in cellular activity that affects practically all important functions in the body.

eicosapentaenoic acid (EPA) An omega-3 fatty acid with 20 carbons and five carbon-carbon double bonds. It is present in large amounts in fatty fish and is slowly synthesized in the body from alpha-linolenic acid.

electrolyte A mineral that separates into positively or negatively charged ions in water. They are able to transmit an electrical current.

elimination diet A restrictive diet that systematically tests foods that may cause an allergic response by first eliminating them for 1 to 2 weeks and then adding them back, one at a time.

embryo In humans, the developing offspring in utero from about the beginning of the third week to the end of the eighth week after conception.

emulsifier A compound that can suspend fat in water by isolating individual fat droplets, using a shell of water molecules or other substances to prevent the fat from coalescing.

endocrine gland A hormone-producing gland.

endocrine system The body system consisting of the various glands and the hormones these glands secrete. This system has major regulatory functions in the body, such as reproduction and cell metabolism.

endometrium The membrane that lines the inside of the uterus. It increases in thickness during the menstrual cycle until ovulation occurs. The surface layers are shed during menstruation if conception does not take place.

endoplasmic reticulum (ER) An organelle composed of a network of canals running through the cytoplasm. Part of the endoplasmic reticulum contains ribosomes.

endorphins Natural body tranquilizers that may be involved in the feeding response and function in pain reduction.

energy balance The state in which energy, calorie intake, in the form of food and

beverages, matches the energy expended, primarily through basal metabolism and physical activity.

energy density A comparison of the calorie (kcal) content of a food with the weight of the food. An energy-dense food is high in calories but weighs very little (e.g., potato chips), whereas a food low in energy density has few calories but weighs a lot (e.g., an orange).

enterohepatic circulation A continual recycling of compounds such as bile acids between the small intestine and the liver.

environmental assessment Includes details about living conditions, education level, and the ability of the person to purchase, transport, and cook food. The person's weekly budget for food purchases is also a key factor to consider.

enzyme A compound that speeds up the rate of a chemical reaction but is not altered by the reaction. Almost all enzymes are proteins (some are made of genetic material).

eosinophil This white blood cell is a type of phagocyte that increases in number during allergic reactions.

epidemiology The study of how disease rates vary among different population groups.

epigenetics Heritable changes in gene function that are independent of DNA sequence. For example, malnutrition during pregnancy may modify gene expression in the fetus and affect long-term body weight regulation in the offspring.

epigenome A network of chemical compounds surrounding DNA that modify the genome without altering the DNA sequences and have a role in determining which genes are active (expressed) or inactive (silenced) in a particular cell.

epiglottis The flap that folds down over the trachea during swallowing.

epinephrine A hormone also known as *adrenaline*; it is released by the adrenal glands (located on each kidney) at times of stress. It acts to increase glycogen breakdown in the liver, among other functions.

epithelial tissue The surface cells that line the outside of the body and all external passages within it.

ergogenic Work-producing. An ergogenic aid is a mechanical, nutritional, psychological, pharmacological, or physiological substance or treatment intended to directly improve exercise performance.

erythrocyte Mature red blood cell. These have no nucleus and a life span of about 120 days; they contain hemoglobin, which transports oxygen and carbon dioxide.

erythropoiesis Formation of red blood cells.

erythropoietin A hormone secreted mostly by the kidneys that enhances red blood cell synthesis and stimulates red blood cell release from bone marrow.

esophagus A tube in the GI tract that connects the pharynx with the stomach.

essential amino acids The amino acids that cannot be synthesized by humans in sufficient amounts or at all and therefore must be included in the diet; there are nine essential amino acids. These are also called *indispensable amino acids*.

essential fatty acids Fatty acids that must be supplied by the diet to maintain health. Currently, only linoleic acid and alpha-linolenic acid are classified as essential.

essential nutrient In nutritional terms, a substance that, when left out of a diet, leads to signs of poor health. The body either cannot produce this nutrient or cannot produce enough of it to meet its needs. If added back to a diet before permanent damage occurs, the affected aspects of health are restored.

Estimated Energy Requirement (EER) Estimate of the energy (kcal) intake needed to match the energy use of an average person in a specific life stage.

ethanol Chemical term for the form of alcohol found in alcoholic beverages.

exercise Physical activities that are planned, repetitive, and intended to improve physical fitness.

extracellular fluid Fluid found outside the cells; it represents about one-third of body fluid.

extracellular space The space outside cells; represents one-third of body fiuid.

facilitated diffusion Movement of a substance across a semipermeable membrane from an area of higher solute concentration to an area of lower solute concentration. This type of transport does not require energy, but it does require a carrier.

failure to thrive Condition of inadequate growth during infancy or early childhood caused by poor nutritional intake, inefficient nutrient absorption, or excessive energy expenditure; commonly defined as weight-for-age below the fifth percentile on multiple occasions or weight declining two or more major percentile lines on a standardized growth chart.

famine An extreme shortage of food, which leads to massive starvation in a population; often associated with crop failures, war, and political unrest.

fat adaptation Manipulating the diet and physical training regimen so that muscles become more efficient at metabolizing fat as fuel during aerobic activity.

fat-soluble Soluble in fats, oils, or fat solvents.

fat-soluble vitamins Vitamins that dissolve in fat and some chemical compounds but not readily in water. These vitamins are A, D, E, and K.

fecal impaction The presence of a mass of hard, dry feces that remains in the rectum as a result of chronic constipation.

feces Mass of water, fiber, tough connective tissues, bacterial cells, and sloughed intestinal cells that passes through the large intestine and is excreted through the anus; also called *stool.*

female athlete triad A condition characterized by low energy availability, lack of menstrual periods (amenorrhea), and osteoporosis.

fermentation The conversion of carbohydrates to alcohols, acids, and carbon dioxide without the use of oxygen.

ferritin A protein that stores iron and releases it in a controlled manner. Acts as a buffer against iron deficiency and iron overload.

fetal alcohol spectrum disorders (FASDs) A group of irreversible physical and mental abnormalities in the infant that result from the mother's consumption of alcohol during pregnancy.

fetal alcohol syndrome (FAS) Severe form of FASD that involves abnormal facial features and problems with development of the nervous system and overall growth as a result of maternal alcohol consumption during pregnancy.

fetal origins hypothesis A theory that links nutritional and other environmental insults that occur during gestation to the future health of the offspring.

fetus The developing life form from about the beginning of the ninth week after conception until birth.

fiber Indigestible substances in plant foods that add bulk to feces. Fiber naturally found in foods is also called *dietary fiber.*

flavonoids Most common group of polyphenol phytochemicals; found in citrus fruits, berries, red onion, tea, red wine, and dark chocolate.

fluorosis Discoloration of tooth enamel sometimes accompanied with pitting due to consuming a large amount of fluoride for an excessive period.

foam cells Lipid-loaded white blood cells that have surrounded large amounts of a fatty substance, usually cholesterol, on the blood vessel walls.

FODMAPs **F**ermentable **o**ligosacchardes, **d**isaccharides, **m**onosaccharides, **a**nd **p**olyols. These carbohydrates may be poorly digested and lead to GI symptoms such as bloating, gas, and diarrhea in some people.

folate term to describe a variety of forms of this B vitamin found in foods and in the body.

food allergy An adverse reaction to food that involves an immune response; also called *food hypersensitivity.*

food deserts Urban neighborhoods and rural towns without ready access to fresh, healthy, and affordable food.

food insecure The state of being without reliable access to a sufficient quantity of affordable, nutritious food.

food insecurity A condition of anxiety regarding running out of either food or money to buy more food.

food intolerance An adverse reaction to food that does not involve an allergic reaction.

food jag A period of time (usually a few days or weeks) during which a person will eat only a limited variety of foods.

food lists A system for classifying foods into numerous lists based on the foods' macronutrient composition, and establishing serving sizes, so that one serving of each food on a list contains the same amount of carbohydrate, protein, fat, and calorie content; also called *exchange lists.*

food waste Food that is edible or fit for consumption being discarded as plate waste by consumers and by retailers due to color or appearance.

foodborne illness Sickness caused by the ingestion of food containing harmful substances.

foodborne infection Occurs when a person eats food containing harmful microorganisms, which then grow in the intestinal tract and cause illness.

foodborne intoxication Results when a person eats food containing toxins that cause illness.

free radical An unstable atom with an unpaired electron in its outermost shell; also called *reactive oxygen species.*

fructose A six-carbon monosaccharide that usually exists in a ring form; found in fruits and honey; also known as *fruit sugar.*

fruitarian A person who primarily eats fruits, nuts, honey, and vegetable oils.

functional fiber Fiber added to foods that has been shown to provide health benefits.

functional foods Foods that have health benefits beyond basic nutrition.

fungi Simple parasitic life forms, including molds, mildews, yeasts, and mushrooms. They live on dead or decaying organic matter. Fungi can grow as single cells, like yeast, or as a multicellular colony, as seen with molds.

galactose A six-carbon monosaccharide that usually exists in a ring form; closely related to glucose.

gallbladder An organ attached to the underside of the liver; site of bile storage, concentration, and eventual secretion.

gastroesophageal reflux disease (GERD) Disease that results from stomach acid backing up into the esophagus. The acid irritates the lining of the esophagus, causing pain.

gastrointestinal (GI) tract The main sites in the body used for digestion and absorption of nutrients. It consists of the mouth, esophagus, stomach, small intestine, large intestine, rectum, and anus. Also called the *digestive tract.*

gene A specific segment on a chromosome. Genes provide the blueprint for the production of cell proteins.

gene expression Use of DNA information on a gene to produce a protein. Thought to be a major determinant of cell development.

generally recognized as safe (GRAS) A list of food additives that in 1958 were considered safe for consumption. Manufacturers were allowed to continue to use these additives, without special clearance, when needed for food products. The FDA bears responsibility for proving they are not safe and can remove unsafe products from the list.

genetic engineering Manipulation of the genetic makeup of any organism with recombinant DNA technology.

genetically modified organism (GMO) Any organism created by genetic engineering.

genomics The study of the function and structure of the complete set of DNA within a single cell of an organism, known as the genome.

gestation The period of intrauterine development of offspring, from conception to birth; in humans, normal gestation is 38 to 42 weeks.

gestational diabetes A high blood glucose concentration that develops during pregnancy and returns to normal after birth; one cause is the placental production of hormones that antagonize the regulation of blood glucose by insulin.

gestational hypertension Blood pressure of 140/90 mmHg or higher that is first diagnosed after 20 weeks of gestation. This may evolve into preeclampsia or eclampsia.

global maternal mortality ratio The number of maternal deaths per 100,000 live births.

glucagon A hormone made by the pancreas that stimulates the breakdown of glycogen in the liver into glucose; this ends up increasing blood glucose. Glucagon also increases the generation of glucose from noncarbohydrate substances.

glucose A six-carbon sugar that exists in a ring form; found in blood and in table sugar bound to fructose; also known as *dextrose,* it is one of the simple sugars.

glutathione peroxidase An antioxidant enzyme system that converts certain free radicals (peroxides) into less harmful compounds (alcohols and water).

gluten Poorly digested protein found in wheat, barley, and rye.

glycemic index (GI) The blood glucose response of a given food, compared to a standard (typically, glucose or white bread). Glycemic index is influenced by starch structure, fiber content, food processing, physical structure, and macronutrients in the meal such as fat.

glycemic load (GL) A measure of both the quality (GI value) and quantity (grams per serving) of a carbohydrate in a meal.

glycerol A three-carbon alcohol used to form triglycerides.

glycogen A carbohydrate made of multiple units of glucose with a highly branched structure. It is the storage form of glucose in humans and is synthesized (and stored) in the liver and muscles.

glycosylation The process by which glucose attaches to (glycates) other compounds, such as proteins.

goiter An enlargement of the thyroid gland; this is often caused by insufficient iodine in the diet.

Golgi complex The cell organelle near the nucleus that processes newly synthesized protein for secretion or distribution to other organelles.

gout A form of arthritis caused by the buildup of uric acid crystals in the joints.

green revolution Refers to increases in crop yields that accompanied the introduction of new agricultural technologies in less-developed countries. The key technologies were high-yielding, disease-resistant strains of rice, wheat, and corn; greater use of fertilizer and water; and improved cultivation practices.

gruel A thin mixture of grains or legumes in milk or water.

gums Polysaccharides occurring naturally that cause an increase in solubility; used as thickeners, gels, emulsifiers, and stabilizers.

gut-associated lymphoid tissues (GALT) Clusters of lymphoid cells located throughout the gastrointestinal tract that destroy pathogens.

hard water Water that contains high levels of calcium and magnesium.

hazard Chance that injury will result from use of a substance.

heart attack Rapid fall in heart function caused by reduced blood flow through the heart's blood vessels. Often part of the heart dies in the process. Technically called a myocardial infarction.

heavy drinking Any pattern of alcohol consumption in excess of 4 drinks in 1 day or 14 drinks per week for men or 3 drinks in 1 day or 7 drinks per week for women.

helminth Parasitic worm that can contaminate food, water, feces, animals, and other substances.

hematocrit The percentage of blood made up of red blood cells.

heme iron Iron provided from animal tissues in the form of hemoglobin and myoglobin. Approximately 40% of the iron in meat is heme iron; it is readily absorbed.

hemicellulose A nonfermentable fiber containing xylose, galactose, glucose, and other monosaccharides bonded together.

hemochromatosis A disorder of iron metabolism characterized by increased iron absorption and deposition in the liver and heart. This eventually poisons the cells in those organs.

hemoglobin The iron-containing part of the red blood cell that carries oxygen to the cells and carbon dioxide away from the cells. The heme iron portion is also responsible for the red color of blood.

hemolytic uremic syndrome (HUS) Disease characterized by anemia caused by destruction of red blood cells (hemolytic), acute kidney failure (uremic), and a low platelet count.

hemopoietic Stem cells in the bone marrow that are capable of developing into blood cells.

hemorrhage An escape of blood from blood vessels.

hemorrhagic stroke Damage to part of the brain resulting from rupture of a blood vessel and subsequent bleeding within or over the internal surface of the brain.

hemorrhoid A pronounced swelling of a large vein, particularly veins found in the anal region.

hemostasis The process of stopping blood loss.

hepatic portal circulation The portion of the circulatory system that uses a large vein (portal vein) to carry nutrient-rich blood from capillaries in the intestines and portions of the stomach to the liver.

hepatic portal vein Large vein that carries absorbed nutrients from the gastrointestinal tract to the liver.

high-density lipoprotein (HDL) The lipoprotein in the blood that picks up cholesterol from dying cells and other sources and transfers it to the other lipoproteins in the bloodstream, as well as directly to the liver; low HDL increases the risk for cardiovascular disease.

high-fructose corn syrup (HFCS) Corn syrup that has been manufactured to contain between 42% and 90% fructose.

high-intensity interval training (HIIT) Short, intense aerobic workout that alternates short periods of intense anaerobic exercise with less-intense recovery periods to provide improved athletic capacity and condition, improved glucose metabolism, and improved fat burning.

high-quality (complete) proteins Dietary proteins that contain ample amounts of all nine essential amino acids.

homocysteine An amino acid that arises from the metabolism of methionine. Vitamin B-6, folate, vitamin B-12, and choline are required for its metabolism. Elevated levels are associated with an increased risk of cardiovascular disease.

hospice care A program offering care that emphasizes comfort and dignity at the end of life.

human immunodeficiency virus (HIV) The virus that leads to acquired immune deficiency syndrome (AIDS).

hunger The primarily physiological (internal) drive to find and eat food.

hydrogenation The addition of hydrogen to a carbon-carbon double bond, producing a single carbon-carbon bond with two hydrogens attached to each carbon.

hydrolyzed protein formula Infant formula in which the proteins have been broken down into smaller peptides and amino acids to improve digestibility and reduce exposure to potential food allergens; sometimes called *predigested* or *hypoallergenic infant formula.*

hydroxyapatite Crystalline compound containing calcium, phosphorus, and sometimes fluoride, also known as bone mineral.

hygiene hypothesis Assumption that reduced exposure to microorganisms in the environment (e.g., as a result of overuse of antibacterial soaps and antibiotics) impairs proper development of the immune system, making a person more susceptible to allergies and autoimmune diseases.

hyperglycemia High blood glucose, above 125 milligrams per 100 milliliters of blood.

hypertension A condition in which blood pressure remains persistently elevated. Obesity, inactivity, alcohol intake, excess salt intake, and genetics may each contribute to the problem.

hypertonic Having high concentration of solutes.

hypochromic Pale in color (in reference to red blood cells), as could occur with inadequate hemoglobin content.

hypoglycemia Low blood glucose, below 40 to 50 milligrams per 100 milliliters of blood for nondiabetics.

hyponatremia Dangerously low blood sodium level.

hypothalamus A region at the base of the brain that contains cells that play a role in the regulation of energy intake, respiration, body temperature, satiety, and other body functions.

hypotheses Tentative explanations by a scientist to explain a phenomenon.

hypotonic Having low concentration of solutes.

identical twins Two offspring that develop from a single ovum and sperm and, consequently, have the same genetic makeup.

ileocecal sphincter The ring of smooth muscle between the end of the small intestine and the beginning of the large intestine.

ileum Last segment of the small intestine; approximately 5 feet in length.

immunoglobulins Proteins found in the blood that bind to specific antigens; also called antibodies. The five major classes of immunoglobulins play different roles in antibody-mediated immunity.

incidental food additives Additives that appear in food products indirectly, from environmental contamination of food ingredients or during the manufacturing process.

indirect calorimetry A method to measure energy use by the body by measuring oxygen uptake and carbon dioxide output. Formulas are then used to convert this gas exchange value into energy use, estimating the proportion of energy nutrients that are being oxidized for energy in the fuel mix.

infertility Inability of a couple to conceive after 1 year of unprotected intercourse.

inflammatory response A response that occurs when tissues are injured, causing the damaged cells to release chemicals that result in blood vessels leaking fluid into the tissues, causing swelling and inflammation.

inorganic Any substance lacking carbon atoms bonded to hydrogen atoms in the chemical structure.

insoluble fiber A fiber that is not easily metabolized by intestinal bacteria; also called nonfermentable *fiber.*

insulin A hormone produced by the pancreas. Insulin allows for the movement of glucose from the bloodstream into body cells and signals the synthesis of glycogen.

intentional food additives Additives knowingly (directly) incorporated into food products by manufacturers.

international unit (IU) A crude measure of vitamin activity, often based on the growth rate of animals in response to the vitamin. Today IUs have largely been replaced by more precise milligram or microgram measures.

intracellular fluid Fluid contained within a cell; it represents about two-thirds of body fluid.

intrinsic factor A protein-like compound produced by the stomach that enhances vitamin B-12 absorption in the ileum.

ion A positively or negatively charged atom.

irradiation A process in which radiation energy is applied to foods, creating compounds (free radicals) within the food that destroy cell membranes, break down DNA, link proteins together, limit enzyme activity, and alter a variety of other proteins and cell functions of microorganisms that can lead to food spoilage. This process does not make the food radioactive.

isoflavones Phytochemicals produced in legumes, with soybeans being the most common source of isoflavones in food.

isotonic Having equal concentration of solutes.

jejunum Middle segment of the small intestine; approximately 4 feet in length.

ketone bodies Partial breakdown products of fat that contain three or four carbons.

ketosis The condition of having a high concentration of ketone bodies and related breakdown products in the bloodstream and tissues.

kidney nephrons The units of kidney cells that filter wastes from the bloodstream and deposit them into the urine.

kilocalorie (kcal) Heat energy needed to raise the temperature of 1000 grams (1 L) of water 1 degree Celsius.

kwashiorkor A disease occurring primarily in young children who have an existing disease and consume a marginal amount of calories and insufficient protein in relation to needs. The child generally suffers from infections and exhibits edema, poor growth, weakness, and an increased susceptibility to further illness.

kyphosis Abnormally increased bending of the spine.

lactase An enzyme made by absorptive cells of the small intestine; this enzyme digests lactose to glucose and galactose.

lactation The period of milk secretion following pregnancy; typically called *breastfeeding.*

lacteal Lymphatic vessel that absorbs fats from the small intestine.

lactic acid A three-carbon acid formed during anaerobic cell metabolism; a partial breakdown product of glucose; also called *lactate.*

lactic acid bacteria Strains of bacteria that produce lactic acid from fermentation of dairy products; may confer health benefits when consumed as probiotics.

lactoovovegetarian A person who consumes plant products, dairy products, and eggs.

lactose Glucose bonded to galactose; also known as *milk sugar.*

lactose intolerance A condition in which symptoms such as abdominal gas and bloating appear as a result of severe lactose maldigestion.

lactovegetarian A person who consumes plant products and dairy products.

lanugo Downlike hair that appears after a person has lost much body fat through semistarvation. The hair stands erect and traps air, acting as insulation for the body to compensate for the relative lack of body fat, which usually functions as insulation.

laxative A medication or other substance that stimulates evacuation of the intestinal tract.

lean body mass Body weight minus fat storage weight equals lean body mass. This includes organs such as the brain, muscles, and liver, as well as bone and blood and other body fluids.

lecithin A group of phospholipid compounds that are major components of cell membranes.

leptin A hormone made by adipose tissue in proportion to total fat stores in the body that influences long-term regulation of fat mass. Leptin also influences appetite and the release of insulin.

let-down reflex A reflex stimulated by infant suckling that causes the release (ejection) of milk from milk ducts in the mother's breasts; also called *milk ejection reflex.*

leukocyte White blood cell; cell of the immune system.

life expectancy The average length of life for a given group of people born in a specific year.

life span The potential oldest age a person can reach.

lignin A nonfermentable fiber made up of a multiringed alcohol (noncarbohydrate) structure.

limiting amino acid The essential amino acid in lowest concentration in a food or diet relative to body needs.

linoleic acid An essential omega-6 fatty acid with 18 carbons and two double bonds.

lipase Fat-digesting enzyme produced by the salivary glands, stomach, and pancreas.

lipid A compound containing much carbon and hydrogen, little oxygen, and sometimes other atoms. Lipids do not dissolve in water and include fats, oils, and cholesterol.

lipoprotein A compound found in the bloodstream containing a core of lipids with a shell composed of protein, phospholipids, and cholesterol.

lipoprotein lipase An enzyme attached to the cells that form the inner lining of blood vessels; it breaks down triglycerides into free fatty acids and glycerol.

lobules Saclike structures in the breast that store milk; also called *alveoli.*

locavore Someone who eats food grown or produced locally or within a certain radius such as 50, 100, or 150 miles.

long-chain fatty acid A fatty acid that contains 12 or more carbons.

low birth weight (LBW) Referring to any infant weighing less than 2.5 kilograms (5.5 pounds) at birth; most commonly results from preterm birth.

low-density lipoprotein (LDL) The lipoprotein in the blood containing primarily cholesterol; elevated LDL is strongly linked to cardiovascular disease risk.

lower esophageal sphincter A circular muscle that constricts the opening of the esophagus to the stomach. Also called the *gastroesophageal sphincter* or the *cardiac sphincter.*

lower-body (gynoid) obesity The type of obesity in which fat storage is primarily located in the buttocks and thigh area. Also known as gynoid or gynecoid obesity.

lower-quality (incomplete) proteins Dietary proteins that are low in or lack one or more essential amino acids.

lumen The hollow opening inside a tube, such as the GI tract.

lymph A clear fluid that flows through lymph vessels; carries most forms of fat after their absorption by the small intestine.

lymph nodes Clusters of lymphoid tissue, situated along the lymph vessels, that trap and destroy pathogens.

lymphatic system A system of vessels and lymph that accepts fluid surrounding cells and large particles, such as products of fat absorption. Lymph eventually passes into the bloodstream from the lymphatic system.

lymphocyte The white blood cell responsible for the immune response; regulates antibody production.

lymphoid tissue Specialized cells that participate in the immune response; includes the thymus, spleen, lymph nodes, and white blood cells.

lysosome A cellular organelle that contains digestive enzymes for use inside the cell for turnover of cell parts.

lysozyme An enzyme produced by a variety of cells; it can destroy bacteria by rupturing their cell membranes.

macrocytic (megaloblastic) Large cell size.

macronutrient A nutrient needed in gram quantities in a diet.

macrophages Large white blood cells that arise from monocytes; one of several types of white blood cells that phagocytize pathogens and signal other white blood cells to mount an immune response.

major mineral Vital to health, a mineral that is required in the diet in amounts greater than 100 milligrams per day.

malignant Malicious; in reference to a tumor, the property of spreading locally and to distant sites.

malnutrition Failing health that results from longstanding eating practices that do not coincide with nutritional needs.

maltase An enzyme made by absorptive cells of the small intestine; this enzyme digests maltose to two glucoses.

maltose A disaccharide consisting of glucose bonded to glucose.

marasmus A disease resulting from consuming a grossly insufficient amount of protein and calories; one of the diseases classed as protein-calorie malnutrition. Victims have little or no fat stores, little muscle mass, and poor strength. Death from infections is common.

market basket Food the FDA buys, prepares, and analyzes as part of the ongoing Total Diet Study, which monitors levels of about 800 contaminants and nutrients in the average U.S. diet; the number varies slightly from year to year. About 280 kinds of foods and beverages from representative areas of the country are included four times a year.

megadose Large intake of a nutrient well beyond estimates of needs or what would be found in a balanced diet; 2 to 10 times above human needs is typically a starting point.

megaloblast A large, immature red blood cell that results from the inability of the cell to divide normally (*megalo* = large; *blast* = primitive or immature).

megaloblastic (macrocytic) anemia Anemia characterized by the presence of abnormally large red blood cells.

Menkes syndrome An inherited X-linked recessive pattern disorder that affects copper levels in the body.

menopause The cessation of the menstrual cycle in women, usually beginning at about 50 years of age.

metabolic syndrome A condition in which a person has poor blood glucose regulation, hypertension, increased blood triglycerides, and other health problems. This condition is usually accompanied by obesity, lack of physical activity, and a diet high in refined carbohydrates. Also called Syndrome X.

metabolic water Water formed as a by-product of carbohydrate, lipid, and protein metabolism.

metabolism Chemical processes in the body by which energy is provided in useful forms and vital activities are sustained.

metastasize The spreading of disease from one part of the body to another, even to parts of the body that are remote from the site of the original tumor. Cancer cells can spread via blood vessels, the lymphatic system, or direct growth of the tumor.

methotrexate A drug used to treat cancer, because it interferes with the growth of cells that reproduce quickly.

methyl group In chemistry, a carbon atom that shares bonds with three hydrogen atoms. The methyl group is the omega end of a fatty acid.

microbiome Entire collection of microorganisms, their genes, and their environment.

microbiota Community of microorganisms living in a particular region; with regard to our discussion of probiotics, the community of microorganisms coexisting on and within the human body.

microcytic Small cell size.

micronutrient A nutrient needed in milligram or microgram quantities in a diet.

microvilli Extensive folds on the muscosal surface of the absorptive cells.

mineral Element used in the body to promote chemical reactions and to form body structures.

mitochondria Organelles that are the main sites of energy production in a cell. They contain the pathway for oxidizing fat for fuel, among other metabolic pathways.

moderate drinking For men, consuming no more than 4 drinks in 1 day AND no more than 14 drinks per week; for women, consuming no more than 3 drinks in 1 day AND no more than 7 drinks per week.

moderate-intensity aerobic physical activity Aerobic activity that increases a person's heart rate and breathing to some extent (4–6 on RPE scale). Examples include brisk walking, dancing, swimming, or bicycling on level terrain.

monocyte The white blood cell that ingests foreign cells; also called a phagocyte.

monoglyceride A breakdown product of a triglyceride consisting of one fatty acid attached to a glycerol backbone.

monosaccharide Simple sugar, such as glucose, that is not broken down further during digestion.

monounsaturated fatty acid A fatty acid containing one carbon-carbon double bond.

motility Generally, the ability to move spontaneously. It also refers to movement of food through the GI tract.

mucilage A soluble fiber consisting of chains of galactose, mannose, and other monosaccharides; characteristically found in seaweed.

mucus A thick fluid secreted by many cells throughout the body. It contains a compound that has both carbohydrate and protein parts. It acts as a lubricant and means of protection for cells.

multiple sclerosis An unpredictable disease of the central nervous system that can range from relatively benign to somewhat disabling to devastating, as communication between the brain and other parts of the body is disrupted.

muscle tissue A type of tissue adapted to contract to cause movement.

muscle-strengthening activity Physical activity that increases skeletal muscle strength, power, endurance, and mass. Examples include lifting weights, using weight machines, and calisthenics (e.g., push-ups).

myelin A combination of lipids and proteins that covers nerve fibers.

myocardial infarction Death of part of the heart muscle. Also termed a *heart attack*.

myoglobin Iron-containing protein that binds oxygen in muscle tissue.

negative energy balance The state in which energy intake is less than energy expended, resulting in weight loss.

negative protein balance A state in which protein intake is less than related protein losses, such as often seen during acute illness.

neotame General-purpose, nonnutritive sweetener that is approximately 7000 to 13,000 times sweeter than table sugar. It has a chemical structure similar to aspartame.

nervous system The body system consisting of the brain, spinal cord, nerves, and sensory receptors. This system detects sensations, directs movements, and controls physiological and intellectual functions.

nervous tissue Tissue composed of highly branched, elongated cells that transport nerve impulses from one part of the body to another.

neural tube defect A defect in the formation of the neural tube occurring during early fetal development. This type of defect results in various nervous system disorders, such as spina bifida. Folate deficiency in the pregnant woman increases the risk that the fetus will develop this disorder.

neuron The structural and functional unit of the nervous system. Consists of a cell body, dendrites, and an axon.

neurotransmitter A compound made by a nerve cell that allows for communication between it and other cells.

neutrophil A common white blood cell that fights infections; levels rise during bacterial or fungal infections.

night blindness Vitamin A–deficiency disorder that results in loss of the ability to see under low-light conditions.

night eating syndrome Eating a lot of food in the late evening and nocturnal awakenings with ingestion of food.

nitrosamine A carcinogen formed from nitrates and breakdown products of amino acids; can lead to cancer.

nonceliac gluten sensitivity (NCGS) One or more of a variety of immune-related conditions with symptoms similar to celiac disease that are precipitated by the ingestion of gluten in people who do not have celiac disease.

nonessential amino acids Amino acids that can be synthesized by a healthy body in sufficient amounts; there are 11 nonessential amino acids. These are also called *dispensable amino acids.*

nonheme iron Iron provided from plant sources and animal tissues other than in the forms of hemoglobin and myoglobin. Nonheme iron is less efficiently absorbed than heme iron; absorption is closely dependent on body needs.

nonspecific immunity Defenses that stop the invasion of pathogens; requires no previous encounter with a pathogen; also called *innate immunity.*

norepinephrine A neurotransmitter from nerve endings and a hormone from the adrenal gland. It is released in times of stress and is involved in hunger regulation, blood glucose regulation, and other body processes.

NSAIDs Nonsteroidal anti-inflammatory drugs; include aspirin, ibuprofen (Advil),® and naproxen (Aleve).®

nutrient density The ratio derived by dividing a food's nutrient content by its calorie content. When the food's contribution to our nutrient need for that nutrient exceeds its contribution to our calorie need, the food is considered to have a favorable nutrient density.

nutrients Chemical substances in food that contribute to health, many of which are essential parts of a diet. Nutrients nourish us by providing calories to fulfill energy needs, materials for building body parts, and factors to regulate necessary chemical processes in the body.

nutrigenetics Study of the effects of genes on nutritional health, such as variations in nutrient requirements and responsiveness to dietary modifications.

nutrigenomics Study of how food impacts health through its interaction with our genes and its subsequent effect on gene expression.

nutrition security Secure access to a nutritious diet coupled with a sanitary environment and adequate health services and care.

nutritional genomics Study of interactions between nutrition and genetics; includes nutrigenetics and nutrigenomics.

nutritional state The nutritional health of a person as determined by anthropometric measurements (height, weight, circumferences, and so on), biochemical measurements of nutrients or their by-products in blood and urine, a clinical (physical) examination, a dietary analysis, and economic evaluation; also called nutritional status.

obesity Disorder involving excessive body fat that increases the risk of health problems.

oleic acid An omega-9 fatty acid with 18 carbons and one double bond.

oleogustus A taste for fat. The presence of fatty acids in foods stimulates taste receptors in the mouth; this sensation is unpleasant.

omega-3 (ω-3) fatty acid An unsaturated fatty acid with the first double bond on the third carbon from the methyl end ($-CH_3$).

omega-6 (ω-6) fatty acid An unsaturated fatty acid with the first double bond on the sixth carbon from the methyl end ($-CH_3$).

organ A group of tissues designed to perform a specific function; for example, the heart, which contains muscle tissue, nerve tissue, and so on.

organ system A collection of organs that work together to perform an overall function.

organelles Compartments, particles, or filaments that perform specialized functions within a cell.

organic food Food grown without use of pesticides, synthetic fertilizers, sewage sludge, genetically modified organisms, antibiotics, hormones, or ionizing radiation.

osmosis The passage of water through a membrane from a less concentrated compartment to a more concentrated compartment.

osteoarthritis A degenerative joint condition caused by a breakdown of cartilage in joints. It often results from "wear and tear" due to repetitive motions or the pressure of excess body weight.

osteoblast Bone cells that initiate the synthesis of new bone.

osteocalcin Small protein in the organic matrix of bone.

osteoclast Bone cells that break down bone and subsequently release bone minerals into the blood.

osteocyte Osteoblast embedded into the bone matrix.

osteomalacia Adult form of rickets. The bones have low mineral density and subsequently are at risk for fracture.

osteopenia A bone disease defined by low mineral density.

osteoporosis The presence of a stress-induced fracture or a T-score of −2.5 or lower. The bones are porous and fragile due to low mineral density.

ostomy Surgically created short circuit in intestinal flow where the end point usually opens from the abdominal cavity rather than the anus; for example, a colostomy.

overnutrition A state in which nutritional intake greatly exceeds the body's needs.

ovum The egg cell from which a fetus eventually develops if the egg is fertilized by a sperm cell.

oxalic acid (oxalate) An organic acid found in spinach, rhubarb, beet greens, chard, and sweet potatoes. It can depress the absorption of certain minerals, such as calcium, but only in the food itself.

oxidation The process of losing an electron during a chemical reaction.

oxidative stress Imbalance between the production of reactive compounds and the body's ability to protect against their adverse effects.

oxidize In the most basic sense, the loss of an electron or gain of an oxygen by a chemical substance. This change typically alters the shape and/or function of the substance.

oxytocin A hormone secreted by the pituitary gland. It causes contraction of the musclelike cells surrounding the ducts of the breasts and the smooth muscle of the uterus.

parasite An organism that lives in or on another organism and derives nourishment from it.

parathyroid hormone (PTH) A hormone made by the parathyroid glands that increases synthesis of the vitamin D hormone and aids calcium release from bone and calcium conservation by the kidneys, among other functions.

Parkinson's disease Disease that belongs to a group of conditions called motor system disorders, which are the result of the loss of dopamine-producing brain cells. The four primary symptoms of PD are tremor, or trembling in hands, arms, legs, jaw, and face; rigidity, or stiffness of the limbs and trunk; bradykinesia, or slowness of movement; and postural instability, or impaired balance and coordination.

passive diffusion Movement of a substance across a semipermeable membrane from an area of higher solute concentration to an area of lower solute concentration. This type of transport does not require a carrier and does not require energy.

pasteurizing The process of heating food products to kill pathogenic microorganisms and reduce the total number of bacteria.

pectin A soluble fiber containing chains of galacturonic acid and other monosaccharides; characteristically found between plant cell walls.

pellagra Niacin-deficiency disease characterized by dementia, diarrhea, and dermatitis, and possibly leading to death.

pepsin A protein-digesting enzyme produced by the stomach.

peptide bond A chemical bond formed between amino acids in a protein.

peer review Evaluation of work by professionals of similar competence (peers) to the producers of the work to maintain standards of quality and credibility. Scholarly peer review is used to determine if a scientific study is suitable for publication.

percentile Classification of a measurement of a unit into divisions of 100 units.

perforation A hole made by boring or piercing. With reference to the gastrointestinal tract, the hole is in the wall of the esophagus, stomach, intestine, rectum, or gallbladder. Complications include bleeding and infection.

periodization Cycling the volume, intensity, and activities of workouts throughout the training season.

periosteum A specialized connective tissue covering all bones and having bone-forming potential.

peristalsis A coordinated muscular contraction used to propel food down the gastrointestinal tract.

pernicious anemia The anemia that results from a lack of vitamin B-12 absorption; it is pernicious because of associated nerve degeneration that can result in eventual paralysis and death.

peroxisome A cell organelle that destroys toxic products within the cell.

pescovegetarian A person who eats aquatic animal protein.

pH A measure of relative acidity or alkalinity of a solution. The pH scale is 0 to 14. A pH of 7 is neutral; a pH below 7 is acidic; a pH above 7 is alkaline.

phagocytes Immune cells (e.g., neutrophils and macrophages) that engulf substances.

phagocytosis A process in which a cell forms an indentation, and solid particles enter the indentation and are engulfed by the cell.

pharynx The organ of the digestive tract and respiratory tract located at the back of the oral and nasal cavities, commonly known as the throat.

phenylketonuria (PKU) Disease caused by a genetic defect in the liver's ability to metabolize the amino acid phenylalanine into the amino acid tyrosine; untreated, toxic by-products of phenylalanine build up in the body and lead to brain damage and severe health issues.

phlebotomy Therapeutic blood removal, as a blood donation, for the purpose of ridding the body of excess iron.

phosphocreatine (PCr) A high-energy compound that can be used to reform ATP. It is used primarily during bursts of activity, such as lifting and jumping.

phospholipid Any of a class of fat-related substances that contain phosphorus, fatty acids, and a nitrogen-containing component. Phospholipids are an essential part of every cell.

photosynthesis Process by which plants use energy from the sun to synthesize energy-yielding compounds, such as glucose.

physical activity Any movement of skeletal muscles that requires energy.

physical fitness The ability to perform moderate to vigorous activity without undue fatigue.

physiological anemia The normal increase in blood volume in pregnancy that dilutes the concentration of red blood cells, resulting in anemia; also called *hemodilution*.

phytic acid (phytate) A constituent of plant fiber that chemically binds minerals and prevents their absorption. Phytic acid can depress calcium absorption from other foods present in the GI tract.

phytochemical A chemical found in plants. Some phytochemicals may contribute to a reduced risk of cancer or cardiovascular disease in people who consume them regularly.

pica The practice of eating nonfood items, such as dirt, laundry starch, or clay.

pinocytosis A process in which a cell forms an indentation, and fluid enters the indentation and is engulfed by the cell.

placebo Generally, an inactive medicine or treatment used to disguise the treatments given to the participants in an experiment.

placenta An organ that forms in the uterus in pregnant women. Through this organ, oxygen and nutrients from the mother's blood are transferred to the fetus, and fetal wastes are removed. The placenta also releases hormones that maintain the state of pregnancy.

plaque A cholesterol-rich substance deposited in the blood vessels; it contains various white blood cells, smooth muscle cells, various proteins, cholesterol and other lipids, and eventually calcium.

plasma The fluid, extracellular portion of blood.

platelet A protoplasmic disc smaller than a red blood cell that promotes coagulation; also called *thrombocyte*.

polycystic ovary syndrome (PCOS) A condition of hormonal imbalance (e.g., elevated testosterone and insulin) in a woman that can lead to infertility, weight gain in the abdominal region, excessive growth of body hair, and acne.

polypeptide A group of 10 to 2000 or more amino acids bonded together to form proteins.

polysaccharides Carbohydrates containing many glucose units, from 10 to 1000 or more.

polyunsaturated fatty acid A fatty acid containing two or more carbon-carbon double bonds.

pool The amount of a nutrient stored within the body that can be mobilized when needed.

positive energy balance The state in which energy intake is greater than energy expended, generally resulting in weight gain.

positive protein balance A state in which protein intake exceeds related protein losses, as is needed during times of growth.

prebiotic Selectively fermented ingredient that results in specific changes in the composition and/or activity of the gastrointestinal microbiota, thus conferring benefits upon the host.

preeclampsia A form of gestational hypertension characterized by protein in the urine.

preservatives Compounds that extend the shelf life of foods by inhibiting microbial growth or minimizing the destructive effect of oxygen and metals.

preterm An infant born before 37 weeks of gestation; also referred to as *premature*.

primary hypertension Blood pressure of 140/90 mmHg or higher with no identified cause; also called *essential hypertension*.

primary lactose maldigestion Develops at about age 3 to 5 years when the production of the enzyme lactase decreases.

probiotics Live microorganisms that, when administered in adequate amounts, confer health benefits on the host.

progression Incremental increase in frequency, intensity, and time spent in each type of physical activity over several weeks or months.

prolactin A hormone secreted by the pituitary gland that stimulates the synthesis of milk in the breast.

prostate gland A solid, chestnut-shaped organ surrounding the first part of the urinary tract in the male. The prostate gland secretes substances into the semen.

protein Food and body compounds made of more than 100 amino acids; proteins contain carbon, hydrogen, oxygen, nitrogen, and sometimes other atoms in a specific configuration. Proteins contain the form of nitrogen most easily used by the human body.

protein equilibrium A state in which protein intake is equal to related protein losses; the person is said to be in protein balance.

protein turnover The process by which cells break down old proteins and resynthesize new proteins. In this way, the cell will have the proteins it needs to function at that time.

protein-calorie malnutrition (PCM) A condition resulting from regularly consuming insufficient amounts of calories and protein. The deficiency eventually results in body wasting, primarily of lean tissue, and an increased susceptibility to infections. Also known as *protein-energy malnutrition (PEM)*.

proton pump inhibitor A medication that inhibits the ability of gastric cells to secrete hydrogen ions.

protozoa One-celled animals that are more complex than bacteria. Disease-causing protozoa can be spread through food and water.

provitamin A A substance that can be converted into vitamin A.

purging disorder An eating disorder characterized by repeated purging (e.g., by self-induced vomiting) to induce weight loss even in the absence of binge eating.

pyloric sphincter Ring of smooth muscle between the stomach and the small intestine.

pyruvic acid A three-carbon compound formed during glucose metabolism; also called *pyruvate*.

R-proteins Proteins produced by the salivary glands that bind to free vitamin B-12 in the stomach and protect it from stomach acid.

radiation Literally, energy that is emitted from a center in all directions. Various forms of radiation energy include X rays and ultraviolet rays from the Sun.

rancid Containing products of decomposed fatty acids that have an unpleasant flavor and odor.

receptor A site in a cell at which compounds (such as hormones) bind. Cells that contain receptors for a specific compound are partially controlled by that compound.

Recommended Dietary Allowance (RDA) Nutrient intake amount sufficient to meet the needs of 97% to 98% of the individuals in a specific life stage.

rectum Terminal portion of the large intestine.

reduction The process of gaining an electron during a chemical reaction.

registered dietitian (RD) A person who has completed a baccalaureate degree program approved by the Accreditation Council for Education in Nutrition and Dietetics (ACEND), performed at least 1200 hours of supervised professional practice, passed a registration examination, and complies with continuing education requirements.

registered dietitian nutritionist (RDN) The RDN is the updated credential formerly abbreviated RD. The credential was updated to better reflect the scope of practice of the dietitian and to align with the new name of the professional organization for dietitians, the Academy of Nutrition and Dietetics.

relapse prevention A series of strategies used to help prevent and cope with weight-control lapses, such as recognizing high-risk situations and deciding beforehand on appropriate responses.

repolarization During nerve impulse transmission, the restoration of the resting state of the nerve cell membrane.

reserve capacity The extent to which an organ can preserve essentially normal function despite decreasing cell number or cell activity.

resorption The process of losing substance. Bone resorption is part of the initial process for remodeling and growth.

resting metabolism The amount of calories the body uses when the person has not eaten in 4 hours and is resting (e.g., 15 to 30 minutes) and awake in a warm, quiet environment. It is usually slightly higher (10%) than basal metabolism due to the less strict criteria for the test; often referred to as *resting metabolic rate (RMR)*.

retina A light-sensitive lining in the back of the eye. It contains retinal.

retinal Aldehyde form of vitamin A.

retinoic acid Acid form of vitamin A.

retinoids Chemical forms of preformed vitamin A; one source is animal foods.

retinol Alcohol form of vitamin A.

retinyl Storage form of vitamin A.

rheumatoid arthritis A degenerative joint condition resulting from an autoimmune disease that causes inflammation in the joints and other sites of the body.

ribonucleic acid (RNA) The single-stranded nucleic acid involved in the transcription of genetic information and translation of that information into protein structure.

ribosomes Cytoplasmic particles that mediate the linking together of amino acids to form proteins; may exist freely in the cytoplasm or attached to endoplasmic reticulum.

rickets A disease characterized by poor mineralization of newly synthesized bones because of low calcium content. Arising in infants and children, this deficiency is caused by insufficient amounts of vitamin D in the body.

risk factors A term used frequently when discussing the factors contributing to the development of a disease. A risk factor is an aspect of our lives, such as heredity, lifestyle choices (e.g., smoking), or nutritional habits.

saccharin Alternative sweetener that yields no energy to the body; 200 to 700 times sweeter than sucrose.

safety Relative certainty that a substance will not cause injury.

saliva Watery fluid, produced by the salivary glands in the mouth, that contains lubricants, enzymes, and other substances.

sarcopenia In general, loss of muscle tissue. Among older adults, this loss of lean mass greatly increases their risk of illness and death.

sarcopenic obesity Loss of muscle mass accompanied by gains in fat mass.

satiety A state in which there is no longer a desire to eat; a feeling of satisfaction.

saturated fatty acid A fatty acid containing no carbon-carbon double bonds.

scavenger cells Specific form of white blood cells that can bury themselves in the artery wall and accumulate LDL. As these cells take up LDL, they contribute to the development of atherosclerosis.

scurvy The vitamin C–deficiency disease characterized by weakness, fatigue, slow wound healing, bone pain, fractures, sore and bleeding gums, diarrhea, and pinpoint hemorrhages on the skin.

secondary hypertension Blood pressure of 140/90 mmHg or higher as a result of disease (e.g., kidney dysfunction or sleep apnea) or drug use.

secondary lactose maldigestion Occurs when production of the enzyme lactase declines for unknown reasons. When significant symptoms develop after lactose intake, it is then called *lactose intolerance.*

secretory vesicles Membrane-bound vesicles produced by the Golgi complex; contain protein and other compounds to be secreted by the cell.

self-monitoring Tracking foods eaten and conditions affecting eating; actions are usually recorded in a diary, along with location, time, and state of mind. This is a tool to help people understand more about their eating habits.

sequestrants Compounds that bind free metal ions. By so doing, they reduce the ability of ions to cause rancidity in foods containing fat.

serum Protein-rich portion of blood that separates out when blood coagulates.

set-point Theory of weight status that refers to the close regulation of body weight. It is not known what cells control this set point or how it functions in weight regulation. There is evidence, however, that complex mechanisms exist that help regulate weight.

sickle cell disease (sickle cell anemia) An illness that results from a malformation of the red blood cell because of an incorrect structure in part of its hemoglobin protein chains.

sigmoid colon Last segment of the large intestine that carries feces from the descending colon to the rectum.

simple sugar Monosaccharide or disaccharide in the diet. These simple carbohydrates are broken down and digested very quickly. Most contain refined sugars and very few essential vitamins and minerals.

small for gestational age (SGA) Referring to infants who weigh less than the expected weight for their length of gestation. This corresponds to less than 2.5 kilograms (5.5 pounds) in a full-term newborn.

soft water Water that contains a high level of sodium.

soluble fiber A fiber that is readily fermented by bacteria in the large intestine; also called *viscous fiber*.

solvent A liquid substance in which other substances dissolve.

sorbitol Alcohol derivative of glucose that yields about 3 kcal/g but is slowly absorbed from the small intestine; used in some sugarless gums and dietetic foods.

specific immunity Function of white blood cells directed at specific antigens; also called *adaptive immunity*.

spina bifida Birth defect resulting from improper closure of the neural tube during embryonic development. The spinal cord or fluid may bulge outside the spinal column.

spleen Lymphoid organ located near the stomach that filters aged and dead cells and foreign proteins out of blood.

spontaneous abortion Cessation of pregnancy and expulsion of the embryo or nonviable fetus prior to 20 weeks' gestation. This is the result of natural causes, such as a genetic defect or developmental problem; also called *miscarriage*.

starch A carbohydrate made of multiple units of glucose attached together in a form the body can digest; also known as *complex carbohydrate*.

sterol A compound containing a multi-ring (steroid) structure and a hydroxyl group (–OH). Cholesterol is a typical example.

stevia Alternative sweetener derived from South American shrub; 200 to 400 times sweeter than sucrose.

stimulus control Altering the environment to minimize the stimuli for eating such as removing foods from sight by storing them in kitchen cabinets.

stress fracture A fracture that occurs from repeated jarring of a bone. Common sites include bones of the foot and shins.

stroke A decrease or loss in blood flow to the brain that results from a blood clot or other change in arteries in the brain. This in turn causes the death of brain tissue. Also called a *cerebrovascular accident*.

stromal Stem cells that can produce bone, cartilage, and fat.

subclinical Stage of a disease or disorder not severe enough to produce symptoms that can be detected or diagnosed.

sucralose Alternative sweetener that has chlorines in place of 3 hydroxyl (–OH) groups on sucrose; 600 times sweeter than sucrose.

sucrase An enzyme made by absorptive cells of the small intestine; this enzyme digests sucrose to glucose and fructose.

sucrose Fructose bonded to glucose; also known as *table sugar.*

sugar A simple carbohydrate with the chemical composition $(CH_2O)n$. The basic unit of all sugars is glucose.

superoxide dismutase Antioxidant enzyme system that converts certain free radicals (superoxide anions) into less damaging products (oxygen and hydrogen peroxide).

sustainable agriculture Agricultural system that provides a secure living for farm families; maintains the natural environment and resources; supports the rural community; and offers respect and fair treatment to all involved, from farm workers to consumers to the animals raised for food.

sustainable development Economic growth that will simultaneously reduce poverty, protect the environment, and preserve natural capital.

symptom A change in health status noted by the person with the problem, such as stomach pain.

synapse The space between one neuron and another neuron (or cell).

synbiotic Combination of pro- and prebiotics taken to confer health benefits on the host.

systolic blood pressure The pressure in the arterial blood vessels associated with the pumping of blood from the heart.

teratogen A compound (natural or synthetic) that may cause or increase the risk of a birth defect. Exposure to a teratogen does not always lead to a birth defect; its effects on the fetus depend on the dose, timing, and duration of exposure.

tetany A body condition marked by sharp contraction of muscles and failure to relax afterward; usually caused by abnormal calcium metabolism.

theory An explanation for a phenomenon that has numerous lines of evidence to support it.

therapeutic phlebotomy Periodic blood removal, as a blood donation, for the purpose of ridding the body of excess iron.

thermic effect of food (TEF) The increase in metabolism that occurs during the digestion, absorption, and metabolism of energy-yielding nutrients. This represents 5% to 10% of calories consumed.

thrifty metabolism A genetic tendency toward efficient use of energy that results in below-average energy requirements and increased storage of calories as fat.

thrombocyte (platelet) A protoplasmic disc smaller than a red blood cell; promotes coagulation.

thymus Lymphoid organ located near the heart that participates in maturation of white blood cells.

thyroid hormones Hormones produced by the thyroid gland that regulate growth and metabolic rate.

tissue saturation The limited storage capacity of water-soluble vitamins in the tissues.

tissues Collections of cells adapted to perform a specific function.

tocopherols The chemical name for some forms of vitamin E. The alpha form is the most potent.

Tolerable Upper Intake Level (UL) Maximum chronic daily intake level of a nutrient that is unlikely to cause adverse health effects in almost all people in a specific life stage.

tolerance Needing more of a substance to achieve the desired effect (e.g., intoxication) or experiencing diminished effects of a given amount of a substance after repeated use.

toxicity Capacity of a substance to produce injury or illness at some dosage.

toxicology Scientific study of harmful substances.

toxin-mediated infection Occurs when a person eats food containing harmful bacteria. While in the intestinal tract, the bacteria produce toxins that cause illness.

toxins Poisonous compounds produced by an organism that can cause disease.

trabecular bone The less dense, more open structure bone found in the inner layer of bones.

trace mineral Vital to health, a mineral that is required in the diet in amounts less than 100 milligrams per day.

trachea The airway that extends from the throat, down the neck, to the lungs; also called the *windpipe.*

trans fatty acid A form of an unsaturated fatty acid, usually a monounsaturated one when found in food, in which the hydrogens on both carbons forming the double bond lie on opposite sides of that bond.

transcription Process by which genetic information stored as DNA within the nucleus is copied to RNA during protein synthesis.

transferrin Iron-binding protein; controls the level of free iron in blood.

translation Process by which genetic information copied into RNA dictates the amino acid sequence to form a protein.

transverse colon Segment of the large intestine that carries feces from the ascending colon, from right to left across the top of the abdomen, to the descending colon.

triglyceride The major form of lipid in the body and in food. It is composed of three fatty acids bonded to glycerol.

trimesters Three 13- to 14-week periods into which the normal pregnancy (on average, 40 weeks) is divided somewhat arbitrarily for purposes of discussion and analysis.

Development of the offspring, however, is continuous throughout pregnancy, with no specific physiological markers demarcating the transition from one trimester to the next.

trypsin A protein-digesting enzyme secreted by the pancreas to act in the small intestine.

tumor Mass of cells; may be cancerous (malignant) or noncancerous (benign).

type 1 diabetes A form of diabetes characterized by total insulin deficiency due to destruction of insulin-producing cells of the pancreas. Insulin therapy is required.

type 1 osteoporosis Porous trabecular bone characterized by rapid bone demineralization following menopause.

type 2 diabetes A form of diabetes characterized by insulin resistance and often associated with obesity. Insulin therapy can be used but is often not required.

type 2 osteoporosis Porous trabecular and cortical bone observed in men and women after the age of 70.

ulcer Erosion of the tissue lining, usually in the stomach or the upper small intestine. As a group these are generally referred to as peptic ulcers.

ultra-high temperature (UHT) processing Method of sterilizing food by heating it above 275°F (135°C) for 1 to 2 seconds. Also called *ultra-heat treatment.*

ultratrace mineral A mineral present in the human diet in trace amounts but that has not been shown to be essential to human health.

umami A brothy, meaty, savory flavor in some foods. Monosodium glutamate enhances this flavor when added to foods.

undernutrition Failing health that results from a long-standing dietary intake that is not enough to meet nutritional needs.

underwater weighing Also known as hydrostatic weighing or hydrodensitometry, this is a method of estimating total body fat by weighing the individual on a standard scale and then weighing him or her again submerged in water. The difference between the two weights is used to estimate total body volume.

underweight A BMI below 18.5. The cutoff is less precise than for obesity BMI classifications because this condition has been less studied.

upper-body (android) obesity The type of obesity in which fat is stored primarily in the abdominal area; defined as a waist circumference more than 40 inches (102 centimeters) in men and more than 35 inches (88 centimeters) in women; closely associated with a high risk for cardiovascular disease, hypertension, and type 2 diabetes. Also known as android obesity.

urea Nitrogenous waste product of protein metabolism; major source of nitrogen in the urine.

ureter Tube that transports urine from the kidney to the urinary bladder.

urethra Tube that transports urine from the urinary bladder to the outside of the body.

urinary system The body system consisting of the kidneys, urinary bladder, and the ducts that carry urine. This system removes waste products from the circulatory system and regulates blood acid–base balance, overall chemical balance, and water balance in the body.

vasoconstriction The narrowing of blood vessels. As part of hemostasis, this temporarily reduces the flow of blood to the site of injury while a clot is being formed.

vegan A person who eats only plant foods.

vein A blood vessel that carries blood to the heart.

very-low-calorie diet (VLCD) This diet allows a person fewer than 800 calories per day, often in liquid form. Of this, 120 to 480 calories are typically from carbohydrate, and the rest are mostly from high-quality protein.

very-low-density lipoprotein (VLDL) The lipoprotein created in the liver that carries cholesterol and lipids that have been taken up or newly synthesized by the liver.

vigorous-intensity aerobic physical activity Aerobic activity that greatly increases a person's heart rate and breathing (7–8 on RPE scale). Examples include jogging, singles tennis, swimming continuous laps, or bicycling uphill.

villi (singular, villus) The fingerlike protrusions into the small intestine that participate in digestion and absorption of food.

virus The smallest known type of infectious agent, many of which cause disease in humans. A virus is essentially a piece of genetic material surrounded by a coat of protein. They do not metabolize, grow, or move by themselves. They reproduce only with the aid of a living cellular host.

vitamin An essential organic (carbon-containing) compound needed in small amounts in the diet to help regulate and support chemical reactions and processes in the body.

vitamin D_2 (ergocalciferol) Form of vitamin D found in nonanimal sources, such as in some mushrooms.

vitamin D_3 (cholecalciferol) Previtamin form found naturally in some animal sources, including fish and egg yolks.

water The universal solvent; chemically, H_2O. The body is composed of about 60% water. Water (fluid) needs are about 9 (women) or 13 (men) cups per day; needs are greater if one exercises heavily.

water intoxication Potentially fatal condition that occurs with a high intake of water, which results in a severe dilution of the blood and other fluid compartments.

water-soluble Capable of dissolving in water.

water-soluble vitamins Vitamins that dissolve in water. These vitamins are the B vitamins and vitamin C.

white blood cells One of the formed elements of the circulating blood system; also called *leukocytes.* White blood cells are able to squeeze through intracellular spaces and migrate. They phagocytize bacteria, fungi, and viruses, as well as detoxify proteins that may result from allergic reactions, cellular injury, and other immune system cells.

whole grains Grains containing the entire seed of the plant, including the bran, germ, and endosperm (starchy interior). Examples are whole wheat and brown rice.

Wilson's disease A genetic disorder that results in accumulation of copper in the tissues; characterized by damage to the liver, nervous system, and other organs.

withdrawal Physical symptoms related to cessation of substance use, such as sweating, rapid pulse, shakiness, insomnia, nausea and vomiting, anxiety, and even seizures.

xerophthalmia Hardening of the cornea and drying of the surface of the eye, which can result in blindness.

xylitol Alcohol derivative of the five-carbon monosaccharide xylose.

zoochemicals Chemicals found in animal products that have health-protective actions.

zygote The fertilized ovum; the cell resulting from the union of an egg cell (ovum) and sperm until it divides.

Index

Page numbers followed by f and t indicate figures and tables, respectively.